Estimated Sodium, Chloride, and Potassium Minimum Requirements of Healthy Persons

Age	Weight (kg)	Sodium (mg)[a,b]	Chloride (mg)[a,b]	Potassium (mg)[c]
Months				
0-5	4.5	120	180	500
6-11	8.9	200	300	700
Years				
1	11.0	225	350	1,000
2-5	16.0	300	500	1,400
6-9	25.0	400	600	1,600
10-18	50.0	500	750	2,000
>18[d]	70.0	500	750	2,000

[a] *No allowance has been included for large, prolonged losses from the skin through sweat.*

[b] *There is no evidence that higher intakes confer any health benefit.*

[c] *Desirable intakes of potassium may considerably exceed these values (~13,500 mg for adults).*

[d] *No allowance included for growth. Values for those below 18 years assume a growth rate at 50th percentile reported by the National Center for Health Statistics and averaged for males and females.*

Estimated Safe and Adequate Daily Dietary Intakes of Selected Vitamins and Minerals[a]

		Vitamins		Trace Elements[b]				
Category	Age (years)	Biotin (μg)	Pantothenic Acid (mg)	Copper (mg)	Manganese (mg)	Fluoride (μg)	Chromium (μg)	Molybdenum (mg)
Infants	0-0.5	10	2	0.4-0.6	0.3-0.6	0.1-0.5	10-40	15-30
	0.5-1	15	3	0.6-0.7	0.6-1.0	0.2-1.0	20-60	20-40
Children and adolescents	1-3	20	3	0.7-1.0	1.0-1.5	0.5-1.5	20-80	25-50
	4-6	25	3-4	1.0-1.5	1.5-2.0	1.0-2.5	30-120	30-75
	7-10	30	4-5	1.0-2.0	2.0-3.0	1.5-2.5	50-200	50-150
	11+	30-100	4-7	1.5-2.5	2.0-5.0	1.5-2.5	50-200	75-250
Adults		30-100	4-7	1.5-3.0	2.0-5.0	1.5-4.0	50-200	75-250

[a] *Because there is less information on which to base allowances, these figures are not given in the main table of RDA and are provided here in the form of ranges of recommended intakes.*

[b] *Since the toxic levels for many trace elements may be only several times usual intakes, the upper levels for the trace elements given in this table should not be habitually exceeded.*

CONTEMPORARY NUTRITION

issues and insights

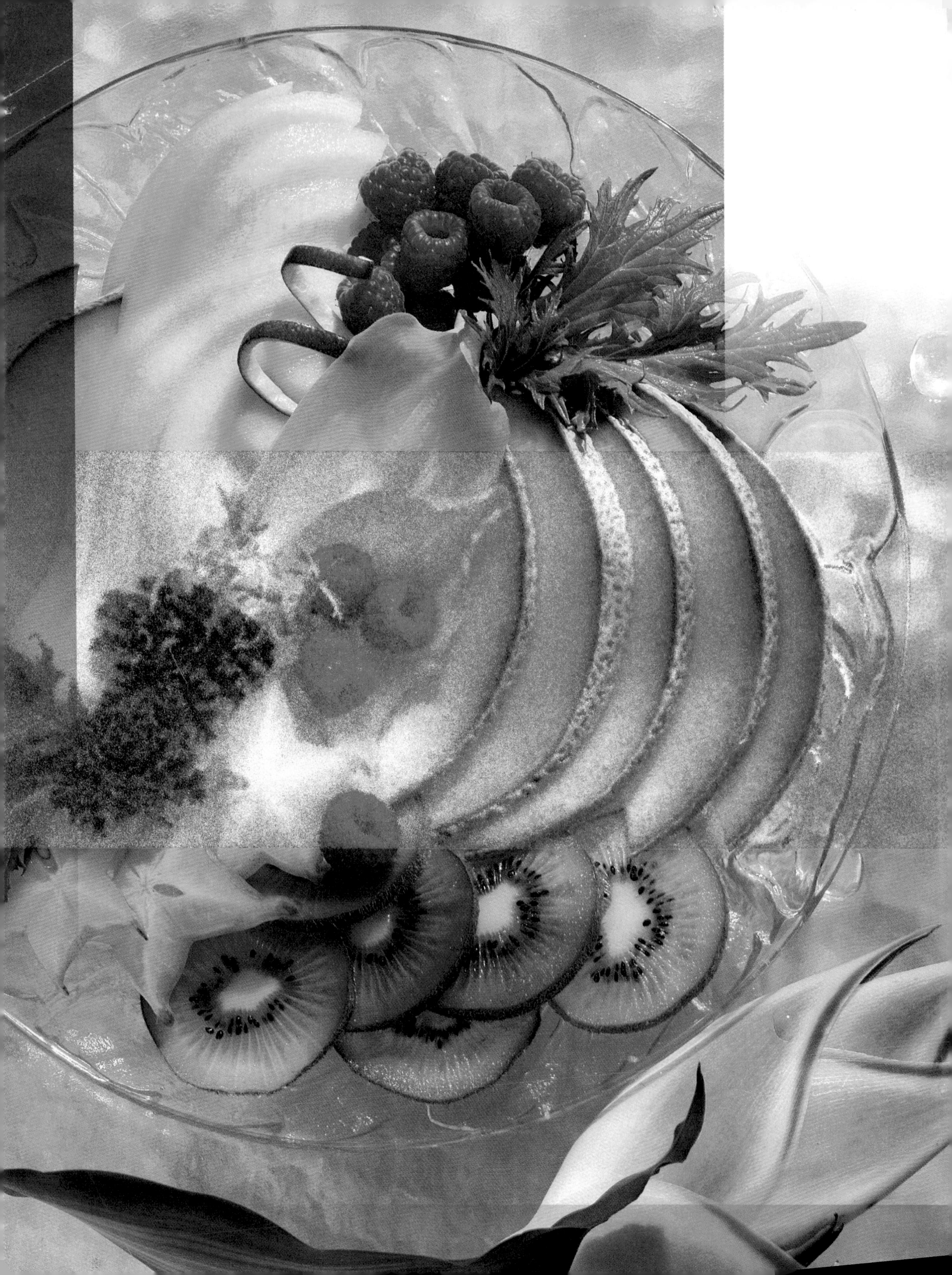

CONTEMPORARY NUTRITION

issues and insights

second edition

GORDON M. WARDLAW, Ph.D., R.D., L.D.
Division of Medical Dietetics
The Ohio State University

PAUL M. INSEL, Ph.D.
Stanford University School of Medicine

MARCIA F. SEYLER, M.Phil.

with 352 illustrations

Illustrations by
Medical and Scientific Illustration:
William C. Ober, M.D.
Claire Garrison, R.N., B.A.

Mosby

St. Louis Baltimore Boston Chicago London Madrid Philadelphia Sydney Toronto

Mosby
Dedicated to Publishing Excellence

Editor-in-Chief: James M. Smith
Acquisitions Editor: Vicki Malinee
Developmental Editor: Loren Stevenson
Project Manager: Patricia Tannian
Production Editor: Ann E. Rogers
Design: Studio Montage
Manufacturing Supervisor: Kathy Grone
Cover photo: Kathy Sanders

SECOND EDITION

Printed in the United States of America
Composition by Clarinda Company
Printing/binding by Von Hoffmann Press, Inc.

Mosby–Year Book, Inc.
11830 Westline Industrial Drive
St. Louis, Missouri 63146

Library of Congress Cataloging in Publication Data
Wardlaw, Gordon M.
Contemporary nutrition: issues and insights/Gordon M. Wardlaw, Paul M. Insel, Marcia F. Seyler, —2nd ed.
ISBN 0-8016-7760-2
1. Nutrition. I. Insel, Paul M. II Seyler, Marcia F. III. Title
QP141.W378 1994 93-29783
613.2—dc20 CIP

93 94 95 96 97 / 9 8 7 6 5 4 3 2 1

About the AUTHORS

GORDON M. WARDLAW, Ph.D., R.D., L.D., teaches nutrition to a variety of students at The Ohio State University. Dr. Wardlaw is the author of numerous articles in prominent nutrition, biology, physiology, and biochemistry journals and was the 1985 recipient of the Mary P. Huddleson Award from the American Dietetic Association. Dr. Wardlaw is a full member of the American Institution of Nutrition and the American Society for Clinical Nutrition, and is certified as a specialist in Human Nutrition by the American Board of Nutrition.

PAUL M. INSEL, Ph.D., is currently Clinical Associate Professor of Psychiatry and Behavioral Sciences at Stanford University. He has been the principal investigator on numerous NIH studies, is the senior author of a leading introductory health text, and is Editor-in-Chief of *Healthline* magazine.

MARCIA F. SEYLER, M.Phil., is a freelance science writer and editor. She has been involved in the development of many college textbooks, specifically *Perspectives in Nutrition* by Gordon M. Wardlaw and Paul M. Insel. She has written numerous articles for *Healthline* magazine and other publications.

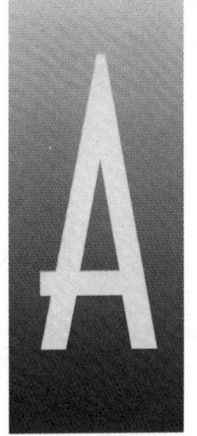

CONTENTS in brief

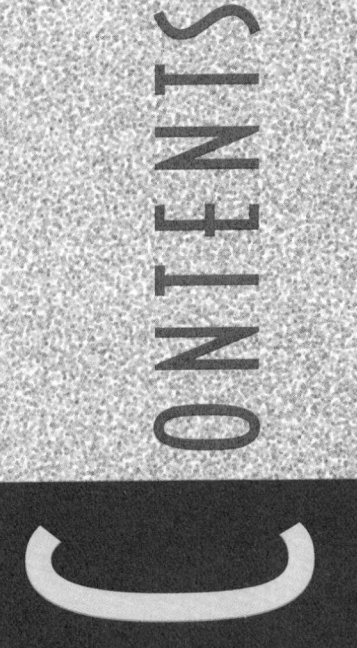

CONTENTS

▸ PART 1 NUTRITION: A KEY TO HEALTH

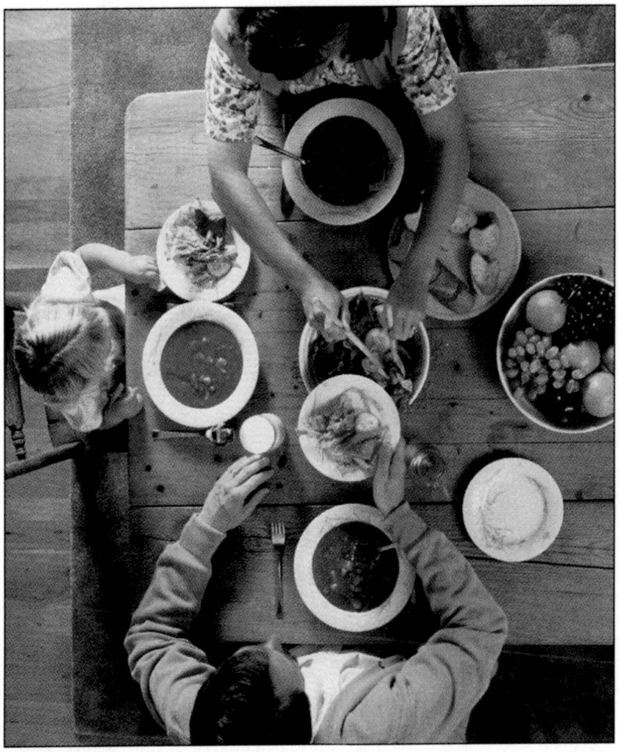

PART 2 NUTRIENTS: THE HEART OF NUTRITION

4 THE HUMAN BODY: A NUTRITION PERSPECTIVE, 96

5 CARBOHYDRATES, 122

6 LIPIDS, 154

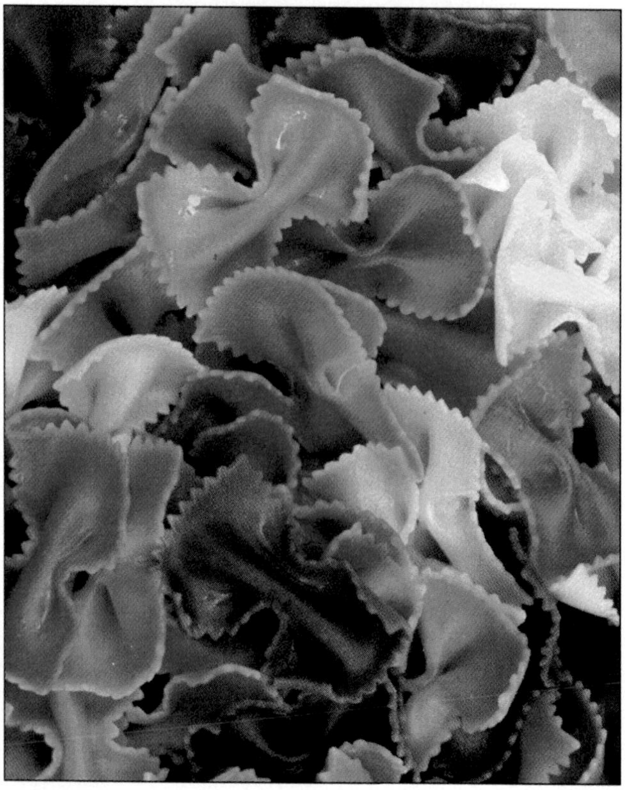

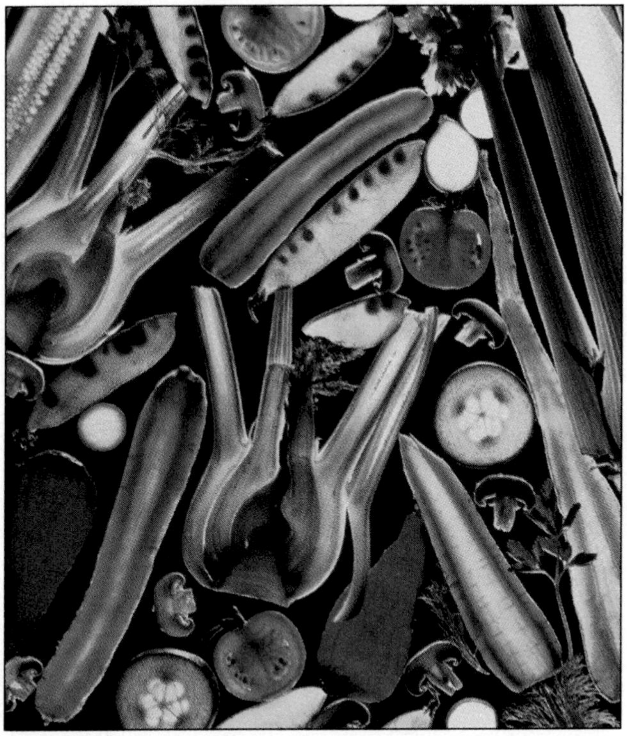

PART 3 ENERGY: BALANCE AND IMBALANCE

10 WEIGHT CONTROL, 310

11 NUTRITION: ATHLETICS AND FITNESS, 351

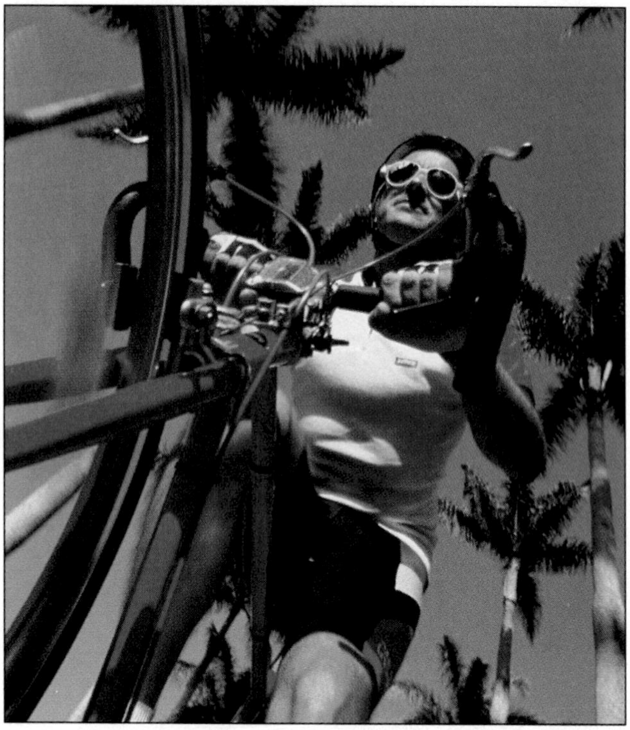

12 ANOREXIA NERVOSA AND BULIMIA, 379

PART 4 NUTRITION: A FOCUS ON LIFE STAGES

13 PREGNANCY AND BREAST-FEEDING, 408

14 NUTRITION FROM INFANCY THROUGH ADOLESCENCE, 441

15 NUTRITION DURING ADULTHOOD, 477

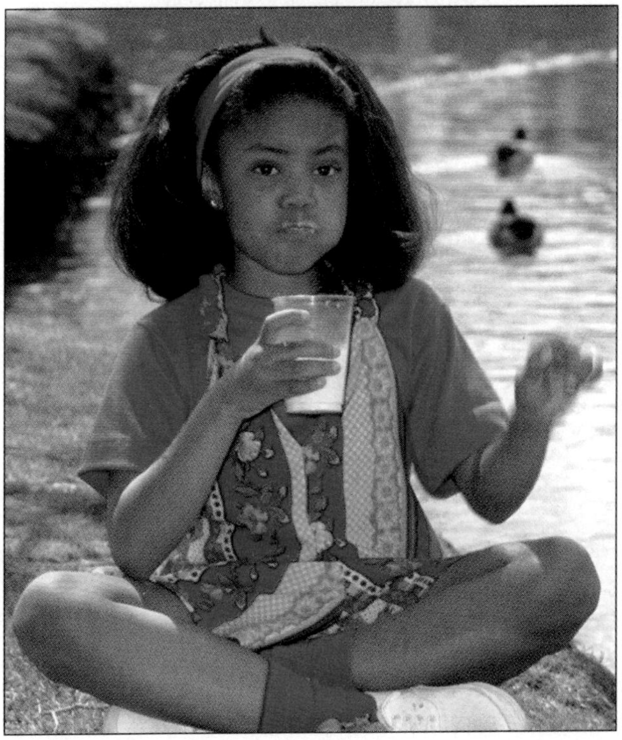

PART 5 NUTRITION: BEYOND THE NUTRIENTS

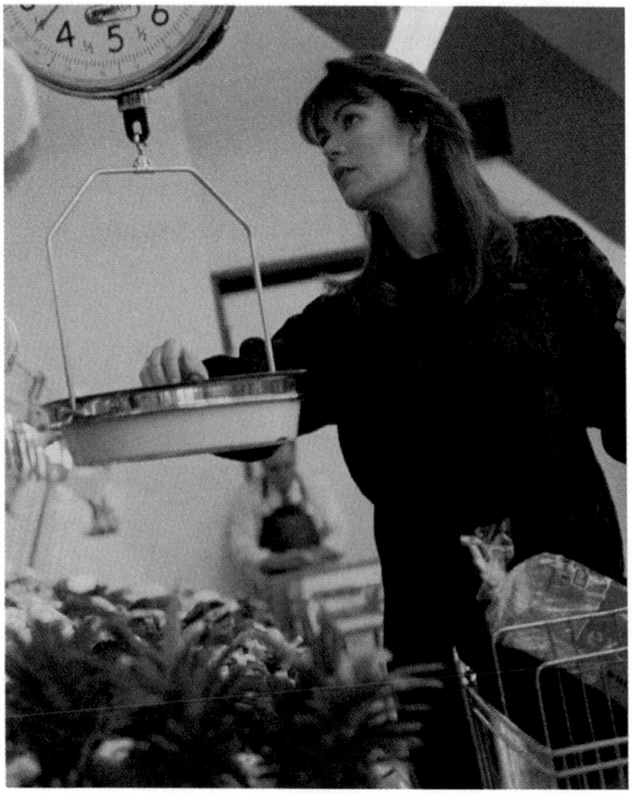

APPENDIXES

PREFACE

As a professor, you undoubtedly already find nutrition a fascinating topic. However, it can also be quite frustrating to teach. There are countless claims and counter-claims about the need for certain constituents in our diet, such as sodium. One group of researchers promotes a reduction in dietary intake by all American adults, while other researchers show that many people can consume sodium freely without significantly increasing their blood pressure above desired levels.

We, too, are frustrated by conflicting data in our field, and so have continued to draw on as many sources as possible in writing the second edition of this textbook. Many major publications have guided us, such as the Surgeon General's Report on Nutrition and Health, the latest National Academy of Sciences Reports: Diet and Health, Nutrition During Pregnancy, and the tenth edition of the RDA. We have incorporated much of the material from these sources, as well as information from many current review articles and basic scientific reports.

We feel this textbook continues to make a break from all others in the field. Like any textbook should, it focuses on the latest research. But it goes further to document important recent research studies and list those references at the back of the chapters. Nutrition Issues in each chapter then reexamine the most controversial nutrition topics of our day. In all, we provide students with a well-rounded view of contemporary nutrition research so that they can more clearly understand and take part in the debate over current nutrition issues.

PERSONALIZING NUTRITION

One overriding theme in nutrition research today is individuality. Not all of us find that saturated fat in our diets raises our blood cholesterol levels over recommended standards. Sugar does not raise everyone's blood glucose levels above accepted guidelines. We often respond in an idiosyncratic manner to nutrients, a fact that is constantly pointed out in this textbook.

Even at this basic level we do not try to put every nutrition student through the same square hole. We constantly ask students to learn more about themselves and their health status and suggest they apply the information given in a manner appropriate to improving their health. After reading this textbook, students will have a much clearer understanding of how the nutrition information given on the evening news, on cereal box labels, in popular magazines, and by government agencies applies to them. Most importantly, they will become knowledgeable consumers of nutrients and nutrition information. They will come to understand that nutrition knowledge allows them to personalize their diet, rather than follow every guideline issued to a population—which by definition actually consists of separate individuals with separate genetic backgrounds and responses to diet.

instructor

In addition, we cover important questions that students often raise concerning vegetarianism, diets for athletes, the safety of our food supply, and fad diets. We emphasize the importance of behavior in terms of understanding one's food choices and changing one's diet. We discuss food behaviors in Chapter 1, behaviors that contribute to weight control in Chapter 10, and behavior modification in detail in Chapter 16.

AUDIENCE

This book has been designed for a nonmajors audience. The chemistry has been kept to a bare minimum. This book will be most suitable as a beginning textbook for any student interested either in an introduction to nutrition or in fulfilling a general science requirement. Health majors, Home Economics majors, Nursing students, Physical Education students, and students in other health-related areas will also find this text quite appropriate. Because of the flexibility of chapter organization and content, this book can be adapted to students of diverse backgrounds.

While the book is most suitable for a semester-length course, it can also be used in a quarter-length course by omitting chapters or multiple sections within chapters. A unique feature of this text is that it is presented in five segments:

PART I	NUTRITION: A Key to Health
PART II	NUTRIENTS: The Heart of Nutrition
PART III	ENERGY: Balance and Imbalance
PART IV	NUTRITION: A Focus on Life Stages
PART V	NUTRITION: Beyond the Nutrients

This organization facilitates tailoring the text to your specific course needs.

NEW TO THIS EDITION

The second edition of CONTEMPORARY NUTRITION incorporates several new features to enhance student learning:

Introduction of digestion and absorption. The discussion of digestion and absorption (in Chapter 4) continues to precede the energy-yielding nutrient chapters but is scaled down to include only the body functions involved in the digestion and absorption process. The digestion and absorption of the energy-yielding nutrients are discussed in the appropriate nutrient chapter to help students better understand these areas in the proper context.

New information from the U.S. Government. New information recently handed down from FDA on food labeling and USDA on the Food Guide Pyramid are discussed in detail to provide students with the most current nutrition information.

Later introduction of behavior change strategies. Chapter 16 encourages the student to plan his or her own diet to enhance health maintenance and then outlines how to do so. This chapter has been moved to the latter half of the text so students gain a full understanding of the major concepts in nutrition before considering strategies for behavior change.

New food composition tables. The food composition tables in Appendix A have been expanded to include more than 700 new foods (more than 1600 in all), which will give students an excellent resource within the text to use for diet analysis exercises.

ADDITIONAL FEATURES

We have organized this text in response to the needs of current instructors and students:

Detailed discussion of consumerism. In Chapter 2 the student will learn how to decipher the new food label. Chapter 3 discusses nutrition fads and fallacies in detail. These topics are often poorly covered by other nutrition textbooks.

Separate chapters on weight control and eating disorders. The student receives a thorough discussion on these very controversial and current topics.

Summary tables. The chapters dealing with vitamins and minerals contain detailed summary tables that include the major points made in the chapters. These tables provide convenient capsules for reference.

Content and controversial topics are well referenced. Approximately 80% of the referenced material is from sources published since 1990. As professors, we demand the latest information to present to our students. Providing this up-to-date research will not only give students the most accurate picture of nutrition today, but will also point them to current materials for further study.

DESIGN

Organizing the illustration program for this textbook continues to be quite exciting. We have drawn heavily from the nutrition expertise of Mosby, and especially from the illustrators under the direction of William Ober, M.D. This textbook remains far ahead of any in the field in depicting important nutrition-related phenomena—such as emulsification, vitamin D metabolism, digestion and absorption, the progression of cancer, and fetal development—in a nonthreatening way. The extensive, three-dimensional graphic presentations in this book will make nutrition come alive for students.

In addition, we draw on many sources to provide what we consider the best photographic program in any nutrition text. The numerous four-color photos for this text were researched and selected to reflect a modern view of food presentation and food consumption. This provides the student with the most outstanding and timely view of the nutrition arena today.

Humor again has been sprinkled throughout the text to aid the learning process. We have combed recent newspapers for the best work of our nation's leading cartoonists. The cartoons make important nutrition points in a way students will remember, such as Gary Larson's wolves hesitating to eat raw pork in Chapter 17.

PEDAGOGY

The following extensive pedagogical features were designed not only to interest the student but also to constantly reinforce the learning process:

Assess Yourself. This exercise at the beginning of each chapter helps students explore their food habits and ideally peaks their interest in the nutritional information in the chapter. For example, the assessment in Chapter 6 is on saturated fat and cholesterol intake, which is a key discussion point in the chapter.

Another Bite. These are short paragraphs spaced throughout the book that examine the application of the material or provide another vantage point from which to view, and possibly better appreciate, the text material.

Margin Definitions. Important key terms are boldfaced at first mention. The more difficult terms are defined in the text's margin. All boldfaced terms are included in the glossary at the back of the text.

Margin Notes. A liberal use of margin notes appears throughout the book. These notes provide clinical examples, references to other chapters, clarification of ideas, and further details for important concepts.

Concept Check. This material summarizes recent chapter content every few pages, providing the student with the opportunity to monitor his or her understanding of the material presented.

Rate Your Plate. This activity at the end of each chapter provides the student with an opportunity to put theory into practice. The suggested assignments generally ask students to carefully analyze part of their current diet or nutrition-related lifestyle.

Nutrition Insight. Each chapter contains one or two short boxed essays, often on controversial topics in nutrition, such as bottled water and fat replacements.

Summary. Chapter content is summarized by highlighting 7 to 10 major points. This feature, together with the Concept Checks, should help students to study for examinations.

Study Questions. Five or so questions at the end of each chapter encourage the student's to probe deeper into the chapter content, helping them make connections and experience new insights.

References. Each chapter contains approximately 20 current references, most published since 1990.

Nutrition Issue. This essay at the end of each chapter extends the chapter content by adding more detailed material on a specific topic.

Glossary. A comprehensive glossary of more than 500 words is included for the student's reference. The glossary contains a list of common medical terms and their root definitions, as well as pronunciation guides for many unfamiliar terms.

SUPPLEMENTARY MATERIALS

Both the student and the instructor are provided with the latest materials to make better use of the text and the concepts of the course:

Instructor's Manual and Test Bank. Prepared by Jeffrey Harris, D.H.Sc., R.D., this comprehensive teaching aid includes chapter summaries with suggestions for teaching difficult material; activities; suggested readings; nutrition assessments; source lists of supplementary materials; and a unique "Survival" chapter addressed to the novice instructor that discusses class organization, scheduling, and problem areas such as cheating.

Extensively reviewed for clarity and accuracy, the test bank features approximately 1400 test items (multiple-choice, short-answer, and matching) coded for level of difficulty, the kind of knowledge being tested, topic, and text page reference. Test items in each chapter follow the sequence of chapter discussions to make selection easy. The resource manual also includes 75 transparency masters of key illustrations from the text and other sources.

Computest computerized test bank. Qualified adopters of the text receive a computerized test bank package compatible with the IBM and Macintosh computers. This software provides a unique combination of user-friendly aids and enables the instructor to select, edit, delete, or add questions, and to construct and print tests and answer keys.

Study guide. Prepared by Gordon M. Wardlaw, this student aid has been thoroughly reviewed by experienced instructors. This comprehensive guide reinforces concepts presented in the text and integrates them with study activities, such as the use of flash cards to reinforce key concepts. It features vocabulary review and sample exams structured to reflect the actual examinations students will face in the classroom. An ongoing dietary analysis highlights the content of each chapter.

Mosby Diet Simple 2.0 nutrient analysis software. This interactive software includes a unique food list with more than 2250 items, selected activities, and food exchange lists. The disk allows students to input food intake and physical activities to determine total kcalories consumed and expended in multiple 24-hour periods.

Transparency Acetates. Seventy-two full-color transparency acetates feature key illustrations from the text with large, easy-to-read labels.

ACKNOWLEDGMENTS

Text development

Barbara Fredin, M.S. aided the authors in the difficult task of tailoring the first edition content for a nonmajors audience. A scientist herself, she has extensive experience editing biology and general science textbooks. Sally Smith, R.D., L.D., took over this role for the second edition, especially helping the authors sift through the vast scientific literature published since the previous edition.

Reviewers

As with the first edition, our goal is to provide the most accurate, up-to-date, and useful introductory nutrition text available. We would like to recognize and thank those people whose direction and insight guided us in the first and second editions.

For the second edition:

Sandra L. Andrews, Ph.D.
Michigan State University

Liz Applegate, Ph.D.
University of California–Davis

Brenda Breeding, M.S.
Oklahoma City Community College

Faye C. Stucy Johnson, Ed.D., R.D., C.H.E.
California State University–Chico

Michael K. McIntosh, Ph.D., R.D., L.D.N.
University of North Carolina–Greensboro

Dorice M. Narins, Ph.D.
Texas Woman's University

Marcia Nahikian-Nelms, M.Ed., R.D.
Southeast Missouri State University

Samuel C. Smith, Ph.D.
University of New Hampshire

Shirley Snarr, Ph.D.
Eastern Kentucky University

Wendy M. Stephens, M.S.
Luther College
(Appendix A)

Maureen C. Zimmerman, M.P.H.
Mesa Community College

For the first edition:

Sara Anderson, Ph.D., R.D.
Southern Illinois University–Carbondale

Joan Benson, M.S., R.D.
University of Utah

Effie Creamer, Ph.D.
Eastern Kentucky University

Julie Ray Friedman, Ph.D.
State University of New York–Farmingdale

Deloy Hendricks, Ph.D.
Utah State University

Michael Hudecki, Ph.D.
State University of New York–Buffalo

Wendy Hunt, M.S., R.D.
American River College

Gladys Jennings, M.S., R.D.
Washington State University

Nelda Loper, M.S., R.D.
Seminole Community College

Margaret Ann McCarthy, M.P.H., R.D.
Eastern Kentucky University

Marsha Read, Ph.D.
University of Nevada

Joanne Spaide, Ph.D.
University of Northern Iowa

Diana Spillman, Ph.D., R.D.
Miami University

Kay Stanek, Ph.D., R.D.
University of Nebraska

Ann Stasch, Ph.D.
California State University–Northridge

SPECIAL ACKNOWLEDGEMENTS

We would like to thank our developmental editor, Loren Stevenson, who nurtured and assisted us every step of the tortuous journey. Vicki Malinee, Acquisitions Editor, and Jim Smith, Editor-in-Chief, facilitated the difficult decisions that frequently arose. Ann Rogers provided excellent and careful copyediting and production work, and Trish Tannian managed the text through the production schedule.

CONTEMPORARY NUTRITION first began with a commitment to simplify nutrition science for the nonmajor student. This remains our goal. We feel that we are succeeding in reestablishing an innovative and exciting text that continues to set a standard for nonmajors nutrition textbooks.

GORDON M. WARDLAW
PAUL M. INSEL
MARCIA F. SEYLER

PREFACE

Oat bran, saturated fat, vegetarianism, high-fiber diets, cholesterol, anorexia nervosa, and Salmonella food poisoning—we suspect you have heard these terms. Which of these are important enough to be a consideration in your life? Americans pride themselves on being individuals. Nutritional advice should be given in that manner. Not all of us have high cholesterol levels, and so don't face a high risk for heart disease. The need to tailor dietary advice to our individual nature is the basic philosophy behind this book. First, we give you a brief introduction to the study of nutrition and give you information on how to be a knowledgeable consumer. With so much information floating around—both accurate and inaccurate—you need to know how to make informed decisions about your nutritional well-being. Then, we give you the basics of nutrition and encourage you to discover how they specifically pertain to you.

We think you will find the study of nutrition fascinating. The text combines some of the most interesting and important aspects of nutrition and food consumption to help you understand both how your body works and how what you eat affects your health.

Features

We have included some features in this book that you should find especially interesting and valuable:

Becoming an informed consumer. In Chapter 3, we discuss the critical information you will need to sort nutritional advice. With so much misleading information being published today, this chapter gives you, the consumer, the tools you will need to separate nutrition fact from fiction.

Planning a new way of eating. Chapter 16 provides you with useful advice on how to improve your dietary patterns. You will follow Alan, a typical college student, as he attempts to improve his diet. We'll show you how to set nutritional goals and design a diet plan to help you attain those goals.

Understanding the world around us. In a college environment, it is often difficult to envision how real the problem of world hunger is. Chapter 18 examines the problem of undernutrition and the conditions that create it. The chapter allows you to examine possible solutions and visualize hope for the future of our planet.

Pedagogy

Contemporary Nutrition: Issues and Insights incorporates some important tools (called pedagogy) to help you learn nutrition. The next few pages graphically point out how to use these study aids to your best advantage.

student

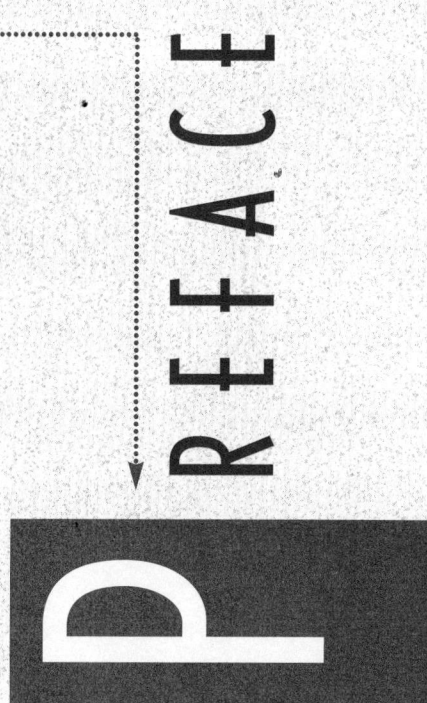

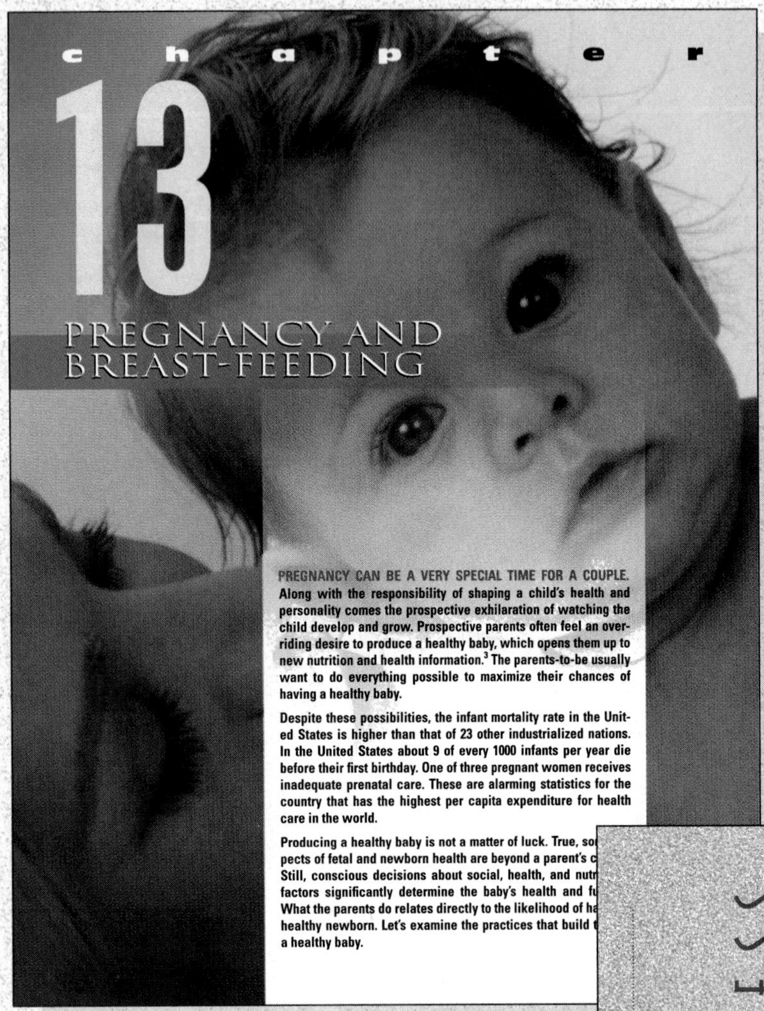

c h a p t e r

13

PREGNANCY AND BREAST-FEEDING

PREGNANCY CAN BE A VERY SPECIAL TIME FOR A COUPLE. Along with the responsibility of shaping a child's health and personality comes the prospective exhilaration of watching the child develop and grow. Prospective parents often feel an overriding desire to produce a healthy baby, which opens them up to new nutrition and health information.[3] The parents-to-be usually want to do everything possible to maximize their chances of having a healthy baby.

Despite these possibilities, the infant mortality rate in the United States is higher than that of 23 other industrialized nations. In the United States about 9 of every 1000 infants per year die before their first birthday. One of three pregnant women receives inadequate prenatal care. These are alarming statistics for the country that has the highest per capita expenditure for health care in the world.

Producing a healthy baby is not a matter of luck. True, so
pects of fetal and newborn health are beyond a parent's c
Still, conscious decisions about social, health, and nutr
factors significantly determine the baby's health and fu
What the parents do relates directly to the likelihood of ha
healthy newborn. Let's examine the practices that build t
a healthy baby.

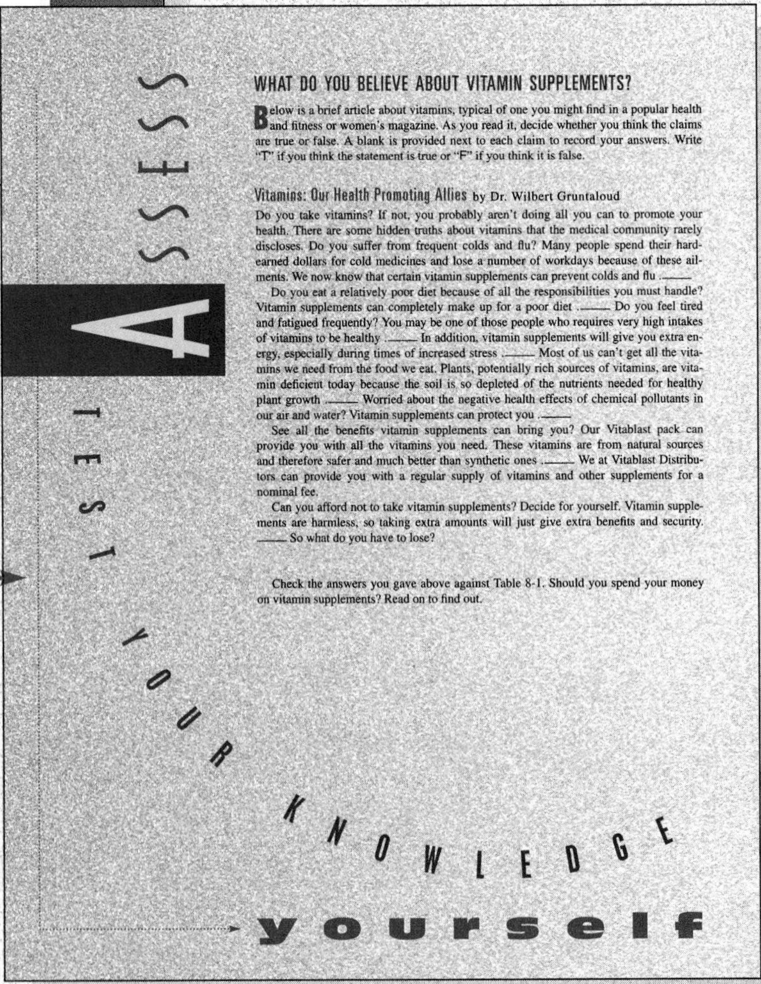

ASSESS yourself

TEST YOUR KNOWLEDGE

WHAT DO YOU BELIEVE ABOUT VITAMIN SUPPLEMENTS?

Below is a brief article about vitamins, typical of one you might find in a popular health and fitness or women's magazine. As you read it, decide whether you think the claims are true or false. A blank is provided next to each claim to record your answers. Write "T" if you think the statement is true or "F" if you think it is false.

Vitamins: Our Health Promoting Allies by Dr. Wilbert Gruntaloud

Do you take vitamins? If not, you probably aren't doing all you can to promote your health. There are some hidden truths about vitamins that the medical community rarely discloses. Do you suffer from frequent colds and flu? Many people spend their hard-earned dollars for cold medicines and lose a number of workdays because of these ailments. We now know that certain vitamin supplements can prevent colds and flu . ____

Do you eat a relatively poor diet because of all the responsibilities you must handle? Vitamin supplements can completely make up for a poor diet . ____ Do you feel tired and fatigued frequently? You may be one of those people who requires very high intakes of vitamins to be healthy . ____ In addition, vitamin supplements will give you extra energy, especially during times of increased stress . ____ Most of us can't get all the vitamins we need from the food we eat. Plants, potentially rich sources of vitamins, are vitamin deficient today because the soil is so depleted of the nutrients needed for healthy plant growth . ____ Worried about the negative health effects of chemical pollutants in our air and water? Vitamin supplements can protect you . ____

See all the benefits vitamin supplements can bring you? Our Vitablast pack can provide you with all the vitamins you need. These vitamins are from natural sources and therefore safer and much better than synthetic ones . ____ We at Vitablast Distributors can provide you with a regular supply of vitamins and other supplements for a nominal fee.

Can you afford not to take vitamin supplements? Decide for yourself. Vitamin supplements are harmless, so taking extra amounts will just give extra benefits and security. ____ So what do you have to lose?

Check the answers you gave above against Table 8-1. Should you spend your money on vitamin supplements? Read on to find out.

Each chapter begins with an **ASSESS YOURSELF.** This exercise will help you determine how much you already know about the chapter content. Review this again when you finish the chapter and you will see how much you have learned or how your opinions have changed.

RATE

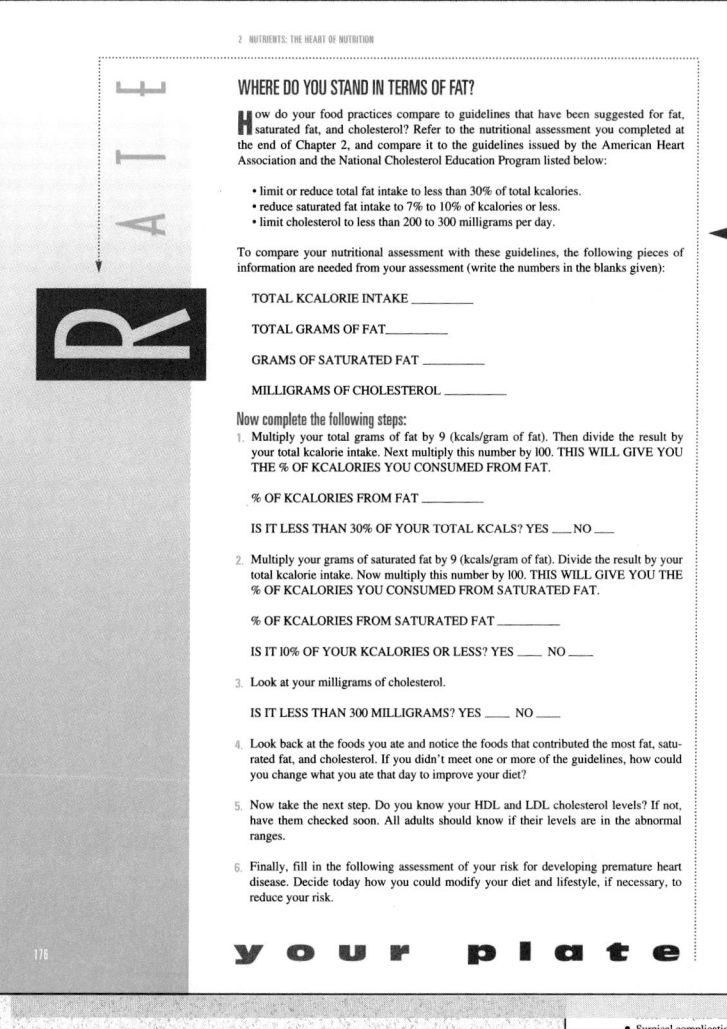

WHERE DO YOU STAND IN TERMS OF FAT?

How do your food practices compare to guidelines that have been suggested for fat, saturated fat, and cholesterol? Refer to the nutritional assessment you completed at the end of Chapter 2, and compare it to the guidelines issued by the American Heart Association and the National Cholesterol Education Program listed below:

- limit or reduce total fat intake to less than 30% of total kcalories.
- reduce saturated fat intake to 7% to 10% of kcalories or less.
- limit cholesterol to less than 200 to 300 milligrams per day.

To compare your nutritional assessment with these guidelines, the following pieces of information are needed from your assessment (write the numbers in the blanks given):

TOTAL KCALORIE INTAKE _________

TOTAL GRAMS OF FAT_________

GRAMS OF SATURATED FAT _________

MILLIGRAMS OF CHOLESTEROL _________

Now complete the following steps:

1. Multiply your total grams of fat by 9 (kcals/gram of fat). Then divide the result by your total kcalorie intake. Next multiply this number by 100. THIS WILL GIVE YOU THE % OF KCALORIES YOU CONSUMED FROM FAT.

   % OF KCALORIES FROM FAT _________

   IS IT LESS THAN 30% OF YOUR TOTAL KCALS? YES ___ NO ___

2. Multiply your grams of saturated fat by 9 (kcals/gram of fat). Divide the result by your total kcalorie intake. Now multiply this number by 100. THIS WILL GIVE YOU THE % OF KCALORIES YOU CONSUMED FROM SATURATED FAT.

   % OF KCALORIES FROM SATURATED FAT _________

   IS IT 10% OF YOUR KCALORIES OR LESS? YES ___ NO ___

3. Look at your milligrams of cholesterol.

   IS IT LESS THAN 300 MILLIGRAMS? YES ___ NO ___

4. Look back at the foods you ate and notice the foods that contributed the most fat, saturated fat, and cholesterol. If you didn't meet one or more of the guidelines, how could you change what you ate that day to improve your diet?

5. Now take the next step. Do you know your HDL and LDL cholesterol levels? If not, have them checked soon. All adults should know if their levels are in the abnormal ranges.

6. Finally, fill in the following assessment of your risk for developing premature heart disease. Decide today how you could modify your diet and lifestyle, if necessary, to reduce your risk.

your plate

At the end of each chapter is a **RATE YOUR PLATE** section that will help you put a major concept in each chapter into focus for your own life. The activity encourages you to look more carefully at your diet, examine your family history, or apply information learned to help others.

besity—the major type of energy imbalance in America—go a (Table 10-1). Since 1948 the Framingham Heart Study has thousand residents of Framingham, a small Massachusetts ed that carrying an excess of 20% or more above one's desir- ks. And the greater the degree of obesity, (1) the more likely roblems and (2) the more serious these problems generally tudy supports other studies that show excess weight raises the

- pendent) diabetes
- Surgical complications
- Hypertension
- Heart disease
- Arthritis
- Gallstones
- Various forms of cancer—colon, rectal, and prostate cancer in men and breast, uterine, and ovarian cancer in women
- Pregnancy risks
- Sleep disturbances
- Early death

The numerous **tables** throughout the text provide convenient capsules of information for your reference.

TABLE 10-1

Health Problems Associated with Excess Body Fat

Health Problem	Partially Attributed To:
Adult-onset diabetes (NIDDM)	Enlarged fat cells, which then poorly bind insulin and also poorly respond to the message insulin sends to the cell
Surgical risk	Increased anesthesic needs and greater risk of wound infections
Pulmonary disease	Excess weight over lungs
Hypertension	Increased miles of blood vessels found in the fat tissue; however, no validated cause is yet known
Coronary heart disease	Increases in serum cholesterol and triglyceride levels, as well as a decrease in physical activity
Bone and joint disorders	Excess pressure put on knee, ankle, and hip joints
Gallbladder stones	An increase in cholesterol content of bile
Skin disorders	The trapping of moisture and microbes in fat folds
Various cancers	Estrogen production by fat cells; animal studies suggest excess energy intake encourages tumor development
Shorter stature (in some forms of obesity)	An earlier onset of puberty
Pregnancy risk	More difficult delivery and increased anesthetic needs (if the latter is used)
Early death	A variety of risk factors for disease listed above

The greater the degree of obesity, the more likely and the more serious these health problems generally become. They are much more likely to appear in people who are greater than twice their desirable body weight.

The **CONCEPT CHECKS** list the major points made in each chapter section. If you don't understand what the Concept Check says, you should reread the preceding section in the textbook.

CONCEPT CHECK

Genetic background plays a role in obesity via body shape and rate of basal metabolism. The role of nurture is exhibited in similar eating habits, activity levels, and degrees of fatness in families. Men's tendency to develop obesity after age 30 and women's pattern of having both childhood and adult roots for obesity suggest the powerful influence of nurture in men. Because both factors have an impact, we speculate that nurture may serve as a catalyst for expressing or denying a genetic tendency toward obesity.

You'll find that the numerous full-color, 3-dimensional **illustrations** almost jump off the page. No other nutrition textbook provides you with such effective, detailed drawings that virtually "come alive."

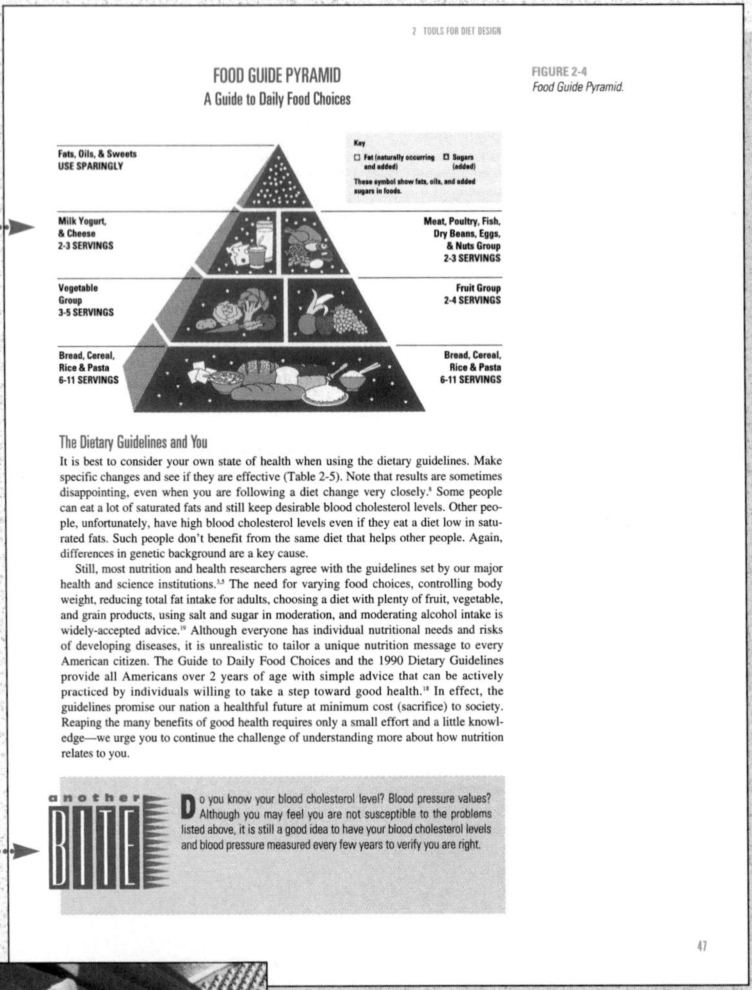

2 TOOLS FOR DIET DESIGN

FOOD GUIDE PYRAMID

A Guide to Daily Food Choices

Fats, Oils, & Sweets
USE SPARINGLY

Key
Fat (naturally occurring and added) Sugars (added)
These symbol show fats, oils, and added sugars in foods.

Milk Yogurt, & Cheese 2-3 SERVINGS

Meat, Poultry, Fish, Dry Beans, Eggs, & Nuts Group 2-3 SERVINGS

Vegetable Group 3-5 SERVINGS

Fruit Group 2-4 SERVINGS

Bread, Cereal, Rice & Pasta 6-11 SERVINGS

Bread, Cereal, Rice & Pasta 6-11 SERVINGS

FIGURE 2-4
Food Guide Pyramid.

The Dietary Guidelines and You

It is best to consider your own state of health when using the dietary guidelines. Make specific changes and see if they are effective (Table 2-5). Note that results are sometimes disappointing, even when you are following a diet change very closely.[8] Some people can eat a lot of saturated fats and still keep desirable blood cholesterol levels. Other people, unfortunately, have high blood cholesterol levels even if they eat a diet low in saturated fats. Such people don't benefit from the same diet that helps other people. Again, differences in genetic background are a key cause.

Still, most nutrition and health researchers agree with the guidelines set by our major health and science institutions.[3,5] The need for varying food choices, controlling body weight, reducing total fat intake for adults, choosing a diet with plenty of fruit, vegetable, and grain products, using salt and sugar in moderation, and moderating alcohol intake is widely-accepted advice.[19] Although everyone has individual nutritional needs and risks of developing diseases, it is unrealistic to tailor a unique nutrition message to every American citizen. The Guide to Daily Food Choices and the 1990 Dietary Guidelines provide all Americans over 2 years of age with simple advice that can be actively practiced by individuals willing to take a step toward good health.[18] In effect, the guidelines promise our nation a healthful future at minimum cost (sacrifice) to society. Reaping the many benefits of good health requires only a small effort and a little knowledge—we urge you to continue the challenge of understanding more about how nutrition relates to you.

another BITE

Do you know your blood cholesterol level? Blood pressure values? Although you may feel you are not susceptible to the problems listed above, it is still a good idea to have your blood cholesterol levels and blood pressure measured every few years to verify you are right.

47

ANOTHER BITE boxes are short paragraphs within the text designed to provide you with a different perspective on chapter material. You'll discover new and different ways to apply information.

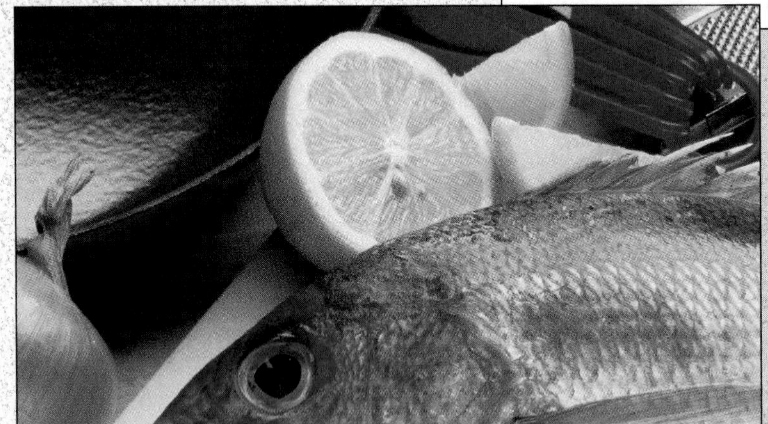

The full-color **photos** reflect a modern view of food consumption and food presentation.

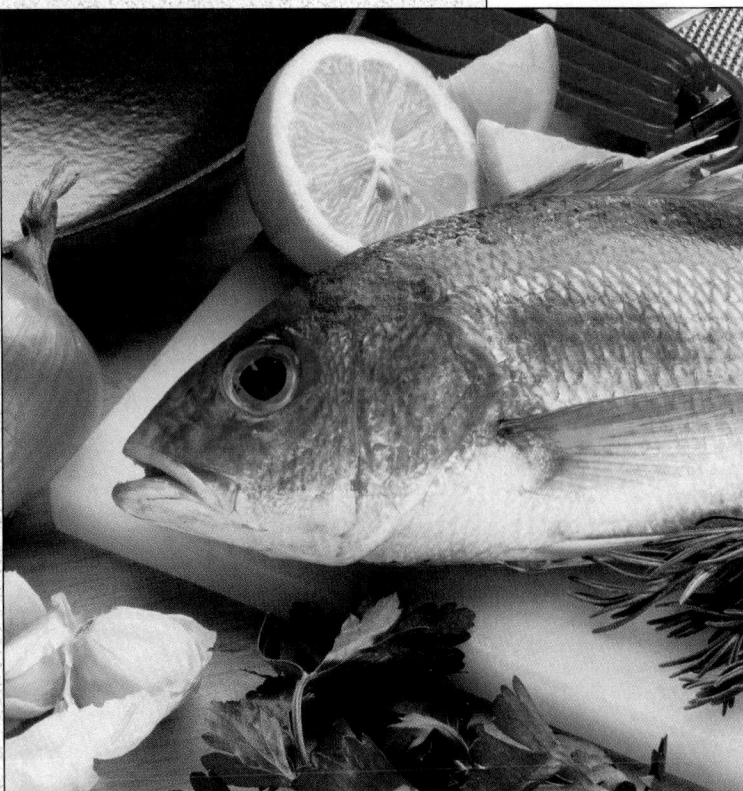

Study Questions

1. John walks into physician's office and his body status is assessed using the 1983 Metropolitan Life Insurance Table. Provide one advantage and one disadvantage of using this method.
2. What are the two most convincing pieces of evidence that both genetic and environment factors play significant roles in the development of obesity?
3. What are the major psychological and physiological problems associated with rapid weight loss?
4. When searching for a sound weight-loss program, what six characteristics would you look for? Give four characteristics of fad diets for weight loss.
5. You are following a nutritional plan for weight loss. What are five specific ways you could save kcalories?
6. Describe the term *behavior modification.* Relate it to the terms *stimulus control, self-monitoring, chain-breaking, relapse prevention,* and *cognitive restructuring.* Give examples of each in the latter group.

We also include approximately five **STUDY QUESTIONS** per chapter. These provide an excellent review for studying for examinations.

References

1. Anderson JW and others: Benefits and risks of an intensive very-low-calorie diet program for severe obesity, *The American Journal of Gastroenterology* 87:6, 1992.
2. Atkinson RL and others: Combination of very-low-calorie diet and behavior modification in the treatment of obesity, *American Journal of Clinical Nutrition* 56:199S, 1992.
3. Bjorntorp P: Metabolic implications of body fat distribution, *Diabetes Care* 14:1132, 1991.
4. Booth DA: Integration of internal and external signals in intake control, *Proceedings of the Nutrition Society* 51:21, 1992.
5. Bray GA: An approach to the classification and evaluation of obesity. In Bjorntorp B, Brodoff BN, editors: *Obesity,* Philadelphia, 1992, JB Lippincott.
6. Bray GA: Drug treatment for obesity, *American Journal of Clinical Nutrition* 55:538S, 1992.
7. Castonguay TW, Stern JS: Hunger and appetite. In Brown ML, editor: *Present knowledge in nutrition,* Washington, DC, 1990, International Life Sciences Institute.
8. Dattilo AM: Dietary fat and its relationship to body weight, *Nutrition Today,* p. 13, January/February 1992.
9. Diaz EO and others: Metabolic response to experimental overfeeding in lean and overweight healthy volunteers, *American Journal of Clinical Nutrition* 56:641, 1992.
10. Forbes GB: Exercise and lean weight: the influence of body weight, *Nutrition Reviews* 50:157, 1992.
11. Forbes JM: Metabolic aspects of satiety, *Proceedings of the Nutrition Society* 51:13, 1992.
12. Gastrointestinal surgery for severe obesity: National Institutes of Health Consensus Development Conference Statement, *American Journal of Clinical Nutrition* 55:615S, 1992.
13. Kushner RF: Bioelectrical impedance analysis: a review of principles and applications, *Journal of the American College of Nutrition* 11:199, 1992.
14. Leibel RL: Fat as fuel and metabolic signal, *Nutrition Reviews* 50:12, 1992.
15. Lichtman SW and others: Discrepancy between self-reported and actual caloric intake and exercise in obese subjects, *The New England Journal of Medicine* 327:1893, 1992.
16. Luke A, Schoeller DA: Basal metabolic rate, fat-free mass, and body cell mass during energy restriction, *Metabolism* 41:450, 1992.
17. National Institutes of Health Technology Assessment Conference Statement: Methods for voluntary weight loss and control, *Nutrition Reviews* 50:340, 1992.
18. Nelson KM and others: Effect of weight reduction on resting energy expenditure, substrate utilization, and the thermic effect of food in moderately obese women,

Throughout each chapter are **boldfaced key terms**. These are terms you will need to be familiar with throughout your study. The more difficult terms will include a definition in the text's margins. All boldfaced terms will appear with their definitions and pronunciations in the **glossary** at the end of the text.

U.S. Recommended Daily Allowances (U.S. RDAs) *Nutrient standards established by the FDA for use on nutrition labels. Generally, the four existing versions use the highest nutrient recommendation in the appropriate age and gender category from the 1968 publication of the RDA. The version that includes children over 4 years of age and adults is most commonly seen on nutrition labels.*

RDAs AND RDIs

...ne practical application of the RDA is the ***U.S. Recommended Daily Allowances (U.S. RDAs)***. Note the "D" stands for "daily," not "dietary" as in RDA. This standard ...as first set in 1974 by the U.S. Food and Drug Administration (FDA) to be used on ...utrition labels on foods and vitamin/mineral supplements (Figure 2-2). It replaced the ...minimum daily requirements (MDR). The U.S. RDAs for adults are primarily based on the highest RDA values determined in 1968 for this specific age-group. For example, the 1968 RDA for iron for adult men was 10 milligrams per day; for adult women it was 18 milligrams per day. The U.S. RDA for adults uses the higher value of 18 milligrams per day. Appendix D lists U.S. RDA values. The values set for children over 4 years of age and adults are commonly listed on food products.

Mainly for economic reasons, the U.S. RDAs have not been updated since they were first set, but new food labeling laws will soon lead to changes.[14] The National Labeling and Education Act of 1990 established the task for our government to increase regulati...n of food labels.[4] As part of this process, the U.S. RDAs will be updated and the new name will be Reference Daily Intakes (RDIs). RDI values will be based on the 1989 RDAs and represent an average value of the RDAs for that nutrient (rather than the highest RDA ...) over the age range to which the RDIs are applied (Appendix D). In addition, ... Values (DRVs) will be set for some nutrients that don't have an RDA, ...ate. RDI and DRV will be combined under one heading on new

...n the current RDAs, especially for vitamin ... RDI values will average 10% to ... the current RDAs. Not ... (as compared ... Some

NUTRITION INSIGHTS are boxes within the text that allow you to explore timely topics that should be of interest to you.

NUTRITION insight

DIET PILLS

Over-the-counter medications that claim to help weight loss sell briskly. Though some can be effective, none matches diet moderation and physical activity for long-term weight loss. Diet aids include caffeine, fiber pills, phenylpropanolamine, and benzocaine. Caffeine tends to blunt appetite. Benzocaine numbs the tongue and affects the sense of taste, so a person tends to eat less. Fiber pills can increase bulk in the stomach and ideally lead to satiety. A typical side effect is significant intestinal gas. Can you guess why? (See Chapter 5.)

Phenylpropanolamine is an epinephrine-like drug that can cause a slight decrease in food intake.[17] At a typical dose of 76 milligrams per day, the degree of appetite suppression varies among people. FDA recommends phenylpropanolamine be used with caution in people with hyperthyroidism, cardiovascular disorders (including hypertension), and diabetes. Adverse reactions may also occur among those taking various other medications at the same time.

Prescription medications

Physicians sometimes prescribe amphetamines for weight loss.[35] Amphetamines decrease appetite, but they can have a hook: addiction. In addition, amphetamines can increase heart rate and nervousness and lead to insomnia. Thyroid hormone preparations, once popular, caused significant loss of lean tissue.

Fenfluramine and fluoxetine have been prescribed by physicians to promote weight loss. By increasing the action of a neurotransmitter in the brain, they may lead to less food craving, especially for high-carbohydrate foods. Note some people complain of rapid weight gain after discontinuing the drug, and fenfluramine worsens depression in those people who already show signs of this disorder.

The experimental medications naloxone and naltrexone significantly decrease food intake in laboratory animals. Results from human studies, however, have proved discouraging. Development of related drugs is continuing.

Overall, in skilled hands, prescription medications can aid weight loss when coupled with diet control; however, they do not substitute for the more conservative approaches of reducing energy intake, modifying problem behaviors, and increasing physical activity.

A history of yo-yo dieting, the repeated loss and regain of weight, also bears consideration. This pattern can predispose a person to subsequent heart disease.

Useless medications

The hormone cholecystokinin (CCK) may regulate food intake within the body, but bought in a bottle, it wastes money. It is widely available in health-food stores in the form of ground up animal intestines (recall CCK is produced in the small intestine). However, the amount of CCK in each pill is almost too small to detect, let alone suppress appetite. In addition, CCK is a protein and so is destroyed by digestion in the stomach; little is absorbed as such from an oral dose. It must be injected to be effective, and you can't buy a form that is safe to inject.

Another class of useless and potentially harmful diet aids is diuretics or "water pills." They have a legitimate medical use in the treatment of hypertension, but they cannot control body fatness. Obesity is not primarily caused by excess water accumulation in healthy people.

310

To briefly clarify and expand concepts presented, **margin notes** are provided for you. These help reinforce concepts you'll learn in every chapter.

17 FOOD SAFETY

SUMMARY

- Bacteria and other microbes in foods are the agents most likely to cause food-borne illness. To guard against this in the past, people used salt, sugar, smoke, fermentation, and drying to preserve foods. Today, we also recognize the importance of proper cooking and of keeping hot foods hot and cold foods cold. Pasteurization has also greatly improved the safety of dairy products.
- Cross-contamination commonly causes food-borne illness. It occurs when bacteria on raw animal products reach other foods that can support bacterial growth. Because of the risk of cross-contamination, no food should be kept at room temperature for more than 2 hours if it has come in contact with raw animal products and can support bacterial growth.
- Treatment for food-borne illness usually requires drinking a lot of fluids, avoiding food handling while diarrhea is present, thorough hand washing, and bed rest.
- The major causes of food-borne illness today are the bacteria *Salmonella*, *Staphylococcus aureus*, and *Clostridium perfringens*. To protect against these agents, cover cuts on the hands, do not sneeze on foods, avoid contact between raw meat or poultry products and other food products, and rapidly cool and then thoroughly reheat leftovers. Thorough cooking of foods and the use of pasteurized dairy products further protects against other problem microbes. Viruses, molds, and parasites also account for many cases of food-borne illness. Again, taking care to select, handle, and cook foods properly can prevent problems.
- Food additives are used primarily to extend shelf life by preventing microbial growth and destruction of food components by oxygen, certain chemical ions, and other substances. Food additives are classed as those intentionally added to foods and those that incidentally end up as contaminants in foods. An additive to a food is limited by the FDA to at most 1/100 of the greatest amount that causes no observable effects in animals. In most cases, the Delaney Clause bans the use of any intentional food additive introduced after 1958 in the United States if it causes cancer.
- Antioxidants, such as vitamin E and sulfites, prevent oxygen and enzyme destruction of food products. Emulsifiers suspend fat in water, improving the uniformity, smoothness, and body of foods, such as ice cream. Common antimicrobial agents include sodium benzoate and sorbic acid, which prevent bacterial growth. Sequestrants bind free chemical ions, preventing them from causing fats to become rancid.
- A variety of environmental contaminants can be found in food. Because most of them dissolve in fat, trimming fat from meats and discarding fat that is rendered during cooking of meats, fish, and poultry are good steps to minimize exposure. In addition, it is helpful to wash fruits and vegetables thoroughly and to discard the outer leaves of leafy vegetables.
- Toxic substances occur naturally in a variety of foods, such as green potatoes, moldy grains, raw soybeans, and raw egg whites. Cooking foods limits their toxic effects. Over the centuries, people have purposely avoided some of these foods, such as moldy grains and the green parts of potatoes.

537

Each chapter ends with a **SUMMARY**. These summary points convey the major ideas of each chapter.

14 NUTRITION FROM INFANCY THROUGH ADOLESCENCE

Nutrition ISSUE

FOOD ALLERGIES AND INTOLERANCES

Adverse reactions to foods—indicated by sneezing, coughing, nausea, vomiting, diarrhea, hives and other rashes—are broadly classed as food allergies or food intolerances.[15] Allergies are reactions linked to immune system responses, such as the rapid increase in heart rate and shortness of breath that occur when susceptible people eat shrimp. The immune system senses what it considers "foreign proteins" and attempts to eliminate these. The symptoms experienced are the result of the battle.

On the other hand symptoms of food intolerances—which include many of those listed above—are not linked to immune system processes. For example, symptoms of foodborne illness, such as Salmonella from infected egg products, are caused by toxins produced by bacteria in food. These toxins directly affect intestinal cells, for example. The immune system is not part of the process. Let's examine each process, allergies and intolerances, separately so you can learn how to reduce your risk of becoming a victim.

Allergic reactions to foods are commonly reported, and more frequently by females. The most common ages for food allergies are infancy and young adulthood. Allergic-related disease appears in about 30-40 million Americans. Types of reactions associated with food ingestion are:

Classic allergy—Itching, reddening skin, asthma, and a runny nose.

Gastrointestinal—Nausea, vomiting, diarrhea, intestinal gas, bloating, pain, constipation, and indigestion.

General—Headache, skin reactions, tension and fatigue, tremors, and psychological problems.

Allergic reaction symptoms vary with the location in the body as noted above. Timelines include from seconds to a few days. A generalized, all-systems reaction is called anaphylactic shock. This severe allergic response results in lowered blood pressure and respiratory and gastrointestinal tract distress. This can be fatal. A person with extreme sensitivity to a food may not be able to touch the food or even be in the same room where it is being cooked without responding to it.

About 90% of food allergies (also called hypersensitivities) are caused by milk, eggs, nuts (especially peanuts), corn, seafood, soy, and wheat. Other foods frequently identified with adverse reactions include alcoholic beverages, meat and meat products, vegetables, sugars, cereals, fish, fats and oils, fruits, chocolate, and cheese.[15] A family history of allergies greatly increases the risk.

Why do food allergies occur?

A food allergy is caused by an immune response to a food substance. *Food sensitivity* is a term often used today to describe milder reactions. Again, the word *allergy* specifies a disorder of the immune system. Allergens are usually large proteins with specific sizes and configurations.

When an allergen enters an allergic-prone host for the first time, a specific immune reaction takes place, although it is not apparent. Subsequent exposures can then trigger various muscles to contract, increase permeability of blood vessels, and lead to nasal secretions, itching, and changes in dilation of the airways.

459

NUTRITION ISSUES are boxes at the end of chapters that develop current topics in nutrition in greater detail than the chapter can. Topics include nutrition and alcohol, heart disease, cancer, fad diets, and nutrition labeling.

STUDY AIDS

A Student Study Guide and Mosby Diet Simple 2.0 software are available for use with *Contemporary Nutrition: Issues and Insights, second edition.* These instructional aids are designed to help you practice the major concepts developed in each chapter and prepare for classroom examinations.

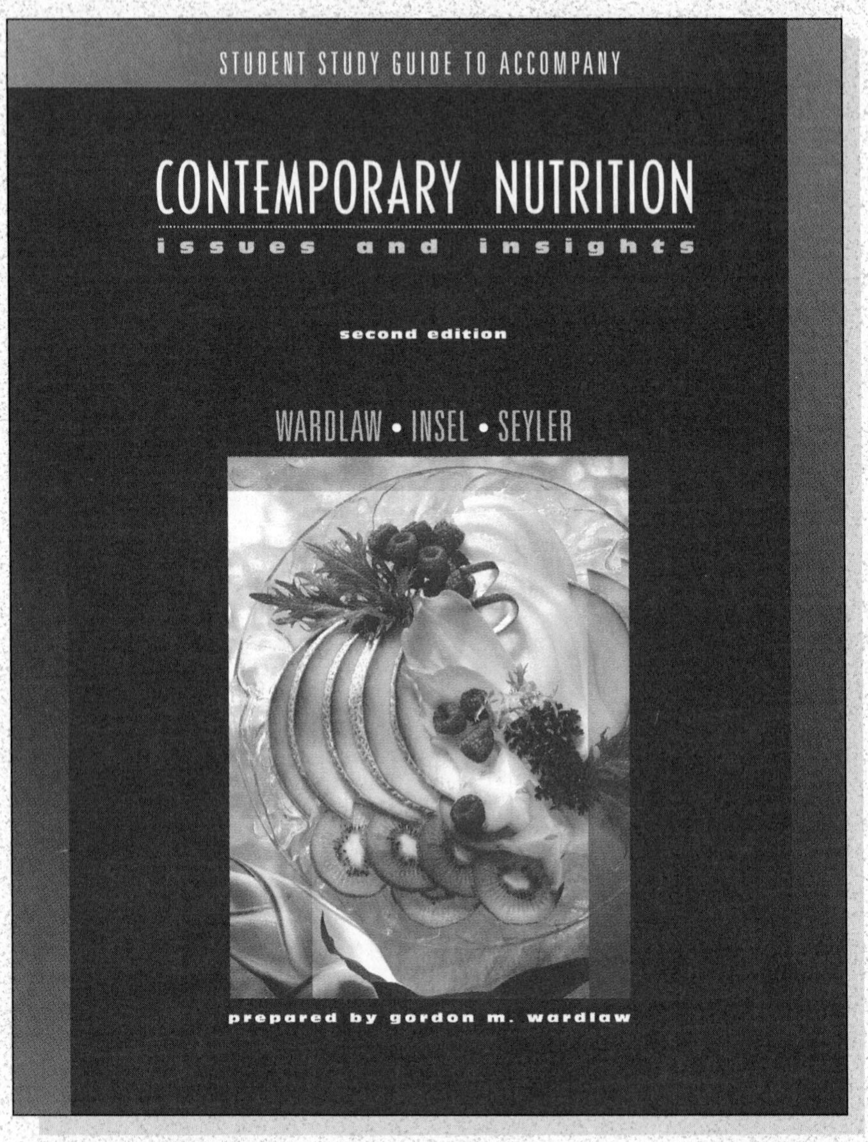

Student Study Guide

Reviewed by instructors and developed in consultation with a learning theory expert, this valuable Study Guide by Gordon M. Wardlaw reinforces concepts presented in the text and integrates them with activities to facilitate learning.

- Sample examinations reflect the actual tests you will face in the classroom.
- Vocabulary review exercises increase your knowledge of terminology.
- Flash cards help you practice explaining the major concepts in the chapter to yourself, and in turn test your understanding of these important concepts.
- Activities include fill-in tables, labeling, and matching terms. These activities follow the text discussion and are anchored with quotations and page citations from the text. An ongoing dietary analysis highlights the content of many chapters.

Mosby Diet Simple 2.0 nutrient analysis software

Created by N-Squared Computing, the nutrient analysis computer software is designed to help you quickly calculate the nutrient content of your diet, learn more about the exchange system, and calculate how many kcalories you use each day. You will find that learning to use this software will help you analyze your diet more efficiently.

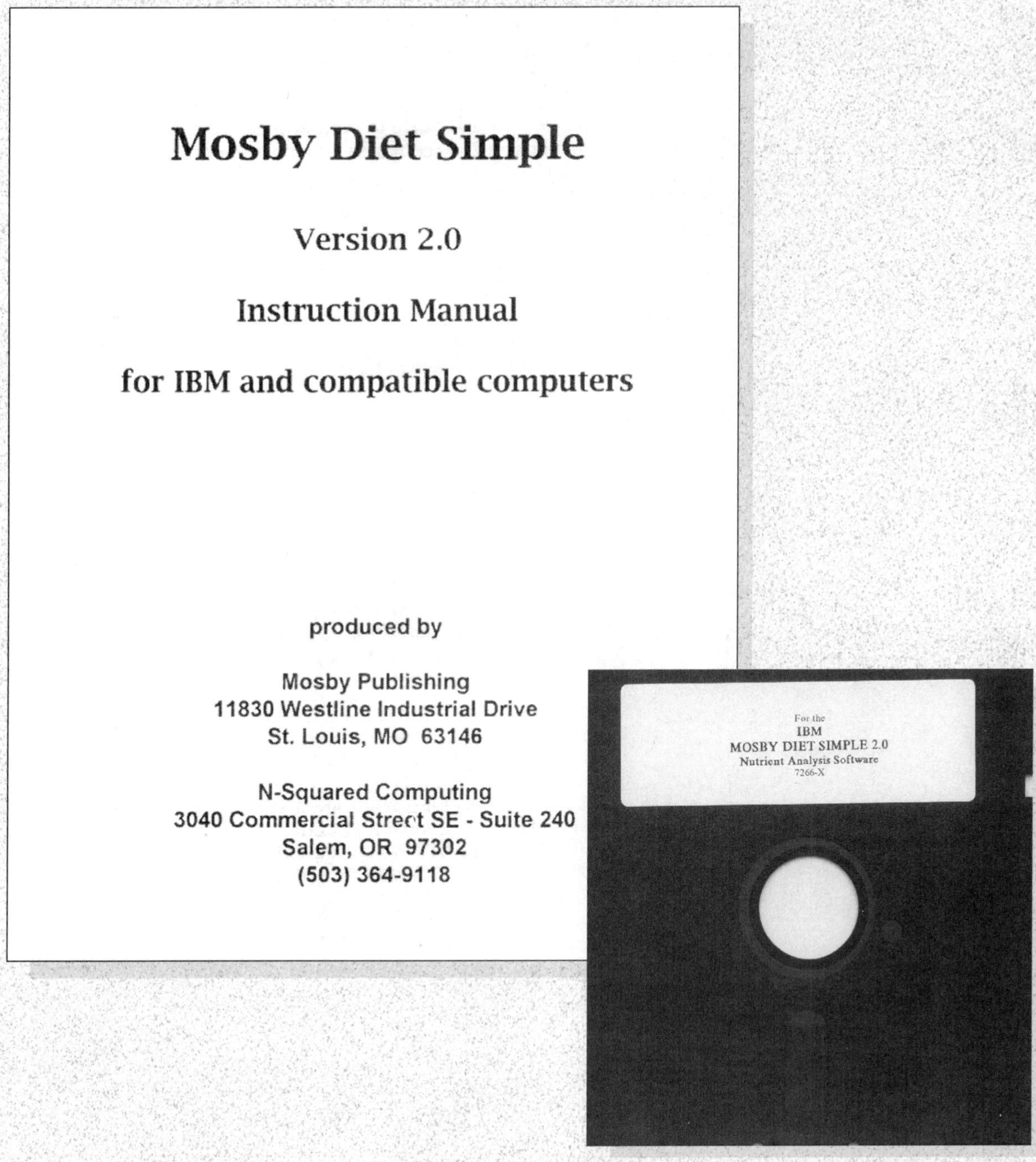
Mosby Diet Simple
Version 2.0
Instruction Manual
for IBM and compatible computers
produced by
Mosby Publishing
11830 Westline Industrial Drive
St. Louis, MO 63146
N-Squared Computing
3040 Commercial Street SE - Suite 240
Salem, OR 97302
(503) 364-9118
For the
IBM
MOSBY DIET SIMPLE 2.0
Nutrient Analysis Software
7266-X

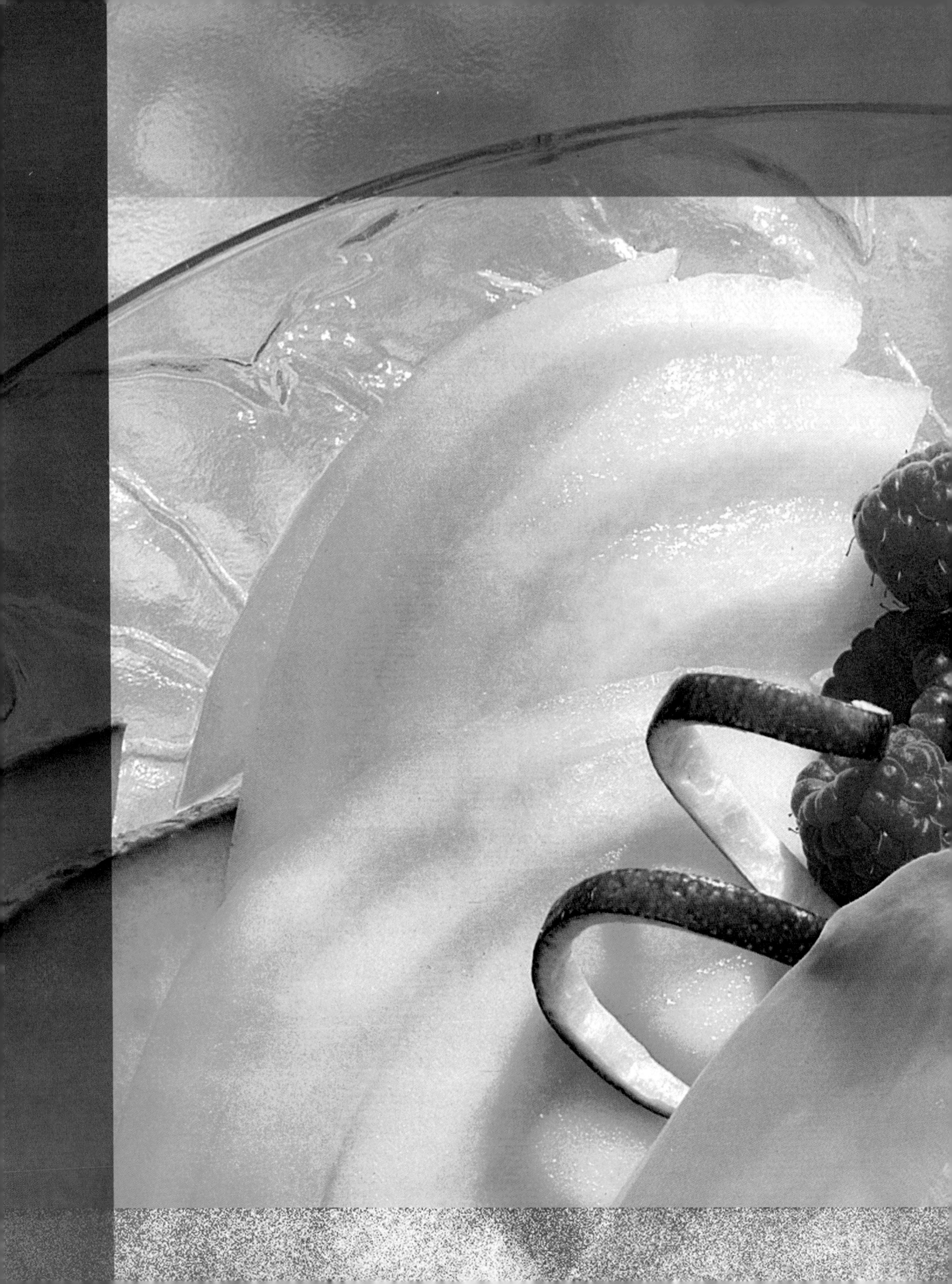

NUTRITION: A KEY TO HEALTH

1

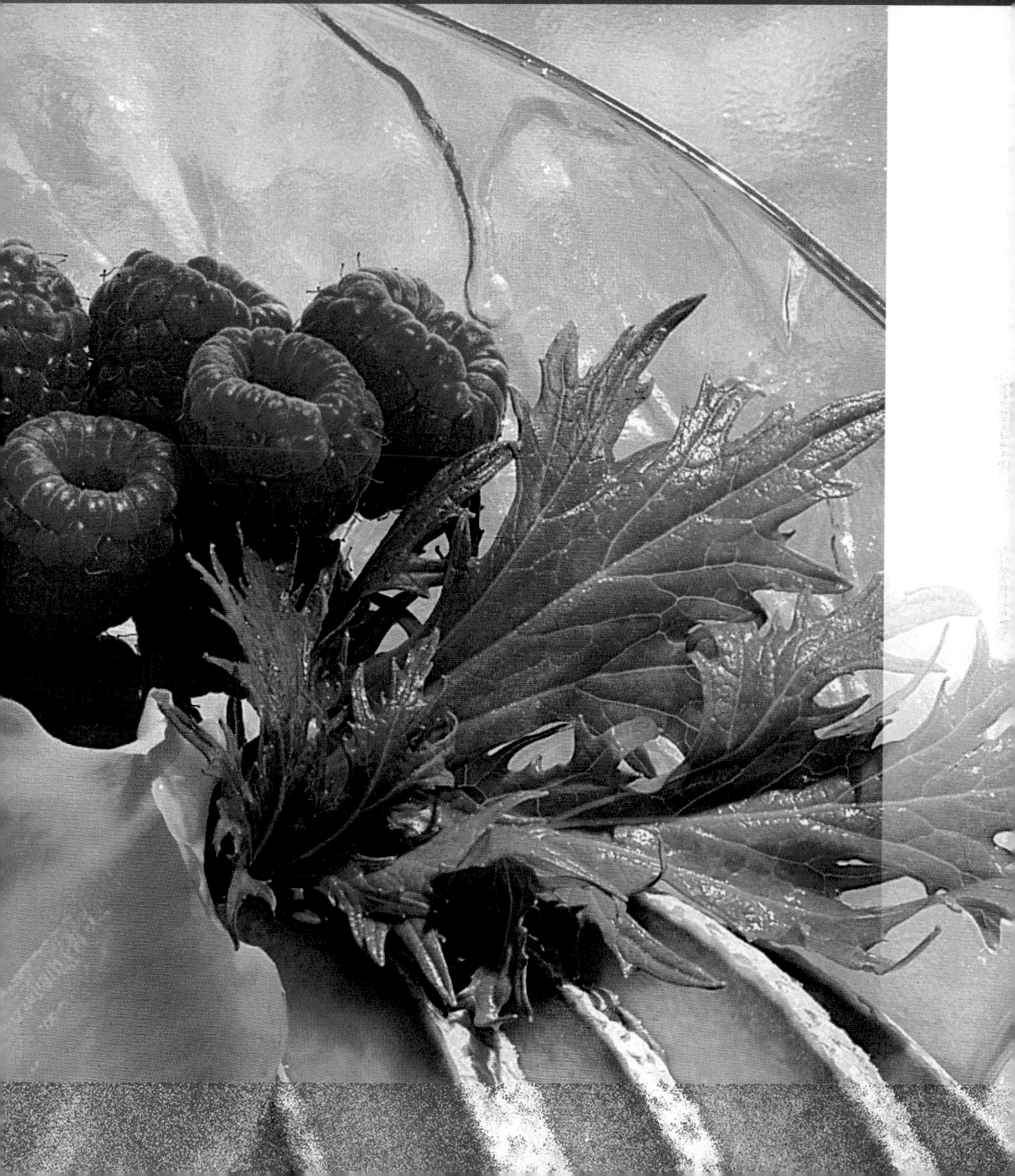

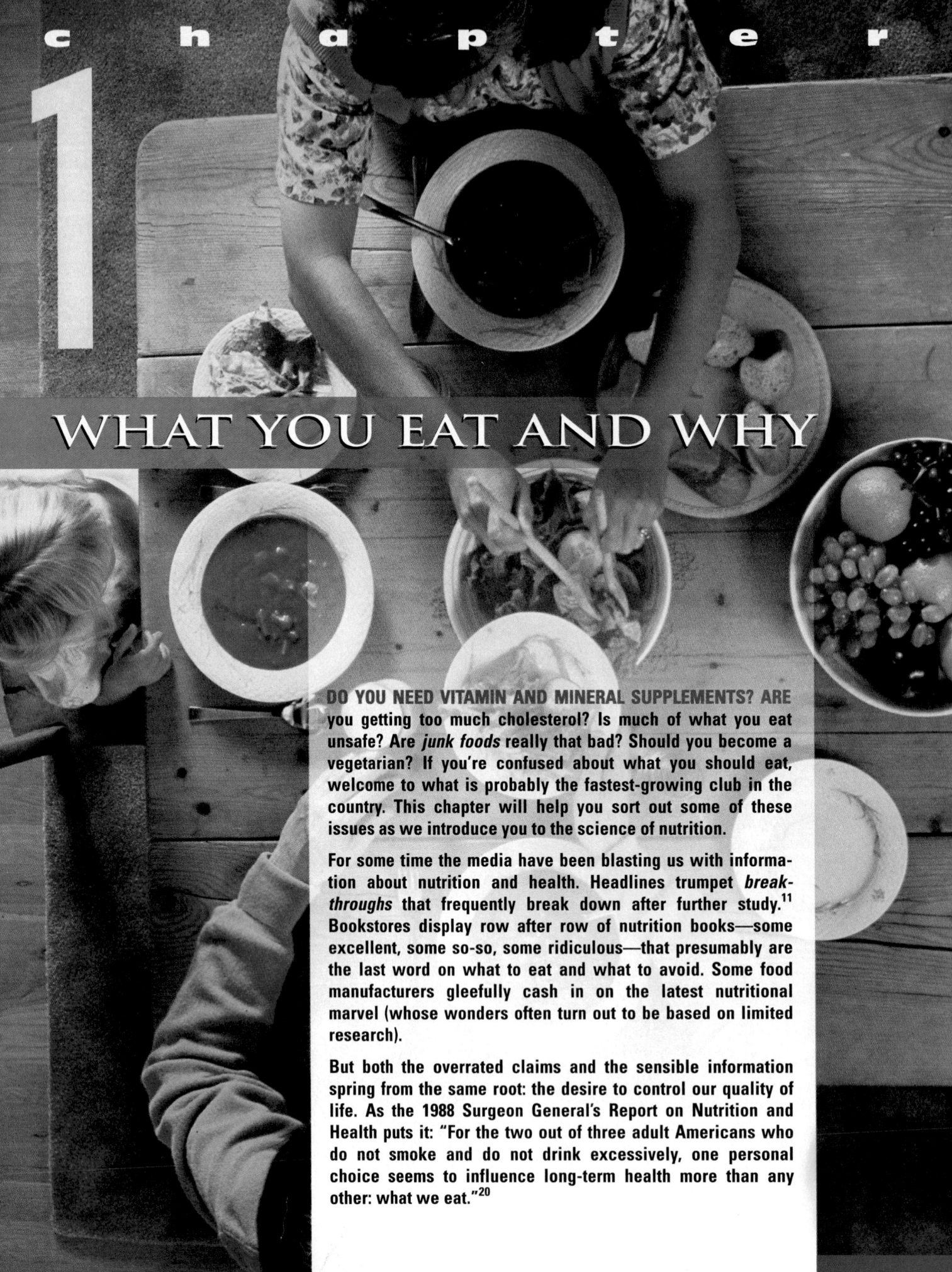

chapter 1

WHAT YOU EAT AND WHY

DO YOU NEED VITAMIN AND MINERAL SUPPLEMENTS? ARE you getting too much cholesterol? Is much of what you eat unsafe? Are *junk foods* really that bad? Should you become a vegetarian? If you're confused about what you should eat, welcome to what is probably the fastest-growing club in the country. This chapter will help you sort out some of these issues as we introduce you to the science of nutrition.

For some time the media have been blasting us with information about nutrition and health. Headlines trumpet *breakthroughs* that frequently break down after further study.[11] Bookstores display row after row of nutrition books—some excellent, some so-so, some ridiculous—that presumably are the last word on what to eat and what to avoid. Some food manufacturers gleefully cash in on the latest nutritional marvel (whose wonders often turn out to be based on limited research).

But both the overrated claims and the sensible information spring from the same root: the desire to control our quality of life. As the 1988 Surgeon General's Report on Nutrition and Health puts it: "For the two out of three adult Americans who do not smoke and do not drink excessively, one personal choice seems to influence long-term health more than any other: what we eat."[20]

WHAT FACTORS DETERMINE YOUR FOOD CHOICES?

What are your favorite foods? Why do you like them? If only the taste buds determined food preferences, you probably wouldn't try strong tasting or spicy foods. Which foods do most of the members of your family enjoy together? Which foods are consistently excluded, if any? Use the following survey to discover how significantly the factors listed determine why you eat the way you do. Circle the number reflecting the most appropriate answer.

	Not significant at all					Very significant
1. Weight control	0	1	2	3	4	5
2. Health	0	1	2	3	4	5
3. Food costs	0	1	2	3	4	5
4. Convenience/Time	0	1	2	3	4	5
5. Family background	0	1	2	3	4	5
6. Advertisements (TV or radio)	0	1	2	3	4	5
7. Emotions	0	1	2	3	4	5
8. Peers (friends, co-workers)	0	1	2	3	4	5
9. Customs/Ethnic background	0	1	2	3	4	5
10. Physical activity level	0	1	2	3	4	5

Interpretation

Take note of the factors that scored 4 or 5. These are your most significant influences. Next to these put a PLUS (+) or MINUS (–) sign to indicate whether you feel they have been a positive or negative influence on your health.

In this chapter we want you to examine what you eat and why, so you understand the origins of your eating habits. We begin with a general discussion of why we eat what we do. Then we ask you to complete an activity that focuses on your reasons for choosing certain foods in a day's menu.

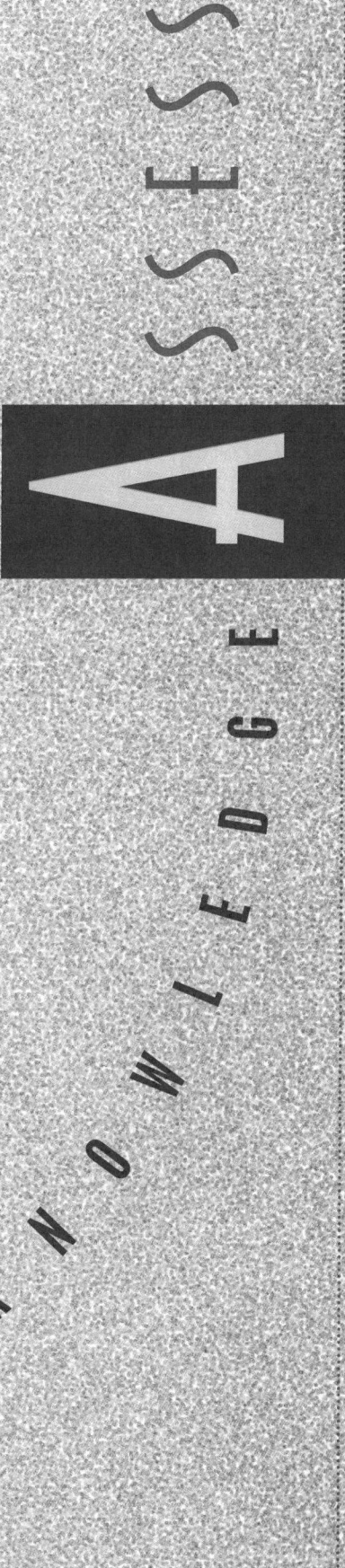

ASSESS YOUR KNOWLEDGE

TEST YOURSELF

Nutrition *The Council on Food and Nutrition of the American Medical Association defines nutrition as "the science of food, the nutrients and the substances therein, their action, interaction, and balance in relation to health and disease, and the process by which the organism (i.e., body) ingests, digests, absorbs, transports, utilizes, and excretes food substances."*

Risk Factor *A term used frequently when discussing diseases and factors contributing to their development. A risk factor is an aspect of our lives—such as hereditary, lifestyle choices (i.e. smoking), or nutritional habits—that may make us more likely to develop a disease.*

Nutrients *Chemical substances in food that are essential parts of a diet. Nutrients nourish us by providing energy, materials for building body parts, and factors to regulate needed chemical processes in the body. The body either can't make these nutrients or can't make them fast enough for its needs.*

YOUR INTRODUCTION TO NUTRITION

Although the science of ***nutrition*** is relatively young, we already know much about what nutrients are needed for an adequate diet and the foods that provide them. In a lifetime you will eat about 70,000 meals and 60 tons of food. In this opening chapter we encourage you to take a close look at your eating habits and discover the underlying reasons for them. This is an important first step. If you make even small changes in your behavior toward food, you can increase your chances for enjoying a long and vigorous life.[20] The more you know about nutrition and your health risks, the better you can plan diets to meet your nutritional needs.

Recent evidence points to poor diet as a ***risk factor*** for ***chronic*** diseases that are the leading causes of adult deaths: ***heart disease, stroke, hypertension, diabetes,*** and some types of ***cancer.***[20] Together, these disorders account for two thirds of all deaths in North America (Table 1-1).[16] Not consuming enough ***nutrients*** also makes us more likely to suffer later bone fractures (from the disease ***osteoporosis***) and iron-deficiency ***anemia.*** At the same time, taking too much of a nutrient supplement—such as vitamin A, vitamin B-6, or copper—can be harmful. Another dietary problem, drinking too much alcohol, is associated with ***cirrhosis*** of the liver, some forms of cancer, accidents, and suicides.[20] As you gain understanding about your nutritional habits and increase your knowledge about nutrition, you have the opportunity to dramatically cut your risk for many of these problems.

As you begin to study nutrition in this chapter, you will learn the names of the nutrients you need. Then you will discover what those nutrients do in your body. Later you will learn how to evaluate a person's nutritional health, as well as evaluate how healthful the current American diet is. Finally, you will discover why people eat the things they do and how to apply the scientific method to nutritional concepts.

TABLE 1-1

Ten Leading Causes of Death in the United States

Rank Order	Cause of Death	Percent of Total Deaths
. . .	All causes	100.0
1	Diseases of heart*	34
2	Malignant neoplasms, including neoplasms of lymphatic and hematopoietic tissues (cancer)*	23
3	Cerebrovascular diseases (stroke)*	7
4	Accidents and adverse effects†	4
. . .	Motor vehicle accidents	(2)
. . .	All other accidents and adverse effects	(2)
5	Chronic obstructive pulmonary diseases and allied conditions (lung diseases)	4
6	Pneumonia and influenza	4
7	Diabetes*	2
8	Suicide†	1
9	Homicide and legal intervention†	1
10	Chronic liver disease and cirrhosis†	1

From National Center for Health Statistics: Annual summary *39(13), 1990.*
NOTE: Acquired immunodeficiency syndrome (AIDS) is ranked no. 11.
**Causes of death in which diet plays a part.*
†Causes of death in which excessive alcohol consumption plays a part.

NUTRIENTS COME FROM FOOD

What is the difference between food, nutrients, and nutrition? Food provides both the energy and the materials needed to build and maintain all body cells. ***Nutrients*** are the nourishing substances we must obtain from food. These essential substances are vital for growth from infancy to adulthood and the maintenance of body functions that keep us alive.[16] Nutrition is the study of nutrients and nourishment: what nutrients consist of, how the body ***metabolizes*** them, and what they finally do in the body to keep us healthy.

Classes of Nutrients

You have probably heard the terms ***carbohydrates, proteins, lipids*** (fats and oils), ***vitamins,*** and ***minerals.*** These, plus ***water,*** make up the six classes of nutrients found in food (Table 1-2). Today we know that the minimum diet for human growth and development must contain about 45 essential nutrients. They are *essential* for a diet, because again, we must get these substances from food. With few exceptions, our bodies cannot manufacture them. This means that if an essential nutrient is left out of a diet, aspects of human health decline. Then if the nutrient is later added back to the diet before permanent damage occurs, those aspects of human health hampered by lack of the nutrient return to normal function. In other words, lost aspects of health can be restored when the essential nutrient is consumed in time.

Nutrients can be sorted into three groups: (1) those that primarily provide us with energy ***(kcalories)***, (2) those that are important for growth and maintenance, and (3) those that act to keep body functions running smoothly. Some overlap exists between these groupings. The energy-yielding nutrients, which make up a major portion of most foods, are introduced first.

Carbohydrates. Carbohydrates provide a major source of fuel for your body. Small carbohydrate forms are called sugars or simple sugars. Table sugar is an example. Simple sugars, such as glucose, can chemically link together to form large storage carbohydrates called complex carbohydrates. One example is ***starch*** in potatoes.

Sugars impart sweetness to many foods. Aside from enjoying this taste, we need sugars or other carbohydrates in our diets primarily to satisfy the energy needs of body ***cells.*** When you do not eat enough carbohydrate to supply one particular sugar (glucose) to your cells, your body will be forced to take what it can from storage and also make this sugar from other important body structures. However, because we generally eat enough carbohydrate each day, this rarely happens.

We begin digesting some of the starches in our diets as soon as we put them into our mouths. The process continues until starches and large sugars break down into single sugar ***molecules*** (like glucose) for absorption into the bloodstream. The links between the sugar molecules in certain complex carbohydrates cannot be broken down by human digestive processes. These carbohydrates are part of what is called ***dietary fiber.*** These fibers then pass down the intestinal tract to provide bulk for the stool (feces) formed in the large intestine (colon). Chapter 5 focuses on the family of carbohydrates.

Lipids. Lipids are a second general class of nutrients that contain the familiar fats and oils. These supply another major fuel for the body. By common definition, fats are solid at room temperature and oils are liquid. The fatty acid is the basic structural unit of most lipids, just as sugars make up most carbohydrates.

There are two basic types of fatty acids found in lipids: saturated and unsaturated. (We will discuss these chemical definitions in greater detail in Chapter 6.) Fats and oils in foods are always a combination of both saturated and unsaturated fatty acids. The dominant type of fatty acid determines the lipid's characteristics, such as whether it's solid or liquid at room temperature. Saturated fatty acids, such as those found dominantly in animal fats, generally form lipids that are solid or semisolid at room temperature. Unsaturated fatty acids, such as those found dominantly in plant oils, form lipids that are liquid at room temperature.

Certain unsaturated fatty acids are essential nutrients in a diet. They help regulate some important body functions, such as blood pressure. They are also needed for the syn-

Metabolism
Chemical processes in the body that allow for life.

Kcalorie
A kcalorie is actually a measure of the energy content in foods. It is the heat needed to raise the temperature of 1000 grams (1 liter) of water to 1 degree C. This is the same as raising the temperature of about 4 cups of water to 2 degrees F.

Cell
The basic structural unit of all living organisms. Cells living and working together compose our bodies. Each body cell metabolizes nutrients in order to stay alive. Inside each cell, tiny structures known as "organelles" are individually responsible for different cell processes, such as respiration, tissue synthesis, and reproduction.

Molecule
A group of like or unlike atoms chemically linked together. It is similar to a compound, which is a group of different types of atoms bonded together in definite proportion.

TABLE 1-2

Essential Nutrients* in the Human Diet and Their Categories

Energy Nutrients			
Carbohydrate	**Fat (lipid)†**	**Protein (Amino Acid)**	**Vitamins Fat-Soluble**
Glucose‡ (or a carbohydrate that yields glucose)	Linoleic acid (omega-6)	Histidine	A
	α-Linolenic acid (omega-3)	Isoleucine	D§
		Leucine	E
		Lysine	K
		Methionine	
		Phenylalanine	
		Threonine	
		Tryptophan	
		Valine	

Vitamins Water-Soluble	Minerals: Major	Minerals: Trace	Minerals: Questionable	Water
Thiamin	Calcium	Chrominum	Arsenic	Water
Riboflavin	Chloride	Copper	Boron	
Niacin	Magnesium	Cobolt	Nickel	
Pantothenic acid	Phosphorus	Fluoride‖	Silicon	
Biotin	Potassium	Iodide		
B-6	Sodium	Iron		
B-12	Sulfur	Manganese		
Folate		Molybdenum		
C		Selenium		
		Zinc		

This table includes nutrients that the current RDA publication lists for humans. Some debate exists over the questionable minerals and other substances that are not listed.

**Dietary fiber could be added to the list of essential substances, but it is not a nutrient (see Chapter 5).*

†The lipids listed are needed in only slight amounts, about 2% of total energy needs (see Chapter 6).

‡In order to prevent ketosis and thus the muscle loss that would occur if protein was used to synthesize carbohydrate (see Chapter 5).

§Sunshine on the skin also allows the body to make vitamin D for itself (see Chapter 8).

‖Primarily for dental health.

Enzyme *A compound that speeds the rate of a chemical process but is not altered by the process. Almost all enzymes are proteins (see Chapters 4 and 7).*

Hormone *A compound secreted into the bloodstream that acts to control the function of distant cells.*

thesis and repair of vital cell parts. You need only about 1 tablespoon of a common vegetable oil (like those found in supermarkets) per day to supply your body with essential fatty acids. The average American diet supplies about 3 times the amount needed. Chapter 6 focuses on lipids, especially their connection to heart disease.

Proteins. Proteins are a third class of nutrients. These form a major part of the body structure. Muscles contain much protein. A major part of bones is also protein. Important parts of blood, most ***enzymes,*** some ***hormones, cell membranes,*** and components of the immune system come from proteins. The basic unit of protein structure is the ***amino acid.*** Amino acids join together to form proteins. Twenty common amino acids are found in food; nine of these are essential parts of an adult's diet.

Most of us eat about one and a half to two times more protein than the body needs to maintain health. In a healthy person this amount of extra protein in the diet is generally not harmful—it simply reflects the standard of living and the dietary habits that most Americans enjoy. The excess is used for fuel or made into fat or carbohydrate. Chapter 7 focuses on proteins.

another BITE

Nutrients such as carbohydrates, fats, and proteins contain carbons attached to hydrogens. This attachment by definition makes these nutrients *organic* compounds in strict chemical terms. Because minerals and water do not contain carbons attached to hydrogens, they are called *inorganic* compounds. These terms are part of the language of nutrition and are based on simple chemistry concepts. Note that they have little to do with organic gardening (see Chapter 3).

Organic *Anything that contains carbon linked to hydrogen in the chemical structure.*

Inorganic *Anything that is free of carbon linked to hydrogen in the chemical structure.*

The fourth and fifth classes of nutrients are vitamins and minerals. These nutrients form key regulators and structural parts in the body. While vitamins and minerals are vital to good health, they are needed only in small amounts in our diet. In fact, large amounts of some can cause harmful effects, as we will point out throughout this book.

Vitamins. Vitamins are carbon-containing compounds that enable many ***chemical reactions*** to occur in the body, some of which release the energy stored in carbohydrates, fats, and proteins. The vitamins themselves provide no energy to the body. We need 13 different vitamins; 4 are fat soluble (they dissolve in fat) and 9 are water soluble (they dissolve in water). Vitamins, with a focus on their role in the fight against cancer, are discussed in Chapter 8.

Minerals. Minerals also play an important role in the body's chemical reactions, such as magnesium for carbohydrate use. In addition, minerals help make up the body's structure and form key components of parts of the bloodstream. Minerals by themselves provide no energy to the body. We know of about 17 essential minerals. Minerals are the focus of Chapter 9, especially how they relate to bone health and high blood pressure (hypertension).

Water. Water is the sixth and last class of nutrients. It nourishes us in many ways. It is vital in the body because it dissolves substances, lubricates structures such as joints, and provides a way to transport nutrients and waste. Our body cells are mostly composed of water. The body can even make water as a by-product of chemical reactions in cells. The bulk of our dietary needs comes from water (about 10 cups a day from a combination of foods, fluids, and water itself) and energy. Compare 10 cups of water with our daily needs of 9 tablespoons of protein, ¼ teaspoon of calcium, and 1/1000 teaspoon (a 2-microgram speck) of vitamin B-12 each day. Water is examined in detail in Chapter 9.

CONCEPT CHECK

The food you eat contains six vital classes of nutrients: carbohydrates, lipids (fats and oils), proteins, vitamins, minerals, and water. The energy (kcalories) you need for activity comes mainly from carbohydrates and lipids. Growth and replacement of body cells require proteins and lipids. Vitamins and minerals have many functions, including aiding in the chemical processes of energy production. Water is the medium of life—a liquid that transports the substances in the body.

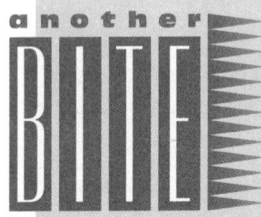

MATH TOOLS FOR NUTRITION

You will use a few mathematical concepts in studying nutrition. Besides performing addition, subtraction, multiplication, and division, you need to know how to calculate percentages and convert English units of measurement to metric units.

Percentages

The term ***percent*** (%) refers to a part of the total when the total represents 100 parts. For example, if you earn 80% on your first nutrition examination, you will have answered the equivalent of 80 out of 100 questions correctly. This equivalent could be 8 correct answers out of 10; 80% also describes 16 of 20 (16/20 = 0.80 or 80%). The best way to master this concept is to calculate some percentages. Some examples are given below:

Question	Answer
What is 6% of 45?	$0.06 \times 45 = 2.7$
What is 32% of 8?	$0.32 \times 8 = 2.6$
What percent of 16 is 6?	$6/16 = 0.375$ or 37.5%
What percent of 99 is 3?	$3/99 = 0.03$ or 3%

Joe ate 15% of the adult recommended dietary allowance (RDA) for vitamin C at lunch. How many milligrams did he eat? (RDA = 60 milligrams)

$$0.15 \times 60 \text{ milligrams} = 9 \text{ milligrams}$$

It is difficult to succeed in a nutrition course unless you know what a percentage means and how to calculate one. Percentages are used frequently when referring to menus and nutrient composition.

The Metric System

The basic units of the metric system are the meter, which indicates length; the gram, which indicates weight; and the liter, which indicates volume. The inside cover of this textbook lists conversions from the metric system to the English system (pounds, feet, cups) and vice versa. Here is a brief summary:

One ***meter*** is 39.4 inches long, or about 3 inches longer than 1 yard (3 feet).

Are You What You Eat?

The amounts of nutrients that your body needs vary widely from one nutrient to another. Nutrient quantities also vary from food to food. Each day we need about 1 pound (500 grams) of energy-yielding substances in the food we eat. Add to this about 5 pounds of water. We need to take in vitamins regularly but in very small amounts—100 milligrams or less. Although we should eat nearly 1 gram of some minerals—such as calcium and phosphorus—each day, many minerals are needed in quantities of only milligrams or less. For example, you need about 10 to 15 milligrams of iron each day, which is just a few grains of zinc oxide. Figure 1-1 shows the proportion of nutrients in a human body, compared with the proportions of the same nutrients in cooked steak and a cooked stalk of

A meter can be divided into 100 units of ***centi***meters,
or into 1000 units of ***milli***meters.

A millimeter is about the thickness of a dime.

There are 2.54 centimeters in 1 inch and about 30 centimeters in 1 foot.

A person 6 feet tall is equivalent to 183 centimeters tall.

A ***gram*** is about $\frac{1}{30}$ of an ounce (28 grams to the ounce).

Five grams of sugar or salt is about 1 teaspoon.

A ***kilo***gram is 1000 grams, equivalent to 2.2 pounds.

A pound weighs 454 grams.

A 154-pound man weighs 70 kilograms (154/2.2 = 70).

A gram can be divided into 1000 milligrams or 1,000,000 ***micro***grams.

15 milligrams of zinc (approximately the adult RDA)
would be a few grains of zinc oxide.

Liters are divided into 1000 units called milliliters.

One teaspoon equals about 5 milliliters, 1 cup is about 240 milliliters,
and 1 quart (4 cups) equals almost 1 liter (0.946 liters to be exact).

If you plan to work in any scientific field, you will need to learn the metric system. For now, remember that a kilogram equals 2.2 pounds, an ounce weighs 28 grams, 2.54 centimeters equals 1 inch, and a liter is almost the same as a quart. In addition, know what the prefixes micro (1/1,000,000), milli (1/1000), centi (1/100), and kilo (1000) represent.

another BITE

For your review, key units in the English system are the following:

3 teaspoons per tablespoon
16 tablespoons per cup
2 cups to a pint
2 pints or 4 cups to a quart
4 quarts to a gallon
16 ounces to a pound

broccoli. Aside from water, food is mostly a mixture of carbohydrates, fats, and proteins. Note how different your body's nutrient makeup is from that of the foods you eat!

A Warning

You may wonder whether what you eat today really does influence your immediate health. The answer is not clear-cut. Often you can go a long time with poor nutritional habits before you see the first outward (clinical) sign of a problem. For example, a person can eat a diet high in saturated fat, which often leads to a high blood ***cholesterol*** level, but not notice any symptoms for years. Eventually, as blood vessels build up deposits of cholesterol and other materials, the person may begin to notice shortness of breath and

Cholesterol
A waxy lipid found in all body cells. It has a structure containing multiple chemical rings that is found only in animal products (see Chapter 6).

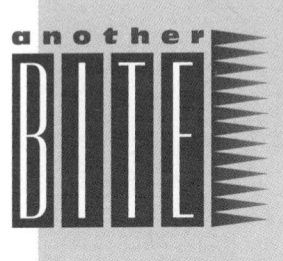

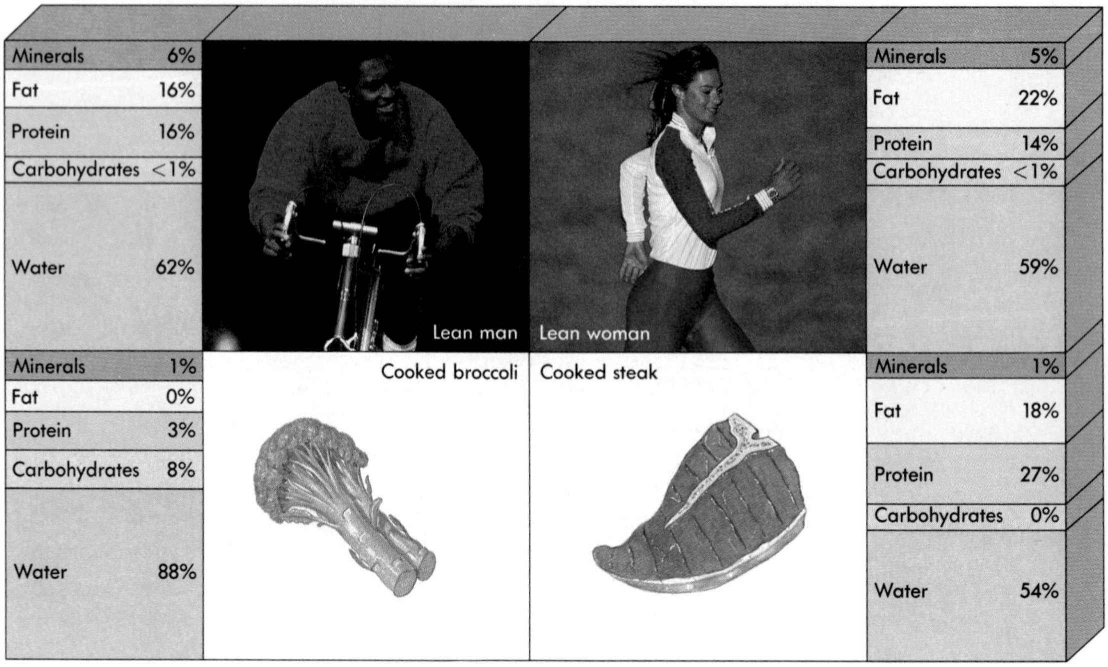

FIGURE 1-1

You aren't what you eat! The proportions of nutrients (nutrient composition) in the human body do not match those found in typical foods—animal or vegetable.

Heart Attack *Rapid fall in heart function caused by reduced blood flow through the heart's blood vessels. Often part of the heart dies in the process (see Chapter 6).*

then chest pain during physical activity. This buildup of fatty substances can one day lead to a ***heart attack*** (see Chapter 6). Thus a person may be on the road to developing a serious disease, but because it progresses slowly, the effects won't be obvious until quite late—perhaps too late.

Furthermore, symptoms of nutritional deficiencies are often not very specific. Typical effects to look for—diarrhea, an irregular walk, facial sores—are symptoms of many different problems. It's often hard to decide whether a problem is caused by poor nutrition or by some other medical disorder. Long lag times and vague symptoms often make it difficult to establish a link between an individual's current diet and his or her overall nutritional state.

Table 1-3 shows the close relationship of nutrition and health. Chapter 2 helps you plan your diet to maximize health and minimize the development of nutrition-related diseases. For now, keep in mind that poor nutrition habits often catch up with us, bringing in turn ill health.[3]

How Could You Measure Your Nutritional State?

Anthropometric, biochemical, clinical, and dietary evaluations make up the ABCD of nutrition assessment.

The measurements of your height, weight, and body circumferences—called ***anthropometry***—reveal something about your current nutritional state (Table 1-4). This type of evaluation is simple but less informative than is a full biochemical evaluation, which measures blood levels of some nutrients and their by-products. Although useful, a biochemical evaluation is an expensive procedure, and most of the tests can be done only in specialized laboratories. Another way to find out about your nutritional state is to get a thorough physical (clinical) examination and make a detailed evaluation of what you eat.

Throughout this book we will point out practical tests that can tell you much about your current nutritional state. We suggest you set a goal to learn as much as you can about your nutritional and total health as you study nutrition.

NUTRITION insight

A FOUNTAIN OF YOUTH?

While most of us wish for long life, we do not like to think of ourselves as suffering poor health when we are old. And rightfully so! We can truly enjoy long life only if we are productive and free of illness. Rather than suffer the ravages of heart disease, stroke, diabetes, osteoporosis, and other chronic diseases from age 50 or 60 years until death, we should strive to be as free of disease as possible and to enjoy vitality even in the last several years of life.[9] Greater physical well-being contributes to a state of physical, mental, and social well-being.

Aging is a natural process: your body cells age no matter what health practices you follow. But to a considerable extent you can choose how fast you age throughout your adult years. Genetic background has a great effect, but you also have some control in the matter (Table 1-3). How you act now is important to your later health. *Successful* aging is the goal. *Age fast or age slow—you choose.*

A Basic Plan for Health Promotion and Disease Prevention

Adults can best promote health and prevent disease by doing the following things:

- Eat a healthful diet—A varied diet that maintains a desirable weight should be a priority. The Food Guide Pyramid, discussed in Chapter 2, is a great place to start. Especially emphasize low-fat dairy products, lean meats, plant proteins, whole grains, plant oils, fruits, and dark green or leafy vegetables.[16,20]
- Exercise—Research suggests that you should spend about 2000 kcalories per week in brisk walking, jogging, swimming, stair climbing, and other activities that stimulate the cardiovascular system. See Chapter 11 for more details.
- Don't smoke—Lung cancer, primarily caused by smoking cigarettes, is the only form of cancer where yearly rates still increase.
- Limit alcohol intake—Don't drink more than 1 to 2 ounces of alcohol per day on a regular basis.[16,20] One 12-ounce beer, a 4-ounce glass of wine, or a mixed drink supplies about ½ ounce (15 grams) of alcohol. Furthermore, women should avoid alcohol during pregnancy, because this can harm the baby (Chapter 14 discusses the disease that can result—fetal alcohol syndrome).
- Limit stress, or adjust to the causes of stress—Practice better time management, relax, listen to music, have a massage, and exercise regularly. Do your favorite things to reduce stress. In addition, maintaining self-esteem and interpersonal relationships contributes to limiting stress and reinforces wellness.
- Consult health care professionals when necessary—Early diagnosis is especially important for controlling the damaging effects of many diseases.

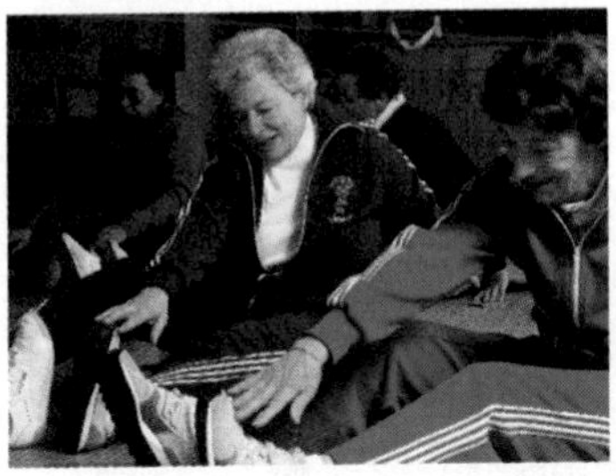

Regular physical activity is one component of a healthful lifestyle.

Your key to optimum health is to discover how to maintain your best physical, mental, psychological, and social states. There is no general formula for achieving this ideal. Each of us must juggle and balance personal goals with opportunities and obstacles we encounter. Proper diet is not the only thing to consider. As we have discussed, other lifestyle choices are also critical. Taking responsibility for yourself is central to achieving long-lasting health. As individuals we can do a lot to improve our health by establishing good health behaviors. Focusing on disease prevention may not allow you to live longer—because heredity, accidents, and other things are outside your control—but you'll probably live a healthier life.[9]

We can begin our journey to better nutrition by looking at what influences our food choices and deciding to take responsibility for making changes in our eating habits that will promote health. This is the goal of Chapters 1 and 2.

TABLE 1-3

What Can We Expect From Good Nutrition and Health Habits?

Diet

Eating enough essential nutrients and meeting energy needs helps prevent:
- Birth defects and low birth weight in pregnancy
- Poor growth and poor resistance to disease in infancy and childhood
- Poor resistance to disease in adult years
- Deficiency diseases, such as cretinism (lack of the mineral iodide), scurvy (lack of vitamin C), and anemia (lack of the mineral iron, the vitamin folate, or other nutrients)

Eating enough of the mineral calcium helps prevent:
- Some adult bone loss

Obtaining adequate intake of the mineral fluoride and minimizing sugar intake helps prevent:
- Dental caries (decay)

Eating enough dietary fiber helps prevent:
- Digestive problems, such as constipation, and possibly some forms of cancer

Eating enough vitamin A and beta-carotene (plant form of vitamin A) may help reduce:
- Susceptibility to some cancers, especially in smokers

Moderating energy intake helps prevent:
- Obesity and related diseases, such as diabetes, hypertension, cancer, and premature heart disease

Limiting intake of the mineral sodium helps prevent:
- Hypertension and related disease of the heart and kidney in susceptible people

Avoiding intake of saturated fat helps prevent:
- Premature heart disease

Moderating intake of essential nutrients by using vitamin and mineral supplements wisely, if at all, prevents:
- Most chances for nutrient toxicities

Exercise

Adequate, regular exercise helps prevent:
- Obesity
- Non–insulin-dependent (adult-onset) diabetes
- Premature heart disease
- Some adult bone loss
- Loss of muscle tone

Lifestyle

Minimizing alcohol intake helps prevent:
- Liver disease
- Fetal alcohol syndrome
- Accidents

In addition, not smoking, minimum use of medications, no illicit drug use, adequate sleep, and limiting stress provide a more complete approach to good nutrition and health.

Alcohol *Ethyl alcohol or ethanol. An energy-yielding substance found in beer, wine, and distilled spirits.*

We Need Energy for Body Functions

We get the energy (again, usually expressed as kcalories) to perform body functions and to do work from carbohydrates, fats, and proteins (Table 1-2). ***Alcohol*** is also an energy source for some of us. It is not considered a nutrient, however, because it has no required function. Still, alcoholic beverages are the third leading contributor of kcalories to the American diet.

Kcalories—A Closer Look

To figure out how many kcalories are in a particular food portion, scientists use an instrument called a ***bomb calorimeter*** (Figure 1-2). Information from the bomb calorimeter is

TABLE 1-4

Components of a Nutrition Assessment

Component	Example
Anthropometry	Assessment of height, weight, body fat composition, etc.
Biochemical evaluation	Assessment of blood, urine, etc.
Clinical examination	Medical history, physical examination, etc.
Dietary evaluation	Detailed assessment of what you eat

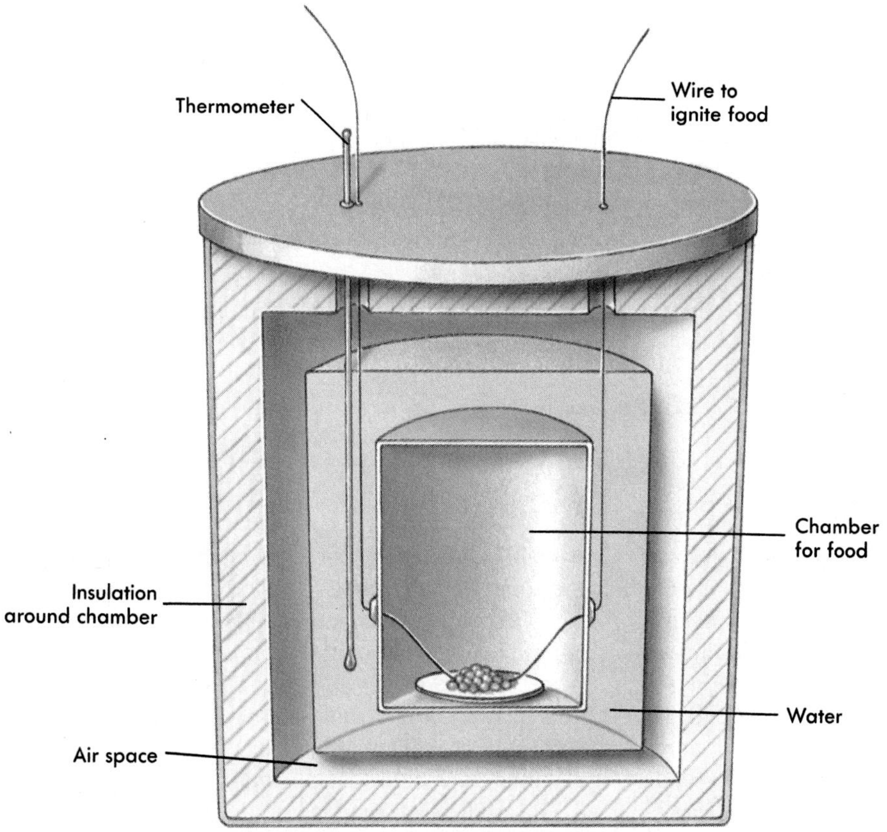

FIGURE 1-2
Cross-section of a bomb calorimeter. To determine energy content, first, a dried portion of food is burned inside a chamber charged with oxygen that is surrounded by water. As the food is burned, it gives off heat. This raises the temperature of the water surrounding the chamber. The increase in water temperature indicates the number of kcalories contained in the food. Recall 1 kcalorie equals the amount of heat needed to raise the temperature of 1 kilogram of water 1 degree Celsius (C).

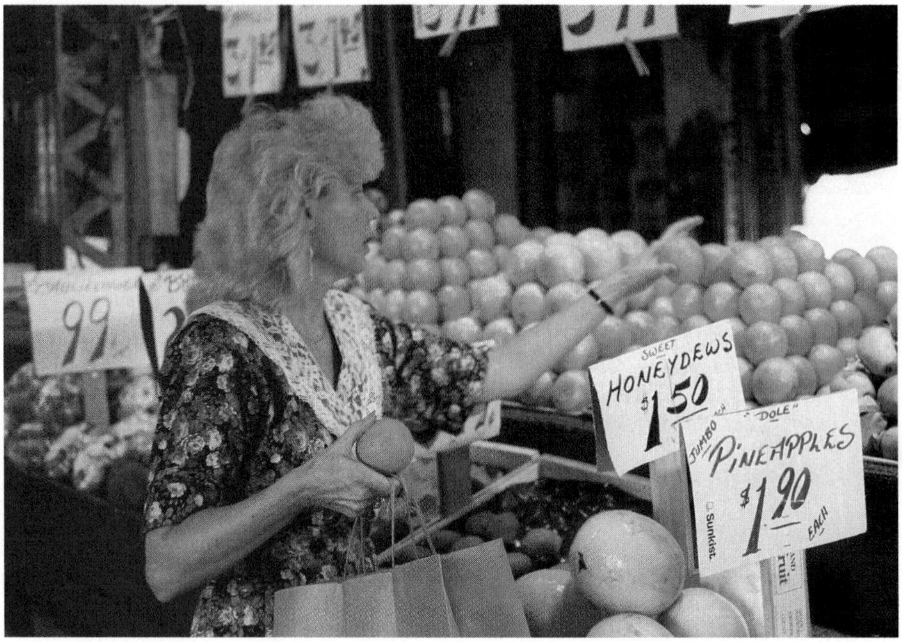

Choose fruits each day as part of your plan for a healthful diet.

Because a calorie is such a tiny unit of heat measurement—like a penny in relation to a 10-dollar bill—we can more efficiently express food energy in terms of kilocalories, which are 1000-calorie units. The abbreviation kcalorie (or kcal) is used throughout this book.

used to calculate the energy available to us from 1 gram of carbohydrate, fat, protein, and alcohol. Specifically, carbohydrates yield 4 kcalories per gram; proteins yield 4 kcalories per gram, fats yield 9 kcalories per gram, and alcohol yields 7 kcalories per gram. From this you can see that fat yields much more energy per gram than do carbohydrates and proteins. Once you know the gram quantities of these substances in a food, it is easy to estimate the total kcalories in that food using the kcalorie values. For example, if Joe ate 200 grams of carbohydrate, 100 grams of fat, and 70 grams of protein yesterday, his intake of kcalories would be calculated as follows:

$$\text{Total kcalories} = (200 \times 4) + (100 \times 9) + (70 \times 4) = 1980$$

The kcalorie breakdown would then be:

$$\%\text{ of kcalories as carbohydrate} = (200 \times 4)/1980 = .404 \text{ or } 40.4\%$$
$$\%\text{ of kcalories as fat} = (100 \times 9)/1980 = .455 \text{ or } 45.5\%$$
$$\%\text{ of kcalories as protein} = (70 \times 4)/1980 = .141 \text{ or } 14.1\%$$

THE AMERICAN DIET

For most of us living in America, our main dietary sources of energy are carbohydrates, fats, and proteins. Without considering alcohol, adults consume about 14% to 18% of their kcalories as proteins, 44% to 47% as carbohydrates, and 35% to 38% as fats. These percentages are estimates and change slightly from year to year. Individual diets also vary widely in composition.[12,13,22]

In the American diet, most protein comes from animal sources; vegetable sources supply only about one third of our protein. In many other parts of the world, vegetable proteins—like those found in rice, beans, and corn—supply most of the protein intake. About half of the carbohydrates in the diets of Americans comes from simple sugars, such as table sugar; the other half comes from starches, such as are found in pasta, bread, other grain products, and potatoes. About 60% of our fats come from animal sources and 40% from vegetable sources.[2]

Profiling the American Diet

Our information about the American diet comes from large surveys[19,22] designed to find out what and when people eat. Results from these surveys and other studies show that we eat a wide variety of foods. Many people are meeting their nutrient needs; others are not. We will look at this situation in more detail in Chapter 2. For now, note that studies show that some of us should choose more foods that are rich in iron, calcium, vitamins A and C, magnesium, zinc, and dietary fiber. Many experts recommend that we eat less fat. Chapter 2 gives specific suggestions on how to do just that. In addition, we should match energy intake with need. Overnutrition usually stems from overindulgence in fat and alcoholic beverages.[16] African-Americans may need to pay special attention to the amount of sodium (***salt*** is a mixture of sodium and chloride) and alcohol in their diets because they have a greater chance of developing hypertension than do other ethnic groups in America, and these substances are linked to that health problem.[20] Actually, a careful look at sodium and alcohol intake—along with fat intake—is a useful task for everyone.

Salt *Generally refers to a compound of sodium and chloride in a 40:60 ratio.*

CONCEPT CHECK

The energy to fuel our bodies comes mostly from carbohydrates, fats, and proteins. Surveys in the United States show that we generally have a variety of food available to us. However, some of us could improve our diets by focusing on good food sources of iron, calcium, vitamins A and C, magnesium, zinc, and dietary fiber. In addition, some of us could use more moderation when consuming energy, fat, sodium, and alcoholic beverages. These recommendations are consistent with an overall goal to attain and maintain good health.

How Aware Are We of Our Nutritional Health?

Judging from the responses of over half of the people in several large surveys, Americans are concerned about good nutrition and have a general awareness of possible health hazards from overeating, especially the dangers of too much fat, sodium, and kcalories.[8, 14] But many people just aren't willing to critically examine their own food habits. While they may be concerned, they don't necessarily make changes to improve their diets. Most people enjoy eating and cooking, but they don't think of or use the principles of nutritional science (Figure 1-3). We hope you will.

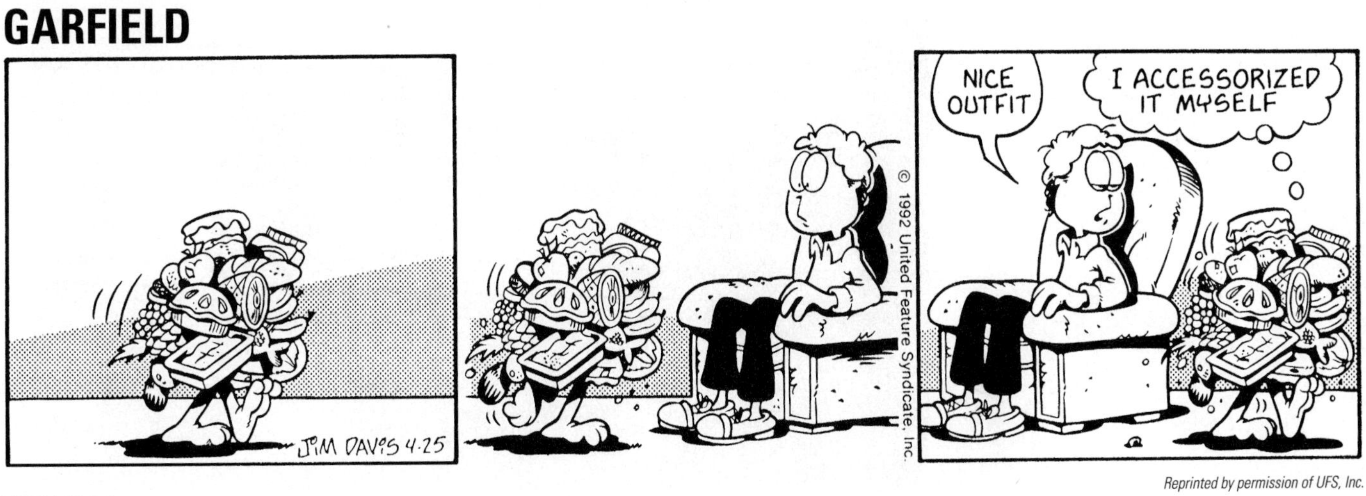

Reprinted by permission of UFS, Inc.

FIGURE 1-3
Garfield.

TABLE 1-5

On a Typical Day in the United States . . .

- 34 new restaurants open and 8 go out of business.
- 134 million people eat out, spending a total of $650 million. Of these people, 16 million eat at McDonald's. Note that McDonald's spends $500 thousand per day to encourage this.
- Each person eats about 4 pounds of food. This includes 16 teaspoons of fat and 32 teaspoons of sugar.
- 11 thousand girls ages 12 to 19 go on a diet, joining the 101 million people already on diets.
- 100 million M&Ms are sold. 2 million Hershey's kisses and 17 million Tootsie Rolls are produced.
- 25 million hot dogs are eaten.
- 524 million Coca-Colas are consumed. To encourage this, Coca-Cola spends $500 thousand per day on advertising.
- $3.5 million are spent on both tortilla chips and vitamin supplements, while $10.4 million are spent on potato chips.
- In total, $22 million are spent on snack foods, while $203 million are spent on low-calorie foods. $1.4 million are spent on laxatives.
- Children see approximately five beer and wine commercials on television. $3 million a day are spent to advertise beer, wine, and other liquors.
- $2 million are spent on baby food.

The United States has about 250 million people.

From Heyman T: On an average day, *New York, 1989, Fawcett Columbine.*

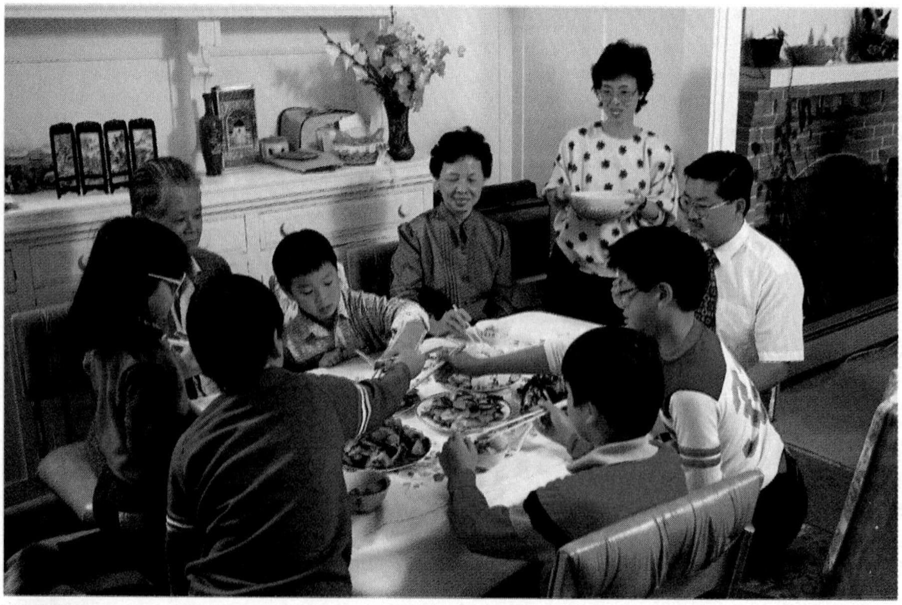

FIGURE 1-4

Meals bring families together. This habit helps create bonds that last a lifetime.

WHAT INFLUENCES OUR FOOD CHOICES?

Does what you eat say something about you? Our daily food choices have a lot to do with our age, gender, genetic makeup, occupation, and lifestyle; where we live; and our family and cultural background (Table 1-5).[15] We eat primarily for nourishment, but food means far more to us than that. Food symbolizes much of what we think about ourselves. We can use it to project a desired image. We bond relationships and express friendships around the dinner table (Figure 1-4). We show our creativity and sensitivity by what we serve to others in our homes. The common use of food as a gift is evidence that food signifies friendliness. We cope with stress and tension by eating or not eating. Food can be used as a reward—a dinner out to celebrate a new job or an ice cream cone for an A on a test. Some of us make special foods and elaborate preparations to observe national holidays and religious feast days.

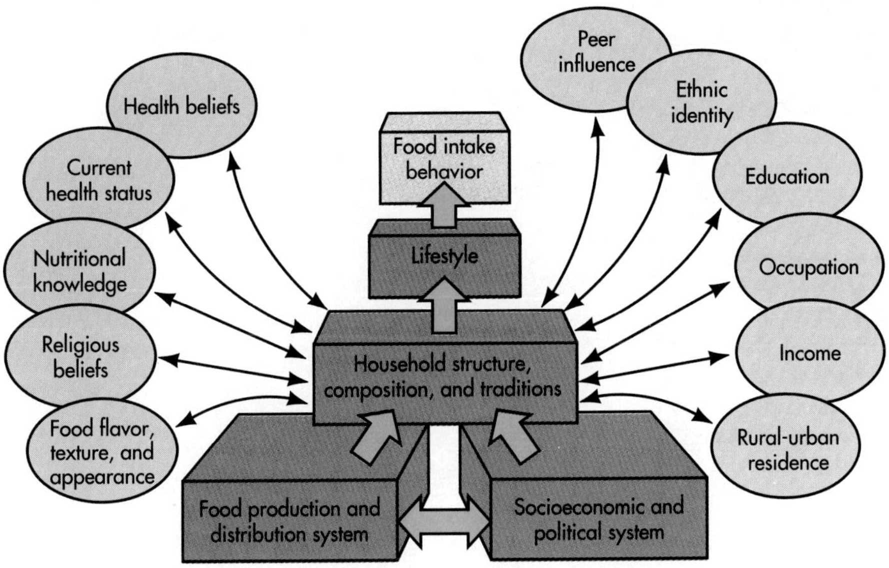

FIGURE 1-5
Food behavior is influenced by many sources. Which are important in your life?

Throughout our lives we spend 13 to 15 years of our waking hours eating. Taste, texture, and appearance are three of the most important things that influence our choice of food. After that we consider the cost of food. What we eat ends up revealing much about who we are—politically, religiously, and socially. Behavior, perception, and environment influence food habits (Figure 1-5).[18] While some people have no concern for nutrition, others will agonize endlessly over the taste, kcalories, fat content, and general nutritional value of everything they eat. Where do you fit into the food and nutrition picture?

Our Early Experiences With Food

Our food preferences begin early in life and then change as we interact with parents, friends, and peers (Figure 1-6).[1] Exposure to people, places, and situations often leads us to expand and change our food patterns. Our earliest food memories may include pancakes on Saturday mornings or hot cocoa on cold winter days. Unfortunately, as young children our food experiences may have been severely limited by parents or other adults responsible for us. Adults may have introduced us to only a small subset of available foods because some excellent foods are often considered inappropriate for children. For example, at what age did you discover lentils, spinach salad, or salmon?

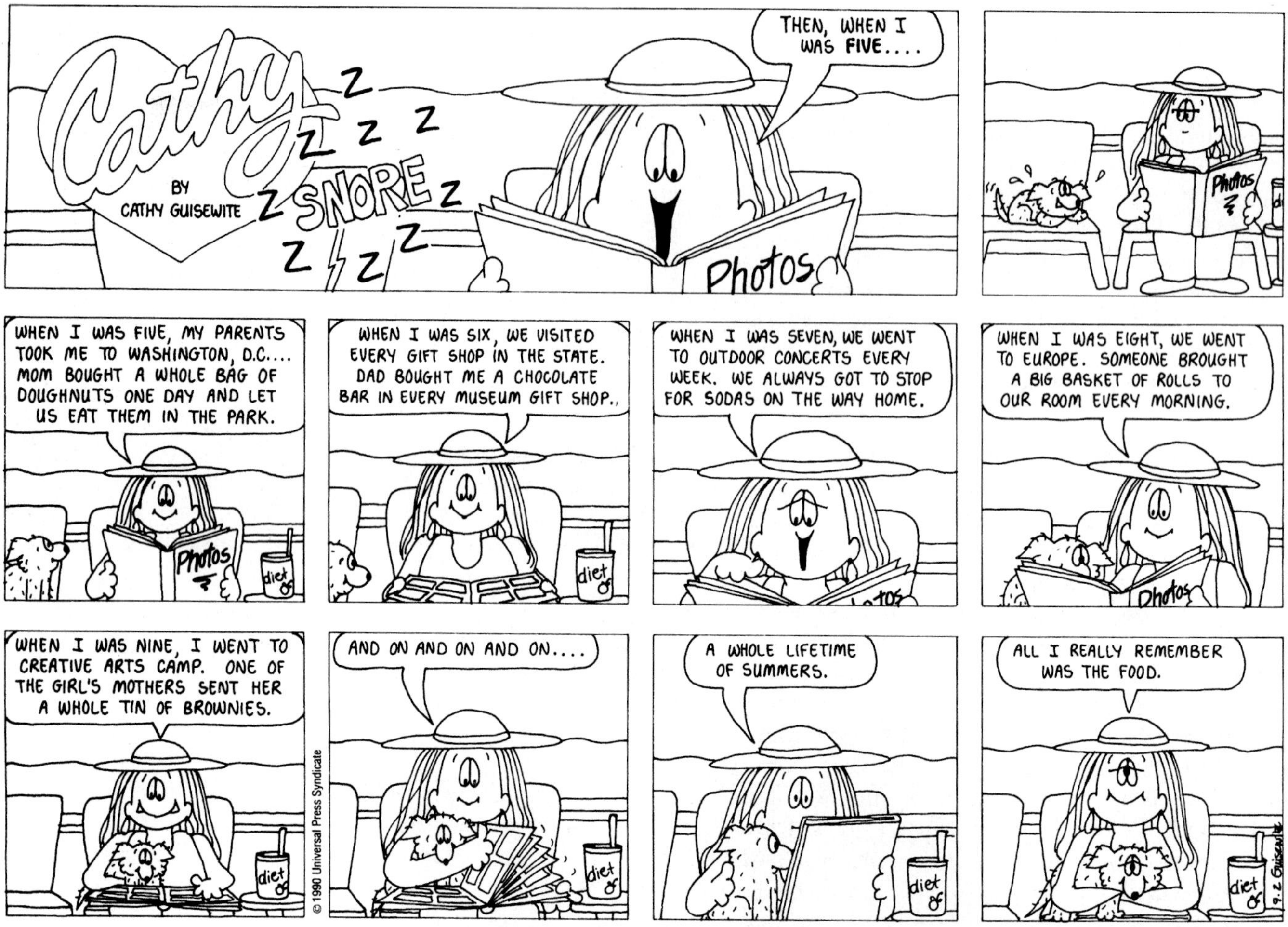

FIGURE 1-6
Cathy.

Just being exposed to a variety of foods can help make us less resistant to try new foods. Young children prefer foods that are sweet or familiar.[1] Preschoolers are usually quite willing to try new things. During school years, children are often strongly influenced by their peers. Adults need to give children under their care a variety of foods to try. It may take time, but children usually come to accept new foods (see Chapter 14).

Some inborn reactions to foods include universal enjoyment of sweet and salty foods and dislike of bitter and sometimes spicy, burning ones.[15] Sweet foods are usually safe to eat. We need to eat *salt* in foods (both the sodium and the chloride in table salt are essential nutrients), although the amount needed is only about ¼ teaspoon a day. Some bitter-tasting foods are poisonous.

However, our inborn responses to some foods can change once we know a food is safe, allowing us to enjoy foods such as jalapeño peppers and fiery curries.

Habit

Some food choices are tied to our routines and habits. The ease with which we can obtain certain foods influences our choices. Most of us eat from a core group of foods. Only about 100 basic items account for 75% of an individual's total food intake. Narrowing our food choices provides us with security. In this context eating quick-service food (often called "fast food") at McDonald's provides common expectations, experiences, and behaviors and can be compared to a *security blanket.*[18]

People often agree that their cooking habits are very similar to those of their mothers. How closely do your habits reflect what your mother taught you? Have you considered taking a cooking class to expand your food choices?

Culture

Religious rules about foods can further influence our diet[18]: Hindus would no more eat beef than you would eat a cat. Some Jewish people do not eat pork or serve milk products and meat at the same meal. There are also ethnic taboos. For example, Swedish people, who regard corn as food for hogs, would not enjoy an ear of sweet corn. In the United States insects are rejected almost entirely as foodstuff, whereas some other cultures regard them as choice foods. We even have fixed ideas about what time of day we eat certain foods. When was the last time you had vegetable noodle soup for breakfast? Many Japanese people prefer it at that time of day. Even where you live can affect food choices. Various foods are available in different areas. For example, it is sometimes difficult to find a wide variety of fresh vegetables in the winter in some areas or ethnic foods in an isolated town.

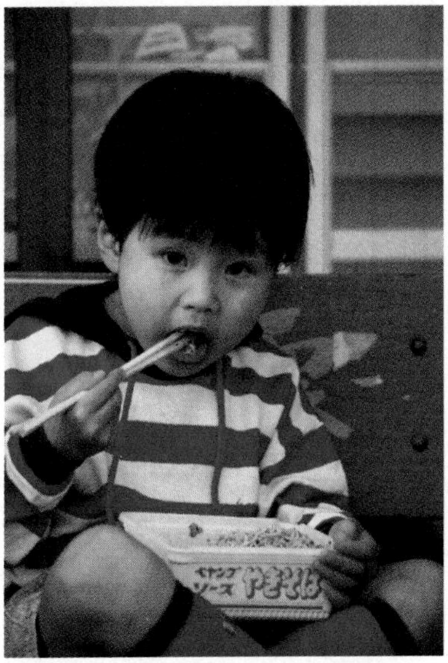

Food likes and dislikes are shaped by early experiences, among other factors.

Health

About half of us consider nutrition, or what we think are good food habits, an important influence on our food purchases. Those Americans who tend to make better food choices are often well-educated, middle-class professionals.[7] These are the same people who often are health oriented and who have an active life-style. Still, all of us should pay attention to nutritional health. In fact, increased health awareness among minority peoples is a major goal of current federal government health strategies.

Sugar used to be the main diet monster; now fat has the limelight.[21] As a result, manufacturers are racing to the market with reduced-fat or nonfat items (many also are lower in cholesterol and sodium), including mayonnaise, salad dressings, cheese, dairy spreads, frozen desserts, luncheon meats, sausage, and butter sprinkles.

Some of us are concerned enough about our health that we want to change our diets. Even so, food tastes and habits still strongly influence us. When people are asked why they don't include foods they know to be healthful in their diets—for instance, yellow vegetables, low-fat milk, margarine, and whole-wheat bread—they say they don't like them. Similarly, people don't want to give up foods such as whole milk, rich cheeses, and fatty meat because they like them too much. This even is the case if they think they should limit fat intake and lower-fat varieties are available.

The modern supermarket is responding to our health concerns by providing fresh, frozen, ready-to-eat, international, gourmet, ethnic, ***vegetarian,*** and even not-so-healthful foods. Salad bars in supermarkets have become a big hit, especially for single people. Stores are stocking more foods lower in fat, salt, and sugar. They are carrying low-fat varieties of cheeses, yogurts, and peanuts; pure fruit juices; high-fiber cereals; whole-grain breads; fruits canned in natural juices; low-sodium soups and sauces; low-fat turkey and chicken franks; and many kinds of fish. We can select from a variety of bulk foods sold in bins, including beans, rice, flours, dried fruits, nuts, and grains. Often market shelves have tags that provide information on the nutritional content of foods, such as kcalories, vitamins, and minerals. There are many options for us as we head down the road to good nutrition. We just have to follow the right directions.[16,20]

Vegetarian
A person who avoids eating animal products to a varying degree, ranging from consuming no animal products to simply not consuming four-footed animal products (see Chapter 7).

Advertising

In recent years some of the most successful food products introduced in the United States are advertised as being healthful.[7] However, many of these new products fail to live up to the claims. Popular products of the 1980s have included fruit rolls and bars, bottled mineral water, granola bars, fruit juices, bulk frozen vegetables without sauce, frozen pasta, soft cookies, microwave popcorn, kiwifruit, Equal ***(aspartame),*** and low-fat foods in general (Figure 1-7). Ice cream lovers have been able to choose frozen yogurt and new fat-free ice creams as alternatives. Are all these good food choices? Chapter 2 will help you decide.

To capture the interest of consumers, food producers spend well over $32 billion annually on advertising and packaging. Some of this advertising is helpful—when it promotes the importance of calcium and dietary fiber in our diets and encourages us to consume

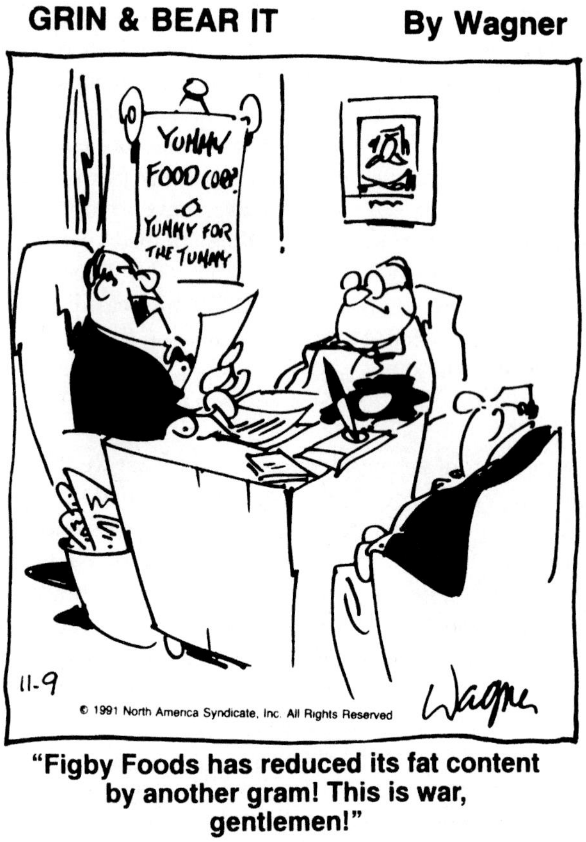
GRIN & BEAR IT
By Wagner
YUMMY FOOD CORP.
YUMMY FOR THE TUMMY
11-9
© 1991 North America Syndicate, Inc. All Rights Reserved
Wagner
"Figby Foods has reduced its fat content by another gram! This is war, gentlemen!"

Reprinted with permission of North America Syndicate, Inc.

FIGURE 1-7
Grin and Bear It.

Confusing and conflicting health messages also hinder diet change. Nutrition science does not have all the answers, but enough is known to (1) help you set a path to good health and (2) put diet-related recommendations you hear in the future into perspective. See Chapter 2 for details.

more low-fat milk products, fruits, vegetables, and lean meats. On the other hand, the current hype of cholesterol-free foods is often quite misleading, as we describe in Chapter 6. Over half of all food references during prime-time television programs are for low-nutrient beverages and sweets. In the supermarket some poor food choices are placed for higher visibility. Highly sweetened cereals, cookies, cakes, pastries, and alcoholic beverages are given choice spots for display. Food manufacturers often pay for the best place in the supermarkets—at the end of the aisle and, depending on the product, at a child's or adult's eye level.

Quick-service restaurants make especially appealing overtures to consumers. Many now offer healthful alternatives to their high-kcalorie and fat-laden foods.[7] Cutting fat has become a major preoccupation. Still, careful choices must be made. Even a salad bar is not always as healthful as it sounds. Many items are loaded with fat, such as potato salad, macaroni salad, nachos, and creamy salad dressings. Portion size then becomes a key decision. For some people—such as traveling sales representatives, students, and truck drivers—it is convenient to stop for quick-service food on a regular basis. For regular consumers of quick-service food, what they choose to eat is crucial if they want to have a nutritious diet (see Chapter 16 for a look at Eating on the Run).

Social Factors

Social changes in recent years have had a strong impact on the food industry. The realities of today's society have an impact people's food choices—homelessness, unemployment, and even divorce must be considered. In addition, growing numbers of working mothers and single parents, both young and old, find less time to prepare meals.[7] A general *time-famine* is emerging. Most people still turn to quick-service–food emporiums, but supermarket food counters are stealing restaurant customers. Microwave ovens and frozen food—often complete meals—have come to the rescue, resulting in a whole new array of products. Even products geared for young children are available. Shopping malls have created a new generation of "mall munchers," who eat everything from ethnic foods to high-priced cookies. Drive-through restaurants are now a large part of our culture, whereas 30 years ago they were much less common. It is convenient to drive through, wolf down 1200 kcalories (about half or more of your daily energy needs) via a burger, fries, and shake, and—you're on your way.

While people have become more educated about nutrition and families are starting to eat more meals together than in the recent past, it is still relatively common to eat out and to skip meals. Over one half of college students report that they eat only two meals a day with many snacks in between. Approximately 30% of adults skip breakfast, a habit that can interfere with proper nutrition. Breakfast is your chance to replace carbohydrate stores used during the night's sleep. You will also most likely get much more accomplished during the day if you just take the 20 minutes to relax and enjoy a morning meal.

another BITE

You eat because you see it, you hear it cooking, you smell it, or it's time to eat. All of these stimuli are concentrated in a mall: the food is there, it smells good, and there's so much to choose from. In addition, food may be the most affordable temptation at the mall. After a few hours of trekking through a mall, you would swear you had walked miles. But you would have to walk almost twice around the average mall to chalk up a mile—and that's only 100 kcalories worth of exercise.

The source of shopper's fatigue is psychological—styles, prices, lines, crowds . . .

Tired and frustrated,

the next step is hungry!

Think about that the next time you go shopping. Eat before you go, take a healthful snack, or be on your guard as you sample the smells.

It also is desirable to try to eat with others often. Meal time is a key social time of the day. The Japanese are ahead of us in recognizing that food's powers go beyond the realm of nutrition. Their national dietary guidelines—which like ours stress the importance of eating a variety of foods, maintaining healthy weight, and limiting fat in the diet—also advise people to make all activities pertaining to food and eating pleasurable.

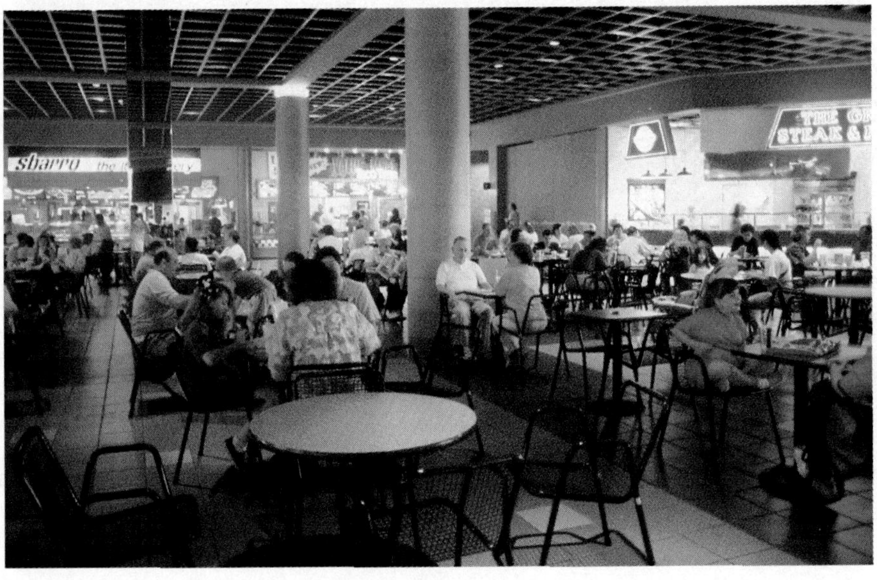

Mall munching can be convenient but costly in terms of the amount of energy consumed.

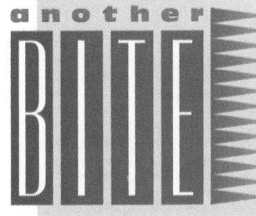

Economics

Food costs affect what we eat. As we make more money, we tend to eat out more often. Two-paycheck households purchase more precooked and prepackaged foods and devote a much larger share of the food budget to eating away from home.[7] However, the relationship between income and overall food consumption is not as strong as you might expect. This is probably because food is relatively inexpensive in the United States, compared with other parts of the world.[1] An average of only 11.8% of after-tax income was spent for food in 1990: 7.3% for food at home and 4.5% for food away from home. Compare this with China or India, where about 50% of income is spent on food. Nevertheless, high beef prices have led people tc choose chicken and turkey as alternatives. The high cost of restaurant meals has made quick-service food an economical choice for families, even though the fare is sometimes limited and of mediocre quality.

CONCEPT CHECK

Our food choices are influenced mainly by taste preferences and habit. Social factors, health concerns, and advertising also enter into the equation. Good food habits, developed and strengthened now, will benefit you in years to come. We encourage you to make this a goal as you pursue your study of nutrition.

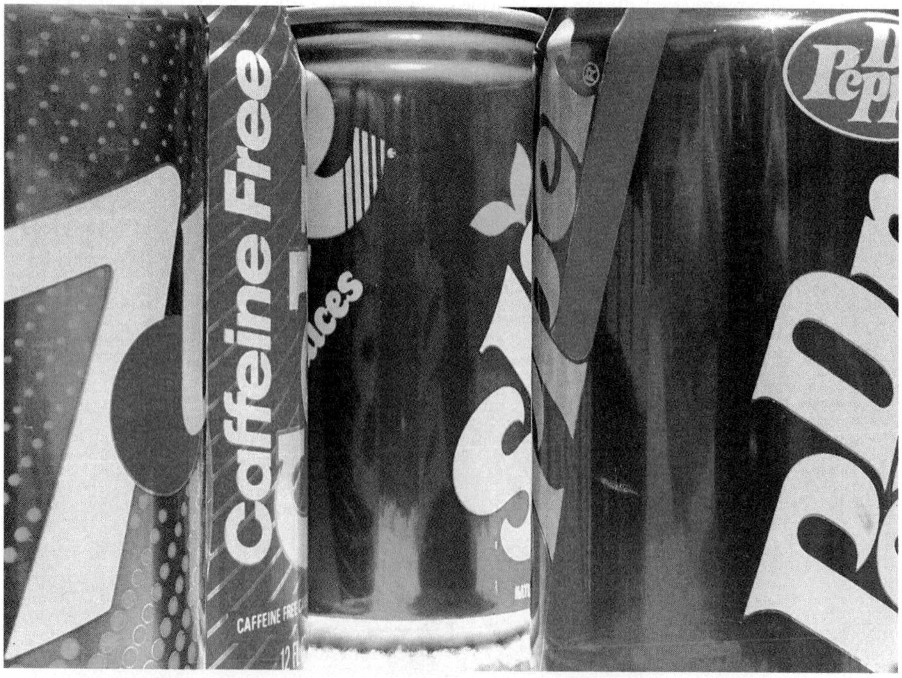

Today, soft drinks are more popular than is milk, although not as beneficial to the diet.

GIVEN OUR FOOD CHOICES, WE CAN DO BETTER

Americans can take pride in their cultural diversity, varied diets, and overall adequate nutritional health. The late 1990s promise a tremendous variety of food choices. Though many recent diet changes are advantageous, some are not. We are eating more fresh and frozen fruits and vegetables than in previous years, but we also drink less milk and more soft drinks. We live longer than ever before and enjoy better general health.[10] Some of us also have more money and time to relax and enjoy life. This can leave us overwhelmed by food and life-style choices.

The final outcome of these trends is not fully known, but deaths from heart disease and stroke have dropped dramatically since the late 1960s.[16] This is partly the result of better medical care and more nutritious diets. On the other hand, affluence can lead us into a sedentary and unhealthful life-style and lull us into alcoholism and/or ***obesity.***[20] Even though a greater variety of available foods makes it easier for us to eat a more nutritious diet than ever before, we must also make careful choices.

Obesity *A condition characterized by excess body fat, often defined as 20% above desirable body weight (see Chapter 10).*

Overall the American diet has improved, but many of us can do better. The goal of this book is to help you find the best path to good nutrition. There are no "junk" or bad foods, but some foods provide relatively few nutrients in comparison to energy content and thus contribute to less nutritious food behaviors. One's overall diet is the proper focus in a nutritional evaluation. Chapter 2 will emphasize this point and show you how to balance your diet.

As you move toward your nutritional goals, remember your health is partly your responsibility. Your body has a natural ability to heal itself. Offer it what it needs, and it will serve you well.[5]

SUMMARY

- Nutrition is the study of what foods are vital for health and how your body uses nutrients to promote and support growth, maintenance, and reproduction of cells.
- The metric system is used throughout science. Lengths are expressed in meters, weights are expressed in grams, and volumes are expressed in liters. A meter equals about 39 inches, a kilogram is about 2.2 pounds, and a liter is about 1 quart.
- There are six classes of nutrients found in foods: (1) carbohydrates, (2) lipids (fats and oils), (3) proteins, (4) vitamins, (5) minerals, and (6) water. Carbohydrates, lipids, and proteins provide energy (kcalories) for the body to use.
- A basic plan for health promotion and disease prevention includes eating a proper diet, exercising regularly, not smoking, limiting alcohol intake, and limiting or coping with stress.
- Good nutrition should be based on eating the right foods rather than taking supplements. Getting necessary nutrients from foods prevents nutrient imbalances.
- Results from large nutrition surveys suggest that some Americans need to consume foods that supply more vitamin A, vitamin C, calcium, magnesium, iron, zinc, and dietary fiber.
- Our food choices are greatly affected by our taste preferences, food habits, culture, upbringing, self-image, and the image we want to present to others. There are no true *junk foods.* The focus should be on balancing a total diet by choosing many nutritious foods.

STUDY QUESTIONS

1. Name some chronic diseases associated with nutrition and a few corresponding risk factors.
2. Outline the concept behind the measurement of kcalories in foods and how these values are determined.
3. Outline the "ABCD" activities often performed to assess current nutritional status.
4. List some changes brought on in your nutritional intake by the recent changes seen in our "modern-age" society (within the past 30 years).
5. If a person needs 2200 calories per day, calculate the actual number of calories provided by 55% of total calories from carbohydrate, 15% from protein, and 30% from lipids. (HINT: refer to the Nutrition Insight on pp. 8-9.)

REFERENCES

1. Birch LL: The acquisition of food acceptance patterns in children. In Boakes RA Pioplewell D, Burton M, editors: *Eating habits: food, physiology, and learned behavior,* New York, 1987, John Wiley & Sons.
2. Block G and others: Nutrient sources in the American diet, *American Journal of Epidemiology* 122:13, 1985.
3. Diet, nutrition, and prevention of chronic diseases—a report of the WHO study group on diet, nutrition, and prevention of noncommunicable diseases, *Nutrition Reviews* 49:291, 1991.
4. Burkitt DP, Eaton SB: Putting the wrong fuel in the tank, *Nutrition* 5:189, 1989.
5. Butrum RR and others: NCI dietary guidelines: rationale, *American Journal of Clinical Nutrition* 48:88, 1988.
6. Callaway CW: The marriage of taste and health: a union whose time has come, *Nutrition Today,* p. 37, May/June 1992.
7. Cassell JA: Commentary: American food habits in the 1980s, *Topics in Clinical Nutrition* 4(2):47, 1989.
8. Checking out the supermarket shopper, *Journal of the American Dietetic Association* 91:1511, 1991.
9. Fries JF: Strategies for reduction of morbidity, *American Journal of Clinical Nutrition* 55:12575, 1992.
10. Garn SM, Leonard WR: What did our ancestors eat? *Nutrition Reviews* 47:337, 1989.
11. Harper AE: Nutrition: from myth and magic to science, *Nutrition Today,* p. 8, January/February 1988.
12. Kant AK and others: Dietary diversity in the U.S. population, NHANES II, 1976-1980, *Journal of the American Dietetic Association* 91:1526, 1991.
13. Kim WW and others: Evaluation of long-term dietary intakes of adults consuming self-selected diets, *American Journal of Clinical Nutrition* 40:1327, 1984.
14. McBean LD: Consumer knowledge and attitudes about diet and nutrition, *Dairy Council Digest* 62:19, 1991.
15. McKee LM, Harden ML: Genetic and environmental origins of food patterns, *Nutrition Today,* p. 26, September/October 1990.
16. National Research Council, National Academy of Sciences: *Diet and health,* Washington, DC, 1989, National Academy Press.
17. Nobmann ED and others: The diet of Alaska native adults: 1987-1988, *American Journal of Clinical Nutrition* 55:1024, 1992.
18. Packard DP, McWilliams M: Cultural foods heritage of middle eastern immigrants, *Nutrition Today* p. 6, May/June 1993.
19. Peterkin BB and others: Nationwide food consumption survey, 1986, *Nutrition Today,* p. 18, January/February 1988.
20. Surgeon General's report on nutrition and health, *Nutrition Today,* p. 22, September/October 1988.
21. Webb L: Changing dietary habits of consumers, *Topics in Clinical Nutrition* 5(3):34, 1990.
22. Wright HS and others: The 1987-88 Nationwide Food Consumption Survey, *Nutrition Today,* p. 21, May/June 1991.

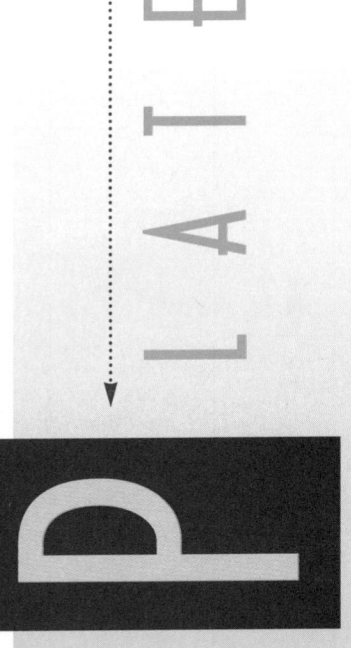

FACTORS AFFECTING EATING

Choose one or more days of the week, as your professor directs, that are typical of your eating pattern. In the table below write down all the foods and drinks you consumed for each day. In addition, write down the approximate amounts you ate in units like CUPS, OUNCES, TEASPOONS, and TABLESPOONS. Figure 16-3 in Chapter 16 provides an example of how to record your intake. A blank form is provided on p. 26 and in Appendix C for your use. Copy either form if you are to record more than 1 day. Check the food composition table in Appendix A for examples of appropriate serving units for different types of food, such as meat and vegetables. After completing this activity you will use this list of foods for future activities.

After you record each food/drink and serving size in the table, indicate why you chose to consume it. Enter the abbreviation given below in the space provided on the form to indicate why you picked that particular food or drink.

TAST	Taste/Texture	HUNG	Hunger
CONV	Convenience	FAM	Family/Cultural
EMO	Emotions	PEER	Peers
AVA	Availability	NUTR	Nutritive value
ADV	Advertisement	$	Cost
WTCL	Weight control	HLTH	Health

You can record more than one reason for choosing a particular food or drink.

Application

Now ask yourself what is your most frequent reason for eating or drinking. To what degree is health a reason for your food choices? Should it be made a greater priority?

Time	Minutes Spent Eating	M or S*	H†	Activity While Eating	Place of Eating	Food and Quantity	Others Present	Reason for Food Choice

*M or S, *meal or snack.*
†*Hunger (0, none; 3, maximum).*

Nutrition ISSUE

ETHNIC INFLUENCES ON THE AMERICAN DIET

As world conditions have changed over the centuries, people of all cultures have migrated to new places. Typically, migrants retain some traditional dietary habits (also known as *foodways*), transform some practices, and abandon others. As people migrate and mingle, their cuisines tend to meld together with other diets. Today technology is responsible for new means of preparing foods, so that many Americans eat in quick-service restaurants. We have seen recent changes in the dietary habits of many nations, for better or for worse.[21]

America—North, South, East, and West—is a unique and exciting "salad bowl" of many different cultures. We are indeed fortunate to experience colorful and tasty diets of many ethnic groups. In this Nutrition Issue, we will examine how various cultures have shaped the American palate. As you continue your study of nutrition, you may come to appreciate the nutrition attributes of many ethnic diets. Remember, the trick to finding healthful food is to carefully evaluate each dish. No single cuisine is all good or bad. Let's look at six diets that have all contributed to food "American-style."

Native Americans

Humans have walked the Earth for about 40,000 years. For 30,000 years, humans survived by hunting wild animals and gathering plants. Early societies, including those in America, were directly affected by the availability of wild game and the seasonal growth of fruits and vegetables. Our early ancestors ate a diet mostly low in fat (especially low-fat wild game) and sodium and high in dietary fiber.[10] Some researchers feel that in modern times we have mistakenly abandoned important aspects of that diet.[4]

Because America is such a large land with varied geography and seasons, diets of native societies consisted of local wild game and vegetation. Native-American civilizations cultivated early forms of such foods as tomatoes, sweet potatoes, squash, peanuts, vanilla, and cocoa. To the far North, Alaska natives—including Eskimos, Indians, and Aleuts—have traditionally subsisted on fish, sea mammals, game, and a few plants, such as seaweed, willow leaves, and berries.

Recent studies have shown that the types of disease that affected these societies differ notably from the diseases common to modern American society. For example, Alaska natives who have eaten the traditional fare have heart disease rates lower than people in the general U.S. population. Younger generations of natives, however, have developed heart disease at rates similar to those in the U.S. mainland.[17] This and other studies indicate that as the world's technology becomes increasingly uniform, so too does the health status of many cultures.

Hispanic-Americans

With the influx of early Spanish inhabitants in what is now Mexico, new foods and flavors were quickly melded into Mexican cooking. For example, we know that Mayans and Aztecs grew corn, beans, and chilies that later formed the basis of Mexican cuisine. They also had orchards of avocados, coconuts, papayas, pineapples, and pears. By the second voyage of Columbus, wheat, chickpeas, melons, radishes, salad greens, grapes, and sugar cane made it to this region. Rice, citrus fruits, and nuts followed closely behind. The Spanish also introduced beef, lamb, and chicken to native civilizations that had thrived on wild game and fish. The spice traders of Europe brought cinnamon, black pepper, cloves, thyme, marjoram, and bay leaves.

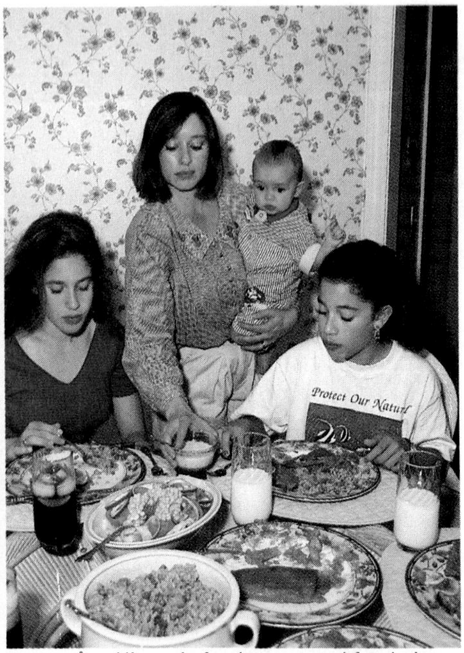

Hispanic foods are noted for their use of grains, vegetables, and beans—rich sources of nutrients

Today, true Mexican cooking bears little resemblance to the foods commonly found in "Mexican" restaurants. It is typically not oily, heavy, or highly seasoned. Mexican cooking offers great regional variety. Southern Mexico stays closer to its native heritage with savory sauces and stews and tortillas made from corn. West-central Mexico is perhaps least identified with ancient native ways—red chili enchiladas, fried tacos, and tequila are among this region's hallmarks. The Gulf states are renowned for delicious seafood dishes prepared with tomatoes, herbs, and olives, whereas the Yucatan holds to Mayan tradition, with such specialties as wild turkey and fish from the peninsula. Fresh produce adds bright color, distinctive flavor, and great nutrition to Mexican dining. Markets in the United States are just beginning to offer more exotic vegetables from south of the border, such as chayote squash and jicama root or cactus and squash blossoms.

European-Americans

Immigrants from North-Central Europe greatly influenced traditional American home cooking. Staples of American fare—such as a hearty portion of fine roast meat with a side dish of mashed potatoes and hot vegetables, hot dogs, french fries, and even many pastry-type desserts—find their origins in East-Central European cuisine. The first large group of settlers from old Europe—the English, French, and German—brought their traditional foodways with them. As all cooks and cultures must do, the Europeans adapted to the vegetation and food availability of the regions in the Americas where they settled. It is not surprising that the menu of North-Central America still retains much of its European heritage—immigrants settled in regions of the "new land" that most closely resembled the landscape, climate, and vegetation of their homelands. Native Americans introduced new foods to the European settlers that are now staples of the American diet—corn and corn products, such as popcorn and hominy, and a variety of squash. Perhaps the European practice most retained in American homes is the traditional method of arranging food on a plate—servings of protein (typically a meat product), vegetables, and starch are separate, instead of combined. For example, a stir fry of rice, protein, and vegetable is a mixture typical of many other ethnic cuisines.

Every eating style has advantages and drawbacks, and the East-Central European style is no exception. This traditional cuisine provides abundant protein and nutrients from dairy and meat products. However, it also delivers a lot of saturated fat and can be short on vitamins, minerals, and dietary fiber typically found in grains, vegetables, and fruits.

African-Americans

The next major migration of a culture, though not by choice, was the import of Africans who were brought to America by European slave traders. Most black Americans descend from ancestors in Western Africa. Though generations of these peoples suffered slavery, segregation, and persecution, their unique culture retained its roots and has strongly influenced today's American culture in its foodways. Enslaved Africans held strongly to familiar, ancient traditions, and, as have other cultures, adapted them to foods encountered in their new environment.

The cuisine perhaps best known to have its roots in the American South is "soul food." If asked to compose a menu of soul food, many would conjure up a feast of barbequed items, fried chicken, sweet potatoes, and chitterlings as representative offerings. Originally soul food was any food available to the black cook in the agrarian South, whether she cooked for her family returning from field work or for the plantation owner and his family. Food available for Southerners of all means consisted primarily of pork and corn products, the basics of soul food. It was not uncommon for the plantation master to eat ribs, pork cutlets, and better cuts of the swine, and for the black slaves and servants to eat the undesirable waste products—entrails, feet, ears, and head.

Vegetable sources in the diet were and have remained primarily turnips, mustard and collard greens, and cabbage. Along with corn, the sweet potato is an important basic. African-American cooks first introduced sweet potatoes and created them into delicacies. Sweet potato pie, for example, is a soul food favorite. Beating grains between stones to form a powder was a technique brought from Africa. The cook would beat corn, add water, and cook the mixture over the hearth of a slave cabin—and viola!—cornbread. Several foods native to Africa that then became part of soul food cuisine are peanuts and peanut paste, okra, and black-eyed peas.

Another exciting development in the history of African-American cuisine was the blending of their food heritage with that of Canadian-French, Spanish, and Native American cuisines. That blend produced a savory menu of what is now recognized as Cajun and Creole food. Cajun and Creole dishes include spicy, thick soups such as gumbo ("gumbo" is derived from "guillobo," which means "okra" in an African language); sausages; Tabasco pepper sauce; red beans; rice; and seafood. More recognizably French are beignets, (sugar-covered doughnuts) and the American favorite, French toast.

Today's traditional African-American cuisine offers nutritional benefits and hazards. It provides ample vitamins, minerals, and dietary fiber in the rich variety of fruits, vegetables, and grain products. Other foods are high in saturated fat, such as the traditional meats and foods flavored or prepared with lard. Dairy products may not be emphasized enough, and that lack may be of concern to African-Americans who continue to practice traditional dietary customs (especially older generations). The roots of this avoidance include difficulty with digestion of milk sugar (lactose) by many African-American adults (see Chapter 5 for details). However, dairy products are an excellent source of calcium. Traditional soul food is still frequently found at special events and holidays in African-American families, and its contributions to the American diet are many and delicious.

Chinese-Americans

Known for its variety, the average Chinese diet consists of about 69% carbohydrate, 10% protein, and 21% fat—similar to proportions some Western nutritionists and cancer experts recommend.[5] There is richness and variety in Chinese cuisine, evidenced by the use of over 200 vegetables. In the Southeastern coastal area around Canton, estimates of the number of dishes range up to 50,000.

Rice is the core of the diet in Southern China, whereas in the temperate North wheat is predominant. This is made into noodles, bread, and dumplings. Common preparations are hot pots—stews consisting of dozens of ingredients—and stir-fried vegetables, meats, and fish, which are cooked almost instantaneously in a lightly-oiled, very hot wok. Bok choy and other forms of Chinese cabbage, perhaps the most widely-consumed vegetables in the world, are high in vitamin C and dietary fiber. When Chinese immigrants first came to America during the mid-1800s gold rush, they brought with them their traditional food preparation methods, which tend to preserve nutrients in foods. Though many traditional characteristics remain, North American restaurant versions of Chinese cooking usually emphasize foods that are not as typical of Chinese food as we like to think. Chinese-American food uses meat and sauces prepared with fats far more than is found in the basic Chinese sauces: oyster, hoisin, soy, and black bean. Other seasonings used are ginger root, scallions, almonds, sesame oil, rice wine, and garlic.

You can still order a healthful meal in a Chinese-American restaurant by choosing dishes that are not deep-fat fried or by substituting a vegetable dish for one meat entree. The average Chinese consumes the same amount of salt as an American does, and it may be wise to limit the amount of soy sauce sprinkled on your rice. Health authorities in China are calling for a cut in salt intake and a switch from saturated to unsaturated fats.

Italian-Americans

Loved for its savory seasonings and pasta dishes, authentic Italian cuisine is much more diverse than an American would expect. Ethnic foods of different regions reflect Italy's varied geography and climate. Northern Italy is the principal producer of meat, butter, and cheese, and rice dishes such as risotto are widely eaten. The Venetian diet, however, differs from that of most other Northern regions: vegetables and fish are plentiful and meat is limited. Foods from the Genoa region share similarities with their neighboring Mediterranean cultures. Fish plays a larger culinary role in cultures closer to the sea, and lighter foods—such as fresh vegetables prepared with herbs and olive oil—are characteristic. The regions south of Rome, such as Sicily, are known for their diet rich in grains, vegetables, dried beans, and fish—with little meat and oil. Compared with Northern Italians of the same economic class, Southern Italians consume only two thirds as much beef and veal, less than half the chicken, and one fifth the butter. Southern Italians eat one fifth more bread, pasta, vegetables, and fruit and twice the fish.

Pasta is still the heart of the Italian diet: Italians eat six times more of this simple wheat and water concoction than do North Americans. Though wheat was introduced to Italy around the sixteenth century from the New World, Americans have learned to love this nutritious Italian invention that is the basic ingredient of Friday night's spaghetti dinner. Italian cuisine in America typically offers those foods more common to the north of Italy, including cheese, cream, and pesto sauces for pasta and pizza made with higher-fat meats such as Italian sausages. A favorite, pizza is quickly becoming the most frequently consumed food in the United States. Though ingredients may differ slightly, the principal components of American pizza do not vary greatly from those of Italian pizza. Garlic and olive oil, prized for their flavor and use in Italian cookery, have become essentials to many American cooks.

Though some aspects of the Italian diet provide substantial amounts of saturated fat, nutrition experts now know that some components of the traditional Italian fare—such as whole-grain pasta, olive oil, and a variety of vegetables—are beneficial to good health. Instead of choosing a cheesy Alfredo sauce on that pasta dish, try pasta topped with fresh tomato sauce and a flavorful entree of fish and vegetables prepared with a small amount of wine, olive oil, and herbs for a simple, nutritious, and delicious meal.

Twentieth-Century Trends and Ethnic Diets

Though we have described only six diets here, a vast number of ethnic cuisines have contributed to the colorful, exotic, and unique culinary experiences possible in America. You may now be more aware of how traditional foods, which use a variety of foods available from the land, can be very healthful. As people of different cultures continue to move, assimilate new cultures, and assert their heritage, we will continue to incorporate new ethnic cuisines into our own. For example, recent social unrest in Russia and Thailand has contributed to an increase in immigrants to the United States. Indeed, restaurants serving traditional Russian and Thai fare, once rare, are now beginning to introduce new foods to those willing to try.

Based on research begun in the 1940s and 1950s, some scientists have developed a formula for a diet they consider the best overall for our bodies. The key is to eat simple foods prepared in simple ways—not elite treats.[4] Scientists discovered that an especially healthful diet consists of components of the inexpensive traditional fare—precisely the diet people abandon as they move into affluence. Simple foods prepared in simple ways have fueled humans for their entire existence on Earth. As we turn toward the twenty-first century, Americans are savoring the roots of their ethnic pasts. It is an exciting choice to experience different cuisines and a challenge worth pursuing to discover each contribution to overall health.[6]

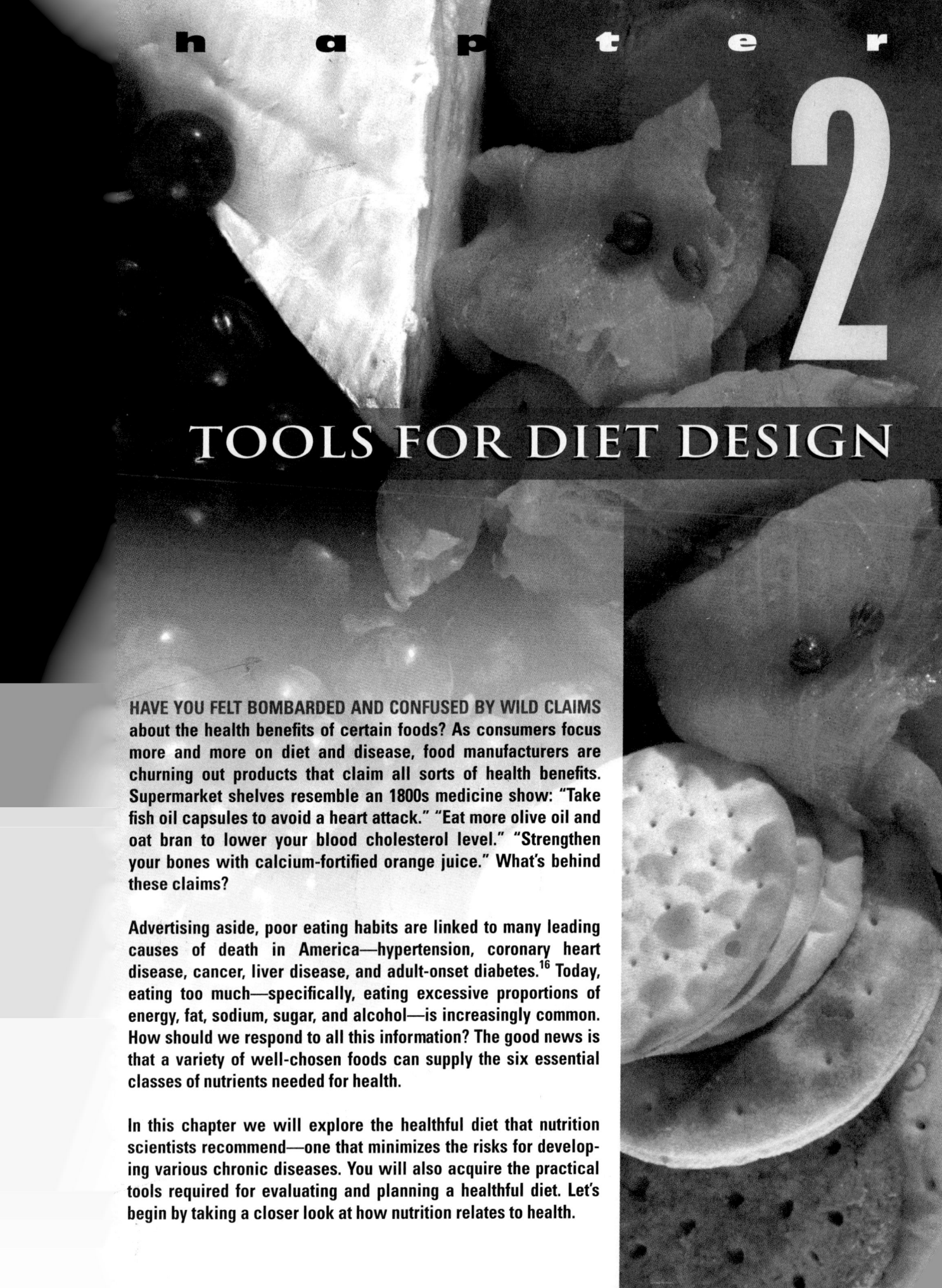

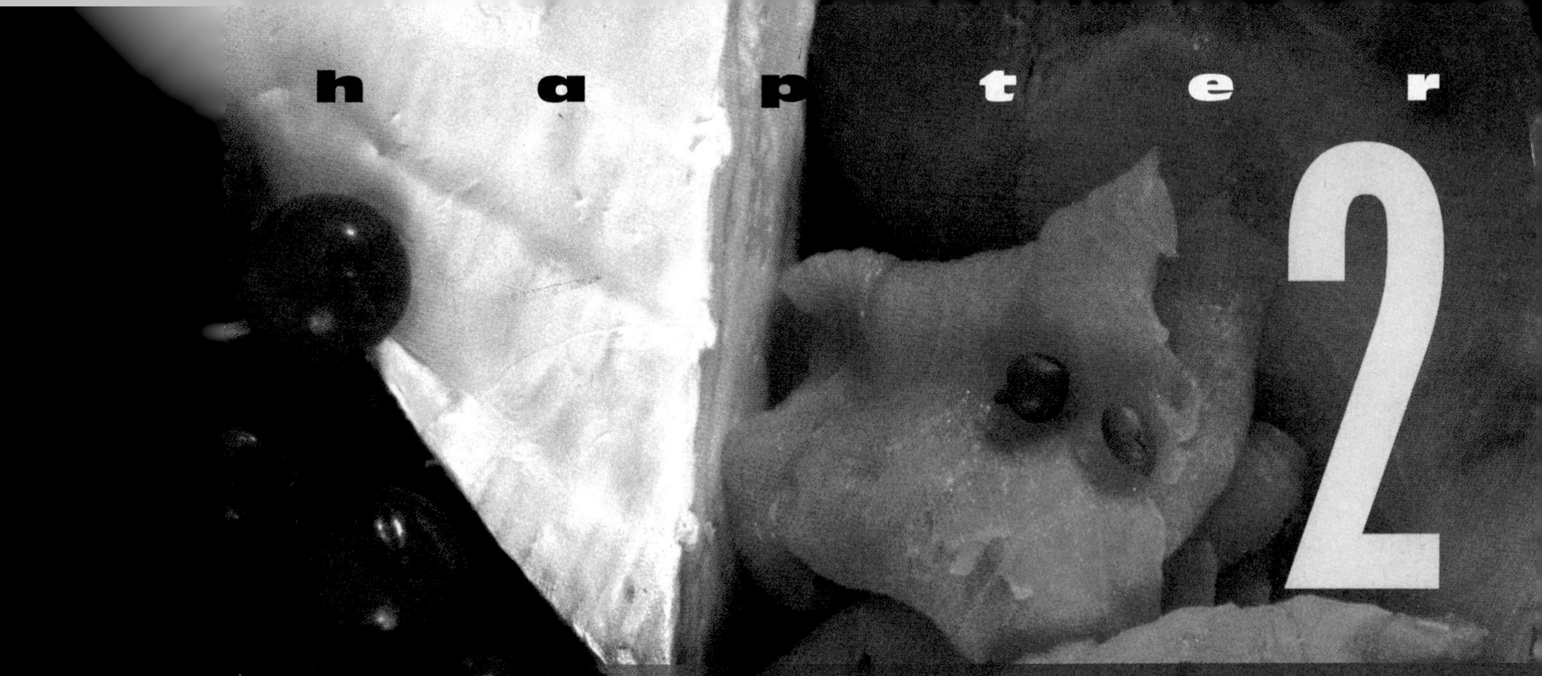

chapter 2

TOOLS FOR DIET DESIGN

HAVE YOU FELT BOMBARDED AND CONFUSED BY WILD CLAIMS about the health benefits of certain foods? As consumers focus more and more on diet and disease, food manufacturers are churning out products that claim all sorts of health benefits. Supermarket shelves resemble an 1800s medicine show: "Take fish oil capsules to avoid a heart attack." "Eat more olive oil and oat bran to lower your blood cholesterol level." "Strengthen your bones with calcium-fortified orange juice." What's behind these claims?

Advertising aside, poor eating habits are linked to many leading causes of death in America—hypertension, coronary heart disease, cancer, liver disease, and adult-onset diabetes.[16] Today, eating too much—specifically, eating excessive proportions of energy, fat, sodium, sugar, and alcohol—is increasingly common. How should we respond to all this information? The good news is that a variety of well-chosen foods can supply the six essential classes of nutrients needed for health.

In this chapter we will explore the healthful diet that nutrition scientists recommend—one that minimizes the risks for developing various chronic diseases. You will also acquire the practical tools required for evaluating and planning a healthful diet. Let's begin by taking a closer look at how nutrition relates to health.

ASSESS

TEST YOUR KNOWLEDGE

yourself

HOW DOES YOUR DIET RATE FOR VARIETY?

Directions: Check the box that best describes your eating habits.

How Often Do You Eat:	Seldom or Never	1 or 2 Times a Week	3 to 4 Times a Week	Almost Daily
1. At least six servings of bread, cereals, rice, crackers, pasta, or other foods made from grains (a serving is one slice of bread or ½ cup cereal, rice, etc.) per day?	☐	☐	☐	☐
2. Foods made from whole grains?	☐	☐	☐	☐
3. Three different kinds of vegetables—about ½ cup each—per day?	☐	☐	☐	☐
4. Two servings of 2-3 ounces of lean meat, poultry, fish, eggs, dry beans, or nuts per day?	☐	☐	☐	☐
5. A dark green leafy vegetable, such as spinach or broccoli?	☐	☐	☐	☐
6. Two kinds of fruit (whole piece) or fruit juice (¾ cup) per day?	☐	☐	☐	☐
7. Two servings (three if teenager, pregnant, or breast feeding) of a combination of milk, (1 cup) yogurt (1 cup), or cheese (1 ounce) per day?	☐	☐	☐	☐

SCORING: Compare your behaviors with the preferred practices.

Question 1: Almost Daily

Eating breads and cereals will not make you fat. Extra kcalories often come from the fat and/or sugar you may eat with them. Both whole-grained and enriched breads and cereals provide starch and essential nutrients.

Question 2: Almost Daily

Whole-grained breads and cereals contain vitamins, minerals, and dietary fiber that are lacking in the diets of some Americans. Select whole-grain cereals and bakery products, or make your own and use whole-wheat flour.

Question 3: Almost Daily

Vegetables vary in the amounts of vitamins and minerals they contain. So it's important to include several kinds every day.

Question 4: Almost Daily

Most Americans include some meat, poultry, or fish in their diets regularly. Dry beans and peas, peanuts (including peanut butter), nuts and seeds, and eggs can be used as alternatives.

Question 5: 3 to 4 Times a Week

Spinach and other dark green leafy vegetables are excellent sources of some nutrients and are lacking in many diets.

Question 6: Almost Daily

Fruits taste good and are good for you. Choose several different kinds each day.

Question 7: Almost Daily

Adults as well as children need the calcium and other nutrients found in milk, cheese, and yogurt.

DOES WHAT YOU EAT MAKE ANY DIFFERENCE TO YOUR HEALTH?

Let's take a closer look at how nutrition relates to health. You may wonder why some people show no outward symptoms of poor health even though they eat very poor diets. We don't always know the answer to this question. Given time, though, problems often appear, as discussed in Chapter 1. We can usually distinguish between people who are well-nourished and those who have endured prolonged poor nutrition, but the gray area—the gradual slide from a good to a poor nutritional state—can be difficult to detect. A lot of current nutrition research aims to develop better methods for early detection of nutritional problems.

Current methods for evaluating nutritional status focus on classifying a person in one of four stages of nutritional health: overnutrition, desirable status, undernutrition, and state of body deficiency. Table 2-1 shows how this general scheme relates to the function of a familiar essential nutrient, iron, in our bodies.

A CLOSER EXAMINATION OF THE STATES OF NUTRITIONAL HEALTH

Overnutrition

One nutritional state that is reaching epidemic proportions in Western society today is ***overnutrition.***[16] Many of us simply overeat. This overloads the body mostly with too many kcalories, but excesses of certain nutrients can build up as well. Overnutrition over a 1- or 2-week period generally causes no symptoms. But keep it up, and blood levels of some nutrients increase along with body weight. The average adult gains 15 to 20 pounds from ages 18 to 54 years.[11] In the long run, an overweight condition can lead to serious diseases, such as adult-onset diabetes and hypertension.

Overnutrition
A state in which nutritional intake exceeds the body's needs.

TABLE 2-1

States of Nutritional Health With Respect to Iron

General Conditions	Conditions With Respect to Iron
Overnutrition	
Nutrients consumed in excess of body needs (degree of toxicity varies for each nutrient)	Results in toxic damage to liver cells and possibly increased risk for heart disease
Desirable Nutritional State	
Sufficient amount of nutrients to support body functions and stores of nutrients for times of increased need	Body has desirable liver stores of iron and normal values for iron-related compounds
Undernutrition	
Stores depleted; tissue levels fall	Serum* ferritin, an iron-containing protein in the blood, drops below normal levels
Body Deficiency	
Reduced biochemical function	Hemoglobin, an iron-containing pigment in red blood cells, drops below normal levels
Clinical symptoms	Pale complexion, greatly increased heart rate during activity, and poor body temperature regulation

**Serum is the liquid portion of blood present after blood clots.*
This general scheme can apply to all nutrients. We have chosen iron because you are likely to be familiar with this nutrient. More details can be found in Chapters 6 (on heart disease) and 9 (iron in general).

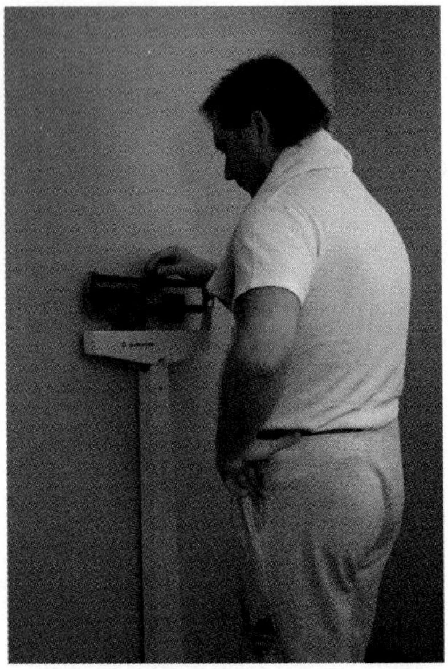

Body weight is a key component of a nutrition assessment.

Recently, another type of overnutrition has surfaced as a result of the ingestion of too many vitamin and mineral supplements. For most nutrients there is a wide gap between the right amount and too much. A typical multivitamin and mineral supplement taken daily probably won't supply a harmful amount of any nutrient. However, if a healthful diet is eaten, a general supplement is not needed. Intake of specific supplements—vitamins A and D and iron, for example—can be harmful unless supervised by a physician. Recent studies indicate that very high doses of vitamin B-6 and niacin can also cause health problems. If supplements are routinely taken in high doses, toxic levels usually build up in the body. This can lead to serious medical consequences. Chapter 8 discusses in greater detail some potential problems with supplement use.

In the past, people often didn't get enough of the essential nutrients in their diets. Undernutrition was the nutritional battle cry at the beginning of the twentieth century. Today problems arise mostly from overnutrition, combined with too little physical activity. Many of us end up taking in more kcalories than we need. Others of us eat too much sodium and saturated (mostly animal) fats. Both of these habits can jeopardize heart health.

Some of us should monitor what we eat more carefully, because our biological make-up is more susceptible to some diseases.[15] Otherwise, health problems can result. This is an issue we will help you focus on throughout the book.

Desirable Nutritional State

You reach a desirable status with respect to the amount of a nutrient in the body when the body tissues have enough of that nutrient for both routine chemical processes and surplus stores of it for use during times of increased need (Table 2-1). A desirable nutritional state can be achieved by obtaining essential nutrients from a variety of foods. This then contributes to maintenance of a healthy body.

Undernutrition

If you don't eat enough nutrients to support cell activities and maintain body functions, surplus stores of nutrients soon become used up. This is the path to ***undernutrition,*** which results in a state in which the body cannot function appropriately. Although body stores of nutrients can make up for a poor diet over a short time, they do not last indefinitely. Once stores are depleted, the body attempts to obtain essential nutrients from itself. This continues to drain nutrients from vital tissues. Eventually some body processes slow down or even stop. Biochemical changes then occur, resulting in ***biochemical deficiency symptoms.*** For example, when the body does not have enough iron, the level of the red blood cell protein *hemoglobin* falls because iron is needed to make hemoglobin. Serious problems, such as iron-deficiency anemia, can then arise. Women especially tend to develop anemia, because they often do not consume enough iron and so eventually deplete their iron stores (see Chapter 9 for details).

Undernutrition *Failing health that results from a long-standing dietary intake that does not meet nutritional needs.*

Biochemical deficiency symptoms *Nutrition deficiency symptoms observed in the blood or urine, such as low levels of nutrient by-products or low enzyme activities. These indicate reduced biochemical functioning in the body.*

Clinical symptoms *Generally, a change in health status noted by the individual (such as stomach pain) or noticed by a clinician during physical examination (the latter is technically called a clinical* sign).

Body Deficiency

If a biochemical change that results from depleted nutrients becomes severe, ***clinical symptoms*** eventually develop. Changes can be seen in the body: skin, hair, nails, tongue, and eyes. Perhaps you have noticed people who appear unhealthy; they lack the vigorous glow that comes with good health. In the case of iron deficiency, the person may appear very pale and may have a much faster heart rate during even moderate activity.

Just not feeling well, let alone the long-term effects of poor nutrition, is unpleasant. It's wise for you to begin understanding how diet relates to health now—sound nutrition practices will move you toward your goal of good health for the rest of your life. Now that you know that foods supply you with the essential nutrients needed to help reach and maintain good health, let's take a closer look at a healthful diet.

WHAT SHOULD I EAT TO MAINTAIN NUTRITIONAL HEALTH?

You may be surprised to learn that what you should eat is exactly what you've heard many times before—a great variety of foods balanced in moderation with each other.

However, a recent survey conducted by the American Dietetic Association showed that two of five people in the United States believe that following a healthful diet means giving up foods they enjoy. To the contrary, a healthful diet requires only some simple planning and doesn't have to mean deprivation and misery. Besides, eliminating favorite foods typically doesn't work for "dieters" in the long run. The best plan consists of learning what the basics of a healthful diet are—a variety of foods from all food groups that provides a balance of foods within each food group, and eating all foods in moderation. We shall continually stress these aspects of a healthful diet—variety, balance, and moderation—throughout this book.

Many people would like to live on pizza alone. What are pizza's nutrient strengths and inadequacies? Check the food composition table in Appendix A for the vitamin C content of pizza. How many slices would you need to eat to yield the RDA of 60 milligrams? (ANSWER : 25 slices).

A Food Philosophy That Works

Recall that no one natural food meets all your nutrient needs. Human milk, for example, comes close to meeting the needs of an infant, except for its low amounts of iron and vitamin D. Cow's milk also contains very little iron. Meat provides protein but little calcium. Eggs have no vitamin C, and the calcium is mostly in the shell. This is why you need a variety of foods—the nutrients you need are scattered among many foods.

One good way to achieve balance in the diet is to select foods from the five major food groups every day. These groups are as follows:

1. Breads, cereals, and other grain-based products
2. Vegetables
3. Fruits
4. Milk, cheese, and other dairy products, such as yogurt
5. Meats, fish, poultry, and dry beans and peas

Foods are classified according to their many similar nutrient contents. By including foods from all five groups, different types of foods are eaten. You then are more likely to meet your overall nutrient needs.[17] For example, a meal consisting of a bean burrito with tomatoes, a glass of milk, and an apple takes care of all five food groups. Fats, oils, and sweets can also be added to the diet in moderation to increase desirability.

Choosing a variety of foods within each food group also helps ensure that we receive essential nutrients. For example, carrots may be your favorite, but if you choose carrots every day as a vegetable, you may miss out on vitamin C. Other vegetables such as broccoli are rich sources of this nutrient. This concept is true of all foods that compose the five different food groups. Different foods within each food group vary some in the nutrients they provide, but they generally provide similar types of nutrients. Incorporating variety can make eating fun too—no one ever said that we have to eat the same foods and meals that we've eaten since childhood. We can obtain our vitamin C not only from orange juice and citrus fruit, but also from potatoes.

The foundation of good dietary habits is to eat food in moderation—eating enough but not too much of any one food. How much is enough? Later in this chapter, we will discuss the amounts of foods that generally are needed to meet a person's nutrient requirements and how that relates to the five food groups. An overall goal is to moderate—not eliminate—the intake of foods available to us. By thinking about our food choices, it is possible to enjoy all foods; we can plan ahead on how to juggle nutrient sources. For example, when you plan to eat something relatively high in fat and salt, such as a bacon cheeseburger, eat other foods that are lower in the same nutrients, like fruits and salad greens, on the same day. If you prefer whole milk to low-fat or skim milk, choose lower-fat alternatives elsewhere in your meals. Try low-fat salad dressings or use jam instead of butter or margarine on your toast.

Balance—Choose foods from all five food groups.

Variety—Choose different types of foods within each food group.

Moderation—Control portion size so balance and variety are possible in a diet.

Most important, when considering variety, balance, and moderation, eat foods that appeal to you. Remember that there are no "good" or "bad" foods. Focus on your total day's intake when you make a "health" evaluation. Fortunately, our food supply is abundant and safe. For most of us a good diet is affordable, and we have a huge variety of food choices. A well-balanced and healthful diet can be planned to match your family and cultural traditions, lifestyle, and budget. Even so, white bread, whole milk, doughnuts, cookies, French fries, hot dogs, hamburgers, and meat loaf—many of which are high in fat—

and sugared soft drinks make up a major part of the American diet. As a nation, we have our work cut out for us to improve our nutrition and health habits. Health professionals have recommended the same basic diet plan for the last 10 years: watch how much you eat, focus on the major food groups, and stay physically active.[6] Let's now fine-tune this advice, beginning with a look at how scientists establish our nutrient needs.

CONCEPT CHECK

Foods are preferred over supplements as a source of nutrients, primarily because each food contains a wide variety, and rarely a potentially toxic amount, of nutrients. One's nutritional state affects biochemical processes in the body. Serious health problems can result from excess, as well as poor, nutrient intake. The most important principles of sound dietary habits are to include variety, balance, and moderation in food choices. No foods are "good" or "bad"—the focus of a healthful diet should be the entire day's intake, and not necessarily on one specific food choice.

Recommended Dietary Allowances (RDAs) *Recommended nutrient intakes that meet the needs of essentially all people of similar age and gender. These are established by the Food and Nutrition Board of the National Academy of Sciences.*

The RDA assumes we eat a wide variety of foods (mixed diet), experience no temperature extremes, and do not participate in long, strenuous physical activity.

RECOMMENDED DIETARY ALLOWANCES

Before designing a diet, we must determine what frequency and amount of each nutrient is needed. People have puzzled over this question for centuries. During World War II, when many men were rejected from military service because of the effects of poor nutrition on their health, the need for official dietary recommendations was recognized. In 1941 a group of 25 scientists formed the first Food and Nutrition Board. They established dietary standards for evaluating the nutritional intakes of large populations and for planning agricultural production. This board developed the first ***Recommended Dietary Allowances (RDAs).*** They left open the option to revise the RDAs as better scientific evidence became available. Every 4 or 5 years the RDAs are revised using the following guidelines[5]:

1. Estimate how much of each essential nutrient the average person requires to be healthy and how those requirements vary among people.
2. Increase the average requirement by about 30% to 50% to cover the needs of almost all members of the population. For example, if the average requirement for a vitamin is found to be 20 milligrams per day, the RDA may be approximately 28 milligrams per day (40% higher).
3. Increase the RDA again to make up for cooking losses and inefficient use by the body, as well as for cases in which greater nutrient needs are placed on the body, such as in pregnancy.
4. Use scientific judgment to interpret and establish allowances when specific data are limited.

Using this process the Food and Nutrition Board determines RDAs for healthy males and females of various age-groups. See the inside cover of this book for the specific recommendations.

The RDAs are your guide for estimating your nutritional needs. However, make sure these nutrients come from foods, rather than mainly from vitamin and mineral supplements. Using foods is important because as a whole they contain all essential nutrients. Only 19 of approximately 45 necessary nutrients—not counting certain essential amino acids that make up food protein—have an RDA. Not enough is known about many nutrients for the Food and Nutrition Board to establish an RDA. However, all essential nutrients should be part of your diet.

The RDAs Are Not for Amateurs

One common misconception about the abbreviation RDA is that the "D" stands for "daily." It stands instead for "dietary." We don't need to eat the RDA for each nutrient every day, because our bodies store nutrients for later use. Think instead of averaging the RDA for vitamins and minerals over a week's time: some days you eat more, and some days you eat less, but the average for 3 to 7 days should meet the RDA. That can be extended to months for vitamin A and vitamin B-12, because they are not readily excreted by the body.

Notice also that the "R" does not stand for "required," but "recommended." Because the RDAs actually apply to groups rather than to individuals, they should be used primarily to plan and evaluate diets for groups of people.[5] They are not to be interpreted as specific personal nutritional requirements for individuals. Those values can be scientifically determined only in a laboratory. Because the allowances are set quite high, healthy people should not expect their health to improve if they eat more than RDA levels of various nutrients.[7,10] The Food and Nutrition Board's goal in establishing RDAs is to protect Americans from getting either too much or too little of the needed nutrients. Too often people think that if a little of something is good, a lot must be better. This can lead to trouble with some nutrients, as you will see in Chapters 8 and 9. The Rate Your Plate activity at the end of this chapter will help you evaluate how well you are meeting the RDAs for your age and gender.

While the original purpose of the RDAs was to plan and evaluate soldiers' diets, its scope now includes all healthy groups of Americans, such as college students eating in a campus dormitory cafeteria.

A Close Look at One RDA: Protein

Eating protein regularly is critical to maintaining your health. The RDA for protein is 0.8 grams per kilogram of desirable body weight (or about 0.35 grams per pound) for an adult.[5] That amount allows daily protein intake to balance the body's normal protein losses from hair, skin, stool, and so on, and allows the body to maintain protein ***equilibrium*** (Figure 2-1). (Chapter 7 contains more details on proteins in the body.) The recommenda-

Equilibrium
In nutritional terms, a state in which nutrient intake equals nutrient losses. This allows the body to maintain a stable condition.

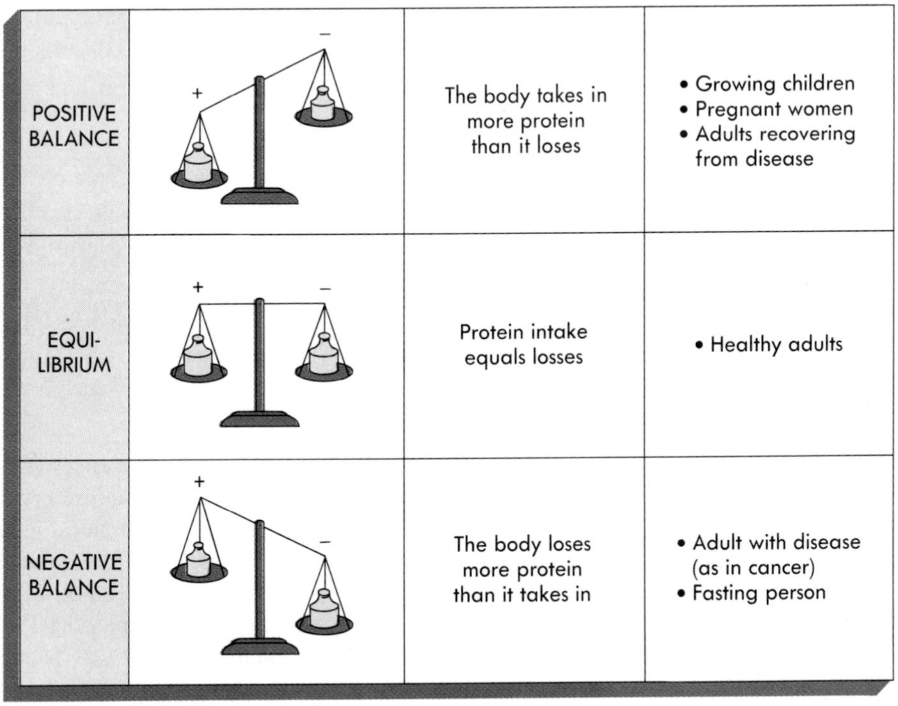
POSITIVE BALANCE
+
−
The body takes in more protein than it loses
• Growing children
• Pregnant women
• Adults recovering from disease
EQUILIBRIUM
+
−
Protein intake equals losses
• Healthy adults
NEGATIVE BALANCE
+
−
The body loses more protein than it takes in
• Adult with disease (as in cancer)
• Fasting person

FIGURE 2-1
Nutrient balance using protein as an example. This balance concept can be applied to all nutrients.

tion also allows for some extra protein to stock the body's protein stores. In this way protein status of the body should stay about the same each day.

When setting the RDA for children, scientists add extra protein to accommodate daily growth needs in new cells. For children it is not enough to balance daily protein losses and store a little extra; to provide for growth, children must regularly take in more protein than they lose. The RDA is adjusted to account for this.

If you total the amount of protein you eat in 1 week and divide by seven, you will have your average daily protein consumption. If that value is close to the RDA, you are most likely eating enough protein. Even if you eat less protein than the RDA, you might not suffer ill effects, because your needs are most likely less than the RDA.[5] As a general rule, however, the further you stray below the RDA—particularly as you approach less than half the recommendation—the greater your risk of a nutritional deficiency.

Symptoms of nutritional deficiencies may be subtle and develop slowly. It takes a long time to detect problems such as a weakened immune system, reduced chemical processing in body cells, or an impaired ability to carry oxygen in the blood. If you suspect that your diet is not nutritious enough, don't wait for warning signs to develop. Start eating a diet that meets your RDAs for all listed nutrients rather than risk developing health problems from poor nutrition.

Estimated Safe and Adequate Daily Dietary Intakes

The Food and Nutrition Board sets ***Estimated Safe and Adequate Daily Dietary Intakes (ESADDI)*** for several nutrients that have no true RDA. These include copper, biotin, and chromium (see the inside cover for values). The Board feels that information on these nutrients is too incomplete to set an RDA but detailed enough to set a range for a reasonable group intake.[5] By providing a range, the ESADDI not only recommend intake to meet nutritional needs, but also discourage people from eating too much of these nutrients. The Board also sets ***minimum requirements for health*** for sodium, potassium, and chloride. Note that these nutrients do not have RDA or ESADDI.[5]

Some nutrients—carbohydrates and fats, for example—still have no RDA, ESADDI, or minimum requirement for health. Still, our needs for these nutrients can easily be met by eating a diet that meets our established nutrient needs. Chapters 5 and 6 discuss this issue in more detail.

Estimated Safe and Adequate Daily Dietary Intake (ESADDI) *Nutrient intake recommendations made by the Food and Nutrition Board that give a range for intake of some nutrients, because insufficient information is available to set an RDA.*

Minimum Requirements for Health *Nutrient intake standards set by the Food and Nutrition Board for sodium, potassium, and chloride.*

U.S. Recommended Daily Allowances (U.S. RDAs) *Nutrient standards established by FDA for use on nutrition labels. Generally, the four existing versions use the highest nutrient recommendation in the appropriate age and gender category from the 1968 publication of the RDA. The version that includes children over 4 years of age and adults is most commonly seen on nutrition labels.*

RDA for Energy Needs

The RDA for energy estimates average energy needs for physically active people of various age-groups and then suggests a wide range for the allowance (see the inside cover for recommendations). Note that no extra amount is added for human variabilities, as is done for nutrient RDAs.

The energy RDAs provide only rough estimates. Energy intake really should depend on energy use.[5] For most adults, weight maintenance is the best indicator of energy balance—energy intake matching energy output.

U.S. RDAs and RDIs

One practical application of the RDA is the ***U.S. Recommended Daily Allowances (U.S. RDAs).*** Note the "D" stands for "daily," not "dietary" as in RDA. This standard was first set in 1974 by the U.S. Food and Drug Administration (FDA) to be used on nutrition labels on foods and vitamin/mineral supplements (Figure 2-2). It replaced the Minimum Daily Requirements (MDRs). The U.S. RDAs for adults are primarily based on the highest RDA values determined in 1968 for this specific age-group. For example, the 1968 RDA for iron for adult men was 10 milligrams per day; for adult women it was 18 milligrams per day. The U.S. RDA for adults uses the higher value of 18 milligrams per day. Appendix D lists U.S. RDA values. The values set for children over 4 years of age and adults are commonly listed on food products.

Mainly for economic reasons, the U.S. RDAs have not been updated since they were first set, but new labeling laws will likely lead to changes.[14] The National Labeling and

Education Act of 1990 increased government regulation of food labels and called for the reexamination of the U.S. RDA.[9] Many scientists support a reevaluation because a number of nutrients have lower RDAs today than they had in 1968.[1] However, some scientists and the vitamin industry in general oppose lowering the nutrient levels in the U.S. RDA because either they believe the public generally underconsumes some of the nutrients covered, such as vitamin E, or they cite purely economic grounds. Nevertheless, U.S. RDA will undergo a name change to ***Reference Daily Intakes (RDIs)*** to reduce confusion with the RDAs. Whether the nutrient levels will be lowered compared with the U.S. RDA is now an open question. FDA is currently evaluating the pros and cons. Appendix D lists proposed RDIs based on the 1989 RDA.

New labeling laws will also create a new category called ***Daily Reference Values (DRVs).*** These will be set for some nutrients that don't have RDAs, such as fat and carbohydrate. The RDIs and DRVs will be combined under one heading on new food labels—***Daily Values (DVs).***

Under the new law, the nutrition label format on food products will change as well. Figure 2-2, *A* shows a typical nutrition label currently in use that lists nutrients in terms of percentages of the U.S. RDA for the adult category.

The label shown in Figure 2-2, *A* states that one serving of this food contains 30% of the U.S. RDA for iron. Because the U.S. RDA for iron is 18 milligrams, this product contains about 5.4 milligrams of iron per serving ($0.3 \times 18 = 5.4$). The label also states that one serving contains 20% of the U.S. RDA for the vitamin niacin. Because the U.S. RDA for niacin is 20 milligrams, the niacin content is 0.20×20, or 4 milligrams.

The other label in Figure 2-2, *B* shows the new nutrition labels that appeared in 1993. After May 1994 this is the only format that will be allowed. Note the listing of DVs instead of the U.S. RDAs. Again, RDIs and DRVs are combined under the DVs heading. Note in addition that the DRV standards for fat, saturated fat, cholesterol, and sodium are not seen as goals to shoot for. Rather, the DRVs generally represent limits we should try to stay below. In practice, the percent values for DRVs for fat, saturated fat, cholesterol, and sodium for all food consumed in a day should add up to less than 100% for each of these nutrients.[8] The Nutrition Issue on p. 59 details these and other new regulations that apply to nutrition labels on foods.

Reference Daily Intakes (RDIs) *New term for expressing nutrient content on nutrition labels. For the present time, these will be the same as the U.S. RDAs. A proposal has been made for RDIs to be based on average 1989 RDA values set for a nutrient that is applicable for a parrticular age-group, such as from children over 4 years through adults. A decision on this proposal is pending.*

Daily Reference Values (DRVs) *Reference values for some nutrients that don't have a 1989 RDA value, such as sodium, carbohydrate, fat, and dietary fiber. DRVs and RDIs will help consumers evaluate individual food choices and how they fit into a total diet as they combine to form the standard or Daily Values (DVs).*

CONCEPT CHECK

Recommended Dietary Allowances (RDAs) are designed to meet the nutrient needs of groups—not individuals. RDAs are established for specific age and gender categories. No one knows personal nutritional requirements unless these have been scientifically measured in a laboratory. But RDAs are good diet benchmarks. The further you stray below the RDA for your age and gender, the greater the chance of experiencing a nutritional deficiency. In 1974 FDA designed the U.S. RDA as a means of expressing nutrient content of foods on nutrition labels. Nutrient content is listed on labels as a percentage of the U.S. RDA. Soon the term *Reference Daily Intakes* (RDIs) will replace the U.S. RDAs. It is likely that RDIs will eventually reflect the nutrient recommendations made in the 1989 RDAs. Daily Reference Values (DRVs) have been set for some nutrients that don't have an RDA, such as fat, cholesterol, and dietary fiber. The Daily Values (DVs) to be listed on new nutrition labels will use the RDI or DRV standards, whichever is appropriate.

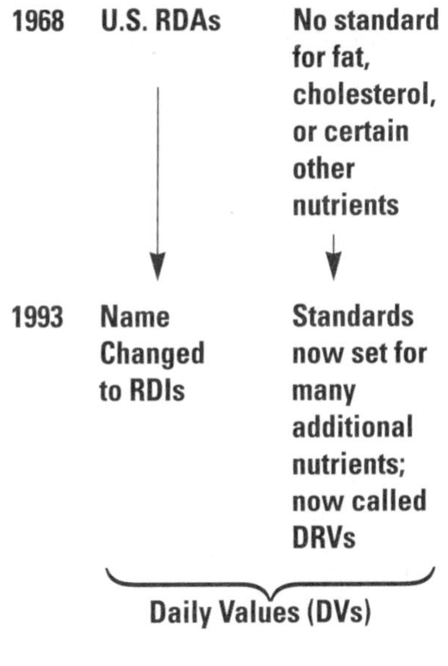

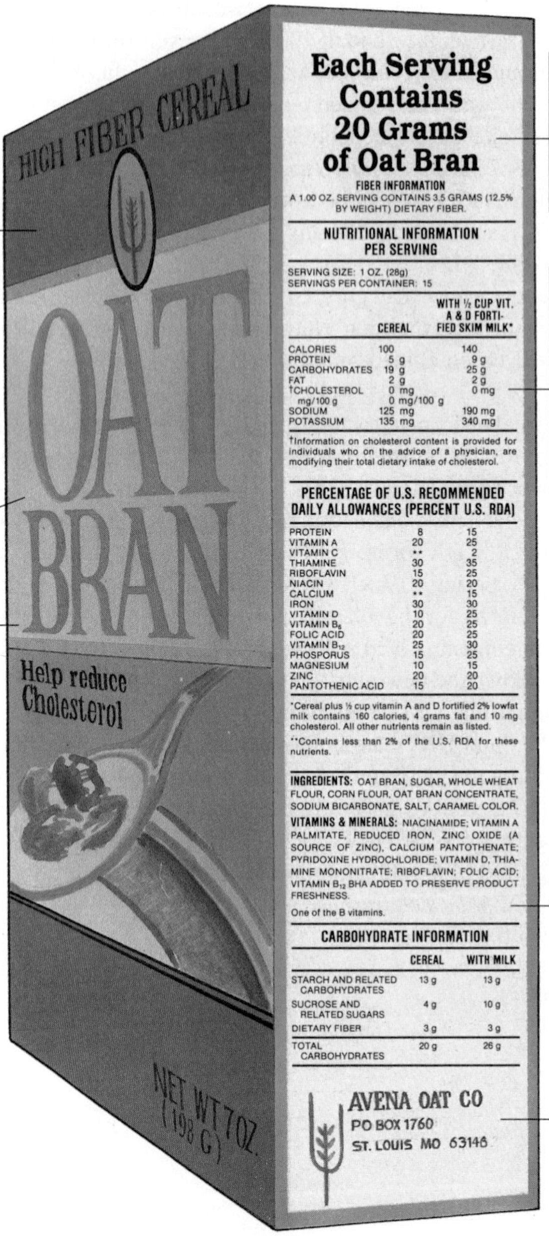
HIGH FIBER CEREAL
OAT BRAN
Help reduce Cholesterol
NET WT 7 OZ (198 G)
Each Serving Contains 20 Grams of Oat Bran
FIBER INFORMATION
A 1.00 OZ. SERVING CONTAINS 3.5 GRAMS (12.5% BY WEIGHT) DIETARY FIBER.
NUTRITIONAL INFORMATION PER SERVING
SERVING SIZE: 1 OZ. (28g)
SERVINGS PER CONTAINER: 15
CEREAL
WITH ½ CUP VIT. A & D FORTIFIED SKIM MILK*
CALORIES 100 140
PROTEIN 5 g 9 g
CARBOHYDRATES 19 g 25 g
FAT 2 g 2 g
†CHOLESTEROL 0 mg 0 mg
mg/100 g 0 mg/100 g
SODIUM 125 mg 190 mg
POTASSIUM 135 mg 340 mg
†Information on cholesterol content is provided for individuals who on the advice of a physician, are modifying their total dietary intake of cholesterol.
PERCENTAGE OF U.S. RECOMMENDED DAILY ALLOWANCES (PERCENT U.S. RDA)
PROTEIN 8 15
VITAMIN A 20 25
VITAMIN C ** 2
THIAMINE 30 35
RIBOFLAVIN 15 25
NIACIN 20 20
CALCIUM ** 15
IRON 30 30
VITAMIN D 10 25
VITAMIN B_6 20 25
FOLIC ACID 20 25
VITAMIN B_{12} 25 30
PHOSPORUS 15 25
MAGNESIUM 10 15
ZINC 20 20
PANTOTHENIC ACID 15 20
*Cereal plus ½ cup vitamin A and D fortified 2% lowfat milk contains 160 calories, 4 grams fat and 10 mg cholesterol. All other nutrients remain as listed.
**Contains less than 2% of the U.S. RDA for these nutrients.
INGREDIENTS: OAT BRAN, SUGAR, WHOLE WHEAT FLOUR, CORN FLOUR, OAT BRAN CONCENTRATE, SODIUM BICARBONATE, SALT, CARAMEL COLOR.
VITAMINS & MINERALS: NIACINAMIDE; VITAMIN A PALMITATE, REDUCED IRON, ZINC OXIDE (A SOURCE OF ZINC), CALCIUM PANTOTHENATE; PYRIDOXINE HYDROCHLORIDE; VITAMIN D, THIAMINE MONONITRATE; RIBOFLAVIN; FOLIC ACID; VITAMIN B_{12} BHA ADDED TO PRESERVE PRODUCT FRESHNESS.
One of the B vitamins.
CARBOHYDRATE INFORMATION
CEREAL WITH MILK
STARCH AND RELATED CARBOHYDRATES 13 g 13 g
SUCROSE AND RELATED SUGARS 4 g 10 g
DIETARY FIBER 3 g 3 g
TOTAL CARBOHYDRATES 20 g 26 g
AVENA OAT CO
PO BOX 1760
ST. LOUIS MO 63146

Nutritional information is required on all products that make a nutritional claim or add a nutrient.

Making Sense of the U.S. RDAs
U.S. RDAs are recommended daily nutrient standards developed for use in the nutrition labeling of food products. Because nutrient needs vary among individuals, the U.S. RDAs are set high enough to cover the needs of nearly everyone.

To calculate the amount of iron in one serving, multiply 0.30 times the U.S. RDA of 18 milligrams (see Appendix D): 0.3 × 18 = 5.4 milligrams of iron per serving.

Oat Bran Per Serving
Label lists the grams of oat bran per serving. The serving size of ready-to-eat Oat Bran cereal is 28 grams (1 ounce or 3/4 cup). The serving size is set arbitrarily by the manufacturer.

Fat
There are 9 kcalories in each gram of fat. The percentage of kcalories from fat is determined by multiplying the number of fat grams by nine, dividing that by the number of kcalories, and then multiplying by 100. This cereal derives 18% of its kcalories from fat.

Sodium
Sodium is frequently listed on food product labels. Sodium occurs naturally in some foods and is frequently added for taste by a manufacturer.

Ingredients
For most foods, the ingredients must be listed on the label. The ingredient present in the largest amount, by weight, must be listed first, followed by other ingredients in descending order. However, an ingredient label doesn't tell you how much of an ingredient is actually in the product. For example, although sugar is listed as the second ingredient, it is actually a relatively small portion of the ingredients.

Manufacturer's Name and Address
The manufacturer's name and address appears on the package.

FIGURE 2-2
A, *Our current nutrition label. This label is a source of detailed nutrient information on about half of all foods. See the Nutrition Issue on p. 59 for details about the parts of this label.*

MEAL PLANNING TOOLS

Throughout the twentieth century, nutritionists have worked to clarify nutrition concepts so that people can estimate whether their food selections supply enough of all essential nutrients. Many approaches have been tried, with various numbers of food groups (Figure 2-3). By the mid-1950s, various food plans evolved into a plan that consisted of four food groups: (1) milk, two to three servings; (2) meat, two servings; (3) fruits and vegetables, four servings; and (4) breads and cereals, four servings. In 1979 the U.S. Department of Agriculture (USDA) revised the names of the groups, and a fifth group composed of fats, sweets, and alcoholic beverages was added as part of the "Hassle-Free Daily Food Guide." People were urged to use caution in consuming items from the fifth group and to add them sparingly to their diet.

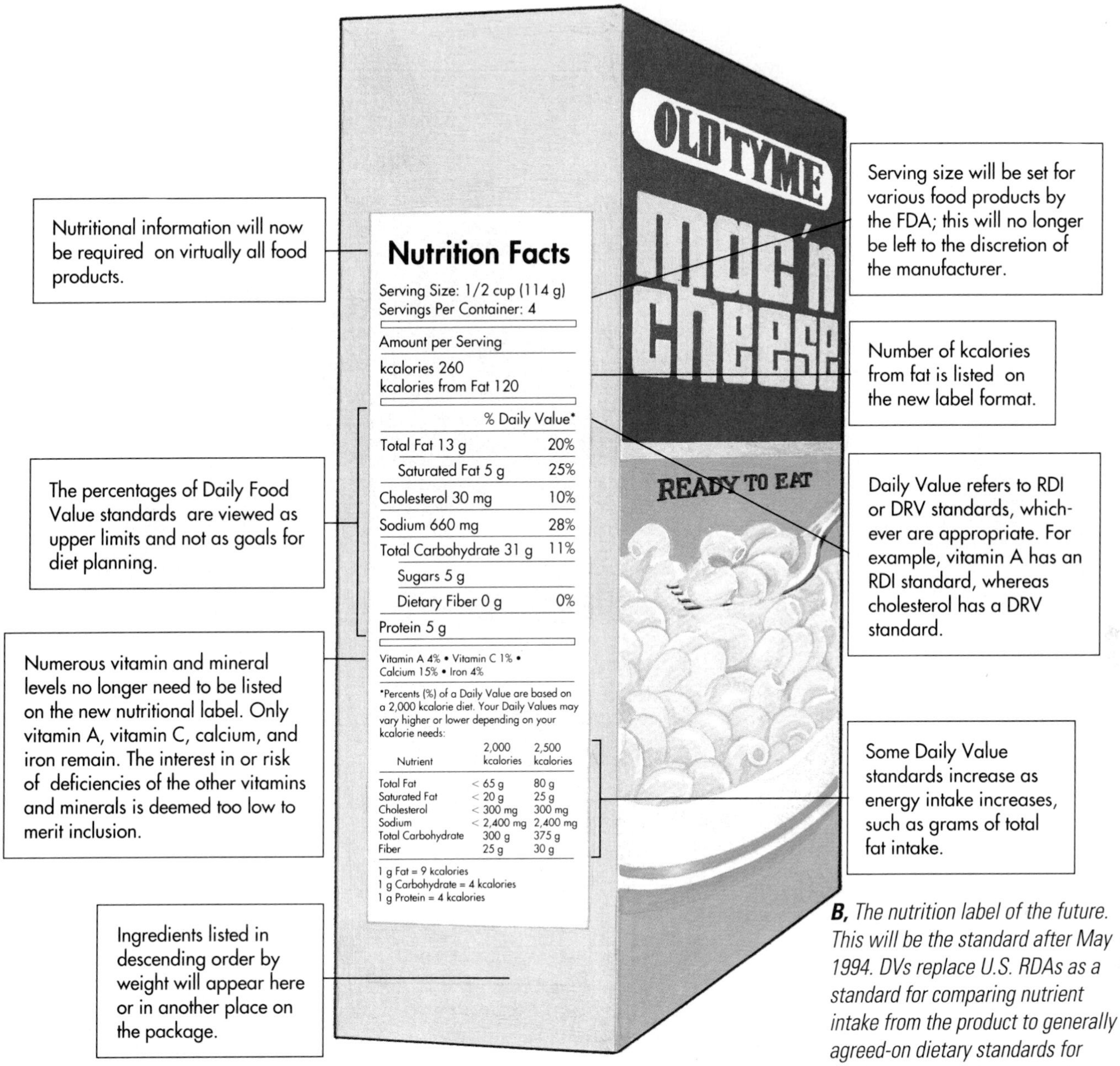
Nutritional information will now be required on virtually all food products.
The percentages of Daily Food Value standards are viewed as upper limits and not as goals for diet planning.
Numerous vitamin and mineral levels no longer need to be listed on the new nutritional label. Only vitamin A, vitamin C, calcium, and iron remain. The interest in or risk of deficiencies of the other vitamins and minerals is deemed too low to merit inclusion.
Ingredients listed in descending order by weight will appear here or in another place on the package.
OLD TYME
mac 'n cheese
READY TO EAT
Nutrition Facts
Serving Size: 1/2 cup (114 g)
Servings Per Container: 4
Amount per Serving
kcalories 260
kcalories from Fat 120
% Daily Value*
Total Fat 13 g 20%
Saturated Fat 5 g 25%
Cholesterol 30 mg 10%
Sodium 660 mg 28%
Total Carbohydrate 31 g 11%
Sugars 5 g
Dietary Fiber 0 g 0%
Protein 5 g
Vitamin A 4% • Vitamin C 1% • Calcium 15% • Iron 4%
*Percents (%) of a Daily Value are based on a 2,000 kcalorie diet. Your Daily Values may vary higher or lower depending on your kcalorie needs:
Nutrient 2,000 kcalories 2,500 kcalories
Total Fat < 65 g 80 g
Saturated Fat < 20 g 25 g
Cholesterol < 300 mg 300 mg
Sodium < 2,400 mg 2,400 mg
Total Carbohydrate 300 g 375 g
Fiber 25 g 30 g
1 g Fat = 9 kcalories
1 g Carbohydrate = 4 kcalories
1 g Protein = 4 kcalories
Serving size will be set for various food products by the FDA; this will no longer be left to the discretion of the manufacturer.
Number of kcalories from fat is listed on the new label format.
Daily Value refers to RDI or DRV standards, whichever are appropriate. For example, vitamin A has an RDI standard, whereas cholesterol has a DRV standard.
Some Daily Value standards increase as energy intake increases, such as grams of total fat intake.

B, *The nutrition label of the future. This will be the standard after May 1994. DVs replace U.S. RDAs as a standard for comparing nutrient intake from the product to generally agreed-on dietary standards for nutrient intake. Other innovations make the label more consumer-oriented, such as listing the percentage of kcalories from fat.*

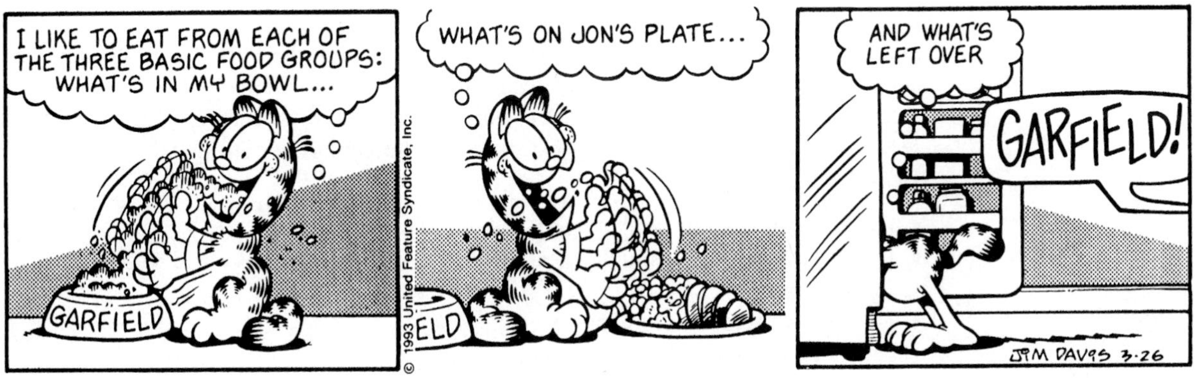

Reprinted by permission of UFS, Inc.

FIGURE 2-3
Garfield.

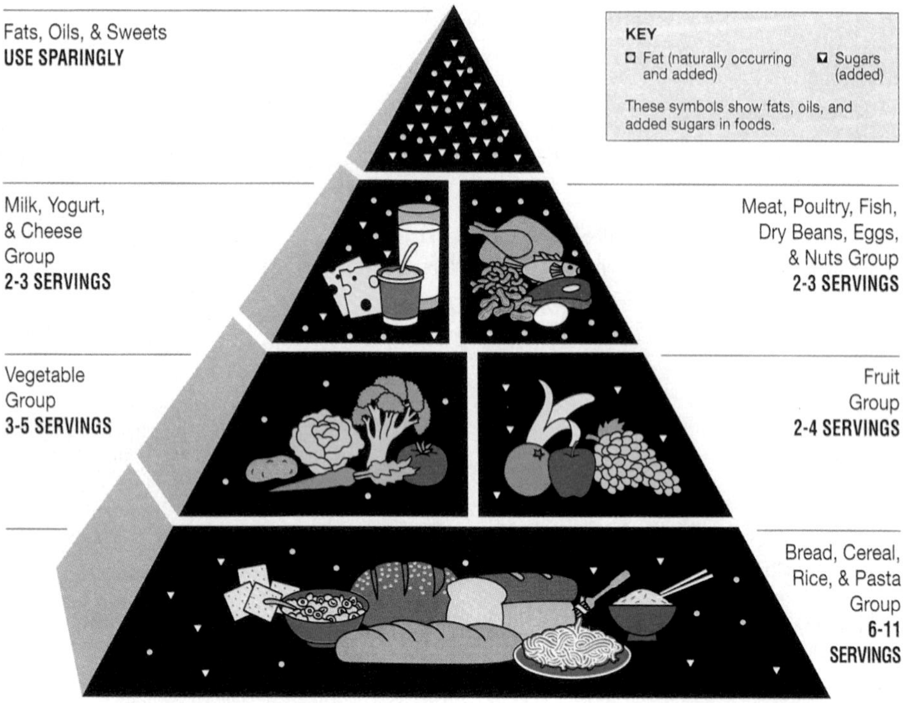

FIGURE 2-4
USDA's Food Guide Pyramid. This guide lists the food groups and the number of servings to consume of each. Note that children, teenagers, and adults under age 25 should choose three servings from the milk, yogurt, and cheese group.

The USDA recently revised the Hassle-Free Daily Food Guide to represent a total diet, rather than simply a foundation for a diet, as was the intention of earlier guides.[17] This latest plan is called "USDA's Food Guide Pyramid" (Figure 2-4). The major changes in this Food Guide Pyramid are an increase in total fruit and vegetable servings from four per day to five to nine per day and an increase in bread and cereal servings from four per day to six to eleven per day. One goal of these changes is to provide the bulk of dietary energy intake from carbohydrate while limiting fat intake. This is reflected in the placement of food groups in the pyramid—grains, fruits, and vegetables form the foundation.

Using the Food Guide Pyramid

The number of servings required from each food group in the Food Guide Pyramid depends on a person's age and energy needs. Table 2-2 lists a summary of the food groups, recommended servings per day, major nutrient contributions of each food group, and the serving sizes of sample foods. Basically, the plan for adults over the age of 25 consists of the following:

- Two servings from the milk, yogurt, and cheese group
- Two to three servings from the meat, poultry, fish, dry beans, eggs, and nuts group (5 to 7 ounces total)
- Three to five servings from the vegetable group
- Two to four servings from the fruit group
- Six to eleven servings from the bread, cereals, rice, and pasta group

TABLE 2-2

The Food Guide Pyramid—a Summary

Food Group	Serving	Major Contributions	Foods and Serving Sizes*
Milk, yogurt, and cheese	2 (adult‖) 3 (children, teens, young adults, and pregnant or lactating women)	Carbohydrate Calcium Riboflavin Protein Potassium Zinc	1 cup milk 1½ ounces cheese 2 ounces processed cheese 1 cup yogurt 2 cups cottage cheese 1 cup custard/pudding 1½ cups ice cream
Meat, poultry, fish, dry beans, eggs, and nuts	2-3	Protein Niacin Iron Vitamin B-6 Zinc Thiamin Vitamin B-12†	2-3 ounces cooked meat, poultry, or fish 1-1½ cups cooked dry beans 2 tablespoons peanut butter 2 eggs ½-1 cup nuts
Fruits	2-4	Carbohydrate Vitamin C Dietary fiber	¼ cup dried fruit ½ cup cooked fruit ¾ cup juice 1 whole piece of fruit 1 melon wedge
Vegetables	3-5	Carbohydrate Vitamin A Vitamin C Folate Magnesium Dietary fiber	½ cup raw or cooked vegetables 1 cup raw leafy vegetables 3-4 small crackers
Bread, cereals, rice, and pasta	6-11	Carbohydrate Thiamin Riboflavin§ Iron Niacin Folate Magnesium‡ Dietary fiber‡ Zinc‡	1 slice of bread 1 ounce ready-to-eat cereal ½-¾ cup cooked cereal, rice, or pasta
Fats, oils, and sweets		Foods from this group should not replace any from the other groups. Amounts consumed should be determined by individual energy needs.	

This is a practical way to turn the RDA into food choices. You can get all essential nutrients by eating a balanced variety of foods each day from the food groups listed here. Eat a variety of foods in each food group to reach and maintain desirable weight. The minimum number of servings of each food group provides approximately 1600 to 1800 kcalories. Most adults require this amount of kcalories to meet their RDAs for nutrients.

*May be reduced for child servings.
†Only in animal food choices.
‡Whole grains especially.
§If enriched.
‖≥ 25 years of age.

A final group that requires cautious use includes fats, oils, and sweets. Some population groups—children, teenagers, adults under age 25, and pregnant or lactating women—need three servings of the milk, yogurt, and cheese group. Take a minute to note the similarities and differences between the various food groups.

Here are several points to keep in mind when you use this plan:

1. The guide does not apply to infants nor to children under 2 years of age.
2. No one food provides all essential nutrients. Each food is low in at least one essential nutrient.
3. No one food group provides all essential nutrients adequately. Each food group offers some important nutrients.
4. Variety is the key to the plan. Variety is guaranteed by choosing foods from all groups and selecting different foods within each group.

TABLE 2-3

Putting the Food Guide Pyramid Into Practice

Breakfast

1 peeled orange
1½ cup Special K cereal with ½ cup 1% milk
1 slice raisin toast with 1 teaspoon margarine
Optional: coffee or tea

Lunch

Ham sandwich
  2 slices whole-wheat bread
  2 ounces ham
  2 teaspoons mustard
Apple
2 oatmeal raisin cookies (small)
Optional: diet soda

3 PM Study Break

1 whole bagel
1 tablespoon peanut butter
½ cup 1% milk

Dinner

Lettuce salad
  1 cup romaine lettuce
  ½ cup sliced tomatoes
  1 tablespoon 1000 Island dressing
  ½ grated carrot
3 ounces broiled salmon
½ cup rice
¾ cup green beans with teaspoon margarine
Optional: coffee or tea

Late Night Snack

1 cup fruited low-fat yogurt

Nutrient Breakdown:

1800 kcalories

Carbohydrate	55% of kcalories
Protein	20% of kcalories
Fat	25% of kcalories

Meets RDA/ESADDI values for all vitamins and minerals for a 25-year-old adult. For adolescents and adults under age 25, add one additional serving from the milk, yogurt, and cheese group.

Again, the foundations of nutrition are variety, balance, and moderation. Choosing from every group and varying choices within groups allows a healthful variety in food choices.

By following the Food Guide Pyramid, you can easily plan a diet for a typical intake of kcalories and still meet the adult RDAs for protein, thiamin, niacin, riboflavin, calcium, and other important nutrients. Table 2-3 puts the Guide into practice for an 1800-kcalorie diet and reflects the recommended servings of foods from the five food groups for this kcalorie amount. Keep in mind that 1800 kcalories is not enough for most active adults, though it may be sufficient for some sedentary adults or elderly people. The minimum recommended servings in Table 2-2 provide approximately 1600 to 1800 kcalories, which is the minimum amount of foods needed to obtain the RDA for most adults. If an adult is active, 2200 to 3400 kcalories more likely will be needed in a day's time. The minimum recommended servings then must be increased to meet greater energy needs, with emphasis on the bottom part of the pyramid.

To ensure that enough vitamin E, vitamin B-6, magnesium, iron, zinc, and dietary fiber are present in a diet based on the Food Guide Pyramid, we recommend the following:

1. Make sure to regularly include servings of vegetable protein sources.
2. For vegetables, include a dark green variety almost every day.
3. Choose whole-grain varieties of breads, cereals, rice, and pasta often.

Not following this advice can leave a diet of 1600 to 1800 kcalories short on the nutrients just mentioned. Recall that excessive consumption of any one food is also not desirable and can be risky. Overall, our diets must continue to be balanced, though with less of a bias toward meat and high-fat dairy products—which are staples of the American diet—to moderate fat intake.[19]

If an energy intake of 1800 kcalories is too much for you to maintain a desirable body weight, the first step to offset the excess is to increase your level of physical activity rather than eat less. Once again, it is difficult to consume enough nutrients from a daily diet that contains fewer than 1600 to 1800 kcalories. It is not necessary to meet the RDAs for all nutrients every day, but you may not know what nutrients you can eat less of on a regular basis and still remain healthy. If you can't increase your energy output, you should consider including some nutrient-fortified foods in your diet, such as ready-to-eat breakfast cereals. Chapter 8 discusses whether nutrient supplements are a wise choice; they are usually not needed. In addition, if your diet does not include meat or other animal products, see the Nutrition Issue on vegetarianism in Chapter 7.

Using Nutrient Density as a Diet-Planning Tool

Today, kcalories are a concern for many of us. How can we evaluate foods so that we know we are choosing good sources of nutrients for the amount of energy (kcalories) they provide?

The concept of ***nutrient density*** is one means. This is a measure that compares the vitamin or mineral content of a food with its number of kcalories. The higher the nutrient density in the food, the more nutrient there is per kcalorie and the better the food source is for that particular nutrient. Oranges are a nutrient-dense source of vitamin C, whereas carrots are a nutrient-dense source of vitamin A (see Chapter 8 for more details). Still, the focus in menu planning is on the total diet, not whether one food is the key to an adequate diet.[7] Nonetheless, nutrient-dense foods help balance less nutrient-dense choices, such as cookies and chips. The latter are often called "empty-calorie foods," because they supply energy and few other nutrients.

Nutrient density *The ratio formed by dividing a food's contribution to the needs for a nutrient by its contribution to energy needs. When the contribution to nutrient needs exceeds that to energy needs, the food is considered to have a favorable nutrient density for that nutrient.*

Searching for nutrient-dense foods is important in some cases. This can aid diet planning for people who tend to consume little food energy, including some elderly people and those following weight-loss diets. Examples of nutrient-dense choices include fruits and vegetables in general. Most breakfast cereals are fortified with vitamins and minerals and so also provide a nutrient-dense boost to a diet. Adding low-fat or non-fat milk contributes even more nutrients for a low energy cost.

CONCEPT CHECK

The Food Guide Pyramid translates nutrient needs into a food plan. This guide recommends that adults over age 24 consume the following:

- Two servings from the milk, yogurt, and cheese group (three if age 24 or younger, pregnant, or lactating)
- Two to three servings from the meat, poultry, fish, dry beans, eggs, and nuts group
- Three to five servings from the vegetable group
- Two to four servings from the fruit group
- Six to eleven servings from the bread, cereals, rice, and pasta group
- Cautious use of fats, oils, and sweets

At least 1600 to 1800 kcalories are recommended for most adults to receive adequate nutrients, which can be achieved by using the Guide. The concept of nutrient density provides another diet-planning tool. So evaluate nutrient contributions of a food by comparing its energy value for a specific nutrient with its contribution to total energy needs. Nutrient-dense foods provide a high amount of one or more nutrients in comparison with energy content.

Goiter An enlargement of the thyroid gland (located in the neck area) often caused by insufficient iodide in the diet.

Dietary Guidelines General goals for nutrient intakes and diet composition set by the USDA and the Department of Health and Human Services (DHHS).

Further Guidelines to Help You Plan Your Meals

The Food Guide Pyramid primarily focuses on supplying enough essential nutrients to keep our body systems functioning well. Yet, many deficiency diseases that were common in years past, such as ***goiter*** (iodide deficiency) and pellagra (niacin deficiency), are no longer a big problem. In fact most chronic "killer" diseases prevalent in America—such as heart disease, cancer, diabetes, and cirrhosis of the liver—are not associated with nutrient deficiencies or general poor body function. The real problems in the American diet are excess kcalories, saturated fat, alcohol, and sodium (salt)[11,16] (Figure 2-5). For some people, too little calcium, iron, zinc, or dietary fiber in the diet is also a problem.[9]

In response to concerns about diet-related disease patterns in the United States, the federal government has issued ***Dietary Guidelines*** for people over 2 years of age. The latest version (1990) states the following[12]:

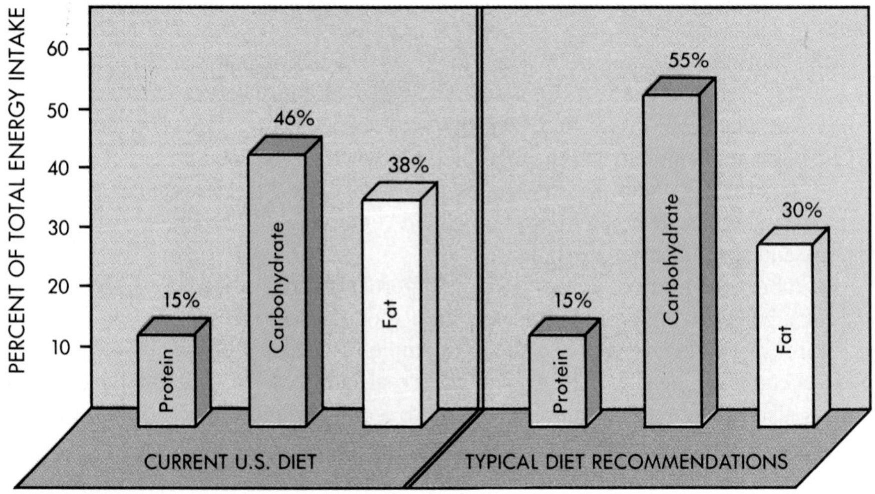

FIGURE 2-5
Is our current diet in our best interests? Many scientists evaluating the relationship between diet and health have concluded that we should eat more carbohydrate-rich foods and fewer fat-rich foods.

1. Eat a variety of foods.
2. Maintain healthy weight.
3. Choose a diet low in fat, saturated fat, and cholesterol.
4. Choose a diet with plenty of vegetables, fruits, and grain products.
5. Use sugars only in moderation.
6. Use salt and sodium only in moderation.
7. If you drink alcoholic beverages, do so in moderation.

These guidelines refer to your total day's or week's intake, not to one meal or a certain food choice. Overall, the plan aims to ensure you get ample vitamins and minerals by eating a variety of foods. By following the guidelines, you can reduce your risk for obesity, hypertension, heart disease, diabetes, and alcoholism. If you eat the typical American diet, which is high in saturated fat (provided mostly by high-fat meats and high-fat dairy products), you will need to make a few changes to follow this plan.[11] In general, you would eat more vegetables, fruits, and grain products (Table 2-4). This plan is easily incorporated into the Food Guide Pyramid.

TABLE 2-4

Putting Dietary Guidelines Into Practice

For Variety:

- Include a number of foods from all food groups every day: breads, cereals, and other grain products; fruits; vegetables; meat, poultry, fish, and alternates; milk, cheese, and yogurt.

To Maintain Healthy Weight:

- The inside cover contains one possible standard to use for healthy weight.
- Choose a variety of foods that provide needed nutrients.
- Go easy on foods that supply mainly calories—sugars, sweets, fats and oils, foods high in sugars and fats, and alcoholic beverages.

To Choose a Diet Low in Fat, Saturated Fat, and Cholesterol:

- Choose lean meat, fish, poultry, and dry beans and peas as protein sources.
- Use skim or low-fat milk and milk products.
- Use egg yolks and organ meats in moderation.
- Use fats and oils in moderation, especially those high in saturated fat, such as cream, lard, and butter.
- Use foods high in fat in moderation, such as deep-fried or breaded foods.
- Trim fat off meats; remove skin from poultry.
- Broil, bake, boil, steam, or microwave, rather than fry.
- Read labels carefully to determine both amount and type of fat present in foods.

To Consume Alcoholic Beverages in Moderation, if at all:

- Men should limit intake to two servings per day. Women should limit intake to one serving per day.
- A serving is 12 ounces of beer, 5 ounces of wine, or 1½ ounces of distilled spirits.

To Choose a Diet with Plenty of Vegetables, Fruits, and Grain Products:

- Choose foods that are good sources of starch—breads, cereals, pasta, rice, dry beans and peas, and starchy vegetables, such as potatoes, corn, and lima beans.
- Choose foods that are good sources of fiber, such as whole-grain breads, cereals, and pasta; vegetables and fruits with edible skins; and dry beans and peas.

To Use Sugars Only in Moderation:

- Use less of all sugars and foods containing large amounts of sugars, including white sugar, brown sugar, raw sugar, honey, and syrups. Examples include soft drinks, candies, cakes, and cookies.
- Remember, how often you eat sugar and sugar-containing food is as important to the health of your teeth as how much sugar you eat. It will help to avoid eating sweets between meals.
- Read food labels for clues on sugar content. If the name sugar, sucrose, glucose, maltose, dextrose, lactose, fructose, or syrups appears first, then there is a large amount of sugar.
- Select fresh fruits or fruits processed without syrup or with light, rather than heavy, syrup.

To Use Salt and Sodium Only in Moderation:

- Learn to enjoy the flavors of unsalted foods.
- Cook without salt or with only small amounts of added salt.
- Try flavoring foods with herbs, spices, and lemon juice.
- Add little or no salt to food at the table.
- Limit your intake of salty foods, such as potato chips, pretzels, salted nuts and popcorn, condiments (soy sauce, steak sauce, garlic salt), pickled foods, cured meats, some cheeses, and some canned vegetables and soups.
- Read food labels carefully to determine the amounts of sodium.
- Use lower-sodium products, when available, to replace those you use that have higher-sodium content.

NUTRITION insight

GENETICS AND NUTRITION

The genetic code in cells directs cell growth and development. The genes that form this code establish your individual traits, such as height and eye color. Most chronic diseases in which nutrition plays a role are also influenced by genetic background.[15] The risk for developing heart disease, high blood pressure (hypertension), obesity, diabetes, cancer, and osteoporosis is influenced by interactions between genetic and nutritional factors. Studies of families, including those with twins and adoptees, provide strong support for the effect of genetic background in the aforementioned disorders. In fact, family history is considered to be one of the greatest risk factors for many key diseases that influence human health (see Figure 2-6).

Heart Disease

Present in about 1 of every 500 persons in the general North American population is a genetic defect that results in greatly slowing cholesterol removal from the bloodstream. As you will learn in Chapter 6, this leads to a high risk for developing heart disease at a young age. Diet changes can help these people, but medications and surgery are sometimes needed in addition to address this problem.

Hypertension

An estimated 10% to 15% of individuals are very sensitive to salt intake. When these salt-sensitive people consume too much salt, their blood pressure values tend to climb out of the desirable range. The fact that more of these people are African-Americans than Caucasian suggests a genetic link to the problem.[16] At present, there is no certain method for identifying which persons with hypertension are salt-sensitive. A salt-restricted diet needs to be followed to determine the effect it has on an individual's blood pressure.

Obesity

Most obese people have at least one parent who is obese. Findings from many human studies suggest that a variety of genes are involved in the regulation of body weight. Little is known, however, about the specific nature of these genes or how the actual changes in body metabolism, such as a lower energy use at rest, are produced. Some people may be genetically predisposed to store body fat, but whether they actually do depends on how much excess energy—above energy needs—they ultimately consume. Lifestyle affects whether genetic inheritance is expressed. Not every person with a genetic tendency toward obesity develops the problem, but for some individuals a lifetime risk most likely exists.

Diabetes

Both of the two common types of diabetes—insulin-dependent and non–insulin-dependent—have genetic links, as shown by studies of families and twins. Only sensitive and expensive testing can determine who is at risk. The major form of diabetes that leads to 80% to 90% of all cases has a strong link to obesity.[11] Again, we see lifestyle affecting nature. A genetic tendency for the major form of diabetes will be expressed once the person becomes obese, but often not before.

Cancer

A few cancers have a strong genetic link, such as some forms of colon cancer.[11] Still, cancer provides another example of the interaction of genetic tendency with environmental factors, such as diets high in energy and fat. Obesity raises the risk for many forms of cancer. One third of all cancers result from smoking. Again, often a genetic tendency is not enough to bring on all cases of the disease—environment must also contribute to the risk profile.

Osteoporosis

Twins and mother-daughter pairs show similarities for bone mineral density, and thus bone strength. The relative importance of genetic versus dietary factors is unknown. Scientists strongly support the need to consume enough calcium in childhood and adolescence to build a strong bone structure. Still, genetic background does influence the overall risk for developing osteoporosis in later life. Note in Chapter 9 we cover the good news—this disease can be virtually prevented by a combination of medical and nutritional means if therapy is started at least by mid-life.

Implications

The fact that genetic background influences disease risk means that not all people will benefit equally from the same dietary measures. Recommendations to consume more calcium or less salt are more important for people who have a genetic risk profile and so especially require this advice. It is not presently possible, given the resources allocated to medical care in America, to identify all people at genetic risk for the major chronic "killer" diseases. Thus many health authorities feel it is reasonable to give a general nutrition message to everyone, noting that some people will benefit from the advice much more than will others.[13] In an ideal world, dietary advice would be tailored to one's unique health-risk profile—pointing out how to avoid the "controllable" risk factor(s) that make genetically linked diseases more likely to appear in one's life.[7]

Throughout this book we will try to point out how you can personalize nutrition advice based on your genetic background. Overall, keep in mind that a family history for certain diseases should raise your awareness for the potential of developing that disease and desire to prevent this from happening. Consider discovering what your family history is for the diseases listed in Table 1-1 on p. 4 (consider siblings, parents, and grandparents for a start).

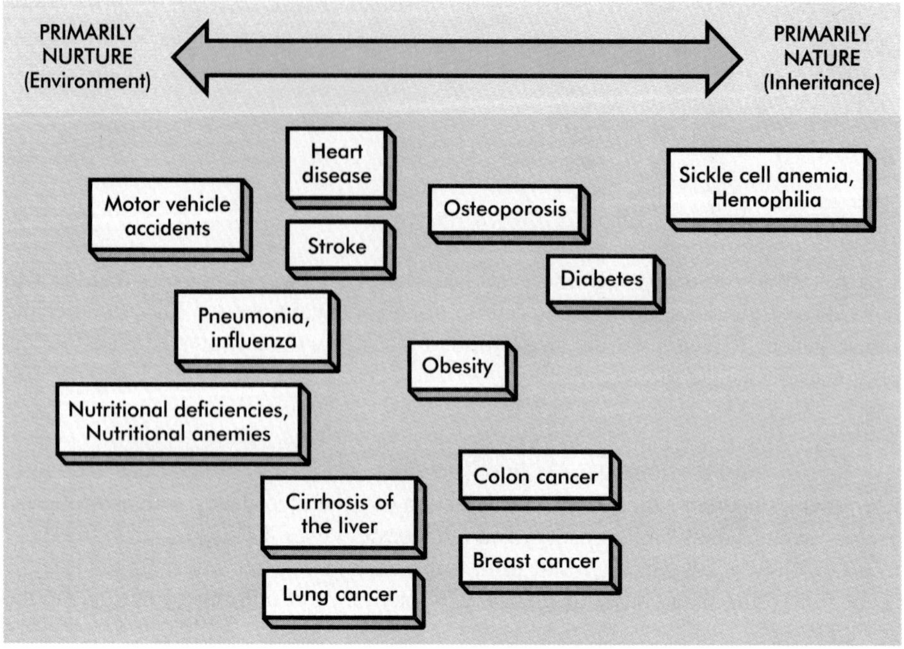

FIGURE 2-6

Common causes of death and illness in our population vary in their links to genetic background versus environmental influences. We must consider both influences as we study each disease.

Putting Dietary Guidelines into Perspective

The Dietary Guidelines suggested for Americans have disturbed some nutritionists. They think many of the guidelines are too general to meet specific individual nutrition needs. As individuals, we vary in our tendencies toward developing high blood cholesterol levels, hypertension, obesity, cancer, and other health problems that the guidelines are designed to prevent.[15] Genetic background is one key reason for the variation (Figure 2-6).

another BITE

Do you know your blood cholesterol level? Blood pressure values? Although you may feel you are not susceptible to the problems listed previously, it is still a good idea to have your blood cholesterol levels and blood pressure measured every few years to verify you are right.

The Dietary Guidelines and You

It is best to consider your own state of health when using the dietary guidelines. Make specific changes and see whether they are effective (Table 2-5). Note that results are sometimes disappointing, even when you are following a diet change very closely. Some people can eat a lot of saturated fats and still keep desirable blood cholesterol levels. Other people, unfortunately, have high blood cholesterol levels, even if they eat a diet low in saturated fats. Such people don't benefit from the same diet that helps other people. Again, differences in genetic background are a key cause.

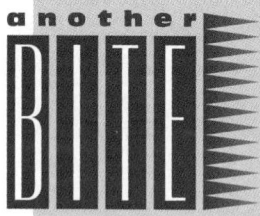

TABLE 2-5

Advice for Applying the Dietary Guidelines to Practical Situations

You Usually Eat This:	Reconsider and Eat This:
White bread	Whole-wheat bread—not as many nutrients have been lost in refinement/processing
Sugared breakfast cereal	Low-sugar cereal; use the kcalories you save for a side dish of fruit
Cheeseburger and French fries	Hamburger (hold the mayonnaise) and baked beans (for less fat and the benefits of plant proteins)
Potato salad at the salad bar	Three-bean salad
Doughnut	Bran muffin or bagel (no cream cheese)
Soft drinks	Water, diet soft drinks, or iced tea (save the kcalories for more nutritious foods)
Boiled vegetables	Steamed vegetables (more nutrient retention)
Canned vegetables	Frozen vegetables (less nutrients lost in processing)
Fried meats	Broiled meats (watch the fat drain away)
Fatty meats, such as ribs	Lean meats, such as ground round; also, eat chicken and fish often
Whole milk and ice cream	1% Milk and sherbet or frozen yogurt (to reduce saturated fat intake)
Mayonnaise or sour cream salad dressing	Oil and vinegar dressings or diet varieties (to save kcalories and limit intake of saturated fats)
Cookies	Popcorn (air popped with minimal margarine)

Still, most nutrition and health researchers agree with the guidelines set by our major health and science institutions.[3,5] The need for varying food choices; controlling body weight; reducing total fat intake for adults; choosing a diet with plenty of fruits, vegetables, and grain products; using salt and sugar in moderation; and moderating alcohol intake is widely accepted advice.[19] Although everyone has individual nutritional needs and risks of developing diseases, it is unrealistic to tailor a unique nutrition message to every American citizen. The Food Guide Pyramid and the 1990 Dietary Guidelines provide all Americans over 2 years of age with simple advice that can be actively practiced by individuals willing to take a step toward good health.[18] In effect, the guidelines promise our nation a healthful future at minimal cost (sacrifice) to society. Reaping the many benefits of good health requires only a small effort and a little knowledge—we urge you to continue the challenge of understanding more about how nutrition relates to you.

CONCEPT CHECK

The 1990 Dietary Guidelines issued by the federal government are designed to minimize the risk of developing obesity, hypertension, heart disease, diabetes, and alcoholism. To accomplish these goals, the Dietary Guidelines encourage people to eat a variety of foods. Further, the guidelines suggest that we maintain a healthy weight and moderate our intake of saturated fat, salt, sugar, and alcohol, while eating more fruits, vegetables, and grain products. Genetic background causes variation in each individual's disease risk, but in general, following the Dietary Guidelines reduces one's risk for developing these diseases and is cost-beneficial for the individual and for our nation as a whole.

NUTRITION insight

WHERE TO GET RELIABLE NUTRITION ADVICE

If you have a question about nutrition, the most convenient person to ask is probably your professor or another nutrition faculty member on your campus. Local ***registered dietitians (RDs)*** and your family physician are also good resources.

When you are seeking nutrition counseling, it is important to find an RD. They are specially trained to help you meet your nutritional needs through healthful, tasty diets. Hospitals and health departments are good places to begin your search. A person obtains RD certification by earning a bachelor's degree in nutrition, completing extensive professional practice under expert supervision, and successfully passing a comprehensive examination.

People who do not have the appropriate training and education sometimes claim to be nutrition professionals. They may have a doctorate degree in a non-nutrition field or a mail-order diploma, but they are not qualified to give nutritional advice (Figure 2-7). Although some of these people may give sound advice, others may promise results that sound too good to be true. They may encourage the use of bogus tests, such as inappropriate allergy tests or hair analyses. They may promote pills, gimmicks, and gadgets and boast success with numerous testimonials from other clients. They may refuse to consult with your physician and try to convince you that no medical doctor has the answer for your ailment. The consumer must be wary of such claims.

FRANK & ERNEST ® by Bob Thaves

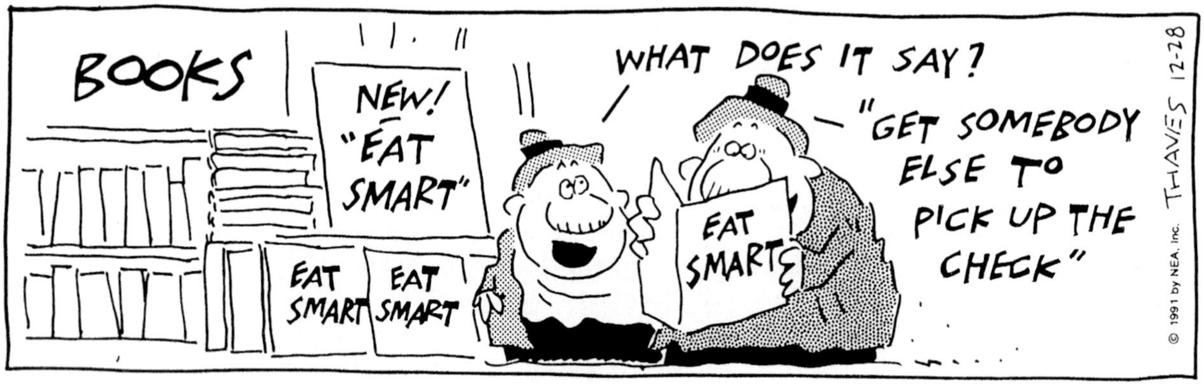

Reprinted by permission of NEA, Inc.

FIGURE 2-7
Frank and Ernest.

Currently about half of all states license the right to use the title *dietitian*. In other states, however, people can legally call themselves dietitians or nutritionists even though they have no training in those fields. An RD credential guarantees that the holder has a good background in nutrition that is based on education in the sciences and has had work experience under the supervision of other dietitians.

When you meet with a nutrition professional, you should expect that he or she will do the following:

- Ask questions about your medical history, lifestyle, and current eating habits. The professional may ask you to keep a detailed diet diary to establish a baseline before making major diet changes or recommendations.
- Formulate a diet plan tailored to your needs, as opposed to simply tearing a form from a tablet that could apply to almost anyone.
- Schedule follow-up visits to track your progress, answer any questions, and help keep you motivated.
- Involve family members in the diet plan, when appropriate.
- Consult directly with your physician, and readily refer you back to the physician for health problems a nutritionist is not trained to treat.

Usually you first need a physician's diagnosis for conditions requiring detailed nutrition advice. An exception to this might be losing weight when you are otherwise healthy. An accurate diagnosis by a physician is needed because you could have a condition that actually results from another disease. A physician needs to evaluate your total health to properly diagnose problems. The next step is to consult a registered dietitian to help you design an appropriate diet.

When evaluating a new diet in your favorite magazine, check for the author's credentials and evaluate the advice using tools learned in this chapter, including the Food Guide Pyramid, the Dietary Guidelines, and the principles of variety, balance, and moderation.

Steer clear of nutritionists who say that everyone needs vitamin and mineral supplements to get enough essential nutrients. Likewise, avoid the advice of anyone who suggests that most diseases are caused by faulty nutrition or that large doses of vitamins and minerals will cure many diseases. And, above all, beware of any practitioner—licensed or not—who sells vitamins in his or her office. We discuss nutrition fraud further in Chapter 3. Chapter 10 gives tips for separating facts from fiction regarding weight loss diets.

What Is the Exchange System?

The ***exchange system*** is another valuable diet planning tool. It was developed by the American Dietetic Association and the American Diabetes Association. With this system you can quickly estimate the energy, protein, carbohydrate, and fat content of a food or meal. The exchange system is also a convenient way for a person to plan kcalorie-controlled diets. Weight Watchers uses a system based on exchanges.

The exchange system arranges food into six different categories: milk, fruit, vegetables, starch/bread, meat, and fat. Given the appropriate serving size, each food within a category provides about the same amount of carbohydrate, protein, fat, and kcalories. For instance, in the bread group, one slice of bread is equivalent to ½ cup of bran flakes or 2½ tablespoons of cornmeal in providing energy-yielding nutrients. Thus, as you select servings from each group, foods within a category can be *exchanged* for each other.

The exchange system was developed in the 1950s for planning diabetic diets. It is easier for a person with diabetes to control the disease if the diet contains about the same proportion of energy-yielding nutrients day after day. By using a set number of choices (or exchanges) from each of the six categories, a person can achieve regularity more easily.

In addition, because the exchange system also provides a quick way to estimate the content of energy and carbohydrate, protein, and fat in a food or meal, it has a more general use. You can use it to design meal patterns containing specified amounts of protein, carbohydrate, fat, and kcalories. As in learning a foreign language, you need some practice before you feel comfortable with the exchange system. Appendixes E and F describe the system fully and demonstrate how to use it.

A B C

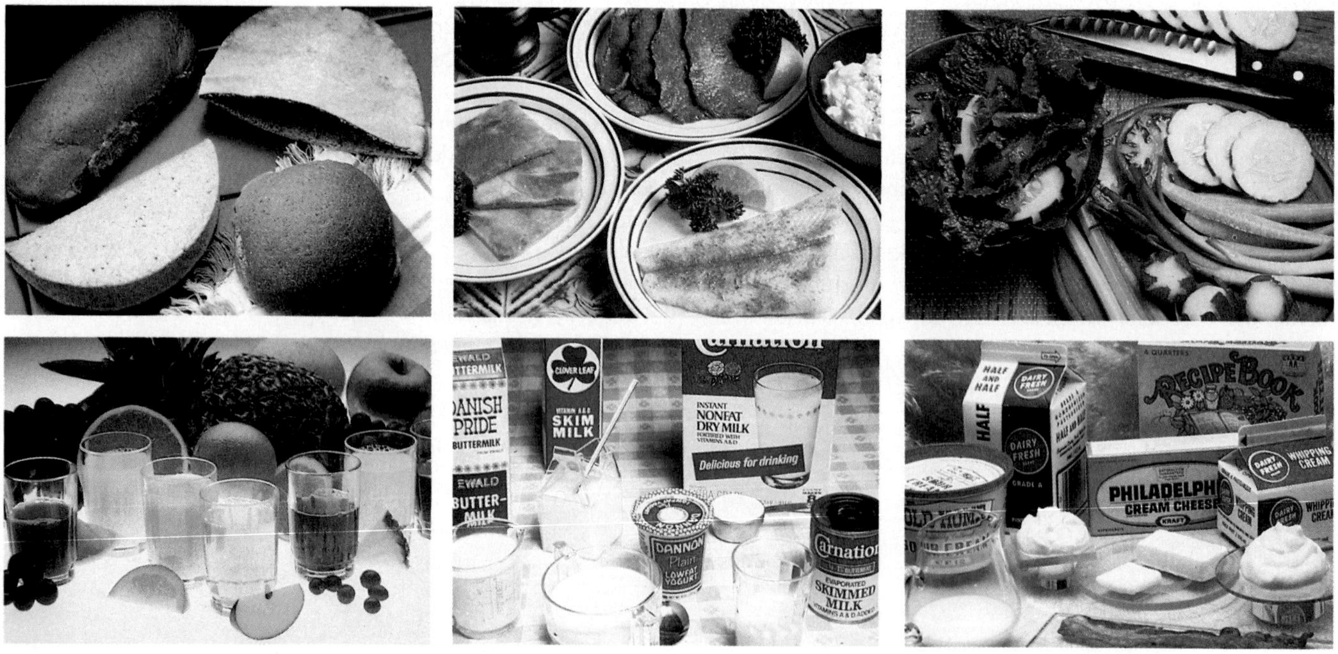

D E F

A, *The starch/bread exchange group;* ***B,*** *the meat exchange group;* ***C,*** *the vegetable exchange group;* ***D,*** *the fruit exchange group;* ***E,*** *the milk exchange group; and* ***F,*** *the fat exchange group.*

SUMMARY

- As nutritional health diminishes, nutrient stores in the body are depleted. Biochemical reactions in the body then slow down. Finally, outward clinical symptoms appear as a state of nutritional deficiency develops.
- Overnutrition is a problem in the United States today. This is a condition in which too much energy, too much fat, or too much of certain vitamins and minerals is consumed.
- Recommended Dietary Allowances (RDAs) are set for many nutrients. These levels represent the amount of a nutrient that healthy people should consume regularly to meet their needs for that nutrient. RDA guidelines differ for men and women and for various age-groups. The further you stray below RDA values, the greater your chance of developing a nutrient deficiency. At half the RDAs, your nutritional needs are unlikely to be met.
- The U.S. RDAs are based primarily on the highest RDA levels found in the 1968 publication. The U.S. RDAs form the basis for listing nutrient levels on food labels.
- As a part of new government regulations, the U.S. RDAs have undergone a name change to Reference Daily Intakes (RDIs). Daily Reference Values (DRVs) have also been set for nutrients not having an RDI. The RDIs and DRVs will be combined under one category called Daily Values (DVs) on the new nutrition labels, which appeared on products in the United States in late 1993.
- The Food Guide Pyramid provides a way to convert nutrient recommendations from the RDA into a food plan. We should emphasize low-fat (or nonfat) milk, yogurt, and cheese products; proteins from vegetables, as well as from lean meat; and liberal intake of fruits, vegetables, and whole-grain forms of breads, cereals, rice, and pasta.
- Nutrient density reflects the nutrient content of a food in relation to its energy (kcalorie) content. Nutrient-dense foods are relatively rich in nutrients, in comparison with energy content.
- The Dietary Guidelines help individuals plan a menu pattern to reduce the risk of developing chronic "killer" diseases. These guidelines emphasize eating a variety of foods; maintaining a healthy weight; moderating intake of fats, cholesterol, sugar, salt, and alcohol; and including ample vegetables, fruits, and grains in the diet.
- The exchange system provides a powerful tool for estimating the carbohydrate, fat, protein, and energy content of a food or meal.

Study Questions

1. What three key points would you make as you explained to a friend what the RDAs represent?
2. How do the RDAs differ from U.S. RDA (and now RDI) in intention and application? Which standard more accurately reflects the needs of people your age and gender?
3. Put the term *nutrient density* into common language. For instance, how would you explain the concept to a fourth-grade class?
4. Describe how use of the exchange system would aid the control of a disease process, based on what the system can predict and monitor.
5. Nutritionists encourage all people to read nutrition labels to learn more about what they eat. What four nutrients could easily be tracked in your diet if you regularly read nutrition labels? What do the standard Daily Values (DVs) represent in this context?

References

1. ADA reports: ADA timely statement on proposed revision of U.S. RDAs for use on food labels, *Journal of the American Dietetic Association* 92:361, 1992.
2. American Dietetic Association: Nutrition and health information on food labels, *Journal of the American Dietetic Association* 90:583, 1990.
3. Anonymous: Diet, nutrition and the prevention of chronic diseases—a report of the WHO study group on diet, nutrition and prevention of noncommunicable diseases, *Nutrition Reviews* 49:291, 1991.
4. FDA's final regulations on health claims for foods, *Nutrition Reviews* 51:90, 1993.
5. Food and Nutrition Board, National Academy of Sciences—National Research Council: *Recommended dietary allowances, revised,* Washington, DC, 1989, The Board.
6. Goldberg JP: Nutrition and health communication: the message and the media over half a century, *Nutrition Reviews* 50:71, 1992.
7. Hegsted DM: Nutrition standards for today, *Nutrition Today,* p. 34, March/April 1993.
8. Kurtzweil P: Nutrition facts to help consumers eat smart, *FDA Consumer,* p. 27, May 1993.
9. Mandatory nutrition labeling—FDA's final rule, *Nutrition Reviews,* 51:101, 1993.
10. Monsen ER: The 10th edition of the recommended dietary allowances: what's new in the 1989 RDAs, *Journal of the American Dietetic Association* 89:1748, 1989.
11. National Research Council: *Diet and health,* Washington, DC, 1989, National Academy Press.
12. Peterkin BB: Dietary guidelines for Americans, 1990 edition, *Journal of the American Dietetic Association* 90:1725, 1990.
13. Rosenberg IH: Health claims on foods: American style, *Nutrition Reviews* 50:148, 1992.
14. Rosenberg IH: The new reference daily intakes: for better or for worse? *Nutrition Reviews* 50:119, 1992.
15. Sucher KP, Kittler PG: Nutrition isn't color blind, *Journal of the American Dietetic Association* 91:297, 1991.
16. Surgeon General's report on nutrition and health, *Nutrition Today,* p. 22, September/October 1988.
17. Welsh S and others: Development of the food guide pyramid, *Nutrition Today,* p. 12, November/December 1992.
18. Woteki CE, Thomas PR: *Eat for life,* Washington, DC, 1991, National Academy Press.
19. Wynder EL and others: Nutrition: the need to define optimal intake as a basis for policy decisions, *American Journal of Public Health* 82:346, 1992.

DOES YOUR DIET MEET THE RDAs?

Instructions: Perform either part I or part II. Then perform part III. (For assistance in following the instructions for this activity, see the sample Assessment in Appendix C.)

Part I.

A. Take the information from the 1-day food intake record you completed in Chapter 1 and record it on the blank form provided in Appendix C. Make sure to record the food or drink ingested and the amount (weight) consumed. NOTE: Your professor may require you to keep the food record for more than 1 day.

B. Review the 1989 RDAs on the inside cover of the book and choose the appropriate recommendations for your gender and age. Write the appropriate value for each nutrient on the line labeled "Your RDA." NOTE: The values for sodium and potassium from the table on the inside cover of the book are labeled "Estimated Sodium, Chloride, and Potassium Minimum Requirements of Healthy Persons."

C. Look up the foods and drinks you've listed on the form in the food composition table, Appendix A. Record on the form the amounts of each nutrient and kcalories present in them.

D. For each food and drink, add the amounts in each column and record the results on the line labeled "Totals."

E. Compare the totals to your RDAs. Divide the total for each nutrient by the specific RDA or minimum requirement and multiply that by 100. Record the result on the line labeled "% of your RDA."

F. Hold on to this assessment for use in subsequent activities for other chapters.

Part II.

A. Obtain copies of the computer software Mosby Diet Simple from your instructor, as well as directions for using it. Follow the instructions and load the software into the computer.

B. Choose your RDA category based on your age and gender.

C. Enter the information from the 1-day food intake record you completed in Chapter 1. Make sure to enter each food and drink and the appropriate serving size.

D. This software program will give you the following results:
   a. Your 1989 RDA value for each nutrient.
   b. The total amount of each nutrient and kcalories consumed for the day.
   c. The percentage of the RDA 1989 values you consumed for each nutrient.

E. Hold on to this assessment for use in subsequent activities in other chapters.

Part III. Evaluation

Remember that you don't necessarily need to consume 100% of the 1989 RDA values, but this is a good goal to strive for over a 3- to 5-day period. It would be best not to exceed 150% of any RDA value to avoid potential toxic effects. There is no proven advantage in exceeding 100%.

A. For which nutrients do you fall below the RDA?

B. Did you exceed the minimum requirements for sodium? To what degree?

C. For which nutrients did you exceed the RDA by greater than 50% (1.5 times greater)?

D. What dietary changes could you make to correct or improve your dietary profile? If you are unsure, future chapters will help guide your decisions.

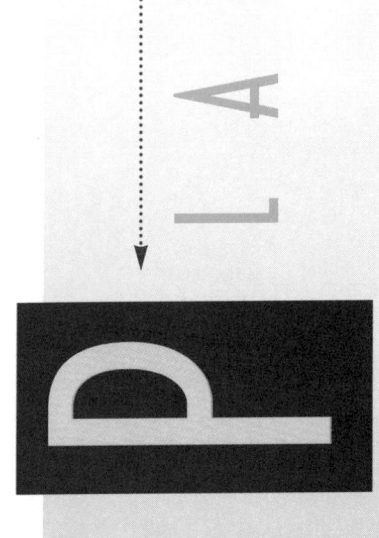

Part IV.

A. Take the information from the 1-day food record you completed in Chapter 1 and record it on the blank form entitled "Food Guide Pyramid," Appendix C. Make sure to record all food and drinks ingested and the amount consumed. Then specify the number of servings of each item consumed under the appropriate food group column. NOTE : You may want to refer to Table 2-2 (The Food Guide Pyramid—a Summary) to estimate serving size.

B. Total the number of servings you consumed for each food group and record amounts on the line labeled "Group Totals."

C. Review the Food Guide Pyramid in Table 2-2 and list the minimum recommended servings on the line labeled "Food Guide Pyramid."

D. Compare the number of servings you received with the minimum recommended servings of the Food Guide Pyramid. Remember that the recommended minimum servings represent 1600 to 1800 kcalories and that your energy needs may be greater than this.

E. Now evaluate your intake for variety, balance, and moderation. How did you do?

F. Hold on to this assessment for use in subsequent activities in other chapters.

Nutrition ISSUE

WHAT'S ON THE LABEL?

In the United States the U.S. Food and Drug Administration (FDA) is responsible for most food labeling. Exceptions are meat and poultry products, which are regulated by the USDA, and alcoholic beverages, which are regulated by the Bureau of Alcohol, Tobacco and Firearms. The Federal Trade Commission (FTC) regulates the advertising of food products and has authority to take action against unsubstantiated claims with enforcement by FDA.

Most foods packaged and sold in the United States must be labeled with the product name, the manufacturer's name and address, the amount of product in the package, and the ingredients.[8] Note the ingredients are listed in order of amount from most to least by weight. So, when you buy a breakfast cereal, for example, choose one that has a whole grain listed first (such as whole wheat or oatmeal).

Since 1973, if manufacturers (1) add a nutrient to a food product or (2) make a nutritional claim about the product, they must provide a *nutrition label.* The next time you see a food package that announces the product is "low in sodium" or "high in fiber," check the nutrition label for more specific information. Today 60% of the foods under FDA control carry a nutrition label. Of those, about half are voluntary—no nutrition label is legally required. Many foods, however, give us no nutrient information aside from contents. This will change soon because a new law passed in 1990, The National Education and Labeling Act, requires most foods to be so labeled.[4] Exceptions will include foods sold in restaurants and cafeterias; food served on airplanes; medical foods, specific foods such as plain coffee and tea, and some spices, among others; and foods produced by small businesses or packaged in small containers. These foods can carry nutriton information voluntarily.[9]

An example of a traditional nutrition label is shown in Figure 2-2, *A.* The label lists serving size of the product, servings per package, kcalories, protein, carbohydrate, fat, and sodium content. If the product contains more than 2% of the U.S. RDA for certain nutrients, the percentages of the U.S. RDA must be listed. These nutrients include protein, vitamins A and C, thiamin, riboflavin, niacin, calcium, and iron. Additional information may be provided on other vitamins and minerals, dietary fiber, and the amount of sugar, types of fats, and cholesterol.

Always check serving sizes when comparing nutrition labels because currently manufacturers determine their own serving sizes, and these vary from product to product. Until new labels are in place, a product may be lower in kcalories than another similar one because the manufacturer simply listed a smaller serving size. Don't be fooled (Figure 2-8).

As mentioned previously, FDA is the midst of changing labeling regulations. Nutrition labels appearing in late 1993 and to become standard by May 1994 are required to list the following:[9]

- Serving size
- Servings per container
- Total kcalories and kcalories from fat per serving
- Total fat, saturated fat, cholesterol, sodium, protein, and total carbohydrates in sugars and dietary fiber

FRANK & ERNEST® by Bob Thaves

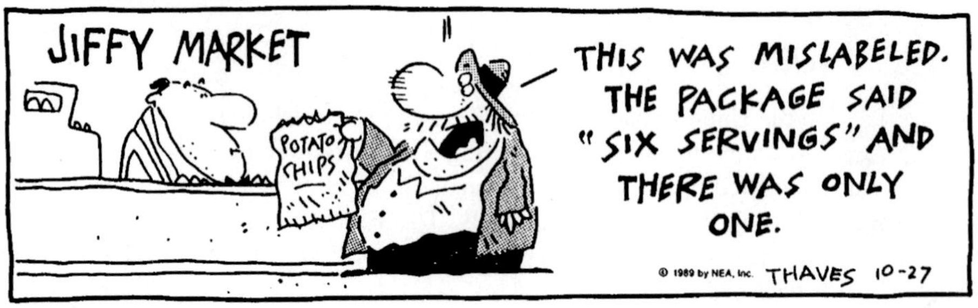
JIFFY MARKET
POTATO CHIPS
THIS WAS MISLABELED. THE PACKAGE SAID "SIX SERVINGS" AND THERE WAS ONLY ONE.
© 1989 by NEA, Inc. THAVES 10-27

Reprinted by permission of NEA, Inc.

FIGURE 2-8
Frank and Ernest.

- Amount of vitamins A and C, calcium, and iron; other vitamins and minerals are not required to be listed
- How the nutrients fit into a daily diet based on 2000 kcalories
- Exactly how many grams and milligrams of total fat, saturated fat, cholesterol, sodium, carbohydrates, and dietary fiber are allotted to a 2000- and 2500-kcalorie diet
- How to convert 1 gram of fat, carbohydrate, or protein into kcalories

In addition, the U.S. RDAs will undergo a name change to RDIs as noted earlier and are likely to eventually be updated to more closely conform to the current RDAs. Serving size will follow more uniform patterns. FDA has also set *Daily Reference Values (DRVs)* for certain parts of a diet not covered by the 1989 RDA, such as carbohydrate, fat, and dietary fiber. RDIs and DRVs will be listed under one category, *Daily Values (DVs),* on the label.

Figure 2-2, *B* shows an example of the new labels, which will list serving size and servings per package. The new labeling legislation will require that serving sizes for similar products be uniform. For example, for all boxed macaroni and cheese products, the serving size must be ½ cup, as shown in Figure 2-2, *B*.

The DVs listed will be based on a 2000-kcalorie diet. In Figure 2-2, *B*, the amount of total fat in one serving (½ cup) provides 20% of the DV (which is 65 grams, as listed on the label) for a 2000-kcalorie diet. For active people, the DVs for a 2500-kcalorie diet are also provided. A goal of the new labels is to aid consumers in fitting nutrient contributions of products into their entire day's diet. In addition, FDA has provided a "dictionary of terms," which contains legal definitions for content claims on food products (such as "free" or "low") and for comparative claims (such as "reduced" or "less"). Fuller disclosure of ingredients is also required, such as for sugar substitutes or various preservatives added to a product.[8]

Labeling Pitfalls

Food marketers are happy to satisfy our cravings for *healthful* foods with healthful-sounding food choices labeled "no cholesterol," "low fat," "organic," and "sugar free." How trustworthy are these claims? Though technically true, many of the claims are irrelevant; others are misleading or only paint part of the picture.[13] Table 2-6 lists today's most-used labeling buzzwords.

Health Claims on Labels

Authorities are still debating the limits to the claims of health benefits that manufacturers can make on a food product label. Today manufacturers are allowed to state that a food

TABLE 2-6

Definitions for Terms on Food Labels—Examples of the Meanings of Some Key Descriptive Words for Specific Nutrients Used on Nutrition Labels

Sugar

- ***Sugar Free:*** Less than 0.5 grams (g) per serving.
- ***No added sugar, Without added sugar, No sugar added:***
  - No sugars added during processing or packing, including ingredients that contain sugars (for example, fruit juices, applesauce, or dried fruit).
  - Processing does not increase the sugar content above the amount naturally present in the ingredients. (A functionally insignificant increase in sugars is acceptable for processes used for purposes other than increasing sugar content.)
  - The food that it resembles and for which it substitutes normally contains added sugars.
  - If the food doesn't meet the requirements for a low- or reduced-calorie food, the product bears a statement that food is not low-calorie or calorie-reduced and directs consumers' attention to the nutrition panel for further information on sugars and calorie content.
- ***Reduced sugar:*** At least 25 percent less sugar per serving than reference food.

Calories

- ***Calorie free:*** Fewer than 5 kcalories per serving.
- ***Low calorie:*** 40 kcalories or less per serving and if the serving is 30 g or less or 2 tablespoons or less, per 50 g of the food.
- ***Reduced or Fewer calories:*** At least 25 percent fewer kcalories per serving than reference food.

Fiber

- ***High fiber:*** 5 g or more per serving. (Foods making high-fiber claims must meet the definition for low fat, or the level of total fat must appear next to the high-fiber claim.
- ***Food source of fiber:*** 2.5 g to 4.9 g per serving.
- ***More or added fiber:*** At least 2.5 g more per serving than reference food.

Fat

- ***Fat free:*** Less than 0.5 g of fat per serving.
- ***Saturated fat free:*** Less than 0.5 g per serving and the level of trans fatty acids does not exceed 1 percent of total fat.
- ***Low Fat:*** 3 g or less per serving and if the serving is 30 g or less or 2 tablespoons or less, per 50 g of the food.
- ***Low saturated fat:*** 1 g or less per serving and not more than 15 percent of kcalories from saturated fatty acids.
- ***Reduced or less fat:*** At least 25 percent less per serving than reference food.
- ***Reduced or less saturated fat:*** At least 25 percent less per serving than reference food.

Cholesterol

- ***Cholesterol Free:*** Less than 2 milligrams (mg) of cholesterol and 2 g or less of saturated fat per serving.
- ***Low Cholesterol:*** 20 mg or less and 2 g or less of saturated fat per serving, and if the serving is 30 g or less or 2 tablespoons or less, per 50 g of the food.
- ***Reduced or less cholesterol:*** At least 25 percent less and 2 g or less of saturated fat per serving than reference food.

Sodium

- ***Sodium free:*** Less than 5 mg per serving.
- ***Low sodium:*** 140 mg or less per serving and, if the serving is 30 g or less or 2 tablespoons or less, per 50 g of the food.
- ***Very low sodium:*** 35 mg or less per serving and, if the serving is 30 g or less or 2 tablespoons or less, per 50 g of the food.
- ***Reduced or less sodium:*** At least 25 percent less per serving than reference food.

Other Terms:

- ***Enriched:*** The vitamins thiamin, riboflavin, and niacin and the mineral iron have been added to the product to replace (and in some cases augment) what is lost in processing.
- ***Fortified:*** Vitamins and/or minerals have been added to the product in amounts in excess of at least 10 % of that normally present in the reference product.
- ***Healthy:*** FDA is proposing a definition for "healthy." The term would be applicable to foods low in fat and saturated fat and having not more than 480 mg. of sodium or 60 mg. of cholesterol per serving.
- ***Light or Lite:*** The descriptor "light" or "lite" can mean two things; first that a nutritionally altered product contains one-third fewer kcalories or half the fat of the reference food (if the food derives 50% or more of its kcalories from fat, the reduction must be 50% of the fat); and second, that the sodium content of a low-calorie, low-fat food has been reduced by 50%.

  In addition, "light in sodium" may be used for food in which the sodium content has been reduced by at least 50%. The term "light" may still be used to describe such properties as texture and color, so long as the label explains the intent; for example, "light brown sugar" and "light and fluffy".
- ***Diet:*** A food may be labeled with terms such as "diet," "dietetic," "artificially sweetened," or "sweetened with nonnutritive sweetener" only if the claim is not false or misleading, and the food can also be labeled "low calorie" or "reduced calorie."
- ***Good source:*** "Good source" means that one serving of a food contains 10% to 19% of the Daily Value for a particular nutrient.
- ***Organic:*** FDA has deferred rulemaking regarding the use of the term "organic" until USDA has adopted appropriate regulations. At that time, FDA will determine whether any regulations governing the term "organic" are necessary.
- ***Natural:*** Food must be free of food colors, synthetic flavors, or any other synthetic substance.

Many definitions are from FDA's Dictionary of terms, as established in conjunction with the 1990 NELA.

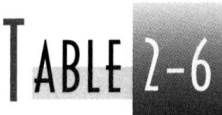

contains certain nutrients, as long as a nutrition label backs up the claim. The actual debate is about whether a manufacturer can state that these nutrients provide specific health benefits, such as saying that dietary fiber in food helps prevent some types of cancer.[13] Manufacturers want to make health claims to sell their products. Since 1984 the Kellogg Company has marketed its high-fiber cereals as a possible preventive measure against some forms of cancer. The extent to which this should be allowed is far from settled.

The FDA traditionally has viewed health-related messages as drug claims, meaning that foods making these claims should be regulated as drugs. This status would require manufacturers to prove that the food does what it is advertised to do and is safe to use at advertised dosages. However, manufacturers simply want to promote products that are healthful and think consumers want such information to help them select healthful foods. After relaxing rules to allow for this in 1987, government agencies are now not sure how far they should let manufacturers go. Currently FDA allows listing the following nutrient–disease relationships on food labels:

- Calcium and osteoporosis
- Fat and cancer
- Saturated fat and cholesterol and heart disease
- Fiber-containing fruits, vegetables, and grain products and cancer
- Fiber-containing fruits, vegetables, and grain products and heart disease
- Sodium and hypertension
- Fruits and vegetables and cancer

A "may" or "might" qualifier must be used in the statement.[4]

A major problem that likely will continue is that a *good food/bad food* comparison is promoted by many claims on labels, and the emphasis on total diet is ignored. As we have discussed, one's total meal plan and nutrient intake should be the focus because nutrients work together—not as separate entities existing in a vacuum—to maintain health. Protein metabolism needs vitamin B-6, glucose metabolism needs the vitamin thiamin, and fat metabolism needs the vitamins niacin and riboflavin.

The American Dietetic Association (ADA) believes health claims are permissible as part of a labeling or marketing system, as long as the claims are presented in the context of total diet recommendations and are generally supported by the scientific community.[2] But, too often, these claims deceive us by leaving out information (for example, not pointing out missing nutrients or high amounts of ingredients that can be harmful). The consumer can't choose wisely if information is missing. The ADA endorses claims that support the recommendations of the Dietary Guidelines. The ADA also supports listing both positive and negative health claims on food labels so that the public will not be misled. For example, a label that claims a food is high in fiber should also state whether the food is high in fat. In this way, important information about the food is not hidden from the consumer.

The bottom line for health claims on food packages is honesty. The whole story needs to be told.[2] Exactly how federal agencies in the United States intend to make sure this happens is not yet fully known. Your best tactic is to read the small print and question what it says. In Appendix D we have included a brief exercise to help you sharpen your label-reading skills.

c h a p t e r 3

NUTRITIONAL ADVICE: FACTS AND FALLACIES

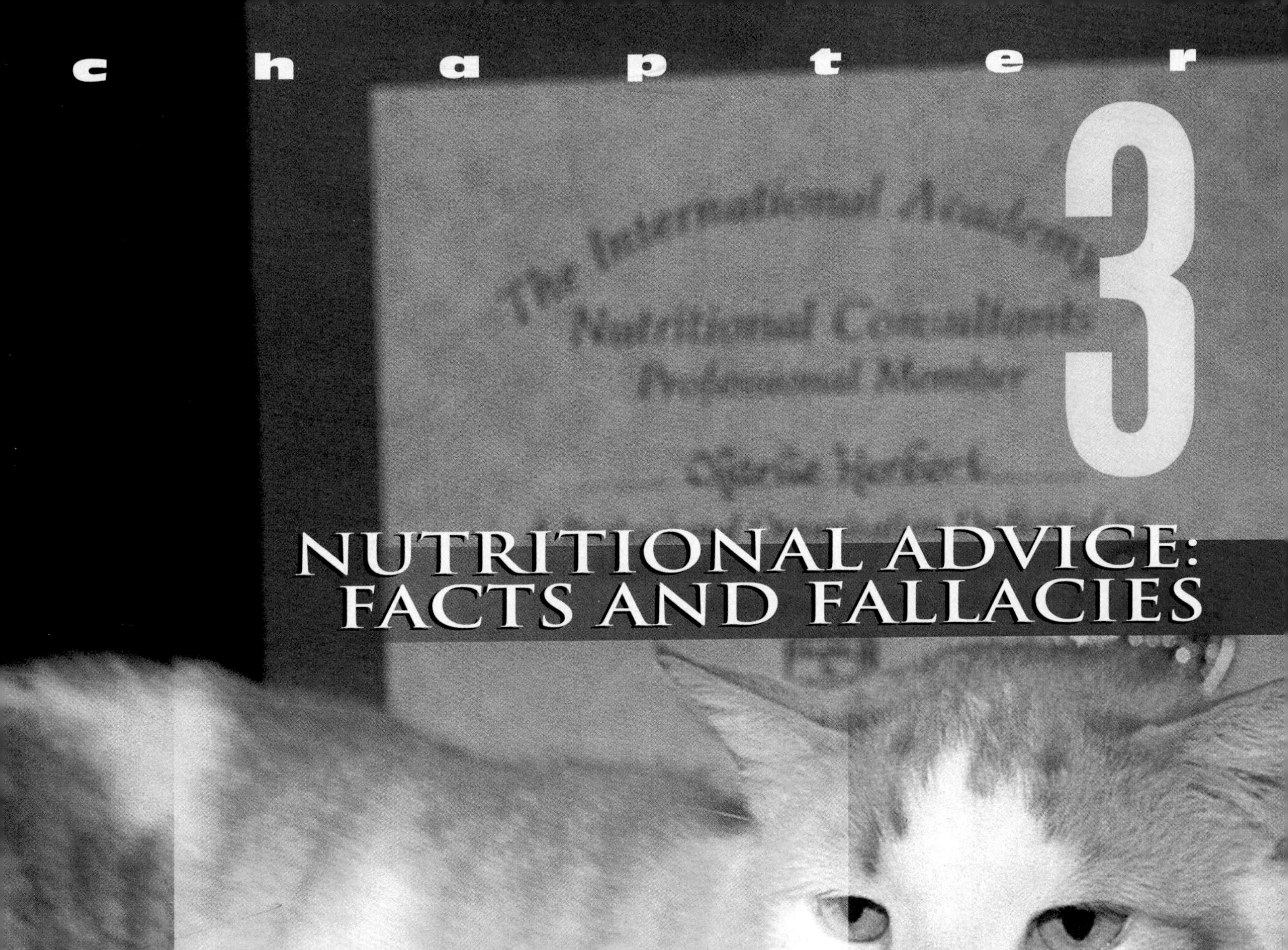

ADVICE ABOUT FOODS TO EAT AND AVOID IS OVERWHELMING:

- Eat organic produce to avoid pesticides.
- Don't eat processed foods that contain preservatives.
- Take large doses of vitamin C to cure colds.
- Eat foods that contain oat bran.
- Choose baked goods made with honey instead of sugar.
- Eat brown rice for perfect nutrition.
- Take large doses of laetrile (a compound found in apricot pits) to cure cancer.
- An apple a day keeps the doctor away.

Sound convincing? Have you heard these statements argued both ways? Contradictory advice can be confusing. How do you distinguish food fact from fiction? Many food products and legitimate businesses ride a nutritional bandwagon. Unfortunately, so do quacks.[1] This chapter presents popular nutrition myths and misconceptions. Familiarity with the claims and methods of quackery can help you distinguish between sound and unsound nutritional advice. If you can spot a myth, you can protect yourself from pretentious health claims and fraudulent food promotions and practices.[2] More information on fad diets can be found in Chapter 10. For now, let's sort out the credible nutrition advice from common fallacies.

Consumers need to be wary of people with credentials from "diploma mills." Charlie Herbert (the cat) is a nutrition consultant, according to the diploma purchased by his owner.

ASSESS

TEST YOUR KNOWLEDGE

yourself

CAN YOU SPOT A QUACK?

Quacks are people who exaggerate health claims. Every day, people fall prey to quackery. By following quack advice you can lose considerable money. You can also damage your health. Americans spend at least $14 billion a year on quackery. Protect yourself by knowing what to look for.

Put a "Q" in blanks preceding statements that describe behaviors of quacks. Write "E" before statements that describe behaviors of reliable nutrition experts.

____ 1. They use anecdotes and testimonials to support their claims. They refer to stories of people being cured of cancer or arthritis by using product X as proof of the effectiveness of the product.

____ 2. They promise quick, dramatic, miraculous cures.

____ 3. They display credentials recognized by responsible scientists or educators.

____ 4. They say that most disease is caused by faulty diet and can be treated with "nutritional" methods.

____ 5. They support the pros and cons of a claim with scientific studies and evidence.

____ 6. In literature they use or write, they cite few if any scientific studies to support the product or claims.

____ 7. They claim that most food additives and preservatives are safe; however, some still require further testing and study.

____ 8. They claim that "natural" vitamins are better than synthetic ones.

____ 9. They say you can get all foods necessary for a healthful diet from the supermarket.

____ 10. They tell you not to trust the medical community.

____ 11. They tell you that no food is really good or bad, but that all foods provide some nutritional value—some more than others.

____ 12. They claim that modern food processing methods and storage remove all nutritive value from food.

____ 13. They say that organically grown foods are not necessarily superior to plants cultivated using chemical fertilizers.

____ 14. They claim that they are being persecuted by orthodox medicine and that their work is being suppressed because it is controversial.

____ 15. They recommend that everybody take vitamins, eat health foods, or both because diet alone does not supply enough nutrients.

Interpretation

Characteristics of a quack: 1, 2, 4, 6, 8, 10, 12, 14, 15
Characteristics of an expert: 3, 5, 7, 9, 11, 13

Put the total number you answered correctly in this blank ____
Were you able to tell the difference between a quack and a reliable expert? ____

From Herbert V, Barrett S: Twenty-one ways to spot a quack, *Nutrition Forum*, p. 65, September 1986.

QUACKERY

Dictionaries define ***quack*** as "a pretender of medical skill; a charlatan" and "one who talks pretentiously without sound knowledge of the subject discussed." Quackery encompasses fraudulent actions, claims, and practices. These definitions suggest deliberate deception.[2] However, many promoters of ineffective and unproven remedies sincerely believe in their products. They may be victims of quackery themselves or may merely wish to believe in something they hope will make them better. In their naivete and enthusiasm they pass on misinformation.

Quack ■ *A person who does not have the medical skills or knowledge that he or she claims to have.*

Americans spend billions of dollars every year on quackery, many times in search of a "quick fix" and sometimes in a desperate attempt to cure themselves of illness.[19] Over $2 billion is spent on unnecessary vitamin and mineral supplements. Another $1 billion is spent on unfounded cancer cures. Can you say you were never a victim of quackery? Health fraud and quackery fool many people, not just gullible or ignorant people. Quackery also preys on the unsuspecting.

Most fraudulent health claims cost only the money lost. But if trying a quack remedy delays needed medical treatment, the cost may be needless physical harm.[6] Until something bad happens, we usually don't recognize dishonest treatment. When we get "burned" by "hot" health frauds, a wiser skepticism results.

Elderly persons are particularly vulnerable to quackery. Their wish to relieve pain and heal failing bodies can be a powerful force.[14] Access is easy; invitations to be healed are everywhere. It's even cheaper than seeing a physician.[3] Hope of such relief offered with naive sincerity sells many useless, expensive cures to frightened and weary elderly persons.

People tend to believe what they hear repeatedly. As with any type of brainwashing, a repeated claim can seem real even when it has no basis in fact. Nutritional brainwashing floods the media, the food shelves, and the conversations of those seeking good health. Quack ideas are everywhere, but repetition does not make them valid.[9]

another BITE

Will the government protect you from false advertising and misleading health claims? Despite its broad powers, it often does not. However, you possess that power, given some basic knowledge. The following pages will alert you to a truer picture of reality:

"LET THE BUYER BEWARE"

Sources of Nutrition Quackery

Unsound nutrition claims enter your world daily through radio, television, newspapers, books, and magazines.[1,19] You need not seek fringe health sources for this false information. A well-meaning but poorly informed medical reporter on the nightly news may mislead you unknowingly. Separating fact from fiction can stump even health professionals. A product effective in relieving one ailment may be worthless for another. Often only intricate knowledge can distinguish fact from food fad. That's where nutrition studies come in.

Most medical schools offer minimal nutrition education. Physicians graduate with impressive skills in diagnosing and treating illnesses. But when patients need dietary advice after a physician's careful diagnosis of a problem, consultation with a registered dietitian is advisable.[14] All in all, healthy skepticism may be our best guide in the often expensive arena of alternative food choices.

Fad is a shortened version of fiddle-faddle, which means to "play with" and then "cast aside."

Miracle cures are myths. If a cure has not been reported in a scientific journal and if physicians are not familiar with it, the cure is probably no miracle.[2,19] Most cures are discovered in steps over long periods—rarely in a miraculous flash.

Let's now look specifically at the many forms of quackery and food fads. Has quackery infiltrated your daily life?

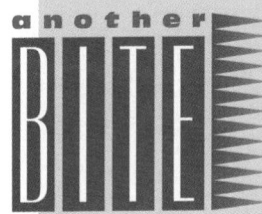

ALTERNATIVE FOOD CHOICES

Whether a product or practice defies convention tells you nothing of its usefulness. The risks and benefits of any product or practice should be ascertained before we embrace any decision.

Organically Grown Produce

Pesticide scares crop up in the news as regularly as a harvest season. One year we hear apples are unsafe; the next year it may be that grapes can kill. The public listens. To please the public, supermarket aisles are now stocked with produce once found only in health food stores. Today, organic food is a $3 billion industry. Though large, it still represents only about 2% of the U.S. food production, partly because of its higher price.

Just what is organically grown food? Recently, Congress passed a farm bill that called for a federal standard defining organic farming methods. By September 1993 we will have a national definition of "organic" as part of the National Organic Standards Law in the 1990 Farm Bill. Both USDA and FDA will enforce these standards once in place. But until new laws are in place, no federal standard controls the production methods of such foods. Organic farmers usually reject ***pesticides*** and use natural soil improvers, such as compost, instead of manufactured fertilizers.[18] They rotate crops to enrich soil further and may control pests with biological intervention. But still, even state requirements for organic foods are inconsistent. Currently, some states require no pesticide use for 3 years before foods can be labeled "organic." Other states require 1 year, and some states either have not delineated the time or have no specific laws on this issue.

Pesticide ■
A general term for an agent that can destroy bacteria, fungi, insects, rodents, or other pests.

Organic food advocates claim these crops offer more nutrition and fewer health hazards than does conventionally grown food. Nutrition scientists find such claims inherently misleading for the following reasons:

1. Surveys find similar pesticide levels in both organically and conventionally grown foods. Cross-contamination from wind and groundwater partly accounts for this. Washing fruits and vegetables removes some external pesticide residue from conventional foods. Still, according to FDA, tiny amounts of pesticides that remain in conventional foods pose no significant health risk for the average person (see Chapter 17 for a detailed discussion). Most dangerous pesticides have been banned in this country. Those currently used are regulated so that even if consumed over a lifetime, the chances of inducing cancer in a person would be less than one in a million.
2. Soil nutrients from natural fertilizers, such as manure, are no different from those in chemical fertilizers made in factories. Furthermore, nutrients from organic fertilizers can't be absorbed until the organic material decomposes. The key issue is whether specific nutrients are present in a fertilizer—not whether natural or manufactured fertilizer is used.[4]
3. Genetic makeup determines a plant's nutrient content and needs. Plants thrive when soil offers a nutritious fare. Long-term studies find no nutritional differences between organic crops and those grown under standard conditions.[18]
4. Freshness, hereditary makeup, and harvest time determine a plant food's flavor. Organic food moves through an entirely separate distribution and marketing system to avoid any possibility that it could lose its identity by being commingled with nonorganic food. Producers, distributors, and retailers tend to market goods less efficiently than do large grocery chains, where centralized distribution systems are the rule. This can translate to poorer-quality produce and more spoilage, because organic food tracks slowly through distribution en route to stores. A large-scale study compared 25 types of organic foods with their ordinary supermarket counterparts for taste and eye appeal. In general, the ordinary produce won both the taste and beauty contests.[4]

However, dangerous pesticides may not be outlawed in other countries, and we may be consuming them in imported produce.

Organically grown produce costs more. Are you wasting your money? We suggest using your money to buy the freshest foods. These will have the best taste and highest vitamin level. If eating organic food holds high value for you, then the extra dollars may give you peace of mind. If so, try to find out your store's current standards for labeling foods "organic." You may be paying more for an organic tomato that was actually grown very much like its counterpart on the next counter. Often a special label certifies the food as organic. Still, it is not guaranteed to be free of pesticide residues or grown without chemical fertilizers until new laws are enacted.

"Natural" Foods

Decades ago a walk down your main street may have taken you past a health food store that offered mainly vitamins and other supplements. Today's health food industry goes beyond organic foods and herbal remedies and is much more visible. Like local grocery stores, health food stores offer produce and breads. Their proprietors promise ***natural*** products, which supposedly are minimally processed and have no additives or other artificial ingredients. But can a line be drawn between processed and unprocessed foods? For example, consider a cracker. Making a single cracker requires grinding, mixing, boiling, baking, and pressing—a lot of processing. Yet health food crackers get a "natural" label (and price tag), because they contain no artificial coloring or preservatives. Is this fair? How natural are the ingredients once they become a cracker?

Ask questions when you see bold exclamations of natural foods.[2] Some foods, whether bought in a health food store or a grocery store, contain naturally occurring toxins: aflatoxins in grains, solanine in potatoes, goitrogens in some raw vegetables, and other poisons in mushrooms and herbs (see Chapter 17). Think first before buying a product that touts that it is natural, compared with its poison-filled grocery store counterpart. Many naturally occurring toxins are harmless when eaten in small amounts in foods as part of a balanced diet. In addition, some highly touted natural and health food snacks—while they may contain dietary fiber and other good things—are notoriously high in fat.

Recall from Chapter 2 that current labeling laws only narrowly restrict the use of the word "natural" for most foods. Any food can claim to be so if free of food colors, synthetic flavors, or any other synthetic substance. What are your criteria for a natural food?

Are There True Health Foods?

We consider even the term "health food" inherently misleading. All foods eaten in moderation can be healthful in the context of a balanced diet.[19] And all foods, even Popeye's spinach, can be unhealthful when eaten in excess.

Some food products have taken on almost a magical aura (Figure 3-1). Is it true that some foods can offer "super nutrition" and are better than others? Some foods, such as brown rice and whole-wheat flour, do offer more dietary fiber, protein, and certain vita-

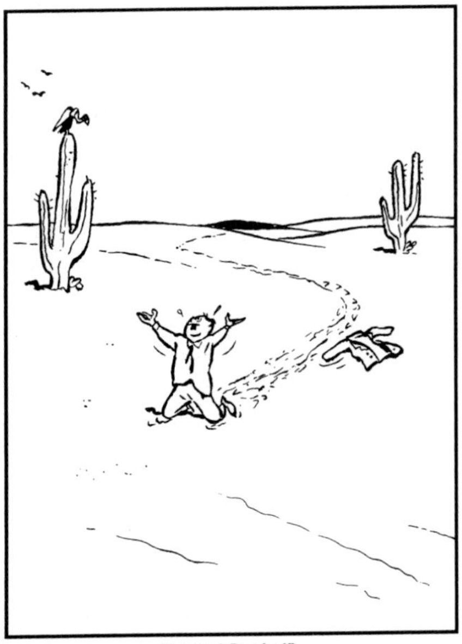

"Perrier! Perrier!"

FIGURE 3-1
Grin and Bear It.

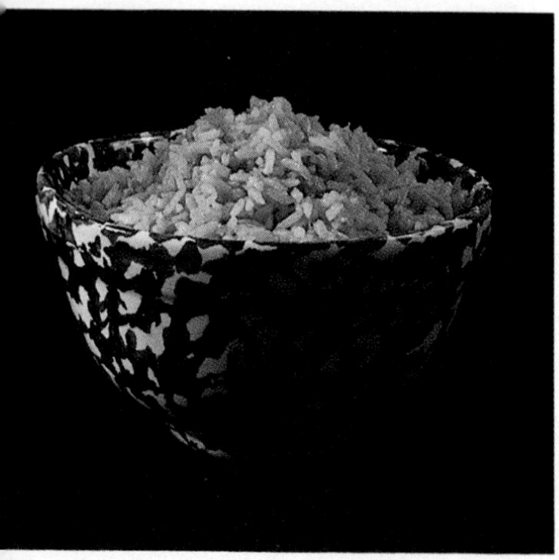

Rice is often given high status in health food circles.

mins and minerals than their more highly processed counterparts. Still, most grocery stores stock these staples. Rice, wheat, and all grains—the seeds of grasses—have a germ (seed) surrounded by starch. The starch provides nourishment once the seed sprouts. A layer of bran and an outer, inedible hull protect the germ and starch. Edible whole grains, such as rice and whole wheat, contain everything but the hull.

Most grain processing strips away some nutrient content. The valuable dietary fiber of bran and the important nutrients of the germ are removed at the mill to produce the white rice and flour many desire. Food processors ***enrich*** some white rice and flour by adding the significant nutrients lost. And ***converted*** white rice can claim a few higher nutrient values than ordinary enriched rice. But both enriched and converted foods lack the fiber and some nutrients contained in the whole food. Overall, it is whole grains rather than refined grains that best offer us the good nutrition we should strive for.

However, food processing does not always mean removing healthful ingredients. And sometimes nutrients are added through fortification to such foods as breakfast cereals. This makes the food more nutritious in some regards. Sometimes processing means safer food. For example, unprocessed (raw) milk can contain microorganisms that cause disease. Pasteurizing milk (heating it to high temperatures for a short time) kills microorganisms capable of causing disease, such as bacteria and viruses. Even when produced under high standards of cleanliness, raw milk is not safe. Each processed food, then, deserves a separate evaluation. As we said in Chapter 2, it is the total diet that deserves the main focus. How do your food choices fit into a diet plan to meet your nutrient needs?

Preservatives
Compounds that extend the shelf life of foods by inhibiting microbial growth or minimizing the destructive effect of oxygen and metals.

Rancid
Having a disagreeable odor or taste, usually caused by fat breakdown.

Toxic
Poisonous; caused by a poison.

What if a Food Contains Additives?

The practice of adding preservatives and other additives to foods commercially tends to evoke strong feelings among some consumers. In other words, controversy surrounding this issue is far more widespread than are the facts about the usefulness and safety of food additives. The most widely used additives are sugar, salt, and corn syrup—all found naturally. These three—plus citric acid (found naturally in oranges and lemons), baking soda, vegetable colors, mustard, and pepper—account for 98% by weight of all food additives used in the United States. Additives are used in food processing to retard the growth of microorganisms, prevent off flavors in fat by reducing the incidence of rancidity, keep mixtures from separating, and retain food crispness. Some preservatives are nutrients, like vitamin C, or potentially beneficial, like BHA and BHT, which may prevent cancer-causing chemicals from forming. Other types of additives can raise the nutrient value, as they do in enriched rice, or they may enhance eye appeal and flavor (see Chapter 17).

FDA checks additive safety. But some people are skeptical. Still, it is important to consider that food additives not only contribute nutrients and enhance food safety, but also prevent quick spoilage. This helps minimize food waste both while on the way to market and at home. From this perspective, having additive-free foods would likely mean higher prices for the consumer.[18] Even without additives, some unprocessed foods contain natural—yet potentially toxic—substances, as we just pointed out. Our body's defense mechanisms help guard against harm from additives and other foreign compounds. Liver enzyme systems and the constant shedding of the intestinal tract are two of many means by which our bodies defend themselves.

Overall, most scientific experts believe the food safety and nutritional and price benefits that result from the use of additives far outweigh the minimal risk of health damage—if any—caused by them.

Health Food Stores in Perspective

Do some foods in the health food store serve important nutritional roles? Whole-grain products, the most popular candidates, are followed in sales by fruits and vegetables, juices, yogurt, tofu, and nut butters. Though of nutritional value, these products often can be bought at a grocery store, generally at lower cost. And, one in three shoppers in health food stores spends money on dubious nutritional products. For example, digestive enzymes, amino acid supplements, bee pollen, ginseng, protein supplements, and primrose oil play no important nutritional role in diet planning despite promotions as cures for all kinds of ailments.[4] Table 3-1 lists common foods that are sold individually or as an ingredient in many health food store concoctions.

The health food industry, with its many dubious products, costs Americans billions of dollars and can be dangerous and even illegal. FDA works hard to investigate complaints of quackery and harm to individuals caused by fraudulent nutrition products, but it does not have enough time or money to investigate all leads. The fact remains that many Americans are willing to try bogus health food products and to believe their miracle

TABLE 3-1

Dubious Claims for Nutrition Products

Food	Claims	Facts
Acidophilus milk (contains bacteria that ferment milk sugar)	Aids digestion; promotes health of digestive tract	Few bacteria survive the production process; bacteria also may not survive acidic stomach environment; may be of value to people who cannot readily digest milk sugar (lactose) or need to reestablish intestinal bacteria after long-term antibiotic therapy
Alfalfa sprouts	Have nutrients not available in other vegetables	Have less nutritional value than broccoli, carrots, and spinach; alfalfa tea can disturb digestion and respiration
Amino acid tablets	Help build muscle mass	Amino acids make up proteins; an abundant level is supplied by diets following the Guide to Daily Food Choices
Bee pollen	A perfect food; can help athletic and sexual performance; prevents cancer, infection, and allergy; prolongs life; promotes both weight loss and gain	Its nutrients are found in conventional foods; no evidence shows that it helps athletes; people allergic to specific pollens can develop severe allergic reactions after ingestion
Bioflavonoids ("vitamin P")	Essential for good health; provides resistance to colds and flu	Bioflavonoids are not vitamins or essential nutrients; no evidence that they are useful for treating any health condition
Blackstrap molasses (less refined form of molasses)	Wonder food that can restore hair and cure anemia	Contributes to iron intake; has no effect on hair color and does not cure anemia
Bone meal	A rich source of calcium	Calcium in bone meal is poorly absorbed; can contain high levels of lead
Brewer's yeast	Excellent diet supplement	Good source of protein and several B vitamins, but adds nothing to a balanced diet; unsavory taste for some
Brown rice	Most perfect food; improves health even if eaten exclusively	A nutritious food, but lacks some needed nutrients; must be complemented by other foods to maintain health
Cider vinegar	Keeps body in balance; thins blood; aids digestion	No evidence to support these claims
Fertile eggs	Nutritionally superior to unfertilized eggs; have fewer unnatural hormones	Fertilization does not add to an egg's nutritional value; if hens are not given hormones, their eggs may have fewer unnatural hormones
Fish oil capsules	Lowers blood cholesterol levels	Can be used to lower some levels of blood lipids (only cholesterol when given in very high doses), but can also make control of blood sugar in diabetes more difficult (see Chapter 6)
Garlic	Purifies blood; reduces high blood pressure; prevents diabetes and heart disease	Garlic and onion contain substances that help prevent blood cells from clumping into blood clots
Kelp (type of seaweed)	Good source of iodine; energy booster	A good source of iodine, but is more expensive than iodized salt
Lecithin	Reduces heart disease risk	Only flawed research supports lecithin's effectiveness in reducing heart disease; the body makes lecithin
Oat bran	Superior food ingredient for lowering blood cholesterol	Only effective in high doses (80-100 grams/day), while people usually eat much less; reducing saturated fat in the diet is a more reliable way to lower blood cholesterol levels (see Chapter 6)
Para-aminobenzoic benzoic acid (PABA)	Oral doses can prevent or reverse graying in hair	PABA is a vitamin for bacteria but not for humans; useful ingredient in sunscreens
Spirulina (blue-green algae)	Helps you lose weight; helps people with diabetes, liver disease, and ulcers	Good source of protein, but is more expensive than conventional foods; no evidence that it promotes weight loss or has medical value

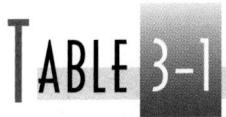

NUTRITION insight

COLORFUL CHARACTERS IN THE HEALTH FOOD MOVEMENT

Chapter 6 introduces you to Sylvester Graham, of cracker fame, and to the rival cereal barons C.W. Post and the Kellogg brothers. Other men and women may not have left breakfast industries in their wake, but these men made waves worth noting. Each presented promises of health that captivated consumer food habits.[4]

James Caleb Jackson, a farmer turned doctor, attributed his health to gulping 30 to 40 glasses of water daily. In 1858 he opened a women's sanitarium that advocated frequent walks and naps, each minus the cumbersome corsets and petticoats of the times. Mealtime specialties included fresh fruit, whole-grain bread, Mr. Graham's crackers, and Mr. Jackson's own specialty, rock-hard bits of baked wheat softened in water. He called this appetizing mixture Granula, later marketing it through "Our Home Granula Company." Mr. Jackson's mixture is resurrected today as "granola."

Bernarr Macfadden, born in 1868, preached exercise. Today scientists agree with this basic concept. But most of Mr. Macfadden's beliefs were unfounded. He advocated the following:

- Fasting to cure some 30 diseases, including heart disease
- Walking to work, preferably barefoot
- Eating a *perfect* diet of nuts and fruits
- Eating when hungry and drinking ½ gallon of water each morning to strengthen the heart and prevent constipation
- Exercising the teeth by eating hard crackers or zwieback
- Sleeping on the floor

In 1890 Macfadden's *Physical Culture* magazine hit the newsstands. Within 2 years 100,000 subscribers were following his bare footsteps, and readership eventually ballooned to 1 million. By 1931 he had an estimated $31 million in revenues. He lived to the age of 87, still downing ½ gallon of water before breakfast.

Horace Fletcher, the high priest of mastication, chewed his way to fame and fortune. He believed large chunks of food interfered with digestion and advocated chewing until the food "swallowed itself." This meant approximately 30 to 70 chomps per mouthful, which reduced the food to near liquid form. Fletcher practiced what he preached, eventually taking nothing but liquids and purees. His death by heart failure in 1916 saddened many followers, including the editors of *The Ladies Home Journal.* Two years previously, in 1914, the popular magazine had begun promoting Fletcher's chew-your-food teachings to its readers.

Adelle Davis received a degree in dietetics from the University of California, Berkeley, and a master of science degree in biochemistry from the University of Southern California School of Medicine. Her four books sold 10 million copies. Davis accused the American diet of being excessively high in salt, loaded with refined sugar, and contaminated by pesticides, growth hormones, and preservatives. She claimed modern food processing destroyed vital nutrients. She advocated vitamin supplements, organic fruits and vegetables, wheat germ, certified raw milk, fresh stone-ground 100% whole-grain bread or cereal, and many other health food products.

Three documented cases revealed harm to children when their mothers followed advice in Davis' book *Let's Have Healthy Children.* In one incident, a mother, following the book's recommendation, gave her 2-month-old infant liquid potassium for colic. After the second dose he became listless and blue, stopped breathing, and was rushed to a hospital where he died the next day. High blood potassium levels interfered with proper heart function.[4]

After filing suit against the publisher, the estate of Adelle Davis, and the store where the potassium supplement was purchased, the infant's parents received a total of $160,000 in out-of-court settlements. The publisher withdrew the book from the marketplace but reissued it with changes made by a physician aligned with the health food industry.

Carlton Fredericks, described on his early book jackets as "America's Foremost Nutritionist," often diagnosed patients and prescribed vitamins to remove the aches and pains of illness. But according to FDA, Fredericks had virtually no nutrition or health science training. In 1945 he was charged with practicing medicine without a license. Fredericks pleaded guilty, paid a small fine, and went back to work. For 30 years, beginning in 1957, he hosted Design for Living, a daily radio show. For several years before his death in 1987, he performed nutrition consultations for $200 each in the offices of Robert Atkins, M.D. (author of *Dr. Atkins' Diet Revolution*). We discuss this fad diet in Chapter 10.[4]

Dr. Lendon H. Smith is a pediatrician who claimed with essentially no scientific proof that allergies, insomnia, hyperactivity in children, and a variety of other ailments are the result of enzyme disturbances that can be helped by dietary changes. He recommends a variety of food supplements and avoidance of white sugar, white flour, pasteurized milk, and other foods that are not "natural." His ideas were promoted widely on his own syndicated TV program and through guest appearances on other shows. His books include *Feed Your Kids Right, Feed Yourself Right,* and *Improving Your Child's Behavior Chemistry.*

In 1973 the Oregon State Board of Medical Examiners placed Smith on probation, because he prescribed medication that was "not necessary or medically indicated" for six adult patients, one diagnosed as hyperactive and the other five as heroin addicts. He remained on probation until 1981. Then in 1987 Smith permanently surrendered his medical license rather than face Board action on charges of insurance fraud.[4]

American opinions about diet and health change when colorful figures such as these clamor their way to national attention. Hard crackers were big sellers at the turn of the century thanks to Bernarr Macfadden's belief in strong teeth. Chewing foods completely became a rage in the early 1900s when Horace Fletcher's teachings swept the homefront. Adelle Davis' devotion to organic foods changed the thrust of the health food industry in the 1960s. And people increased their intake of vitamin capsules when Carlton Fredericks' radio show echoed across the airwaves. Parents around the country responded to the advice of Lendon Smith and kept sugar and treats away from their children. Have any of your beliefs about nutrition been influenced by these popular trendsetters?

Be assured that if all the health food stores in the United States were closed, no one's health would necessarily suffer. The stores serve no essential function as far as we know—grocery stores and supermarkets can supply all our nutrient needs.

actions. More than 70 million Americans take vitamin supplements they do not need, and an estimated $14 billion per year is spent by the American public on products that amount to pure quackery.[4]

Popular products that are frequently sold at health food stores claim to increase muscle growth, enhance sexuality, boost energy, reduce body fat, increase strength, provide missing nutrients to allow you to live longer, and even improve brain function. For example, a popular supplement fad of the 1990s has been "smart drugs" that claim to allow you to think more clearly. Some "smart drugs" are herb mixtures, and others are prescription drugs that are sold illegally by foreign mail-order distributors. It's good to remember that unless any product making a fantastic claim has undergone extensive research by reputable scientists, you take a dangerous risk of ill health when you embark on a self-cure by means of health food store products.[2]

Many ingredients in health food store products have not been tested.[12] Some have undergone testing and are known to be unsafe. For example, the blossoms of the germander plant (*Teucrium chamaedris*) have been sold in North American pharmacies and health food stores and are touted as a remedy for weight loss and anal itching. Researchers have shown that *Teucrium* causes liver damage, and seven cases of hepatitis (liver inflammation) have been reported in people taking germander for 3 to 18 weeks. Though germander in capsule and tea bag form is no longer being marketed, crude germander is still sold in health food stores. Our federal government must spend billions of dollars annually investigating and researching questionable health food store products—money that could be spent on developing scientifically sound cures.

CONCEPT CHECK

Quackery is at work whenever the promises for a food or medical regimen go beyond its scientifically established benefits. The victim pays in dollars and cents and sometimes physical harm. Choosing organically grown and natural foods to avoid pesticides, chemical fertilizers, additives, and artificial ingredients costs more. Studies show no higher nutritional value in organic foods than in ordinary foods. In some cases, choosing processed foods buys safer nourishment. FDA, the nation's federal food regulatory watchdog, requires testing of all food additives when safety is questioned. The grocery store, not the health food store, is the place to seek the foods you need to nourish your body.

VITAMIN AND MINERAL SUPPLEMENTS

If you check the grocery carts of health food shoppers, you often find bottles of vitamin and mineral supplements tucked amid the breads and grains. The yearly expense totals about $3 billion. The two most popular purchases are vitamin C and multiple vitamin and mineral products. People often buy these supplements, fearing that their normal diets fail to provide sufficient nourishment. You now know that this typically need not be the case. In Chapter 2 you learned that a balanced diet offers the nutrition you need. Table 3-2 analyzes common sales pitches for vitamin supplements. Do any look familiar?

Do you take vitamin supplements? Why? If not, why not?

Nutrition experts believe that a diet following the Food Guide Pyramid provides the best diet for a healthy person.[19] The Guide encourages a balanced diet containing a wide variety of foods, including some whole grains and fresh or frozen fruits and vegetables. Does your daily food intake meet the Food Guide standards? To find out, keep a record of every nibble, snack, and meal for a few days, as we suggested in Chapter 1. Then compare your choices with those in the Food Guide, or analyze your diet with the computer

TABLE 3-2

Analysis of Scare Tactics Used to Promote Vitamins

Claim	Comment
"Remember that the health of your eyes, teeth, bones, and internal systems depends on a sufficient intake of these vital nutrients."	Messages of this type, intended to make a person nutrient conscious, are true but misleading. They never say how to tell whether a person is getting enough.
"Of the approximately 40 nutrients that are considered essential in meeting daily body requirements, many cannot be manufactured or stored by the body. These nutrients must be ingested daily."	This claim subtly exaggerates the likelihood of deficiency. The body's storage of water-soluble vitamins is limited, but occasional low dietary intake poses no danger.
"How much of your vitamin C gets lost on the way to the table? Picking, packing, processing—all these plus transportation can lead to the destruction of part of the vitamin C in your foods."	The real issues are how much vitamin C remains in one's diet and whether it is enough. Following the Food Guide Pyramid ensures an adequate intake of vitamin C.
"No matter how hard you try, in our fast-paced society, it's often difficult to make sure you're getting enough essential vitamins and minerals in the food you eat."	This claim exaggerates the difficulty of balancing one's diet.
"Most packaged foods have many, if not all, of the natural nutrients removed during processing and replaced with chemicals."	This statement greatly exaggerates the amount of nutrients lost in processing and exploits public fear that our foods contain too many chemicals.
"Our soils are depleted."	This claim falsely suggests that adequate nutrition can be obtained only by ingesting food supplements or special foods.
"I take my vitamins every day. Just to be on the safe side." (Said by man pictured climbing a steep mountain.)	This is a misleading comparison of the dangers of mountain climbing and of not taking daily vitamin pills.

From Cornacchia HJ, Barrett S: Consumer health, *St. Louis, 1993, Mosby–Year Book.*
We discuss these vitamin-related issues further in Chapter 8.

software available for this book. (Chapter 2 and Appendix C contain directions for completing a diet analysis.)

When survey respondents are asked to state their most important reason for taking vitamins, the answers generally fall into the following categories[4]:

- **To supplement the diet (31%):** "I don't get a balanced diet at all times"; "I don't eat right"; "I don't get enough vitamins during the day"; "I'm an irregular eater."
- **Healthful/makes me feel better (30%):** "To be healthy"; "As a health supplement"; "They're good for you"; "For general health reasons."
- **For energy/strength (12%):** "Give me pep"; "To keep going"; "I am run down"; "As a pick-me-up."
- **Doctor recommended/prescribed (17%)**
- **Pregnant (5%)**

Some vitamin manufacturers advertise that stress raises vitamin needs. For these hucksters, stress can mean physical demands, overwork, or mental burdens. A vitamin vendor might suggest you raise your intake around examination time or before a big date. Other supplement companies pursue athletes, homemakers, and busy executives by plugging products for each group's special needs.[2,16] Some companies make no health claims at all and rely on the product's name or fast-talking salespeople to sell it.

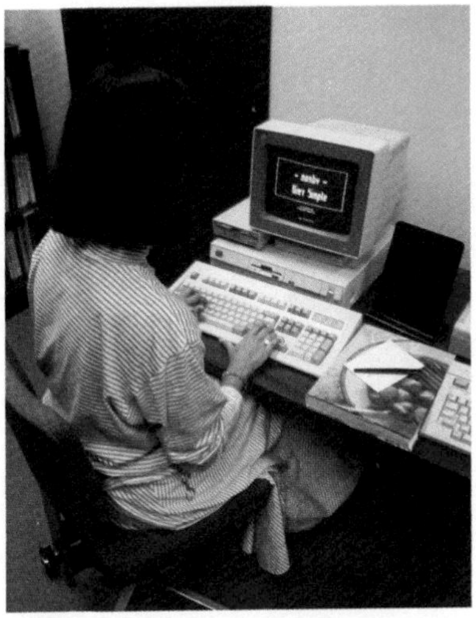

Make sure you need that vitamin supplement—analyze your typical intake first.

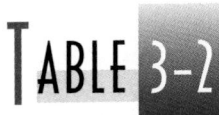

Stress vitamins typically contain several B vitamins and 10 or more times the RDA for vitamin C. No scientific evidence demonstrates we need more vitamins during emotional stress.

Advertisements claim that strenuous physical activity increases vitamin needs, implying that the athlete or fitness enthusiast should shovel in supplements. A vigorous workout increases the need for kcalories, carbohydrates, and water. The body's natural instinct to eat will ensure that the nutrients are replaced. As we discuss in Chapter 8, extra vitamins do not provide extra energy.

When Are Supplements Warranted?

In some specific cases, use of vitamin and mineral supplements should be considered. However, a medical doctor's recommendation should be sought in most cases. Recently a panel of scientists from the American Institute of Nutrition and the American Society for Clinical Nutrition suggested that the following conditions may merit supplementation:

Lactation
The period after childbirth during which milk is produced in the woman's breasts.

Diuretic
A substance that, when ingested, increases the flow of urine.

- Women who bleed excessively during menstrual periods may need more iron.
- Pregnant or ***lactating*** women may need extra iron, calcium, and the vitamin folate.
- People with low energy intakes (1200 kcalories or less) need the range of vitamins and minerals. This can include elderly people who perform little physical activity.
- Some vegetarians may need extra calcium, iron, zinc, and vitamin B-12. Vitamin B-12 is found in appreciable amounts only in animal products.
- Newborns, under the direction of a physician, need a single dose of vitamin K to last until diet and synthesis by intestinal bacteria suffice.
- People with specific illnesses or diseases and those on certain medications may need supplementation of specific vitamins and minerals at the direction of a physician. Examples include extra potassium for someone using thiazide ***diuretics*** and possibly extra vitamin D for someone being treated for osteoporosis.

Supplementation during illness or drug therapy should be directed by a physician, because some vitamins and minerals counteract the effect of certain medications. Professional advice should be sought to help you evaluate whether supplementation is in your best interest. Chapter 8 discusses this point in greater detail.

another BITE

In 1990 Miles Laboratories (makers of *One-A-Day* products) signed a 3-year "assurance of discontinuance" order with the attorneys general of New York, California, and Texas and agreed to pay $10,000 to each of these three states. Without admitting wrongdoing, the company pledged not to claim that (1) the average consumer needs a supplement to prevent mineral and vitamin loss, (2) vitamins can prevent or reverse lung damage caused by pollution, (3) routine daily stress depletes vitamins, and (4) routine physical exercise (such as the aerobics shown in Miles' television ad) depletes essential minerals.[4]

Natural Versus Synthetic Vitamins

Are natural vitamins superior to the synthetic variety? No.[2] Vitamins are specific molecules. The slightly different structures of a few synthetic vitamins do not decrease their value inside the body. Your body cannot tell a natural vitamin from a synthetic one. The only real difference is price—natural vitamins cost more.

Buyer Beware!

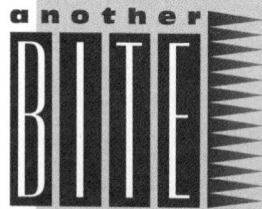

FDA does not regulate all vitamin and mineral supplements closely. The Proxmire Amendment to the 1938 Food, Drug, and Cosmetic Act prevents regulation of supplements unless they are known to be inherently dangerous or marketed with illegal claims. FDA is in the process of trying to set standards for health claims made for supplements. A final draft is due by December 1993. The industry resents this greater scrutiny of its practices and is using its political muscle to limit FDA regulation. Therefore Americans cannot currently depend on the federal government to protect them from vitamin and mineral supplement overuse. For health's sake, people should know what they are ingesting and preferably should seek the advice of physicians and registered dietitians. In cases where vitamin and mineral supplements are necessary, professional guidance is advised.

"ALTERNATIVE" THERAPIES

Meganutrient Therapies

Nutrition therapy can occasionally fight a disease, but not most diseases. Touting nutrients as a cure for many diseases is quackery. About 35 years ago a few physicians began treating schizophrenic patients with ***megadoses*** of vitamins (quantities of more than 10 times the RDA). Today this approach is used by a tiny minority of physicians, who call it meganutrient, orthomolecular, or nutritional therapy.[4]

Megadose ■ *Quantity of nutrient greater than 10 times one's RDA value listed in the 1989 publication.*

Will large doses of vitamin C cure your cold? Members of many households supplement morning orange juice with megadoses of vitamin C, a treatment touted by Dr. Linus Pauling. Cold symptoms are just slightly less severe (see Chapter 8). But as we just pointed out, excess vitamins and minerals can harm your body. Although chemical imbalances in the body contribute to many diseases, meganutrient therapies have not been accepted as remedies to these imbalances.[4] The risk of such therapies outweighs dubious benefits. In addition, high doses of the vitamins A, D, and B-6 and the minerals iron and copper—to name a few—can all cause harmful side effects.

Herbal Therapies

Throughout history, healers have gone to the garden, the forest, and the sea to seek herbal remedies. Largely by trial and error, certain roots, plants, barks, and seeds were found to possess medicinal properties. As early as the second century BC, the Egyptians used myrrh, cumin, peppermint, caraway, fennel, and clove oil for various ailments. In sixteenth-century Europe, physicians began experimenting with sarsaparilla, the dried root of the smilax plant, in attempts to cure venereal disease. Later the root was gathered as a cure for chronic rheumatism and skin disease. When late-nineteenth-century physicians abandoned belief in its medicinal powers, sarsaparilla found new life as a syrup for soft drinks.

In 1989 Americans spent an estimated $500 million for herbal teas, bulk herbs, and other herbal products. Many people choose herbal products for flavor; some choose them for healing. Today most plant substances, however, remain in the forest. Pharmaceutical companies have replaced them with synthetic medicines. For example, reserpine, found naturally in snakeroot (rauwolfia), was used effectively and extensively to treat high blood pressure during the 1950s and 1960s. Today synthetic drugs more effectively lower blood pressure. Companies run their synthetic drugs through rigorous FDA-approved tests to determine safety, effectiveness, and side effects. The controlled testing offers consumers information not available for herbal remedies.

Printed promotion for herbal therapies may be as simple as a cheaply printed flyer or as elaborate as an attractive, finely bound catalog. Don't be fooled by the cover.[4] Use your consumer knowledge to check the following points:

1. Like megavitamin recommendations, megaherb recommendations have no basis in fact. Hearsay, folklore, and tradition keep herbal-healing practices active. Some herbs have yielded valuable substances for modern medical care. However, scientific evidence that establishes their effectiveness, such as double-blind studies, is lacking for most herbal remedies.
2. Many claims are based on treatises written by the sixteenth-century herbalist John Gerard or the seventeenth-century apothecary-astrologer Nicholas Culpepper. Many herbs recommended by their writings contain compounds that can cause cancer.
3. Though some herbs are dangerous, no warning labels accompany herbal remedies. Some herbalists claim that magical properties of a natural herb prevent it from harming people. No evidence supports this claim.

4. Many herbs contain hundreds or even thousands of chemicals that have not been completely cataloged. We may someday find that these chemicals serve useful medicinal purposes. But others could prove toxic.[10] Moreover, many conditions for which herbs are recommended (such as diabetes mellitus and arthritis) are not suitable for self-treatment.

If an herb contains a needed drug, pharmacists can provide the drug in a purer form and in a more controlled dosage than in herbal preparations or teas. With safe and effective medicines available, would you choose herbal treatment?

Promoters claim herbal teas offer therapeutic value. However, these teas—often blends of up to 20 kinds of leaves, seeds, and flowers—can produce unpredictable and potentially serious side effects. The following substances in herbal teas can cause problems: juniper berries, shave grass, horsetail, buckthorn bark, senna leaves, burdock root, catnip, ginseng, hydrangea, lobelia, jimsonweed, wormwood, nutmeg, chamomile, licorice root, devil's claw root, sassafras root bark, Indian tobacco, mistletoe, chaparral, groundsel, comfrey, heliotropium, pulmonaria, and pokeweed (especially the root).[4,12]

The California-based company Herbalife International manufactures and markets a line of herb-based powders, pills, and other concoctions. In the past few years, several legal actions have been taken against this company because of potentially harmful herbs present in its products. In 1982 Herbalife responded to an FDA "Notice of Adverse Findings" by removing two unsafe herbs, mandrake and pokeroot, from its products. FDA documented 100 cases of adverse reactions to Herbalife products. This example illustrates the danger of irresponsible herbal promotions.

Our knowledge of herbs is based largely on folklore and tradition rather than on reliable safety testing. The uses and dangers of these herbs are unexplored territory. For treating serious illnesses we must consider that the poisons of some herbal substances can be dangerous. It is best to see a medical doctor for advice and check with the local poison control center before self-medicating.

another BITE

Today the American public can buy herbs in pill form. Nature's Sunshine Products packages over 70 different herbs singly and encapsulates about 60 herbal combinations, some containing as many as 18 different herbs. The capsules have the safe appearance of traditional medicines. A little pill seems more legitimate than the mixing of magic potions. Same potions, different packages. Estimated yearly sales of Nature's Sunshine Products exceeded $60 million.

Macrobiotics
A food plan that emphasizes vegetable foods over animal foods, often with heavy use of brown rice.

Macrobiotics

Macrobiotics, a quasireligious/philosophical way of life founded by the late Japanese philosopher George Ohsawa, advocates a mainly vegetarian diet. Foods of animal origin get shifted from main course to condiment. Ohsawa outlined a 10-stage Zen macrobiotic diet, with each stage being more restrictive. In the highest state, followers consumed only brown rice and water. This eating plan was purported to overcome many illnesses attributed to excesses in diet. Though no scientific evidence supports the claims, proponents believe macrobiotics cures anemia, arthritis, appendicitis, cancer, cataracts, tuberculosis, diabetes, epilepsy, heart disease, hernia, leprosy, and schizophrenia.[15]

Today, under the leadership of Michio Kushi, Ohsawa's followers promote macrobiotics as a cancer cure. In fact, this diet can interfere with legitimate cancer treatment because patients lose their appetite, as well as weight. Also, the diet may not meet the increased nutritional needs of some cancer patients.

To compare this food plan with a recommended vegetarian diet, see Chapter 7.

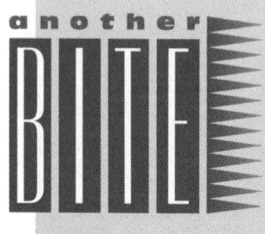

Current macrobiotic diets are less restrictive than earlier versions. Proponents now recommend whole grains (50% to 60% of each meal), vegetables (25% to 30% of each meal), whole beans or soybean-based products (5% to 10% of daily food), nuts and seeds (small amounts as snacks), miso soup, herbal teas, and small amounts of white meat or seafood once or twice weekly. Do you see any important foods missing from this diet?

The American Academy of Pediatrics cautions that a macrobiotic diet is especially hazardous to children. Recently some children following macrobiotic diets were diagnosed with ***rickets.*** This bone disease was linked in these cases to poor vitamin D and calcium intake.[6] Vitamin D–fortified milk in the diet would add these nutrients. This diet may also stunt growth by discouraging children from getting needed calories and protein. Children may not be able to eat enough of these bulky foods to meet their nutrient needs (see Chapter 14).

Rickets *A disease characterized by softening of the bones because of poor calcium deposition. This deficiency disease arises from insufficient vitamin D activity in the body.*

CONCEPT CHECK

We can meet vitamin and mineral requirements by eating a balanced diet. Mental stress does not create a need for nutritional supplements, nor do vitamins give extra energy. Therapies based on herbs or megadoses of vitamins and minerals lack scientific endorsement and may be dangerous. Likewise, macrobiotic diets do not cure disease. Such diets can even harm children through inadequate nutrient intake.

HOW TO EVALUATE CLAIMS

The opening exercise in this chapter contains many tips for spotting quackery. The following suggestions should help you make healthful and economical nutrition decisions:

1. Apply the basic principles of nutrition as outlined in Chapters 1 and 2 to any nutrition claim. Do you note any inconsistencies? Do reliable references support the claims? (See Appendix O for reliable sources of nutrition information.) Beware of the following:
   - Testimonials about personal experience
   - Disreputable publication sources
   - Lack of evidence of supporting studies made by other scientists
2. Examine the background philosophy of the individual, organization, or publication making a nutritional claim. Usually a reputable author is one whose educational background and/or present affiliation is with a nationally recognized university or medical center that offers programs or courses in the field of nutrition, medicine, or a closely allied specialty. The philosophy will be based on scientific validation when possible.
3. Be wary of anyone who promotes the fads and fallacies identified in this chapter. Consider whether:
   - The pros balance the cons. (Are advantages and disadvantages discussed?)
   - Conclusions are overstated. (Are claims made about curing disease?)
   - Extreme bias is aimed against the medical community or traditional medical treatments.
   - Fear-arousing techniques are used.
   - The cure is quick and painless.
   - The product promoted applies to a wide variety of diseases and conditions.
   - The claim is touted as a new or secret scientific breakthrough (Figure 3-2).
4. Avoid practitioners who prescribe vitamin supplements for everyone or who sell them in connection with their practice.[2]
5. Examine product labels carefully. Be skeptical of any product promotion not clearly stated on the label. Remember, federal laws require that health products be truthfully labeled and carry adequate directions for use. A product is not likely to do something that is not specifically claimed on its label or package insert (legally part of the label).
6. Keep in mind that nutrition scientists normally report their studies in reputable scientific journals. Top-notch research journals require every article to be reviewed by other scientists. Follow-up studies are then demanded before hypotheses can be supported. Again, testimonials do not count as scientific evidence or support.[2]

The Nutrition Issue in this chapter discusses how to apply the scientific method to nutrition claims.

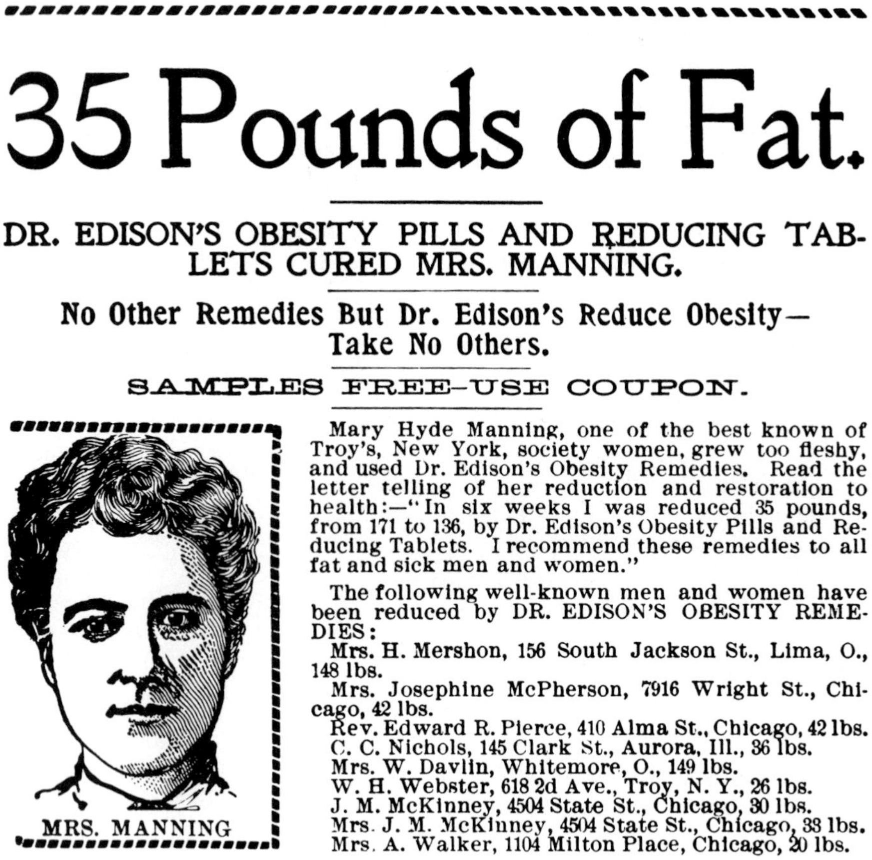

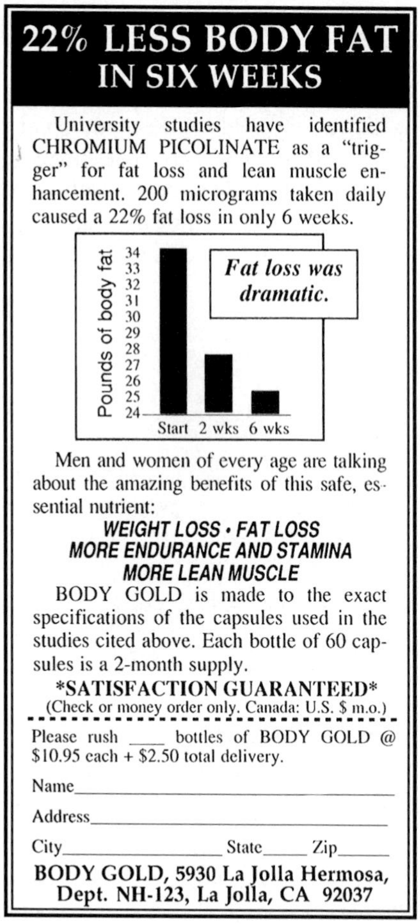

FIGURE 3-2

Quackery has been with us for ages. **A,** *Even at the turn of the century, people wanted to believe that fat could be lost without changing habits or without much effort, and,* **B,** *they still do.*

HOW DO QUACKS PROMOTE QUESTIONABLE NUTRITION?

Quackery is easier to perpetuate than you might think. Overall, the reality is "let the buyer beware."

Skirting the Law Is Easy

How can freedoms of speech and press harm the consumer and protect the phony-food promoter? If you falsely promote a product but are not the actual vendor, you cannot be charged. Thus, while it is illegal to label a vitamin as a cure for cancer, a TV talk show guest can testify to wonder cures without facing prosecution. Retailers can then refer to the talk show (or magazine article, etc.) and take advantage of misinformation. They can refer customers to more misinformation in popular literature or materials distributed by supplement manufacturers (Table 3-3).[4] Storekeepers attending seminars sponsored by trade organizations can gather these illegal claims and pass them on in the privacy of health food stores. Practitioners' offices and customers' homes also serve as pulpits for pandering such misinformation.[7]

TABLE 3-3

Advertising Claims Used to Promote Quack Products and Services and Rebuttals

"Our product has FDA approval."

Manufacturers are prohibited by law from claiming to have FDA approval.

"Our case histories and testimonials are reliable and useful."

Such testimonials may come from people with chronic ailments who (1) have had a symptom-free period, (2) have had a spontaneous remission, (3) have experienced a placebo effect, or (4) have been misdiagnosed. Celebrities and sports heroes often give testimonials in exchange for payment.

"The medical profession's attempts to persecute our company hides the truth."

The medical/scientific community uses the scientific method when testing validity of health claims. Double-blind studies prevent the results from being biased. The medical profession seeks truth; it does not bear grudges.

"Words like wondrous, breakthrough, ancient, secret, and revolutionary **herald a reevaluation we should all consider."**

True medical breakthroughs are never secret. They are reported in medical journals and the general media, not in the back sections of magazines or in leaflets.

"Our product cures many ailments overnight."

No single product can be effective for a wide variety of ailments; any claim for a quick and painless cure is usually too good to be true.

Recognizing the Quack

Beware of promoters who profess the following without scientific evidence[2]:

1. Particular foods can cure specific diseases.
2. Many harmful foods should be eliminated from your diet.
3. Only natural foods should be eaten.
4. Modern processing methods strip the nutritional value from foods.
5. Sugar is a deadly poison.
6. Stress greatly increases your need for nutrients.

Food Fads Are Irresistible to Many

There are many reasons that people fall unsuspecting prey to food faddism. Some food-fad victims may be fulfilling certain behavior needs (Table 3-4). Food faddists may be trying to use foods to achieve control over their lives. Some aspects of food quackery even evolve into social movements or rebellions against authority, society-at-large, or some imagined enemy, such as the medical profession or the government.[3] Food faddism can take on an almost hysterical tone in reaction to fears of chemicals, pesticides, and preservatives in food. Although real health problems can arise from the use of certain foods, small unscientific groups guided by folklore, wishful thinking, and hearsay will not be the ones to separate fact from fiction. Choosing reliable sources and reading widely and skeptically will be your best guide to eating well.

Where do quacks find their victims? Enough people reject conventional medical and nutritional advice to create a booming market for alternative advice, alternative foods, and supplements.[13] Finding someone who seemingly listens and cares enough to try to help hooks many victims. Some quacks sincerely want to help. They offer their time along with their own innocence and ignorance. Alternative practitioners in one study spent about eight times as much time with their patients as did medical doctors. Con-

TABLE 3-4

Types of Food-Fad Victims and the Behavior Needs These Practices Serve

Victims	Need Served by Fad
Miracle-seeker	Seeks diets promising eternal youth in an attempt to believe in self-worth
Rebel	Chooses foods that fit into antisocial belief system
Mr. Atlas	Seeks diets promising to slow aging to fit with self-image of super strength and perfect health
Skeptic	Rejects traditional medical and nutritional advice to establish appearance of control and independence
Food Fashion Groupie	Buys into any popular diet to fit in and to gain approval and acceptance
Ms. Know-It-All	Reads extensively and makes food choices to confirm own nutrition know-how
Analyzer	Challenges all input to protect self from feared manipulation
Worrier	Seeks certainty in food choices in attempt to find certainty and stability in the world

From Schafer R, Yetley EA: Social psychology of food faddism, Journal of the American Dietetic Association *66:129, 1975.*

sumers praise "the helpful people at the health food store because they take time to share the latest discoveries in the health field." Thus an important aspect of their success seems to be the "healer's" marketing of tender loving care.[3]

What motivates these scam peddlers? In many cases, particularly with mail-order crooks, it is profit—pure and simple. Quackery schemes are a very lucrative business. Quack practitioners connect with something basic in human nature. Beyond the quest for good health, people fall prey to scams in their search for a stable, predictable life pattern. By offering hope of good health and beauty, quacks play on what people want to believe. They repeatedly echo their sales pitch, knowing that what is repeated becomes truth in people's minds.

In the 1970s, laetrile promoters waged a vigorous and constant propaganda campaign, never feeling obligated to prove their claims of a cancer cure. Sales then peaked.[2]

Most of us are pushovers for hope. When the orthodox medical community offers no present hope for a cure to such diseases as multiple sclerosis, acquired immunodeficiency syndrome (AIDS), and advanced stages of certain cancers, an unorthodox "healer's" promises and attention seem very inviting, as we noted at the outset of this chapter.[12] Feeling abandoned by personal physicians while living with pain and fear leaves patients vulnerable to quackery.[3]

If you felt left by the wayside and someone offered a magical drink of life for a price, would you choose to buy hope?

another BITE

Let terms such as *alternative* and *holistic* serve as warning flags when they are used to promote treatments. Quacks are experts at "bio babble." Think twice when you hear buzzwords such as homeopath, naturopath, nutripath, clinical ecology, cytotoxic testing, and psychic surgeon. Worthless diagnostic methods and treatments include saliva tests, iridology (close examination of the eye), cellulite removal, applied kinesiology, metabolic therapy, hair analysis done by mail-order laboratories, coffee enemas, and colonic irrigation/detoxification.[2] Rigorous scientific testing has disproved the effectiveness of many of these.

Hair analysis is an experimental research tool used in mineral research. It has little or no place in clinical practice.[4]

Some quacks are impostors who purchase bogus credentials. Dr. Victor Herbert, a noted "quack buster" and nutrition scientist, purchased two diplomas—one from the American Association of Nutrition and Dietary Consultants, the other from the equally "prestigious" International Academy of Nutritional Consultants—by submitting the name and address of the applicant, along with a check for $50. The first certificate was inscribed with the name of Dr. Herbert's pet poodle, Sassafras; the other belongs to his cat, Charlie (see chapter photo, p. 63).[8]

Using Popular Books

The health food industry's well-organized promotion machine capitalizes on popular books. In 1991 more than $100 million was spent on books purchased in health food stores. Nutri-Books, the largest distributor, stocks more than 2000 titles, most of which promote questionable health ideas and products. *Life Extension,* a 1982-1983 best-seller, based its theme on a medically unacceptable premise: building on animal experiment data that showed that underfeeding extends life span, the authors generalize that underfed humans might live to 150 years of age. (Chapter 15 discusses the research behind this premise.) According to the publisher's promotions, the authors appeared on national TV more than a dozen times. The magazine *Health Foods Business,* which reports industry trends, noted that sales of "antioxidants, moisturizers, and anti-aging products" promoted by the book jumped after its publication. A number of companies even designed new products to take advantage of the book's popularity.[4]

Meganutrient therapy is described in such books as *Orthomolecular Psychiatry: A Treatment Approach,* by Drs. Linus Pauling and David Hawkins; *Mega-Nutrition,* by Dr. Richard Kunin; and *Dr. Pfeiffer's Total Nutrition,* by Dr. Carl C. Pfeiffer. Dr. Kunin's book claims that a balanced diet is a practical impossibility and that "the nutrition-prescription movement is . . . a new direction toward which all of medicine is moving."[4]

Coinciding with public concern about AIDS, the 1985 publication of *Dr. Berger's Immune Power Diet* sparked the marketing of many health food products promising to boost the immune system. In fact, any aid beyond a balanced diet amounts to quackery.[2]

Michio Kushi's books touting macrobiotics as a "nutritional cure" for cancer and heart disease continued to be best-sellers throughout the 1980s and 1990s. Books supporting herbal therapy instead of traditional medicine—such as those by James Balch, M.D.—are commonplace on the health food store bookshelf, alongside numerous books on weight loss.

Using Sales Pyramids

Many companies market food supplements, diet plans, and other health products using person-to-person sales. Anyone can become an *independent distributor.* Simply complete an application form, pay a small fee for a sales kit of product literature, and practice the pitch. Companies require no knowledge of nutrition or health care. Pitch the product with personal testimonials and persuade others to become distributors. This type of distribution system, known as a sales pyramid, is a typical get-rich-quick scam. When sales mount, distributors make money from a percentage of the sales of those below them in the pyramid. Like many such scams, promises of profits that continually multiply are rarely fulfilled.[7]

Health Food Stores as an Outlet

Health Foods Business estimated 1991 gross sales for the 7300 health food stores in the United States at $3.9 billion. This included $1.5 billion for vitamins and supplements (Figure 3-3). Although it is illegal for storekeepers to diagnose or prescribe, it is common for them to do both.[4] No special knowledge or training is required to become a salesperson at a health food store. Personnel in these stores typically obtain information by reading books and magazines that promote supplement products for the treatment of virtually all health problems. Investigators from the American Council on Science and Health uncovered the following practices with 105 inquiries at stores in a three-state area:

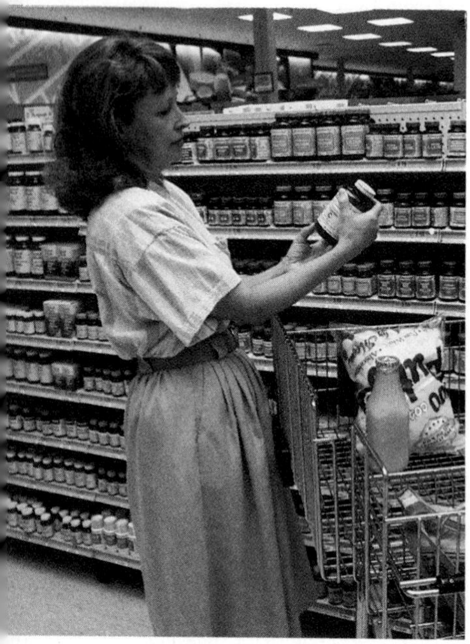

FIGURE 3-3
Health food stores sell billions of dollars in vitamin supplements each year.

- When asked about eye symptoms characteristic of glaucoma, 17 of 24 storekeepers suggested a wide variety of products; none recognized that urgent medical care was needed.
- When asked over the telephone about a sudden, unexplained 15-pound weight loss in 1 month, 9 of 17 storekeepers recommended products sold in their store; only 7 suggested medical evaluation.
- Seven of 10 stores carried *starch blockers,* despite an FDA ban in 1982.
- Nine of 10 storekeepers recommended bone meal and dolomite, products considered hazardous from lead contamination.
- Nine stores made false claims for the effectiveness of bee pollen.
- Ten stores made false claims about RNA (ribonucleic acid, a part of almost all cells).

The investigators concluded that most health food store clerks give advice that is irrational, unsafe, and illegal.[4] As we noted earlier, a person need never enter a health food store in an effort to maintain health. They provide no pivotal or even needed role in the maintenance of health in our nation.

Pharmacies Can Contribute to the Problem

Pharmacies typically carry hundreds of supplements, many completely useless. Many pharmacies display posters or flyers that tell what vitamins do in the body. These tend to promote sales by inducing customers to think that if a little is good, more is better. Pharmacy schools generally teach the facts needed to advise customers that "nutrition insurance" is not usually needed, that "stress" supplements are a scam, and that doses above the RDA are rarely appropriate. Yet pharmacists throughout the United States seem to profit from public confusion by marketing supplements in their stores.

Using Bogus Organizations

Some organizations with scientific-sounding names actually jeopardize public health with misleading nutritional information. One organization, the National Health Federation (NHF), promotes the gamut of alternative health methods with its theme of "freedom of choice" in health matters. Actually NHF just about locks out one choice—medically acceptable types of treatment. Their underlying message implies that anyone opposing NHF ideas is part of an anticonsumer conspiracy controlled by the government, organized medicine, and big business.[4]

NHF publications criticize such proven public health measures as pasteurizing milk, vaccinating for polio, and fluoridating water. This group, based in Monrovia, California, stretches its influence to Washington, D.C., filing lawsuits against government agencies and helping defend people prosecuted for selling questionable "health" products or services.[4]

It is not always easy, even for health care professionals, to tell the difference between a reputable and a bogus organization. More than once, slipshod organizations have billed themselves as scientific "foundations" working for the public good, while they actually sell enticing cure-alls for common ailments. Often such pseudoprofessional organizations list an impressive board of "scientific advisors" bearing Ph.D. degrees or with positions in universities and research centers across the world. When such lists have been investigated, many members of the scientific advisory committees do not even exist.[19]

Clues can tell us more about the nature and intent of an organization. Frequently, pseudoscientific organizations whose intent is to dupe the public and make a profit will advertise their "comprehensive plan" or "health package" that conquers such common ailments as arthritis or perhaps such chronic diseases as diabetes or cancer. Organization members can purchase nutrition products at "discount" prices. In researching a questionable organization, check to see what information about the company and scientific studies of its product can be provided and at what cost.

WHAT ACTIONS CAN YOU TAKE?

If you suspect false claims about a product or service, seek answers from reputable sources. Choices include the following:

- The local public health department
- Medical societies
- Other professional organizations (Table 3-5)
- Registered dietitians in hospitals and private practice (the Nutrition Insight on p. 52 discussed the RD's qualifications.)
- The medical or nutrition department of a university or college

FDA also responds to inquiries about product claims. A local FDA office may be listed in the telephone book under Health and Human Services in the U.S. Government listings. False or misleading advertising about nutrition products is handled by the Federal Trade Commission (FTC), not FDA. In addition, the Postal Service can act against persons making false claims for products sold through the mail. Postal prosecution has been fairly effective in curbing this type of quackery.

You can also fight quackery through the media—where it speaks loudest. If you notice a newspaper article, radio or television broadcast, or advertisement that contains health misinformation, complain to the source. Call the station or paper. Consider enlisting the help of the National Council Against Health Fraud, Inc. (Box 1276, Loma Linda, Calif. 92354). Some people fear that speaking out against quackery will put them in legal jeopardy. It won't if they stick to the facts and avoid name-calling. You need not label someone a "quack" to speak out against false claims for a product. Remember, if it sounds too good to be true, it likely is.[4]

TABLE 3-5

Where to Complain About Quackery and Health Fraud

In matters of health there should be no tolerance for deception. A small effort in opposing quackery may save many people from being hurt—and may even save a life. If more than one agency seems appropriate for a problem, contact each one.

Problem	Agencies to Contact
False advertising	FTC Bureau of Consumer Protection* Regional FTC office Editor or station manager of media outlet where ad appeared
Product marketed with false or misleading claims	FDA national or regional office* State attorney general State health department Local Better Business Bureau Congressional representatives
Bogus mail-order promotion	Chief Postal Inspector, U.S. Postal Service*
Improper treatment by licensed practitioner	Local or state professional society (if practitioner is a member) Local hospital (if practitioner is a staff member) State licensing board National Council Against Health Fraud Task Force on Victim Redress
Improper treatment by unlicensed individual	Local district attorney State attorney general National Council Against Health Fraud Task Force on Victim Redress

From Barrett S: Nutrition quackery—a brief look at the marketplace, Healthline, *p. 2, October 1991.*
**Federal agency addresses: FDA, 5600 Fishers Lane, Rockville, MD 20857; FTC Bureau of Consumer Protection, Washington, DC 20580; Chief Postal Inspector, Washington, DC 20260–1100; regional offices are listed in the blue pages of telephone directories in the areas where they are located.*

HOW TO SPOT FRONT-PAGE FALLACIES

By Anthony Schmitz

1. Study: Eating Citrus Can Help Against Cholesterol

Associated Press

MIAMI—Eating citrus can reduce cholesterol plaque in clogged arteries and help reverse atherosclerosis, a leading cause of heart attacks and strokes, researchers said Wednesday.

2. A two-year experiment with pigs found that citrus pectin—the sticky substance that's used to make jelly—reduces the formation of fatty plaque in coronary arteries, said D. Sigurd Normann of the University of Florida.

3. The practical impact of our investigation is that we can tell a patient with severe atherosclerosis all is not lost," said fellow researcher Dr. James Cerda. "Based on this research, I would advise my patients with high cholesterol levels to eat a low-fat diet, get some exercise, and eat at least one grapefruit or several fresh oranges every day."

4. The researchers emphasized that citrus juice doesn't have the same beneficial effects because pectin is found only in the rind and in the pulp.

5. Normann, chief of cardiac pathology at the university's college of medicine, presented the study Thursday to the Federation of American Societies of Experimental Biology in Atlanta.

6. The primary grant for the research came from the Florida Citrus Commission, a state-appointed, industry-funded panel, but the commission played no role in reviewing the results, university officials said.

Norman said the study used pigs because their arteries and susceptibility to atherosclerosis are similar to humans'.

7. Dr. Margo Denke, a specialist with the Center for Human Nutrition at the University of Texas's Southwestern Medical Center in Dallas, said she was impressed with the research. The findings fit in with previous studies showing pectin, a type of soluble fiber, can reduce cholesterol levels.

"They saw the change in a very short period of time, which is quite dramatic," she said. "But I think that more research is going to need to be done, and we might not expect such a dramatic effect in humans."

The study indicated as little as one grapefruit a day was enough to show results, but Denke said some other research has suggested that higher amounts might be necessary.

Dr. George Lumb, a scholar in residence at Duke Medical School who has conducted research on heart disease for 30 years, questioned whether people would be willing to eat that much fresh citrus fruit every day. He said his research team is conducting studies on 24 volunteers with high cholesterol levels to test the effects of pectin-enriched fruit punch.

YOUR NEWSPAPER probably prints some type of food news every day. It may be important; it may be meaningless. Don't count on the editors' knowing the difference. You can defend yourself against half-baked findings and wild advice—if you read carefully. Here's how to skeptically evaluate a food news piece, one that hit the pages of the *Minneapolis Star Tribune* on April 26, 1991. The Nutrition Issue on p. 89 covers the application of research to human health in detail.

1. The bold, beckoning words at a newspaper story's top are usually cranked out by a special headline writer whose familiarity with the subject can be measured in minutes. If eating citrus can help against cholesterol, your first questions should be "How much citrus? Whom does it help?"

2. Now you know they're talking about pigs. Even if you have four legs and a snout, you shouldn't go for the pectin quite yet. The writer left out the study size—seven control pigs, seven pigs on pectin—which is too small to make the results widely applicable *even for pigs.* For humans, the conclusions are shakier still. That's not to say the research is irrelevant. Human arteries harden about the same way pigs' do. But the story doesn't say what else the pigs ate. Pigs are more sensitive to food's cholesterol; we're more sensitive to fat. Animal studies alone can't prove anything about human nutrition and health.

3. Did the pigs eat an amount of pectin that a reasonable pig, or a reasonable person, might eat? The answer (not that it's here) is no. Researchers fed 60-pound Yucatan micropigs half an ounce of pure pectin a day. Chances are you weigh two or three times more than a micropig. To have any hope of a cholesterol drop like that of the pigs, you'd have to eat at least *two dozen* grapefruits a day.

4. Great news if you eat grapefruit *rind.* Most people don't.

5. There's a big difference between papers delivered at a conference, such as this one, and papers published in the *Journal of the American Medical Association,* the *New England Journal of Medicine, Science, Nature,* and the like. Journal articles are usually reviewed by experts who help editors toss out the scientific chaff. Presentations at conferences aren't as carefully winnowed and shouldn't be taken as seriously.

6. If the bills are paid by the citrus industry, wouldn't the researchers inevitably find *something* good to say about grapefruits and oranges? Maybe; maybe not. You can't jump to conclusions about bias, warns *Washington Post* science writer Victor Cohn. Some crooked researchers *do* get money from corporations, he notes. "But the peddler of a biased point of view is as likely to be an anti-establishment crusader or an academic ladder-climber as a corporate darling." You have to judge each study on its own merits.

7. The last paragraphs are often more helpful than the first. This is usually where outside experts comment, putting the finding in perspective. In this case Margo Denke, a member of the American Heart Association's nutrition committee, makes three good points: This study confirms others showing that soluble fiber lowers cholesterol. Humans, however, aren't the same as pigs. And there ought to be more research done before anyone warms up the citrus bandwagon.

Anthony Schmitz is a contributing editor to Health magazine.

When a friend, relative, or fellow student is buying into quackery, consider the following tactics:

1. Ask whether the claim or product has scientific studies to support its message. If it does, take the literature to a reputable source (such as those listed previously) for evaluation and share the professional's opinion with your friend.
2. If the product is a diet, evaluate the diet as compared with the Food Guide Pyramid. Does the diet stand on its own for balance, variety, and moderation?
3. Remember that people try new things for a number of reasons. The best you may be able to do is to provide an objective opinion and then let your friend make his or her own decision.

CONCEPT CHECK

Quacks promote their ideas through salespeople and mainstream media—print, radio, and television. As long as people seek eternal health and quick cures, dubious health practitioners will thrive. Health food retailers often suggest remedies for illnesses best treated by a medical professional. Protect yourself by being an informed and skeptical consumer.

SUMMARY

- Though capable of causing bodily harm, quackery hits most people in the pocketbook. However, abandoning medical therapy for a quack remedy can have serious physical consequences.
- Organically grown and natural foods provide alternatives to foods that contain artificial ingredients and additives and to foods grown with chemical fertilizers and pesticides. But the nutritional benefits are few, if any.
- Quacks often suggest that the average diet lacks vitamins and minerals and should be supplemented with their products. Choosing whole grains, fruits and vegetables, and other selections from the Food Guide Pyramid provides excellent nutrition. An excess of certain vitamin and mineral supplements, such as vitamins A and D and the minerals iron and copper, can cause harm.
- Herbal remedies and megadose vitamin and mineral therapies are not reliable and may be dangerous.
- Consumers who feel shortchanged by orthodox health care provide a large and willing market for those promoting questionable and dangerous nutritional advice. Before accepting alternative health products or suggestions, check for supporting evidence and reputable credentials. If in doubt, check with a physician or registered dietitian.

STUDY QUESTIONS

1. What is the difference between a "natural" and an "organic" product? What do these terms have in common?
2. What products are typically sold in health food stores? Which products are harmless? Which may be potentially harmful?
3. List some common claims for vitamin and mineral supplements. Evaluate these claims—why or why aren't such claims accurate? In what situations are vitamin or mineral supplements sometimes warranted?
4. List three "alternative" therapies and provide a brief explanation of each therapy's approach. Why might these therapies be potentially dangerous?
5. What groups of people in the United States do you think may be more susceptible to nutrition fraud? Why? What products are frequently sold to such groups of people?

REFERENCES

1. ADA Reports: Position of the American Dietetic Association: Identifying food and nutrition misinformation, *Journal of the American Dietetic Association* 88:1589, 1988.
2. Barrett S: *Health schemes, scams, and frauds,* Mt Vernon, NY, 1990, Consumer Reports Books.
3. Campion EW: Why unconventional medicine? *The New England Journal of Medicine* 283:282, 1993.
4. Cornacchia HJ, Barrett S: *Consumer health,* ed 4, St Louis, 1993, Mosby–Year Book.
5. Cramer T: Cal-Ban banned, *FDA Consumer,* p. 39, June 1992.
6. Dagnelie PC and others: High prevalence of rickets in infants on macrobiotic diets, *American Journal of Clinical Nutrition* 51:202, 1990.
7. Gelb L: Hope hoax? Unproven cancer treatments, *FDA Consumer,* p. 10, March 1992.
8. Goldman B: American crusader brings message about health care fraud to Canada, *Canadian Medical Association Journal* 140:1189, 1989.
9. Green S: A critique of the rationale for cancer treatment with coffee and diet, *Journal of the American Medical Association* 268:3224, 1992.
10. Haller JS: A short history of the quack's materia medica, *New York State Journal of Medicine,* p. 520, September 1989.
11. Johnson GC, Gottesman RA: The health fraud battle, *Postgraduate Medicine* 85:289, 1989.
12. Kassler WJ and others: The use of medicine herbs by human immunodeficiency virus–infected patients, *Archives of Internal Medicine* 151:2281, 1991.
13. King L: Quackery, *Journal of the American Medical Association* 261:1979, 1989.
14. Kleiner SM: Beware of nutrition quackery, *Physician and Sportsmedicine* 18:46, 1990.
15. Kuske TT: Fads and quackery in nutrition, *Journal of the Medical Association of Georgia* 80:159, 1991.
16. Philen RN and others: Survey of advertising for nutritional supplements in health and body building magazines, *Journal of the American Medical Association* 268:1008, 1992.
17. Richmond C: The campaign against health fraud, *Practitioner* 233:1329, 1989.
18. Simko MD, Jarosz L: Organic foods: are they better? *Journal of the American Dietetic Association* 90:367, 1990.
19. Stare FJ: Combatting misinformation—a continuing challenge for nutrition professionals, *Nutrition Today,* p. 43, May/June 1992.

RATE

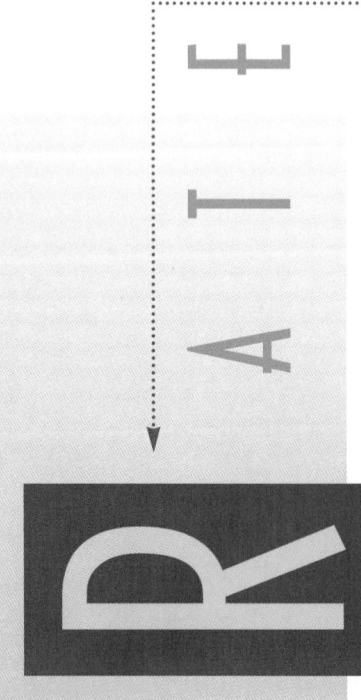

SHOULD I BAG THE BROWN FOOD?

Many articles in popular magazines have provocative titles such as the following: "Newest Nutrition Breakthroughs"
"The Latest Secret to Weight Control"
"Exclusive Formula for Building Your Largest Muscles"
"The Only Diet to Conquer Chronic Fatigue"

Finding truth amid this hype is a challenge. Your powers to evaluate such claims should have been sharpened with this chapter. These consumer skills will save money, disappointment, and wasted time. The following article simulates those found in popular health and fitness magazines. Using information from this chapter, critically evaluate the article's claims and air of authority.

Conquering the Blues with Brown Food

By Wilma Fuzzlenuts, N.D.C.

Do you often feel like you are living in slow motion? Are you always tired? Is fun the last thing on your mind? You might be suffering from what doctors now call Chronic Fatigue Syndrome—also called "Yuppie Flu." Many respectable scientists and doctors attribute the syndrome to a continual viral infection. Dr. Mickey Fibernugget, an endocrinologist, commented, "I was seeing so many tired patients in my practice that I knew it had to have some medical cause."

Would you like to have more energy? Feel sexier? Recapture that ambition to succeed in life? Well, a little known medical breakthrough may be the stroke of luck to lead you from your troubles. Recently discovered in a small laboratory and medical clinic in Bentenhausen, Norway, this miracle diet has not yet reached the desks of most physicians, nutritionists, and scientists.

When Dr. Val Hornwhipper, Ph.D., noted psychologist, fed his tired patients a diet of only brown food, their energy level and vigor vastly improved. Dr. Hornwhipper claims his Brown Food Empowerment Diet changes lives after only 2 weeks.

How does the brown food diet restore vigor? According to Dr. Nord Viplaugher, noted scientist of the Chocolate Guild in Norway, this exciting new diet speeds up your metabolic rate. You immediately feel energized. Viplaugher refers to this biochemical effect as "catalytic kinetics." In addition, brown food naturally causes your body's immune cells to destroy many different viruses.

By properly incorporating foods like brown rice, chocolate, brown bean soup, brown bread, and coffee, you can eliminate fatigue problems. Helen Howrowitz says, "After following the Brown Food Empowerment Diet for 1 week I felt like I could run a marathon." Vird Veerplank, world-class cross country skier, raved, "I've never performed like this in my sport." Over 20 psychologists and physicians now promote this exciting fatigue-buster.

Why feel tired for even 1 more day? Buy Dr. Hornwhipper's book, *The Brown Food Empowerment Diet* and begin waking up to high energy days. You have discovered a future your physician probably never dreamed of.

Wilma Fuzzlenuts is a National Dietary Consultant for the Wambaugh Holistic Eating Center. She has run five marathons and has worked in nutrition for 10 years. Much of her knowledge comes from personally experimenting with foods to improve her athletic performance.

Evaluation

1. Evaluate this article using characteristics of food faddists (p. 79) and "How to Evaluate Claims" (p. 77). In your critique include aspects of the article that intrigued you and aspects that made you suspicious.
2. After critiquing Fuzzlenut's article, would you buy Hornwhipper's book or follow his brown food diet?

your plate

Nutrition ISSUE

APPLYING LOGIC TO NUTRITION

Like other sciences the study of nutrition has developed by using the scientific method, a procedure for testing that is designed to detect and eliminate error. Scientists begin by observing life. They speculate about the causes of phenomena and suggest possible explanations called ***hypotheses*** for what they observe. Hypotheses must then be tested in controlled, scientific ***experiments.*** The data gathered from these experiments may either support or refute each hypothesis. If data or evidence from many experiments supports a hypothesis, it becomes generally accepted by scientists and can be called a ***theory*** (such as the theory of gravity). Very often, the results from one experiment suggest a new set of questions to be answered.

A scientist must be skeptical of hypotheses and theories by not accepting them immediately when there is little evidence and rejecting those that fail to pass critical analyses (Figure 3-4). In the science of nutrition we must keep a healthy skepticism and be very critical of many current ideas about nutrition.[19]

Where Do Hypotheses Come From?

By studying the history of diseases and specific health disasters, such as the large outbreaks of scurvy during the fifteenth through nineteenth centuries, scientists observe clues to causes of poor health. Other clues come from seeing general patterns of diseases and diet habits in whole populations of people in various parts of the world. The study of disease patterns in populations is called ***epidemiology.***

When European explorers left Europe to come to the Americas in the fifteenth and sixteenth centuries, many developed ***scurvy*** while at sea. The sailors developed scurvy but their land-dwelling counterparts didn't. This was an epidemiological observation. Only after many years was scurvy proven to result from a vitamin deficiency. The sailors weren't getting enough vitamin C from the few fruits and vegetables available aboard the ship.

In the 1920s epidemiological studies helped Dr. Joseph Goldberger determine that the disease ***pellagra*** was caused by a dietary deficiency rather than by an infection. He noticed that prisoners in jail—but not their jailers—suffered from pellagra. If pellagra were an ***infectious disease,*** the prisoners would pass the infection to their jailers and the disease would occur in both populations.

During World War II, the German army blockaded the Russian city of Leningrad and the people began to suffer from undernutrition. Along with widespread undernutrition there was an increase in infant deaths during childbirth, an occurrence that had been much rarer when the population was able to eat a nutritious diet. Scientists in North America later speculated that pregnant women might benefit from food supplements in terms of survival for their infants.

Epidemiology
The study of how disease rates vary between different population groups—for example, a comparison of the rates of stomach cancer in Japan and in Germany.

Scurvy
The deficiency disease that results after a few months of not consuming enough vitamin C (see Chapter 8).

Infectious Disease
Any disease caused by an invasion of the body by microorganisms, such as bacteria, fungi, or viruses.

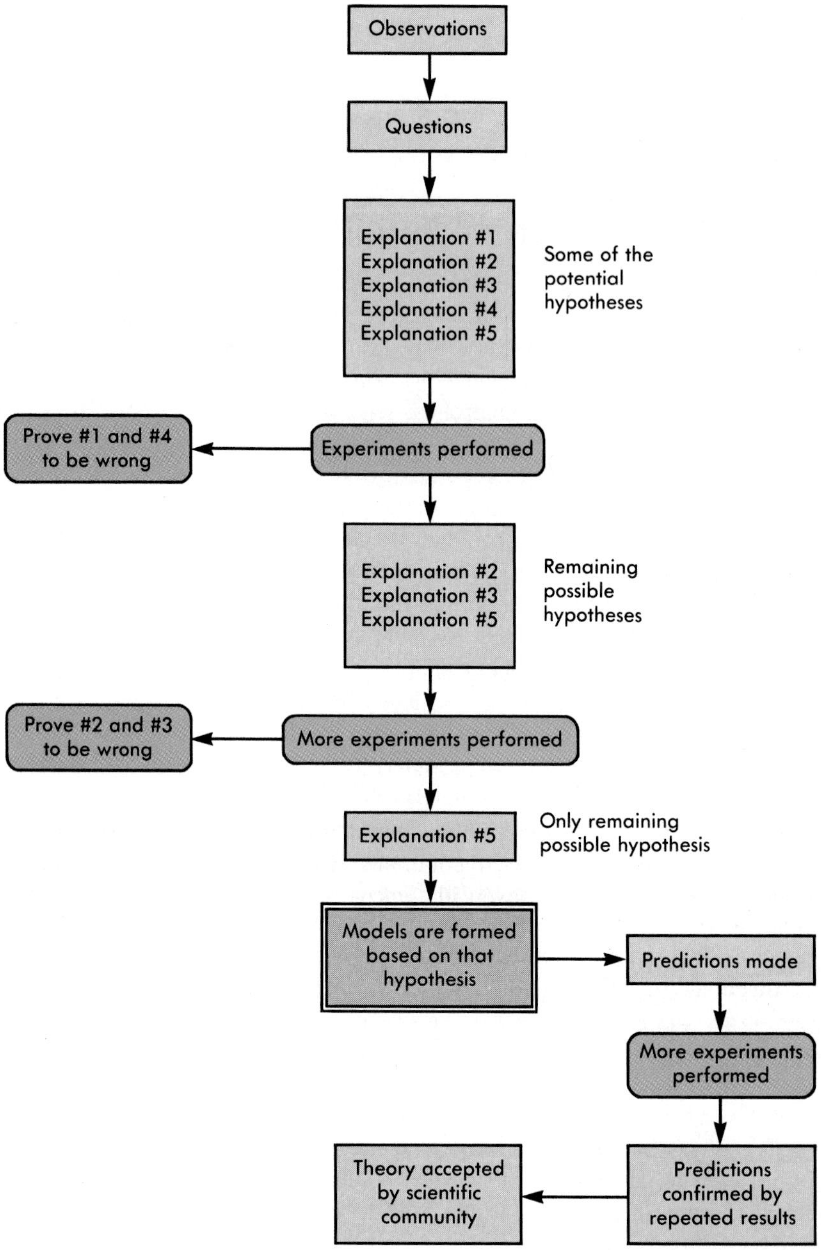

FIGURE 3-4
From question to theory—the process of science applied to nutrition. Only after careful and thorough analysis does a research finding deserve to influence our food choices.

In the 1970s Dr. Denis Burkitt noted that Africans had a low rate of intestinal problems, as compared with North Americans and Europeans. Burkitt speculated that the large amount of dietary fiber eaten by Africans led to greater intestinal health, whereas the little amount of dietary fiber eaten by many North Americans and Europeans caused intestinal problems and might be related to cancer development.

Testing the Assumptions of Epidemiology

Epidemiological observations by themselves do not establish that a dietary problem causes a certain disease. We need better evidence. This requires experimental testing. In the case of scurvy, British scientists eventually discovered that lime juice cured the scurvy.

But it wasn't until about 300 years later that vitamin C, the crucial substance in citrus fruit that prevents scurvy, was discovered.

As science grew more sophisticated, so did experimental tests. In the 1920s various foods were fed to people in mental asylums who suffered from pellagra. The experiment showed that yeast and high-protein foods could cure pellagra. In another experiment, food supplements were given to poor women in Boston and Toronto who were at risk for nutrient deficiencies to see what effect supplements had on their pregnancies. Results of this experiment showed that food supplements did increase the chances of having a healthy baby.

Experiments in these cases have shown without a doubt that dietary deficiencies can cause scurvy and pellagra and impair pregnancy outcome. However, it is not always so easy to prove a cause and effect relationship. For example, the importance of dietary fiber is still being established. So far, experiments have shown that adding fiber to your diet will often improve the health of your intestines, but more testing with regard to cancer prevention is still needed. This is discussed in Chapter 5.

Using Animal Experiments to Study Epidemiology

When scientists cannot test their hypotheses on humans, they often use animals. Much of what we know about human nutritional needs and functions derives from animal experiments. In the 1930s scientists showed that a pellagra-like disease seen in dogs, called blacktongue, was cured by nicotinic acid. But only when nicotinic acid actually cured the related disease pellagra in humans were scientists convinced that nicotinic acid, later called niacin (a vitamin), was the critical dietary factor. Thus when a disease found in animals mimics a particular human disease, the ***animal model*** can be used to test the human hypothesis.

Today we know that low doses of the mineral fluoride in the diet can strengthen teeth (see Chapter 9). It can also stimulate growth in rats. However, we still don't have experimental evidence for its effect on growth in humans. While some speculate that fluoride might stimulate growth in humans, there is no real proof.

In addition, there are ethical considerations in animal and human experiments. Some people think it is reasonable to feed rats a low-copper diet to study copper's importance in the formation of blood vessels, while others argue that animal experiments are unethical. Almost universally, however, people would find it unethical to study how a copper deficiency, which is potentially deadly, influences the formation of blood vessels in infants.

Ethical considerations, lack of animal models for specific human diseases, and insufficient funds are all reasons that scientists are often unable to test hypotheses that are suggested by epidemiological evidence.

another BITE

Throughout this book we will point out areas where more research is needed to answer important nutritional questions. Some of these questions arise from epidemiological studies or observations of scientists, which await testing in an experimental setting (either in an animal model or, even better, in the human clinical laboratory). Until overwhelming evidence supports a hypothesis, it should not be considered a nutrition "fact."

Conducting Experiments—Using Human Subjects to Answer Research Questions

An important type of experimental approach used to test hypotheses is the ***double-blind study.*** This starts with a group of ***subjects*** who follow specific instructions, such as eating certain foods. In addition, the experiment must balance this experimental group against a ***control group*** of subjects who do not change their normal pattern of living. Scientists

Double-Blind Study
An experiment where the subjects and researchers are unaware of the actual subject assignment and outcomes until the study is completed.

Control Group
Participants in an experiment whose habits are not altered.

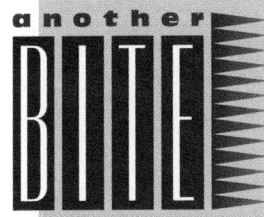

then observe the experimental group over time to see whether there are changes in this group that are not found in the control group. Sometimes subjects are used as their own control: first, they are observed for a period of time, and then they are observed after being treated to see what changes occur.

The bias (prejudice) of the subject or the experimenter can easily affect the outcome of an experiment. Either may have a stake in the outcome. Thus researchers need to limit the amount of bias they and their subjects bring to the experiment. The best way to do that is to *blind* the subjects and the scientific investigators so that neither knows which subjects are in the experimental group and which are in the control group. In addition, the outcome of the experiment is not disclosed until the entire study has been completed. Now we have all parts of a double-blind study: experimental group, control group, and "blinding" of all parties. This approach avoids the chance that the subjects may begin to feel better, for example, simply because they know they are part of an experimental group rather than a control group. Also, it avoids the possibility that researchers may see the change they want to see in the subjects in order to prove a certain hypothesis, even though the change did not actually occur. The effect of mere suggestion is referred to as the placebo effect. The Latin word placebo means "I shall please." The placebo effect cannot be accounted for on the basis of pharmacological or other direct physical action. Feeling better when the physician walks into the room is a common example of the placebo effect.

In a double-blind experiment, a ***placebo*** (fake medicine) is often given to the control group to camouflage who is in what group. Until the experiment is complete, only a third party knows which group is which. For some experiments, only a single-blind setup is possible. In single-blind experiments, either the subjects or the researchers are kept in the dark, but not both.

Vitamin experiments are often double-blind, because it is easy to develop a placebo that looks like a vitamin pill. However, food studies often cannot be placebo-controlled. It is hard to disguise a diet high in fruits and vegetables from one that has none. In such cases the experimenters should try to keep the results from the blood studies or other samples a secret until the end of the study. This way much of the bias can be eliminated. The less bias in an experiment, the more confidence we can have in the results.

Another type of experimental approach with humans is the case-control study, which can be considered almost a microscopic epidemiological study. It is a study wherein one looks at individuals with the condition in question, such as breast cancer, and compares them with a group without the condition but having similar characteristics not under study, such as age and gender. This comparison may point out factors, other than the condition in question, that differ between the two groups. Such knowledge may enable the researchers to determine the possible cause of the condition.

Sharing Experimental Results with Other Scientists

Once scientists complete an experiment, they summarize the findings and publish the results in a scientific journal. At the end of each chapter in this book you'll find a list of references for important experiments that have been published in scientific journals. Most of these journals are ***peer-reviewed.*** This means other scientists have been asked to review and judge the quality of the research; this is designed to ensure that only high-quality research findings are published. Because of peer review, research results published in the *American Journal of Clinical Nutrition,* the *New England Journal of Medicine,* or the *Journal of the American Dietetic Association* are much more reliable than those found in popular magazines, newspapers, and health newsletters, or promoted on television talk shows.

The Need for Follow-Up Studies

Even if a study follows all the rules and is accepted by the scientific community, one set of experimental results is not enough. Results from one laboratory must be confirmed by other laboratories (Figure 3-5). Only then can we really trust and use the results. We don't advise accepting new nutritional ideas as fact or applying them in your life until they are proven by several lines of evidence. Instead of drastically changing your diet in response to new scientific evidence, your best approach, in general, is to eat a variety of foods in moderate amounts.[19] See the discussions on olive oil and oat bran in Chapter 6 for further elaboration of this point. New diet recommendations may be made in the future, but these must be supported by multiple lines of evidence and ideally double-blind human trials before the public need take note.

FIGURE 3-5
Frank and Ernest.

FRANK & ERNEST ® by Bob Thaves

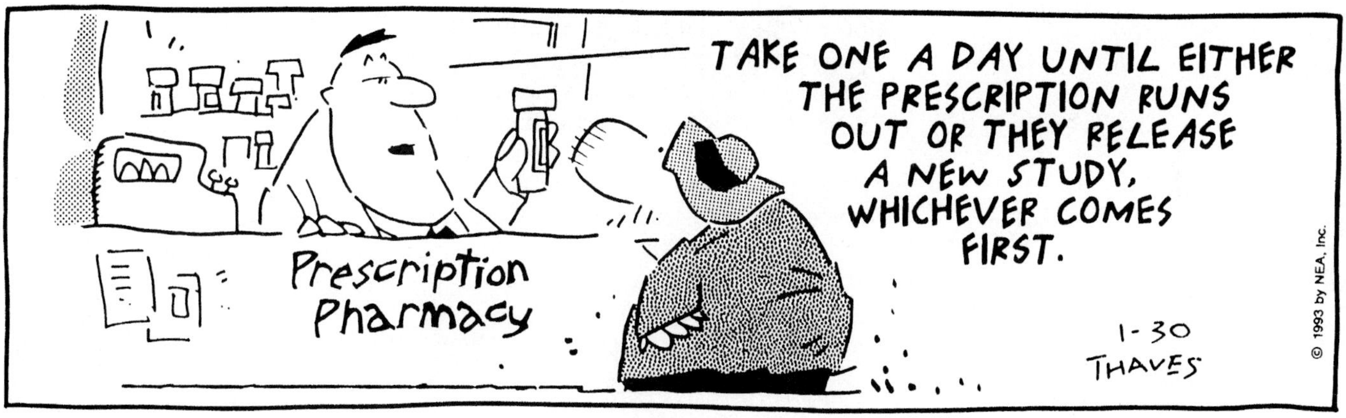

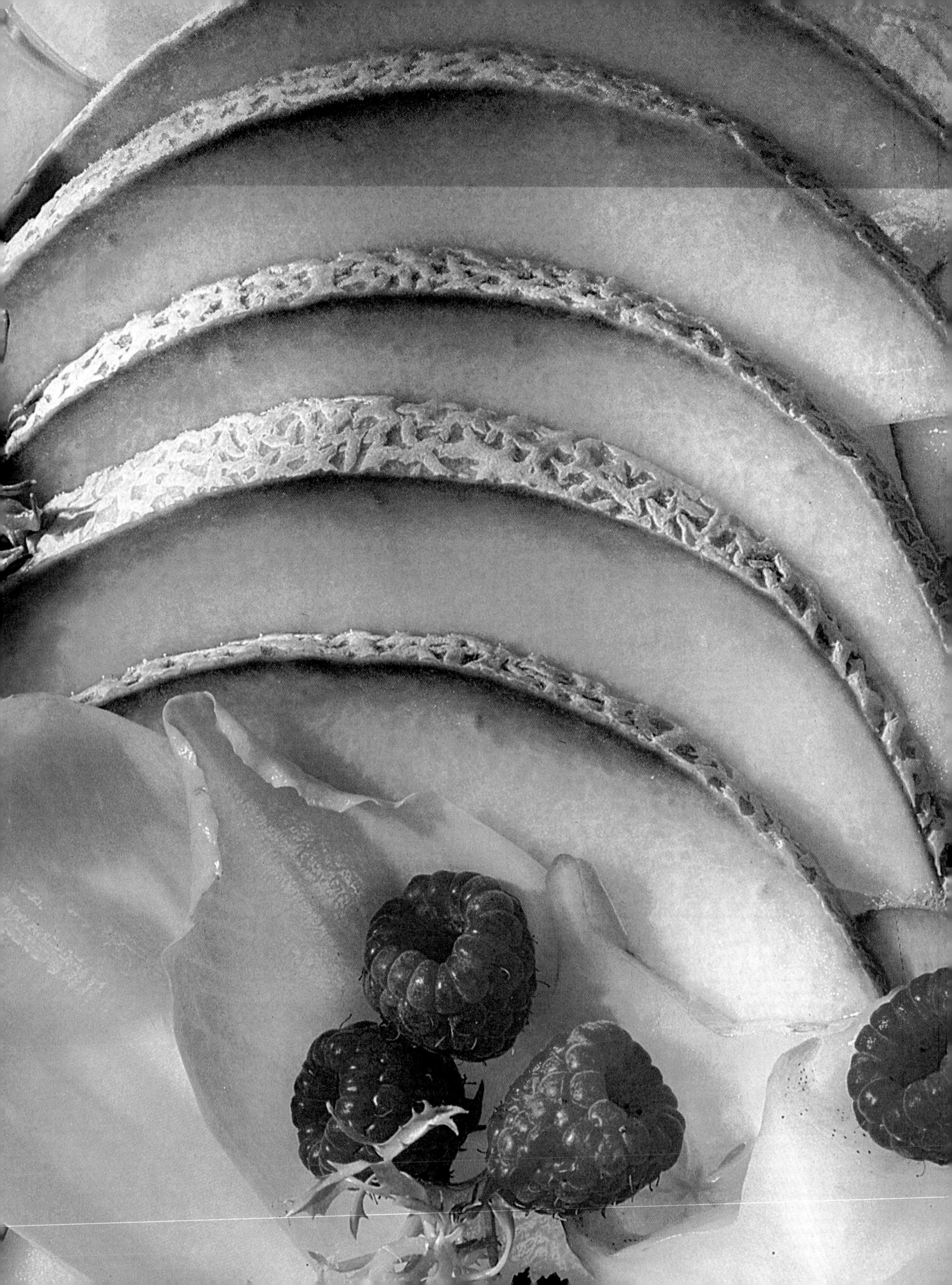

NUTRIENTS: THE HEART OF NUTRITION 2

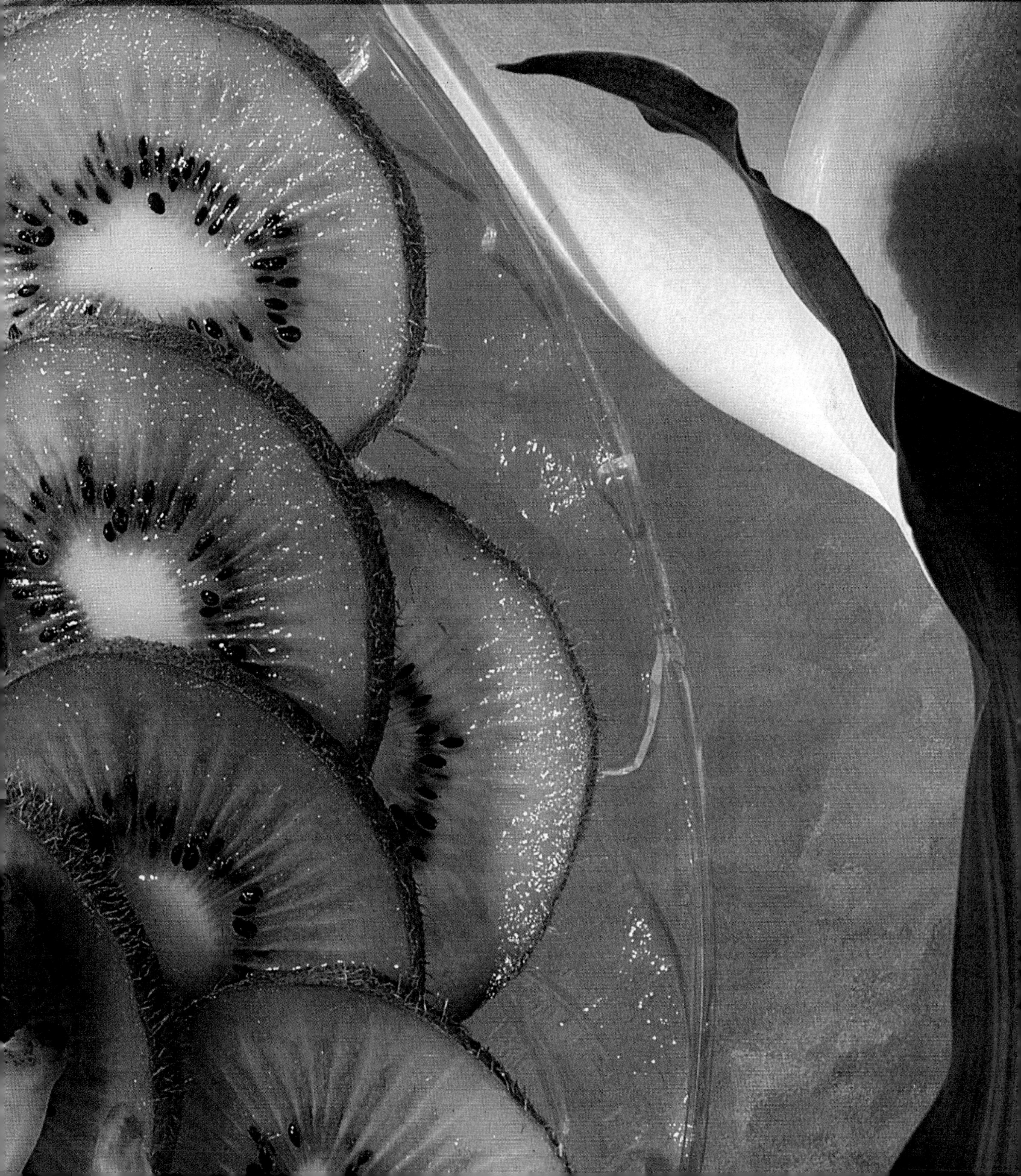

chapter

4

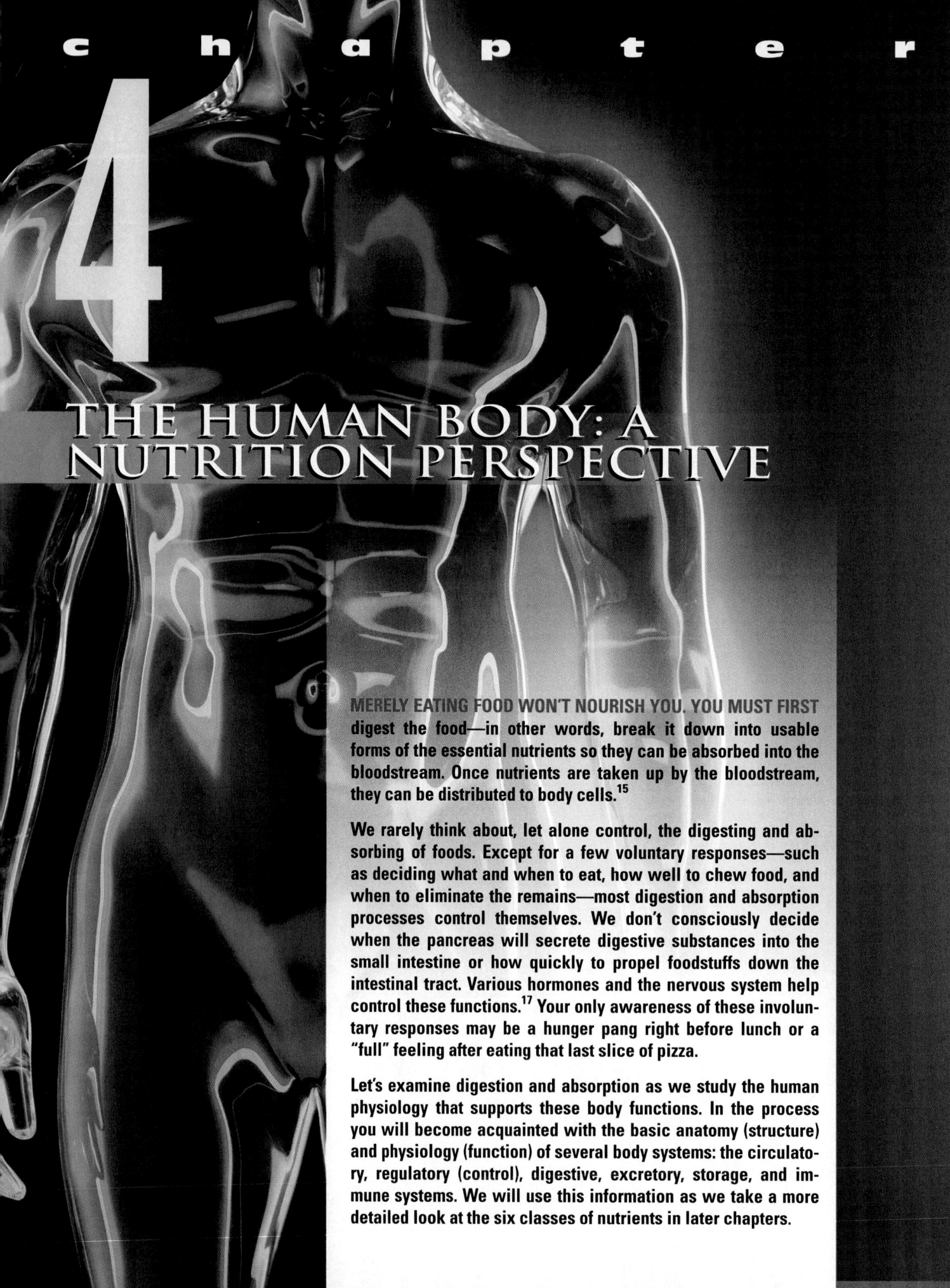

THE HUMAN BODY: A NUTRITION PERSPECTIVE

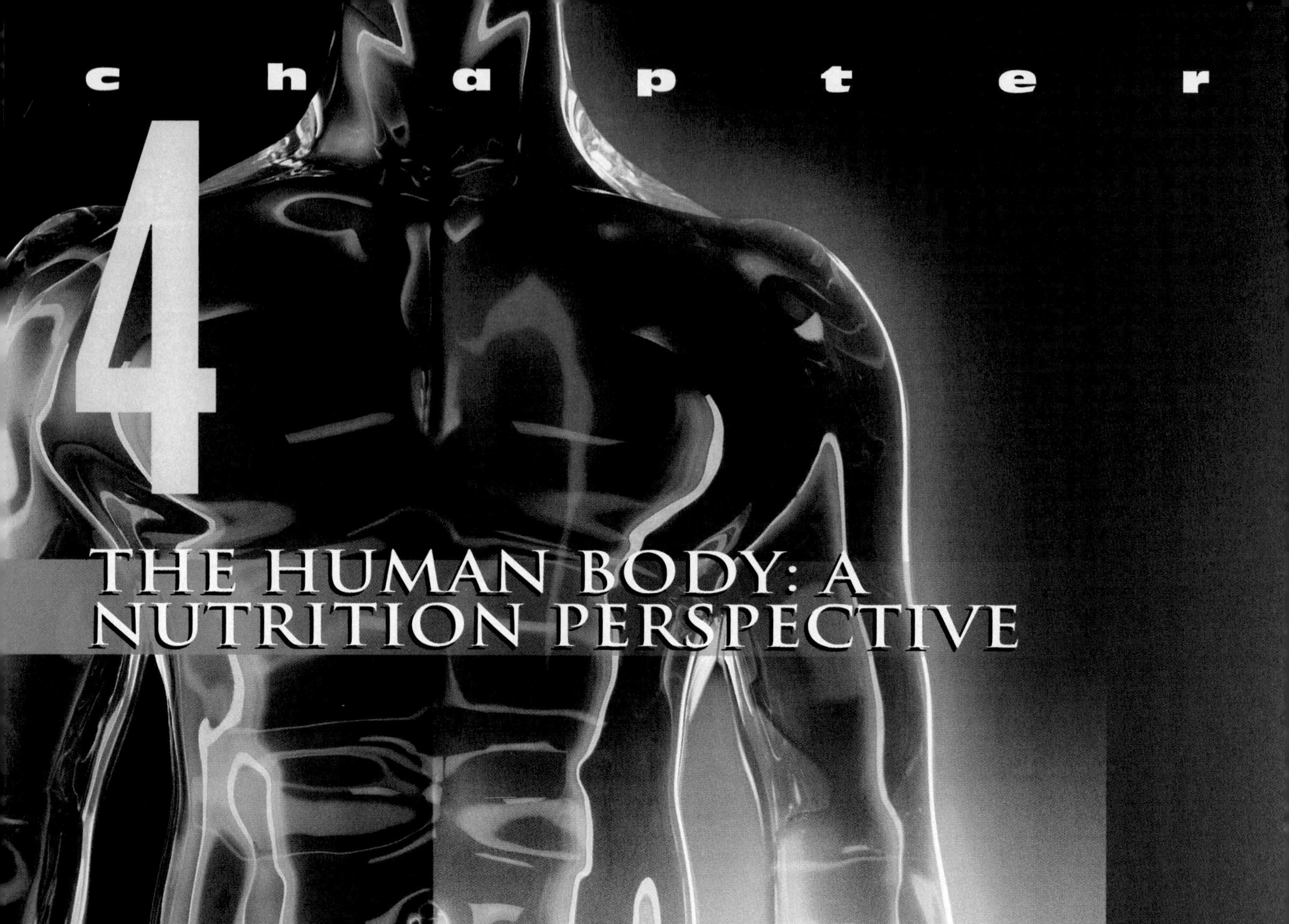

MERELY EATING FOOD WON'T NOURISH YOU. YOU MUST FIRST digest the food—in other words, break it down into usable forms of the essential nutrients so they can be absorbed into the bloodstream. Once nutrients are taken up by the bloodstream, they can be distributed to body cells.[15]

We rarely think about, let alone control, the digesting and absorbing of foods. Except for a few voluntary responses—such as deciding what and when to eat, how well to chew food, and when to eliminate the remains—most digestion and absorption processes control themselves. We don't consciously decide when the pancreas will secrete digestive substances into the small intestine or how quickly to propel foodstuffs down the intestinal tract. Various hormones and the nervous system help control these functions.[17] Your only awareness of these involuntary responses may be a hunger pang right before lunch or a "full" feeling after eating that last slice of pizza.

Let's examine digestion and absorption as we study the human physiology that supports these body functions. In the process you will become acquainted with the basic anatomy (structure) and physiology (function) of several body systems: the circulatory, regulatory (control), digestive, excretory, storage, and immune systems. We will use this information as we take a more detailed look at the six classes of nutrients in later chapters.

HOW HEALTHY IS YOUR DIGESTIVE TRACT?

We rarely think about our digestive tract until we notice an unpleasant symptom. But there are eating routines we can practice to keep this system functioning efficiently. The following assessment is designed to get you to examine your habits and symptoms associated with the health of your digestive tract. Put a "Y" in the blank to the right of the question to indicate a yes and an "N" to indicate a no.

1. Are you currently experiencing greater than normal stress and tension? ______
2. Do you have a family history of digestive tract problems such as ulcers, hemorrhoids, diverticulosis, constipation, or lactose intolerance? ______
3. Do you feel pain in your stomach region about 2 hours after you eat? ______
4. Do you smoke cigarettes? ______
5. Do you take aspirin frequently? ______
6. Do you feel the gnawing pain of heartburn in your upper chest at least once a week? ______
7. Do you frequently lie down immediately after eating? ______
8. Do you feel abdominal pain, bloating, and gas about 30 minutes to 2 hours after consuming milk products? ______
9. Do you often have to strain while having a bowel movement? ______
10. Do you drink less than 6 to 8 cups of water or other fluids per day? ______
11. Do you exercise aerobically (jog, swim, walk briskly, row, stairclimb) for less than 20 to 30 minutes, three times per week? ______
12. Do you eat a diet relatively low in dietary fiber? (A diet high in dietary fiber contains liberal quantities of whole fruits, vegetables, legumes, nuts and seeds, whole-grain breads, and cereals.) ______
13. Do you frequently experience diarrhea? ______
14. Do you frequently use laxatives or antacids? ______

Interpretation

Add up the number of Y's and record the total in the blank to the right. ______

If you score between 8 and 14, your habits and symptoms suggest that digestive problems are present and/or you risk experiencing digestive tract problems in the future. This chapter examines the processes of digestion and absorption. How these normal processes can be disrupted will be discussed. Take particular note of the habits you can adopt to cooperate with your digestive tract.

ASSESS YOUR KNOWLEDGE

TEST YOUR

yourself

BODY SYSTEMS USED IN DIGESTION AND ABSORPTION

The body is composed of millions of cells (see Appendix G for a review of the parts and structure of a cell if you do not recall this from previous coursework). Each is a self-contained, living entity. Cells represent the basic building blocks of the body, ultimately forming all body structures.

From Cells to Organ Systems

When cells of the same type work together for a common purpose—bound together by intercellular substances—they form ***tissues,*** such as bone, cartilage, muscle, and nerve. Often two or more tissues combine in a particular way to form more complex ***organs,*** such as skin, kidneys, and liver. At still higher levels of coordination, several organs can cooperate for a common purpose to form an organ system, such as the respiratory system or the digestive system. The human body is a coordinated unit of many such organ systems and is called an ***organism*** (Figure 4-1).[15]

Tissue
A group of cells designed to perform a specific function; muscle tissue is an example.

Organ
A group of tissues designed to perform a specific function—for example, the heart. It contains muscle tissue, nerve tissue, and so on.

Organism
A living thing. The human body is an organism consisting of many organs acting in a coordinated manner to support life.

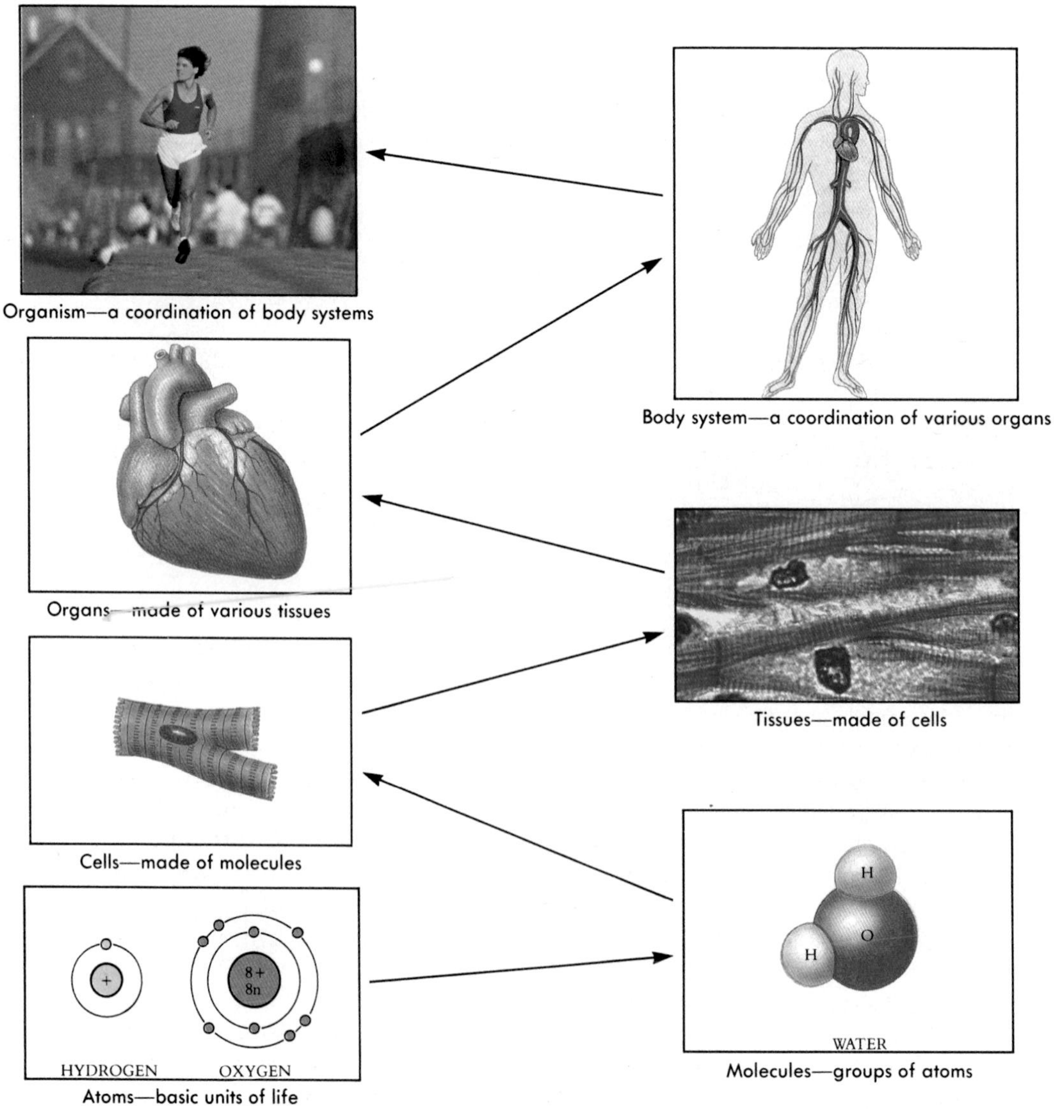

FIGURE 4-1
The levels of human biological organization. We are as simple as a collection of atoms and as complex as a whole organism.

Every cell in the human body performs a specialized job. A cell's master plan for its work and for generating the corresponding machinery necessary to do its work is encoded into the cell's genetic material, the ***deoxyribonucleic acid (DNA).*** The DNA acts as a blueprint for synthesizing specific proteins required to perform specific tasks in the body. Although most cells in our bodies contain the same DNA information, each cell is programmed to use only the subsets of DNA instructions that are applicable to perform its own tasks, depending on the type of tissue it is part of.[15] For example, stomach cells and bone marrow cells receive the same master plan. However, stomach cells use only a subset of the DNA code to make ***mucus,*** while cells in the bone marrow that make the oxygen-carrying protein hemoglobin use a different subset of the DNA code.

Chemical processes occur all the time in every living cell: the chemical synthesis of new substances is balanced by the chemical breakdown of other materials into smaller units. For these reactions to occur, the cell requires a continuous supply of energy and oxygen. Cells also need water, the medium in which they live. They further need their own building blocks, especially the materials they can't make themselves—the essential nutrients supplied from food. These substances enable the tissues, composed of individual cells, to function properly.

Healthful nutrition can supply adequate nutrients to all body cells. But to ensure the best use of these nutrients by cells, the following organ systems must also be healthy and working efficiently.

Mucus DNA
A thick fluid secreted by glands throughout the body. It contains a compound that is both carbohydrate and protein in nature. Mucus acts as both a lubricant and a means of protection for cells.

Lymphatic System
System of vessels that can accept fluid surrounding cells and large particles, such as products of fat absorption. This lymph fluid eventually passes into the bloodstream via the lymphatic system.

CIRCULATORY SYSTEM

Blood travels two basic routes. It circulates between the right side of the heart and the lungs (the pulmonary circuit) and between the left side of the heart and all other body parts (the systemic circuit) (Figure 4-2). The heart is a muscular pump that normally contracts and relaxes 50 to 90 times per minute while the body is at rest. This continuous pumping keeps blood moving through these circuits.

The circulatory system distributes nutrients yielded from digestion and absorption, along with oxygen from the air, to all body cells. All blood goes to the lungs to pick up oxygen and release carbon dioxide. The oxygenated blood then returns to the heart to be pumped to all other body tissues. In the capillaries, cells exchange nutrients and wastes with the blood: cells empty their waste products into the blood and take nutrients from it.[15] Capillaries, networks of tiny blood vessels, service every region of the body via individual capillary beds that are only one cell layer thick. Nutrients, gases, and other substances can pass through capillary cells to both enter into and exit out of other body cells. In this way, cells can take up needed nutrients and oxygen from the bloodstream and return waste products to the bloodstream for later external excretion.

Portal and Lymphatic Circulation Plays an Important Role in Nutrient Absorption

Fluids and particles, once absorbed through the intestinal wall, travel two different routes. One pathway is the bloodstream. As we noted, the blood—laden with oxygen and nutrients—leaves the heart and enters the arteries. Some of this blood travels to the intestine and ends up in capillary beds inside the intestine. From there, some nutrients are taken up by intestinal cells for nourishment, while much of the nutrients from foods recently eaten transfers into the bloodstream. The actual transfer points are the capillary beds. The blood then passes into veins and eventually collects in a very large vein, called the ***portal vein*** (see Figure 4-2).[15] This vein leads directly to the liver. Most veins in the body double back directly to the heart. However, by going first to the liver, the portal vein enables the liver to process absorbed nutrients before they enter the general circulation of the bloodstream. Most nutrients—such as glucose and amino acids—are water-soluble, and so they enter the bloodstream through the portal vein.

The ***lymphatic system*** is the second system of circulatory vessels that serves the body. It carries lymph, which is mostly made up of a clear fluid that forms between cells (see Figure 4-2). This fluid filters into tiny lymphatic vessels that compose a one-way network

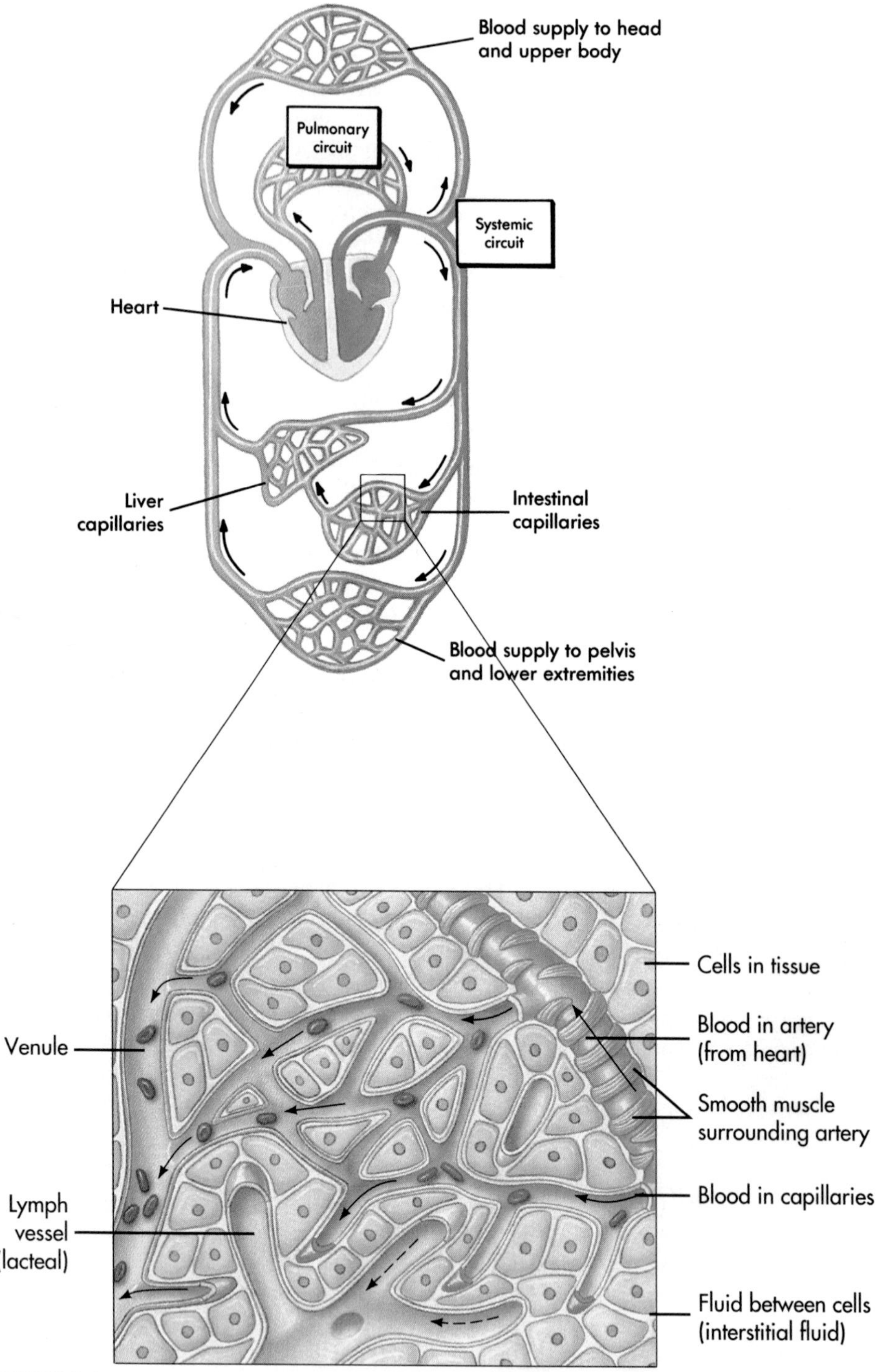

FIGURE 4-2

Blood circulation throughout the body. This represents the route blood takes through the two circuits that begin and end at the heart. The red color indicates blood that is richer in oxygen; blue is for blood carrying more carbon dioxide. Oxygen and nutrients are exchanged for carbon dioxide and waste products in the capillaries, the points at which the arteries and veins merge. A key player in this system is the portal vein, because it supplies the liver with nutrients absorbed from the intestinal tract. The box at the bottom shows a close up of a capillary bed in the small intestine, including the location of the lymphatic vessels. This second set of circulatory vessels—part of the lymphatic system—picks up fluid that builds up between cells (interstitial fluid) and large particles, such as some fats. This fluid and the particles become lymph. *This travels through further lymph vessels to reach the bloodstream. Lymph vessels in the intestine are also called* lacteals.

where they produce & what they do? < Hormon >

that funnels lymph from all over the body into large lymphatic vessels. From these vessels, the lymph fluid empties into major veins returning to the heart. The lymphatic system thereby serves as a second route to return fluids that eminate from the capillaries and ultimately must return to the circulatory system.

Lymphatic vessels that serve the small intestine have an important role in nutrition.[4] These vessels pick up and transport the majority of products yielded from fat absorption—those substances too large to enter the bloodstream directly. The lymphatic vessels from the intestine drain into a large duct that stretches from the abdomen to the neck. This duct connects with the bloodstream through a vein near the neck. It is in this way that the majority of absorbed fat products eventually enter the bloodstream. Other parts of the lymphatic system play a key role in our immune system.[5]

REGULATORY (CONTROL) SYSTEMS

The hormonal and nervous systems form two regulatory mechanisms that greatly influence nutrient use in the body.[4] The hormone insulin helps control blood glucose levels, and thyroid hormones help control the body's metabolic rate. Hormones that are especially important in regulating digestive processes include ***gastrin, secretin,*** and ***cholecystokinin (CCK)*** (Table 4-1). Gastrin primarily influences digestive processes in the stomach, whereas secretin and CCK act primarily on the pancreas and gallbladder, two organs that participate in the digestive processes. Insulin and CCK also are involved in hunger regulation (see Chapter 10).

Nerves influence acid ***secretion*** in the stomach and regulate intestinal muscle action. The senses of sight, hearing, touch, smell, and taste all use nerve pathways to communicate information—such as the availability of food or the need for it—to the brain. Some nutrients are important in nerve functioning, especially the vitamins thiamin and niacin.

Gastrin *A hormone that stimulates enzyme and acid secretion by the stomach.*

Secretin *A hormone that both causes the pancreas to release bicarbonate ion and slows stomach emptying.*

Cholecystokinin (CCK) *A hormone that stimulates enzyme release from the pancreas and bile release from the gallbladder.*

Secrete *To produce and then release a substance, generally called a secretion, from a cell into the body.*

Gastrointestinal (GI) Tract *The main sites in the body used in nutrient digestion and absorption. It consists of the mouth, esophagus, stomach, small intestine, large intestine, rectum, and anus.*

Digestion *The process whereby food is broken down into forms that can be taken up by the GI tract.*

CONCEPT CHECK

Digestion and absorption require the coordinated efforts of many body systems. These processes aid in supplying energy, oxygen, water, and essential nutrients to all body cells. The circulatory and lymphatic systems transport nutrients throughout the body. The hormonal and nervous systems are two regulatory (control) mechanisms that help direct nutrient use and the digestive process.

THE PHYSIOLOGY OF DIGESTION

The ***gastrointestinal (GI) tract,*** also known as the ***alimentary canal*** or digestive tract, is a long tube stretching from the mouth to the anus (Figure 4-3). Nutrients from the food we eat must pass through the walls of this tube—from the inside to the outside— to be absorbed into the bloodstream. The GI tract promotes ***digestion*** and absorption through a variety of functions: it simultaneously moves and "grinds" foods (a process called "motility"). This is the "physical" phase of digestion. The GI tract also secretes chemical substances to promote the breakdown of foods. This is the "chemical" phase of digestion. Finally, the GI tract eliminates wastes. Adding to this, the GI tract also promotes nutrient production; the bacteria living in the intestine make certain vitamins we can then use.[4]

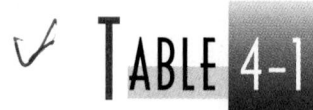

TABLE 4-1

Some Hormones That Regulate Digestion

Hormone	Origin	Stimulus to Secretion	Action
Gastrin	Lower region of the stomach	Food and other substances in the stomach, especially proteins, caffeine, spices, alcohol; nerve input	Stimulates flow of stomach enzymes and stomach acid
Cholecystokinin (CCK)	Upper small intestine	Food, especially fat and protein in upper small intestine	Causes contraction of gallbladder and in turn flow of bile to upper small intestine; causes secretion of enzyme-rich pancreatic juice and bicarbonate-rich pancreatic juice into upper small intestine
Secretin	Upper small intestine	Acid stomach contents entering the small intestine	Causes secretion of bicarbonate-rich pancreatic juice into upper small intestine and reduces stomach contractions

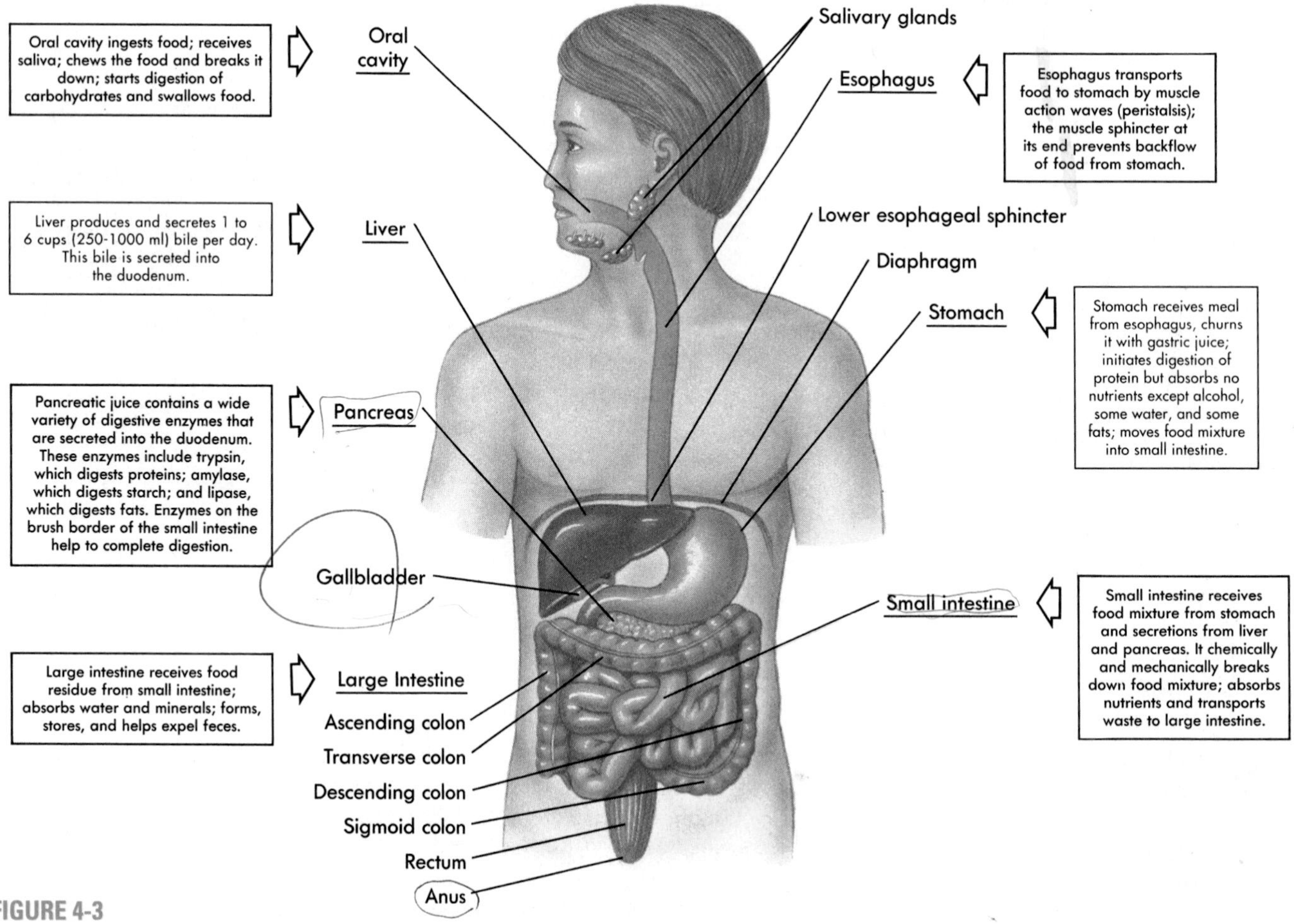
Oral cavity ingests food; receives saliva; chews the food and breaks it down; starts digestion of carbohydrates and swallows food.
Oral cavity
Salivary glands
Esophagus
Esophagus transports food to stomach by muscle action waves (peristalsis); the muscle sphincter at its end prevents backflow of food from stomach.
Liver produces and secretes 1 to 6 cups (250-1000 ml) bile per day. This bile is secreted into the duodenum.
Liver
Lower esophageal sphincter
Diaphragm
Stomach
Stomach receives meal from esophagus, churns it with gastric juice; initiates digestion of protein but absorbs no nutrients except alcohol, some water, and some fats; moves food mixture into small intestine.
Pancreatic juice contains a wide variety of digestive enzymes that are secreted into the duodenum. These enzymes include trypsin, which digests proteins; amylase, which digests starch; and lipase, which digests fats. Enzymes on the brush border of the small intestine help to complete digestion.
Pancreas
Gallbladder
Small intestine
Small intestine receives food mixture from stomach and secretions from liver and pancreas. It chemically and mechanically breaks down food mixture; absorbs nutrients and transports waste to large intestine.
Large intestine receives food residue from small intestine; absorbs water and minerals; forms, stores, and helps expel feces.
Large Intestine
Ascending colon
Transverse colon
Descending colon
Sigmoid colon
Rectum
Anus

FIGURE 4-3

The organization and function of organs of the gastrointestinal (GI) tract. Many organs work in a coordinated fashion to digest food, absorb nutrients, and eliminate waste products.

TABLE 4-2

Important Secretions of the Digestive Tract

Secretion	Site of Production	Purpose
Saliva	Mouth	Contributes to starch digestion, lubrication
Mucus	Mouth, stomach, small intestine, large intestine	Protects cells, lubricates
Enzymes	Mouth, stomach, small intestine, pancreas	Promotes digestion of foodstuffs in particles small enough for absorption
Acid	Stomach	Promotes digestion of protein among other functions
Bile	Liver (stored in gallbladder)	Suspends fat in water to aid fat digestion in the small intestine
Bicarbonate	Pancreas	Neutralizes stomach acid when it reaches the small intestine

The Flow of Digestion

Let's review the major body parts of the GI tract, starting with the mouth. Even before you put food into your mouth, you may experience a sudden rush of ***saliva*** in response to the mere sight or smell of food. This saliva, secreted by special glands in the mouth, contains ***mucus*** that envelops and lubricates each morsel, easing its passage down the GI tract (Table 4-2). Saliva also contains specific substances that break down large carbohydrates into small units. Chewing breaks food into small pieces, exposing more food surface to digestive action. The more surface exposed, the more efficient digestion is in the mouth and throughout the entire GI tract as well.[4]

Saliva *A watery fluid produced by the salivary glands in the mouth; it contains lubricants, enzymes, and other substances.*

The tongue aids chewing and also contains taste sensors for sweet, salt, sour, and bitter.[14] The sweet and salt sensors are near the tip of the tongue; the sour and bitter sensors are near the base. These taste sensors are most sensitive in childhood, and often fade in response in the elderly years.[13]

The mouth and stomach are connected by a tube called the esophagus. At its top is a flap of tissue (called the epiglottis) that prevents food from being swallowed into the trachea (windpipe). During swallowing, food lands on the flap, folding it down to cover the opening of the trachea. Breathing also automatically stops. These responses ensure that swallowed food will only travel down the esophagus, helped along by the lubricating mucus, muscular contractions, and gravity (Figure 4-4).

The food then enters the stomach, which is basically a 4-cup (1-liter) holding tank. Only proteins are significantly digested in the stomach. This protein digestion proceeds as the stomach secretes digestive acid and enzymes to help break down the food and slowly churns these into the food. (Later sections discuss the role of acid and enzymes in the digestive process in detail.) A meal usually leaves the stomach within 2 to 3 hours of eating.[4] Solids take longer than liquids to leave the stomach, and a fatty meal usually leaves later than a meal containing mostly protein or carbohydrate.

The stomach is connected to the 10 feet of small intestine, which is coiled inside the abdomen. The small intestine is considered "small" only because of its narrow diameter. Its considerable length provides ample opportunity for digestion to occur.

At death, the muscles of the small intestine relax, allowing the small intestine to lengthen to about 23 feet as measured at autopsy. This 23-foot length is a figure that is often cited in textbooks.

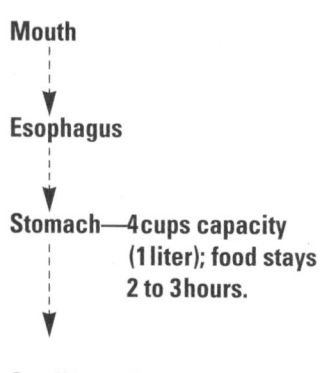

Colon Another name for the large intestine.

Bile A substance secreted by the liver and stored in the gallbladder; it is released into the small intestine to aid fat absorption by suspending fat in tiny droplets within a watery fluid.

Sphincter A muscular valve; these valves help control flow of foodstuffs in the GI tract.

Heartburn A pain emanating from the esophagus due to stomach acid backing up into the esophagus and irritating its tissue.

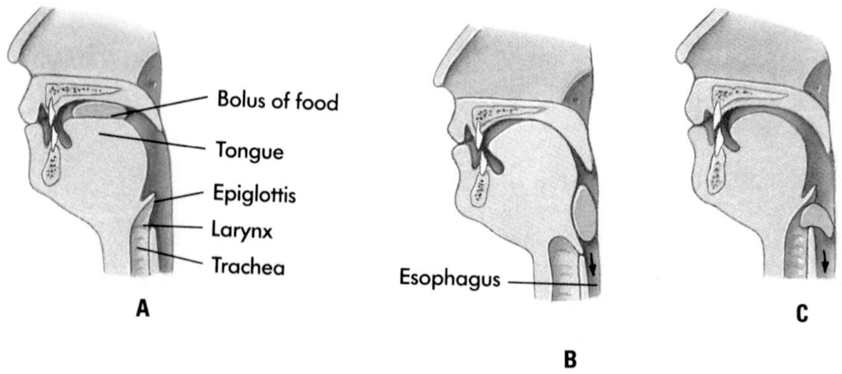

FIGURE 4-4
The process of swallowing. During swallowing, food cannot normally enter the trachea because the epiglottis closes over the larynx. The arrow shows that this allows food to head down the esophagus **(A, B).** *When a person chokes, food becomes lodged in the trachea, thereby blocking airflow to the lungs* **(C).** *The food should have gone down the esophagus to prevent choking.*

Muscular contractions constantly mix the food in the small intestine. This churning enhances digestive action, because it exposes more food surface to enzyme action. A meal remains in the small intestine about 3 to 10 hours. About 95% of a total meal has been digested by the time it leaves.[15] Most digestion is completed in the upper half of the small intestine.

From the small intestine, food moves into the large intestine, also called the ***colon.*** This organ is about 3½ feet long. Bacteria in the large intestine digest mostly leftover plant fibers[9]; little else remains to be digested. The food remnants and wastes stay in the large intestine for about 24 to 72 hours before being eliminated.

The large intestine ends in a cavity called the rectum, which connects to the anus, the end of the GI tube. These final sections work with the large intestine to prepare the feces for elimination.

As we have mentioned before, other organs associated with the GI tract aid digestion in the small intestine (see Figure 4-3). The liver secretes ***bile*** needed to digest fat. Bile helps suspend fat in the watery digestive mixture, making the fat more available to the digestive processes. The body stores bile in the gallbladder until it is needed.[12] The pancreas secretes enzymes that aid digestion and bicarbonate (the chemical in baking soda) to neutralize the acid that was produced earlier in the stomach. Ducts leading from the pancreas and gallbladders merge, allowing the pancreatic juices and bile to blend as they are released into the upper small intestine for digestion.[15] In this way the liver, pancreas, and gallbladder work with the GI tract, but are not actually part of it.

GI Tract Flow

Mouth
↓
Esophagus
↓
Stomach—4 cups capacity (1 liter); food stays 2 to 3 hours.
↓
Small Intestine—10 feet long; food stays 3 to 10 hours.
↓
Large Intestine (Colon)—3½ feet long; food can remain up to 72 hours.

GI Tract Control Valves: Sphincters

A variety of ringlike muscles form valves, called ***sphincters,*** all along the GI tract (Figure 4-5). They retard or prevent backflow of partially digested food. These sphincters respond to various stimuli, such as signals from the nervous system, hormones, and the pressure that builds up around them.[4] A sphincter in the lower esophagus is critical for preventing backflow of stomach contents up into the esophagus. If highly acidic stomach contents come in contact with the esophagus, they can cause pain, known as ***heartburn.***[6]

The pyloric sphincter, located at the base of the stomach, controls the flow of processed foodstuffs from the stomach into the small intestine. Only about a teaspoon (a few milliliters) at a time of acidic stomach contents squirt into the small intestine. Such small amounts enable bicarbonate from the pancreas to efficiently neutralize the acid coming from the stomach.

At the end of the small intestine, another sphincter prevents the contents of the large intestine from reentering the small intestine. At the end of the large intestine are two final sphincters, one of which is under voluntary control. Once a child is toilet trained, he or

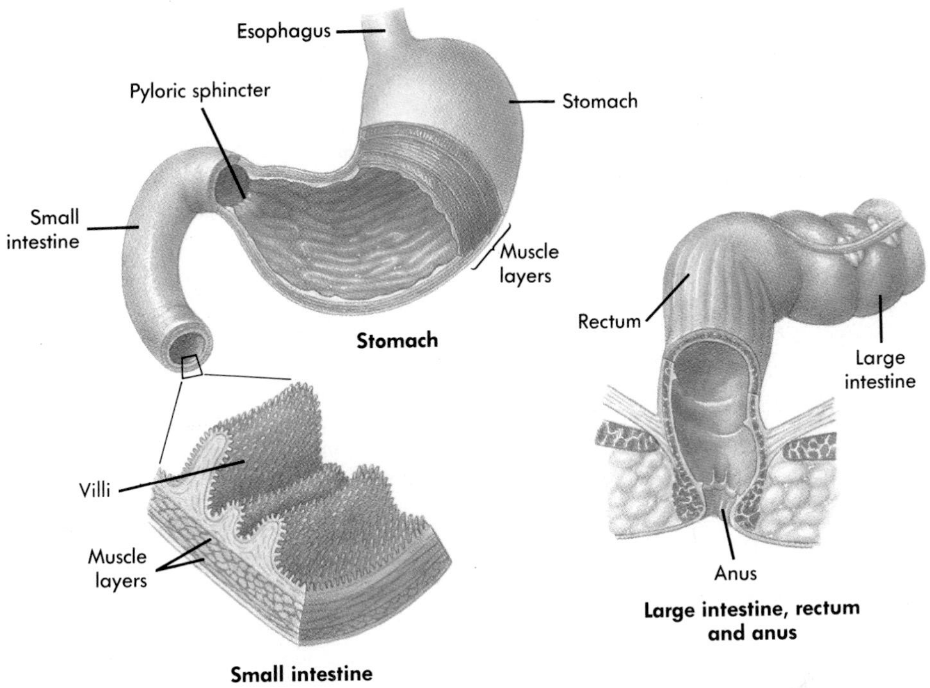

FIGURE 4-5

A close-up view of the intestinal tract—muscles, sphincters, and villi. These features of the GI tract perform key roles in digestion, absorption, and elimination.

she can fairly well determine when the outer sphincter will relax and when it will stay rigid, in turn affecting whether elimination occurs. Relaxation of the sphincter allows for elimation.

GI Tract Propulsion: Peristalsis

Food is propelled down the GI tract mainly by a wavelike process called ***peristalsis.*** Groups of muscles encircle the GI tract, while other groups run along its length (see Figure 4-5). When food is swallowed, coordinated squeezing and shortening by the muscle groups in the esophagus create two waves closely following each other. In the stomach, the same muscle action creates a mixing and grinding motion as often as three times each minute during digestion. More active peristaltic waves occur in the small intestine, about every 4 to 5 seconds.[15] In contrast, the large intestine has very sluggish peristalsis, using occasional large contractions—called ***mass movements***—to help eliminate the feces.

Peristalsis A coordinated muscular contraction that serves to propel food down the GI tract.

Mass Movements Peristaltic waves that are simultaneously coordinated over a large area of the colon. These move matter from one portion of the colon to another and from the colon into the rectum.

Enzymes Play a Vital Role in Digestion

As we noted earlier, enzymes play a key part in digestion. These substances essentially enhance digestion by making chemical breakdown more likely to happen. Enzymes bring specific chemicals close together and then create an environment that allows the chemicals to change forms (Figure 4-6). Almost every chemical process in the body, and especially digestive processes, requires an enzyme to hasten the event. The pancreas and small intestine produce most digestive enzymes. A few are secreted by the mouth and stomach (Table 4-3). Each type of enzyme can speed only one specific type of chemical process. For example, enzymes that recognize and digest table sugar (sucrose) ignore milk sugar (lactose). The body can even increase the synthesis of certain digestive enzymes in response to the type of diet consumed, for example, producing more fat-digesting enzymes in response to a high-fat diet.[17]

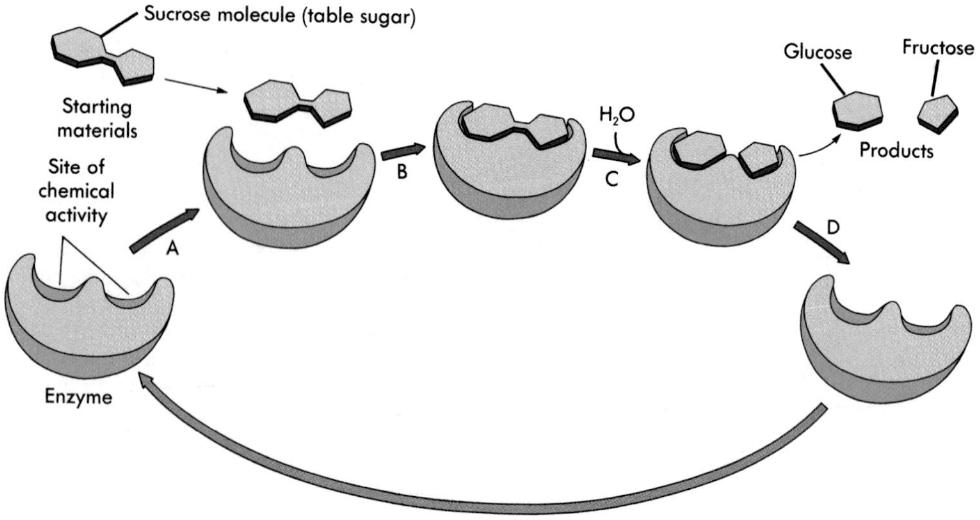

FIGURE 4-6

A model of enzyme action. With some enzymes, the chemical reaction can go both ways. Sometimes energy input is needed to help the enzyme push the reaction along.

TABLE 4-3

Examples of Key Digestive Enzymes

Secretion Origin	Enzyme	Target
Salivary glands	Salivary amylase	Starch
Stomach glands	Pepsin	Protein
Pancreas	Trypsin Chymotrypsin Pancreatic amylase Lipase	Protein Protein Starch Fat
Intestinal wall	Peptidases Maltase Sucrase Lactase	Small proteins Maltose Sucrose Lactose

Cystic Fibrosis
A disease that often leads to overproduction of mucus, among other effects. Mucus can invade the pancreas, decreasing enzyme output. The lack of lipase enzyme output then contributes to severe fat malabsorption.

Enzyme actions occur only under rather specific conditions. Besides working only on particular types of chemicals, enzymes are sensitive to acid and base conditions, temperature, and the types of vitamins and minerals they require. Digestive enzymes that work in the acid environment of the stomach do not work well in the alkaline (basic) environment of the small intestine.

Again, the pancreas is a major site of production for digestive enzymes. In ***cystic fibrosis***—an inherited disease of infants, children, and sometimes adults—the pancreas is often affected. It develops thick mucus that blocks its ducts, and active cells then die. As a result, the pancreas is not able to effectively deliver its digestive enzymes into the small intestine. Digestion of carbohydrate, protein, and—most notably—fat is impaired because the needed enzymes are not released in adequate amounts. Often these enzymes then must be ingested in capsule form with meals to aid in digestion, thereby preventing abdominal discomfort from malabsorption.[20] If much undigested protein, carbohydrate, or fat makes it into the large intestine, bacteria there make these into acids and gas (see the discussion on the large intestine on p. 109).

CONCEPT CHECK

The gastrointestinal (GI) tract consists of the mouth, esophagus, stomach, small intestine, large intestine (colon), rectum, and anus. Organs associated with the GI tract are the liver, gallbladder, and pancreas. Together these organs perform the digestion needed to extract nutrients from food and funnel them into the bloodstream. In the GI tract, peristalsis propels food from the esophagus to the anus. During this journey, digestion is aided by enzymes produced by the mouth, stomach, pancreas, and small intestine cells. The transit time between eating food and eventually eliminating the indigestible remains is usually about 1 to 3 days.

A CLOSER LOOK AT THE DIGESTIVE PROCESS

Even before we eat a morsel of many foods, the work of digestion—the breakdown of foods into usable forms we can absorb—is often partially accomplished for us. Cooking or other preparations—such as marinating, pounding, or dicing—have often begun the process. Starch granules in foods swell as they soak up water during cooking, making them much easier to digest. Cooking also softens the tough connective tissues in meats and the fibrous tissue of plants, such as is found in broccoli stalks. As a result, the food is easier to chew, swallow, and break down during later digestion. As you will see in Chapter 17, cooking also makes many foods—such as eggs, meats, fish, and poultry—much safer to eat.

Key Digestive Processes in the Stomach

The stomach secretes ***pepsin,*** a major enzyme used for protein digestion.[17] The release of pepsin is controlled by the hormone gastrin (see Tables 4-1 and 4-3). Just thinking about food or chewing food stimulates nerves in the brain that control special gastrin-producing cells in the base of the stomach. The release of gastrin then signals cells in the stomach to begin producing pepsin. Gastrin also stimulates other cells in the stomach to produce acid.

The stomach is protected from digesting itself—called ***autodigestion***—in several ways. Because the hormone gastrin is released only when we eat or think about eating, acid production is limited to these times. Furthermore, as the stomach becomes strongly acidic, gastrin release stops. The stomach also protects itself by secreting a thick layer of mucus that lines and insulates it from the acid and pepsin produced for digestion.

Key Digestive Processes in the Small Intestine

All liquids consumed with a meal combine with stomach acid to form a very watery food mixture called ***chyme.*** As this chyme squirts into the upper small intestine (called the duodenum), the acid in the chyme triggers the release of the hormone secretin. That hormone stimulates the pancreas to release bicarbonate, which neutralizes the acid, as we mentioned earlier. If the chyme is not neutralized, it corrodes the wall of the duodenum. This could quickly lead to an ***ulcer,*** because—unlike the stomach—the small intestine lacks a protective layer of mucus.[17] This form of protection is not possible, because it would impede nutrient absorption. Secretin also acts to reduce stomach peristalsis (motility), helping to prevent the stomach from overwhelming the small intestine with lots of chyme over a short period.

When food enters the small intestine, the hormone CCK is also released from the wall of the upper small intestine into the bloodstream.[16] This hormone then travels to the pan-

Pepsin *A protein-digesting enzyme produced by the stomach.*

Chyme *A mixture of stomach secretions and partially digested food.*

Ulcer *Erosion of the tissue lining in either the stomach or upper small intestine; generally referred to as a peptic ulcer.*

creas and gallbladder and causes these organs to release their products—namely, such enzymes as ***lipase*** from the pancreas and bile from the gallbladder (see Tables 4-1 and 4-3). Note that both lipase and bile are needed for fat digestion.

SMALL INTESTINE: SITE FOR MOST NUTRIENT ABSORPTION

Most nutrient absorption—that is, the transfer of nutrients from the intestine to the bloodstream—occurs in the small intestine; little is absorbed in the stomach or large intestine.[15] The small intestine can absorb about 95% of the kcalories it receives in the form of protein, carbohydrate, fat, and alcohol (Figure 4-7). The mouth and/or stomach absorb only water, small amounts of alcohol, certain types of minor fats, and some glucose. The large intestine absorbs some minerals, water, and some fat and carbohydrate by-products (produced by bacterial action).

Alcohol is not a nutrient per se, because it performs no essential role in the body. But as we mentioned in Chapter 1, alcohol does supply energy and is a common source of this in adult diets. Chapter 15 discusses alcohol in detail, especially as it relates to nutrition and overall health.

FRANK & ERNEST® by Bob Thaves

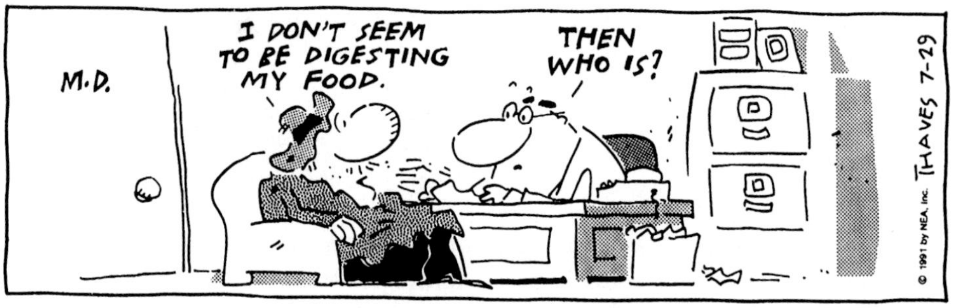

FIGURE 4-7
Frank and Ernest.

Lipase
Fat-digesting enzymes; lipase produced by the pancreas to act in the small intestine is the most important form used in digestion.

Villi
Fingerlike protrusions in the small intestine that participate in digestion and absorption of foodstuffs.

The enormous surface area of the small intestine promotes efficient nutrient absorption. The wall of the small intestine is folded, and within the folds are fingerlike projections called ***villi*** (see Figure 4-5). These "fingers" trap foodstuffs between each other to enhance absorption. Each villus "finger" is made up of numerous absorptive cells, and each of these cells has a highly folded cap, known as the brush border, or microvilli. The combined folds, fingers, and microvilli in the small intestine increase its surface area 600 times beyond that of a simple tube. New absorptive cells are constantly produced and appear daily along the surface of each villus "finger," most likely because absorptive cells are subjected to a harsh environment. This environment demands constant renewal of the intestinal lining as a biological necessity, and it leads to a high nutrient demand from the small intestine. The health of these cells is further enhanced by the various hormones and other substances that participate in or are produced as part of the digestive process.[9,11]

another BITE

Cancer treatments often involve the use of medications (chemotherapy) to prevent rapid cell growth. Cancer cell growth is the intended target. But, although the medications can slow the growth of rapidly-dividing cancer cells, they also affect other body cells that normally reproduce rapidly, such as the absorptive cells in the small intestine. This is why diarrhea is a common side effect of chemotherapy.

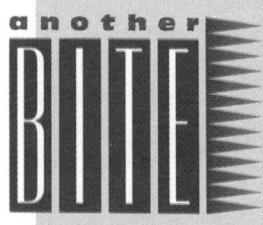

Types and Means of Absorption

The small intestine absorbs nutrients into the intestinal cells through various means and processes. For such nutrients as fats the intestine is easily permeable. When the nutrient concentration is higher in the inside cavity (***lumen***) of the smaller intestine than in the ***absorptive cells,*** the difference in nutrient concentration drives absorption because nutrients naturally move from higher to lower concentration. Fats and other nutrients now enter the absorptive cells from the lumen of the small intestine via this ***passive absorption*** route. Water and some minerals also are absorbed in this way.[3]

Another absorption mechanism uses both a carrier and energy input to actively pump nutrients from the lumen of the small intestine into the absorptive cells. This makes it possible for the body to take up nutrients even when they are not concentrated in the diet. Some sugars, for example, follow this route—called ***active absorption.*** The sugar glucose is much more concentrated in the absorptive cells than in the chyme in the small intestine, because the absorptive cells are bathed by the glucose-rich bloodstream. To get glucose into the absorptive cells—given the high concentration already present (an uphill battle, so to speak)—it must be pumped in using energy.[15]

A further means of active absorption entails the absorptive cells' literally engulfing compounds or liquids. A cell membrane can form an indentation itself, so that when particles or fluids move into the indentation, the cell membrane surrounds and engulfs them. This process is used when an infant absorbs immune substances from human milk (see Chapter 13).

The Large Intestine Completes Absorption

When the intestinal contents enter the large intestine, little of the original foodstuff eaten still remains. Only a minor amount (5%) of carbohydrate, protein, and fat has escaped absorption.[15] Some water is still present, because the small intestine absorbs only 85% to 90% of the fluid it receives, which includes large amounts of GI tract secretions produced during digestion. The remnants of the meal also include some minerals and food fibers (Figure 4-8).

In the upper half of the large intestine, much of the remaining water and the minerals—mostly sodium and potassium—is absorbed. The unabsorbed water now amounts to only a few ounces. Products from the metabolism of certain plant fibers and small amounts of undigested starches are also absorbed. The contents of the large intestine are semisolid by the time they have passed through the first two thirds of it. The stool remains in the last third until muscular movements push it into the rectum to be eliminated.

The presence of feces in the rectum stimulates elimination. As previously mentioned, this process involves powerful muscular reflexes in the large intestine and rectum, as well as relaxation of the anal sphincters. What remains in the feces—besides water—are indigestible plant fibers, tough connective tissues (from animal foods), bacteria from the large intestine, and some body wastes, such as parts of dead intestinal cells.[4]

When either the small intestine or the pancreas is diseased, it may not produce enough of the important enzymes, as we noted may occur in persons with cystic fibrosis. This lack of enzymes can result in poor digestion and, consequently, very poor absorption of nutrients into the bloodstream. This condition accompanies many intestinal diseases. In such cases the foodstuffs travel into the large intestine, rather than being absorbed mostly into the bloodstream from the small intestine. Once the foodstuffs are in the large intestine, bacteria metabolize them into acids and gas. A person with poor intestinal function often experiences abdominal discomfort caused by intestinal gas. Insufficient enzyme production or not enough time for complete enzyme action is often at the root of these problems.[20]

Absorptive Cells *A class of cells that line the villi (fingerlike projections in the small intestine) and participate in nutrient absorption.*

Passive Absorption *Absorption that requires (1) permeability of the absorptive surface to the substance and (2) a higher concentration of the substance in the intestinal lumen than is in the absorptive cells. The higher concentration of the substance in the lumen of the intestine in comparison with that in the absorptive cells promotes the absorption of the nutrient.*

Active Absorption *Absorption using a carrier and expending energy. In this way the absorptive cell absorbs nutrients, such as glucose, when a high concentration of the nutrient is already present in the absorptive cells.*

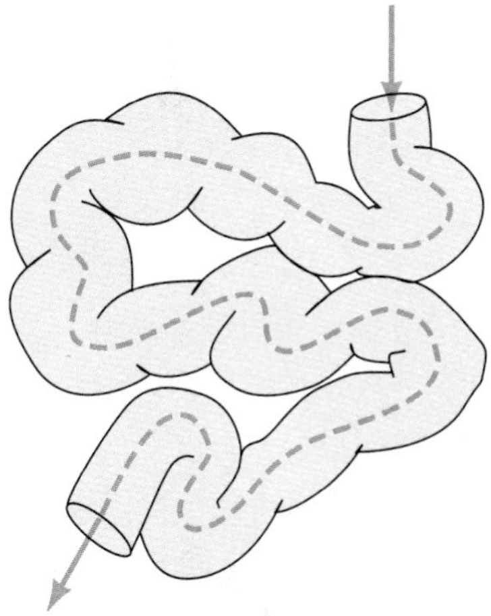

Lumen. *The inside of a tube, such as the inside cavity of the GI tract.*

FIGURE 4-8
Major sites of absorption along the GI tract. The size of the arrow indicates the relative amount of absorption at that site.

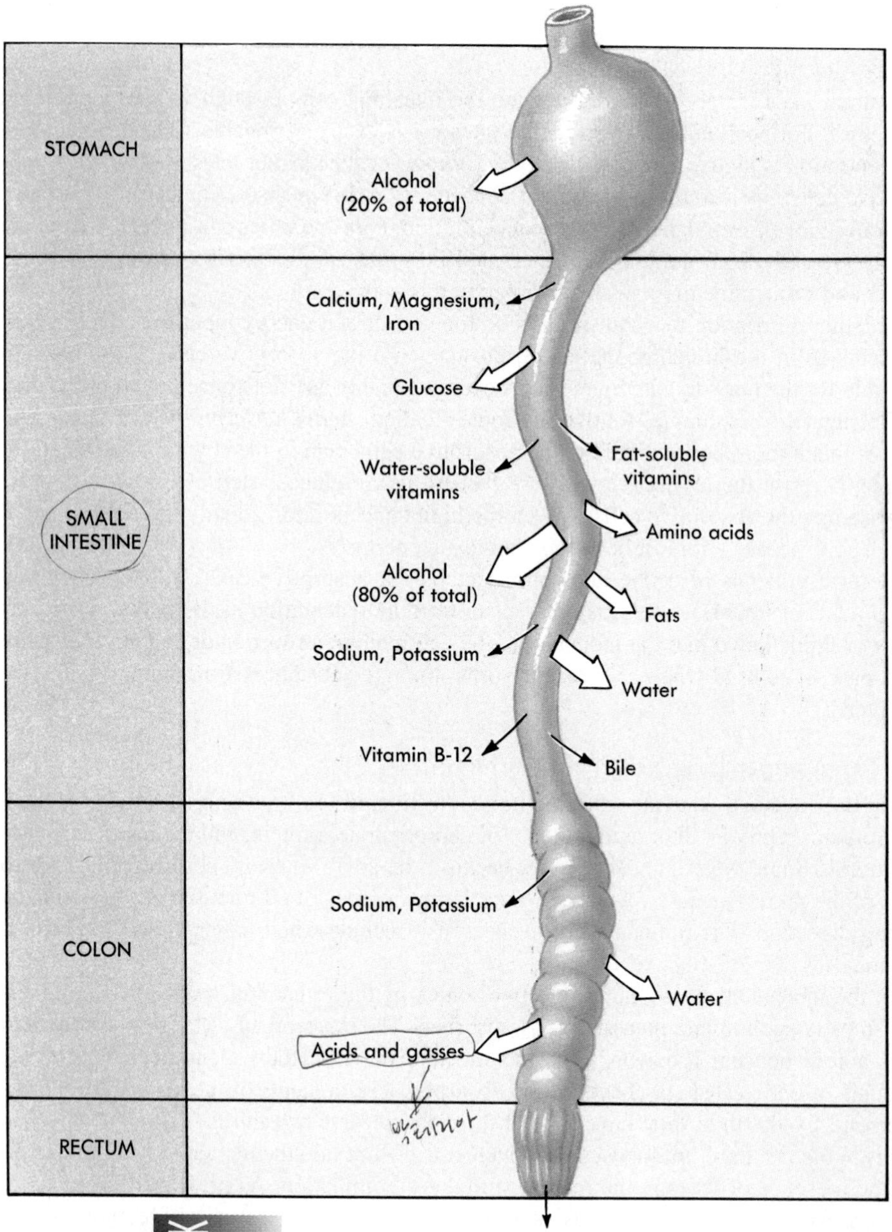

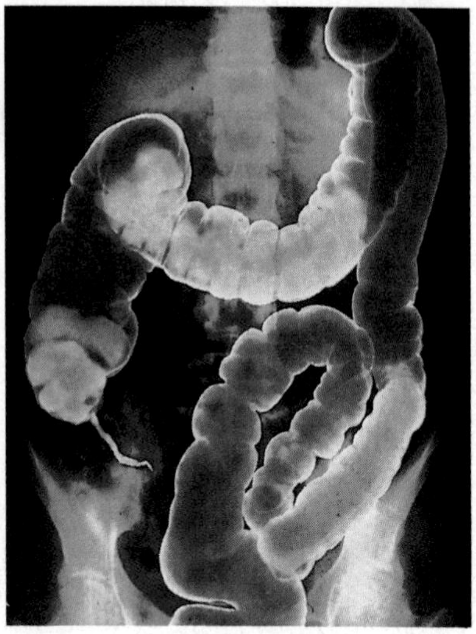

The colon has a large diameter and no villi.

CONCEPT CHECK

Some food preparation methods, such as dicing and cutting, aid digestion by breaking down foods into smaller, more digestible products. Mucus in the stomach helps prevent autodigestion. Control mechanisms—such as hormones, bicarbonate, and sphincters—also help regulate the rate of digestion and in turn help protect the digestive tract from acid corrosion. Stomach acid and enzymes also contribute to digestion of foodstuffs. The small intestine is the major site for nutrient absorption. Numerous folds and fingerlike projections create a large amount of absorptive surface for nutrient absorption. Absorptive cells have a life span of a few days, and so the lining of the small intestine is constantly renewed. These cells can perform passive types of absorption, which are promoted by a concentration difference that is greater in the lumen of the intestine than in the absorptive cell. They also perform more active forms of absorption by either overcoming the resistance of high concentration through the use of carrier and energy input or physically engulfing compounds.

NUTRITION insight

THE IMMUNE SYSTEM—WITH A NUTRITION FOCUS

Many types of body cells work in cooperation to maintain a defense against infection.[5] We know of the importance of good nutrition for immune function. Early humans were plagued by famine, infections, and death. Today, because of better nutrition, many of us avoid that cycle. In striving for good nutrition, however, it is easy to go too far. While a proper nutrient intake is needed to maintain immune function, excess quantities can in fact jeopardize it. In reviewing some major components of the immune system—the skin, intestinal cells, and white blood cells—let's also consider how nutrient intake affects each component (Figure 4-9).

Skin

The skin forms an almost continuous barrier surrounding the body. Invading microbes have difficulty penetrating the skin. However, if the skin is split by lesions, bacteria can easily penetrate this barrier. Skin health is hampered by deficiencies of such nutrients as essential fatty acids, vitamin A, niacin, and zinc. Vitamin A deficiency also decreases gland secretions in the skin—necessary secretions that contain enzymes capable of killing bacteria. Bacterial eye infections in citizens of poorer countries are also often due to vitamin A deficiency.

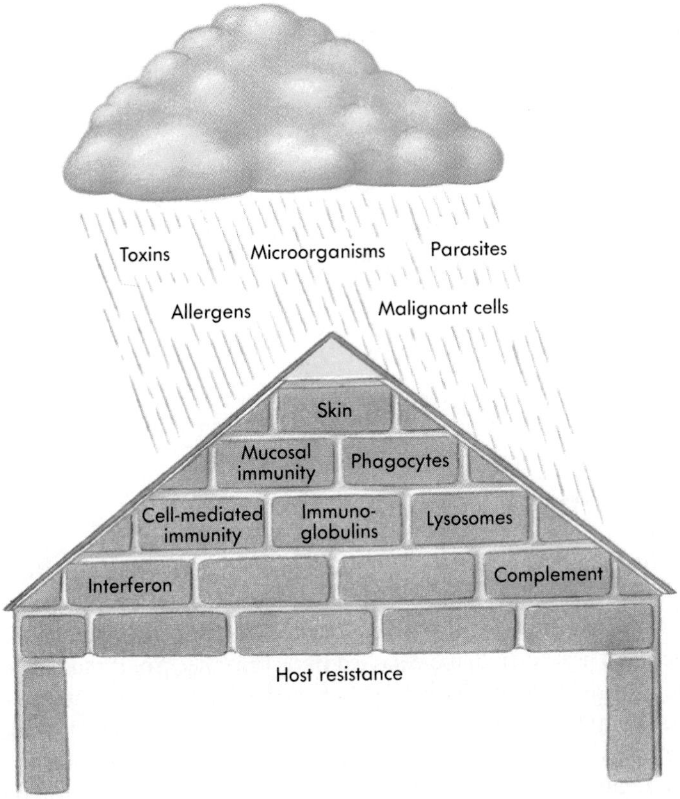

FIGURE 4-9
Host protective factors. The immune system has many components, all influenced by nutrient intake.

Intestinal Cells

The cells of the intestines form an important barrier to invading microbes. Not only are the cells closely packed together, but specialized cells that produce immune bodies—such as immunoglobulins—are also scattered throughout the intestinal tract. These immune bodies bind to the invading microbes, preventing them from entering the bloodstream. This process is called "mucosal immunity."[5] When both protein and vitamin A are deficient, the specialized cells produce fewer immune bodies.

For a person in a nutritionally deficient state, the intestinal cells break down so that microbes more easily enter the body and cause infections. Two common results of undernutrition are diarrhea and bacterial infections of the bloodstream. To protect the health of the intestinal tract, an adequate nutrient intake is necessary—especially of protein; vitamins A, B-6, B-12, and C; folate; zinc; and other nutrients needed for intestinal cell synthesis and maintenance.

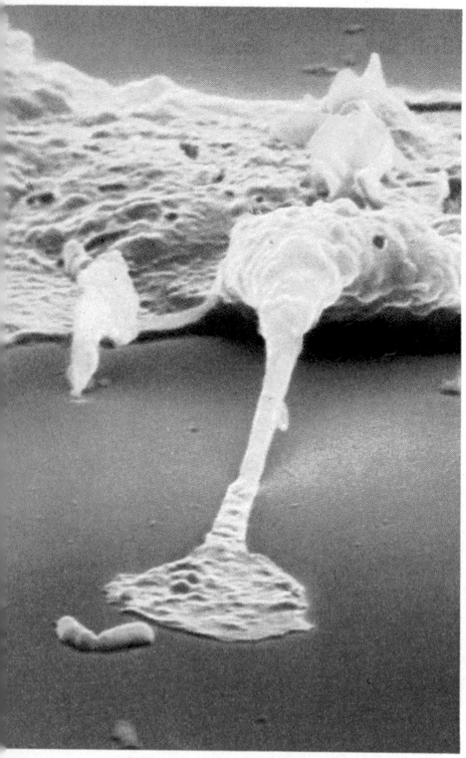

Proteins allow immune processes—like this white blood cell attacking a bacterium—to take place in the body.

White Blood Cells

Once a microbe enters the bloodstream, white blood cells move in to attack it. A variety of types of white blood cells participate in this response and function in unique ways (see Figure 4-9). For example, a class called phagocytes circulates throughout the circulatory system, along with other immune system cells, and ingests and sometimes digests microbes and foreign particles.[5] Other white blood cells participate in cell-mediated immunity, achieved when certain immune cells recognize foreign cells and attack and destroy them. White blood cells, along with proteins in the blood called immunoglobulins and complements, contribute to an antibody response that binds microorganisms, engulfs and digests them, and then creates a template (memory) that allows future recognition of the microbe. Recognition allows more rapid attacks in the future.

One class of white blood cells matures in the thymus gland. Certain immune components are notably less active in elderly people, partly because the thymus gland—which processes a class of immune cells—shrinks after sexual maturity.

Your nutrient intake affects these white blood cells and protein factors. Some white blood cells live only a few days. Their constant resynthesis requires a steady nutrient input. The immune system needs (1) iron to produce an important killing factor that is used, (2) copper for the synthesis of a specific type of white blood cell, and (3) adequate amounts of protein; vitamins B-6, B-12, and C; and folate for general cell synthesis and, later, cell activity. Zinc and vitamin A are also needed for the overall growth and development of the immune cells.

One proof that nutrition is important to immune status is the body's response to microbes: microbes normally present in the body usually cause disease only in severely un-

EXCRETORY SYSTEM

Urea ■ *Nitrogen-containing waste product found in urine. Most nitrogen excreted from the body leaves in this form.*

The kidneys, digestive tract, skin, and lungs all remove wastes from the body. For example, as blood passes through the kidneys, body wastes like ***urea*** are removed and shunted into the urine to be excreted (Figure 4-10). Excess intakes of water-soluble nutrients and other substances are also filtered and excreted in that manner. So, if the body already has enough vitamin C, for example, the kidneys screen the extra amount out of the blood and redirect it into the urine. The skin excretes body wastes, along with perspiration, through the pores. The lungs remove the carbon dioxide produced during the metabolism of energy-yielding nutrients, including carbohydrates, fats, and proteins. The carbon dioxide is then exhaled into the air.

dernourished people. A good example is measles. Your parents probably had this viral infection and survived. (You were probably vaccinated against measles.) However, many undernourished children who contract it die. Thus the presence of a virus or microbe in the body does not guarantee its triumph over the immune system. But if a person's health is already compromised through undernutrition, the chances of a destructive microbe's winning are greater.

An infection that occurs primarily in undernourished people is called an ***opportunistic infection.*** Opportunistic infections are also characteristic of acquired immunodeficiency syndrome (AIDS), a disease in which one class of white blood cells becomes severely depleted. A type of pneumonia that rarely occurs in people with normal immune function is often able to take hold in people with AIDS.[20]

Opportunistic Infection ■
An infection that arises primarily in people who are already ill because of another disease.

Adipose (Fat) Tissue ■
A grouping of fat-storing cells.

another BITE

In the early 1970s, physicians began providing nutritional care to patients with major body burns much sooner after the incident than they had in the past. This earlier feeding dramatically reduced (by 80%) the number of infections that burn patients suffered and thus greatly improved their chances of surviving. A major reason for this improved survival is the earlier supply of nutrients to support immune function.

A Note of Caution

Many studies show that good nutritional status is associated with good immune status. However, other studies also show that an overabundance of certain nutrients can actually harm the immune system. Too many polyunsaturated fatty acids and too much vitamin E have been implicated in a decreased immune response in mice. Taking too much zinc also appears to decrease immune function. This decrease may be partially due to zinc's interfering with copper absorption. The copper deficiency contributes to decreased synthesis of a specific class of white blood cells.

The message here is that eating a balanced diet will help us maintain the health of all components of our immune systems. Our bodies need this system to continuously defend us from harmful microbes in the environment. The diets of some elderly people are a concern in this context since energy intakes may be too low to meet all nutrient needs. Careful nutrient supplementation then deserves consideration (see Chapter 8 for a discussion of supplement use and abuse). However, keep in mind that consuming more nutrients than needed is not going to boost the immune system to even higher abilities. In fact, it can harm certain aspects of immune function.

STORAGE SYSTEMS

The human body must maintain reserves of nutrients. Otherwise, we would need to eat continuously. Storage capacity varies for each different nutrient. Most fat is stored at sites designed specifically for this—***adipose (fat) tissue.*** Short-term storage of carbohydrate occurs in muscle and liver, and the blood maintains a small reserve of amino acids.[20] The many vitamins and minerals stored in the liver make animal liver a rich food source. Other nutrient stores are found in individual cells themselves.

When a person is not meeting his or her nutrient needs, some nutrients are obtained by breaking down a tissue that contains high concentrations of the nutrient. Calcium is taken from bone, and protein is taken from muscle. But neither bones nor muscles are meant to act as nutrient reserves. Rather, nutrient losses in cases of deficiency harm these tissues.

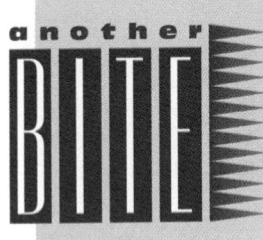

Many people believe that if too much of a nutrient is obtained, for example from a vit-

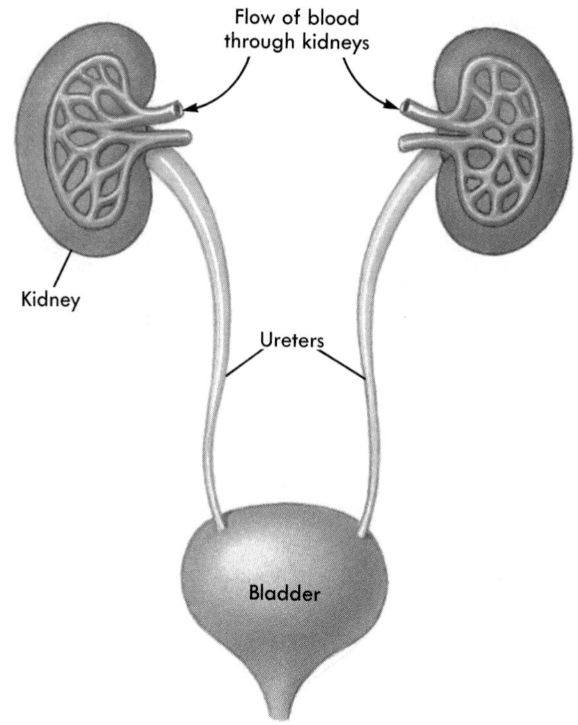

FIGURE 4-10
The urinary tract. Blood enters the kidney by way of the arteries. The kidney filters waste from the blood and sends it as urine to the bladder. The bladder then periodically eliminates the urine.

amin or mineral supplement, only what is needed is stored and the rest is excreted by the body. Though partially true, as with vitamin C, the large dosages found frequently in supplements, such as vitamins A and D, can cause harmful side affects because these are not readily excreted. This is one reason why getting your nutrients from a balanced diet is the safest means for obtaining the building blocks you need to maintain good health of all body systems.

• • • •

This review of human anatomy and physiology from a nutrition perspective sets the stage for developing a more detailed understanding of nutrition science. We will build on this information as we study the nutrients in greater detail.

CONCEPT CHECK

The kidneys, skin, and lungs all perform excretory functions for the body. The health of these organ systems depends on a sufficient and appropriate supply of nutrients. Nutrients are constantly present in the blood for immediate use and are stored to a greater or lesser extent in body tissues for later use when sufficient food is unavailable. But when the body suffers a nutrient deficiency caused by a poor diet, it breaks down vital tissues for their nutrients, which can lead to ill health. As well, too much of any nutrient can be detrimental. It's best to get all essential nutrients from a balanced diet.

SUMMARY

- The cell is the basic building block of body tissues. DNA is the blueprint found in all cells. This determines the cell type, its functions and structures, and the kind of chemicals each type of cell will produce.
- Blood travels the pulmonary circuit, picking up oxygen at the lungs. Then via the systemic circuit, the blood delivers essential nutrients, energy, oxygen, and water to all body cells. Nutrients and wastes are exchanged between the blood and cells across the cell membrane.
- Water-soluble compounds in the villi enter the portal vein and travel to the liver. Fat-soluble compounds enter the lymphatic system, which eventually connects to the bloodstream.
- The gastrointestinal (GI) tract consists of the mouth, esophagus, stomach, small intestine, large intestine (colon), rectum, and anus. Most digestion and absorption of nutrients occur in the small intestine.
- The liver, gallbladder, and pancreas participate in digestion and absorption. Products from these organs, such as enzymes and bile, enter the small intestine and play important roles in digesting protein, fat, and carbohydrates.
- Along the GI tract are ringlike valves (sphincters) that control the flow of foodstuffs. Muscular contractions, called peristalsis, propel the foodstuffs down the GI tract. A variety of nerves, hormones, and other substances control the activity of sphincters and peristaltic muscles.
- Digestive enzymes are secreted by the mouth, stomach, wall of the small intestine, and pancreas. Pancreatic enzyme release is controlled by the hormone cholecystokinin (CCK). The presence of food in the small intestine stimulates the release of this hormone. Bile needed for fat digestion is synthesized by the liver, stored in the gallbladder, and released in digestion, as directed by the action of CCK.
- The major absorptive sites consist of fingerlike projections called villi, located in the small intestine. Absorptive cells cover the villi. This intestinal lining is continually renewed. Absorptive cells can perform passive and active forms of absorption, and they are able to absorb substances by physically engulfing them.
- Most digestion and absorption occurs in the small intestine. Little digestion and absorption occurs in the stomach or large intestine, but some protein is digested in the stomach. Some plant fibers and undigested starch are digested by bacteria in the large intestine; undigested plant fibers are eliminated in the feces.
- Final water and mineral absorption takes place in the large intestine. Products from bacterial breakdown of some plant fibers and other substances are also absorbed here. The presence of feces in the rectum provides a strong impetus for elimination.

STUDY QUESTIONS

1. Describe the nervous and hormonal systems' interactions that regulate the digestive tract.
2. Depict the key mechanisms that protect the health and absorptive abilities of the cells of the small intestine.
3. Explain why the small intestine is better suited than the other organs of the digestive tract to carry out the bulk of the absorptive process.
4. Why do different types of cells generally need to perform different tasks? Provide examples of cells in the digestive system that carry out different tasks. Name the necessary components that cells generally need to survive.
5. What two sets of circulatory systems play important roles in digestion? Provide a brief description of how these systems work.
6. How can a poor diet affect the health of organ systems in the body? Provide two examples.

REFERENCES

1. Allison MC and others: Gastrointestinal damage associated with the use of nonsteroidal antiinflammatory agents, *New England Journal of Medicine* 327:749, 1992.
2. Anda RF and others: Self-perceived stress and the risk of peptic ulcer disease, *Archives of Internal Medicine* 152:829, 1992.
3. Caspray WF: Physiology and pathophysiology of intestinal absorption, *American Journal of Clinical Nutrition* 55:299S, 1992.
4. Cashman MD: Principles of digestive physiology for clinical nutrition, *Nutrition in Clinical Practice* 1:241, 1986.
5. Claman HN: The biology of the immune system, *Journal of the American Medical Association* 268:2790, 1992.
6. Cramer T: When do you need an antacid, *FDA Consumer,* p. 19, January/February 1992.
7. Cummings M: Laxatives rarely needed, *FDA Consumer,* p. 33, April 1991.
8. Ebell MH: Peptic ulcer disease, *American Family Physician* 46:217, 1992.
9. Evans MA, Shrouts EP: Intestinal fuels: glutamine, short-chain fatty acids, and dietary fiber, *Journal of the American Dietetic Association* 92:1239, 1992.
10. Hill P: It is not what you eat, but how you eat it: Digestion, life-style, nutrition, *Nutrition* 7:385, 1991.
11. Jackson WD, Grand RJ: The human intestinal response to enteral nutrients: a review, *Journal of the American College of Nutrition* 10:500, 1991.
12. Lewis R: The gallbladder, an organ you can live without, *FDA Consumer,* p. 13, May 1991.
13. Lewis R: When smell and taste go awry, *FDA Consumer,* p. 29, November 1991.
14. Mattes RD, Mela DJ: The chemical senses and nutrition, *Nutrition Today,* p. 19, May/June 1988.
15. Mayes PA: Nutrition, digestion, and absorption. In Murray RK and others, editors: *Harper's biochemistry,* East Norwalk, Conn, 1990, Appleton & Lange.
16. Ransohoff DF: Gastroenterology, *Journal of the American Medical Association* 270:206, 1993.
17. Schneeman B: Nutrition and gastrointestinal function, *Nutrition Today* p. 20, January/February 1993.
18. Stehlin D: No strain no pain, the bottom line in treating hemorrhoids, *FDA Consumer,* p. 31, March 1992.
19. Wilson JD and others: *Harrison's principles of internal medicine,* ed 12, New York, 1991, McGraw-Hill.
20. Zeman FJ: *Clinical nutrition and dietetics,* ed 2, New York, 1991, Macmillan.

The Processes of Digestion and Absorption

Label each organ shown in the figure below, and note if (and if so, how) it participates in digesting, absorbing, and/or ultimately excreting the remains of what you ate for dinner last night. Later chapters cover the digestion and absorption of each nutrient in detail. Use this exercise to build your knowledge.

pancreas	anus
trachea	salivary glands
appendix	mouth
esophagus	large intestine (colon)
liver	rectum
stomach	small intestine
epiglottis	gallbladder
pyloric sphincter	common bile duct

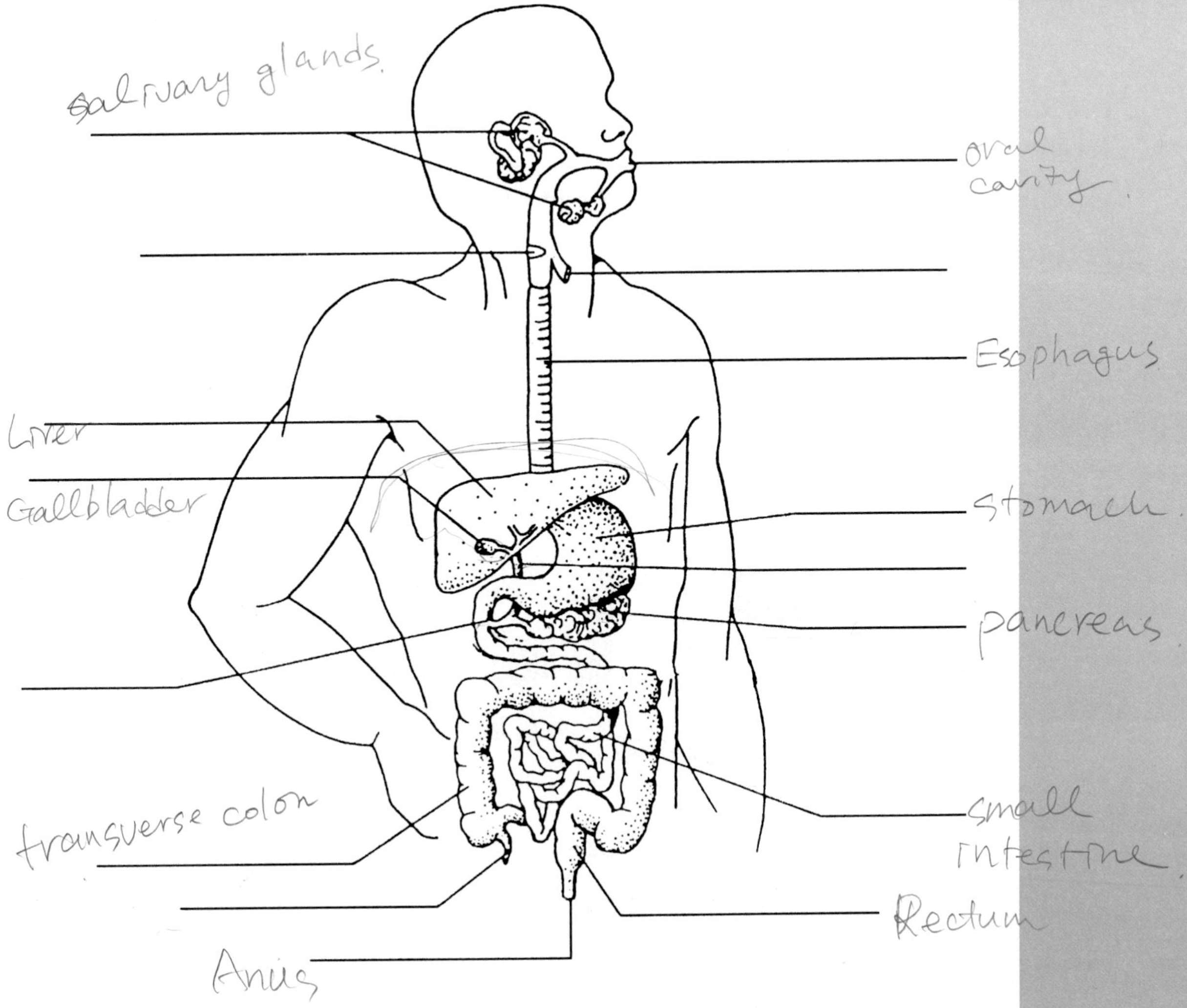

Nutrition ISSUE

WHEN DIGESTIVE PROCESSES GO AWRY

Ulcers

An unfortunate sign of success can be an ulcer. For some people, stress and tension greatly excite the nerves that control the stomach.[2] This in turn increases acid secretion by the stomach's acid-producing cells. More tension means more acid. Eventually the acid erodes through the stomach's mucous layer into the stomach wall. Acid can also erode the wall of the upper small intestine. Either way, the result is an ulcer. Some people are more susceptible to ulcers than are others, because their stomach and intestinal cells can't sufficiently protect themselves from the acid. Recent research also links certain bacterial infections in stomach cells to ulcers, and current therapies are beginning to address the potential cause, such as use of certain antibiotics.[16]

The typical symptom of an ulcer is pain about 2 hours after eating. Digestive acids that work on a meal irritate the ulcer after most of the meal moves down into the small intestine.

The primary risk posed by an ulcer is the possibility that it will eat entirely through the stomach or intestinal wall. The GI tract contents could then spill into the body cavity, causing a massive infection. In addition, an ulcer may erode a blood vessel, leading to massive blood loss (hemorrhage).

In the past, milk and cream therapy was used to help cure ulcers. Today we know that milk and cream are two of the worst foods for an ulcer. The calcium in these foods stimulates gastrin, the hormone that increases stomach acid secretion. Thus this therapy actual-

TABLE 4-4

Recommendations to Prevent Ulcers and Heartburn from Recurring

Ulcers

1. *Stop smoking, if you are now a smoker.*
2. Avoid aspirin, ibuprofen, and other aspirin-like compounds when you can.
3. Minimize the use of coffee, tea, and alcohol (most notably, wine), especially between meals.
4. Limit use of pepper, chili powder, and other strong spices, if this helps.
5. Eat nutritious meals on a regular schedule.
6. Chew foods well.
7. Lose weight if you are now overweight.

Heartburn

1. Wait about 3 hours after a meal before lying down.
2. Don't overeat at mealtime.
3. Observe the recommendations for ulcer prevention.

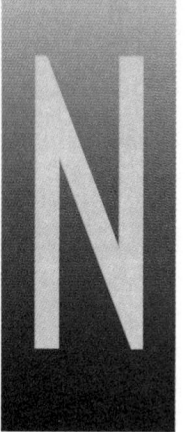

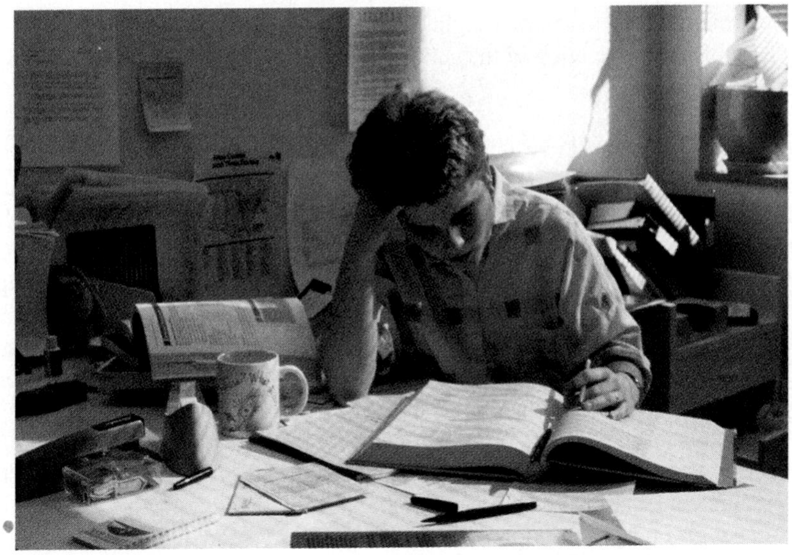

Stress can bring on an ulcer in some of us.

ly impedes ulcer healing. Instead, antacid medications are the first line of medical treatment for ulcers. In this instance, however, antacids should be taken only under a physician's supervision, because side effects—such as kidney damage—are also possible with prolonged use. In addition to antacids, the physician may prescribe other medications that reduce stomach acid secretion or protect the ulcer from further erosion by acid.[8] By minimizing the presence of effects of stomach acidity, the medications greatly speed ulcer healing and so have greatly reduced the need for surgical treatment.

A person who is prone to developing ulcers should not smoke.[19] Minimizing the use of aspirin and other aspirin-like compounds is also important, because these irritate the stomach and small intestine.[1] The combination of not smoking, avoiding aspirin, and taking antacids and other anti-acid medications has so revolutionized ulcer therapy that changing one's diet is of secondary importance (Table 4-4).

Heartburn

Some people are very susceptible to heartburn. The gnawing pain in the upper chest is caused by acid flowing back into the esophagus from the stomach. Unlike the stomach, the esophagus has no mucous lining to protect it. The acid quickly erodes the esophageal wall, causing pain.

An important dietary measure in preventing heartburn is to eat smaller, low-fat meals. Large meals containing much fat remain in the stomach longer and create more pressure in the stomach than do the smaller, low-fat meals. This can force the stomach contents up into the esophagus. Someone who suffers from heartburn should not smoke, not lie down after eating, and avoid foods and other substances that can specifically contribute to heartburn, such as chili powder, onions, garlic, caffeine, alcoholic beverages, and chocolate.[10] Each person must discover which foods bother him or her and tailor the diet accordingly.

Certain physical conditions can lead to heartburn. For example, for pregnant women and obese people, production of the hormones progesterone and/or estrogen increases. These hormones relax the sphincter in the esophagus, making backflow from the stomach into the esophagus more likely. Pregnancy also increases pressures in the abdomen, which makes heartburn more likely.[19] A pregnant woman may find it helpful to eat smaller, more frequent meals until she gives birth. An obese person can try to lose weight, so that blood levels of these hormones decrease.

Heartburn that recurs several times a week for a month should be investigated by a physician. Long-term heartburn—especially when associated with difficult or painful

Constipation ■
A condition in which bowel movements are infrequent.

Laxative ■
A medication or other substance that stimulates evacuation of the intestinal tract.

swallowing, blood in the stool, or weight loss—may require aggressive medical therapy, because it can lead to alteration in the cells of the esophagus. This increases the risk of a rare form of cancer.[19]

Constipation and laxatives

Difficult or infrequent evacuation of the bowels is known as ***constipation.*** It is caused by slow movement of feces through the large intestine. The feces become dry and hard as fluids are increasingly absorbed during their extended time in the large intestine. Constipation can result from irregular elimination patterns that develop when people regularly inhibit their normal bowel reflexes for a long period. People tend to ignore normal urges when they don't want to interrupt occupational or social activities. Muscle spasms of an irritated large intestine can also slow the movement of feces and contribute to constipation. Even such medications as antacids can cause constipation.[20]

Constipation is difficult to diagnose. Normal stool frequency ranges from 3 to 12 times per week. However, definitions of "normal" vary from person to person. The best guide for recognizing constipation is the presence of unusually hard, dry stools at infrequent intervals—not a general prescription of "once a day." Any sudden, prolonged changes in stool frequency should be evaluated by a physician. This may be a warning that a more serious intestinal disorder is developing.

Eating dietary fiber, such as is found in whole-grain breads and cereals, is the best alternative for treating typical cases of constipation (see Chapter 5 for a detailed discussion). Dietary fibers stimulate peristalsis by helping form a bulky stool. In addition to consuming more dietary fiber, a person with constipation should drink more fluids. Eating dried fruits can also help. The person may need to develop more regular bowel habits; designating the same time each day for a bowel movement can help train the large intestine to respond routinely. Finally, relaxation facilitates regular bowel movements, as does regular exercise.[7]

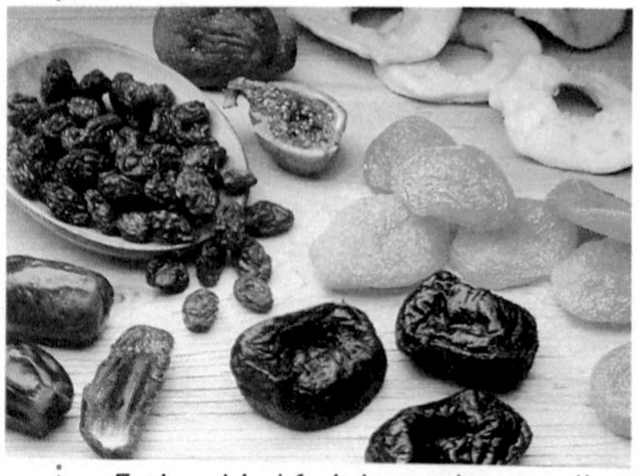
Eating dried fruit is another excellent way to increase your dietary fiber intake.

Laxatives can also lessen constipation. They work either by irritating the intestinal nerve junctions, which stimulates the peristaltic muscles, or by drawing water into the intestine to enlarge the stool. A larger stool stretches the peristaltic muscles, making them rebound and then constrict. Regular laxative use, especially of the irritating varieties, can decrease muscle action in the large intestine, causing more constipation in the future. In time the GI tract can actually become dependent on laxatives for functioning.[7] Thus it is unwise to use laxatives routinely, although people in certain circumstances—those who are bedridden or quite elderly—may need periodic help from laxatives to relieve constipation.

another BITE

Perhaps you have heard that taking laxatives after overeating prevents fat gain from the excess kcalories. This erroneous and dangerous premise has gained popularity among followers of numerous fad diets. It is true that you may temporarily feel less full after using a laxative. That is because laxatives hasten emptying of the large intestine and increase fluid loss. Note, however, that most laxatives do not actually hurry the passage of food through the small intestine, where digestion and most nutrient absorption take place. As a result, laxatives do not prevent your getting most of the kcalories you would have gotten without using the laxative.

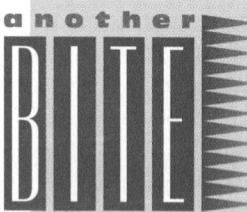

Hemorrhoids

Hemorrhoids, also called piles, are swollen veins of the rectum and anus. The blood vessels in this area are subject to intense pressure, especially during bowel movements. Added stress to the vessels from pregnancy, obesity, prolonged sitting, violent coughing or sneezing, or straining at the toilet can lead to a hemorrhoid.[19]

Hemorrhoids can develop unnoticed until a strained bowel movement precipitates symptoms. These may include pain, itching, and bleeding. Itching caused by moisture in the anal canal, swelling, or other irritation is perhaps the most common symptom. Pain, if present, is usually aching and steady. Bleeding may result from an internal hemorrhoid and appear in the toilet or as a streak in the feces. The blood is bright red. Protrusion, or the sensation of a mass in the anal canal after a bowel movement, is symptomatic of an internal hemorrhoid that protrudes through the anus.

Anyone can develop a hemorrhoid. Pressure from prolonged sitting or exertion is often enough to bring on symptoms, although diet, lifestyle, and possibly heredity play a role. If you think you have a hemorrhoid, you should consult your physician. Rectal bleeding, although usually caused by hemorrhoids, may also indicate other problems, such as cancer.

Your physician may also suggest a variety of other self-care measures. The best treatment for hemorrhoids is prevention. The suggestions for relieving constipation help prevent the formation of hemorrhoids.[18] Drinking liquids is important for maintaining the digestive tract. Pain can be lessened by warm, soft compresses or sitz baths several times a day. A sitz bath requires sitting in a tub of warm water for 15 to 20 minutes. Over-the-counter remedies can also offer relief of symptoms. Ask your physician for advice.

Hemorrhoids
Swollen veins of the rectum and anus, often protruding into the anus.

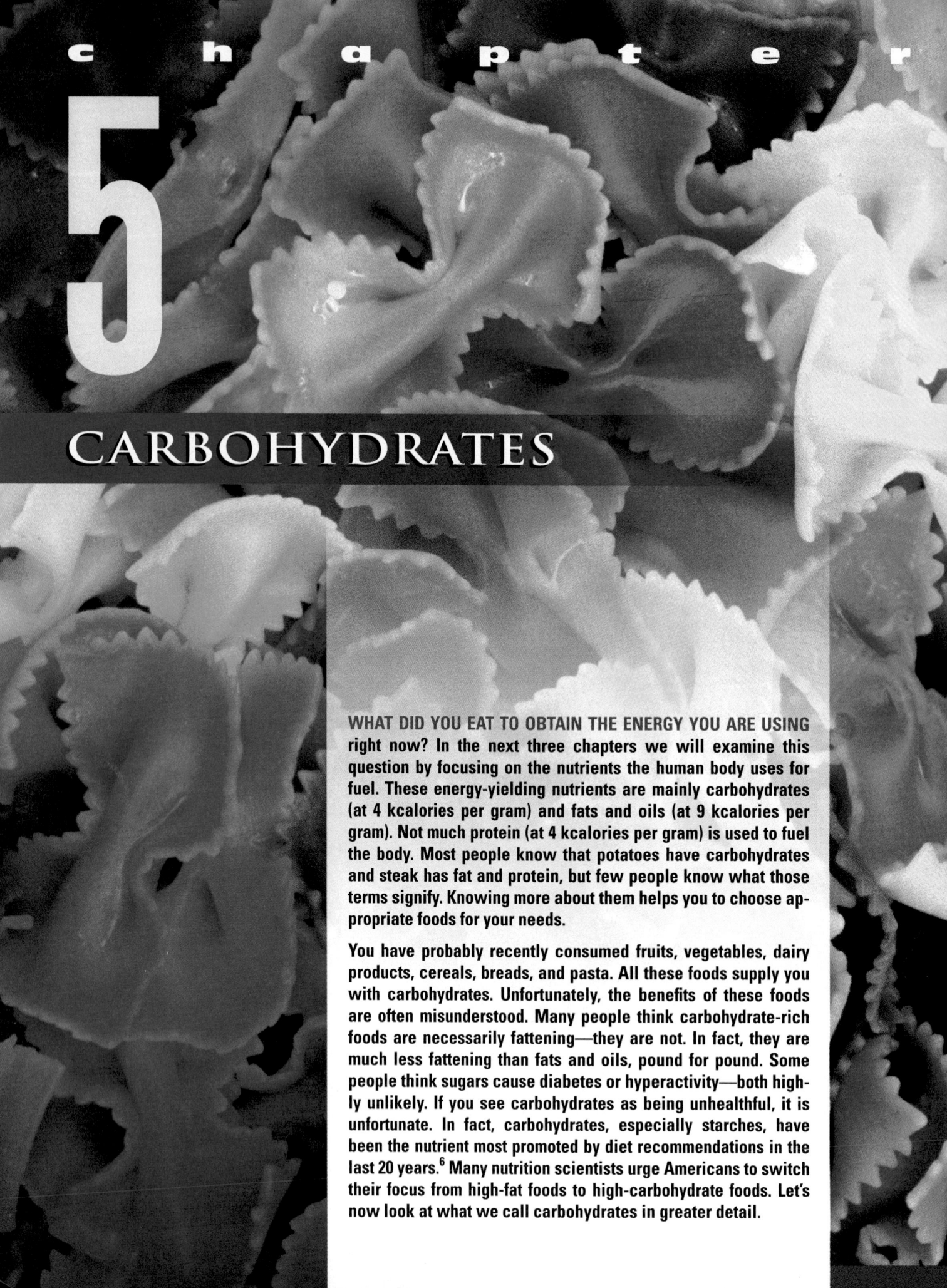

chapter

5

CARBOHYDRATES

WHAT DID YOU EAT TO OBTAIN THE ENERGY YOU ARE USING right now? In the next three chapters we will examine this question by focusing on the nutrients the human body uses for fuel. These energy-yielding nutrients are mainly carbohydrates (at 4 kcalories per gram) and fats and oils (at 9 kcalories per gram). Not much protein (at 4 kcalories per gram) is used to fuel the body. Most people know that potatoes have carbohydrates and steak has fat and protein, but few people know what those terms signify. Knowing more about them helps you to choose appropriate foods for your needs.

You have probably recently consumed fruits, vegetables, dairy products, cereals, breads, and pasta. All these foods supply you with carbohydrates. Unfortunately, the benefits of these foods are often misunderstood. Many people think carbohydrate-rich foods are necessarily fattening—they are not. In fact, they are much less fattening than fats and oils, pound for pound. Some people think sugars cause diabetes or hyperactivity—both highly unlikely. If you see carbohydrates as being unhealthful, it is unfortunate. In fact, carbohydrates, especially starches, have been the nutrient most promoted by diet recommendations in the last 20 years.[6] Many nutrition scientists urge Americans to switch their focus from high-fat foods to high-carbohydrate foods. Let's now look at what we call carbohydrates in greater detail.

SHARING YOUR SUGAR HABITS

One of the Dietary Guidelines for Americans you learned about in Chapter 2 says, "Use sugars only in moderation." In this chapter you will learn about facts and fallacies regarding why we are to do this. Complete this quiz about your sugar habits. Put a "Y" in the blank to the right of the questions to indicate yes and an "N" to indicate no. Don't answer the questions in the way you think they should be answered, but according to what you generally do.

1. Do you read the ingredient labels to identify added sugars in a product? ____
2. Do you try to select items lower in sugar when possible? ____
3. Do you buy fresh fruits or fruits packed in water, juice, or light syrup, rather than those in heavy syrup? ____
4. Do you generally avoid or limit the serving size of foods high in sugar, such as prepared baked goods, candies, sweet desserts, soft drinks, and fruit-flavored punches? ____
5. Do you purposely try to reduce the sugar in foods you prepare at home? ____
6. Do you experiment with spices—such as cinnamon, nutmeg, and ginger—to enhance the flavor of foods, rather than using a lot of sugar? ____
7. Do you use home-prepared items (with less sugar) when possible instead of commercially prepared ones that are higher in sugar? ____
8. Do you try to use less of all sugars (white and brown sugar, honey, molasses, and syrups)? ____
9. Do you reach for fresh fruit instead of sweets for dessert or when you want a snack? ____
10. Do you try to minimize the addition of sugar to foods, such as coffee, tea, cereal, or fruit? ____

INTERPRETATION

For every "Y" give yourself 1 point and every "N" 0 points. Record your total points (from 0 to 10) in this blank. ____

The Dietary Guideline "Use sugars only in moderation" encourages Americans to evaluate their total intake of sweetened foods and sugar. The higher your score on the quiz, the more you should reevaluate your sugar intake in an effort to comply with the Dietary Guideline. Although a current emphasis in diet planning is placed on increasing the total amount of carbohydrate in the diet, this should come mainly from grain, fruit, and vegetable sources. It's wise to limit carbohydrate intake from sugar sources. Look through your answers and see how you could reduce your sugar intake. In the space below, indicate one easy way.

____

____

As you read this chapter, you will find out how to and why you should examine your sugar intake, as well as reasons to examine whether you need to increase your starch and dietary fiber intake.

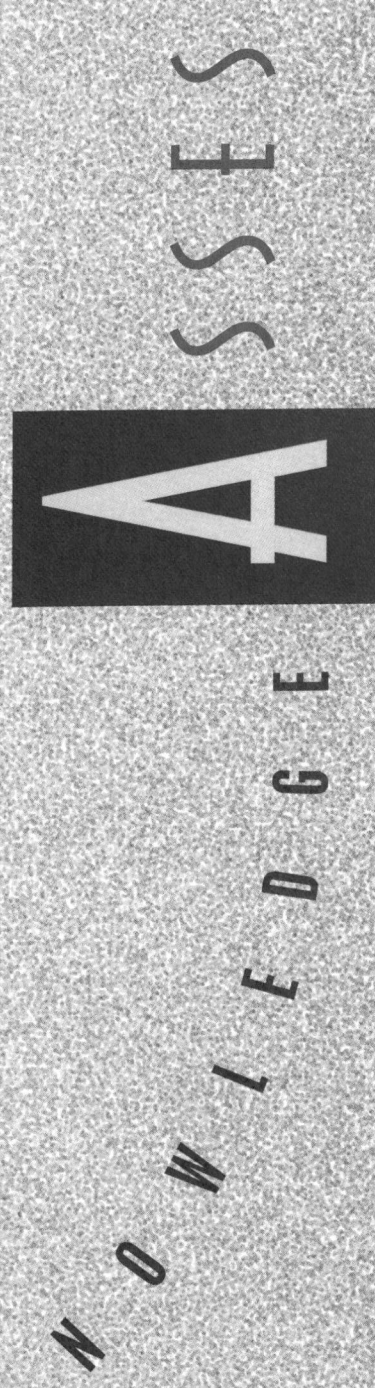

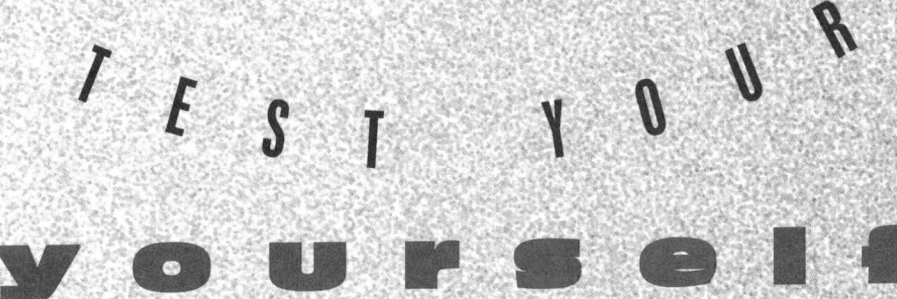

ASSESS

4

TEST YOUR KNOWLEDGE

yourself

Photosynthesis Process by which plants use energy from the sun to synthesize energy-yielding compounds, such as glucose.

Monosaccharide A single sugar, such as glucose, that is not broken down further during digestion.

FORMS OF SIMPLE CARBOHYDRATES

Carbohydrates in our foods are made by green plants. Leaves capture the sun's heat and light in special areas of their cells and transform them to chemical energy. This energy then is used to produce glucose from the carbon dioxide that leaves take from the air and the water that roots bring up from the soil. This complex process is called ***photosynthesis.***[20]

$$\underset{(CO_2)}{\text{6 Carbon dioxide}} + \underset{(H_2O)}{\text{6 Water}} \longrightarrow \underset{(C_6H_{12}O_6)}{\text{The carbohydrate glucose}} + \underset{(O_2)}{\text{6 Oxygen}}$$

As the name suggests, most carbohydrate molecules are composed of carbon, hydrogen, and oxygen atoms. Simple forms of carbohydrates are called sugars, whereas larger, more complex forms are called either starches or dietary fibers.

Monosaccharides—Glucose, Fructose, and Galactose

Monosaccharides are the single sugar forms (*mono* means one) that are the basic unit of all sugar structures. Glucose is the major monosaccharide found in the body (Figure 5-1). Glucose is also known as dextrose or blood sugar, because it is the major form of sugar found in the bloodstream. Glucose is a primary source of energy for human cells. Most sugars in foods are converted to glucose in the liver and thus readily serve as a source of cellular energy.[20]

Fructose, also called levulose or fruit sugar, is another common sugar. After it is consumed, fructose is absorbed by the small intestine and then transported to the liver. There it is quickly metabolized; some is converted to glucose, while the rest goes on to form other compounds.[20]

The sugar ***galactose*** has nearly the same structure as glucose. It does not exist free in nature in large quantities. Instead, galactose usually is found attached to glucose in lactose, a sugar found in milk and other dairy products. After it is absorbed, galactose arrives in the liver. There it is either transformed into glucose per se, or further metabolized. One product of this conversion is glycogen, a special storage form of glucose found in liver and muscle.[20]

PHOTOSYNTHESIS

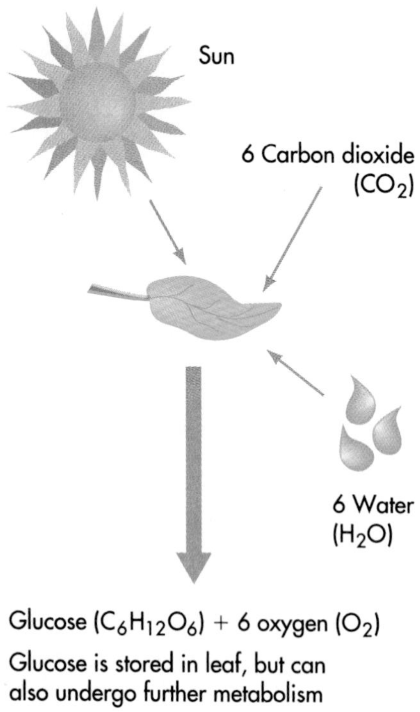

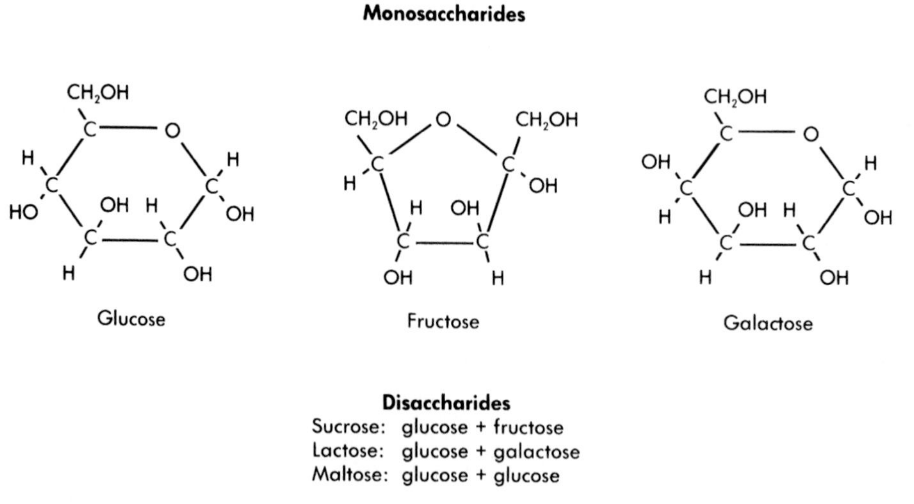

FIGURE 5-1
Some common sugars. Sucrose and fructose are the most common sugars in our diets.

Disaccharides—Sucrose, Lactose, and Maltose

Disaccharides are formed when two monosaccharides combine (*di* means two). The most common disaccharides in foods are sucrose, lactose, and maltose.

Sucrose—ordinary table sugar—forms when the two sugars glucose and fructose join together. Sucrose is found in sugar cane, sugar beets, honey, and maple sugar. Animals do not produce it.

Lactose forms when glucose joins with galactose. Again, our major food source for lactose is milk products. An accompanying Nutrition Focus discusses the problems that result when we can't readily digest lactose.

Maltose forms when two glucose molecules combine. Our major food source for maltose is produced when grains sprout (germinate). As the starch in grains breaks down during germination, maltose forms. To brew beer, grains are first germinated. The yeast can then metabolize the maltose, or malt, produced. We have few other sources of maltose in our diets.

Monosaccharides and disaccharides are often referred to as simple sugars, because each contains few sugar units. Food labels sometimes lump all these sugars under one category, listing them as "sucrose and other sugars."

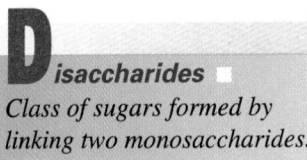

Disaccharides ■ *Class of sugars formed by linking two monosaccharides.*

CONCEPT CHECK

Monosaccharides are single sugar forms. Important monosaccharides in the diet are glucose, fructose, and galactose (the latter as part of lactose). Glucose is a primary energy source for body cells. Disaccharides form when two single sugars combine. Important disaccharides in the diet are the table sugar sucrose (glucose joined with fructose), maltose (glucose joined with glucose), and the milk sugar lactose (glucose joined with galactose). Once digested into monosaccharide forms and absorbed, most carbohydrates are transformed into glucose in the liver.

MAKING CARBOHYDRATES AVAILABLE FOR BODY USE

As we pointed out in Chapter 4, simply eating a food does not supply nutrients to body cells. Digestion and absorption must first take place.

Carbohydrate Digestion

Carbohydrate digestion actually begins before we start eating. Preparing food can be viewed as the first step in digestion. Cooking softens tough connective tissues in the fibrous tissue of plants, such as broccoli stalks. When starches are heated, the starch granules swell as they soak up water, making them much easier to digest. All these effects of cooking generally make food easier to chew, swallow, and break down during digestion.

Digestion of the large carbohydrates—starches—begins as these mix with saliva during the chewing of food. Saliva contains an enzyme called *salivary amylase.* This enzyme breaks down starch (a chain of thousands of monosaccharide units) into many smaller sugar units (disaccharides, such as maltose) (Figure 5-2). You can observe this conversion while chewing a saltine cracker. Prolonged chewing of the cracker causes it to taste sweeter as some starch breaks down into the sweeter sugars.

Salivary amylase does not work in an acidic environment. Once food moves down the esophagus into the stomach, the stomach's acidity halts further salivary amylase action and subsequently any starch digestion. However, salivary amylase is not so important, because the enzyme pancreatic amylase finishes in the small intestine what salivary amylase does not finish in the mouth.[14]

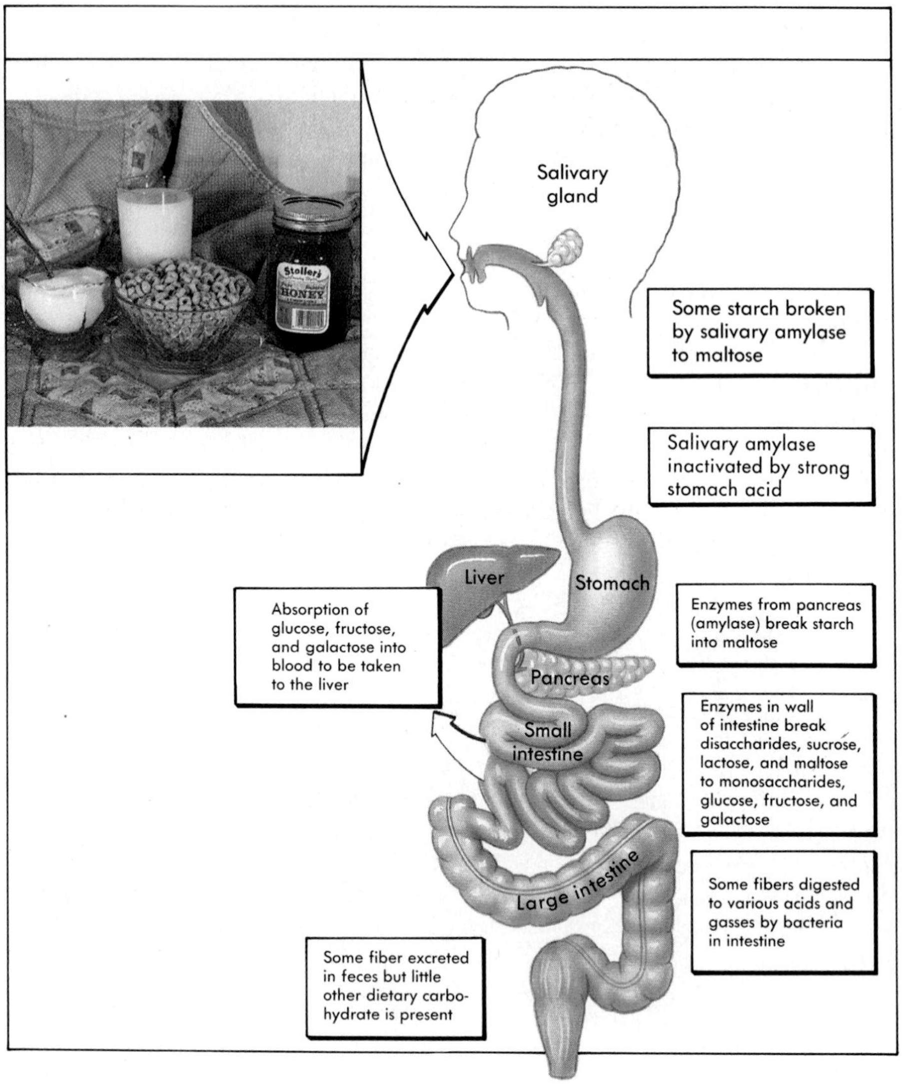
Salivary gland
Some starch broken by salivary amylase to maltose
Salivary amylase inactivated by strong stomach acid
Liver
Stomach
Enzymes from pancreas (amylase) break starch into maltose
Absorption of glucose, fructose, and galactose into blood to be taken to the liver
Pancreas
Small intestine
Enzymes in wall of intestine break disaccharides, sucrose, lactose, and maltose to monosaccharides, glucose, fructose, and galactose
Large intestine
Some fibers digested to various acids and gasses by bacteria in intestine
Some fiber excreted in feces but little other dietary carbohydrate is present

FIGURE 5-2

Carbohydrate digestion and absorption. Enzymes made by the mouth, pancreas, and small intestine participate in the process of digestion. Most carbohydrate digestion and absorption takes place in the small intestine.

After the carbohydrates are in the intestine and pancreatic amylase has had time to act, the original carbohydrates in a food are now present as monosaccharides (mostly any glucose and fructose obtained as such from the food), as well as disaccharides (maltose from starch breakdown, lactose mainly from dairy products, and sucrose from food preparation and that added at the table). Eventually all the disaccharide forms are digested to their monosaccharide forms by specialized enzymes attached to the cells of the small intestine. The enzyme maltase acts on maltose to produce two glucose molecules. Sucrase acts on sucrose to produce glucose and fructose. Lactase acts on lactose to produce glucose and galactose.

When considering carbohydrate digestion, it is important to remember that key digestive enzymes come from both the pancreas and the cells of the intestinal wall.[14] Intestinal diseases can interfere with the production of the intestinal wall enzymes. Such conditions may interfere with the efficient digestion of the sugars maltose, lactose, and sucrose. The portion of these carbohydrates that is not fully digested will not be absorbed. When they eventually end up in the large intestine, the bacteria there will use the sugars to produce acid and gas. If produced in large amounts, these can cause abdominal discomfort. People

NUTRITION insight

LACTOSE INTOLERANCE

Lactose intolerance is a common intestinal problem. If the enzyme lactase is not produced in sufficient quantity in the small intestine, then lactose in the diet travels into the large intestine. There bacteria break down the lactose into acids and gas. About 30 minutes to 2 hours after consuming milk products, the person with lactose intolerance experiences abdominal distention and gas symptoms. This decrease in lactose digestion does not reduce calcium absorption from milk, but it does create annoying problems.

Lactose intolerance is common in Native Americans, African-Americans, Asians, Hispanics, and people of Mediterranean descent.[10] People who historically raised dairy herds, as did Northern Europeans, show the lowest rates. But even though lactose intolerance is more common in some races than in others, almost anyone is susceptible. Probably 70% of adults worldwide experience a large decrease in their abilities to synthesize lactase as they age. This loss of lactase activity is not due to disease; it happens naturally.

The ability to tolerate lactose is not "all or none."[10] In addition, tolerance can be improved when food choices are changed appropriately. A person with lactose intolerance should not necessarily give up all milk and milk products, because these are very good sources of calcium, the vitamin riboflavin, and the minerals potassium and magnesium. All four of these nutrients are present in other foods in the American diet, but even so, some groups of people don't consume enough of these nutrients. Diet planning for these nutrients is much easier if one uses milk and milk products. A better option for lactose-intolerant people is the consumption of smaller servings of milk products and also taking these with other foods. This often works because the digestive systems of such persons can digest some lactose but not large loads. Fat in a meal also slows digestion, leaving more time for lactase action. Affected people can also eat cheese. Much lactose is lost when milk is made into cheese. Some lactose-intolerant people can tolerate yogurt, because the bacteria in yogurt provide their own lactase activity. Thus if the yogurt contains active bacteria cultures, the lactose present is essentially digested by the yogurt.[13] Freezing destroys the bacteria's activity, so frozen yogurts—as currently manufactured—may have little remaining lactase activity. In general, foods tolerated best by lactose-intolerant individuals are hard cheeses and regular yogurt.

In the past few years, manufacturers have been producing low-lactose milk. To do this, they treat regular milk with lactase that has been isolated from yeast. Most of the lactose is digested into glucose and then galactose, greatly reducing symptoms of lactose intolerance.[5] This milk tastes a bit sweeter, because the breakdown products—glucose and galactose—are together much sweeter than is lactose. This reduces symptoms in most cases. Low-lactose milk can be made at home by adding commercially available lactase to regular milk. Special lactase pills can also be purchased for use at mealtimes. Thus several options are available to lactose-intolerant people, only one of which is abandoning milk products. People with severe lactase deficiency who avoid all dairy products should seek other sources of calcium (see Chapter 9).

Lactose Intolerance *A condition in which lactose digestion is reduced because lactase production declines. Symptoms include gas and bloating after the consumption of dairy products.*

recovering from intestinal disorders, such as diarrhea or bacterial infections, may need to avoid lactose for a few weeks if temporary lactose intolerance is experienced. Two weeks will be sufficient time for the small intestine to again begin producing enough lactase enzyme to allow for lactose digestion.

Carbohydrate Absorption

Single sugars found naturally in foods and those formed as by-products of earlier starch digestion in the mouth and small intestine generally follow an active absorption process (one that requires energy input) when they are taken up by the absorptive cells in the small intestine. Once glucose, galactose, and fructose enter the villi, they are transported via the portal vein to the liver. The liver then exercises its metabolic options—transforming monosaccharides into glucose and releasing them directly into the bloodstream, producing the storage form of carbohydrate glycogen, or producing fat.[14] Only a minor amount of carbohydrate (5%) escapes absorption.

CONCEPT CHECK

Carbohydrate digestion is the process of breaking down larger carbohydrates into their monosaccharide and disaccharide components. Digestion of starches begins in the mouth with salivary amylase. Enzymes made by the pancreas and small intestine complete the digestion of carbohydrates in the small intestine. Primarily following an active absorption process, the single sugars—either resulting from the digestive process or present in the meal as such—are taken up by absorptive cells in the intestine, enter intestinal villi, and are transported via the portal vein to the liver. Then the liver exercises its metabolic options.

PUTTING SIMPLE CARBOHYDRATES TO WORK IN THE BODY

Simple carbohydrates serve a useful function in the body. They provide a necessary and readily available source of energy. This fuel source is generally available at all times to all body cells.[20]

Ketone *Incomplete breakdown products of fat containing three or four carbons.*

Hyperglycemia *High blood glucose levels, above 140 milligrams per 100 milliliters of blood.*

In digestion, starches—also known as complex carbohydrates—are transformed into single-sugar glucose. Therefore, in the body, the main functions of most carbohydrates—both sugars and starches—are the same as they are for glucose itself. We cover starches in detail later.

Producing Energy

The main function of glucose is to supply energy for the body: 1 gram of carbohydrate yields 4 kcalories.[14] Certain tissues in the body, such as red blood cells, can use only glucose and other simple carbohydrate forms for energy. Most parts of the brain also derive energy only from simple carbohydrates, unless the diet contains almost none. In that case, much of the brain can use partial breakdown products of fat—called ***ketones***—for energy (see p. 131). Simple carbohydrates can also fuel muscle cells and other body cells, but many of these cells also use fat for energy needs (see Chapter 11 for details).

In America, carbohydrates supply about 45% of our dietary energy; sugars and starches contribute about equal amounts. Worldwide, however, carbohydrates account for about 70% of all kcalories consumed. In some countries this percentage climbs as high as 80%. In North America and other industrialized areas where meat and overall fat intakes are high, carbohydrates end up supplying a lower percentage of total kcalories.

Regulating This Energy Source. Under normal circumstances, a person's blood glucose level is regulated within a very narrow range. If blood glucose rises too high, the condition is called ***hyperglycemia*** (*hyper* means high, and *emia* means in the bloodstream). Excess glucose then spills over into the urine.[14] This is what happens in people with poorly controlled or undiagnosed diabetes (see the Nutrition Issue in this chapter). If blood glucose falls too low, a person feels nervous, irritable, and hungry, and may develop a headache. This is referred to as ***hypoglycemia*** (*hypo* means low). It is not too surprising that a headache results, because the brain is fueled almost entirely by glucose.

Recall that when carbohydrates are digested and taken up by the absorptive cells of the intestinal villi, the portal vein then transports the resulting sugars to the liver. The liver is the first organ to screen the absorbed sugars. One of its roles is to guard against excess glucose entering the bloodstream after a meal.

The pancreas works with the liver to control glucose levels. As soon as eating begins, the pancreas releases small amounts of the hormone ***insulin.*** Once much glucose enters the bloodstream, the pancreas releases more insulin. This insulin stimulates the liver to synthesize glycogen—the storage form of glucose in the body—and stimulates muscle cells, fat cells, and other cells to increase glucose uptake. By triggering both glucose storage in the liver and glucose movement out of the bloodstream into certain cells, insulin keeps glucose levels from rising too high in the blood[14] (Figure 5-3).

Other hormones have the opposite effects of insulin. When a person has not eaten for a few hours and the blood glucose level begins to fall, the pancreas releases the hormone ***glucagon.*** This hormone prompts the breakdown of glycogen into glucose, which is then released from the liver into the bloodstream. In this way glucagon keeps blood glucose levels from falling too low.[14]

A different mechanism increases blood glucose levels during times of stress. ***Epinephrine*** (adrenaline) is the hormone responsible for the "flight or fight" reaction. It is released in large amounts from the adrenal gland (located near the kidneys) and various nerve endings in response to a perceived threat, such as a car approaching head-on. Epi-

Hypoglycemia
Low blood glucose levels, below 40 to 50 milligrams per 100 milliliters of blood.

Insulin
A hormone produced by the beta cells of the pancreas. Among other processes, insulin increases the synthesis of glycogen in the liver and the movement of glucose from the bloodstream into body cells.

Glucagon
A hormone made by the pancreas that stimulates the breakdown of glycogen in the liver into glucose; this raises the blood glucose level. Glucagon also performs other functions.

Epinephrine
A hormone also known as adrenaline; it is released by the adrenal gland (located near the kidneys) and various nerve endings in the body. It acts to increase glycogen breakdown in the liver, among other functions.

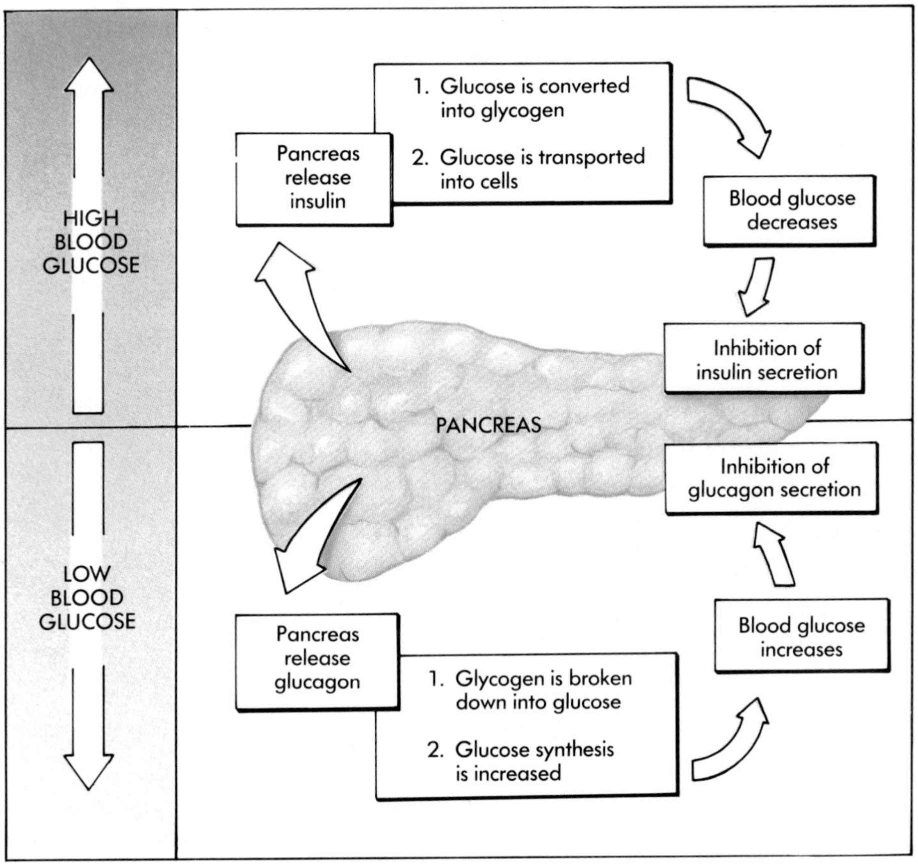

FIGURE 5-3
The regulation of blood glucose. The hormones insulin and glucagon constitute key control points with regard to maintenance of normal blood glucose levels.

In addition, other hormones—such as cortisol, growth hormone, and thyroid hormone—also help regulate the blood glucose level. In essence, the action of insulin to decrease blood glucose is balanced by the actions of glucagon, epinephrine, and these other hormones as they increase blood glucose.

nephrine causes glycogen in the liver to break down into glucose. The resulting rapid flood of glucose into the bloodstream helps promote quick mental and physical reactions.[14]

CONCEPT CHECK

Blood glucose levels are maintained within a very narrow range. When blood glucose levels rise after a meal, the hormone insulin is released in great amounts from the pancreas. Insulin acts to restore normal levels by increasing glucose storage in the liver and glucose uptake by many body cells. If blood glucose levels fall during fasting, then glucagon and other hormones increase the liver's release of glucose into the bloodstream to restore normal levels. In a similar way, the hormone epinephrine can make more glucose available in response to stress. This balance in hormone activity helps maintain blood glucose levels within a healthy range.

TABLE 5-1

The Sweetness of Sugars and Alternative Sweeteners

Type of Sweetener	Relative Sweetness* (Sucrose = 1.0)	Typical Sources
Sugars		
Lactose	0.2	Dairy products
Maltose	0.4	Sprouted seeds
Glucose	0.7	Corn syrup
Sucrose	1.0	Table sugar, most sweets
Invert sugar†	1.3	Some candies, honey
Fructose	1.2 - 1.8	Fruit, honey, some soft drinks
Sugar alcohols		
Sorbitol	0.6	Dietetic candies, sugarless gum
Mannitol	0.7	Dietetic candies
Xylitol	0.9	Sugarless gum
Alternate sweeteners		
Cyclamate	30	Not currently in use in the United States
Aspartame	200	Diet soft drinks, diet fruit drinks, sugarless gum, powdered diet sweetener
Acesulfame-K	200	Sugarless gum, diet drink mixes, powdered diet sweetener, puddings, gelatin desserts
Saccharin (sodium salt)	300	Diet soft drinks

American Dietetic Association, 1993.
**On a per gram basis.*
†Sucrose broken down into glucose and fructose.

Flavoring and Sweetening Foods

Even a young baby responds to sugars with a smile. On the tip of the tongue are sensors for tasting sweetness. The sensors recognize a variety of sugars, and even some noncarbohydrate substances. Some sugars are sweeter than others; per gram, fructose is almost twice as sweet as sucrose under cold and acidic conditions, as found in soft drinks.[2] Glucose and lactose are much less sweet than fructose (Table 5-1).

Sparing Protein and Preventing Ketosis

The importance of carbohydrate fuel for the body cannot be overstated. As a fuel for the brain and red blood cells, it is critical. If you don't eat enough carbohydrates, your body is forced to make glucose from other nutrients, mainly certain amino acids that make up proteins. But then some of the proteins from your diet can't be used to make body tissues and perform other vital functions. Under normal circumstances, sugars in the diet mostly end up as blood glucose to be used by the brain, red blood cells, and most other body cells for fuel. This allows proteins to be saved for their normal functions, like building and maintaining muscles. Therefore sugars are considered protein sparing.

During long-term starvation, proteins in the muscles, heart, liver, kidneys, and other vital organs break down into amino acids, and certain forms are turned into needed glucose.[14] If the process occurs over weeks at a time, these organs become partially weakened. (See Chapters 7 and 18 for discussions of the specific effects of starvation.)

When you don't eat enough carbohydrates, an additional result is that fats don't break down completely in metabolism. In other words, without enough carbohydrate present, fat metabolism is hampered. Partial breakdown products of fats, called ketones, then form. This condition, known as ***ketosis,*** should be avoided, because it disturbs the body's normal acid-base balance and leads to other health problems.[21]

For now, keep in mind that eating at least 50 to 100 grams of carbohydrates per day ensures complete metabolism of fats. It also prevents the body weakness that usually results from needlessly having to use protein to compensate for an insufficient carbohydrate intake. Still, typical adults in the United States need not worry. Our daily carbohydrate intakes usually exceed 100 grams.

Ketosis *The condition of having high levels of ketones in the bloodstream.*

another BITE

The life-threatening wasting of protein that occurs during long-term fasting has prompted companies that produce products used for rapid weight loss, like Optifast,* to include 30 to 120 grams of carbohydrate in the formulation. This significantly decreases protein breakdown, and so helps protect vital tissues and organs, including the heart.

*Most of these products are powders that can be mixed with different kinds of fluids, are consumed five or six times per day, and are very low in kcalories.

CONCEPT CHECK

The major reason to consume carbohydrates is to provide glucose for the energy needs of red blood cells and parts of the brain. Eating less than 50 to 100 grams of carbohydrates per day forces the body to make glucose, using primarily amino acids from proteins found in vital organs. A low glucose supply in cells also inhibits efficient metabolism of fats. Ketosis can then result.

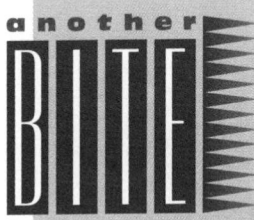

FORMS AND FUNCTIONS OF COMPLEX CARBOHYDRATES

Complex carbohydrates are composed of many units of smaller, simpler carbohydrates. Complex carbohydrates are found primarily in grains, vegetables, and fruits. Scientists recommend that we obtain more complex carbohydrates in our diets as we attempt to moderate use of fat and simple sugars.[6]

Polysaccharides Carbohydrates containing from hundreds to over 3000 or more glucose units; also known as complex carbohydrates.

Amylose A straight-chain digestible polysaccharide made of glucose units.

Polysaccharides

The scientific name for larger complex carbohydrates is ***polysaccharides.*** Polysaccharides are very long carbohydrate chains composed of many monosaccharide units, mainly glucose (*poly* means many). Some polysaccharides have 3000 or more glucose units. These forms include ***amylose*** in plants and glycogen in animal tissues.[20] Amylose is a long, straight chain of glucoses (Figure 5-4). This forms much of the starch found in potatoes, beans, breads, pasta, and rice. In corn, for example, glucose converts to starch as corn ages. This reflects the function of polysaccharides as a carbohydrate storage form in plants.

As noted before, glycogen (animal starch) is a storage form for the glucose we make. This polysaccharide consists of a chain of glucoses with many branches. Enzymes that digest starches can start digestion only at the ends of the molecule. The numerous branches

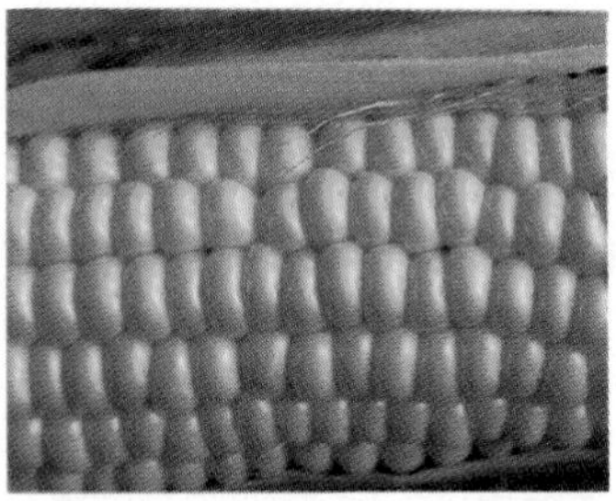

Sugars turn to starch as corn ages.

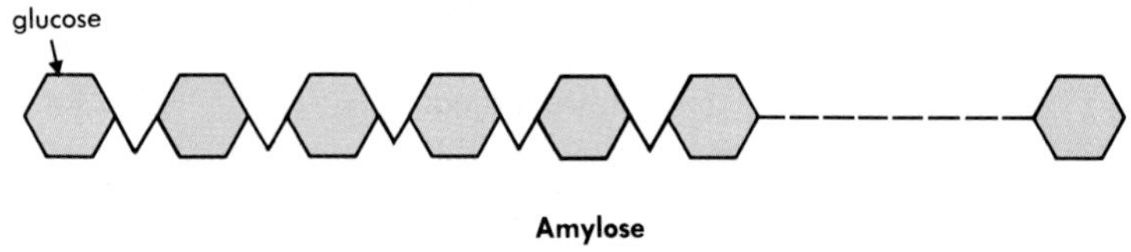

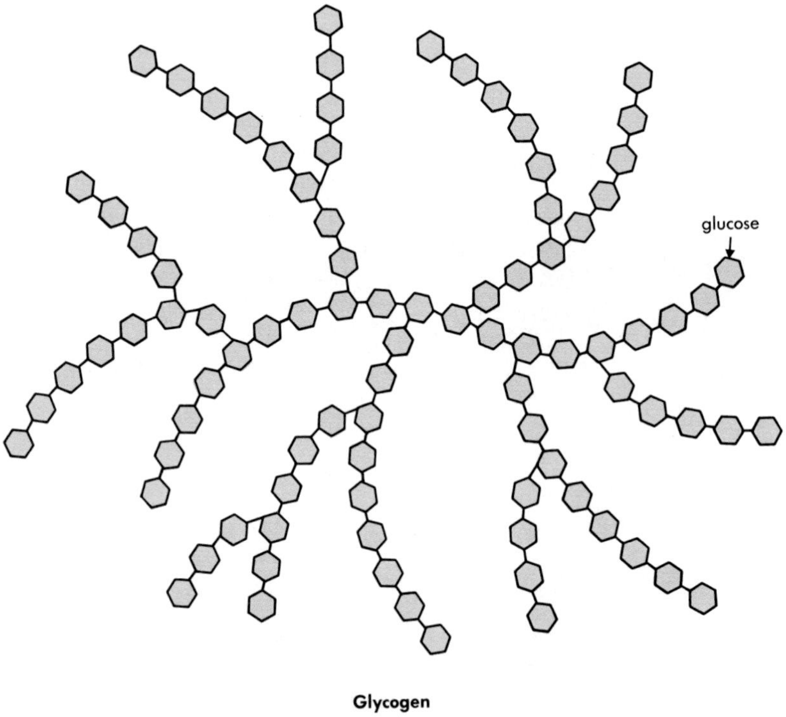

FIGURE 5-4
Some common starches. We consume essentially no glycogen. All glycogen found in the body is made by our cells, primarily in the liver and muscle.

of a glycogen molecule provide many sites (ends) for enzyme action. It is thus an ideal form for carbohydrate storage in the body, because it can be quickly broken down.[14] Because both plant and animal starches yield glucose in digestion, their function in the body is the same as that of simple carbohydrates—to provide energy.

The liver and muscles are the major storage sites for glycogen. Because only about 80 kcalories of glucose are available from the blood, these storage sites for carbohydrate energy—amounting to about 1800 kcalories—are extremely important. The 400 kcalories of liver glycogen can be turned into blood glucose, but the 1400 kcalories of muscle glycogen cannot.[14] Still, glycogen in muscles can supply glucose for muscle use, especially during high-intensity and endurance exercise. (See Chapter 11 for a discussion of carbohydrate use in exercise.)

Dietary Fibers

Dietary fibers are primarily polysaccharides. They differ from starches in that the chemical links that join individual sugar units cannot be digested by human enzymes in the small intestine. This prevents the small intestine from absorbing the sugars that make up dietary fibers. Dietary fiber is not a single substance, but actually a group of substances with similar characteristics (Table 5-2).[19] The group consists of the carbohydrates ***cellulose, hemicelluloses, pectins, gums,*** and ***mucilages,*** as well as the noncarbohydrate ***lignins.***

Cellulose, hemicelluloses, and lignins form the structural parts of plants. A cotton ball is pure cellulose. Bran fiber is rich in hemicelluloses. The woody fibers in broccoli are partly lignins. Because none of these compounds readily dissolves in water, nor is metabolized by intestinal bacteria, they are called ***insoluble fibers.***[19]

Pectins, gums, and mucilages are contained around and inside plant cells. These compounds either dissolve or swell when put into water. So they are called ***soluble fibers.***[19] These exist as gum arabic, guar gum, locust bean gum, and various pectin forms in foods, especially in salad dressings, some frozen desserts, jams, and jellies.

Most foods contain mixtures of soluble and insoluble fibers. A food listed as a good source of one type of fiber usually contains some of the other type of dietary fiber. So when adding fiber-rich foods to your diet, you usually get both types.

Insoluble Fibers
Fibers that mostly do not dissolve in water and are not digested by bacteria in the large intestine. These include cellulose, some hemicelluloses, and lignins.

Soluble Fibers
Fibers that either dissolve or swell when in water or are metabolized by bacteria in the large intestine. These include pectins, gums, mucilages, and some hemicelluloses.

TABLE 5-2

Classification of Dietary Fibers

Type	Component	Examples	Physiological Effects	Major Food Sources
Insoluble				
Noncarbohydrate	Lignins	Wheat bran	Uncertain	All plants
Carbohydrate	Cellulose	Wheat products	Increases fecal bulk	All plants
	Hemicelluloses	Brown rice	Decreases intestinal transit time	Wheat, rye, rice, vegetables
Soluble				
Carbohydrate	Pectins, gums, mucilages	Apples Bananas Citrus fruits Carrots Barley Oats Kidney beans	Delays stomach emptying; slows glucose absorption; can lower blood cholesterol level	Citrus fruits, oat products, beans

Diverticulae *Pouches that protrude through the outside wall of the large intestine. Diverticulosis is the condition of having many diverticula in the colon.*

Diverticulitis *An inflammation of the diverticula caused by acids produced by bacterial metabolism inside the diverticula.*

Mortality *Synonymous with death; number of deaths.*

Whole Grains *Grains containing the entire seed of the plant, including the bran, germ, and endosperm (starchy interior). Examples include whole wheat and brown rice.*

Another term sometimes used for fiber is ***crude fiber.*** This term was coined in the 1800s to reflect the amount of indigestible foodstuff present in animal feed. Using acids and then alkalis to chemically digest the animal feed, the amount of crude fiber was determined by measuring what remained "undigested." This is mostly cellulose and lignins. Because the other types of dietary fibers are destroyed by this type of treatment, it is misleading to substitute the term crude fiber for dietary fiber. If you see the term crude fiber on food composition tables, keep in mind that values reported often bear little resemblance to dietary fiber values. This point is important. When nutrition scientists talk about fiber, they are referring to dietary fiber. Other terms for fiber, such as *roughage* and *bulk,* are also no longer widely used.

We need much more data concerning the dietary fiber content of foods. In fact, researchers still disagree on the best means for determining dietary fiber content.[19] In all analyses used today, some dietary fiber is lost. That explains the occasional discrepancies that can be found between food tables and nutrition labels on foods concerning the amounts of dietary fiber present.

Why Do We Need Dietary Fiber?

Many types of dietary fiber absorb water and hold onto it in the intestine. When enough fiber is consumed, its water-retaining property helps enlarge and soften the stool, easing elimination.[8] Basically the larger stool size stimulates the intestinal muscles that promote peristalsis (see Chapter 4). Consequently, less pressure is necessary to expel the stool. This link between dietary fiber and the health of the intestine has interested people for hundreds of years.

When too little dietary fiber is eaten, the opposite can occur: the stool may be small and hard. Constipation may result, requiring strong pressures to move the stool in the large intestine during elimination. Hemorrhoids then may result from excessive straining.[21] Also, the high pressures can force parts of the large intestine wall to pop out from between the surrounding bands of muscle. This forms small pouches, called ***diverticulae,*** leading to a condition called diverticulosis. About 50% of elderly people have many of these pouches (Figure 5-5). Diverticulae rarely occur in people in Third World countries, probably because of their high dietary fiber intakes. In contrast, people in Western countries often ingest only a small amount of dietary fiber in their diets.[8]

Diverticulosis is normally not noticeable. But if the diverticula become filled with food particles, especially hulls or seeds, bacteria can metabolize them into acids and gases. This irritates the diverticula and may eventually cause inflammation, a condition known as ***diverticulitis.*** Treatment includes taking antibiotics to counter the bacterial action and eating a limited amount of dietary fiber to reduce a food source for bacterial activity. Once the inflammation subsides, a high dietary fiber intake (but free of seeds) is begun to ease elimination and reduce the risk of a future attack.[21]

Insoluble fibers, particularly certain types of hemicelluloses, are the best fibers for increasing stool size.[8] Again, bran—the fibrous covering of grain kernels—is rich in hemicelluloses. Because bran layers form the outer covering of all grains, whole grains are good sources of insoluble fiber. Increasing fluids and getting regular exercise to stimulate peristalsis are also helpful for intestinal health.[21]

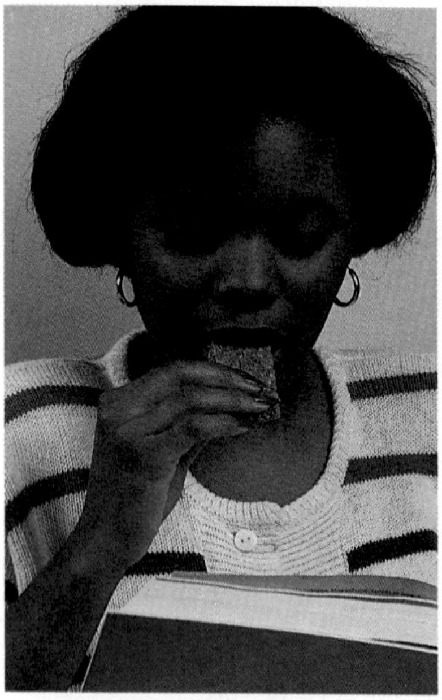

Make high-fiber food choices a regular part of your diet.

Can Dietary Fiber Play Other Roles in Preserving Health?

Dietary fiber may also play a key role in preventing colon cancer.[1,22] Among the deadly cancers, colon cancer ranks second only to lung cancer in occurrence and ***mortality*** in the United States. Dozens of epidemiological studies have linked its occurrence to diets low in ***whole grains,*** fruits, and vegetables—all good sources of dietary fiber—and high in fat, meat, and excess energy intake.[1] Still, researchers are not sure how fiber might affect cancer development. There is a good reason for suggesting that potential cancer-causing compounds in the intestinal contents are being diluted by fluid attracted to the fibers, bound to the fibers, and more rapidly excreted as fibers speed passage of feces through

Bacteria in the large intestine metabolize soluble fibers into such products as acids and gases. These can cause intestinal gas (flatulence). Gas is not harmful but can be inconvenient. However, the body tends to adapt over time and produce less gas.

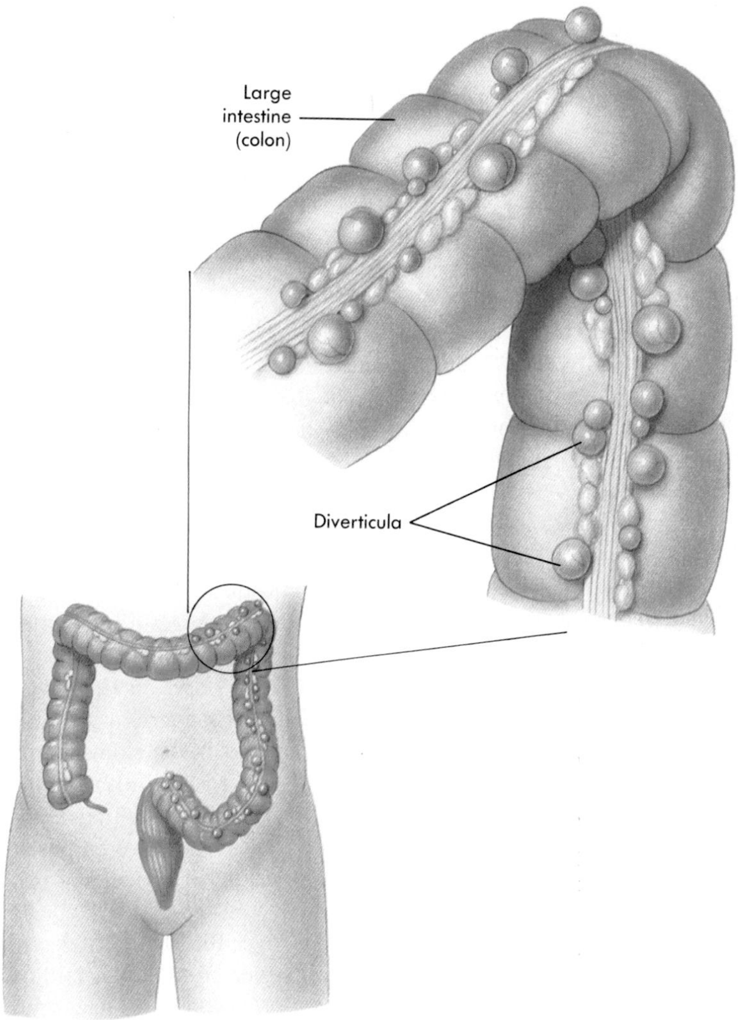

FIGURE 5-5
Diverticulosis in the colon. A low-fiber diet increases the risk of developing this disorder.

the intestinal tract. Colon cancers have been prevented in laboratory animals by dietary fiber. Nevertheless, there is not enough evidence to convince all scientists of this possible effect of fiber.[4] The major protective factors could be increased consumption of compounds such as vitamin C and carotenes in fruits and vegetables, or simply the reduction in meat and fat intake when a high-fiber diet is instituted.

Soluble fibers taken in high amounts in the diet can decrease blood cholesterol levels.[7] The dose, if oat bran is used, needs to be about 80 to 100 grams (about ¾ of a cup) per day—not an easy feat. With cooked beans, about 150 grams (1½ cups) is needed. The effect is partly caused by the binding of cholesterol-rich substances in the intestinal tract. These are pulled into the feces for elimination. Additional mechanisms may be at work as well (see Chapter 6). Other rich sources of soluble fibers include fruits and vegetables in general, soybean fiber, rice bran, and psyllium seeds (found in many commercial fiber laxatives).

NUTRITION insight

HISTORY OF FIBER IN AMERICA

Folklore surrounding dietary fiber has been a part of American culture since the 1800s. Food faddism flourished during this time.

Sylvester Graham, a minister, traveled up and down the East Coast extolling the virtues of fiber in the 1820s and 1830s.[4] Graham claimed that the true cause of disease was the removal of bran from flour during processing. The dark bread (brown bread) he recommended was later called Graham bread. Graham also believed that meat excited vile tempers and drove men to sexual excesses. He claimed that the bacterial infection cholera was the price for too much lewdness and eating chicken pie. He further claimed that people did not bathe enough and needed external applications of cold water at least weekly. Partly as a result of his advocacy, Saturday night baths and sitting-up exercises before open windows became common practices. His legacy to us is the Graham cracker. However, today's graham cracker bears little resemblance to the whole-grain product he promoted.

The next wave of fiber frenzy crested in the mid-1870s. Dr. John Harvey Kellogg was hired by the Seventh Day Adventist Church to manage their health sanitarium in Battle Creek, Michigan. Kellogg claimed that 90% of health ills centered in the stomach and bowels. He advocated ridding the digestive tract of "poisons" derived from meat-eating, drinking, and condiments. He believed that bowel eliminations should occur frequently. Tablespoons of sterilized bran were given to patients at every meal for laxative purposes. Lettuce and bran were commonly given at breakfast. Kellogg said, "Bran does not irritate, it titillates."

Adherents, including many famous people, came from all over the United States to "take the cure" at the sanitarium. Dr. Kellogg became the first person to earn a million dollars from "health foods," and he wrote more than 80 books.

One man who came for a cure in 1891, Charles W. Post, decided he could do what Dr. Kellogg was doing. He created the Post Toasted Cornflakes Company, started producing Postum Cereal Food Coffee, and developed a hard-baked wheat cracker, which he broke into small pieces and called Grape Nuts. Sold as a health food in 1898, it was advocated as a food for the brain and a cure for appendicitis, loose teeth, consumption, and malaria. Post netted $1 million from his products in 1901 alone.

How Much Dietary Fiber Do We Need?

A reasonable goal for dietary fiber intake is 20 to 35 grams per day. The average intake for Americans is closer to half this amount. Men eat more dietary fiber on average than do women, partly because they eat more food. Increasing dietary fiber intake to 20 to 35 grams is not difficult to achieve (Table 5-3). This should prevent much diverticulosis, which typically develops in Western countries.[8] Recall from Chapter 2 that the Food Guide Pyramid suggests we consume 5 to 8 servings of fruits/vegetables and 6 to 11 servings of breads/cereals each day. All of these food choices can provide dietary fiber.

Not to be outdone, William Kellogg—John Harvey Kellogg's brother—began promoting the Kellogg Toasted Corn Flake Company in 1906. Today both companies are active in the breakfast cereal market. True to form, the Kellogg Company is still promoting fiber to Americans.

Fiber finally received its scientific letters in the early 1970s.[19] Dr. Denis Burkitt, a noted British physician, observed that many "Western" diseases did not exist in Africa. These included diverticulitis, colon cancer, appendicitis, hemorrhoids, constipation, and other intestinal disorders. Burkitt surmised that the high-fiber intake of Africans was an important reason these diseases did not occur. He noticed that Africans had very large stools, almost twice the weight of stools from Westerners.

Many researchers followed Burkitt's lead. Soon studies showed that high-fiber intakes decreased the transit time of food through the GI tract. That is, the more fiber eaten, the less time needed to propel the undigested part through the intestinal tract to be eliminated. Researchers suggested that if the stool stayed in the colon for only a short time, less bacterial metabolism of the stool would occur. Thus probably fewer toxins and perhaps fewer carcinogens would form. This faster transit time is especially promoted by insoluble fibers.[8]

As we discussed in Chapter 2, the fiber argument sharpened in the mid-1980s when the Kellogg Company began promoting high-fiber cereals in the war against colon cancer. Actually, the company was following the lead of the National Cancer Institute. Scientists at the National Cancer Institute believed that a verifiable link existed between low-fiber diets and colon cancer and thought the public needed to be alerted.

The bold move by the Kellogg Company to promote fiber to Americans has been criticized as premature by some scientists. They believe that if a low fiber intake is related to colon cancer, it is not a very strong association. Some scientists are still not convinced that a high-fiber diet will prevent enough colon cancer to justify giving fiber much publicity. Fiber is important for regular bowel habits (and is found in some laxatives for that reason). Soluble varieties can help lower blood cholesterol levels.[8] However, scientific research does not support the promotion of fiber to the average person much beyond that.[4]

TABLE 5-3

A 25-Gram Fiber Diet for 1500 kcalories

Menu	Fiber (grams)
Breakfast	
Orange juice, 1 cup	—
Wheaties, ¾ cup	3.0
1% Milk, ½ cup	—
Whole-wheat toast, 1 slice	1.9
Margarine, 1 tsp	—
Coffee	—
Lunch	
Lean ham, 2 oz	—
Whole-wheat bread, 2 slices	3.8
Baked beans, ½ cup	3.5
Mayonnaise, 2 tsp	—
Lettuce, ¼ cup	0.2
Pear (with skin), 1	4.3
Dinner	
Broiled chicken (no skin), 3 oz	—
Baked potato, 1 large (with skin)	3.6
Margarine, 1½ tsp	—
Green beans, 1 cup	2.0
Margarine, ½ tsp	—
1% Milk, 1 cup	—
Apple (with peel), 1	3.0
TOTAL	25 grams

Carbohydrate	*61% of kcalories*
Protein	*19% of kcalories*
Fat	*20% of kcalories*

Increasing Dietary Fiber Intake

Before increasing your dietary fiber intake, first calculate the amount of fiber you are already eating. If it is less than 20 to 35 grams per day, find some foods higher in fiber to substitute for those you already eat, or add some new ones (Table 5-4). Recall from Chapter 2 that eating a high-fiber cereal for breakfast is a good idea. Also, don't remove edible peels from fruits or vegetables unless absolutely necessary.

We suggest whole food sources over bran supplement sources, because foods provide a broader variety of nutrients. This is especially true for many high-fiber foods. Note also that one should drink fluids with fiber-containing foods, because fibers tend to bind with water.

TABLE 5-4

Increasing Dietary Fiber Intake Is Not That Hard to Do

Try This:	Instead of This:	Dietary Fiber Bonus (grams)
Whole-wheat bread, 1 slice	White bread, 1 slice	1.5
Brown rice, ½ cup	White rice, ½ cup	0.5
Baked potato in the skin, 1 medium	Mashed potatoes, ½ cup	1.5
Unpeeled apple (or applesauce made with unpeeled apples), 1 medium	Regular applesauce, ½ cup	1.5
Orange segments, 1 orange	Orange juice, 1 cup	1
Whole-grain cereals (hot or ready-to-eat), 1 cup	Sweetened cereals, 1 cup	2.5
Popcorn (lightly seasoned with butter or salt, if at all), 3 cups	Potato chips, 12	1
Bean dip, ¼ cup	Sour cream dip, ¼ cup	1.5
Kidney beans on salad, 2 Tbsp	Bacon bits on salad, 2 Tbsp	3
Fruit juice, 1 cup	Coffee or tea, 1 cup	1.5
Salad bar, 2 cups	French fries, 12	1.0

By eating whole-grain breads, beans, high-fiber cereals, and fruits and vegetables, it is easy to eat enough dietary fiber. However, some people may need to minimize their intake of foods made with refined flour—doughnuts, sweet rolls, coffee cakes, and white bread—to control energy intake (Figure 5-6).

Read the Label

To check for whole grains, read the label on the food package (Figure 5-7). Note that manufacturers often list enriched white flour as wheat flour on food labels. Most people think that if a product is labeled *wheat,* they are getting a whole-wheat product. However, if the label does not say whole-wheat flour in the ingredient list, it is not a whole-wheat product. Bread made from white (refined) flour lacks the bran that forms a protective coating around the wheat kernel. Bran makes flour coarser, but contains important nutrients, including dietary fiber.

In your search for dietary fiber, must you always avoid white bread, rolls, and fluffy, white pancakes? Must you always choose the whole-grain types? No. You don't have to give up favorite foods, as long as you frequently choose whole-grain alternatives of breads and cereals. Again, the goal of 20 to 35 grams of dietary fiber a day is not that hard to attain (see Table 5-3).

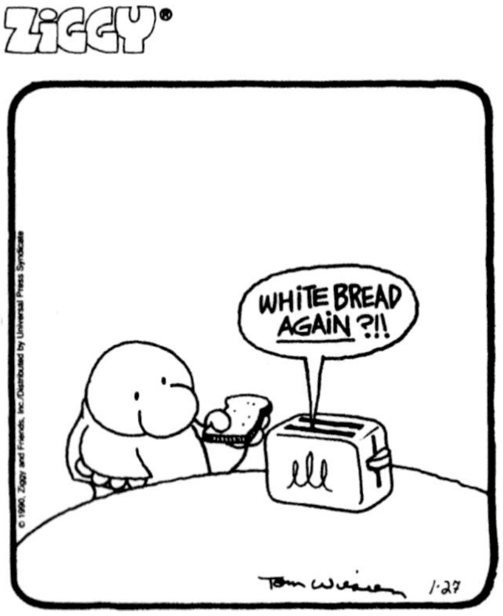

FIGURE 5-6
Ziggy.

Problems with High-Fiber Diets

Very high dietary fiber intakes—for example, 60 grams per day—can pose some health risks. A high dietary fiber intake requires a high water intake. Not consuming enough water with the dietary fiber can leave the stool very hard, making it difficult and painful to eliminate. Intestinal blockage has occurred in people who consume great amounts of wheat bran and oat bran. Large amounts of dietary fiber can also bind important minerals, especially calcium, zinc, and iron, making them less available to the body.[8] More studies are needed concerning the long-term effects of high-fiber diets on mineral status. High-fiber diets also contribute to intestinal gas. Finally, great amounts of dietary fiber can fill up a child before he or she eats enough food to meet energy needs. As with many practices, moderation with dietary fiber is the best approach.

INGREDIENTS: Corn, wheat, and oat flour; sugar; partially hydrogenated vegetable oil (one or more of: cottonseed, coconut, and soybean); salt; color added including yellow #6; natural orange, lemon, and cherry and other natural flavorings;
VITAMINS AND MINERALS: vitamin C (sodium ascorbate and ascorbic acid); niacinamide; zinc (oxide); iron; vitamin B_6 (pyridoxine hydrochloride); vitamin B_2 (riboflavin); vitamin A (palmitate; protected with BHT); vitamin B (thiamin hydrochloride); folic acid; and vitamin D.

CARBOHYDRATE INFORMATION

	Cereal	With 1/2 cup vitamins A & D skim milk
Complex carbohydrates, g	11	11
Sucrose & other sugars, g	13	19
Dietary fibers, g	1	1
Total carbohydrates, g	25	31

INGREDIENTS

Whole wheat, raisins, wheat bran, sugar, natural flavoring, salt, corn syrup and honey.

VITAMINS AND MINERALS

Vitamin A palmitate, niacinamide, iron, zinc oxide (source of zinc), vitamin B_6, riboflavin (vitamin B_2), thiamine mononitrate (vitamin B_1), vitamin B_{12}, folic acid and vitamin D.

CARBOHYDRATE INFORMATION

	Cereal	With skim milk
Dietary fiber	6g	6g
Complex carbohydrate	11g	11g
Natural sugar in raisins	7g	7g
Sucrose and other sugars	7g	13g
Total carbohydrate	31g	37g

FIGURE 5-7
Reading labels helps us choose more nutritious foods. Based on information from their nutrition labels, which cereal is the better choice for breakfast? Especially consider dietary fiber. Did the ingredient list give you any clues?

CONCEPT CHECK

Dietary fiber has been the focus of human attention for centuries. Insoluble fiber forms are a vital part of the diet because they provide mass to the stool, which helps ease elimination and lessen the risk for developing diverticulosis. Fiber in the diet may also reduce the risk of colon cancer. Soluble fiber can aid in decreasing blood cholesterol levels. Whole grains, vegetables, and fruits are excellent sources of both types of dietary fiber.

RECOMMENDATIONS FOR CARBOHYDRATE INTAKE

No RDA for carbohydrate intake has been established. As we discussed before, it is important to consume at least 50 to 100 grams of carbohydrate per day to prevent ketosis. This assumes that the diet also contains enough total kcalories to meet energy needs. It is easy to consume 50 grams of carbohydrate. Just 3 pieces of fruit, 3 slices of bread, or a little more than 3 cups of milk suffice. In fact, it is difficult to eat so little carbohydrate in a diet that it produces ketosis.

Beyond that need, carbohydrates provide important fuel for the body. The average adult American eats more than 130 grams of a combination of all carbohydrates—sugars and starches—per day. This adds up to about 45% of all kcalories eaten. We noted in Chapter 2 that many health authorities recommend that we boost carbohydrate intake to 55% or more of kcalories and reduce fat intake (Figure 5-8).

Most carbohydrates in the American diet are consumed in the form of white breads, sugared soft drinks, baked goods, sugar itself, and milk. The Dietary Guidelines we discussed in Chapter 2 emphasize the importance of starch and fiber in the diet. We suggest that you eat at least one third or more of your kcalories in the form of starches—35% to 45% of total energy intake is a reasonable goal (Figure 5-9). The diet listed in Table 5-3 illustrates one example of this approach.

Each day Americans eat about 80 grams of sugars, not including the lactose in dairy products. This 80 grams is made up of a combination of (1) sugars that naturally occur in foods, such as in fruits and (2) sugars that are added during food processing, such as in jam. This total sugar intake corresponds to about 18% of total energy intake.[2] Most of these sugars are added to foods and beverages during manufacturing. The rest occur naturally in foods or are added from the sugar bowl. Overall consumption of sucrose has dropped in the last 10 years, but consumption of corn sweeteners has increased. This is mostly because corn sweeteners are cheaper to use for food manufacturers than are other forms of sugars.

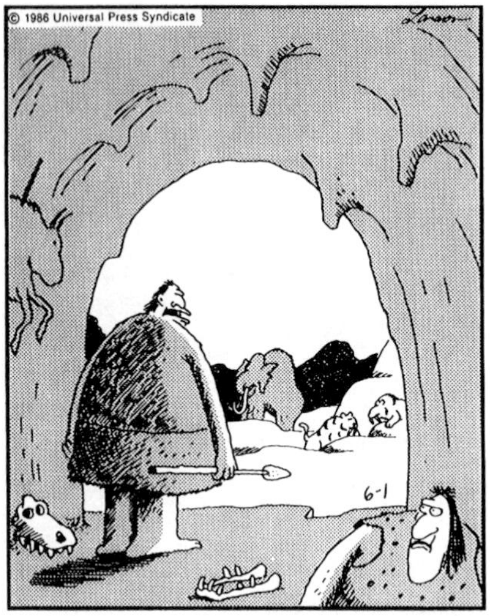
© 1986 Universal Press Syndicate
6-1

"Once in a while couldn't we just have some pasta?"

FIGURE 5-8
The Far Side.

another BITE

During processing of food, the sugar content often is increased. Usually, the more processed the food, the higher the sugar content. An apple has 0 grams of added sugar, canned apples in heavy syrup have 10 to 15 grams, and one sixth of a 9-inch apple pie has 30 grams of added sugar. For comparison purposes, 1 teaspoon of sugar is 5 grams.

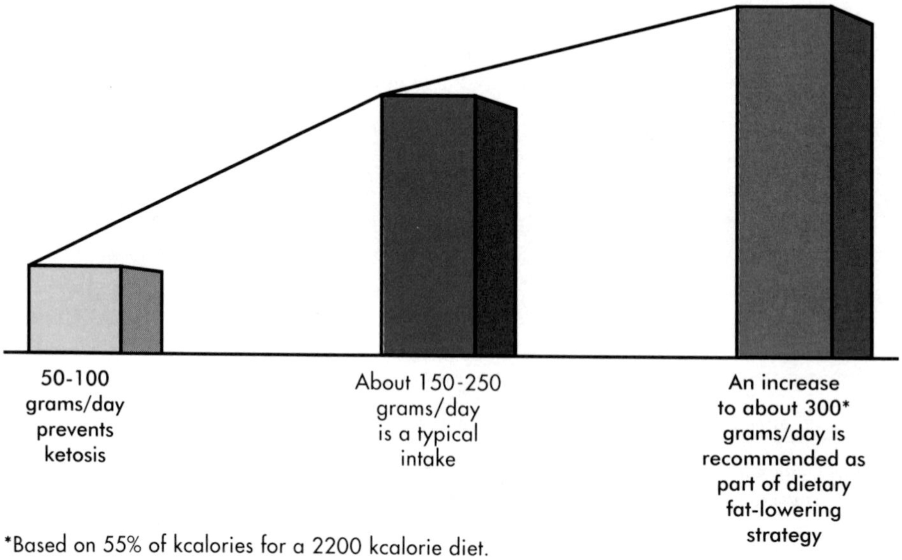
50-100 grams/day prevents ketosis
About 150-250 grams/day is a typical intake
An increase to about 300* grams/day is recommended as part of dietary fat-lowering strategy
*Based on 55% of kcalories for a 2200 kcalorie diet.

FIGURE 5-9
The dietary carbohydrate continuum. Relatively little dietary carbohydrate is needed to prevent ketosis. Much more carbohydrate is advised, especially complex varieties, as we reduce our fat intake and search for kcalories to replace those fat kcalories.

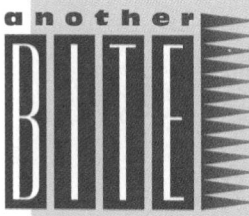

TABLE 5-5

Some Sources of Sugars

Food	Serving	Teaspoons of Sugar
Beverages		
Cola drinks	1 (12-oz bottle or glass)	7
Cordials	1 (3/4-oz glass)	1 1/2
Ginger ale	12 oz	10
Orangeade	1 (8-oz glass)	5
Root beer	1 (10-oz bottle)	4 1/2
Seven-up	1 (12-oz bottle)	7 1/2
Cakes and cookies		
Angel food	1 (4-oz piece)	7
Applesauce cake	1 (4-oz piece)	5 1/2
Banana bread	1 (2-oz piece)	2
Cheesecake	1 (4-oz piece)	2
Chocolate cake, plain	1 (4-oz piece)	6
Chocolate cake, iced	1 (4-oz piece)	10
Coffee cake	1 (4-oz piece)	4 1/2
Cupcake, iced	1	6
Fruit cake	1 (4-oz piece)	5
Jelly-roll	1 (2-oz piece)	2 1/2
Orange cake	1 (4-oz piece)	4
Pound cake	1 (4-oz piece)	5
Sponge cake	1 (1-oz piece)	2
Strawberry shortcake	1 serving	4
Brownies, unfrosted	1 (3/4 oz)	3
Chocolate cookies	1	1 1/2
Fig Newtons	1	5
Dairy products		
Ice cream	1/3 pt (3 1/2 oz)	3 1/2
Ice cream bar	1	1-7 accord. to size
Ice cream cone	1	3 1/2
Ice cream soda	1	5
Ice cream sundae	1	7
Malted milk shake	1 (10-oz glass)	5
Frozen yogurt	3 oz	3

Food	Serving	Teaspoons of Sugar
Jellies and jams		
Apple butter	1 Tbsp	1
Jelly	1 Tbsp	4-6
Orange marmalade	1 Tbsp	4-6
Peach butter	1 Tbsp	1
Strawberry jam	1 Tbsp	4
Candies		
Milk chocolate bar (e.g., Hershey)	1 (1 1/2 oz)	2 1/2
Chewing gum	1 stick	1/2
Fudge	1-oz square	4 1/2
Gumdrop	1	2
Hard candy	1 oz	5
Lifesavers	1	1/2
Peanut brittle	1	3 1/2
Canned fruits and juices		
Canned apricots	4 halves & 1 Tbsp syrup	3 1/2
Canned fruit juices, sweetened	1/2 cup	2
Canned peaches	2 halves & 1 Tbsp syrup	3 1/2
Fruit salad	1/2 cup	3 1/2
Fruit syrup	2 Tbsp	2 1/2
Stewed fruits	1/2 cup	2
Breakfast cereals*		
Cheerios	1 oz	1/5
Special K	1 oz	2/3
Total	1 oz	2/3
Quaker 100% Natural	1 oz	2
Sugar Frosted Flakes	1 oz	2
Sugar Smacks	1 oz	3
Raisin Bran	1 oz	1 1/2
Cracklin' Oat Bran	1 oz	1 1/2
Froot Loops	1 oz	2 1/2
Cap'n Crunch	1 oz	2 1/2
Rice Krispies	1 oz	2/3

**Before milk is added.*

Although a desirable level of sugar intake has not yet been set, less than 10% to 15% of total kcalorie intake is considered a reasonable level.[2] This allows for 10 to 15 teaspoons a day on a 2000-kcalorie diet, including what is added to foods, such as cookies and soft drinks. Table 5-5 shows some common sources of sugars in our diets. Are these foods major players in your diet?

Does This Mean Sugar Is Bad for You?

Some people think it is not healthful to consume sugar at all. It is true foods high in simple sugars may supply few, if any, vitamins, minerals, or proteins compared with the number of kcalories they supply. However, if you can afford to consume some extra kcalories, there is nothing wrong with eating moderate amounts of sugar. Scientists think

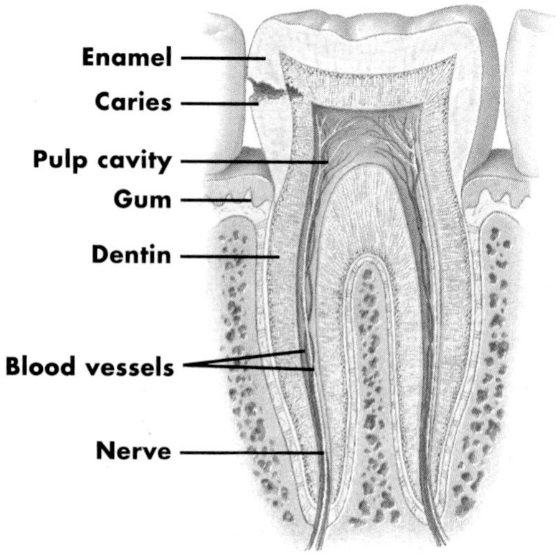

FIGURE 5-10

Dental caries. Bacteria can collect in various areas on a tooth. Simple sugars are used by the bacteria to create acid that can dissolve tooth enamel, leading to caries. The bacteria also produce plaque to adhere themselves to the tooth surface.

that sugar is mostly a problem when it is eaten at the expense of more nutritious foods. When this happens, a person could become deficient in vitamins and other important nutrients.[2]

Dental caries (cavities) is the main problem associated with a high sugar intake.[2] Cavities are formed when bacteria that live on the teeth metabolize sugars to acid. The acid then dissolves the tooth enamel and underlying structure (Figure 5-10). Starches in breads and cakes that stick to the teeth can also cause caries. These starches are metabolized to maltose by saliva in the mouth and then used by bacteria on the teeth.

Tooth decay actually begins with dental plaque, the sticky film that continuously forms in the mouth. Bacteria that produce the plaque are also those responsible for the breakdown of food, particularly sugars, into acids.

another BITE

Research has indicated that certain foods—such as cheese, peanuts, and sugar-free chewing gum—actually can help reduce the amount of acid on teeth. Also, if one rinses after meals and snacks, the acidity level in the mouth is reduced.

Overall, the frequency and amount of time that sugar is retained in the mouth play the greatest role in the cariogenicity of a food. Sticky or gummy foods that are high in sugars—such as caramels and raisins—are the worst caries offenders, whereas liquid sugar sources—like fruit juices—are not nearly so bad. Note also that sugar-containing foods are not the only foods that are turned to acid by the bacteria in the mouth. If held in the mouth for a long time, starch-containing foods (such as saltines and breads) may be acted on by enzymes in the mouth that break down the starch to sugar. The frequency of snacking on sugar-containing foods affects dental health in the absence of good dental hygiene. Snacking regularly allows the bacteria on the teeth to continually make acid. It is best to limit the intake of sweets or to eat them with meals, instead of between meals or by themselves. This way, other foods help to dilute and neutralize the acid that is produced.

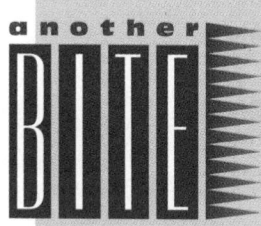

In the last 15 years, dental caries rates have decreased by 30% in the United States, even though simple-sugar consumption has remained about constant. This decline is primarily because of the addition of fluoride to water. When teeth develop in the presence of the mineral fluoride, they become much more resistant to acid (see Chapter 9).

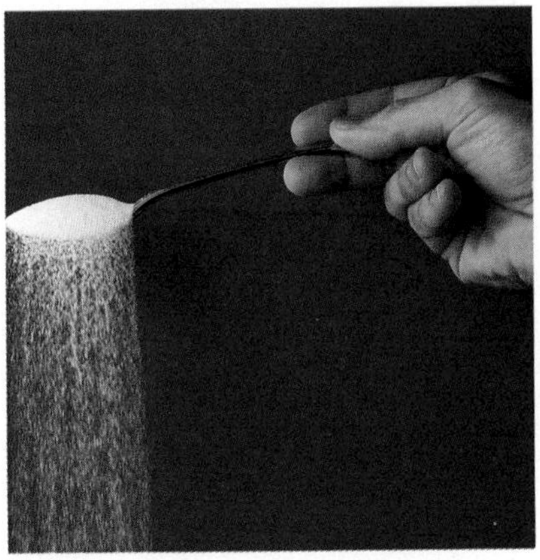

Sugars should be used in moderation, because they provide little else than a source of energy.

Are There Risks Besides Dental Caries?

No credible research supports claims that sugar causes heart disease, diabetes, or other problems. Many major scientific groups have examined the research surrounding sugar and basically have given sugar a clean bill of health, except for its tendency to cause dental caries.[2]

As for sugar's connection to hyperactivity, some researchers have suggested that sucrose affects behavior, especially in children. They claim that sucrose creates an excited—even antisocial—state, which may lead to violence and disruptive behavior. However, most researchers find that sucrose itself is not the villain. It actually has a calming effect on many children.[9] If there is a villain, it is probably the excitement or tension in situations where high-sucrose foods are prevalent, such as at parties and on Halloween. Any improvement in behavior that is seen when a child is put on a relatively sucrose-free diet is probably because of the extra attention received.

In the final analysis, use of sugar should follow the same guideline given for many other food products—moderation. By regularly visiting the dentist, practicing good dental hygiene, and following the Food Guide Pyramid while keeping weight under control, consuming sugar in reasonable amounts poses no health threat. Table 5-6 advises how to reduce sugar intake if you think you eat too much of it.

Names of sugars used in foods

- Sugar
- Sucrose
- Brown sugar
- Confectioners' sugar (powdered sugar)
- Turbinado sugar
- Invert sugar
- Glucose
- Levulose
- Lactose
- Honey
- Corn syrup or sweeteners
- High-fructose corn syrup
- Molasses
- Maple syrup
- Dextrose
- Fructose
- Maltose

TABLE 5-6

Suggestions for Reducing Sugar Intake

At the Supermarket

- Read ingredient labels. Identify all the added sugars in a product. Select items lower in total sugar when possible.
- Buy fresh fruits or fruits packed in water, juice, or light syrup, rather than those in heavy syrup.
- Buy fewer foods that are high in sugar, such as prepared baked goods, candies, sweet desserts, soft drinks, and fruit-flavored punches and soft drinks. Substitute vanilla wafers, graham crackers, bagels, English muffins, and diet soft drinks, for example.
- Buy nuts (dry roasted), sunflower seeds, and popcorn (use hot-air popper) to replace candy for snacks.

In the Kitchen

- Reduce the sugar in foods prepared at home. Try new recipes or adjust your own. Start by reducing the sugar gradually until you've decreased it by one third or more.
- Experiment with such spices as cinnamon, cardamom, coriander, nutmeg, ginger, and mace to enhance the flavor of foods.
- Use home-prepared items (with less sugar) instead of commercially prepared ones that are higher in sugar, when possible.

At the Table

- Use less of all sugars. This includes white and brown sugar, honey, molasses, and syrups.
- Choose fewer foods high in sugar, such as prepared baked goods, candies, and sweet desserts.
- Reach for fresh fruit instead of a sweet for dessert or when you want a snack.
- Add less sugar to foods—coffee, tea, cereal, or fruit. Get used to using half as much, then see whether you can cut back even more
- Cut back on the number of sugared soft drinks and punches you drink. Substitute water, fruit juice, or diet soft drinks.

From the USDA Home and Garden Bulletin No. 232-5, 1986.

CARBOHYDRATES IN FOODS

For foods in general, the greatest nutrient densities for carbohydrates are found in sugars, honey, jams and jellies, fruit, and potatoes. They contain essentially all their energy as carbohydrate (Figure 5-11). Corn flakes, rice, bread, and noodles all contain at least 75% of their energy as carbohydrates. Foods with moderate amounts of carbohydrates are peas, broccoli, oatmeal, pork and beans, cream pies, French fries, and skim milk. In these foods the overall carbohydrate concentration is reduced either by the ample protein content, as in the case of skim milk, or by fat, as in the case of a cream pie.

Chocolate, potato chips, and whole milk contain 30% to 40% of energy as carbohydrates. Again, the carbohydrate content of these foods is overwhelmed by either their fat or protein content. Foods with essentially no carbohydrates include beef, chicken, fish, vegetable oils, butter, and margarine.

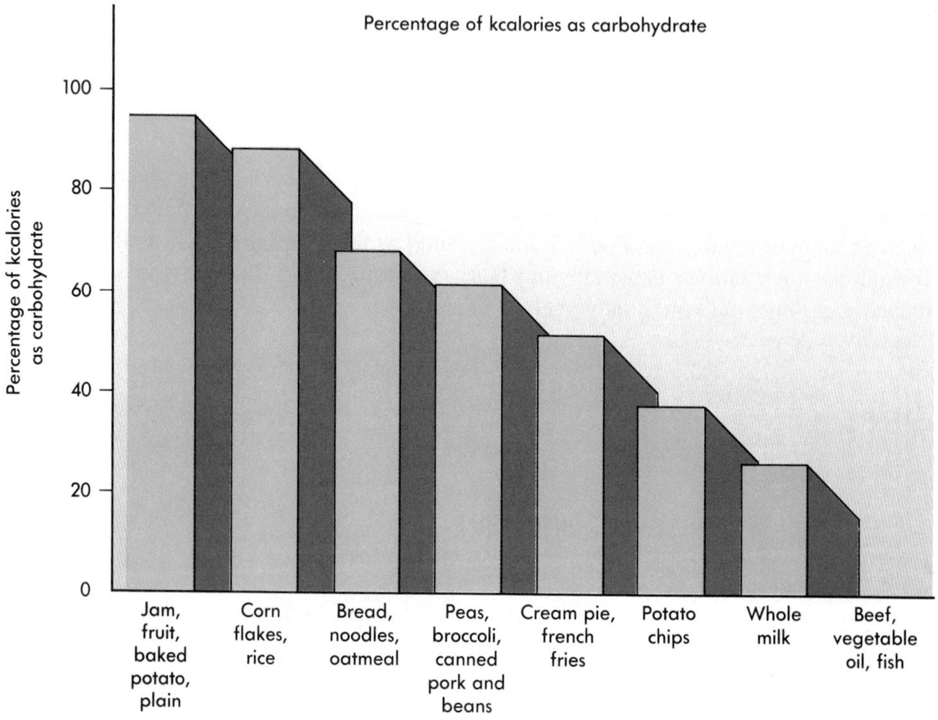

FIGURE 5-11

Percent of kcalories as carbohydrates in foods. Jams, fruits, rice, and many breakfast cereals provide almost all kcalories as carbohydrates. Fruits, vegetables, and grains are often high in complex carbohydrates.

Sweeteners in Foods

Sucrose is the tried-and-true sweetener. A relatively new sweetener in food is ***high-fructose corn syrup,*** which contains 40% to 90% fructose.[2] It is made by treating corn starch with acid and enzymes. Much of the starch is broken down into glucose and then changed into fructose. The syrup is usually as sweet as sugar. Its major advantage is that it is cheaper and can be shipped in a more concentrated form than sugar. Also, it has better freezing properties, because it doesn't encourage the formation of ice crystals. High-fructose corn syrups are used in soft drinks, candies, jams, jellies, other fruit products, and desserts.

High-Fructose Corn Syrup
A corn syrup containing between 40% and 90% fructose.

In addition to sucrose and high-fructose corn syrup, brown sugar, turbinado sugar, honey, maple syrup, and other sugars are added to foods. Raw (unrefined) sugar is generally unavailable in the United States. FDA considers it unfit for human consumption. A partially refined version of raw sugar that can be sold is turbinado sugar. This has a slight molasses flavor. Brown sugar is basically white sugar containing some molasses; either the molasses is not totally removed from the sugar during processing or it is added back to the sucrose crystals.

Maple syrup is made by boiling down the sap from sugar maple trees. Pancake syrup sold in supermarkets is sweetened mostly with corn syrup—not maple syrup.

To make honey, bees alter nectar from plants, breaking down the sucrose into fructose and glucose. Honey offers the same nutritional value as do other simple sugar sources. A common misconception is that honey contains vitamins and minerals. It is a source of energy but little else (see Appendix A). Note that giving honey to infants is risky, because it can contain spores of the bacterium ***Clostridium botulinum.*** These spores can develop into bacteria that cause fatal food-borne illness (see Chapter 17). Adults can safely consume honey because the acidic environment of an adult's stomach inhibits bacterial growth. An infant's stomach is not very acidic, leaving it susceptible to the risks this bacterium poses.

Only the sweetener black strap molasses, a by-product of sugar production, contains any appreciable amount of minerals. However, our consumption of molasses in foods is very low.

Sorbitol ■
An alcohol derivative of glucose that yields about 4 kcalories per gram but is slowly absorbed from the small intestine. It is used in some sugarless gums and dietetic foods.

Saccharin ■
An alternate sweetener that yields no energy to the body; it is 300 times sweeter than sucrose.

Aspartame ■
An alternate sweetener made of two amino acids (part of proteins) and methanol; it is 200 times sweeter than sucrose (table sugar).

Alternate Sweeteners

People who want to limit sugar have two sets of alternate sweeteners to consider. One set is the sugar alcohols: ***sorbitol,*** mannitol, and xylitol.[20] Today the one used in greatest amount in foods is sorbitol. This is found in some sugarless gum and some dietetic foods like dietetic candy. Sugar alcohols yield energy (close to 4 kcalories per gram) but are not readily metabolized by the bacteria in the mouth. Thus they do not promote dental caries. Nor do sugar alcohols cause as rapid a rise in blood glucose as do typical dietary monosaccharides—hence their use in dietetic foods. However, when taken in large amounts, sorbitol and mannitol can cause diarrhea, because they are not readily absorbed from the small intestine.[9] Products whose foreseeable consumption may result in a daily ingestion of 50 grams of sorbitol or mannitol must bear this labeling statement: "Excess consumption may have a laxative effect."

The other major class of alternate sweeteners available in the United States today are saccharin, aspartame, and acesulfame-K. Another alternate sweetener, cyclamate, was banned in 1970 by the FDA because of its link with cancer and birth defects. New research has introduced some questions about the necessity of such a ban. Depending on this reexamination, cyclamate could be back on the grocery shelves soon.[9]

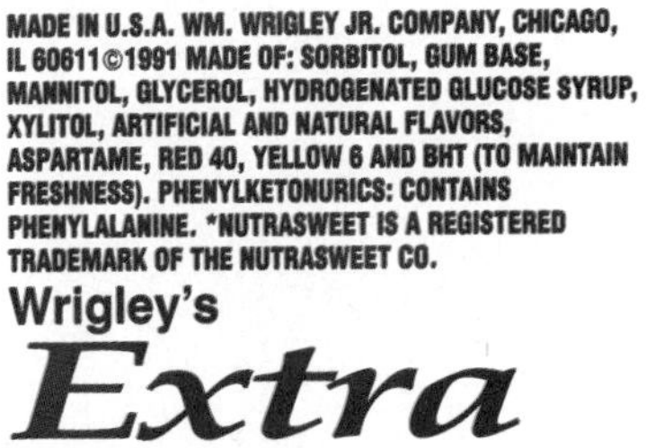
MADE IN U.S.A. WM. WRIGLEY JR. COMPANY, CHICAGO, IL 60611©1991 MADE OF: SORBITOL, GUM BASE, MANNITOL, GLYCEROL, HYDROGENATED GLUCOSE SYRUP, XYLITOL, ARTIFICIAL AND NATURAL FLAVORS, ASPARTAME, RED 40, YELLOW 6 AND BHT (TO MAINTAIN FRESHNESS). PHENYLKETONURICS: CONTAINS PHENYLALANINE. *NUTRASWEET IS A REGISTERED TRADEMARK OF THE NUTRASWEET CO.
Wrigley's
Extra

Sugar alcohols can be found in sugarless gum. Note that aspartame is also used to sweeten this product.

Saccharin. The sweetener ***saccharin*** was first produced in 1879. Although widely used in soft drinks and table sweeteners, it has been recently linked with cancer. Laboratory animals have developed bladder cancer when given high doses of saccharin, especially in the second generation after exposure.[2] Arguments continue concerning the interpretation of data from these experiments, mostly because of saccharin's weak carcinogenic nature, if it is carcinogenic at all. In 1977 FDA attempted to ban saccharin because of this association with cancer. Many saccharin users protested a ban, because it left them with no low-kcalorie sweetener (the others were not available in 1977). Public pressure persuaded Congress to prevent FDA from banning saccharin. In 1991 FDA withdrew its 1977 proposal to ban saccharin. However, products containing saccharin must contain a label of warning of the cancer risk.

Aspartame. In 1981 the alternate sweetener, ***aspartame,*** became available. Its trade name is NutraSweet when added to foods and Equal when sold as powder. Aspartame is composed of the amino acids phenylalanine and aspartic acid, with the addition of methanol. Because amino acids are the building blocks of proteins, aspartame belongs more in the protein class than in the carbohydrate class. Aspartame yields energy—4 kcalories per gram—but is 200 times sweeter than sucrose. This means that much less aspartame yields the same sweetening potency as sucrose. Today aspartame is used mostly in beverages, gelatin desserts, chewing gum, and other food items.[2] Soon it will likely appear in some baked goods, fruit drinks, and other foods as FDA has expanded the allowable uses.

Aspartame is in widespread use throughout the world. It has been approved for use by more than 90 countries, and its use has been endorsed by the World Health Organization, American Medical Association, American Diabetes Association, and American Academy of Pediatrics Committee on Nutrition.[9] Although aspartame never has been linked with cancer, individuals have filed complaints with the FDA claiming adverse reactions to aspartame—headaches, dizziness, seizures, nausea, allergic reactions, and other side effects.

It is important for people who are sensitive to aspartame to avoid it. But the percentage of sensitive people is extremely small. Considering its wide use, the relatively small number of complaints made against aspartame to date suggests most people can use it. In addition, careful research casts doubt on whether it causes headaches or mood swings.[18]

another BITE

You may be left still feeling hungry after consuming an aspartame-sweetened beverage on an empty stomach. This is because you essentially tried to quell hunger with carbonated water. Your usual sugared soft drink would have led to a rise in blood glucose levels and in turn reduced hunger (see Chapter 10 for a look at the glucose-hunger link). A possible solution is to combine a diet beverage with a small meal. This way you can save the kcalories that you would have consumed from the simple sugar-laden beverage and provide energy to quell your hunger from more healthful foods.

Aspartame's high phenylalanine content concerns some people. They feel the blood levels of this amino acid may increase too much, because aspartame is not balanced by the other amino acids normally found in protein foods. This situation can be easily avoided by consuming aspartame with protein foods. Some people also are concerned about aspartame's methanol content. However, the amount of methanol in a soft drink sweetened with aspartame is not more than is found in a cup of many fruit or vegetable juices.

Overall, the scientific community agrees that aspartame itself is safe; as we said, numerous scientific and medical groups support its use. An acceptable daily intake set by the FDA is equivalent to about 14 cans of diet soft drinks a day for an adult, or about 80 packets of Equal. Aspartame is safe for children and pregnant women to consume, but some scientists suggest cautious use by these groups.[12]

One final note about aspartame. A rare disease called ***phenylketonuria (PKU)*** lessens a person's ability to metabolize phenylalanine. We discuss PKU in Chapter 7. For now, note that you were tested for this disease as an infant, probably before leaving the hospital. Labels on products containing aspartame warn people with PKU against using the product (see margin note on p. 145). Individuals carrying only one PKU gene in their DNA do not have the disease and can consume aspartame. Only a person with two PKU genes has inherited the disease and should not use aspartame.

Phenylketonuria (PKU)
A disease in which the liver cannot readily metabolize the amino acid phenylalanine. Toxic by-products of phenylalanine can then build up in the body and lead to mental retardation.

Acesulfame-K
An alternate sweetener that yields no energy to the body; it is 200 times sweeter than sucrose.

Acesulfame-K. The newest alternate sweetener in the United States, ***acesulfame-K*** (Sunette), was approved by the FDA in July 1988. Acesulfame-K is 200 times sweeter than sucrose. Presently, it can be used in chewing gum, powdered drink mixes, gelatins, puddings, and nondairy creamers. It contributes no kcalories to the diet because it is not broken down by the body.

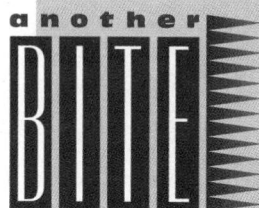

Some studies show that laboratory animals develop cancer after exposure to acesulfame-K. However, the FDA's analysis of these studies suggests that the tumors were not caused by acesulfame-K consumption. They were routinely seen in the untreated animal species studied. Therefore acesulfame-K has FDA approval.[9] It is already used as a sweetener in foods and beverages in at least 40 countries. Acesulfame-K can be used in baking, whereas the current form of aspartame cannot because it breaks down when heated. So acesulfame-K may see wider uses. Currently, little information has been published about acesulfame-K. Some nutrition professionals think the approval of acesulfame-K occurred very rapidly, when compared with other alternate sweeteners, and so still view use of this substance with caution.

On the whole, alternate sweeteners offer many useful benefits: people with diabetes can now enjoy the flavor of sweetness without adding sugar to their diet, and alternate sweeteners can aid in weight loss by providing noncaloric or very low-kcalorie sugar substitutes. There is no conclusive evidence that alternate sweeteners drive hunger or cause weight gain[16]—they do, however, provide individuals who desire to reduce sugar intake with a tasteful alternative.

CONCEPT CHECK

There is no RDA for carbohydrate; nutritionists advise an intake of more than 50 to 100 grams, emphasizing starches, to 55% or more of total kcalories. We should limit consumption of simple sugars to about 10 to 15 teaspoons per day. Most simple sugars are added to foods and beverages during manufacturing or are added from the sugar bowl. To reduce simple sugar consumption, one must eat fewer items that have had a lot of sugar added, such as some baked goods, certain beverages, and some breakfast cereals. Simple sugars contribute to dental caries and provide few vitamins and minerals, if any. There are three major alternate sweeteners available in America today—saccharin, aspartame, and acesulfame-K. These can aid in the goal of reducing simple sugar intake.

SUMMARY

- The monosaccharides in our diet include glucose, fructose, and galactose (the latter as part of lactose). Once absorbed via the small intestine through the portal vein into the liver, much of the fructose and galactose is turned into glucose.
- The major disaccharides are sucrose (glucose plus fructose), maltose (glucose plus glucose), and lactose (glucose plus galactose). When digested, these yield monosaccharide forms. Both monosaccharides and disaccharides are classified as simple sugars.
- Lactose is the sugar found in milk. Lactose intolerance is a condition that results when cells of the intestine wall do not make sufficient or any lactase, the enzyme necessary to digest lactose. Undigested lactose travels to the colon, resulting in such symptoms as abdominal gas, pain, and diarrhea. Some people with lactose intolerance can tolerate cheeses and yogurts, though tolerance to dairy products as a whole varies among affected individuals.
- Some starch digestion occurs in the mouth. In the small intestine, carbohydrate digestion is finished. Some plant fibers are digested by the bacteria present in the colon; undigested plant fibers end up in the feces. Single sugars mostly follow an active absorption process in the intestine. They are then transported to the liver.
- The major digestible polysaccharides—starches—contain multiple glucose units linked together. Glycogen is animal starch and acts as a storage form of glucose in the liver and muscles.

- Carbohydrates provide energy (4 kcalories per gram), protect against needless metabolism of protein for energy, and provide flavor and sweetness to foods. They are not necessarily fattening. Simple carbohydrates can be metabolized to acids by bacteria on teeth. The acid can erode the tooth surface, leading to dental caries.
- Dietary fibers include the indigestible polysaccharides cellulose, hemicelluloses, pectins, gums, and mucilages, as well as the noncarbohydrate lignins. Dietary fiber, especially insoluble varieties, provides mass to the stool, thus easing elimination. It may also decrease the risk for colon cancer.
- There is no RDA for carbohydrate. A minimal intake of 50 to 100 grams is needed; 55% or more of total kcalories is recommended. If carbohydrate consumption is inadequate, the body can make what sugars it needs to support cell metabolism. However, if inadequate carbohydrate intake continues for weeks at a time, the price is a loss of body protein, ketosis, and in turn a general weakening of the body.
- Diets high in complex carbohydrates are encouraged as a replacement for high-fat diets, with an emphasis on starches. Foods to emphasize are potatoes, grains, pastas, fruits, and vegetables. Sugar intake should be limited to 10% to 15% of kcalories. Use of alternate sweeteners, such as aspartame, can help in limiting sugar intake.

Study Questions

1. What are the three major disaccharides? Describe how each plays a part in the human diet.
2. How are amylose and glycogen alike and also different from each other? Why is the difference important in a metabolic sense?
3. What happens in the body if not enough carbohydrate is ingested? What is the recommended amount of carbohydrate per day to prevent these effects?
4. What important role does dietary fiber play in the diet?
5. What, if any, are the ill effects of sugars in the diet?
6. After reading the Nutrition Issue, comment on how insulin-dependent diabetes differs from non-insulin dependent diabetes in cause and treatment.

REFERENCES

1. Alcorn JM: Colorectal cancer prevention: a primary care approach, *Geriatrics* 47(2):24, 1992.
2. American Dietetic Association Reports: Position of The American Dietetic Association: use of nutritive and non-nutritive sweeteners, *Journal of The American Dietetic Association* 93:816, 1993.
3. Anderson JW and others: Metabolic effects of high-carbohydrate, high-fiber diets on insulin-dependent diabetic individuals, *American Journal of Clinical Nutrition* 54:936, 1991.
4. Ausmann, LM: Fiber and colon cancer: does the current evidence justify a preventive policy? *Nutrition Reviews* 51:57, 1993.
5. Brand JC, Holt S: Relative effectiveness of milks with reduced amounts of lactose in alleviating lactose intolerance, *American Journal of Clinical Nutrition* 54:148, 1991.
6. Cronin FJ, Shaw AM: Summary of dietary recommendations for healthy Americans, *Nutrition Today,* p. 26, November/December 1988.
7. DCCT Research Group: Nutrition interventions for intensive therapy in the diabetes control and complications trial, *Journal of The American Dietetic Association* 93:768, 1993.
8. Eastwood MA: The physiological effect of dietary fiber: an update, *Annual Review of Nutrition* 12:19, 1992.
9. Greeley A: Not only sugar is sweet, *FDA Consumer,* p. 17, April 1992.
10. Johnson AO and others: Correlation of lactose maldigestion, lactose intolerance, and milk tolerance, *American Journal of Clinical Nutrition* 57:399, 1993.
11. Leahy JL, Boyd AE: Diabetes genes in non-insulin dependent diabetes mellitus, *The New England Journal of Medicine* 328:56, 1993.
12. London RS: Saccharin and aspartame: are they safe to consume during pregnancy? *Journal of Reproductive Medicine* 33:17, 1988.
13. Martini MC and others: Lactose digestion from yogurt: influence of a meal and additional lactose, *American Journal of Clinical Nutrition* 53:1253, 1991.
14. Mayes PA: Regulation of carbohydrate metabolism. In Murray RK and others, editors: *Harper's biochemistry,* East Norwalk, Conn, 1990, Appleton & Lange.
15. Nelson RL: Hypoglycemia: fact or fiction? *Mayo Clinic Proceedings* 60:844, 1985.
16. Rolls BJ: Effects of intense sweeteners on hunger, food intake, and body weight: a review, *American Journal of Clinical Nutrition* 53:872, 1991.
17. Saudek CD: Recurrent hypoglycemia, *Journal of the American Medical Association* 264:2791, 1990.
18. Schiffman SS and others: Aspartame and susceptibility to headache, *New England Journal of Medicine* 317:1181, 1987.
19. Slavin JL: Dietary fiber: mechanism or magic on disease prevention? *Nutrition Today,* p. 6, November/December 1990.
20. Stryer L: *Biochemistry,* ed 3, New York, 1988, WH Freeman.
21. Wilson JD and others: *Harrison's principles of internal medicine,* ed 12, New York, 1991, McGraw-Hill.
22. Winawer SJ, Shike M: Dietary factors in colorectal cancer and their possible effects on earlier stages of hyperproliferation and adenoma formation, *Journal of the National Cancer Institute* 84:74, 1992.

RATE

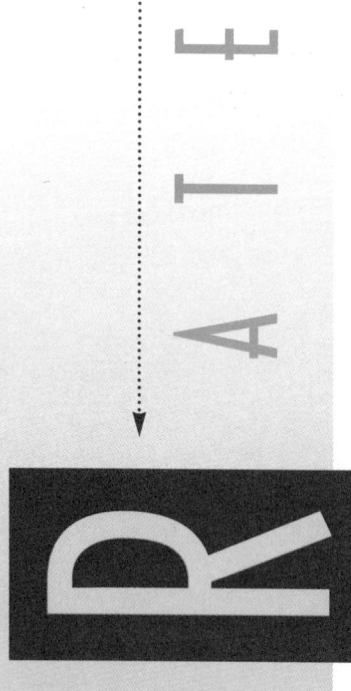

HOW DOES YOUR DIET RATE FOR CARBOHYDRATE AND FIBER?

Remember the nutrition assessment you completed at the end of Chapter 2? That activity includes some information to use for the following diet analysis:

1. Look at your analysis and find the total number of grams of carbohydrate you ate.

TOTAL GRAMS OF CARBOHYDRATE ______________

A. Did you exceed the minimal amount to avoid ketosis—50 to 100 grams?

B. Calculate the percentage of kcalories in your diet from carbohydrate. You will need the total grams of carbohydrate from your assessment, as well as the total kcalories you ate. Use this formula to calculate:

$$\frac{\text{Total grams of carbohydrate} \times 4}{\text{Total kcalories}} \times 100 = \%\text{ of kcalories from carbohydrate}$$

THE % OF KCALORIES FROM CARBOHYDRATE YOU ATE = ______________

Did you approach 55% of kcalories from carbohydrate?
If you didn't, what could you do to increase your carbohydrate intake?

____

____

____

2. Use the list of foods you cited in your nutrition assessment assignment, including the amounts, to calculate fiber consumption. Refer to the software printout for your dietary fiber intake or use the food composition table in Appendix A to look up the fiber content of each food you ate. Take the amount of that food you ate into account. Total the amount of fiber you ate for that day and record it in the blank provided below.

TOTAL AMOUNT OF FIBER CONSUMED______________ grams

A. Did you eat 20 to 35 grams, as suggested in this chapter?

B. If not, what could you do to increase your fiber intake? What foods could you substitute for some of the foods you ate?

____

____

C. Use your computer program to verify that these corrections suffice to increase your fiber intake.

____

3. Finally, use Table 5-6 if you need to reduce your sugar intake, especially if you need to watch your total energy intake to maintain an appropriate body weight.

Nutrition ISSUE

WHEN BLOOD GLUCOSE REGULATION FAILS

The major problem in regulating blood glucose for humans occurs in diabetes. This disease leads to hyperglycemia, a high blood glucose level. The two major forms of diabetes are ***insulin-dependent diabetes*** (Type I) and ***non-insulin dependent diabetes*** (Type II). Both have strong genetic links and so are more likely to be seen in families in which other members have the disease.[11] The symptoms include fasting blood glucose levels above 140 milligrams per 100 milliliters of serum, frequent urination and thirst (the full name *diabetes mellitus* essentially means output of much sweet urine), extreme hunger, rapid weight loss, blurred vision or a sudden change in vision, easy tiring, drowsiness, and general weakness.[21] Many of these symptoms wax and wane or may persist.

Insulin-Dependent Diabetes ■ *A form of diabetes prone to ketosis; it requires insulin therapy.*

Non-Insulin Dependent Diabetes ■ *A form of diabetes in which ketosis is not common and in which insulin therapy may be used but is often not required.*

Insulin-Dependent Diabetes

The insulin-dependent form of diabetes, also referred to as Type I diabetes, often begins in late childhood, from the ages of 8 to 12 years, but it can strike at any age. The hallmark of the disease is the tendency to develop ketosis. Without sufficient insulin, glucose is not taken up by many of the cells that metabolize it. People with diabetes may have a full load of glucose in the bloodstream, but unless that glucose can readily get into body cells, much of it will not be used.[14] Much glucose then spills into the urine. Other hormone shifts cause the liver to respond by producing ketones. In poorly treated insulin-dependent diabetes, the ketone level can rise excessively in the bloodstream. Ketones eventually spill into the urine and can lead to coma and even death.[21] (Coma and/or death will not happen in ketosis caused by starvation, because the ketone levels in the bloodstream do not rise as high.)

A viral infection may play an important part in the development of insulin-dependent diabetes. Some infections are thought to trigger an immune response that attacks the pancreas, especially the cells that make insulin. The pancreas then gradually loses its ability to make insulin. When about 90% of the insulin-producing cells are lost, blood glucose levels are apt to rise very high after eating because not enough insulin is produced. Again, the excess glucose spills over into the urine. Figure 5-12 shows what typically happens to blood glucose levels when a person with diabetes eats a large amount of glucose (glucose tolerance curve).

The disease is treated with diet therapy and insulin injections. The person must eat regular meals and snacks of a precise carbohydrate : protein : fat ratio and replace the missing insulin, either with injections (one to six times a day) or with an insulin pump. The pump dispenses insulin at regular intervals into the body, releasing higher amounts after each meal. Regular meals are especially important for people with diabetes who use insulin, because insulin requires glucose in the bloodstream on which to act.[7] Although these regimented activities may be inconvenient, they are necessary. If the person with di-

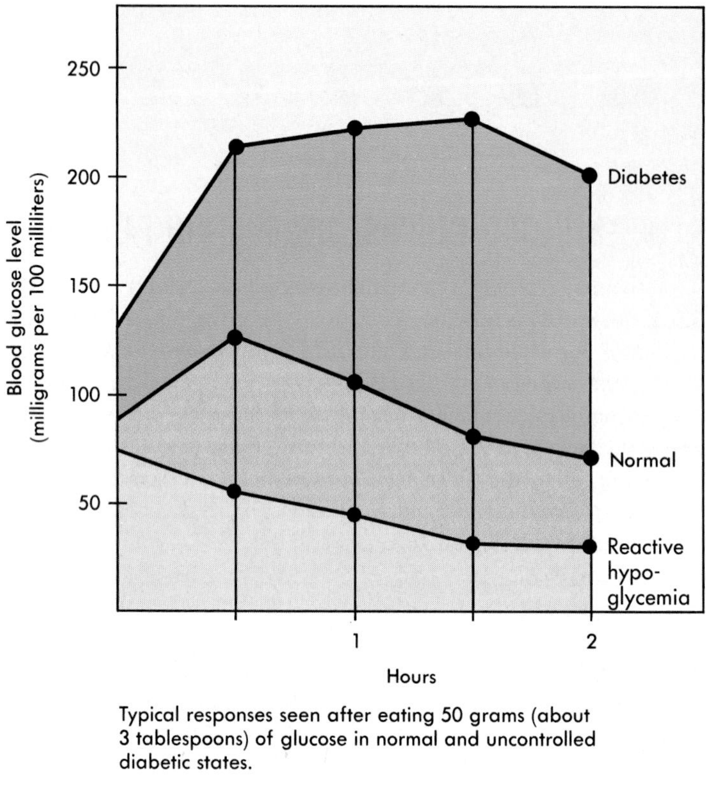

FIGURE 5-12
Glucose tolerance test. These are typical responses after a healthy person, a person with uncontrolled diabetes, and a person with reactive hypoglycemia eat 50 grams of glucose.

abetes doesn't eat, the injected insulin can cause severe low blood sugar levels—hypoglycemia—by acting on whatever little glucose is available.[21] And in the long run, degenerative conditions, such as blindness, heart disease, kidney disease, and numbness from nerve damage, result from poor blood glucose regulation.

Non-Insulin Dependent Diabetes

The non-insulin-dependent form of diabetes, also referred to as Type II diabetes, usually begins in adulthood. It is the most common type of diabetes, accounting for about 90% of cases.[21] In this group, many cases of the non-insulin dependent form of diabetes are associated with obesity, but the hyperglycemia is not necessarily caused by obesity. In fact, there is a growing population of lean people with this type of diabetes. Obesity, with its large fat cells, simply increases the risk for a state of insulin resistance in the body. Overall, liver glucose production rises, the clearance of glucose from the bloodstream falls, and insulin release after a meal is slowed. The main idea to remember is that the pancreas still makes some insulin, but body cells—especially fat cells—resist insulin action. The person then develops hyperglycemia. If obesity is corrected, the diabetes often disappears.

People with non-insulin dependent diabetes mellitus sometimes take oral medications that increase the release of insulin from the pancreas. Regular exercise also helps, because muscles will take up more glucose. In addition, regular meal patterns help minimize the high and low swing in blood glucose levels by spreading food intake throughout the day.[7] High-fiber diets are also helpful, under a physician's scrutiny.[3] Sometimes even insulin injections are used.

Although many cases of the non-insulin dependent form of diabetes can be relieved by losing excess fat stores, many people are not able to lose weight. They continue to show symptoms of diabetes and suffer the consequences of both forms of this disease—blindness, loss of fingers and toes, kidney failure, and heart disease.[21] These problems are caused by nerve deterioration associated with high blood glucose levels and a rapid progression of fatty buildup in blood vessels, which eventually chokes off the blood supply to nearby organs. See Chapter 6 for details of this latter process, called ***atherosclerosis.*** Many specialists in diabetes believe that a substantial amount of the blood vessel and nerve complications of the disease can be prevented with aggressive treatment of both insulin-dependent and non-insulin dependent diabetes directed at keeping blood glucose levels within the normal range.[7]

There is one more diet tool a person with diabetes can use. Research concerning the body's response to various carbohydrates has led to the development of a clinical tool known as the glycemic index.[4] This index compares the total amount of glucose appearing in the bloodstream after eating a food with the total amount of glucose appearing in the bloodstream after eating the same amount of carbohydrate in the form of white bread or glucose. In other words, the glycemic index suggests the degree to which a certain food will cause the blood glucose level to rise.

Several factors must be considered when predicting the glycemic index of a food, including the food's amount of dietary fiber, its digestion rate, and its total fat content. Some foods, such as oatmeal, contain much soluble fiber. Soluble fibers yield a slow increase in blood glucose after a meal.[3] In contrast, such foods as white bread are quickly digested, in turn producing a rapid increase in blood glucose after eating. If a diabetic person eats many foods having low glycemic indexes, then each meal in the entire diet will encourage normal glucose levels.

Hypoglycemia

Another carbohydrate disorder is low blood glucose levels, or hypoglycemia. Blood glucose drops to 40 to 60 milligrams per 100 milliliters of serum (Figure 5-12). This problem comes in two forms, reactive and fasting. ***Reactive hypoglycemia*** is characterized by irritability, nervousness, headache, sweating, and confusion 2 to 4 hours after eating a meal, especially one high in simple sugars.[17] Again, these symptoms make sense when you recall that the brain is particularly dependent on glucose for fuel. It is not clear what causes reactive hypoglycemia. It may be caused by the pancreas' overproduction of insulin in response to rising blood glucose levels.

A second type, ***fasting hypoglycemia,*** is usually caused by a cancer in the pancreas, which can lead to excessive insulin secretion.[21] Blood glucose falls to low levels after fasting for about a day. This form of hypoglycemia is very rare.

Some of us have bouts of low blood sugar and never know it. It is possible, for example, to feel irritable, shaky, and even have a headache if a meal is missed or eaten much later than usual. For a person to be diagnosed with hypoglycemia, however, both a low blood glucose level and the typical symptoms must appear together. People may think they have hypoglycemia, but few actually meet both criteria. Most hypoglycemic symptoms overlap with those of simple anxiety, stress, and depression. On a percentage basis, people complaining of fatigue, shakiness, occasional heavy sweats, and emotional instability rarely have documentable hypoglycemia.[15] Also, for most people in good health, eating simple sugars does not induce hypoglycemia. Unless a metabolic disorder is present, most people's bodies respond adequately to simple sugar and complex carbohydrate intake.

Nevertheless, if you sometimes feel irritable and tired when hungry, simple nutrition therapy often is all that is needed. Eat regular meals, make sure you have some protein and fat in each meal, and eat complex carbohydrates that contain ample soluble fiber—fruits and vegetables, for example. Fat, protein, and soluble fiber in the diet tend to moderate swings in blood glucose.[17]

The glycemic index for common foods

100	**White bread**
90	**Whole-wheat bread, shredded wheat cereal, raisins**
80	**Rice, oatmeal, potatoes**
70	**Bananas, All-Bran cereal**
60	**Orange, baked beans, spaghetti**
50	**Yogurt, apple**
40	**Skim milk, peach**

Atherosclerosis
A buildup of fatty material (plaque) in the arteries, including those surrounding the heart.

Reactive Hypoglycemia
Low blood sugar that follows a meal high in simple sugars, with corresponding symptoms of irritability, headache, nervousness, sweating, and confusion.

Fasting Hypoglycemia
Low blood sugar that follows a day or so of fasting. This is a rare disorder, generally caused by cancer in the pancreas.

chapter 6

LIPIDS

YOUR DOCTOR INFORMS YOU THAT YOUR "TRIGLYCERIDES are up." Your bill from a medical laboratory reads, "Blood lipid profile—$85." Advertisers plug "lowest in saturated fat" or "cholesterol-free." We often hear terms like *triglycerides, blood lipids,* and *cholesterol.* What do they mean?

Lipids—a class of nutrients that includes various fats, oils, and cholesterol—are likely our biggest concern when it comes to diet planning. On the whole, lipids yield 9 kcalories per gram, more than twice as many kcalories as proteins or carbohydrates yield. Eating too much of certain types of saturated fat can boost a person's serum cholesterol over the desired level.[13] This speeds the development of heart disease. But does that mean you must stick to a boring regimen of cottage cheese and grapefruit? Read on and find out.

Although concern about lipids is appropriate, certain varieties play very important roles in the body and in foods. And the diets of some people—for example, young children—benefit from the concentrated source of energy supplied by food fats. Like many other nutrients, too much fat and cholesterol in the diet can cause problems, but not enough of these lipids can devastate the body. Let's look at the various lipids in detail—their functions, metabolism, food sources, and link to heart disease.

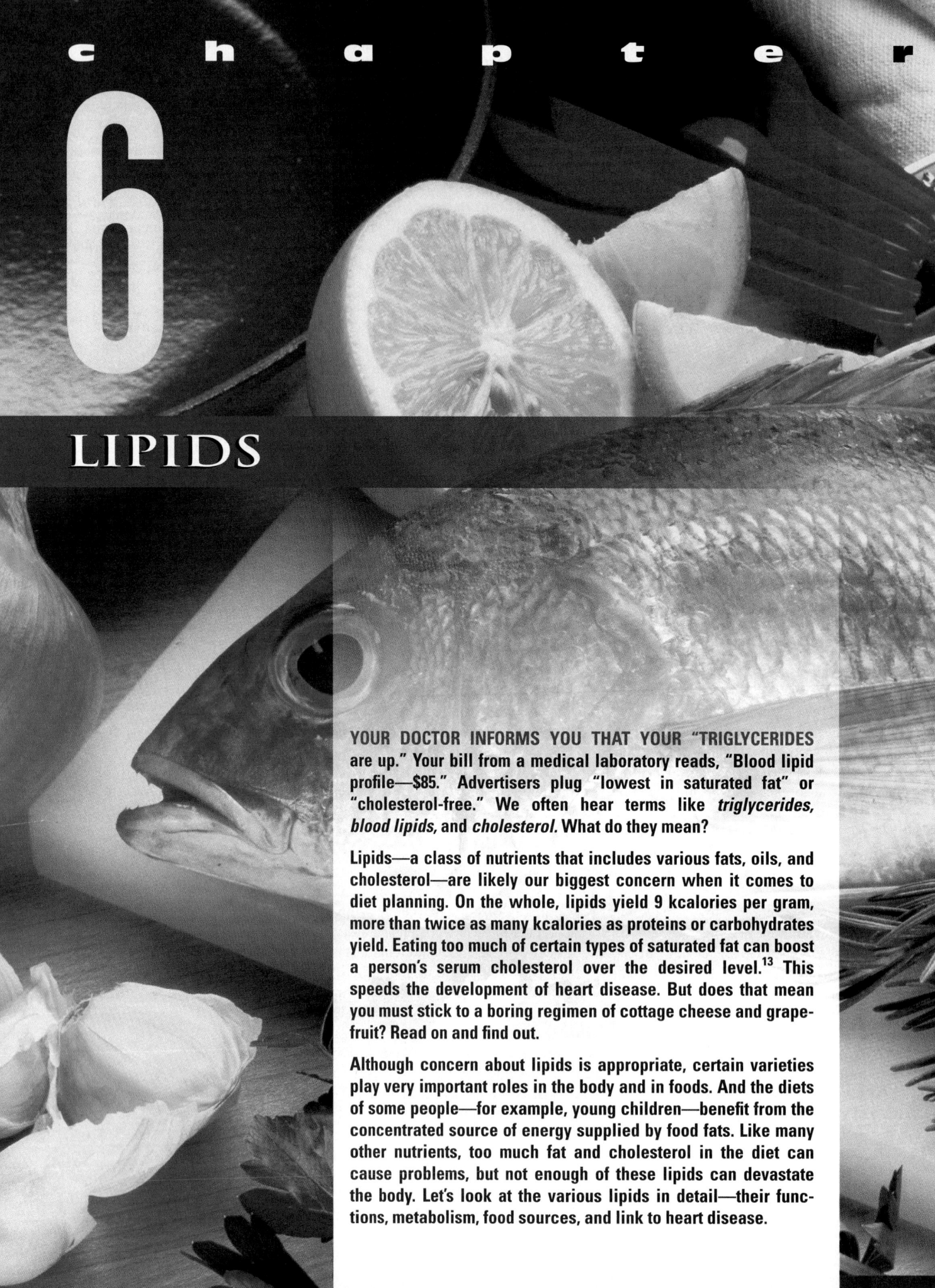

ARE YOU EATING A DIET THAT INCLUDES MANY SATURATED-FAT SOURCES?

Instructions:
Check the food you would typically select from the two choices you are given.

1.	______ Bacon and eggs	______ Ready-to-eat breakfast cereal
2.	______ Doughnut or sweet roll	______ White or whole-wheat roll or bread, no margarine
3.	______ Breakfast sausage	______ Fruit
4.	______ Whole milk	______ Low-fat or nonfat milk
5.	______ Cheeseburger	______ Turkey sandwich, no cheese
6.	______ French fries	______ Baked potato or salad with low-cal or no-oil dressing
7.	______ Meal including fried hamburger or fatty beef	______ Meal including broiled lean hamburger (ground round), chicken, or fish
8.	______ Creamed soup	______ Clear soup (could have meat or vegetables in it)
9.	______ Potato salad	______ Baked potato, plain
10.	______ Fruit or cream pie	______ Graham crackers
11.	______ Ice cream	______ Frozen yogurt, sherbet, or ice milk
12.	______ Butter or stick margarine	______ Soft margarine in a tub

Interpretation

The foods listed on the left are those that tend to be high in saturated fat, cholesterol, and total fat. Those on the right are low. If you want to follow a diet to reduce the risk of heart disease, choose the foods on the right more often than the foods on the left.

ASSESS

TEST YOUR KNOWLEDGE

yourself

LIPIDS IN GENERAL

Lipids are a diverse group of chemical compounds, but they share one main characteristic: they do not dissolve in water. When you compare the structures of the two types of lipids shown in Figure 6-1—a triglyceride *(E)* and cholesterol *(G)*—you will readily see how different they appear. As we noted in Chapter 1, lipids at room temperature that are solid are called fats and lipids that are liquid are called oils.

Most people use the word *fat* to refer to all lipids, because they don't know a difference exists. But as we have already noted, *lipid* is a generic term that includes triglycerides and many other substances, such as cholesterol. To simplify our discussion, we will primarily use the term *fat,* but note that not all the substances we call fats truly are fats. Vegetable oil is one example. When necessary for clarity, we will use the name of a specific lipid, such as cholesterol. Our word usage is consistent with how many people use these terms today.

FATTY ACIDS: THE SIMPLEST FORM OF LIPIDS

The ***fatty acid*** is common to most lipids, both in the body and in foods. It is basically a long chain of carbons linked together and flanked by hydrogens (Figure 6-1, *A*). Fats in foods are not composed of a single type or category of fatty acid. Rather, each dietary fat is a complex mixture of different fatty acids. Butterfat, for example, contains numerous different fatty acids.

If all the links (technically referred to as *chemical bonds*) between the carbons are single connections and the carbons are filled with hydrogen, a fatty acid is said to be ***saturated*** (Figure 6-1, *A*). In other words, it is like a wet sponge saturated (full) with water.

Most fats high in saturated fatty acids remain solid at room temperature. Animal fats, for example, contain a high proportion of saturated fatty acids. The solid fat surrounding a piece of steak at room temperature is a good example. Chicken fat, semisolid at room temperature, contains less saturated fat. Some saturated fats are suspended in a liquid, such as milk, and so the solid nature of these fats at room temperature is not so apparent.

If a fatty acid has one double bond between the carbons, it is ***monounsaturated*** (Figure 6-1, *B*). The term *unsaturated* means the fatty acid could take up more hydrogens. That would then lead to no double bonds between carbons. Olive and canola oils contain a high percentage of monounsaturated fatty acids. If two or more bonds between the carbons are double bonds, the fatty acid is ***polyunsaturated*** and thus even less saturated with hydrogens (Figure 6-1, *C* and *D*). Corn, soybean, and safflower oils are good sources of polyunsaturated fatty acids (Figure 6-2).

The point at which the double bonds begin in the fatty acid is important. If these double bonds start after the third carbon (counting from the end with a $-CH_3$ group), it is an ***omega-3 (w-3) fatty acid.*** If these bonds start after the sixth carbon, it is an ***omega-6 (w-6) fatty acid,*** and so on. ***Alpha-linolenic acid*** is the major omega-3 fatty acid found in food; ***linoleic acid*** is the major omega-6 fatty acid.

Fatty Acid
Acids found in fats. These are composed of a chain of carbon atoms linked together. The chain is flanked by hydrogen atoms and has an acidic chemical group at one end.

Saturated Fatty Acid
A fatty acid with no carbon-carbon double bonds.

Monounsaturated Fatty Acid
A fatty acid containing one carbon-carbon double bond.

Polyunsaturated Fatty Acid
A fatty acid containing two or more carbon-carbon double bonds.

Essential Fatty Acids
Fatty acids that must be present in the diet to maintain health; these consist of linoleic acid and alpha-linolenic acid.

Essential Fatty Acids

Humans can't produce omega-3 and omega-6 fatty acids; we get them only by ingesting them.[4] That is why this structural uniqueness is important. These fatty acids are essential for us to eat, because they participate in immune processes and vision, help form cell membranes, and aid in the production of hormonelike compounds.[3] Because we must get linoleic acid (omega-6) and alpha-linolenic acid (omega-3) from foods, they are called ***essential fatty acids.***

We need to get about 1% to 2% of our total kcalories from linoleic acid. On a 2500-kcalorie diet, that corresponds to 1 tablespoon of plant oil each day. We easily get that much—via mayonnaise, salad dressings, margarine, and other foods—without even noticing. Barring these foods, regular consumption of whole grains and vegetables can also supply enough essential fatty acids.

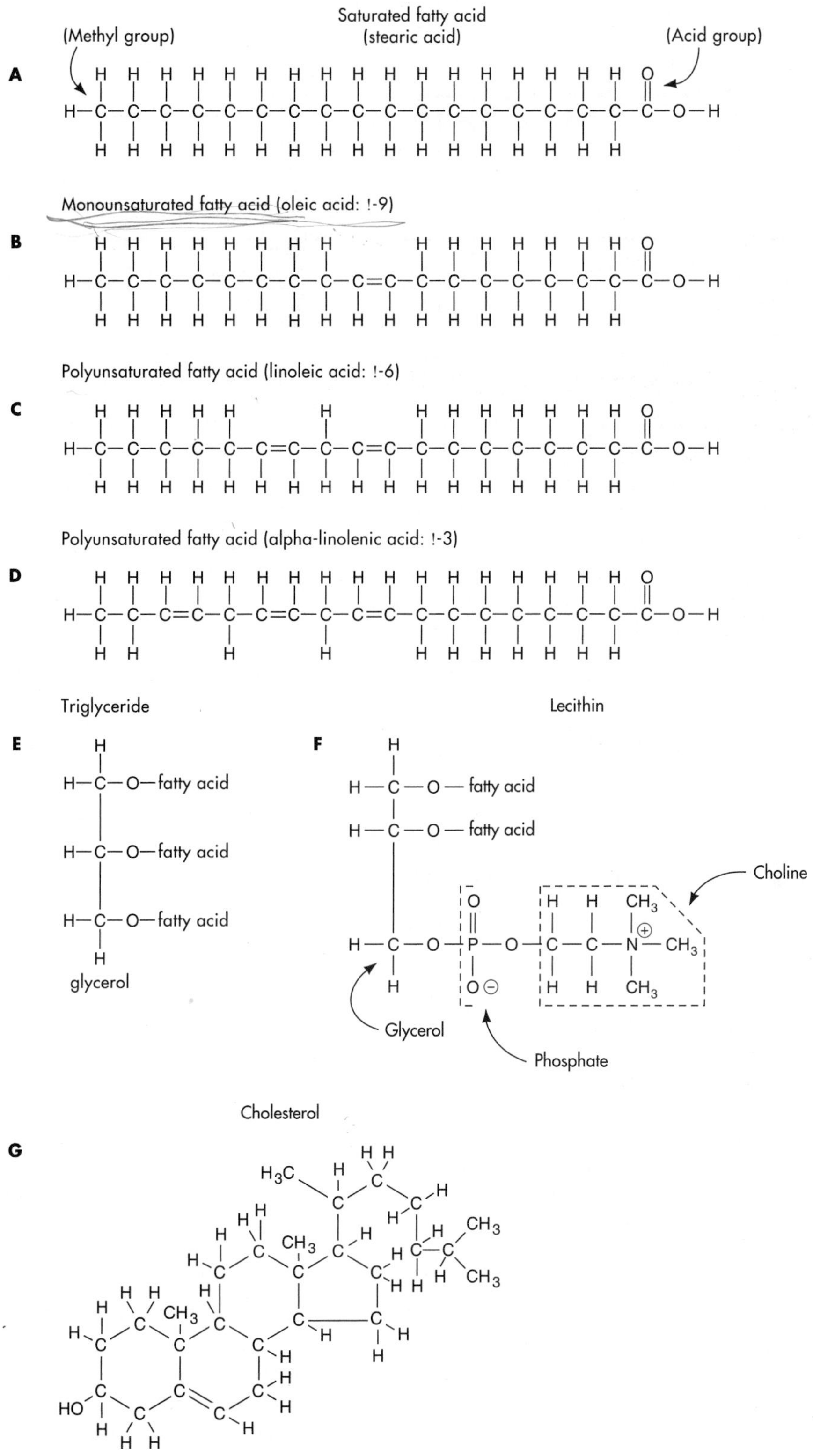

FIGURE 6-1
Examples of lipids found in foods.

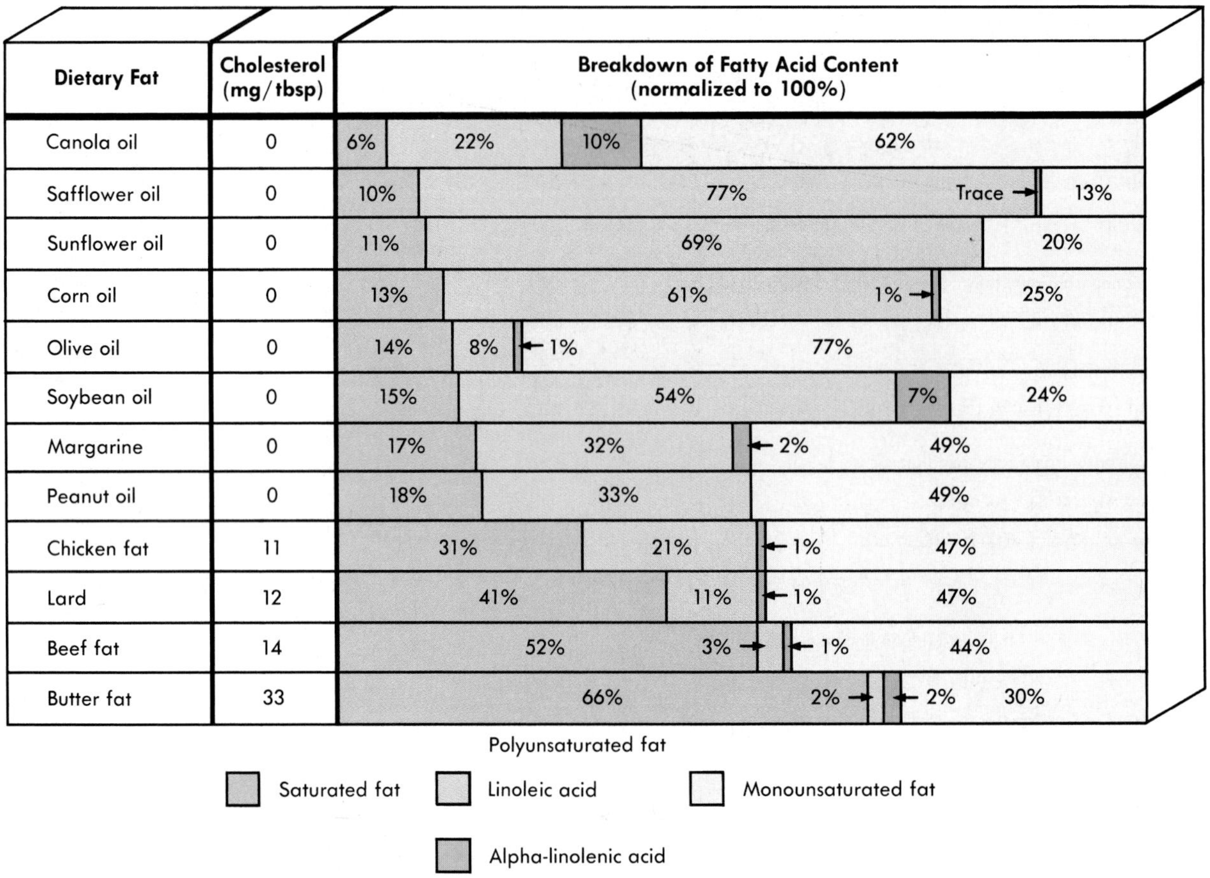
Dietary Fat
Cholesterol (mg/tbsp)
Breakdown of Fatty Acid Content (normalized to 100%)
Canola oil 0 6% 22% 10% 62%
Safflower oil 0 10% 77% Trace 13%
Sunflower oil 0 11% 69% 20%
Corn oil 0 13% 61% 1% 25%
Olive oil 0 14% 8% 1% 77%
Soybean oil 0 15% 54% 7% 24%
Margarine 0 17% 32% 2% 49%
Peanut oil 0 18% 33% 49%
Chicken fat 11 31% 21% 1% 47%
Lard 12 41% 11% 1% 47%
Beef fat 14 52% 3% 1% 44%
Butter fat 33 66% 2% 2% 30%
Polyunsaturated fat
Saturated fat
Linoleic acid
Monounsaturated fat
Alpha-linolenic acid

FIGURE 6-2

Comparison of saturated fat, unsaturated fat, and cholesterol content in food fats. Note that recently manufacturers have been blending canola oil with polyunsaturated vegetable oils to yield a more even balance between monounsaturated and polyunsaturated fats. Later in the chapter we discuss the reasons behind this change.

Eicosapentaenoic Acid (EPA) *An omega-3 fatty acid with 20 carbon atoms and 5 double bonds; present in fish oils.*

Leading researchers also suggest that most diets should include a regular supply of either alpha-linolenic acid or its related omega-3 forms, such as ***eicosapentaenoic acid (EPA).*** This is found in high amounts in fatty, cold-water fish.[12] To get this supply, we need to either eat fish—such as salmon, tuna, and sardines—every week, or regularly use canola or soybean oil. All are good sources of omega-3 fatty acids. This recommendation for consuming omega-3 fatty acids stems from the observation that compounds made from omega-3 fatty acids tend to decrease blood clotting and inflammatory processes in the body, whereas the omega-6 fatty acids generally increase these processes.

Studies from Scandinavia, the Netherlands, and Japan show that people who eat fish about twice a week (total weekly intake: 8 ounces [240 grams]) run lower risks for heart attacks than do people who rarely eat fish. In these cases the omega-3 fatty acids in fish oil probably are acting to reduce blood clotting. In turn, the risk of heart attack decreases, especially for people already at high risk (see the Nutrition Issue at the end of the chapter to learn about the link between blood clots and heart attacks). Greenland Eskimos consume a lot of fish, seal, and whale and also have a greatly reduced risk for heart attacks.

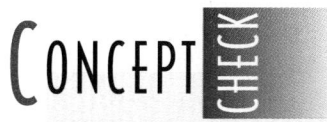

Should We Be Eating "Eskimo Diets"?

We need to remember that blood clotting is a normal body process. Eskimos who eat a lot of seafoods are more likely to have some types of strokes than are other people, because their blood does not clot readily enough. Too much omega-3 fatty acid intake could allow uncontrolled bleeding. A reduction in blood-clotting ability then can act as a double-edged sword. Current studies also show that consuming large amounts of fish oil supplements can impede blood glucose regulation in people who have diabetes and even raise cholesterol levels in people with high blood triglyceride levels. Because of the possibility of harm, we recommend not using fish oil supplements—just stick to eating fish two or three times a week. Atlantic and Pacific herring, sardines, Atlantic halibut and salmon, lake trout, coho, pink and king salmon, blue fish, albacore tuna, and Atlantic mackerel are among the fish with the greatest omega-3 fatty acid contents. Even oysters are a source. New research may soon add more types of fish and seafood to this list.

Effects of a Deficiency of Essential Fatty Acids

If you don't consume enough essential fatty acids, your skin will become flaky and itchy, and diarrhea and other symptoms eventually develop. But because our bodies need the equivalent of only about 1 tablespoon of polyunsaturated plant oil a day, even a low-fat diet, if it follows the Food Guide Pyramid, will provide this much.

CONCEPT CHECK

Lipids are a group of compounds that don't dissolve in water. Fatty acids, the simplest forms of lipids, differ from each other mainly in the number and location of the double bonds between the carbons. Saturated fatty acids contain no carbon-carbon double bonds. This means they are fully saturated with hydrogens. Monounsaturated fatty acids contain one carbon-carbon double bond, and polyunsaturated fatty acids contain two or more. If double bonds begin at the third carbon from the $-CH_3$ end of the chain, the fatty acid is an omega-3 fatty acid. If the double bonds begin at the sixth carbon, it is an omega-6 fatty acid. Humans can't make either omega-3 or omega-6 fatty acids, and so they are essential parts of a diet. Plant oils generally are rich in omega-6 fatty acids. The recommendation to eat fish about twice a week is a good guide to provide omega-3 fatty acids for the body. Products of omega-3 fatty acids tend to reduce blood clotting and inflammatory responses in the body.

Long-Chain Fatty Acids *Fatty acids that contain 12 or more carbon atoms.*

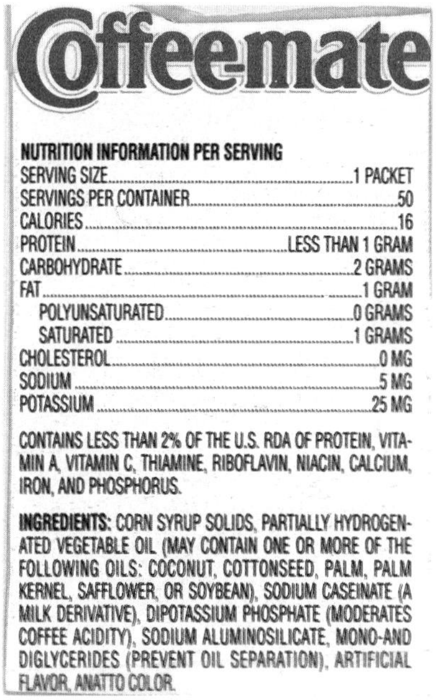
Coffee-mate
NUTRITION INFORMATION PER SERVING
SERVING SIZE 1 PACKET
SERVINGS PER CONTAINER 50
CALORIES 16
PROTEIN LESS THAN 1 GRAM
CARBOHYDRATE 2 GRAMS
FAT 1 GRAM
POLYUNSATURATED 0 GRAMS
SATURATED 1 GRAMS
CHOLESTEROL 0 MG
SODIUM 5 MG
POTASSIUM 25 MG
CONTAINS LESS THAN 2% OF THE U.S. RDA OF PROTEIN, VITAMIN A, VITAMIN C, THIAMINE, RIBOFLAVIN, NIACIN, CALCIUM, IRON, AND PHOSPHORUS.
INGREDIENTS: CORN SYRUP SOLIDS, PARTIALLY HYDROGENATED VEGETABLE OIL (MAY CONTAIN ONE OR MORE OF THE FOLLOWING OILS: COCONUT, COTTONSEED, PALM, PALM KERNEL, SAFFLOWER, OR SOYBEAN), SODIUM CASEINATE (A MILK DERIVATIVE), DIPOTASSIUM PHOSPHATE (MODERATES COFFEE ACIDITY), SODIUM ALUMINOSILICATE, MONO-AND DIGLYCERIDES (PREVENT OIL SEPARATION), ARTIFICIAL FLAVOR, ANATTO COLOR.

Chain Length Affects Fatty Acid Characteristics

Fats in foods that contain primarily saturated fatty acids are solid at room temperature, especially if the fatty acids have a ***long chain*** (12 carbons or longer). ***Medium-chain*** saturated fatty acids (6 to 10 carbons long), such as those in coconut oil, produce liquid oils at room temperature. The shorter chain length overrides the effect of saturation. ***Short-chain*** saturated fatty acids (less than 6 carbons long) also form liquid oils at room temperature. Dairy fats are sources of these short-chain fatty acids. Fats containing primarily polyunsaturated or monounsaturated fatty acids are usually liquid at room temperature. These are not affected by chain length.[15]

The capability of some saturated fatty acids of short-chain or medium-chain lengths to form oils at room temperature is significant. You might assume—incorrectly—that nondairy creamers are a healthful substitute for cream because cream has a high percentage of saturated fat, and saturated fat is something health authorities warn us to eat less of. However, many nondairy creamers contain coconut oil, which is also high in saturated fat, and so becomes a poor food choice as well if used in excessive amounts. Low-fat milk is a much more healthful alternative to both. One reason manufacturers use coconut oil is that it allows the product a long shelf life. You will understand why when we examine the issue of rancidity of fats in a later section.

Hydrogenation of Fatty Acids

In some food preparations, such as pastry making, solid fats work better than do liquid oils. Solid fats yield a flaky product, whereas products made with liquid oils tend to be greasy. To solidify vegetable oils into shortenings and margarines for use in pastries and other products, the polyunsaturated fatty acids must become more saturated. In other words, more hydrogen must be added to turn double bonds between the carbons into single bonds. In the ***hydrogenation*** process, the hydrogens are added by bubbling hydrogen gas into liquid vegetable oils (Figure 6-3). During hydrogenation, changes in the fatty acid occur as well, casting them in a so-called *trans* shape. This structural change also causes the fats to raise serum cholesterol levels just as saturated fats do, which is an important reason for us to limit intake of hydrogenated fat.[24] Generally, the more hydrogenation that occurs, the harder the product is; for example, stick margarine is more hydrogenated (saturated) than is tub margarine. Note that if a liquid oil is listed before any hydrogenated oil on food labels, the food probably contains a greater amount of unsaturated than saturated fat.

Hydrogenation *The addition of hydrogen atoms to the double bonds of polyunsaturated and monounsaturated fatty acids to reduce the extent of unsaturation; this process turns liquid vegetable oils into solid fats.*

It is actually easy to avoid eating too much hydrogenated fat. First, use little or no stick margarine or shortening; instead, substitute limited amounts of softer, tub margarine and vegetable oils. Second, minimize consumption of high-fat foods in restaurants, espe-

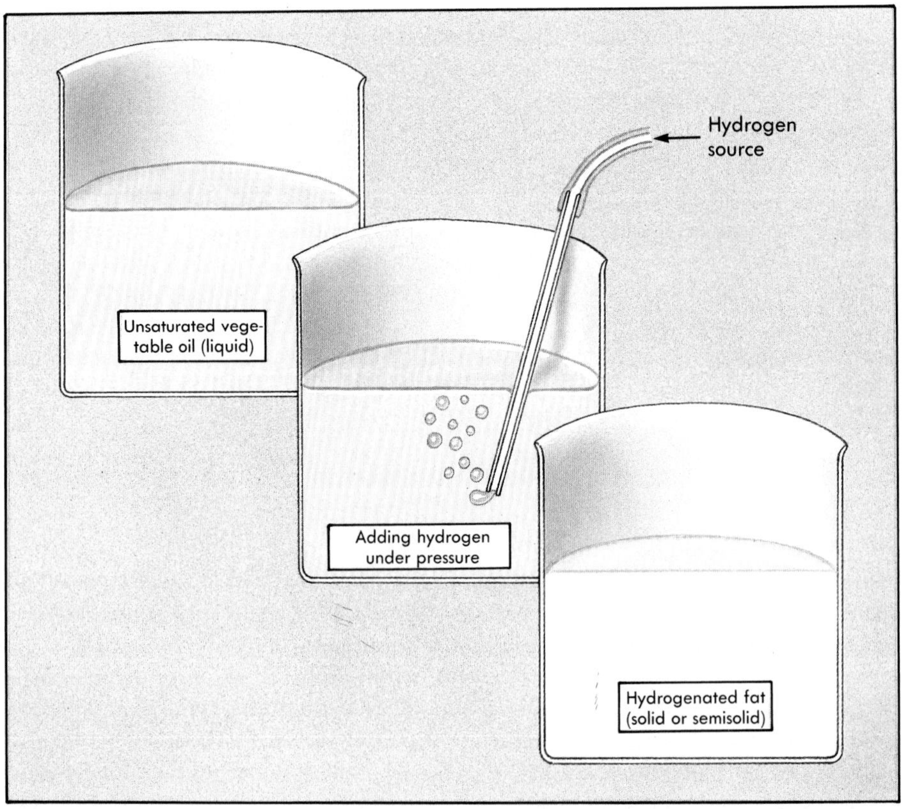

FIGURE 6-3
How liquid oil becomes solid in margarine production. Unsaturated oil starts out in a liquid form. Hydrogen atoms are bubbled in (hydrogenation), changing double bonds to single bonds, as well as producing other changes in fatty acid structure. The hydrogenated product is now either semisolid or solid.

cially those deep fried in hydrogenated fats. For instance, a typical hamburger sandwich, salad (with limited dressing), bowl of chili, soft drink, or milk contain little hydrogenated fat, whereas French fries, fried chicken, and fried pies are often rich sources. Heavy use of commercial cookies, chips, cakes, doughnuts, and high-fat crackers also deserves scrutiny. For now, this approach is a prudent one to take.[10]

Rancidity

Decomposing oils emit a disagreeable odor and taste sour and stale. Stale potato chips are a good example. As double bonds in fatty acids break down, the by-products are said to be ***rancid.*** Ultraviolet rays of light, oxygen, and some chemicals can attack double bonds, break them, and in turn destroy the structure of polyunsaturated fatty acids. Saturated fats can much more readily resist these effects. Why?

Even though eating rancid oils can cause sickness, the odor and taste generally discourage us from eating enough to become sick. However, rancidity is a problem for manufacturers because it reduces a product's shelf life. Therefore manufacturers add hydrogenated plant oils to products to increase shelf life. This again explains why coconut oil—full of saturated fat—is added to nondairy creamers. Foods most likely to become rancid in this manner are fatty fish and fish oil, deep-fried foods, and foods with a large amount of exposed surface (such as powdered eggs or powdered milk).

Vitamin E helps protect foods against rancidity, because it acts as an ***antioxidant.*** It guards against fat breakdown caused by various agents, such as metals found as impurities in vegetable oils. The vitamin E in plant oils reduces the breakdown of double bonds in fatty acids. Chapter 8 discusses this role of vitamin E more fully. When food manufacturers want to prevent rancidity in polyunsaturated fats, they often add ***BHA and BHT.*** (Chapter 17 discusses the safety of these additives.) Look for these food additives in salad dressings, cake mixes, and other products that contain fat. They can even be added to a food's paper packaging. Manufacturers also tightly seal products and use other methods to reduce the presence of oxygen inside packages.

Rancid *Containing products of decomposed fatty acids; they yield unpleasant flavors and odors.*

Antioxidant *A compound that can donate electrons to electron-seeking (oxidizing) compounds. This reduces the destructive nature of oxidizing compounds.*

BHA and BHT *Butylated hydroxyanisol and butylated hydroxytoluene—two common synthetic antioxidants added to foods.*

Glycerol *A three-carbon atom alcohol used to form triglycerides.*

CONCEPT CHECK

At room temperature, saturated fatty acids tend to form solid fats, whereas polyunsaturated and monounsaturated fatty acids tend to form liquid oils. Hydrogenation is the process of turning carbon-carbon double bonds of fatty acids into single bonds by adding hydrogens. This solidifies the fat and reduces rancidity. The presence of vitamin E in oils limits rancidity in the unsaturated fatty acids.

TRIGLYCERIDES

Fats and oils in foods are mostly in triglyceride form. The same is true for fats found in body structures. Some fatty acids are found attached to proteins in the bloodstream as they are being transported, but fatty acids usually do not exist in the body as such. Instead, they form into triglycerides.

Triglyceride molecules contain a simple three-carbon alcohol, ***glycerol,*** which serves as a backbone for the three attached fatty acids (Figure 6-1, *E*). Removing one fatty acid from a triglyceride forms a diglyceride. Removing two fatty acids from a triglyceride forms a monoglyceride. In a later section we note that before most dietary fats are absorbed in the small intestine, the upper and lower fatty acids are typically removed from the triglyceride molecules. This produces fatty acids and monoglycerides. These are absorbed into the intestinal cells. After absorption, the fatty acids and monoglycerides are mostly reformed into triglycerides.[15]

PUTTING TRIGLYCERIDES TO WORK IN THE BODY

Again, many key functions of fat in the body require the use of fatty acids in the form of a triglyceride. In the body, triglycerides are used for fuel, energy storage, insulation, and the transporting of fat-soluble vitamins. In foods, triglycerides impart the taste and texture we consider desirable, and they give us a feeling of satiety (fullness) after eating.

Providing Energy for the Body

The fatty acids supplied by triglycerides both in the diet and stored in fat tissue are the main fuel for muscles while at rest and during light activity. Only in endurance exercises, such as long-distance running and cycling, do muscles burn a lot of carbohydrate in addition to fatty acids. Other body tissues also use fatty acids for energy. Overall, about half of the energy used by the entire body at rest and during light activity comes from fatty acids. On a whole-body basis, the use of fatty acids by muscles is balanced by the use of glucose by the brain and red blood cells. Recall from Chapter 5 that all cells also need carbohydrate to efficiently process fatty acids for fuel.

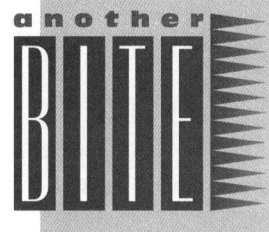

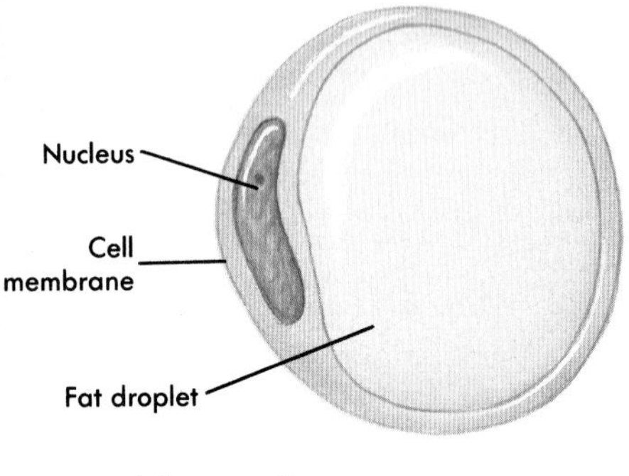

Adipose cell.

Storing Energy

We store energy mainly in the form of triglycerides. The body's ability to store fat is essentially limitless. Its fat storage sites, adipose (fat) cells, can increase about 50 times in weight. If the amount of fat to be stored exceeds the ability of the cells to expand, the body can form new fat cells. (We discuss this further in Chapter 10.)

An important advantage to using triglycerides to store energy in the body is that they are energy dense. Recall that these yield 9 kcalories per gram, whereas proteins and carbohydrates yield only 4 kcalories per gram. In addition, when we store triglycerides in fat cells, we store little else; fat cells contain about 80% lipid and only 20% water and protein. In contrast, imagine if we stored energy as muscle tissue, which is about 73% water. Body weight linked to energy storage would increase dramatically.

Insulating and Protecting the Body

The layer of fat just beneath our skin is made mostly of triglycerides. This fat tissue insulates and protects some organs—kidneys, for example—from injury. We usually don't notice the important insulating function of fat tissue, because we wear clothes and add more as needed. But a layer of insulating fat is quite apparent in animals, particularly in those from cold climates. Polar bears, walruses, and whales all build a thick layer of fat tissue around themselves to insulate against cold-weather environments. The extra fat also provides energy storage for times when food is scarce.

another BITE

We can never be totally fat free, because fat is an essential part of all cells. But people with *anorexia nervosa* often lose 25% or more of body weight and end up about as fat free as is biologically possible. This poses many health risks (see Chapter 12). In addition, in place of the layer of fat tissue under the skin, people with anorexia nervosa often develop downy hair called *lanugo* all over the body. These hairs insulate by standing up and trapping air.

Transporting Fat-Soluble Vitamins

Triglycerides and other fats in foods carry fat-soluble vitamins to the small intestine and aid their absorption. If the small intestine is diseased, however, it may not be able to adequately digest and absorb fat from foods. When this happens, the unabsorbed fat carries the fat-soluble vitamins—A, D, E, and K—into the large intestine. From there they are eliminated with the stool, and the body loses the benefits of the vitamins.

People who generally absorb fat poorly, such as those with the disease cystic fibrosis, are at risk for deficiencies of fat-soluble vitamins, especially vitamin K. A similar risk accrues from taking mineral oil as a laxative at mealtimes. Because the body cannot digest or absorb mineral oil, the undigested oil carries the fat-soluble vitamins from the meal into the large intestine where they are eliminated.

Providing Satiety

If you are fond of cheesecake, you know that a little goes a long way. It's the triglycerides in foods that help give us a full and contented feeling after a meal. The fat we eat triggers hormones that cause the stomach to retain foods longer than when we eat mostly carbohydrate or protein. This is why a high-fat meal allows us to feel full longer.

Many people who want to lose weight cut out much of the fat they eat. However, if dieters cut out too much fat, they lose its satiety value and get hungry quicker. A gradual reduction in fat intake eases the transition to a low-fat diet. Having some low-fat snacks around at times of intense hunger is also a good idea. Fruit is an excellent choice.

Providing Flavor and Texture to Foods

Triglycerides and other fats impart generally desirable textures and flavors to foods. Many flavorings dissolve in fat. Heating spices in oil intensifies the flavors of an Indian curry or Mexican dish far more than simply adding them at the table. The oil then carries these flavors to the sensory cells that discriminate taste and smell in the mouth. We quickly associate *flavorful* with fatty foods. Foods that have had too much fat removed often lack taste and feel dry, as if they need something to bind them together.

If you have ever eaten a high-fat cheese or cream cheese, you probably agree that fat melting on the tongue feels good. This love of fat is universal. Western, Eskimo, and Mediterranean diets are all high in fat. Immigrants to Western cultures, such as many Japanese, quickly embrace the high-fat foods found in the United States. It will likely take a person following a typical American diet some time to adjust to a lower-fat diet. It is possible, but the variety of factors we just reviewed encourages us to move toward the more familiar high-fat diet.

CONCEPT CHECK

Triglyceride is the major form of fat in the body and in food. Triglycerides in the body are used for and stored as energy; they are used to insulate and protect body organs, to transport fat-soluble vitamins, and to provide satiety to a meal. Triglycerides also add flavor and texture to foods.

PHOSPHOLIPIDS

Phospholipids are another class of lipid. Like triglycerides they are built on a backbone of glycerol. However, at least one fatty acid is replaced with a compound containing phosphorus (and often other chemical additions, such as nitrogen) (Figure 6-1, *F*). Many types of phospholipids exist in the body, especially in the brain.[15] They form important parts of cell membranes. ***Lecithin*** is a common example of a phospholipid. It is found in cells and participates in fat digestion in the intestine. Egg yolks contain lecithin in abundance.

Some phospholipids, such as lecithin, function as emulsifiers. Fat and water don't easily mix. By breaking fat globules into small droplets, emulsifiers enable a fat to be suspended in water. To do this, the fatty acid end of lecithin attracts fat. The phosphorus and nitrogen at the other end of lecithin form an area containing positive and negative charges. This area attracts water. When lecithin is added to an oil and water mixture, it

Lecithin *A phospholipid that contains two fatty acids, a phosphate group, and a choline (vitamin-like) molecule.*

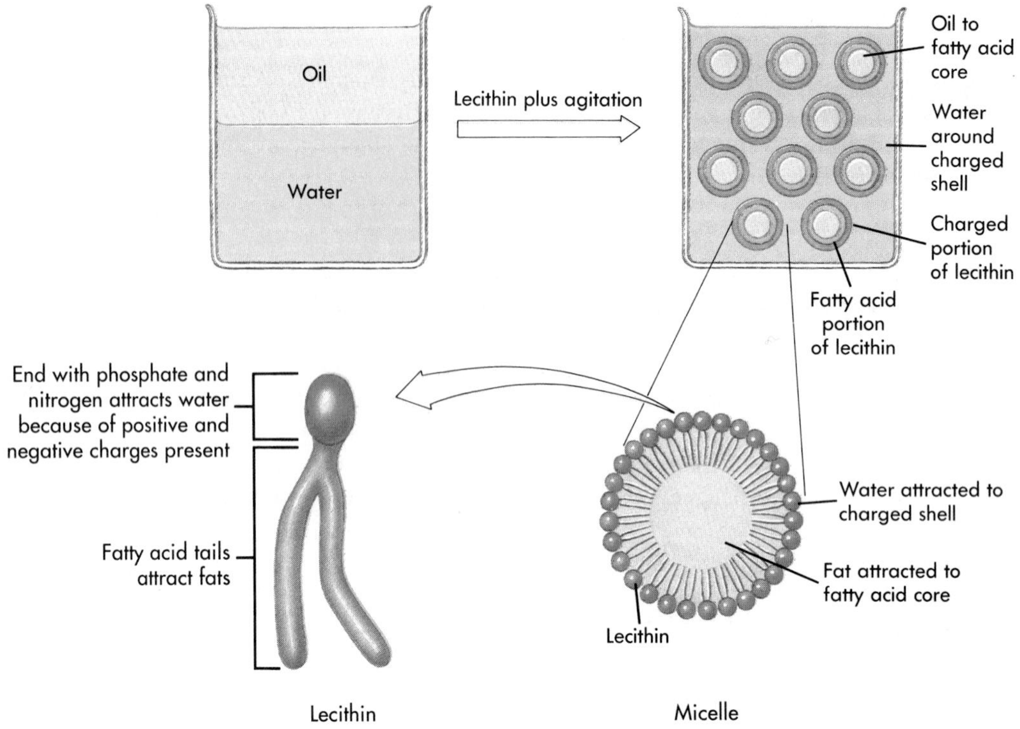

FIGURE 6-4
Emulsification and emulsifiers. Emulsifiers can organize oil and water to form droplets of oil surrounded by shells of water. Using lecithin as an example, the oil is attracted to the fatty acid tails of the emulsifier. The water is attracted to the area with positive and negative charges. Lecithin then ends up forming a bridge between oil and water molecules. Forming oil droplets in water in this manner is a key step in fat digestion.

then acts as numerous bridges that in turn form tiny oil droplets surrounded by thin shells of water. In an emulsified solution, millions of tiny oil droplets are separated by shells of water (Figure 6-4).

Commercial salad dressings find practical use for emulsification. Emulsifiers—such as Polysorbate 60, monoglycerides and diglycerides, and lecithin—are added to salad dressings and other fat-rich products to keep the vegetable oils and other fats suspended in the water. Eggs baked in cakes likewise suspend the fats in the liquid ingredients. The body's main emulsifiers are lecithin and ***bile.*** These are produced by the liver and released into the small intestine via the gallbladder during digestion. By breaking up the fat globules, the emulsifiers create more fat surface for fat-digesting enzymes to act on.

Bile
A substance that is made by the liver and stored in the gallbladder; it is released during digestion to aid in fat digestion and absorption.

Perhaps you've seen health food advertisements touting that it is important to take a lecithin supplement to maintain the health of body cells. This mistaken notion has been encouraged by some popular publications but has no scientific basis. Eating lecithin isn't even an efficient way to obtain it, because the digestive system dismantles most of the lecithin before it even enters the bloodstream. All the lecithin you need for building cell membranes and other functions can be made by your body; in other words, lecithin is not an essential nutrient. Large doses of lecithin can even cause stomach upsets, sweating, salivation, and loss of appetite.

STEROLS

What do sterols have in common with the other lipids we have discussed? Their multi-ringed structure makes them very different from the other lipids you have seen. Consider the important sterol cholesterol (see Figure 6-1, *G*). This waxy substance doesn't look like a triglyceride—it doesn't have a glycerol backbone or any fatty acids. But because it doesn't dissolve in water, it is a lipid.

TABLE 6-1

Cholesterol Content of Common Measures of Selected Foods (in Ascending Order)

Food	Amount	Cholesterol in Milligrams	Food	Amount	Cholesterol in Milligrams
Milk, skim	1 cup	4	Clams, halibut, tuna	3 oz	55
Mayonnaise	1 Tbsp	10	Chicken, turkey, light meat	3 oz	70
Butter	1 pat	11			
Lard	1 Tbsp	12	Beef,* pork*	3 oz	75
Cottage cheese	½ cup	15	Lamb, crab	3 oz	85
Milk, low-fat, 2%	1 cup	22	Shrimp, lobster	3 oz	90-110
Half and half	¼ cup	23	Heart, beef	3 oz	164
Hot dog*	1	29	Egg, yolk*	1 each	213
Ice cream, ≈ 10% fat	½ cup	30	Liver, beef	3 oz	410
Cheese, cheddar	1 oz	30	Kidney	3 oz	587
Milk, whole*	1 cup	34	Brains	3 oz	2637
Oysters, salmon	3 oz	40			

Leading contributors of cholesterol to the U.S. diet.

Cholesterol is used to make some important hormones, such as the estrogens and testosterone. Cholesterol is used to make bile, a key emulsifier needed for digestion.[15] In other words, cholesterol is an essential part of life. We can get cholesterol into our bloodstream either from foods or by manufacturing it ourselves. Each day your liver makes about 500 to 1000 milligrams of cholesterol. About one third is made into bile; the rest circulates through the bloodstream to function as the body needs it. In comparison, we eat about 300 to 500 milligrams per day. When a diet doesn't contain enough cholesterol, the liver makes what the body needs.[15]

Cholesterol is found only in the animal foods we eat (Table 6-1). An egg yolk contains about 220 milligrams of cholesterol. This is our main dietary source of cholesterol. However, humans can make all they need if they don't eat enough of it. Some plants contain related sterols, but none we typically eat contains cholesterol. Manufacturers who advertise peanut butter, vegetable shortening, margarines, and vegetable oils as containing "no cholesterol" are taking advantage of uninformed consumers. Peanut butter and margarine never contain cholesterol—it is not part of their nature!

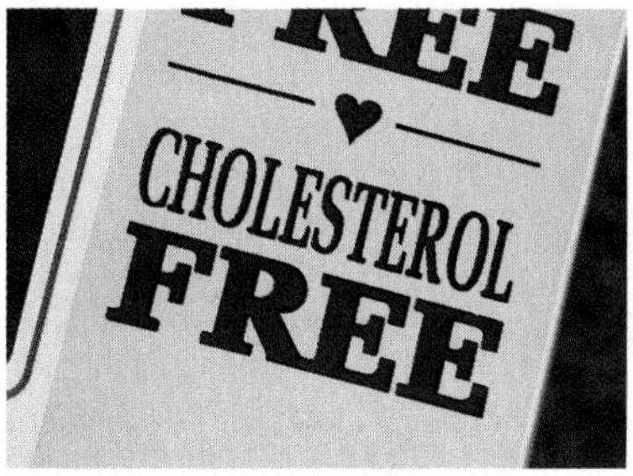

Choosing a diet lower in cholesterol is aided by reading food labels.

CONCEPT CHECK

Phospholipids differ from triglycerides: their glycerol backbone has fatty acids attached, but at least one fatty acid is replaced by another type of compound. Many phospholipids act as emulsifiers. These are compounds that suspend fat as small droplets in water. Phospholipids also form parts of cell membranes and other molecules of the body. Sterols are another class of lipids but are constructed quite differently from either triglycerides or phospholipids. Cholesterol, a sterol, forms hormones and bile; it is essential to the body. Cholesterol is manufactured in the liver, and if sufficient amounts are not ingested, the body makes up the difference. Of the foods we typically eat, cholesterol is found naturally only in those of animal origin.

MAKING FATS AVAILABLE FOR BODY USE

Fat is digested and absorbed primarily in the small intestine.

Fat Digestion

In the first phase of fat digestion, the tongue secretes an enzyme called lingual lipase (*lingual* refers to the tongue). This enzyme acts primarily on triglycerides with fatty acids of short-chain and medium-chain lengths, such as those found in butterfat. The actual digestion occurs in the stomach because lingual lipase requires an acid environment to function. The stomach produces a similar gastric lipase (*gastric* refers to the stomach). The action of both enzymes, however, is usually dwarfed by pancreatic lipase action in the small intestine. Triglycerides and other lipids with long-chain fatty acids, such as those found in common vegetable oils, are generally not digested until they reach the small intestine (Figure 6-5).[15]

The hormone cholecystokinin (CCK), which acts to release enzymes for carbohydrate

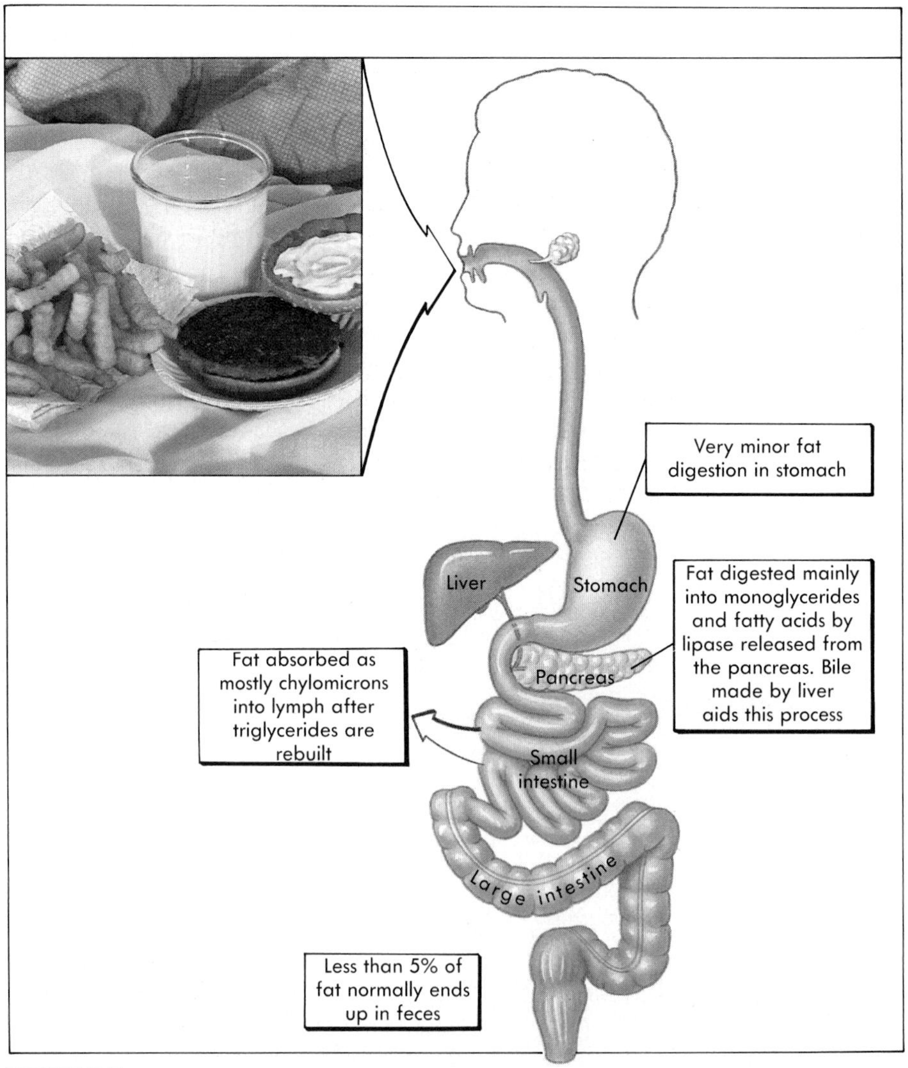

FIGURE 6-5

The primary site for both fat digestion and fat absorption is the small intestine. The enzyme lipase and the emulsifier bile are key participants in fat digestion.

and protein digestion, simultaneously acts to release lipase from the pancreas for fat digestion after eating. In the small intestine, this pancreatic lipase digests the triglycerides into smaller breakdown products, namely monoglycerides (glycerol backbones with single fatty acids attached) and fatty acids. Pancreatic lipase enters the small intestine in a concentration 1000 times greater than needed. This "overkill" makes digestion very rapid and thorough, given the right circumstances. The "right" circumstances include the presence of bile from the gallbladder.[15] Also released in response to CCK, bile helps to emulsify the digestive products of lipase action by forming water-soluble micelles that act like dishwashing detergent breaking up oil spots in dishwater. This improves digestion and absorption, because large fat globules are broken down into smaller ones. The breakdown increases the total surface area for lipase action.

Fats and proteins in the digestive mixture (chyme) also stimulate the release of the hormone gastric inhibitory peptide (GIP) from the walls of the upper small intestine. Release of stomach contents into the small intestine is slowed by GIP. This then helps keep the stomach from overwhelming the upper small intestine with chyme and helps explain why fatty meals cause a feeling of fullness. The chyme remains in the stomach longer, and so we feel full longer. On the other hand, hunger returns quickly after a low-fat meal.

During meals, bile circulates about twice on a path that begins in the liver, and goes on to the gallbladder, through the small intestine, into the portal vein, and then back to the liver. This cycling is called enterohepatic circulation, as we mentioned in Chapter 4. Approximately 98% of the bile is recycled. Only 1% to 2% of the bile ends up in the colon to be eliminated in the stool. In the Nutrition Issue we note that a common way to control very high blood cholesterol levels is to have the person consume resins, which bind bile and draw its constituents into the feces. This treatment reduces bile's enterohepatic circulation. The liver is then forced to make new bile, rather than use recycled bile. The building block for bile synthesis is cholesterol. The liver must take cholesterol out of the bloodstream to make new bile, thus lowering the blood cholesterol level.[6]

Fat Absorption

Most products of fat digestion have been reduced to mere fatty acids and monoglycerides in the small intestine. These are passively absorbed as such into the absorptive cells. One key characteristic of fatty acids and monoglycerides affects their ultimate fate after absorption. If the chain length of a fatty acid is less than 12 carbon atoms (a short-chain or medium-chain variety), it is water-soluble and so will probably travel as such through the portal vein to the liver. If the fatty acid is a long-chain variety (especially 14 or more carbon atoms), then it must eventually be reformed into a triglyceride molecule and enter circulation via the lymphatic system. To travel in the lymphatic system the triglycerides are first combined with cholesterol and other substances and covered with a protein coat. The collective structure of lipid and protein is termed a ***lipoprotein,*** or as in this specific case, a ***chylomicron.*** This chylomicron enters the lymphatic system and eventually the bloodstream to carry most of the absorbed fats yielded from the foods eaten.[15]

Lipoprotein *A compound found in the bloodstream containing a core of lipids with a shell of protein, phospholipid, and cholesterol.*

Chylomicron *Lipoprotein made of dietary fats that are surrounded by a shell of cholesterol, phospholipids, and protein. Chylomicrons are made in the intestine after fat absorption and travel through the lymphatic system to the bloodstream.*

CONCEPT CHECK

In the small intestine, pancreatic lipase digests the triglycerides into smaller breakdown products, namely monoglycerides (glycerol backbones with single fatty acids attached) and fatty acids. The breakdown products then are passively absorbed into the absorptive cells. These products are mostly resynthesized into triglycerides and combined with cholesterol, protein, and other substances to yield a chylomicron. Chylomicrons enter the lymphatic system and eventually the bloodstream.

CARRYING FATS IN THE BLOODSTREAM

Fat and water don't easily mix, as we noted earlier. This incompatibility presents a challenge in transporting fats through the watery mediums of blood and lymph systems.

Carrying Dietary Fats

The whole process of clearing chylomicrons from the bloodstream after eating takes a few hours or longer. Because chylomicrons can affect results of blood tests, people often fast for at least 14 hours before undergoing certain medical tests.

As we just mentioned, once the various dietary fats are digested and absorbed into the small intestine cells, most of these fats are reformed into triglycerides. These combine with phospholipids, protein, and cholesterol to form a chylomicron, one of many types of blood lipoproteins (Figure 6-5). This lipoprotein structure allows fats to float freely in the water-based bloodstream.

Chylomicrons enter the lymphatic system and travel into the bloodstream. Once there, the triglycerides in the chylomicrons are broken down into fatty acids and glycerol by an enzyme on the blood vessel called ***lipoprotein lipase.*** Muscle cells, fat cells, and other cells in the vicinity then absorb most of the fatty acids.[15] Cells can immediately use absorbed fatty acids for fuel, or they can reform them into triglycerides and store them as such. Muscle cells tend to burn the fatty acids, whereas fat cells tend to store them.

Transporting Various Fats Made in the Body

The liver produces more fat and cholesterol than does any other body organ. The source of the needed carbons, hydrogens, and energy to make such things as triglycerides and cholesterol is the carbohydrate and protein the liver takes up from the bloodstream. Any alcohol consumed can also be used as a source. High blood levels of any of these substances encourage the process. The liver coats the cholesterol and triglycerides it makes with a shell of protein and lipids, forming what is called a ***very low-density lipoprotein (VLDL)*** (Figure 6-6).[15]

Very Low-Density Lipoprotein (VLDL) *The lipoprotein that initially leaves the liver; it carries cholesterol and lipids newly synthesized by the liver.*

Low-Density Lipoprotein (LDL) *The product of the VLDL metabolism that contains primarily cholesterol; an elevated level is strongly linked to heart disease.*

When the VLDLs leave the liver, the enzyme lipoprotein lipase on the blood vessels breaks down the triglyceride in the VLDLs into fatty acids and glycerol. Again, these are released into the bloodstream and are taken up by the body cells. Because fats are less dense than water, VLDLs become much heavier—proportionately denser—as triglyceride is released. Much of what remains of these heavy VLDLs becomes particles called ***low-density lipoprotein (LDL).*** LDL is composed primarily of cholesterol.[15]

LDL particles are absorbed from the bloodstream by cells and broken down. Most LDL is taken up by liver cells. Diets low in saturated fat and cholesterol encourage this process, whereas diets high in those lipids can reduce LDL uptake by the liver[12] (see the Nutrition Issue on p. 184). The cholesterol and protein parts then are transported throughout the cell. In this way, liver and other body cells absorb the building blocks used to make bile, sex hormones, and other compounds.

If LDLs are not rapidly taken up by this route, scavenger cells buried in blood vessels detect, alter (or *oxidize*), engulf, and digest the extra circulating LDLs. Over time, cholesterol inundates the scavenger cells.[18]

When scavenger cells have collected and deposited cholesterol for many years at a heavy pace, cholesterol builds up on the inner blood vessel wall—in arteries especially—

another BITE

Some nutrients have antioxidant properties, as we discuss in detail in Chapter 8. These likely can reduce LDL oxidation in the bloodstream and thus slow LDL uptake into plaque.[22] Fruits and vegetables are rich in such antioxidants as beta-carotene and vitamins C and E. Eating fruits and vegetables regularly may then be one positive step we can take to slow the progression of heart disease. On the other hand, an excess intake of iron likely speeds LDL oxidation, making it wise not to take an iron supplement unless a physician prescribes it. People who experience iron storage disease need to pay special attention to this warning[2] (see Chapter 9).

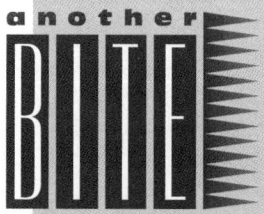

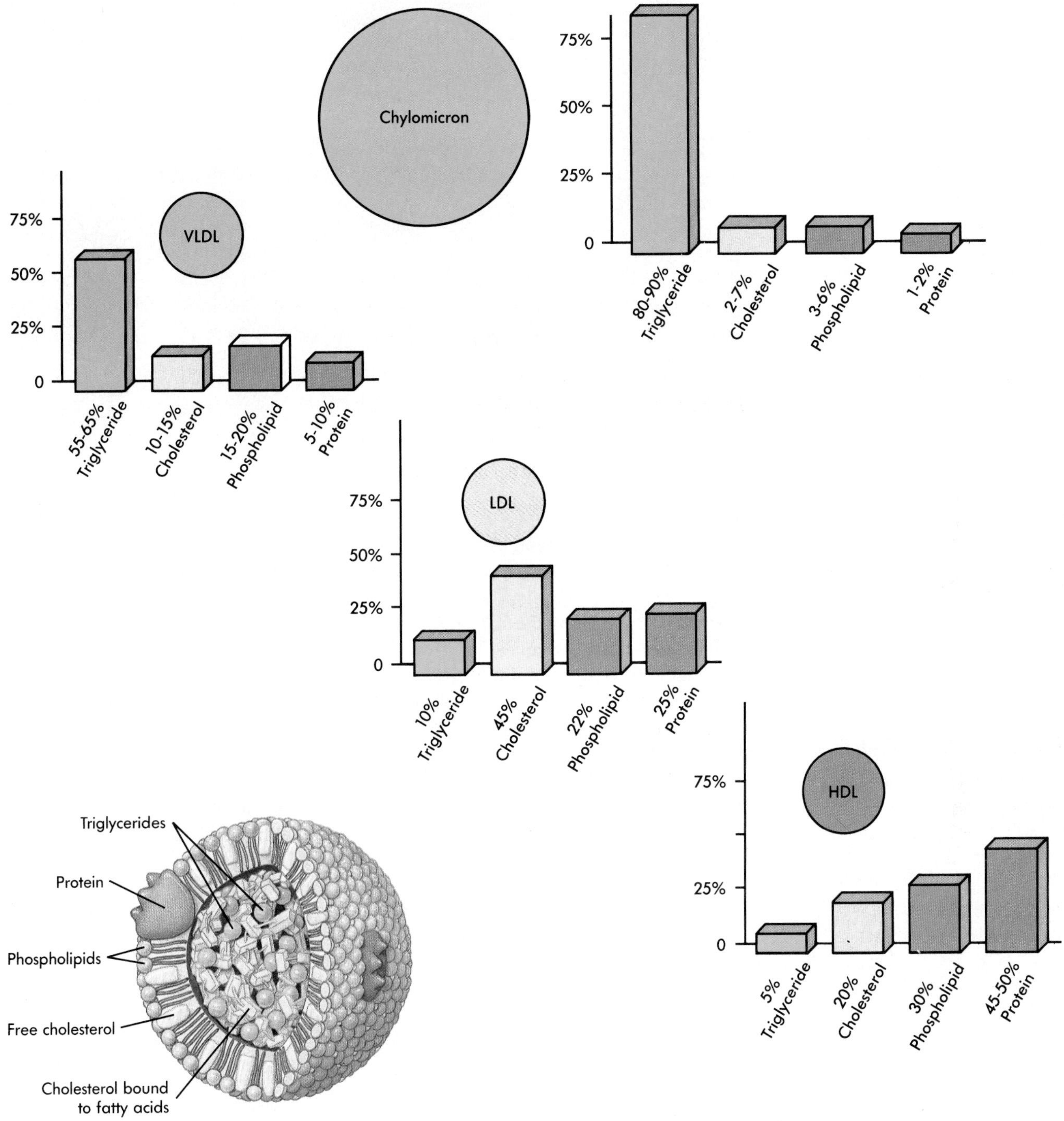

FIGURE 6-6

The structure and composition of the lipoproteins. This structure allows fats to circulate in the water-based bloodstream. Chylomicrons carry fats absorbed from foods through the bloodstream to body cells. VLDLs do the same but carry fats made by the liver. LDLs carry cholesterol to body cells and result from metabolism of VLDLs. HDLs carry cholesterol primarily back to other lipoproteins that in turn are mostly taken up by the liver. Some HDLS also take their cholesterol load directly back to the liver.

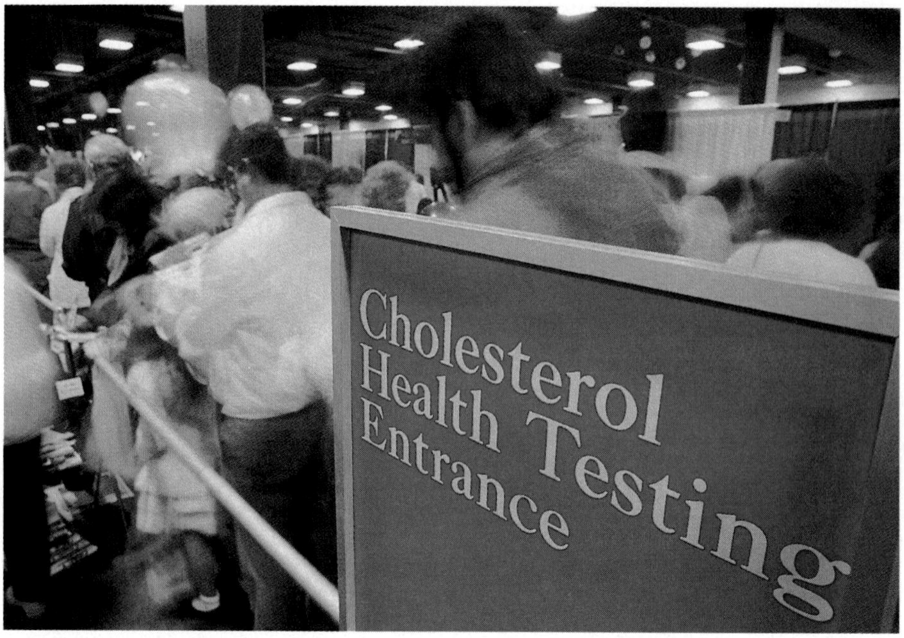

Every adult should know his or her own cholesterol level.

and ***plaque*** develops (Figure 6-7). The plaque eventually mixes with protein and is then covered with a cap of muscle cells and calcium. Atherosclerosis, commonly called hardening of the arteries, develops as plaque grows in the vessel.[11] This chokes off the blood supply to organs, setting the stage for a heart attack and other problems (see the Nutrition Issue at the end of this chapter).[6]

High-Density Lipoprotein (HDL) *A lipoprotein synthesized by the liver and intestine that picks up cholesterol from dying cells and other sources and transfers it primarily to the other lipoproteins in the bloodstream. A low HDL level increases the risk for heart disease.*

A final critical participant in this extensive process of fat transport is the ***high-density lipoprotein (HDL).*** Its high proportion of protein makes it the heaviest (densest) lipoprotein. The liver and intestine produce HDLs that roam the bloodstream, picking up cholesterol from dying cells and other sources. The HDLs donate the cholesterol primarily to other lipoproteins for transport back to the liver to be excreted. Large-scale studies clearly demonstrate that a person's HDL-cholesterol level can closely predict the risk for premature heart disease.[16] The risk increases with low HDL blood levels because little blood cholesterol is transported back to the liver and excreted.

Because a high HDL-cholesterol level slows the development of heart disease, the HDL form of cholesterol is considered the "good" cholesterol. By convention, then, the LDL form would be the bad cholesterol, because a high LDL-cholesterol level speeds the development of heart disease.

CONCEPT CHECK

Most dietary fats are transported in the bloodstream in the form of chylomicrons. Fats and cholesterol synthesized by the liver are carried in the bloodstream as very low-density lipoproteins (VLDLs) and low-density lipoproteins (LDLs). LDLs can be picked up by body cells. Another type of lipoprotein is a high density form, or HDL. It picks up cholesterol from cells and delivers it to other lipoproteins, which transport the cholesterol back to the liver. An elevated LDL-cholesterol level speeds the development of heart disease, as does a low HDL-cholesterol level. Diets rich in saturated fat and cholesterol tend to reduce LDL clearance by the liver.

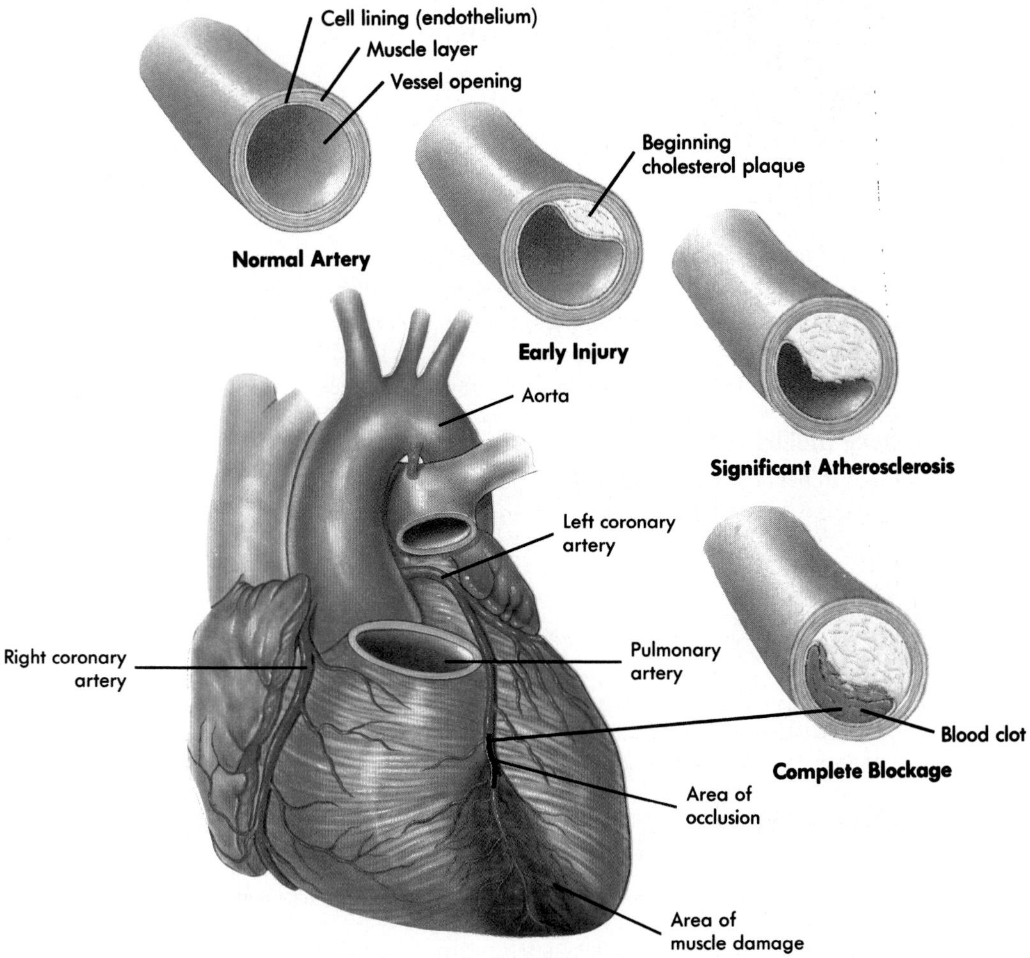

FIGURE 6-7

The road to a heart attack. First, an injury to a blood vessel most likely initiates the process. The process progresses as plaque builds up on the artery walls. The heart attack represents the termination of the process of atherosclerosis—in this case it resulted from blockage of the left coronary artery by a blood clot, the typical cause. The heart muscle that is serviced by the portion of the coronary artery beyond the point of blockage is damaged and may die. This can lead to a significant drop in heart function and often total heart failure.

RECOMMENDATIONS FOR FAT INTAKE

Although we know a great deal about fats, there is no RDA. A good practice, suggested earlier, is to consume at least 1 tablespoon of vegetable oil per day incorporated into foods, such as salad dressings, to obtain the essential fatty acids.

The 1989 RDA publication also states that in the future an allowance for omega-3 fatty acids should be considered. Leading researchers support that suggestion. Currently Canada is the only national government to establish dietary guidelines for omega-3 fatty acids. The Canadian recommendations suggest about 4:1 ratio of omega-6 to omega-3 fatty acids. The current ratio in diets in the United States is about 10:1.

NUTRITION insight

HIDDEN FAT

Some fat in food is obvious: butter on bread, mayonnaise in potato salad, and marbling in raw meat. Fat is harder to detect in other foods that contribute much fat to our diets. Fat is hidden in whole milk, pastries, cookies, cake, cheese, hot dogs, crackers, French fries, and ice cream. When we try to cut down on fat intake, hidden fats need to be exposed and controlled, along with the more obvious sources.

Finding Hidden Fat

A place to begin searching for hidden fat is on the labels of foods you buy in the grocery store. Some words that can alert you to the presence of fat are chocolate; animal fats,

TABLE 6-2

Tips for Avoiding Too Much Fat and Saturated Fat

1. Steam, boil, or bake vegetables. For a change, stir-fry in a small amount of vegetable oil. Consider buying an insert for a pot so you can easily steam your vegetables.
2. Season vegetables with herbs and spices rather than with sauces, butter, or margarine.
3. Try lemon juice on salad or use limited amounts of oil-based salad dressing.
4. To reduce saturated fat, use small amounts of tub margarine instead of butter or stick margarine. In baked products, when possible, use vegetable oil instead of either of these more solid fats or hydrogenated shortenings.
5. Limit baked goods made with large amounts of fat, especially saturated fats: croissants, doughnuts, muffins, biscuits, and butter rolls.
6. Try whole-grain flours to enhance flavors when you bake with less fat and cholesterol-containing ingredients.
7. Replace whole milk with skim or low-fat milk in puddings, soups, and baked products.
8. Substitute low-fat yogurt, blender-whipped low-fat cottage cheese, or buttermilk in recipes that call for sour cream or mayonnaise.
9. Choose lean cuts of meat. Limit bacon, ribs, and meat loaf.
10. Trim fat from meat before and after cooking.
11. Roast, bake, or broil meat, poultry, and fish so fat drains away as the food cooks.
12. Remove skin from poultry before cooking. This eliminates the temptation to eat it along with the meat.
13. Use a nonstick pan for cooking so added fat will be unnecessary; use a vegetable spray for frying.
14. Chill meat or poultry broth until the fat solidifies. Spoon off the fat before using the broth.
15. Eat a vegetarian main dish at least once a week. Include fish (cooked without much added fat) in the diet about two times a week.
16. Choose ice milk, low-fat frozen yogurt, sorbets, and popsicles as substitutes for ice cream.
17. Try angel food cake, fig bars, and ginger snaps as substitutes for commercial baked goods high in saturated fat.
18. Limit high-fat cheese intake.
19. Read labels of commercially prepared foods to find out what type of fat or how much saturated fat they contain.
20. Think about the balance of fats in your menu. If your meal contains whole milk, cheese, ice cream, a higher fat meat, or poultry with skin, use tub margarine and unsaturated vegetable oils for your spreads and dressings. Small amounts of butter, sour cream, or cream cheese can be included if other menu items are low in saturated fat.
21. Use jam, jelly, or marmalade on bread and toast instead of butter or margarine.
22. Buy whole-grain breads and rolls. They have more flavor and do not need butter or margarine to taste good. The dietary fiber present is an added bonus.

such as bacon, beef, ham, lamb, meat, pork, chicken, and turkey fats; lard; vegetable oils; nuts; dairy fats, such as butter and cream; egg and egg-yolk solids; and hydrogenated shortening or vegetable oil. Conveniently, the label lists ingredients by order of weight in the product. If fat is one of the first ingredients listed, you know you are looking at a high-fat product. Whether or not to choose it depends on how you intend to use it in your diet: as a staple item, as an occasional treat, or as a garnish for other foods.

Quick-service foods are notable for their content of hidden fat (see Table 16-2). Quick-service outlets often have nutritional information on their products, but you usually have to ask for it. This literature and your own common sense can help to reduce fat intake from these sources. When you can't find a nutrition label, remember that moderating portion size is a good way to keep fat intake down in foods you suspect are rich in fat.

What to Do

Overall, both visible and hidden sources of fat need to be examined when developing a plan to eat less fat. Consider the practical suggestions we provide in Tables 6-2 and 6-3 for cutting down on visible and hidden fats.

TABLE 6-3

Tips for Avoiding Too Much Fat and Saturated Fat When Dining Out

APPETIZERS			
Best bets:	Vegetable juice, bouillon, fresh fruit, celery, radishes	**Avoid:**	Deep-fried vegetables, creamed soups
MEAT/POULTRY/FISH			
Best bets:	Roasted, baked, broiled—trim off excess fat	**Avoid:**	Fried, sauteed, breaded, gravy, ribs, fatty luncheon meats
EGGS (you may wish to limit as well)			
Best bets:	Poached, boiled; egg whites	**Avoid:**	Fried, scrambled
POTATOES/RICE/PASTA			
Best bets:	Mashed, baked, boiled, steamed	**Avoid:**	Home fried, French fried, creamed, escalloped
VEGETABLES			
Best bets:	Steamed, stewed, boiled	**Avoid:**	Creamed, fried, sauteed
BREADS			
Best bets:	Plain bread, toast, dinner rolls, or muffins	**Avoid:**	Sweet rolls, coffee cake, croissants, biscuits
FATS			
Best bets:	Limited amounts of soft margarine, reduced-calorie salad dressing, low-fat yogurt, low-fat cheeses	**Avoid:**	Gravy, cream sauces, fried foods, heavy-based dressings, sour cream, whole milk cheeses
DESSERTS			
Best bets:	Fresh fruits, nonfat frozen yogurt, sorbet, angel food cake, split a dessert with a friend, new fat-free cake products	**Avoid:**	Pastries, custard, ice cream
BEVERAGES			
Best bets:	Water, coffee, tea, low-fat or nonfat milk, soft drinks	**Avoid:**	Chocolate milk, milk shakes, whole milk

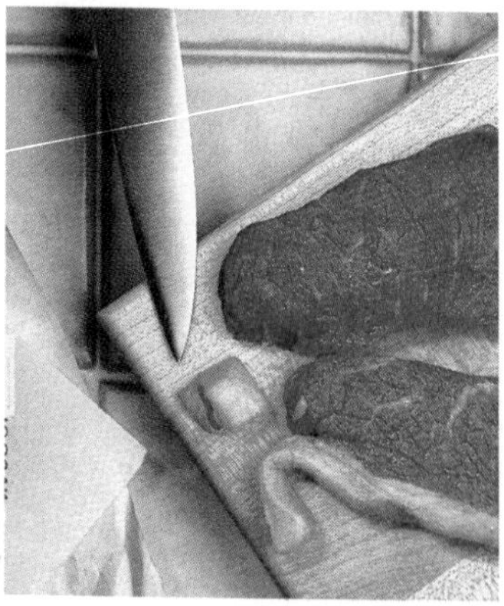

Trim meats before cooking to help reduce your fat intake.

What is actually 30% of kcalories in terms of fat?

Energy (kcalories/day)	Fat (g/day)
1200	40
1500	50
1800	60
1900	63
2100	70
2200	73
2300	77
2600	87
2900	97
3000	100

Americans eat about 36% to 38% of their total kcalories as fat. Vegetable and animal sources each supply about half the fat. Major sources of fat in the American diet are beef products, luncheon meats, whole milk, and pastries.

The American Heart Association (AHA) recommends eating no more than 30% of your total kcalories as fat, using nearly equal amounts of saturated, monounsaturated, and polyunsaturated fatty acids, or a 1:1:1 ratio (Table 6-4). Eating equivalent amounts of the different fatty acids helps control saturated fat intake. Also, reducing fat to 30% of energy intake helps reduce saturated fat consumption and also lowers the chances of creeping weight gain in adulthood. The AHA further recommends eating no more than 300 milligrams of cholesterol a day. Lowering fat intake to 20% of total kcalories in cases where an elevated serum LDL-cholesterol level does not respond to the moderate recommendation is also advised[6] (Table 6-5). One recent study even shows that lowering fat in a diet to only 10% of kcalories and eating essentially NO cholesterol cause plaque in arteries to diminish.[17] More research on this is necessary before we advocate such a severe dietary change—an essentially animal-free diet. Chapter 7 shows how one would plan such a diet, called a vegan diet. The overriding message for most American adults is to eat less fat.

The National Cholesterol Education Program, established in 1985 in the United States, recommends reducing saturated fatty acids even further to 7% of kcalories if a high serum cholesterol level fails to respond to a 10% level.[6] Cholesterol intake should also fall below 200 milligrams per day. We currently eat about 14% of kcalories as saturated fat. Reducing total fat and saturated fat intake is a suggestion that also fits in with the Dietary Guidelines for Americans we reviewed in Chapter 2. Many new fat-free cookies, salad dressings, mayonnaise, cream cheese, crackers, and cakes make this an easier goal to pursue. Tables 6-2 and 6-3 give some further help.

FATS IN FOOD

Salad oils, butter, margarine, and mayonnaise all contain about 100% of kcalories as fat. In other words, they are loaded with fat (Figure 6-8). Walnuts, bologna, avocados, and bacon have about 80% of kcalories as fat. Peanut butter and cheddar cheese have about 75% of their kcalories as fat. Steak and hamburgers have about 60% of kcalories as fat, but this can be reduced by choosing leaner varieties, careful trimming of fat when possi-

TABLE 6-4

Dietary Guidelines for Healthy American Adults: A Statement for Physicians and Health Professionals by the Nutrition Committee, American Heart Association (AHA)

1. Total fat intake should be less than 30% of kcalories.
2. Saturated fat intake should be less than 10% of kcalories.
3. Polyunsaturated fat intake should not exceed 10% of kcalories.
4. Cholesterol intake should not exceed 300 mg/day.
5. Carbohydrate intake should constitute 50% or more of kcalories, with emphasis on complex carbohydrates.
6. Protein intake should provide the remainder of the kcalories.
7. Sodium intake should not exceed 3 g/day.
8. Alcoholic consumption should not exceed 1 to 2 oz of ethanol per day. Two ounces of 100 proof whiskey, 8 oz of wine, and 24 oz of beer each contain 1 oz of ethanol.
9. Total kcalories should be sufficient to maintain the individual's recommended body weight.
10. A wide variety of foods should be consumed.

From Circulation *77:721A, 1988.*

TABLE 6-5

Menus Containing 2000 kcalories and Various Percentages of Fat

30% of Kcalories as Fat	Teaspoons of Fat	20% of Kcalories as Fat	Teaspoons of Fat
Breakfast			
Orange juice, 1 cup	0	Same	0
Shredded wheat, ¾ cup	⅕	Same	⅕
Bagel, toasted	⅕	Same	⅕
Margarine, 2 tsp	1¾	Same	1¾
1% milk, 1 cup	½	Milk, nonfat, 1 cup	⅒
Lunch			
Whole-wheat bread, 2 slices	½	Same	½
Roast beef, lean, 2 oz	1	Ham, boiled, 2 oz	½
Mayonnaise, 2 tsp	1½	Same	1½
Lettuce	0	Same	0
Tomato, sliced	0	Same	0
Animal crackers, 8	⅕	Same	⅕
Snack			
Apple	⅙	Same	⅙
Dinner			
Pork chop, broiled, 3 oz	2⅓	Halibut, broiled, 3 oz	⅔
Pasta, 1½ cup	⅔	Same	⅔
Margarine, 2 tsp	1¾	Margarine, 1 tsp	⅞
Broccoli, ½ cup	0	Same	0
1% milk, 1 cup	½	Milk, nonfat, 1 cup	⅒
		Banana	⅒
Snack			
Raisins, 2 Tbsp.	0	Raisins, ¼ cup	0
Popcorn, air-popped, 6 cups	½	Same	½
With 2 tsp margarine	1¾	With 1 tsp margarine	⅞
TOTALS	14		8½

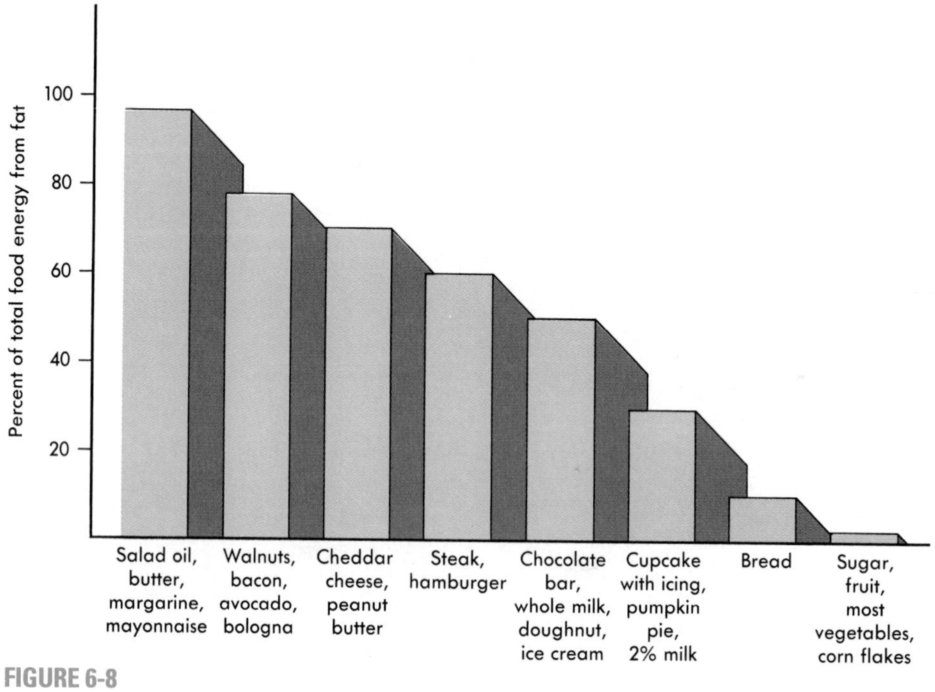

FIGURE 6-8

Percentage of kcalories as fat in foods. Vegetable oils, butter, margarine, and mayonnaise provide almost all energy as fat.

ble, and broiling the meat. Chocolate bars, ice cream, doughnuts, and whole milk have about 50% of kcalories as fat. Pumpkin pie and cupcakes have 35%. Bread contains about 15% of its kcalories as fat. Cornflakes, sugar, and most fruits and vegetables have essentially no fat.

When you read that a certain hot dog is only 27% fat, or 73% fat-free, you might initially be impressed. However, it means that the hot dog is 27% fat by weight, not in terms of kcalories. Actually, 83% of the kcalories come from fat. Remember that water makes up a significant part of the weight of many foods, including a hot dog. So don't be deceived by these kinds of statements. Read the label and calculate the percentage of fat to be sure (Figure 6-9). New nutrition labels now being used will end this consumer deception (see Chapter 2).

The latest fat research points to the 14-carbon myristic acid as the main blood cholesterol–raising fatty acid. This is especially high in dairy fats, such as butter.

We get most of our saturated fats from animal fats. They contain about 40% to 60% saturated fatty acids. Recent evidence suggests that saturated fatty acids with 12 to 16 carbons are the ones that raise serum cholesterol levels.[7] These *problem* saturated fatty acids make up about 25% to 50% of animal fats. Some plant products also contain significant amounts of *problem* saturated fatty acids—for example, cottonseed oil (27%), palm oil (46%), palm kernel oil (71%), and coconut oil (70%). The last three compose a group of what is often called tropical oils, based on their countries of origin. *Trans* fats in hydrogenated vegetable oils further add to the problem fatty acids, as we discussed earlier.[10] It is best to limit, but not necessarily eliminate, consumption of foods rich in all the problem fatty acids.

BEEF FRANKS
73% Fat Free

Ingredients: Beef, Water, Corn Syrup, Salt, Dextrose, Flavorings, Sodium Ascorbate (Vitamin C), Sodium Nitrate, Extract of Paprika.

Nutrition Information Per Serving
Seving Size - 1 link, 1.6 ounces (45 grams)
Servings Per Package - 10

Calories 130	Fat .... 12 Grams
Protein .... 5 Grams	Sodium .... 450 mg (0.45 Grams)
Carbohydrates .... 1 Gram	

On a weight basis: $\frac{\text{fat weight (12 grams)} \times 100}{\text{total weight (45 grams)}} = 27\%$ weight is fat

On a kcalorie basis: $\frac{\text{fat kcalories } (12 \times 9) \times 100}{\text{total kcalories (130)}} = 83\%$ kcalories from fat

FIGURE 6-9
Is this hot dog 27% or 83% fat?

Plant fats contain mostly unsaturated fatty acids, ranging from 76% to 94% (excluding palm and coconut oils). Plant oils supply most of the essential fatty acids in our food supply. Olive oil, canola oil, and peanut oil contain a moderate to high amount of monounsaturated fatty acids (49% to 77%). Some animal fats are also good sources (30% to 48%) (see Figure 6-2). Corn, cottonseed, sunflower, soybean, and safflower oils contain mostly polyunsaturated fat; note that amounts vary (54% to 77%).

Many manufacturers and food growers are trying to devise products that are lower in fats generally, and particularly in saturated fats. During the past several decades, beef producers have altered cattle breeding and feeding practices to increase muscle mass and decrease body fat.

CONCEPT CHECK

There is no recommended dietary allowance for fat. We need the equivalent of about 1 tablespoon of plant oils supplied by foods to provide essential fatty acids. Many health-related agencies recommend a diet containing no more than 30% of energy as fat, and a maximum of one third of that as saturated fat. The American diet contains about 38% of energy as fat. Foods high in fat (over 60% of total kcalories) include plant oils, butter, margarine, mayonnaise, walnuts, bacon, avocados, peanut butter, cheddar cheese, steak, and hamburger. Sources high in saturated fat include animal fats, coconut oil, and palm oil.

NUTRITION insight

FAT REPLACEMENTS

Consumers show great interest in substances that can replace fat in foods and still yield a tasty product. Food manufacturers take basically five different approaches toward that goal.[14] The first method consists of simply adding water to the product, in turn reducing the amount of fat in a serving. A good example is diet margarine. A second method employs starch derivatives to bind water in the food. Typical ingredients include cellulose, N-Oil, Paselli SA2, Sta-Slim, Maltrin, and Oatrim. These ingredients have been used in a variety of foods, including luncheon meats, salad dressings, frozen desserts, table spreads, dips, baked goods, and candies. Third, gums extracted from plants can be added to thicken a product and replace some of the body that fat provided. Diet salad dressings have gums added for this reason.

The fourth and newest type of fat replacement on the market is a protein that has been mixed together in such a way that it produces microscopic, mistlike protein globules. Both egg and milk proteins can be used. Simplesse is a current example.[23] The minute protein globules in Simplesse feel like fat in the mouth, although fatty acids are not present in the product. The texture changes suffice to give the illusion of fat (Figure 6-10). Although it yields energy, Simplesse has only about 1.3 kcalories per gram, much less than regular fat's 9 kcalories per gram. This low kcalorie value is partly because proteins contain 4 kcalories per gram and because of the amount of water incorporated into the product during processing; water accounts for much of its weight.

Currently Simplesse is approved by FDA for use in frozen desserts. It reduces kcalories by about one half and fat content to a negligible amount in these products. Simplesse can also replace fat in mayonnaise, salad dressings, yogurt, cheeses, and other dairy products. Because high temperatures alter the structure of Simplesse so much that it no longer resembles fat, it cannot be used for cooking or frying. People who are allergic to milk

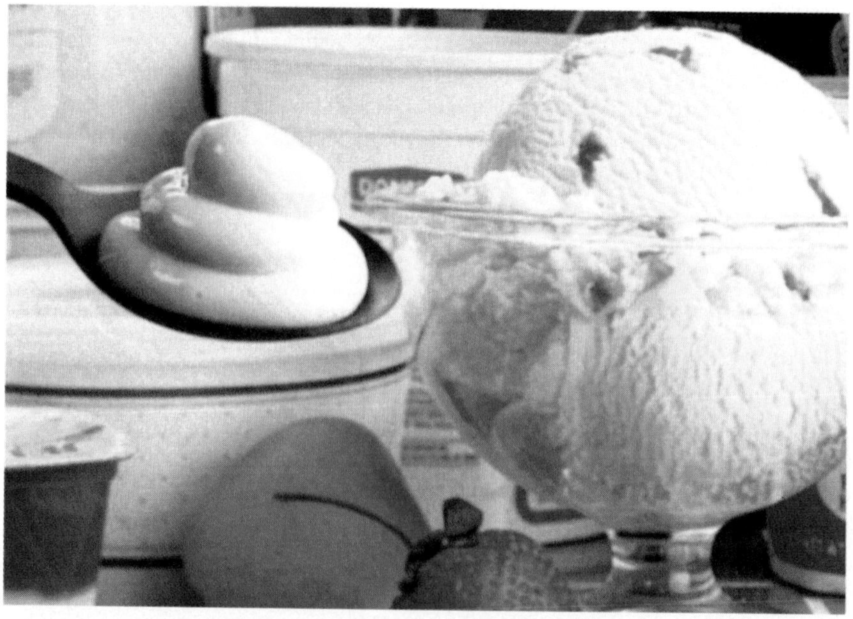

FIGURE 6-10
Simplesse as it appears both in its ingredient form (on the left) and in a frozen dessert.

and/or egg proteins should not consume Simplesse. With extensive use, Simplesse could help reduce total fat intake.

The fifth and final form of fat replacement is the engineered fat. This type of product is synthesized in the laboratory from parts of various food constituents. The experimental product olestra is a good example. It is made by adding fatty acids to a sucrose (table sugar) molecule. Olestra with many fatty acids attached cannot be digested by either human digestive enzymes or bacteria that live in the intestine. Therefore it yields no energy to the body. As it leaves the body, it can even pull cholesterol-containing substances into the intestine with it, thereby lowering the person's blood cholesterol level.

Olestra is quite versatile as an ingredient. The manufacturer feels it can replace up to 35% of the fat in salad dressings and cakes made at home, and it can be used for frying in food manufacturing. But some problems are associated with olestra use. It tends to bind the fat-soluble vitamin E, reducing its absorption. The manufacturer has proposed adding more vitamin E to olestra than the amount it could bind to compensate. Some years ago FDA would not permit the use of mineral oil in foods as a no-kcalorie fat, because it bound up fat-soluble vitamins. For this and other reasons, it is unclear when Olestra will be available. If approved by FDA, Olestra would reduce the fat content of many foods, permit us to eat rich desserts and fried foods, and better control fat intake. Food manufacturers are also working on other types of engineered fats that either wholly or partially escape absorption by the body.

Fat Replacements in Perspective

So far, the effect of fat replacements on the American diet has not been substantial. Current forms are not very versatile. Many foods that are major fat contributors in our diets—hamburgers, hot dogs, whole milk, doughnuts and cake products, and beef steaks and roasts, to name some key players—still remain so. The main benefit of using fat replacements will be cutting some fat from the diet, most importantly saturated fat and cholesterol. The actual energy reduction will probably be less impressive, because people tend to make up the lost energy by eating more of other foods.[23]

We will always need balanced eating habits and moderation in food choice. A diet rich in fruits, vegetables, whole grains, and lean animal products still deserves the most attention. Fat replacements can reduce intake of saturated fat and cholesterol in popular foods Americans are unwilling to relinquish, such as ice cream. But we won't know the true impact of fat replacements on our diets until either more are approved, as in the case of olestra, or existing approaches gain wider use. For now they are of little significance.[14]

SUMMARY

- Lipids are a group of compounds that don't dissolve in water. Fatty acids can be grouped according to the type of bonds between the carbons: saturated fatty acids contain no double bonds, monounsaturated fatty acids contain one double bond, and polyunsaturated fatty acids contain two or more double bonds.
- If the double bonds in a fatty acid begin at the third carbon from the $-CH_3$ end of the chain, the fatty acid is an omega-3 fatty acid. In omega-6 fatty acids the double bonds begin at the sixth carbon. Both omega-3 and omega-6 fatty acids are essential parts of a diet because our bodies need them but don't produce them.

- Body cells use omega-3 fatty acids to synthesize compounds that tend to reduce blood clotting and inflammatory responses. Because many types of fish contain ample amounts of the omega-3 fatty acids, eating fish at least twice a week is a good dietary practice.
- Fats composed of saturated fatty acids tend to be solid at room temperature. Those with polyunsaturated fatty acids are usually liquid at room temperature. However, saturated fatty acids with short chain lengths—coconut oil, for example—are usually liquid. Hydrogenation is the process of adding hydrogens to fatty acids to turn double bonds into single bonds. Manufacturers hydrogenate (increase saturation of) fats to solidify vegetable oils for making shortenings and margarine. This practice also reduces the breakdown of polyunsaturated fatty acids, which lessens rancidity.
- Triglycerides are the major form of fat in food and in our bodies. Besides supplying essential fatty acids to the body, triglycerides supply energy, allow efficient energy storage, insulate and protect the body, transport fat-soluble vitamins, provide satiety, and add flavor and texture to foods.
- Phospholipids are another class of lipids. They are derived from triglycerides. They form important parts of cell membranes. Some act as efficient emulsifiers, allowing fats to disperse in water.
- Cholesterol is in the class of lipids called sterols. It forms part of vital compounds, such as hormones and bile. We eat cholesterol, and cells in the body make it.
- Fat digestion takes place primarily in the small intestine. Pancreatic lipase digests the triglycerides into smaller breakdown products, namely monoglycerides (glycerol backbones with single fatty acids attached) and fatty acids. The breakdown products then are passively absorbed into the small intestine. These products are mostly resynthesized into triglycerides and combined with cholesterol, protein, and other substances to yield a chylomicron. Chylomicrons enter the lymphatic system, in turn passing into the bloodstream.
- Fats are carried in the bloodstream by various lipoproteins: chylomicrons, very low-density lipoproteins (VLDLs), low-density lipoproteins (LDLs), and high-density lipoproteins (HDLs). The greater the amount of triglycerides in the lipoproteins, the less their density. Both an elevated LDL-cholesterol level and a low HDL-cholesterol level speed the development of heart disease.
- There is no RDA for fat. We need to eat at least the equivalent of about 1 tablespoon of plant oils daily in foods to get the needed essential fatty acids. Major contributors of fat to our diets include animal foods, whole milk, and pastries. The fat substitute Simplesse allows us to eat some dairy products—frozen desserts, for example—without consuming much fat.

STUDY QUESTIONS

1. Describe the difference between a saturated and polyunsaturated fatty acid both in foods and in their effects on the human body. Be sure to consider the structure of these two types of fatty acids.
2. Describe the structures and main roles of the four major blood lipoproteins.
3. What do health care professionals recommend regarding fat intake? What does this mean in terms of actual food choices?
4. What are three functions of fat in food? How do these differ from the functions of lipids in the human body?
5. What is the significance of the new fat replacements? List three possible usages.

REFERENCES

1. Anderson JW and others: Prospective, randomized, controlled comparison of the effects of low-fat and low-fat plus high-fiber diets on serum lipid concentrations, *American Journal of Clinical Nutrition* 56:887, 1992.
2. Beard JL: Are we at risk of heart disease because of normal iron status? *Nutrition Reviews* 51:112, 1993.
3. Connor WE and others: Essential fatty acids: the importance of n-3 fatty acids in the retina and brain, *Nutrition Reviews* 50:21, 1992.
4. Drevon CA: Marine oils and their effects, *Nutrition Reviews* 50:38, 1992.
5. Edelstein SL and others: Increased meal frequency associated with decreased cholesterol concentrations; Rancho Bernardo, CA, 1984-1987, *American Journal of Clinical Nutrition* 55:664, 1992.
6. Expert Panel on Detection, Evaluation, and Treatment of High Blood Cholesterol in Adults: Summary of the second report of the National Cholesterol Education Program (NCEP), *Journal of American Medical Association* 269:3015, 1993.
7. Hegsted DM and others: Dietary fat and serum lipids: an evaluation of the experimental data, *American Journal of Clinical Nutrition* 57:875, 1993.
8. Jenkins PA and others: Effect on blood lipids of very high intakes of fiber in diets low in saturated fat and cholesterol, *New England Journal of Medicine* 329:21, 1993.
9. Kang SS and others: Hyperhomocyst(e)inemia as a risk factor for occlusive vascular disease, *Annual Review of Nutrition* 12:279, 1992.
10. Katan MB, Mensink RP: Isomeric fatty acids and serum lipoproteins, *Nutrition Reviews* 50:46, 1992.
11. Klag MJ and others: Serum cholesterol in young men and subsequent cardiovascular disease, *New England Journal of Medicine* 328:313, 1993.
12. McNamara DJ: Coronary heart disease. In Brown ML, ed: *Present knowledge in nutrition,* Washington DC, 1990, ISLI Nutrition Foundation.
13. Manson JE and others: The primary prevention of myocardial infarction, *New England Journal of Medicine* 326:1406, 1992.
14. Mela DJ: Nutritional implications of fat substitutes, *Journal of the American Dietetic Association* 92:472, 1992.
15. Murray RK and others: *Harper's biochemistry,* ed 22, Norwalk, Conn, 1993, Appleton & Lange.
16. NIH Consensus Development Panel: Triglyceride, high-density lipoprotein, and coronary heart disease, *Journal of the American Medical Association* 269:505, 1993.
17. Ornish D and others: Can lifestyle changes reverse coronary heart disease? *Lancet* 336:129, 1990.
18. Parthasarathy S and others: The role of oxidized low-density lipoproteins in the pathogenesis of atherosclerosis, *Annual Reviews of Medicine* 43:219, 1992.
19. Rader DJ, Brewer HB: Lipoprotein(a) clinical approach to a unique atherogenic lipoprotein, *Journal of the American Medical Association* 267:1109, 1992.
20. Renaud SC and others: Alcohol and platelet aggregation: the Caerphilly Prospective Heart Disease Study, *American Journal of Clinical Nutrition* 55:1012, 1992.
21. Rimm EB and others: Prospective study of alcohol consumption and risk of coronary disease in men, *Lancet* 338:464, 1991.
22. Russell RM: Nutrition, *Journal of the American Medical Association* 270:233, 1993.
23. Stern JS, Hermann-Zaidins MG: Fat replacements: a new strategy for dietary change, *Journal of The American Dietetic Association* 92:91, 1992.
24. Troisi R and others: Trans-fatty acid intake in relation to serum lipid concentrations in adult men, *American Journal of Clinical Nutrition* 56:1019, 1992.
25. Virmani R, Farb A: Risk factors in the pathogenesis of coronary artery disease, *Comprehensive Therapy* 18:7, 1992.
26. Wichmann S, Martin DR: Heart disease: not for men only, *The Physician and Sportsmedicine* 20:138, 1992.

RATE

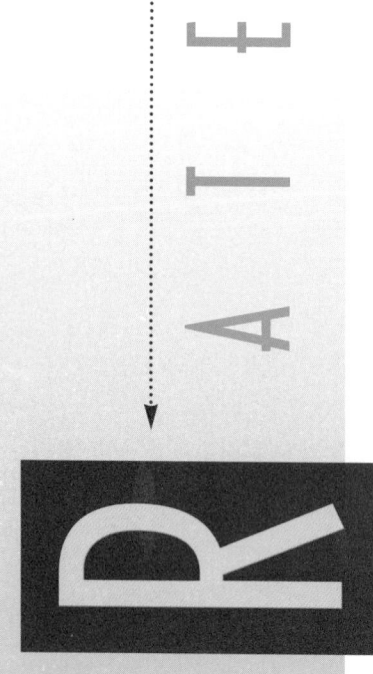

WHERE DO YOU STAND IN TERMS OF FAT?

How do your food practices compare with guidelines that have been suggested for fat, saturated fat, and cholesterol? Refer to the nutritional assessment you completed at the end of Chapter 2, and compare it with the guidelines issued by the American Heart Association and the National Cholesterol Education Program listed below:

- Limit or reduce total fat intake to less than 30% of total kcalories.
- Reduce saturated fat intake to 7% to 10% of kcalories or less.
- Limit cholesterol to less than 200 to 300 milligrams per day.

To compare your nutritional assessment with these guidelines, the following pieces of information are needed from your assessment (write the numbers in the blanks given):

TOTAL KCALORIE INTAKE ___________

TOTAL GRAMS OF FAT ___________

GRAMS OF SATURATED FAT ___________

MILLIGRAMS OF CHOLESTEROL ___________

Now complete the following steps:

1. Multiply your total grams of fat by 9 (kcalories/gram of fat). Then divide the result by your total kcalorie intake. Next multiply this number by 100. THIS WILL GIVE YOU THE % OF KCALORIES YOU CONSUMED FROM FAT.

   % OF KCALORIES FROM FAT ___________

   IS IT LESS THAN 30% OF YOUR TOTAL KCALORIES? YES _____ NO _____

2. Multiply your grams of saturated fat by 9 (kcals/gram of fat). Divide the result by your total kcalorie intake. Now multiply this number by 100. THIS WILL GIVE YOU THE % OF KCALORIES YOU CONSUMED FROM SATURATED FAT.

   % OF KCALORIES FROM SATURATED FAT___________

   IS IT 10% OF YOUR KCALORIES OR LESS? YES _____ NO _____

3. Look at your milligrams of cholesterol.

IS IT LESS THAN 300 MILLIGRAMS? YES ____ NO ____

4. Look back at the foods you ate and notice the foods that contributed the most fat, saturated fat, and cholesterol. If you didn't meet one or more of the guidelines, how could you change what you ate that day to improve your diet?

5. Now take the next step. Do you know your HDL- and LDL-cholesterol levels? If not, have them checked soon. All adults should know if their levels are in the abnormal ranges.

6. Finally, fill in the following assessment of your risk for developing premature heart disease. Decide today how you could modify your diet and lifestyle, if necessary, to reduce your risk.

Do you have . . .	YES	NO
a history of smoking?	____	____
high blood pressure?	____	____
a high LDL-cholesterol level?	____	____
a low HDL-cholesterol level?	____	____
diabetes?	____	____
a history of physical inactivity?	____	____
a family history of premature heart disease?	____	____
a history of obesity?	____	____

Other factors also could be considered, but this provides a good start for assessing your risk.

Nutrition ISSUE

HEART DISEASE

When a heart attack hits, it can strike with the sudden force of a sledgehammer. It can also sneak up on you at night, masquerading as indigestion with slight pain or pressure in your chest.

Heart disease—more precisely termed *cardiovascular disease* —is the major killer of Americans. Each year about 600,000 people die of heart disease in the United States, 60% more than cancer kills. The figure rises to almost 1 million if we include strokes and other circulatory diseases in the more global term cardiovascular disease. The overall male to female ratio for heart disease is about 2:1.[26] For each person in America who dies of heart disease, 10 more (over 6 million people) have heart disease symptoms. And about twice the number who die, 1.5 million, suffer heart attacks each year.

Heart disease is a chronic disease—it takes years to develop symptoms. Sometimes they do not appear until old age. Still, even men under the age of 20 show deposits of atherosclerotic plaque in their arteries, as noted in autopsy data from the Korean and Vietnam wars and automobile accidents. This indicates that plaque buildup often begins in childhood and continues throughout life. It usually goes unnoticed for quite some time.

Preventing premature heart disease—that which appears before age 70 to 80—should be everyone's goal. Although we all die eventually, one key to a better life is to prevent premature death and live in optimal health until essentially the entire body wears out, the heart included. Heart attacks at ages 40 through 60 are closely linked to the risk factors listed below.[11] For most people, there is a good chance to prevent premature heart disease by making some long-term lifestyle changes.

Myocardial Infarction (MI) *Death of part of the heart muscle.*

Cerebrovascular Accident (CVA) *Death of part of the brain tissue caused by a blood clot; also called a stroke.*

Heart disease and strokes are associated with poor blood circulation. Blood supplies the heart muscle with oxygen and nutrients. When blood flow to the heart is interrupted, the heart muscle can be damaged. A heart attack—***myocardial infarction***—may result (see Figure 6-7).[6] This may cause the heart to beat irregularly or to stop altogether. If blood flow to parts of the brain is interrupted long enough, part of the brain dies, causing a ***cerebrovascular accident,*** or stroke. When a stroke causes loss of muscle control, death may occur.

Blood clots can stop blood flow to the heart or brain. Clots form more readily where cholesterol plaque has built up in the arteries that lead to the heart or brain. Small doses of aspirin reduce blood clotting and are now used to treat people at risk for heart attack.[13]

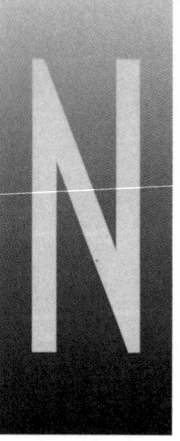

Plaque is probably first deposited to repair injuries in a vessel lining.[25] Hypertension, diabetes, and smoking are agents that lead to injury. Current research also implicates certain bacteria and viruses in the process. Repair of damage is part of the *initiation phase* of atherosclerosis. The rate of further plaque deposition in the next phase—called the *progression phase*—partly depends on the amount of LDL in the bloodstream. The plaque thickens as layers of cholesterol (mostly as part of LDL), protein, muscle, and calcium are laid down. Arteries harden and narrow as plaque builds up, making them less elastic and so unable to expand to accommodate various blood pressures. Then arteries become further damaged as blood pumps through and pressure increases. Finally, in the *termination phase,* a clot or spasm in the plaque-clogged artery leads to the myocardial infarction or cerebrovascular accident. Recent studies show that the risk for this termination phase to develop increases in the few hours after people who have already developed significant atherosclerosis eat a fat-rich meal.

What Is Your Risk for Heart Disease?

Because of rare genetic defects that greatly block clearance of chylomicrons from the bloodstream, reduce LDL uptake by the liver, or limit synthesis of HDL, some people face a much higher risk for premature heart disease than the average American.[13,19] However, for the average person, the most likely risk factors present for premature heart disease are:[6]

- Total blood cholesterol > 200 milligrams per 100 milliliters, and especially ≥ 240 milligrams per 100 milliliters.
- LDL cholesterol >130 milligrams per 100 milliliters and especially ≥ 160 milligrams per 100 milliliters.
- Age: men > 45 years, women ≥ 55 years.
- Family history of premature heart disease.
- Smoking.
- Hypertension.
- HDL-cholesterol level < 35 milligrams per 100 milliliters.
- Diabetes.

Other significant risk factors to consider are a total cholesterol to HDL-cholesterol ratio of > 4.5:1; physical inactivity; an elevated blood triglyceride level; an excessive iron intake[2]; inadequate intakes of vitamins B-6, folate, and B-12[22]; and obesity (especially fat around the waist). However, we should first focus on smoking, hypertension, and high LDL-cholesterol levels—the most widespread contributors—to minimize the risk for premature heart disease. The dietary advice that we offer for minimizing these three main risk factors—along with following the Food Guide Pyramid—is all we can suggest to also address the less widespread causes.[9, 19]

Do you smoke? Chemicals in smoke alter blood vessels, enabling plaque to build up faster. Smoking also makes blood more likely to clot. Do you have hypertension? If your ***systolic blood pressure*** is over 140 (millimeters of mercury) or higher or your ***diastolic blood pressure*** is 90 or more, you have hypertension. Do you have a high LDL-cholesterol level (over 100 to 130 milligrams per 100 milliliters) or total cholesterol level over 200? (If your cholesterol values come out high, have yourself tested at least two more times because the levels vary from day to day.) Is your HDL-cholesterol level low, such that your total cholesterol to HDL-cholesterol ratio is high (greater than 4.5:1)? If this is true or the HDL-cholesterol level alone is below 35 milligrams per 100 milliliters, you have increased risk for heart disease. Add to this your family history and other disease patterns we mentioned to assess whether you are at risk.[6]

LDL-cholesterol and HDL-cholesterol levels and the total cholesterol to HDL-cholesterol ratio, rather than the total cholesterol level, are really the most important values to focus on. If a total cholesterol level is greater than 200 milligrams per 100 milliliters and the higher reading is primarily caused by a high HDL-cholesterol level, especially if more than 60 milligrams per 100 milliliters, the risk of heart disease is still about average or less. That is sometimes the case for women, especially before menopause. It is a good idea for women to have their HDL-cholesterol levels checked to see whether this is why total blood cholesterol is elevated. Unfortunately, men with elevated total cholesterol levels usually have an elevated LDL-cholesterol level. Therefore the total cholesterol to HDL-cholesterol ratio is too high.

Systolic Blood Pressure *The pressure in the bloodstream associated with pumping blood from the heart.*

Diastolic Blood Pressure *The pressure in the bloodstream when the heart is between beats.*

The National Institutes of Health in the United States encourages all people over age 20 to have their total cholesterol and HDL-cholesterol levels checked.[6] Children over 2 years of age with a family history of heart disease deserve similar scrutiny. Heart disease experts also recommend having triglyceride level checked. This value is used to calculate the LDL-cholesterol level. If you don't know your various cholesterol levels and ratio, you don't know your risk of developing premature heart disease. Keep in mind that you have remarkable potential for preventing premature heart disease if you are at risk, but first you must recognize your risk factors.

Reducing an Elevated LDL-Cholesterol Level

Some people exhibit few or none of the major risk factors for heart disease. These people are told simply to eat sensibly, remain physically active, and have their risk factors reevaluated at approximately 5-year intervals. However, if someone discovers that his or her LDL-cholesterol level is high, the first step is to consult a physician. Some diseases raise LDL-cholesterol levels, and treating the disease may remedy the LDL-cholesterol problem as well. If no other disease is present, diet change is advised.[3]

Reducing saturated fat in your diet can lower an elevated LDL-cholesterol level. Although a high blood cholesterol level indicates that an individual is at risk for heart disease, the main food factor associated with a high cholesterol level is eating lots of saturated fat.[6] Eating less saturated fat is more effective for most people than is eating less cholesterol.

Almost everyone who minimizes saturated fat intake can lower an elevated LDL-cholesterol level by about 10% to 20%, especially if the person normally eats lots of foods that are high in saturated fats. About 10% of people have trouble lowering their blood cholesterol level with diet. Genetic defects are the likely reason. On the other hand, about 10% can expect an even bigger drop in LDL-cholesterol levels. Lowering saturated fat in the diet is not so hard, as we pointed out in Table 6-2.

Some recent research with monkeys shows that when they eat essentially no cholesterol, one of the major problem saturated fats in our diet—the 16-carbon palmitic acid—does not induce as high a blood cholesterol level as with typical human cholesterol intakes. This adds another reason to consider eating less cholesterol.

Only about 10% to 25% of people who eat a diet low in saturated fat find that eating less cholesterol lowers their LDL-cholesterol level even more. For some people, even eating six eggs a day for a month does not change their fasting blood cholesterol levels. Still, most authorities encourage us to eat less than 300 milligrams of cholesterol per day,[6] partly to keep blood cholesterol levels as low as possible right after eating. This recommendation for cholesterol intake is close to what most women eat, but most men eat about 100 to 150 milligrams more.

As we mentioned in this chapter, saturated fats from foods probably affect LDL-cholesterol levels by changing uptake of LDLs by the liver. When saturated fat intake is low, more LDLs are cleared from the bloodstream and pulled into the liver for excretion. This causes LDL-cholesterol levels to fall. Reduced lipoprotein synthesis by the liver is also suggested as a mechanism.[12]

A reasonable goal is to eat no more than 7% to 10% of kcalories as saturated fats.[6] Currently we eat about 14%. Limit intake wherever you can, and pay close attention to what you eat. Find substitutes for foods rich in animal fat, butter, coconut oil, palm oil, shortening, and other hydrogenated (solid) fats (see Tables 6-2 and 6-3 and Figure 6-8). Make it a habit to read labels—saturated fats are often hidden in foods.

another BITE

Many people think they need to eliminate beef from their diets to moderate their saturated fat intake. That is not necessary if they choose the right cuts of beef and cook it appropriately, especially trimming the fat off before cooking. If *loin* or *round* is part of its name, the cut is relatively low in fat.

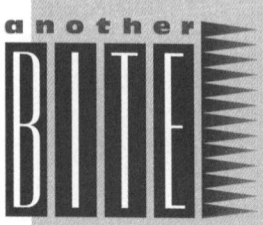

Eating right doesn't mean completely giving up favorite foods, even if they do contain higher-than-desirable levels of saturated fats. If you eat carefully most of the time, you can allow yourself latitude for occasional treats. If you indulge in a high saturated fat meal, it should be balanced by meals of lower-than-usual amounts of saturated fats.

To meet the AHA goal of no more than 300 milligrams of cholesterol per day, decrease the number of egg yolks to four or fewer per week; egg whites have no cholesterol. If you cook for yourself, it is easy to avoid egg yolks. In many recipes—such as those for pancakes, French toast, cookies, and cakes—you can substitute egg whites for whole eggs. Cholesterol-free egg substitutes are also available in the grocery store. These are usually egg whites colored yellow, to which a small amount of fat has been added to improve the flavor. Note again it is the animal foods we eat that supply most of the cholesterol (see Table 6-1).

If fat is trimmed before and after cooking, a 3- to 4-ounce serving of chicken, beef, or pork has surprisingly little cholesterol, roughly a third to half of that in an egg. A 10-ounce portion of meat can contain 260 milligrams of cholesterol, slightly more than in one egg. If meats have a reputation for being high in cholesterol, it is mainly because of an overgenerous portion size, rather than the amount of cholesterol in an ounce of meat—a mere 30 or so milligrams.

Monounsaturated and Polyunsaturated Fats

New observations show that monounsaturated fatty acids in the diet can lower cholesterol levels. Until recently, polyunsaturated fatty acids were recommended as a substitute for saturated fatty acids in the diet to lower LDL-cholesterol levels. However, recent studies show that either monounsaturated or polyunsaturated fatty acids can be used. In fact, monounsaturated fatty acids may be more beneficial, since these do not readily lead to oxidation of LDL.[18] Recall that oxidized LDL is probably most readily taken up by plaque in the arteries, much more so than LDL itself. The presence of much monounsaturated fat in an LDL particle reduces this process. However, aside from moving to Crete or some other Mediterranean country where olive oil is a major part of the diet, there is not much a typical American can do at this point to take advantage of this research on monosaturated fats. Foods rich in this type of fat are not widely available in the United States. For those of us who do much of our own cooking, using canola oil, canola oil blended with other vegetable oils, and olive oil on a regular basis is an option to consider for increasing monounsaturated fat intake.

Fiber and Reduced Heart Disease

Another recent development, as we discussed in Chapter 5, is the connection between eating lots of soluble fiber—found in oatmeal, oat bran, beans, vegetables, and fruits—and lower LDL-cholesterol levels.[1] Again, large amounts must be eaten to have a significant effect. Diets very high in overall fiber (50 to 60 grams per day), especially those that emphasize soluble fibers, work well.[8] Some laxatives with psyllium fiber are also good sources of soluble fiber.

Although it is possible to follow a diet high in soluble fiber, extensive dietary changes would be necessary for most of us. Researchers also now are cautioning people against eating more than 35 grams of dietary fiber a day, primarily because of the potential to bind minerals in the diet. So, consult a physician if you are considering a very high-fiber diet. We think it is easier and safer to cut down on saturated fat than to raise soluble fiber intake dramatically.

Diets high in soluble fiber probably work by binding cholesterol and bile in the small intestine and carrying them into the large intestine for elimination. Removing bile from the body forces the liver to pull more cholesterol out of the bloodstream to make new bile. This action resembles that of some medications that lower LDL-cholesterol levels. Other mechanisms have also been suggested to account for the effects of soluble fibers.[1]

You've probably heard a lot about oat bran. Manufacturers were quick to realize the marketing potential of a product that might lower blood cholesterol levels. But oat bran is not the "magic bullet" manufacturers would have us believe. A person would need to eat about a cup of it a day to reap the desired effect; an oat bran muffin alone won't do it.

Raising the HDL-Cholesterol Level

Although drinking a lot of alcohol can raise a certain type of HDL-cholesterol and likely reduce blood clotting,[20] too many other risks—such as liver and heart muscle damage and accidents—are associated with heavy drinking to justify using it for this purpose. Moderation in use, if used at all, is still the overriding health message.[21]

Physical activity is one method to employ in order to raise HDL-cholesterol levels at the same time. Exercising for at least 45 minutes four times a week can raise the HDL-cholesterol level by about 5 milligrams per 100 milliliters. Losing excess weight and avoiding smoking also help to maintain or raise HDL-cholesterol levels.[13]

In addition, eating regularly (three balanced meals daily), matching the amount of kcalories you eat with those you use up, and eating less total fat often help HDL-cholesterol levels by lowering triglyceride levels. Low triglyceride levels are often associated with high HDL-cholesterol levels. The reason for this is not clear. Nevertheless, the goal is to keep fasting triglyceride levels below 200 milligrams per 100 milliliters. Certain medications also act to lower triglyceride levels. When this happens, HDL-cholesterol levels also often increase.

It is unfortunate that raising an HDL-cholesterol level very much is usually difficult. Lowering LDL-cholesterol levels is usually much easier. And sometimes as LDL-cholesterol levels fall, so do HDL-cholesterol levels. This often the case with very low-fat diets. However, if LDL-cholesterol levels end up around 100 milligrams per 100 milliliters, the drop seen in HDL cholesterol usually is not much of a concern. Researchers note that people of rural Asia who eat low-fat diets generally have low LDL-cholesterol and HDL-cholesterol levels, but also show low risks for premature heart disease.

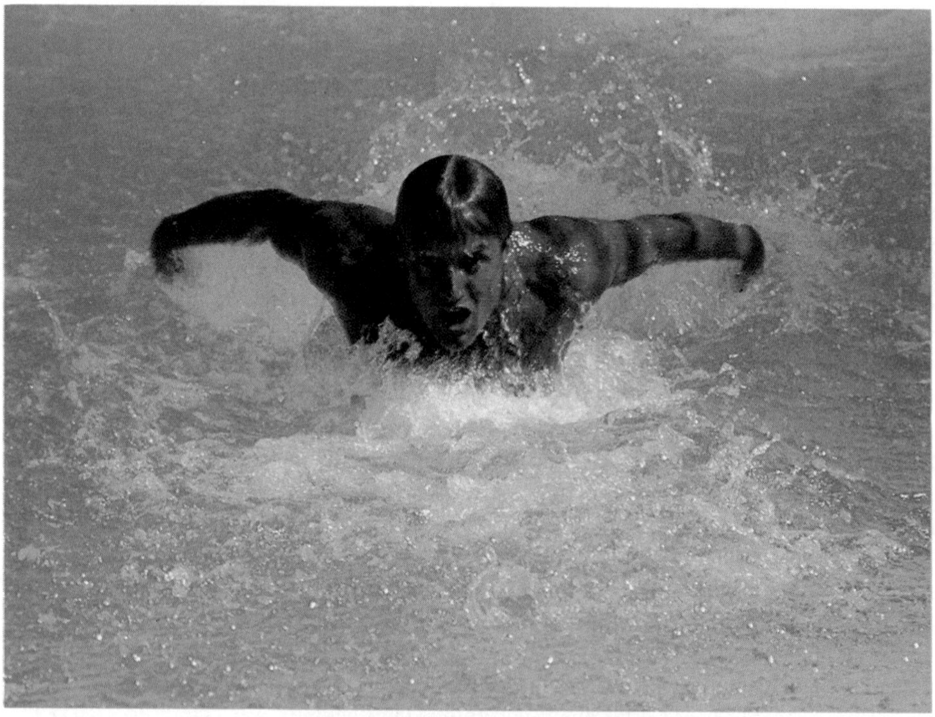

Exercise has been shown to moderately boost HDL-cholesterol levels in some studies.

Diet changes that work for one person may not work for another. Plan to make needed changes and then have your LDL-cholesterol and HDL-cholesterol levels rechecked in a month.

Medications to Lower Serum Cholesterol Levels

Medications are a last resort for treating high LDL-cholesterol or low HDL-cholesterol levels; most are expensive and all have side effects. But sometimes diet changes do not lower high LDL-cholesterol levels enough, especially in people with strong genetic tendencies toward that problem. Current medications to lower LDL-cholesterol levels work in one of two ways. One group inhibits the liver from synthesizing some lipoproteins.[6] These medications include nicotinic acid, lovastatin, probucol, and gemfibrozil. Nicotinic acid and gemfibrozil are also notable for raising HDL-cholesterol levels. The side effects of these medications, however, necessitate a physician's careful evaluation. The other group of medications includes cholestyramine and colestipol; they bind bile in the small intestine and lead to its elimination,[6] forcing the liver to synthesize new bile. The liver pulls LDL cholesterol out of the bloodstream to do this.

All these medications work better when a proper diet is followed; they do not substitute for diet changes.[6]

A controversy currently rages about using medications to combat heart disease. The question is not whether a link exists between a high LDL-cholesterol level or a high total cholesterol to HDL-cholesterol ratio and an increased risk of a heart attack. The question concerns the point at which a person's risk is sufficient to warrant medical treatment. Diet changes are also criticized for the same reason. Still, the sentiment of researchers in the heart disease arena is overwhelming—change the diet and use medications (if needed) to lower an elevated LDL-cholesterol level (ideally to around 100 milligrams per 100 milliliters or less) and to get the total cholesterol to HDL-cholesterol ratio below 4.5:1. This is especially important for people who already show evidence of heart disease. In addition, mortality from all causes, including that resulting from heart disease, is reduced when treatment is followed for a long enough time, approximately 10 years or more.[6] As we mentioned before, new research even shows that plaque regresses in arteries when LDL-cholesterol levels are aggressively lowered with (1) surgery on the intestinal tract, (2) diet plus medications, and (3) even just diet alone, although the diet used was very low in fat and contained essentially no cholesterol.[17]

What Should One Do?

To lower a high LDL-cholesterol level and provide an overall strategy to reduce heart disease risk:

Action	Rationale
• Eat less saturated fat and cholesterol.	This is the first method to employ and should be the overall major dietary focus.
• Exercise regularly.	This may protect and even boost HDL-cholesterol levels.
• Eat regularly spaced meals, not one or two large ones.	The frequency of meals helps determine fasting triglyceride levels. Studies show increasing meal frequency (from three to nine meals per day or so) can even help reduce LDL-cholesterol levels.[5]
• Lose weight to approximate or attain a desirable body weight.	This helps reduce serum triglyceride levels (if elevated), lowers high blood pressure, and can increase HDL-cholesterol levels.

Elevated blood triglycerides (greater than 200 milligrams per 100 milliliters of serum) mostly pose a heart health risk if linked to low HDL-cholesterol levels or diabetes. When serum triglycerides are 500 to 1000, another health risk arises—inflammation of the pancreas.[16]

Action	Rationale
• Eat more soluble fiber.	This binds cholesterol and bile in the small intestine to encourage their elimination via the large intestine, rather than absorption into the bloodstream; other factors may affect the drop in LDL-cholesterol levels.
• Eat less total fat.	This may help achieve the other goals, and it won't hurt anyone who follows the Food Guide Pyramid and meets energy needs.
• Eat fish on a weekly basis.	This tends to reduce blood clotting and so lessens the risk of developing a myocardial infarction. As we mentioned, regular use of aspirin for people at high risk of a myocardial infarction (under a physician's scrutiny) is promoted for the same reason.[13]
• Keep all types of coffee consumption to prudent levels—about two to three cups a day.	Studies show moderate increases in the LDL-cholesterol level with heavy consumption of some types of coffee, including decaffeinated brands (Figure 6-11).

A diet with 30% total kcalories from fat is an appropriate goal for children age 2 or older. Parents shouldn't go overboard with fat restrictions, because children need about 30% fat in their diet to grow properly. Experts do not advise parents to feed fat-restricted diets to children under the age of 2 (see Chapter 14).

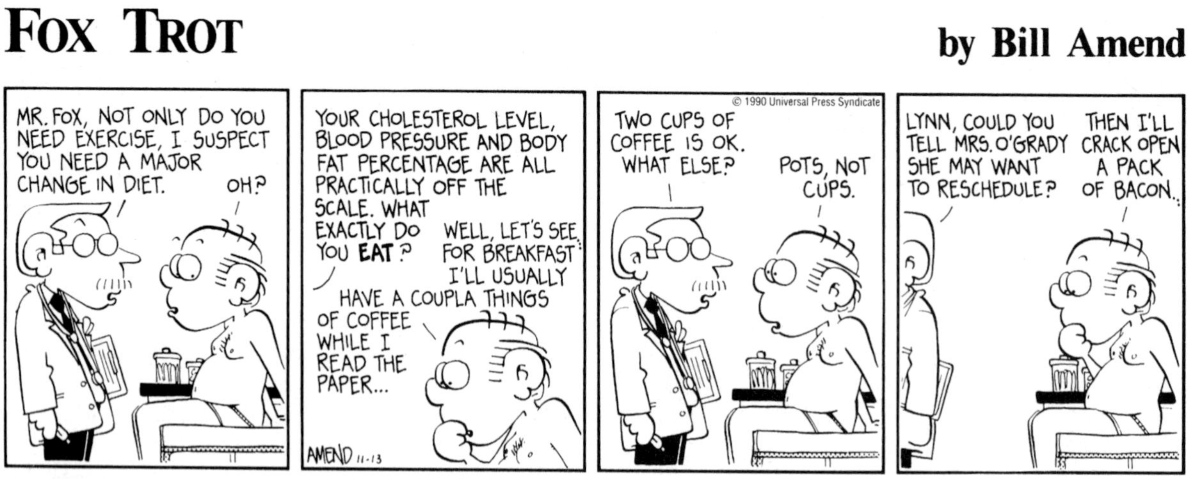

FIGURE 6-11
Fox Trot.

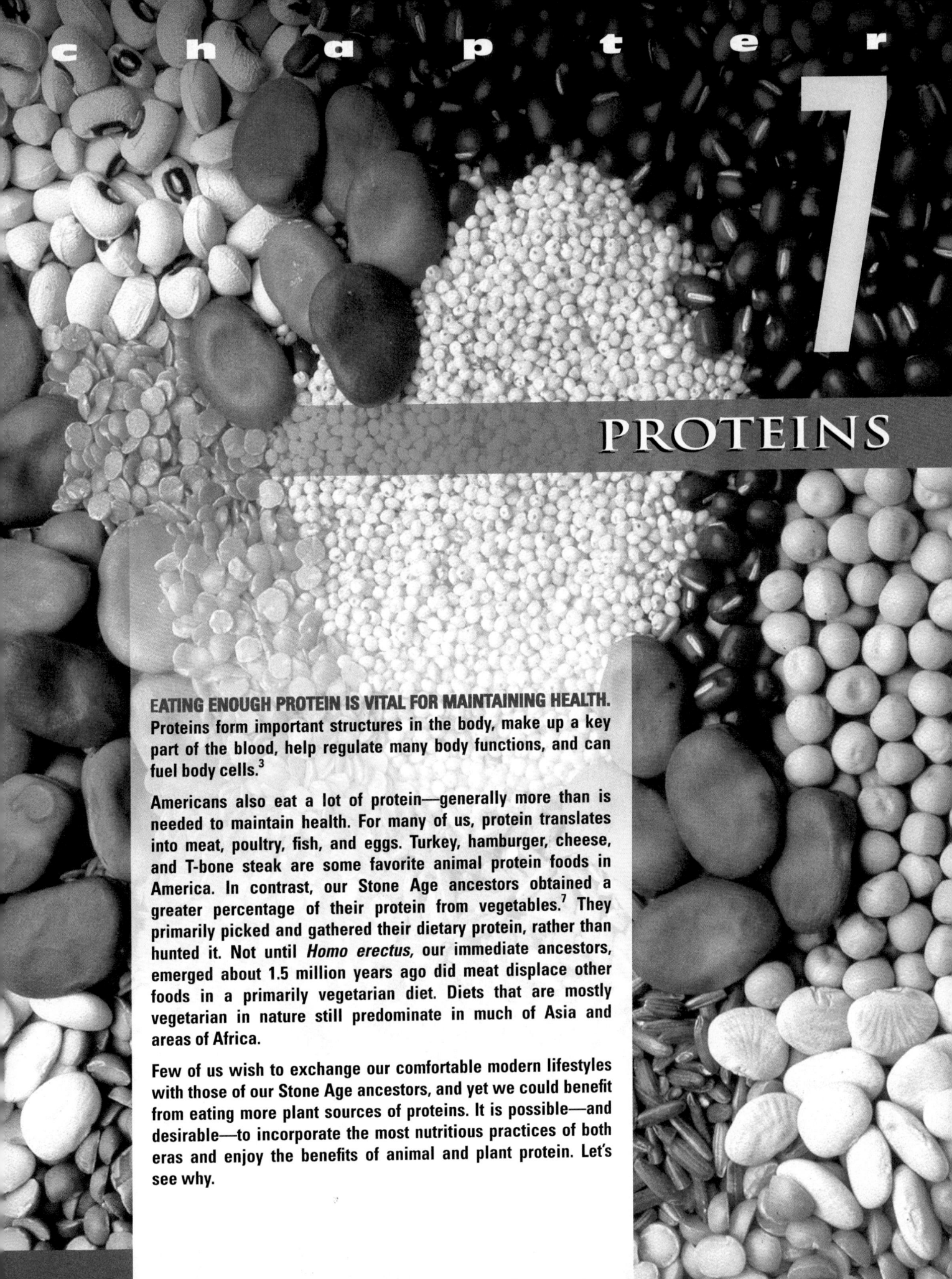

chapter 7

PROTEINS

EATING ENOUGH PROTEIN IS VITAL FOR MAINTAINING HEALTH. Proteins form important structures in the body, make up a key part of the blood, help regulate many body functions, and can fuel body cells.[3]

Americans also eat a lot of protein—generally more than is needed to maintain health. For many of us, protein translates into meat, poultry, fish, and eggs. Turkey, hamburger, cheese, and T-bone steak are some favorite animal protein foods in America. In contrast, our Stone Age ancestors obtained a greater percentage of their protein from vegetables.[7] They primarily picked and gathered their dietary protein, rather than hunted it. Not until *Homo erectus,* our immediate ancestors, emerged about 1.5 million years ago did meat displace other foods in a primarily vegetarian diet. Diets that are mostly vegetarian in nature still predominate in much of Asia and areas of Africa.

Few of us wish to exchange our comfortable modern lifestyles with those of our Stone Age ancestors, and yet we could benefit from eating more plant sources of proteins. It is possible—and desirable—to incorporate the most nutritious practices of both eras and enjoy the benefits of animal and plant protein. Let's see why.

ASSESS

TEST YOUR KNOWLEDGE

yourself

WHAT ARE YOUR PROTEIN PREFERENCES?

Below is a list of various foods that are good sources of protein. Rank your preferences among them from 1 to 11. A ranking of 1 means you like that particular food the best; a ranking of 11 means you like it the least. The letter before the food represents its origin: *(A)*, Animal source; *(P)*, Plant source.

(A) Eggs ________

(P) Beans (e.g., kidney, pinto, navy, or red beans; chick peas) ________

(A) Fish (e.g., salmon, halibut, swordfish, tuna) ________

(A) Beef ________

(P) Grains (e.g., products made from wheat, corn, oats) ________

(A) Poultry (e.g., chicken, turkey) ________

(A) Cheese ________

(P) Nuts and seeds (e.g., almonds, sunflower seeds) ________

(A) Milk and milk products (e.g., yogurt) ________

(A) Pork ________

(A) Processed meats (e.g., pepperoni, bologna, sausage) ________

As we just pointed out, today many rural societies consume more plant than animal sources of protein. This helps diets stay low in fat and cholesterol. In this respect plant proteins add a healthful aspect to many typical American diet patterns because their low saturated fat and cholesterol content helps prevent some chronic diseases. Where did the plant sources of protein rank in terms of your preference—high or low? Do you give excellent sources of plant proteins enough attention?

PROTEINS—A KEY LIFE FORCE

Thousands of various substances in the body are made of ***proteins.*** Aside from water, proteins form the major part of a lean human body, about 16% of body weight. Amino acids—the building blocks for these proteins—contain a special form of nitrogen. This form of nitrogen, essentially a carbon atom linked to a nitrogen atom, is generated by plants. By combining nitrogen from soil and air with carbon and other elements, plants form amino acids. They then form these amino acids into proteins.[20] We ordinarily must get the nitrogen we need by consuming it in the amino acid form found in proteins. This form of nitrogen is something carbohydrates and fats cannot provide us. Proteins thus are very important because they supply nitrogen in a form we can readily use—namely amino acids. Directly using simpler forms of nitrogen is, for the most part, impossible for humans.

Protein ■ *Food components made of amino acids. Proteins contain the form of nitrogen most easily used by the human body.*

Proteins provide a key life force. They are crucial to the minute-by-minute regulation and maintenance of our bodies. Vital body functions—such as blood clotting, fluid balance, hormone and enzyme production, visual processes, and cell repair—require specific proteins. Your body generates proteins in many configurations and sizes so that they can serve these greatly varied functions. All these proteins use the amino acids in protein foods we eat. When we eat proteins, we are really just eating sources of amino acids. Proteins can also supply energy for the body—notably, 4 kcalories per gram.

If you don't regularly eat enough protein, many of your metabolic processes slow down. This is because the body will not have amino acids available to build the proteins it needs. For example, the immune system no longer functions efficiently when it lacks key proteins, thereby increasing the risk of infections, disease, and eventually death.[15] Therefore proteins truly deserve their name, which means "to come first."

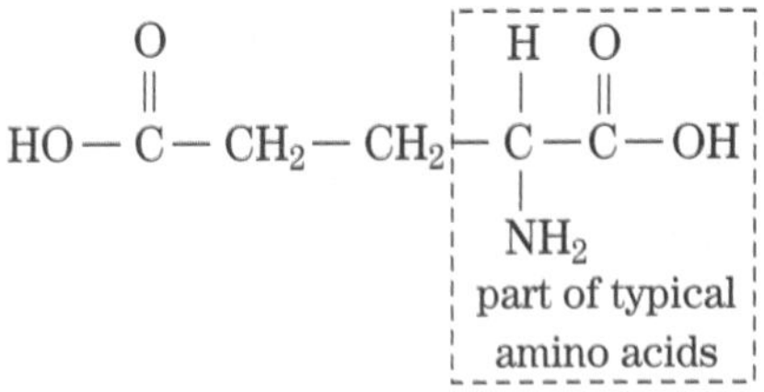

Glutamic Acid.

Amino Acids

Amino acids—again, the building blocks of proteins—are formed mostly of carbon, hydrogen, oxygen, and nitrogen. Note that the key part of an amino acid is nitrogen. The margin diagram shows what a typical amino acid looks like. In this case it is glutamic acid. The amino acids used to make protein show different chemical makeups, but all are slight variations of the amino acid pictured.

TABLE 7-1

Classification of Amino Acids

Essential (Indispensable) Amino Acids	Nonessential (Dispensable) Amino Acids
Histidine	Alanine
Isoleucine	Arginine*
Leucine	Asparagine
Lysine	Aspartic acid
Methionine	Cysteine†
Phenylalanine	(Cystine)
Threonine	Glutamic acid
Tryptophan	Glutamine
Valine	Glycine
	Proline
	Serine
	Tyrosine†

**Arginine may be an essential part of the diet for premature infants.*

†These amino acids are also classed as semiessential. This means they must be made from essential amino acids if not enough is eaten. When that occurs, the body's supply of certain essential amino acids is depleted. Researchers now suggest that some nonessential amino acids even assume an essential status when the body cannot readily generate them. This occurs during some illnesses. Glutamine assumes an essential status after intestinal surgery.

Since two *cysteine* molecules can bind together to form a new amino acid called *cystine,* the number of nonessential amino acids is twelve. If this form of cysteine is not counted as a unique form, then there are 11 nonessential amino acids. Hence we say there are "11 or so" nonessential amino acids.

Nonessential Amino Acids Amino acids that can be synthesized by a healthy body in sufficient amounts; there are about 11 nonessential amino acids. These are also termed dispensable amino acids.

Essential Amino Acids The amino acids that cannot be synthesized by humans in sufficient amounts and therefore must be included in the diet; there are nine essential amino acids. These are called indispensable amino acids.

Your body needs to use 20 or so different forms of amino acids to function. Although they are all important, 11 or so of these amino acids are considered ***nonessential*** (also called ***dispensable***)—it isn't essential to consume them because our bodies make them using other amino acids we consume. In other words, human cells can produce certain amino acids needed to make body proteins as long as the right ingredients are present—the key factor being nitrogen, which is already part of another amino acid (Table 7-1).[21]

The nine amino acids the body cannot make are known as ***essential*** (also called ***indispensable***)—they must be obtained from foods.[21] Both nonessential and essential amino acids are present in foods that contain protein. If you don't eat enough essential amino acids, your body first struggles to conserve what essential amino acids it can.[18] However, eventually your body progressively slows production of new proteins until at some point you will break protein down faster than you can make it. When that happens, as we noted, health deteriorates.

Therefore the two main functions of proteins in our diets are (1) to provide the nine essential amino acids needed by our bodies and (2) to provide either the nonessential amino acids our bodies use or nitrogen from an amino acid, which in turn can be used to make the nonessential amino acids. In a practical sense, a key consideration with respect to protein intake is quantity—getting enough protein via the diet to provide enough essential amino acids and enough of the necessary form of nitrogen for use in the production of any needed nonessential amino acid.[3]

PUTTING ESSENTIAL AND NONESSENTIAL AMINO ACIDS INTO PERSPECTIVE

As noted before, amino acids are the building blocks of proteins. Eating a balanced diet can supply us with both the essential and nonessential amino acids (or building blocks needed) to maintain good health. Let's now look at this concept of essential amino acids, especially in relationship to nonessential amino acids, in more detail.

Physiological Aspects

The disease *phenylketonuria (PKU)* illustrates the importance of one essential amino acid. We mentioned this disease in Chapter 5. Recall that the person with PKU has a limited ability to metabolize the essential amino acid phenylalanine. Normally the body converts much of this essential amino acid consumed in the diet into the nonessential amino acid tyrosine, because the body's need for phenylalanine is easily exceeded by our typical diets. However, enzymes in the liver of a person with PKU vary in their ability to do this conversion. Liver enzyme activity may be grossly or mildly insufficient in processing phenylalanine to tyrosine. When the enzymes cannot synthesize enough tyrosine, both amino acids must be derived from foods. In these cases, consumption of phenylalanine should also be controlled because it can rise to toxic levels in the body. Still, the key point here is that both amino acids now end up to be *essential* in terms of dietary needs. Both must be supplied by the diet.

Dietary Considerations

Animal and plant proteins can differ greatly in proportions of essential and nonessential amino acids. Animal proteins contain ample amounts of all nine essential amino acids. (Gelatin—made from the animal protein collagen—is an exception, because it loses one essential amino acid during processing and is also low in other essential amino acids.) Plant proteins don't match our needs for essential amino acids as precisely as do animal proteins. Many plant proteins, especially those found in grains, are low in one or more of the nine essential amino acids.[14]

As you might expect, human tissue composition resembles animal tissue more than it does plant tissue. The similarities enable us to use proteins from single animal sources more efficiently to support human growth and maintenance than we do those from single plant sources. Again, this is because animal proteins closely match the human pattern of essential amino acid composition. For this reason, animal proteins, except gelatin, are considered ***high-quality*** (also called ***complete) proteins***—they contain all the amino acids we need in sufficient amounts. Individual plant sources of proteins are in turn considered ***low-quality*** (also called ***incomplete) proteins*** because their amino acid patterns are quite different from ours. One single plant protein, such as corn alone, cannot easily support body growth and maintenance. To consume a sufficient amount of amino acids, very large quantities of plant proteins would need to be eaten because each protein lacks adequate amounts of one or more essential amino acids.[14]

If you ate only one food that contained low-quality protein—that is, one not containing an appropriate balance of all nine essential amino acids—you would need to eat much more, compared with eating animal protein sources, to obtain enough of the essential amino acids needed for protein synthesis. And, once any of the nine essential amino acids in the plant protein was used up, protein synthesis would stop. The remaining amino acids present would be used instead for energy or converted to fat and stored as such. Because the absence of just one essential amino acid halts protein synthesis, the process illustrates the *all or none principle:* either all essential amino acids are available or none is used. The essential amino acid in smallest supply in a food or diet becomes the limiting factor (called the ***limiting amino acid***), because it limits the amount of protein the body can synthesize.

For example, assume the letters of the alphabet represent the 20 or so different amino acids we eat. If A represents an essential amino acid, we would need four of these to spell the hypothetical protein ALABAMA. If the body had an L, B, and M, but only 3 As, the "synthesis" of ALABAMA would not be possible. "A" would then be seen as the limiting amino acid, because it is the limiting factor with respect to the body's ability to synthesize ALABAMA.

Most of us eat large enough amounts and such an assortment of protein-rich foods that we easily get a sufficient amount of all nine essential amino acids. That is, Americans eat a diet in which overall protein quality is high. This yields a high-quality (complete) protein diet. Even worldwide, most adults who eat sufficient protein get enough essential

High-Quality (Complete) Proteins ■ *Dietary proteins that contain ample amounts of all nine essential amino acids.*

Low-Quality (Incomplete) Proteins ■ *Dietary proteins that are low in or lack one or more essential amino acids.*

Limiting Amino Acid ■ *The essential amino acid in lowest concentration in a food in proportion to body needs.*

TABLE 7-2

Limiting Amino Acids in Plant Foods

Food	Limiting Amino Acids	Good Plant Source of the Limiting Amino Acids*	Traditional Uses Where the Proteins Complement Each Other
Soybeans and other legumes	Methionine	Grains, nuts and seeds	Tofu (soybean curd) and rice
Grains	Lysine, threonine	Legumes	Rice and red beans, lentil curry and rice
Nuts and seeds	Lysine	Legumes	Soybeans and ground sesame seeds (miso); peanuts, rice, and black-eyed peas; sunflower seeds; green peas
Vegetables	Methionine	Grains, nuts and seeds	Green beans and almonds
Corn	Tryptophan, lysine	Legumes	Corn tortillas and pinto beans

As you might suspect from the information in this table, the amino acids most likely to be low in a diet are lysine, methionine, threonine, and tryptophan. If a diet is low in an amino acid, we recommend finding a good food source to supply it. Forget about amino acid supplements—they can lead to problems, as we discuss later in this chapter.
**Animal products in the diet serve the same purpose, such as when fish is consumed with rice.*

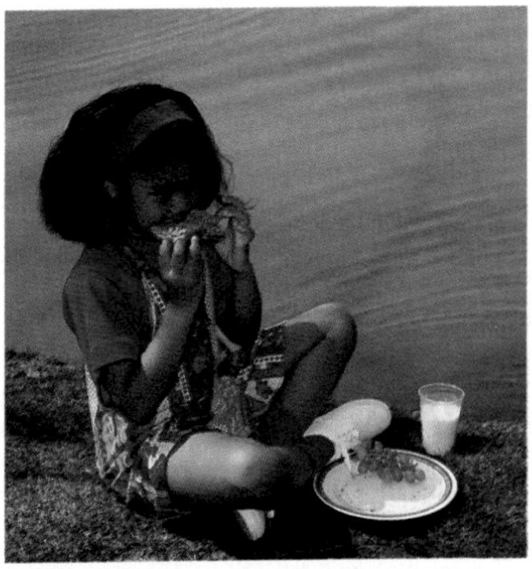

The various plant proteins present in a peanut butter sandwich combine to yield high-quality (complete) protein in the meal.

Complementary Proteins ■ *Two food protein sources that make up for each other's insufficient contribution of specific essential amino acids, so that together they yield a sufficient amount of all nine and so provide high-quality (complete) protein for the diet.*

amino acids to yield a high-quality protein diet, even if the various protein sources in the diet are of low quality. This is because the various low-quality protein sources eaten make up for deficiencies in essential amino acids that each individual protein presents. When two or more proteins combine to compensate for deficiencies in essential amino acid content in each individual protein, the proteins are called ***complementary proteins***[16] (Table 7-2). Mixed diets generally provide high-quality protein because a complementary protein pattern results. Therefore healthy adults should have little concern about balancing foods to yield the proteins needed to obtain all nine essential amino acids.

Infants and preschool children, on the other hand, need much of their protein supplied by essential amino acids.[14] Consequently, food for young children must be carefully planned to make sure enough proteins are present to yield high-quality protein intake. Being sure there are some animal products in the diet helps ensure this is the case. If an infant drinks enough human milk or commercial formula to meet its protein needs, essential amino acid needs are likewise met. Famine situations, where often only one type of grain is available, pose the major health risk for children with respect to protein intake.[18] Famines increase the probability that children will not consume enough of some essential amino acids, leading to poor health. We discuss this in more detail later in the chapter.

another BITE

To get the benefit of a high-quality protein diet, must a person consume all the essential amino acids from plant proteins within one meal? In other words, can plant proteins complement one another's amino acid deficiencies if eaten at separate meals? Research demonstrates that the essential amino acids can be effectively used in adults even when eaten at separate meals in a day.[8] This is primarily because none of the meals will completely lack one or more of the essential amino acids. In addition, some essential amino acids are available from short-term storage in cells, such as in skeletal muscle. However, researchers caution that closer attention needs to be paid to the diets of infants and young children. This is because at these ages the proportion of essential amino acids to total amino acids that must be in a diet is four times greater than for adults (10% for adults versus about 40% for infants and children).

CONCEPT CHECK

The human body uses 20 or so different forms of amino acids from foods. Because a healthy body can synthesize 11 or so of the different amino acids, it is not necessary to get them from foods—only the building blocks for protein synthesis are needed. Nine of the various amino acids used by the body must be consumed and so are termed essential (indispensable) amino acids. Foods that contain all 9 essential amino acids in about the proportions we need are considered high-quality (complete) protein foods. Those low in one or more essential amino acids are low-quality (incomplete) protein foods. When different low-quality protein foods are eaten together, the total intake of amino acids generally makes up for the the individual foods' shortcomings to yield a high-quality protein meal.

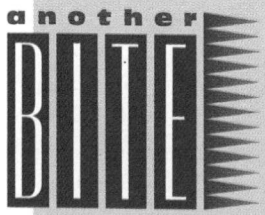

NUTRITION insight

AMINO ACID SUPPLEMENTS HAVE LED TO POISONOUS RESULTS

A rare blood disorder called eosinophilia-myalgia has been linked to the use of supplements of the amino acid tryptophan (L-tryptophan). A contaminant in the product may be the real culprit, but there is some suspicion that tryptophan shares some of the blame.[11] In addition to marked changes in the blood, the condition leads to severe muscle and joint pain, swelling in the limbs, skin rash, and occasionally fever, which can run as high as 105° F. Deaths have been linked to the supplement as well. Of people who exhibit symptoms of this rare blood disease, 99% had taken L-tryptophan. As of August 1, 1992, a total of 1511 cases of toxicity accompanying L-tryptophan use, including 38 deaths, had been reported to the Centers for Disease Control in Atlanta, Georgia. In response to this outbreak the U.S. government ordered a recall of all L-tryptophan supplements.

Though this essential amino acid is normally supplied by protein in the diet, people were using L-tryptophan supplements for a variety of problems, including insomnia, premenstrual syndrome, depression, and attention deficiencies in children. FDA had not approved it for these problems. Tryptophan also is found in many nonprescription and prescription nutritional products used in hospitals. However, these products pose no risk; it is the supplemental form that is linked to problems.[10]

The main point here concerns more than just the risk associated with taking tryptophan supplements. Amino acid supplements are not necessary, because we can easily meet our protein needs through diet. This holds true for all of us, including athletes (see Chapter 11). There are no significant amounts of free amino acids in our food. Nor is there any dietary need for, or unique dietary value from eating free amino acids.[10] The body is designed to handle whole proteins as a dietary source of amino acids. As discussed later in this chapter, the body breaks proteins into manageable pieces, then splits them a few at a time into amino acids, simultaneously absorbing amino acids into the bloodstream. When individual amino acid supplements are taken, they can overwhelm the absorptive mechanism, triggering amino acid imbalances in the body. These imbalances occur because groups of chemically similar amino acids compete for absorption into the bloodstream. An excess of one then can hamper other amino acids from being absorbed.[4]

Every amino acid taken in excess can be harmful. In some cases, excess amounts do not vary much above a normal daily intake. Stick to whole foods as your source for amino acids.

PROTEIN DIGESTION AND ABSORPTION—SUPPLYING AMINO ACIDS TO BODY CELLS

We noted in Chapter 4 that digestion of protein begins in the stomach (Figure 7-1). Certain cells of the stomach secrete pepsin, a major enzyme used for this digestion. Pepsin attacks all proteins and breaks them down into shorter amino acid units, called *peptones.* Pepsin does not completely separate the protein into amino acids, because it can break only a few of the chemical bonds found in protein molecules. Thus it has limited activity. The release of pepsin is controlled by the hormone gastrin. Just thinking about food or chewing food stimulates gastrin release. Gastrin also stimulates other cells in the stomach to produce acid. This acid, in turn, activates pepsin and enhances protein digestion. The partially digested proteins now move with the rest of the nutrients in the foods eaten from the stomach into the small intestine.

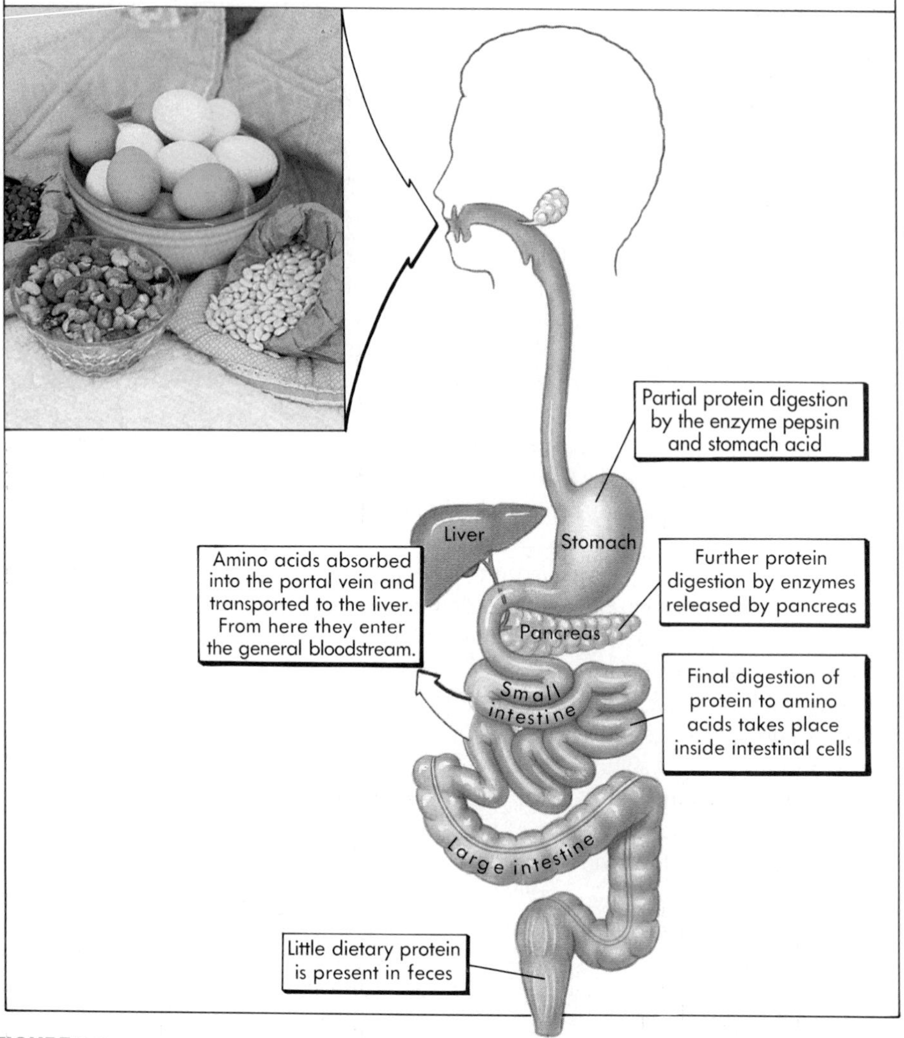

FIGURE 7-1

Protein digestion and absorption. Protein digestion begins in the stomach and ends in the absorptive cells of the small intestine, where the last peptides are broken down into single amino acids. Stomach acid and enzymes also contribute to protein digestion. Absorption from the intestinal lumen into the absorptive cells then requires energy input.

Once in the small intestine, the peptones (and any fats accompanying the incoming peptones produced from a meal) trigger the release of the hormone cholecystokinin (CCK) from the walls of the small intestine. CCK, in turn, travels through the bloodstream to its target organs—the pancreas and the gallbladder. Recall that CCK causes release of bile from the gallbladder and release of enzyme-rich and bicarbonate-rich juice from the pancreas.

The multitude of digestive enzymes released from the pancreas includes the protein-breaking enzymes trypsin and chymotrypsin. Together these and other digestive enzymes divide the peptones into short peptides and amino acids. The eventual digestion of all the peptides into amino acids then occurs inside the absorptive cells of the small intestine. These cells absorb amino acids and peptides through an active process that requires energy input.[4] Few whole proteins are absorbed. The amino acids travel to the liver via the portal vein. There they are either combined into protein, converted into glucose or fat, used for energy needs, or released into the bloodstream.

CONCEPT CHECK

Protein digestion occurs first in the stomach, producing breakdown products called peptones. In the small intestine, peptones separate into small peptides and amino acids. The peptides and amino acids then are absorbed into the absorptive cells by an active process that requires energy input, and are then broken down into single amino acid forms. These enter the portal vein en route to the liver.

PROTEINS—MANY AMINO ACIDS JOINED TOGETHER

Amino acids are joined by chemical links—technically called ***peptide bonds***—to form proteins. These links are difficult to break. However, acids, enzymes, and other agents are able to break these links, as occurs during digestion.

Peptide Bond
A chemical bond formed to link amino acids in a protein.

Protein Organization

By linking various combinations of the 20 or so types of amino acids, the body synthesizes thousands of different proteins. This is the same as using the alphabet to create a dictionary full of words. Amino acids are joined together in specific sequences to form distinct proteins, just as various sequences of letters form specific words. The sequential order of the amino acids determines a protein's configuration. The DNA in a cell directs this ordering during protein synthesis, as we noted in Chapter 4. The key point is that only correctly positioned amino acids can interact and fold properly to form the intended shape for the protein. The resulting unique three-dimensional form dictates the function of each particular protein. If it lacks the appropriate configuration, a protein cannot function.[20]

Sickle cell disease (also called ***sickle cell anemia***) illustrates what happens when amino acids are out of order on a protein. African-Americans are especially prone to this genetic disease. It originates in defective production of the protein chains of hemoglobin, a compound found in red blood cells. In two of its four protein chains, a slight error in the amino acid strings occurs. This small error produces a profound change in hemoglobin structure: it can no longer form the shape needed to carry oxygen efficiently inside the red blood cell. Instead of forming normal circular disks, the red blood cells collapse into cres-

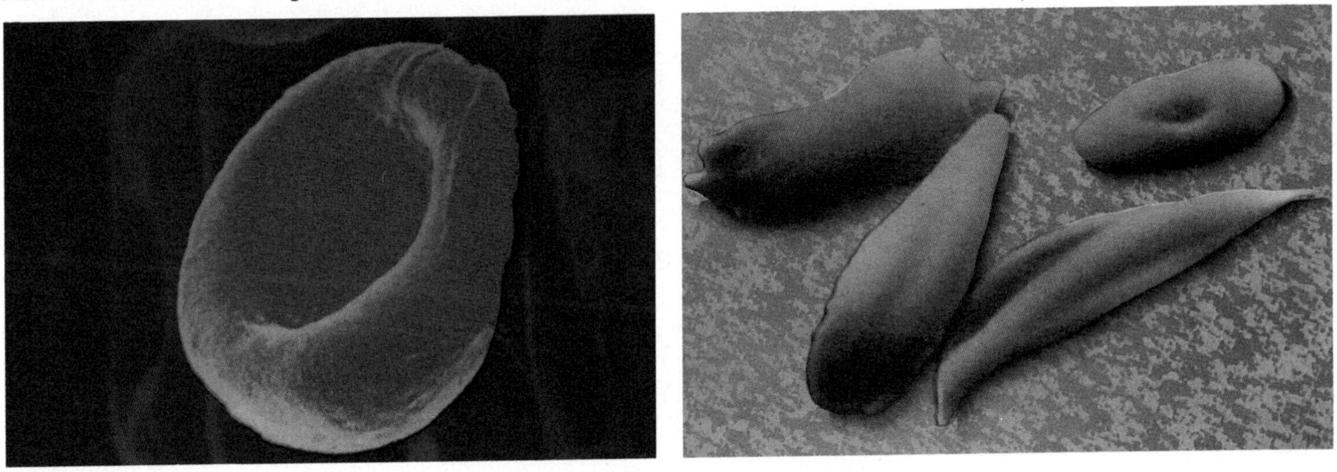

FIGURE 7-2
Sickle-cell disease from the perspective of the red blood cell. **A,** *Normal red blood cell.* **B,** *Blood from a patient with sickle-cell disease. Note the abnormal crescent (sicklelike) shape of the red blood cell near the center.*

cent shapes (Figure 7-2). Health deteriorates, and eventually episodes of severe bone and joint pain, abdominal pain, headache, convulsions, and paralysis may occur.

These life-threatening symptoms are caused by a minute, but critical, error in the hemoglobin amino acid order. Why does this error happen? It results from a defect in a person's genetic blueprint, DNA, which is inherited through one's parents. A defect in the DNA can dictate that a wrong amino acid will be built into the sequence of body proteins.[20] Many diseases stem from incorrect DNA information passed on in the body. Cancer, which we discuss in Chapter 8, is an example.

Denaturation of Proteins

Denature *Alteration of a protein's three-dimensional structure, usually because of treatment by heat, enzymes, acid or alkaline solutions, or agitation.*

Treatment with acid or alkaline substances, heat, or agitation can severely alter a protein's structure, leaving it unfolded and in a ***denatured*** state. The protein can no longer perform its function. For example, once the bacteria in yogurt have synthesized enough acid and enzymes to precipitate some of the milk protein, the product solidifies irreversibly.

Unraveling a protein's shape often destroys its normal functioning. That characteristic is useful for some body processes, such as digestion. As we just covered, when foods reach the stomach, stomach acid is secreted. This denatures some bacteria, plant hormones, many active enzymes, and other forms of proteins in foods. The heat produced during cooking likewise denatures their proteins. Both of these processes render foods safer to eat. Digestion also is enhanced because the unraveling increases exposure of the

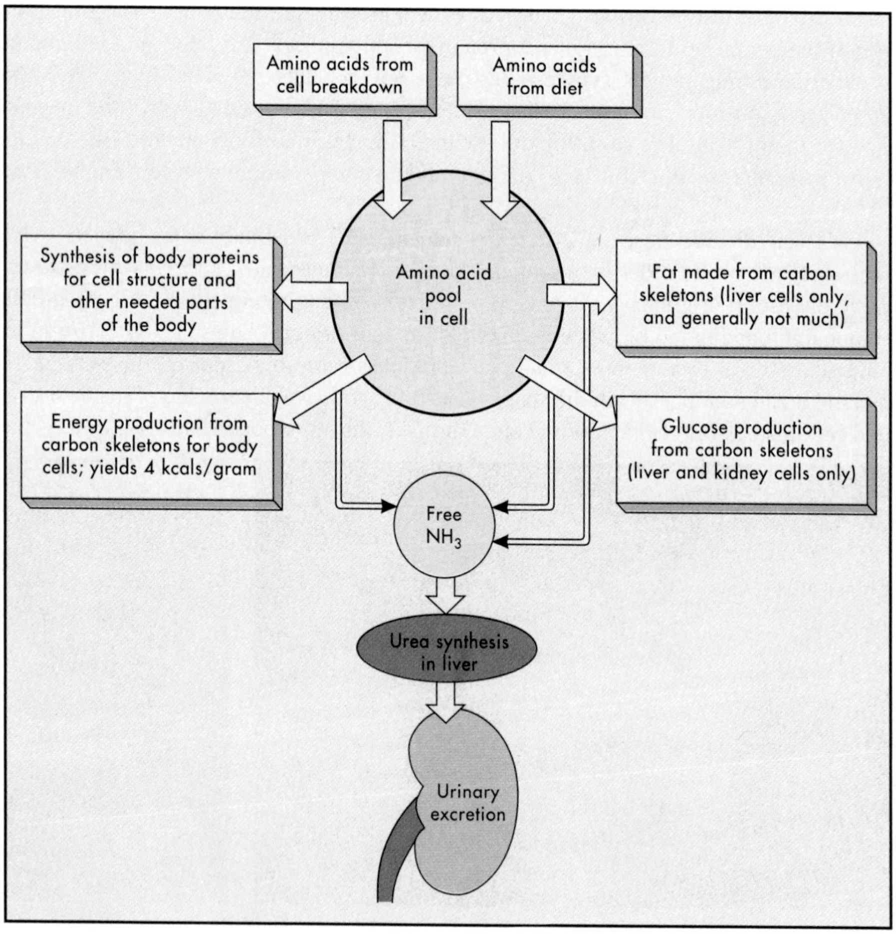

FIGURE 7-3

Amino acid metabolism. This can yield body proteins and a variety of other possible products—from fat and glucose to urea.

food to digestive enzymes. Denaturing proteins in some foods can also reduce their tendencies to cause allergic reactions.

Recall that we need proteins in the diet to supply essential amino acids—not the active proteins themselves. We dismantle the proteins we get from foods and use the amino acids to assemble proteins we need.[20]

FUNCTIONS OF PROTEINS

As we have said, proteins function in a multitude of key roles in human metabolism and in the formation of body structures. We rely on foods to supply the amino acids needed to form these proteins. Note however that only when we also eat enough carbohydrate and fat can food proteins be used most efficiently. If we don't consume enough kcalories to meet energy needs, some amino acids from proteins are broken down to produce needed energy, rather than used to make needed body proteins.[21]

Producing Vital Body Constituents

Every cell contains protein. Muscles, connective tissue, blood-clotting factors, blood-transport proteins, lipoproteins, enzymes, immune bodies, some hormones, visual pigments, and the support structure inside bones are mainly made of protein. Measurements of the amounts of certain body proteins, particularly some of those in the blood, are used as indicators of health or disease. Excess protein in the diet doesn't enhance the synthesis of body components, but eating too little can impede it.

Most vital body proteins are in a constant state of breakdown, rebuilding, and repair, especially in the bone marrow and the intestine. The GI tract lining is constantly ***sloughed*** off. The digestive tract treats sloughed cells just like food particles and absorbs the amino acids released during their digestion. In fact, most protein breakdown products—amino acids—released throughout the body can be recycled and are added to the pool of amino acids available for future protein synthesis (Figure 7-3).[20]

Some protein breakdown products, however, are lost rather than recycled. If a person habitually doesn't eat enough protein to replace this loss, the protein rebuilding and repairing process slows. Thus for body growth and maintenance, amino acids must be supplied constantly from food. Otherwise, skeletal muscles, heart, liver, blood proteins, and other organs decrease in size or amount. Only the brain resists breakdown. To ensure good health a person must eat enough protein.[3]

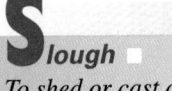

Slough
To shed or cast off.

Edema
The buildup of excess fluid in the spaces surrounding body cells.

Buffer
Compounds that cause a solution to resist changes in acid-base balance.

Maintaining Fluid Balance

Blood proteins—albumins and globulins—help maintain body fluid balance. Blood pressure in the arteries forces blood through blood vessels into capillary beds. The blood fluid then enters from the capillary beds into the spaces between nearby cells to provide nutrients to those cells (Figure 7-4). Proteins in the bloodstream are too large to move out of the capillary beds into the tissues. The presence of these proteins in the capillary beds attracts the fluid back to them, partially counteracting the force of blood pressure. This is especially true of the areas of the capillary beds right next to their venous connections (see Figure 4-2 for a close-up view of a capillary bed).

Unless enough protein is eaten, the level of proteins eventually decreases in the bloodstream. Excessive fluid then builds up in the tissues because the counteracting force produced by the smaller amount of blood proteins is too weak to pull much of the fluid back from the tissues into the bloodstream. As fluids pool in the tissues, the tissues swell. Clinical ***edema*** results.[15] Because edema sometimes leads to serious medical problems, the cause must be identified. In diagnosing the cause, an important step is to measure the level of blood proteins.

Contributing to Acid-Base Balance

Proteins help regulate the degree of acidity—the acid-base balance—in the blood. Special proteins located in cell membranes act to pump chemical ions in and out of cells. The pumping action, among other things, works to keep the blood slightly alkaline. ***Buffers***—

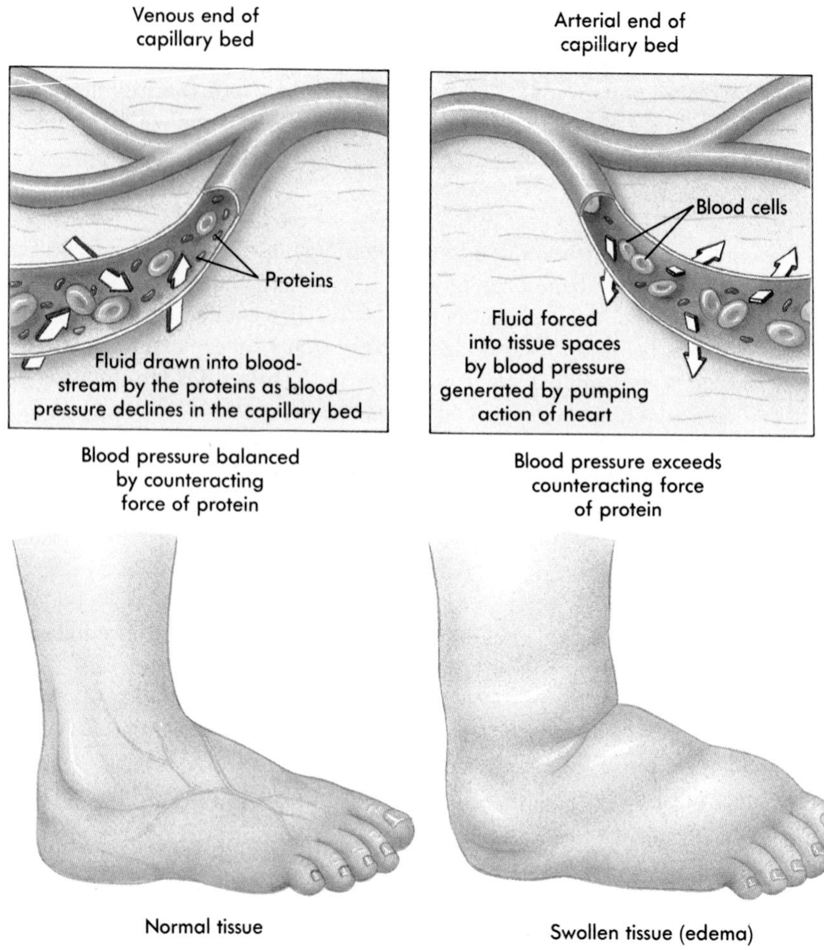

FIGURE 7-4
Blood proteins are important for maintaining the body's fluid balance. Without sufficient protein in the bloodstream, edema develops.

compounds that maintain acid-base conditions within a narrow range—are another means used to regulate acid-base balance in the blood. Some blood proteins are especially good buffers for the body.[20]

Forming Hormones and Enzymes

Protein is required for the synthesis of many hormones—our internal body messengers. Some hormones, such as the thyroid hormones, are made from only one or a few amino acids. Insulin, on the other hand, is composed of 48 amino acids. These and other hormones classified as proteins perform important regulatory functions in the body, such as controlling the metabolic rate and amount of glucose taken up from the bloodstream.

another BITE

Some hormone medicines from the protein class, such as the insulin used to treat some cases of diabetes, must be injected. If taken orally, insulin would be destroyed: the stomach and small intestine would digest the hormone, dismantling it into amino acids.

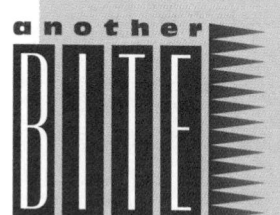

Enzymes are proteins.[20] Recall that enzymes are compounds that speed chemical reactions (see Chapter 4). Occasionally a cell lacks the correct genetic information to make needed enzymes. An infant, for example, who has the disease ***galactosemia*** cannot make an enzyme needed to metabolize the single sugar galactose. If the infant is not put on a galactose-free diet soon after birth—which in practical terms means no cow's milk, human milk, liver, and certain other foods—its growth and mental development will be depressed. A special infant formula must be used. The galactose-free diet is then continued, ideally throughout life. This example again demonstrates the crucial roles that enzymes, and thus proteins, play in cell function.[20]

Galactosemia *A disease characterized by the buildup of the single sugar galactose in the bloodstream, because of the inability of liver to metabolize it. If present at birth and left untreated, it results in severe mental and growth retardation.*

Antibody *Blood proteins that inactivate foreign proteins found in the body. This helps to prevent infections.*

Contributing to the Immune Function

Proteins make up key parts of the cells used by the immune system. Protein ***antibodies*** are produced by one type of immune cell. In an important immune response, the antibodies bind to foreign proteins in the body. Without enough protein from the diet, the immune system will eventually not produce enough of the cells and other tools needed to function properly and resist disease.[15] However, eating more protein than is necessary doesn't boost immune function.

Forming Glucose

In Chapter 5 we noted that the body must maintain a fairly constant level of glucose in the bloodstream to supply energy for red blood cells and nervous tissue. At rest, the brain uses about 35% of the body's energy requirements, and it gets most of that energy from glucose. If you don't eat enough carbohydrate to supply the glucose, your liver (and kidneys to a lesser extent) will be forced to make glucose from amino acids (see Figure 7-3). Many types of amino acids can be used for this purpose.[20]

Making some glucose from amino acids occurs normally. For example, when you skip breakfast and haven't eaten since 7 PM the preceding evening, glucose must be manufactured. Taken to an extreme, however, a constant need to convert amino acids into glucose, such as occurs in starvation, wastes much muscle tissue. This in turn reduces health.

Providing Energy

Proteins supply about 2% to 5% of the energy the body uses (see Chapter 11 for information about the use of amino acids for energy during exercise). Most cells primarily use carbohydrates and fats for energy. Proteins and carbohydrates contain the same amount of usable energy, 4 kcalories per gram. However, proteins are a very costly source of energy, considering the amount of metabolism and processing the liver and kidneys must perform to use this energy source. The monetary cost of protein-rich foods is also a consideration.

CONCEPT CHECK

Amino acids are linked together in specific sequences to form distinct proteins. The amino acid order within a protein determines its ultimate structure. Destroying the shape or structure of a protein denatures it. Acid and alkaline conditions used in the body's digestive processes, heat, and other factors can denature proteins so that they lose their biological activity. Vital body constituents—such as muscle, connective tissue, blood transport proteins, enzymes, hormones, buffers, and immune factors—are mainly proteins. Proteins can also provide fuel for the body and be used for glucose production.

The more precise terminology is used to refer to nitrogen balance rather than protein balance. Recall that proteins supply us with the form of nitrogen we use.

THE RECOMMENDED DIETARY ALLOWANCE FOR PROTEIN

How much protein (actually, amino acids) do we need to eat each day? People who aren't growing need to eat only enough protein to match whatever they lose daily from urine, feces, skin, hair, nails, and so on. In short, people need to balance protein intake with output. This maintains a state of protein equilibrium (Figure 7-5).

When a body is either growing or recovering from an illness, it needs a positive protein balance to supply raw materials needed to build new tissues. To achieve this, a person must eat more protein daily than he or she loses. This positive balance also requires an appropriate hormonal state. The hormones insulin, growth hormone, and testosterone all stimulate positive protein balance. Merely eating more protein does not guarantee a positive balance; building extra body tissues requires the right hormonal condition as well. Weight training also works by itself to enhance muscle mass.

Frequently during semistarvation or illness, the body loses much more protein than is replaced. The body then falls into a negative protein balance.[15]

For healthy people the amount of dietary protein needed to maintain nitrogen equilibrium (where intake equals output) can be determined by increasing protein intake until it just equals losses. Energy needs must be met so that amino acids are not diverted for energy use. Any protein intake above equilibrium also maintains a balance. But to estimate the requirement, we need to determine the least amount of protein intake necessary to balance intake with output.[3]

Edward Smith, a British physician, studied energy and protein metabolism and in 1862 concluded that a physically active man would need 80 grams of protein daily. During the next 40 years, other estimates of protein needs, based on records of protein amounts consumed by healthy working men, ranged up to 150 grams per day. A controversy developed in the early 1900s after Russell Chittenden, an American chemist, concluded from studies on himself, his colleagues, and students at Yale that only 35 to 45 grams of protein daily was required for healthy adults.

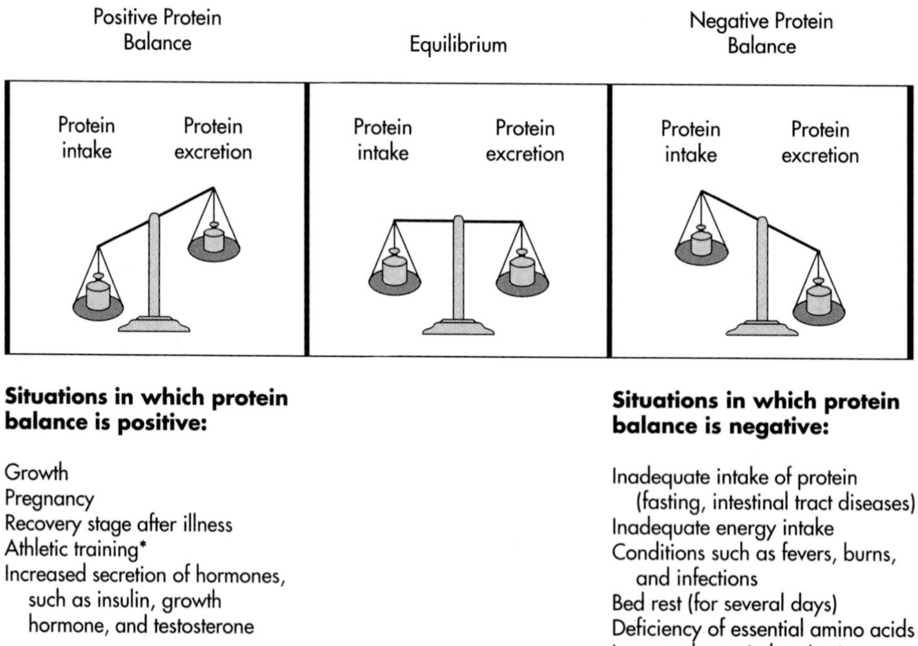

Situations in which protein balance is positive:

Growth
Pregnancy
Recovery stage after illness
Athletic training*
Increased secretion of hormones, such as insulin, growth hormone, and testosterone

Situations in which protein balance is negative:

Inadequate intake of protein (fasting, intestinal tract diseases)
Inadequate energy intake
Conditions such as fevers, burns, and infections
Bed rest (for several days)
Deficiency of essential amino acids
Increased protein loss (as in some kidney diseases)
Increased secretion of certain hormones, such as thyroid hormone and cortisol

*Only when additional lean body mass is being gained. Nevertheless, the athlete is probably already eating enough protein to support this extra protein synthesis: protein supplements are not needed.

FIGURE 7-5
Protein balance in practical terms.

Today the best estimate for the amount of protein required for nearly all adults is 0.8 grams of protein per kilogram of desirable body weight. This amount at least doubles during infancy. (We will discuss specific values for infants and children in Chapter 14 and the concept of desirable weight in Chapter 10). Desirable weight is used as a baseline because excess fat storage doesn't contribute much to protein needs. This recommended amount works out to about 56 grams of protein daily for a 70-kilogram (154-pound) man and about 44 grams of protein daily for a 55-kilogram (120-pound) woman. Approximate protein needs based on the 1989 RDA publication are listed in the inside cover of this textbook. To estimate a recommendation for you, just substitute your body weight in kilograms in the formula listed below. Using either method, it is easy to eat the amount of protein suggested each day to meet body needs (Table 7-3). American men typically consume about 90 grams of protein daily, whereas women typically consume 70 grams daily.

Canadian recommendations for protein are 0.82 grams per kilogram of body weight for adult men, and 0.74 grams per kilogram of body weight for adult women.

0.8 *grams protein per* kg body weight × **70 kilograms body weight** = **56 grams of protein needed**

Recall that an RDA is an allowance, not a requirement. Some people need less than that amount of protein. Yet most of us get much more, because we like many high-protein foods and can afford to buy them. Excess protein eaten cannot be stored as such, so

TABLE 7-3

The Protein Content of a 1200-Kcalorie and a 2400-Kcalorie Diet

This table illustrates how few kcalories can be consumed while still meeting the RDA for protein. It also shows how much protein we eat when we consume typical kcalorie intakes.

1200 Kcalorie Diet	Grams of Protein	2400 Kcalorie Diet	Grams of Protein
Breakfast			
Nonfat milk, 1 cup	8	2% milk, 1 cup	8
Cheerios, ¾ cup	3	Cheerios, ¾ cup	3
Orange	—	Eggs, soft-boiled, 2	12
		Orange	—
Lunch			
Whole-wheat bread, 2 slices	7	Whole-wheat bread, 2 slices	7
Chicken breast, 2 oz	18	Chicken breast, 2 oz	18
Mayonnaise, 1 tsp	—	Provolone cheese, 2 oz	13
Carrot sticks, 1 cup	1	Mayonnaise, 1 tsp	—
Fig	0.5	Oatmeal raisin cookies, 2	2
Diet soda	—	Figs, 2	1
		Diet soda	—
Dinner			
Beef tenderloin, 2 oz	18	Beef tenderloin, 4 oz	36
Spinach pasta, 1 cup with garlic butter, 1 tsp	7	Spinach pasta, 1 cup with garlic butter, 1 tsp	7
Zucchini, ½ cup, sauteed in oil, 1 tsp	0.5	Zucchini, ½ cup, sauteed in oil, 1 tsp	0.5
Nonfat milk, 1 cup	8	2% milk, 1 cup	8
Bagel, toasted, ½	4	Bagel, toasted	7
Margarine, 1 tsp	—	Margarine, 2 tsp	—
TOTAL	75 grams		122 grams

NUTRITION insight

DO YOU NEED TO REDISCOVER LEGUMES?

Legumes are a plant family with seed pods that contain one row of seeds: garden peas; green, lima, pinto, and garbanzo beans; lentils; and soybeans. Dried varieties of the mature seeds—what we know as beans—yield an impressive contribution to the protein, vitamin, mineral, and dietary fiber content of a meal.[16]

Many people dismiss beans from their diets. This unfortunate oversight may be rooted in the Depression of the 1930s when people could afford little else. Beans are such a versatile food. They can anchor or blend into soups, salads, casseroles, sandwich spreads, and cracker dips. They can also be added in small quantities wherever extra body, texture, and/or nutritional value is desired. Incorporating them into your week's menu can add variety and new flavors (Table 7-4).

Most legumes, except lentils, need to be softened before cooking. Soak them overnight, or boil them uncovered for 2 minutes, remove from heat, cover, and let stand 1 hour. Dried beans double or triple in volume as they cook. Because legumes tend to soak up flavors during the cooking process, you can incorporate delicate flavors from combinations of herbs, spices, and broths.

TABLE 7-4

Get to Know the Legumes

Type	Color	Use
Black beans	Black	Baked, soups, stews
Black-eyed peas	White with a black spot	Casseroles
Garbanzo beans (chickpeas)	Brown	Dips, casseroles, salads, soups, stews
Great northern beans	White	Baked, casseroles, chowder, soups, stews
Kidney beans	Red	Casseroles, chili, salads, soups
Lentils	Brown or green	Casseroles, salads, soups
Lima beans	White	Casseroles, soups
Navy beans	White	Baked, soups
Pinto beans	Pink	Baked, casseroles, soups
Red beans	Red	Casseroles, chili
Soybeans	Tan	Casseroles, salads
Split peas	Green or yellow	Soups

From Neiman DC, Butterworth DE, Neiman CN: Nutrition, *1990, William C Brown.*

When you initially add legumes to your diet, they may cause intestinal gas. Split peas, limas, and lentils are less likely to do so than the others, so start with them. Take small servings at first, and give your GI tract a few weeks to adjust. Many people have no trouble with legumes, but it's best to be cautious.

Like all foods, though, legumes do not offer every nutrient, and so they do not make a complete diet by themselves. They contain no vitamin A, C, or B-12, they are low in iron, and their balance of amino acids needs to be improved by eating grains and other vegetables with them. Many traditional ethnic dishes combine legumes with grains and vegetables to yield a high-quality protein balance: lentil curry on rice, pinto beans and corn tortillas, tofu (soybean curd) and rice, and corn and lima beans (succotash).[16] Try these combinations or create your own.

As you prepare foods or order them in a restaurant, look for beans—salad bars usually provide a few choices. Black bean and other bean soups, baked beans, chili, red beans and rice, and soy burgers are other possibilities. Regularly consuming vegetable proteins, as noted in Chapter 2, can add substantial amounts of nutrients to a diet. And as discussed in Chapter 6, the soluble fiber in them can help lower your blood cholesterol level as well, if that is necessary.

An enzyme preparation called Beano is also available to ease gas symptoms from legume consumption. Taken right before a meal, it helps digest the indigestible carbohydrates in beans (and vegetables in general) that contribute to intestinal gas.

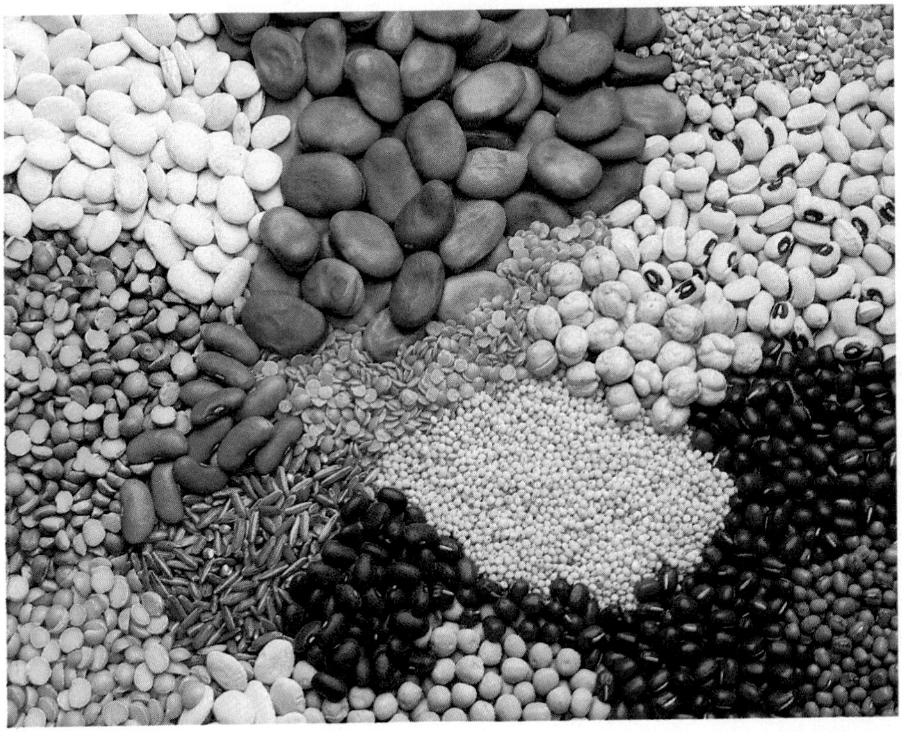

Legumes—another protein source that can meet a body's need. An added bonus is that many other nutrients are also present in legumes.

it is turned into glucose or fat and then either stored or burned for energy needs (see Figure 7-3).[20]

Pregnancy raises protein needs by about 6 grams daily averaged over the 9 months. However, mental stress, physical labor, and routine sports activity do not demand any extra protein allowance. To support either substantial gains in muscle tissue from high-level sports activities or a large muscle mass acquired previously, increasing intake to about 1.3 to 1.5 grams per kilogram of body weight might be considered.[13] However, many Americans eat that much protein already. Adding extra dietary protein to normal adult diets, even for athletes, is usually not needed. In addition, there is no reason for athletes to take either protein or individual amino acid supplements—enough is available in whole foods (Table 7-3).[10]

Instead of protein, it is most important for athletes to emphasize carbohydrate and fluid in the diet (see Chapter 11).

Does Eating a Mainly High-Protein Diet Harm You?

The question is often asked whether the high protein intake of adults in America is harmful. (Getting too much protein can be very harmful to infants. We discuss this in Chapter 14.) The extra vitamin B-6, iron, and zinc that accompany protein foods are often beneficial, but the extra fat—especially saturated fat—found in many high-protein animal foods is not. Research in the 1970s suggested that a high-protein diet might cause greater calcium loss in the urine. This worried researchers because they thought that protein caused calcium to leach out of the bones, setting the stage for osteoporosis, a severe bone disease (see Chapter 9). However, follow-up studies show that if extra

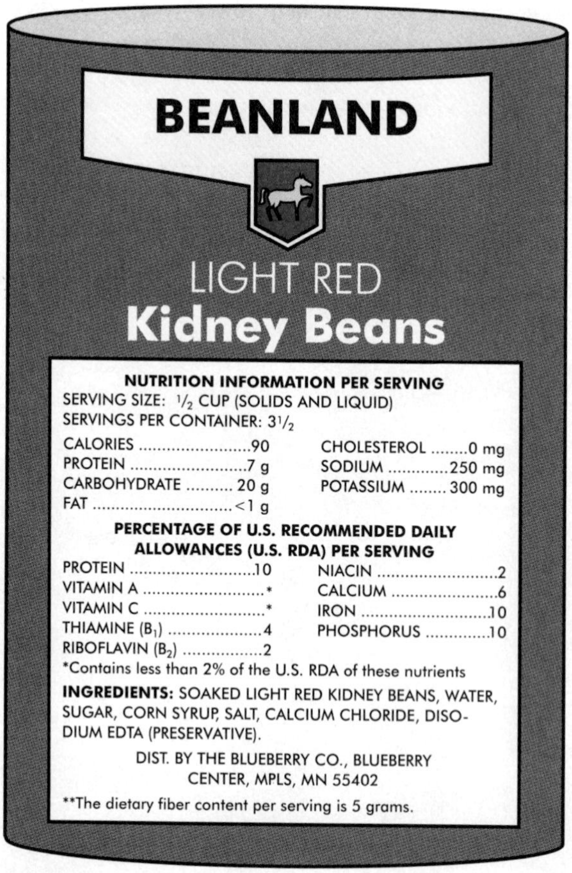

FIGURE 7-6

Legumes are rich sources of protein. One half cup meets about 10% of protein needs, and at a "cost" of only about 5% of energy needs. The addition of dietary fiber to one's diet is an added bonus.

phosphorus is also consumed, urine calcium does not increase so much.[19] Animal foods are excellent sources of both protein and phosphorus. So typical American protein consumption probably doesn't threaten calcium balance as long as it is part of a diet that also meets the RDA for calcium.

There is some concern that a diet high in protein may overwork the kidneys, because they must excrete the excess nitrogen yielded (mostly as urea) into the urine. Laboratory animal studies show that getting just enough protein to meet nutritional needs preserves kidney function over time better than does a high-protein diet. Protecting the kidneys is especially important for people with either diabetes, poor kidney function linked to other disease states, or only one functioning kidney. Presently, many medical centers in the United States are studying whether a conservative protein diet maintains kidney function better than does the typical American protein intake for people with kidney disease. For people without diabetes the overall risk of kidney failure is low, and so the chances of a high-protein diet contributing to kidney disease in later life are slim.[2,17] As we mentioned in Chapter 5, a link between a high meat intake and colon cancer has been seen in epidemiological studies. However, it is not clear if this link is caused by the meat itself or the fat in the meat, or if the finding is even important enough to consider. Overall, we believe the caution against high protein intakes issued by the National Academy of Sciences in their 1989 *Diet and Health Report* deserves consideration. The panel recommended we not consume more than twice the RDA for protein on a regular basis.

The Importance of Plant Proteins

Vegetable sources of proteins deserve more attention from Americans. Many plant foods—in proportion to the amount of energy they supply—provide not only much protein, but also ample magnesium and dietary fiber, along with other benefits.[14] The protein is used somewhat less efficiently by the body than are animal proteins (10% to 20% less), but this drop is not significant enough to influence diet planning. The vegetable proteins we eat also contain no cholesterol and little saturated fat, unless these are added during processing. Regular use of plant foods high in protein makes a valuable addition to the Food Guide Pyramid because these supply a variety of other nutrients. Presently, concentrated sources of plant proteins are not very popular in America, except for maybe peanut butter, baked beans, and refried beans. Should you give them a second look (Figure 7-6)?

CONCEPT CHECK

The Recommended Dietary Allowance (RDA) for adults is 0.8 gram of protein per kilogram of desirable body weight. This adds up to 56 grams of protein daily for a 70-kilogram (156-pound) person. The average American man consumes about 90 grams of protein daily, and a woman consumes about 70 grams. So, typically, we eat more than enough protein to meet our needs. Aside from the fat present in most high-protein diets, current research has not firmly established that this excess poses a major health risk for most of us, but it is also not necessary.

PROTEIN IN FOODS

The most nutrient-dense source of protein is water-packed tuna, which has over 80% of kcalories as protein (Figure 7-7). Notice in Figure 7-7 that all foods with more than 20% of kcalories as protein are animal foods. They are also the major sources of protein in the American diet: we get over two thirds of our protein from animal sources. Worldwide, 54% of the protein consumed comes from animal sources. In Africa and East Asia less than 25% of the protein eaten comes from animals.[15] In the United States, beef still leads

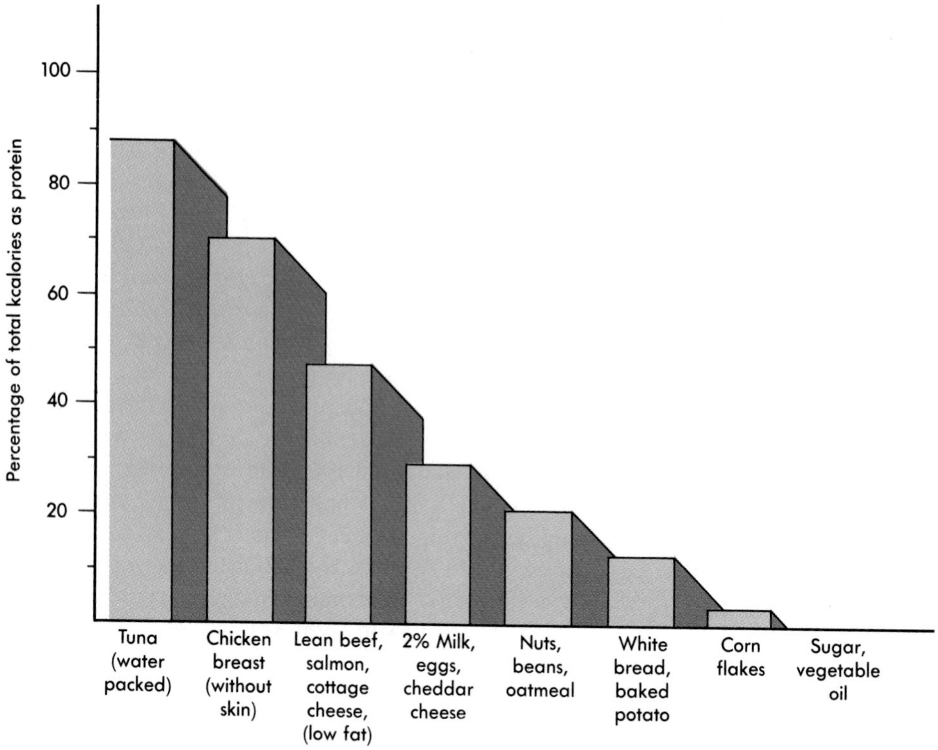

FIGURE 7-7

Percent of kcalories as proteins in foods. Water-packed tuna provides almost all kcalories as proteins. Notice that all foods containing more than 20% of kcalories from protein are of animal origin.

Protein-Energy Malnutrition (PEM) ▪ *A condition resulting from regularly consuming insufficient amounts of energy and protein. The deficiency eventually results in body wasting and an increased susceptibility to infections.*

Marasmus ▪ *A disease that results essentially from starvation—not consuming sufficient protein and energy. Thus it is the equivalent to severe protein-energy malnutrition. The infant or adult will show extremely low weight and have little or no fat stores, little muscle mass, and poor strength.*

Kwashiorkor ▪ *A disease occurring primarily in young children when disease and infections add to the high nutrient demands of growth. If the child also consumes insufficient energy and protein, kwashiorkor may result. Edema, moderate weight deficit, and weakness are common symptoms.*

as an animal protein source, with an annual consumption of 104 pounds per person, but chicken is gaining fast, increasing from 28 pounds per person in 1960 to about 64 pounds currently.

PROTEIN-ENERGY MALNUTRITION

Protein deficiency rarely occurs as an isolated condition. It usually accompanies a deficiency of dietary energy and other nutrients resulting from insufficient food intake. In poorer areas of the world, people often eat diets low in energy and protein. This state of undernutrition stunts their growth in childhood and makes them more susceptible to disease throughout life.[15] (Note that undernutrition is a main focus of Chapter 18.) People who eat too little protein and energy food can go on to develop ***protein-energy malnutrition (PEM),*** also referred to as ***protein-calorie malnutrition (PCM).*** In its milder form, which is most common, it is difficult to tell if a person with PEM is eating too little energy or protein, or both. But if the nutrient deficiency—especially for energy—is quite severe, a deficiency disease called ***marasmus*** can result. On the other hand, when a poor nutrient intake—protein included—is added to other problems from concurrent diseases and infections, a disease called ***kwashiorkor*** can develop.[12] These two diseases form the tip of the iceberg with respect to all states of undernutrition, and symptoms of these two diseases even can be present in the same person (Figure 7-8).

Kwashiorkor

Kwashiorkor is a word from Ghana that means "the disease that the first child gets when the new child comes." From birth the first child is usually breast-fed. By the time the child reaches 1 to 1½ years, the mother is probably pregnant or has already given birth again.

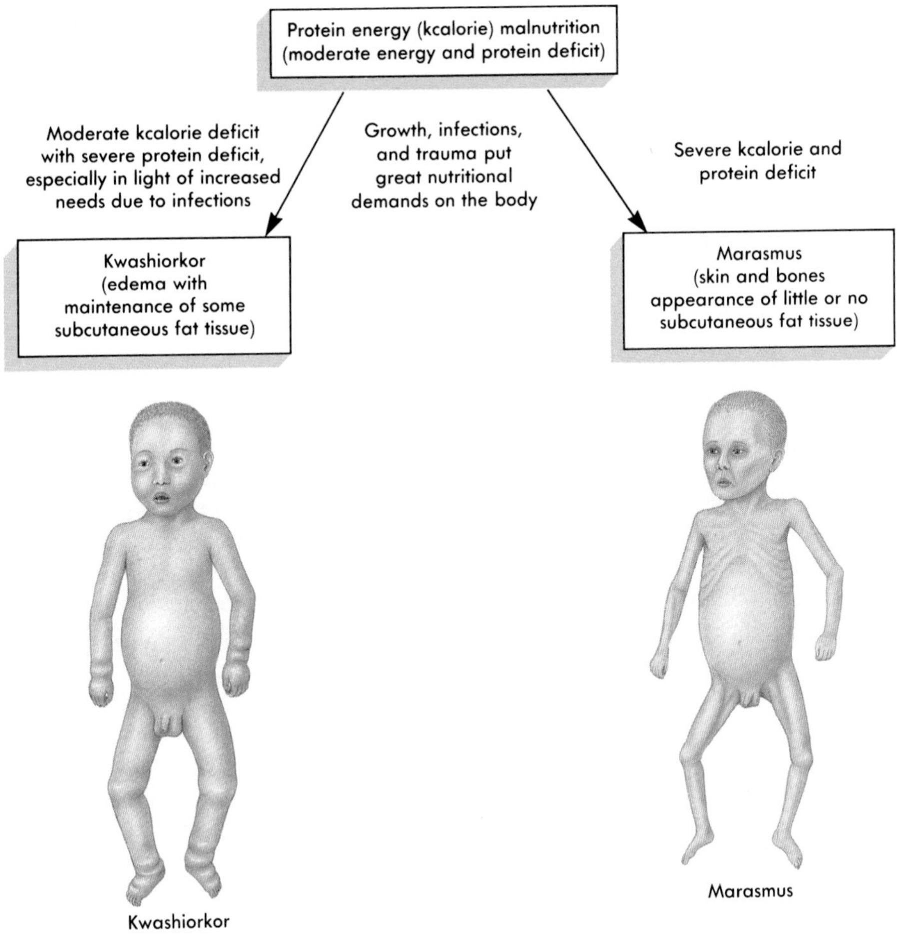

FIGURE 7-8
A schema for classifying undernutrition. The presence of subcutaneous fat (directly underneath the skin) is a diagnostic key for distinguishing kwashiorkor from marasmus.

Breast-feeding is no longer possible for the first child. That child abruptly switches from nutritious human milk to native starchy roots and gruels. These foods have very low protein densities, based on total kcalories. The foods are also often so bulky and full of plant fibers that it is difficult for the child to eat enough of them. So these young children who have high nutrient demands for growth end up consuming some energy, but their protein needs are not met, especially when these needs are also raised by concurrent illnesses, infections, and an insufficient energy intake.[12] Probably many vitamin and mineral needs are also far from being met. Feeding famine victims starchy roots, such as cassava (tapioca), creates the same problem.

The major symptoms of kwashiorkor are apathy, listlessness, failure to grow and gain weight, and withdrawal from the environment. These symptoms are often added to the results of other diseases present. Now measles, a condition that normally makes a healthy child sick for only a week or so, develops into a severely debilitating and even fatal disease. Further effects of kwashiorkor are changes in hair color, flaky skin, fat buildup in the liver, and massive edema in the abdomen and legs. The presence of edema, some visible fat stores, and only a moderate weight deficit are the hallmarks of this disease in children. In addition, a strange behavior among these children is that they hardly move. If you pick them up, they don't cry. When you hold them, you realize you are feeling the plumpness of edema, not lean body tissue.[12]

Although a variety of factors contributes to the clinical picture of kwashiorkor, we can explain some results of kwashiorkor based on what we know about proteins. Proteins play important roles in fluid balance, immune function, lipid transport out of the liver, and production of such tissues as skin and hair. Children deprived of sufficient protein and energy cannot grow and mature normally. And they don't!

If a child with kwashiorkor is helped in time to address medical problems present and fed a diet ample in energy, protein, and other essential nutrients, the disease symptoms reverse. The child begins to grow again and may even show no signs of the previous condition, aside perhaps from shortness of stature. However, by the time many of these children reach a hospital or care center, they already have severe infections. In spite of the best care, they still die. Or, if they survive, they return home only to repeat the cycle.

Marasmus

Marasmus is a disease that occurs when a child basically starves to death.[15,18] The word marasmus means "to waste away." Children do just that. They appear to be "skin and bones," like the figures on posters from relief agencies. Low body weight without edema or fat stores is the hallmark of the disease. A child with marasmus is usually under age 2 and was either not breastfed at all or breastfed for only a few months. In all probability, the weaning formula was improperly prepared, partly because of poor water supplies and partly because the parents couldn't afford enough formula for the child's needs. To stretch the formula out, the parents may have diluted it, providing less nutrients and more water for the child. The parents often have no other alternative.

Marasmus commonly occurs in the large cities of poverty-stricken countries. In the cities it is more common to bottle-feed. When people are poor and live in unsanitary conditions, bottle-feeding often leads to marasmus.[15] A child with marasmus requires large amounts of energy, protein, and other nutrients to attempt to recover from the disease.

Both kwashiorkor and marasmus wreak havoc on infants and children; mortality rates at these ages in poorer countries are often 10 to 20 times higher than in the United States. Over 40,000 infants worldwide die of starvation each year. This high mortality rate in part encourages the high birthrate in poorer countries: If a mother wants 4 children, she had better have 10 to make sure 4 survive. The overload makes infant mortality much

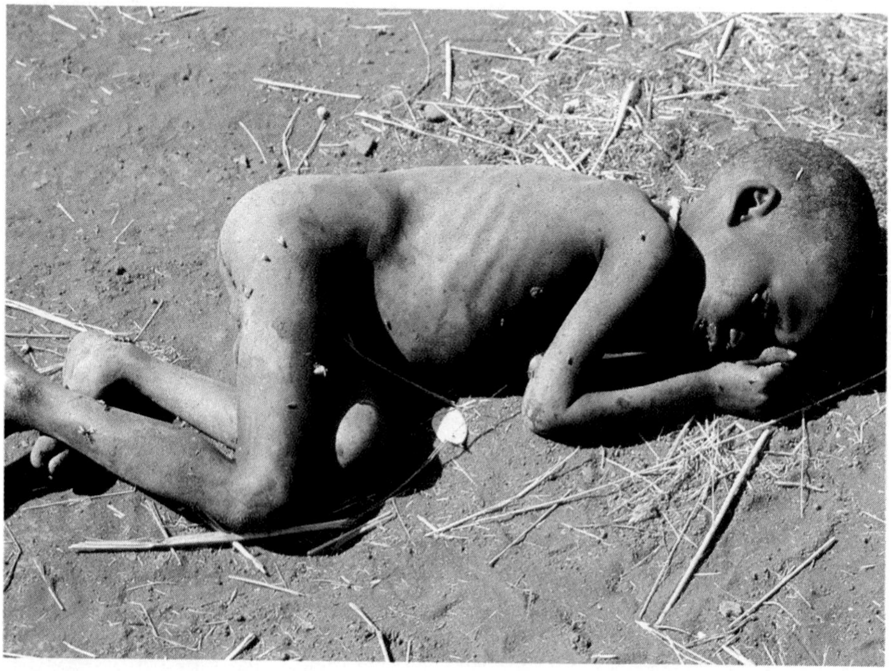

FIGURE 7-9
When undernutrition and people collide, human suffering is a typical result.

more likely. The problem is further fueled by politics and war. In all, the circumstances often create an intolerable environment for raising children (Figure 7-9). Better food availability and improved sanitation would greatly improve the health of many children worldwide. Chapter 18 looks at the issue of undernutrition worldwide in more detail.

CONCEPT CHECK

Most undernutrition worldwide consists of mild deficits in energy, protein, and often other nutrients. If a person needs more nutrients because of disease and infection but does not consume enough energy and protein, a condition known as kwashiorkor can develop. The person suffers from edema and weakness. Children around age 2 are especially susceptible to kwashiorkor, particularly if they already have other diseases. Famine situations where only starchy root products are available to eat can set up this problem. Marasmus is a condition where people—infants especially—essentially starve to death. Symptoms include muscle wasting, absence of fat stores, and weakness. Both an adequate diet and treatment of concurrent diseases must be promoted in poor countries to maintain nutritional health.

SUMMARY

- Amino acids are the building blocks of proteins. Amino acids contain a very useable form of nitrogen for us. Of the 20 or so types of amino acids found in food, 9 are essential to consume and 11 or so can be synthesized by the body.
- High-quality, also called *complete,* protein foods contain ample amounts of all nine essential amino acids. Animal foods typically supply all of them in approximately the right amounts. Low-quality, also called *incomplete,* protein foods lack sufficient amounts of one or more essential amino acids. This is typical of plant foods, especially cereal grains. Plant foods eaten together often complement each other's amino acid deficits, in turn providing a high-quality protein diet. Because supplementing the diet with large amounts of individual amino acids can lead to buildup of harmful levels, their use outside of medical therapy is not advised.
- Protein digestion occurs first in the stomach, producing breakdown products called peptones. In the small intestine, peptones separate into small peptides and amino acids. The amino acids and peptides are then absorbed into the absorptive cells of the villi and travel via the portal vein to the liver.
- Individual amino acids are linked together to form proteins. The sequential order of amino acids determines the protein's ultimate form and in turn function. If the three-dimensional shape of the protein eventually formed is unfolded—denatured—by treatment with heat, acid or alkaline solutions, or other processes, the protein loses its biological activity.
- Important body components—such as muscles, connective tissue, transport proteins, visual pigments, enzymes, some hormones, and immune bodies—are made of proteins. Proteins also provide carbon that can be used to synthesize glucose when necessary.

- The RDA for protein for adults is 0.8 grams per kilogram of desirable body weight. For a 70-kilogram (156-pound) person this corresponds to 56 grams of protein daily. American men consume about 90 grams of protein daily, and women consume closer to 70 grams. Thus the American diet generally supplies plenty of protein. The combined protein intake is also of sufficient quality that most of what is present in the diet can be used to support body functions.
- Animal products are the most nutrient-dense sources of protein. Water-packed tuna contains over 80% of its kcalories as protein. These proteins are of high quality in that we have a great ability to turn them into body proteins. Plant foods generally contain less than 20% of their kcalories as protein; however, legumes provide much protein and contribute high-quality protein to a meal if eaten with grain proteins or animal products.
- Undernutrition occasionally leads to kwashiorkor and marasmus. Kwashiorkor results primarily from a poor energy and protein intake in comparison to needs, which in turn are often raised by concurrent disease and infections. Kwashiorkor often occurs when a child is taken off human milk and fed mostly starchy gruels. Marasmus results primarily from extreme starvation—a negligible intake of both protein and energy. Marasmus commonly occurs in famine conditions, especially in infants.

STUDY QUESTIONS

1. Discuss the relative importance of essential and nonessential amino acids in the diet. Why is it important to replace essential amino acids lost from the body via one's diet?
2. What are four of the functions of proteins? How does the structure of a protein relate to its function?
3. Why is the quality of a protein important? What foods provide high-quality protein?
4. What is the significance of preventing protein-energy malnutrition in children worldwide?
5. What characteristics of legumes could contribute to the improvement of the American diet?

REFERENCES

1. ADA Reports: Position of the American Dietetic Association, vegetarian diets, *Journal of the American Dietetic Association* 88:351, 1988.
2. Blum M and others: Protein intake and kidney function in humans: its effects on normal aging, *Archives of Internal Medicine* 149:211, 1989.
3. Carpenter KJ: Protein requirement of adults from an evolutionary perspective, *American Journal of Clinical Nutrition* 55:913, 1992.
4. Christensen HN: Amino acid nutrition: a two-step absorptive process, *Nutrition Reviews* 51:95, 1993.
5. Clark N: How to pack a meatless diet full of nutrients, *The Physician and Sportsmedicine* 19:31, 1991.
6. Dwyer JT: Nutritional consequences of vegetarianism, *Annual Review of Nutrition* 11:61, 1991.
7. Eaton SB and others: *The Paleolithic prescription,* New York, 1988, Harper Collins.
8. Farley D: Vegetarian diets, *FDA Consumer,* p. 21, May 1992.
9. Freeland-Graves JH: Mineral adequacy of vegetarian diets, *American Journal of Clinical Nutrition* 48:859, 1988.
10. Herbert V: L-tryptophan, *Nutrition Today,* p. 27, March/April 1992.
11. Kamb ML and others: Reply to eosinophilia–myalgia syndrome or fibromyalgia with eosinophilia? *Journal of the American Medical Association* 269:3108, 1993.
12. Latham MC: Protein-energy malnutrition. In Brown ML, editor: *Present knowledge in nutrition,* Washington, DC, 1990, International Life Sciences Institute–Nutrition Foundation.
13. Meredith CN and others: Dietary protein requirements and body protein metabolism in endurance-trained men, *Journal of Applied Physiology* 66:2850, 1989.
14. National Institute of Nutrition (Canada): Risks and benefits of vegetarian diets, *Nutrition Today,* p. 27, March/April 1990.
15. Olson RE: World food production and problems in human nutrition, *Nutrition Today,* p. 15, January/February 1989.
16. Robertson L and others: *The new Laurel's kitchen,* Berkeley, Calif, 1986, Ten Speed Press.
17. Rudman D: Kidney senescence: a model for aging, *Nutrition Reviews* 46:209, 1988.
18. Scrimshaw NS: The phenomenon of famine, *Annual Review of Nutrition* 7:1, 1987.
19. Spencer H and others: Do protein and phosphorus cause calcium loss? *Journal of Nutrition* 118:657, 1988.
20. Stryer L: *Biochemistry,* ed 3, New York, 1988, WH Freeman.
21. Young VR: Kinetics of amino acid metabolism: nutritional implications and some lessons, 1987 McCollum Award Lecture, *American Journal of Clinical Nutrition* 46:709, 1987.

RATE

ARE YOU EATING ENOUGH PROTEIN?

I. How much protein do you eat in a typical day? Look at the nutrition assessment you completed at the end of Chapter 2. Review it closely. Find the figure indicating the amount of protein you consumed on that day, and write it in the space below:

TOTAL PROTEIN ____________

Compare your protein intake with your RDA for protein. Find your desirable weight for height in pounds using the table on the inside cover of this textbook. Choose a midrange value. Divide this number by 2.2 to reveal your desirable weight in kilograms. Next multiply by 0.8 grams per kilogram body weight. This will indicate the RDA for your age and gender. Write it in the space below:

RDA FOR PROTEIN ____________

How does your consumption compare with your RDA?

____

____

____

If you consumed either more or less than the RDA, what foods could you add, subtract, or eat more or less of? (Look at the foods you ate.)

____

____

____

____

Was most of your protein from animal or plant sources?

____

____

II. Plan a day of meatless meals. Can this diet meet your protein needs? A quick calculation using Appendix A or the software for this book will verify the correctness of your assumption.

your plate

Nutrition ISSUE

VEGETARIANISM

The practice of vegetarianism goes back to the time of the Greek philosophers, yet today it is new to many people. Throughout human history, vegetarianism has evolved from a necessity into a personal option (Figure 7-10). Historically, vegetarianism was linked with specific philosophies, religions, or science. Today, vegetarianism in this country usually appeals to a younger segment of people.[8] Overall about 2.7 million Americans call themselves vegetarians.

As nutrition science has grown, new information has enabled us to design adequate vegetarian diets. It is important for vegetarians to take advantage of this information because a diet of only plants can lead to various nutrient deficiencies and poor growth in infants and children. This warning is especially important to note. Multiple nutrient deficiencies and substantial growth retardation from a lack of energy and protein from exclusively plant-based diets have been observed in infants. If you choose to eat a vege-

THE FAR SIDE By GARY LARSON

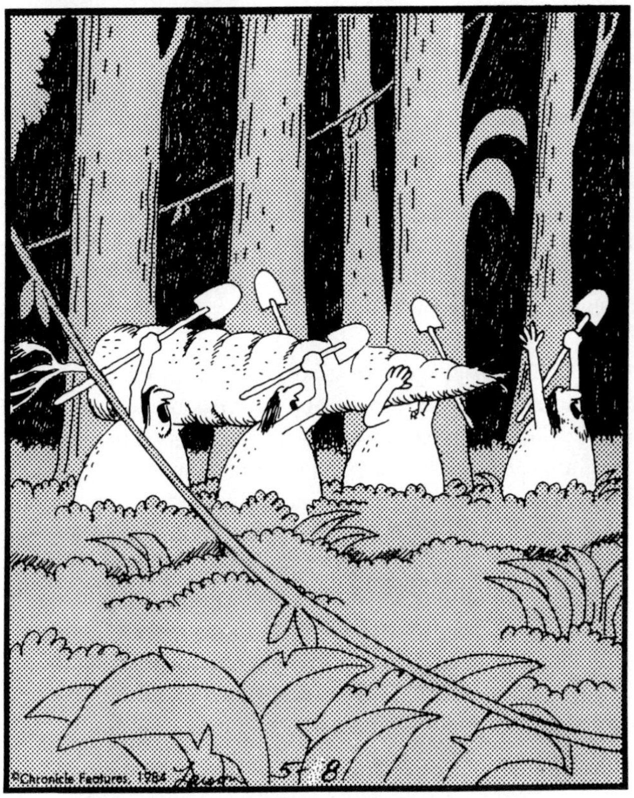

Early vegetarians returning from the kill.

FIGURE 7-10
The Far Side.

tarian diet, you can meet your nutritional needs by following a few basic rules, but it will take some knowledgeable diet planning.

Recent studies show that death rates from some chronic diseases are even lower for vegetarians than for nonvegetarians. Healthful lifestyles (leanness, not smoking, abstinence from alcohol and drugs, and increased physical activity) and social class bias, in addition to the vegetarian diet, probably also account for these findings.[14]

Why Do People Practice Vegetarianism?

People choose vegetarianism for a variety of reasons. Some think it is more ethical not to kill animals for food. Hindus and Trappist monks eat vegetarian meals as a practice of their religion. In the United States, many Seventh Day Adventists base their practice of vegetarianism on biblical texts and believe it is a more healthful way to eat.[8]

A person might choose vegetarianism after realizing that animals are not efficient protein factories. Animals actually use much of the protein they eat just to maintain themselves, rather than using it to synthesize new muscle tissue. A cow eats 21 pounds of plant protein for every pound of meat protein it produces. The ratio for pigs is 8:1; for chickens 5:1. Animals that humans eat sometimes eat grasses that humans cannot digest. However, many also eat grains humans can eat.

People might also practice vegetarianism because the diet encourages a high intake of carbohydrates; vitamins A, E, and C; beta-carotene; magnesium; and dietary fiber, while limiting cholesterol and saturated fat intake.[6] This rationale produces a diet closely resembling that suggested in the Dietary Guidelines for Americans covered in Chapter 2. Studies confirm that vegetarians actually do eat nutritious diets.[14] Some people might pursue vegetarianism because meat is expensive.

Vegan
A person who consumes no animal products.

Lacto-Vegetarian
A semivegetarian food plan where milk products, as well as plant products, are consumed.

Lacto-Ovo-Vegetarian
A semivegetarian food plan where a person consumes plant products, dairy products, and eggs.

Omnivore
A person who consumes both plant and animal food sources.

Food Planning for Vegetarians

There are a variety of vegetarian styles. ***Vegans*** eat only plant foods. ***Fruitarians*** primarily eat fruits, nuts, honey, and vegetable oils. This plan is not recommended, because it can lead to nutrient deficiencies in people of all ages. ***Lacto-vegetarians*** modify vegetarianism a bit—they include dairy products and plant foods. ***Lacto-ovo-vegetarians*** modify the diet even further and eat dairy products and eggs, as well as plant foods.[1] Actually, including these animal products makes food planning easier, because they are rich in some nutrients missing or in low amounts in plants. Overall, the wider the variety of foods eaten, the easier it is to meet nutritional needs. Thus the practice of eating no animal sources of food significantly separates the vegans and fruitarians from all other semivegetarian styles.

Most people who call themselves vegetarians consume at least some dairy products, if not dairy products and eggs. A four-food-group plan has been developed for lacto-vegetarians (Table 7-5).[16] This plan's protein group includes nuts, grains, legumes, and seeds. There is also a vegetable group, a fruit group, and a milk and/or eggs group.

This plan differs a little from the Food Guide Pyramid for ***omnivores,*** but it shares some similarities. The key to this plan is seeking foods other than meats that supply the nutrients contained in meats. It's not nutritionally sound to just cut out meat and to eat everything else without making sure the body's needs are still met. One should eat good-quality plant sources of nutrients to replace those that normally come from meat in the diet.[5] Nuts, grains, legumes, and seeds supply ample nutrients when consumed together; they become the new "meat" group.[16] By following the food plan, a lacto-vegetarian should have no problem eating an adequate diet.

The Vegan

Eating a vegan diet requires some creative planning.[1] First, purchasing some vegetarian cookbooks will simplify the task. They provide numerous ideas for imaginative and nutritious ways to use plant foods. A real effort must be made to use grains and legumes to obtain good-quality protein and other key nutrients in meals. Then if one satisfies energy

TABLE 7-5

A Food Group Plan for Lacto-Vegetarians and Vegans*

Group†	Servings: Lacto-Vegetarian‖	Servings: Vegan§,¶	Key Nutrients Supplied
Grains,‡ legumes, nuts, and seeds	7 or more	11 or more, including 2-3 servings of legumes and 2 servings of nuts/seeds	Protein, thiamin, niacin, vitamins B-6 and E, folate, zinc, magnesium, and fiber
Vegetables	3 or more (include one dark green or leafy)	5 or more (include one dark green or leafy)	Vitamins A and C, folate
Fruits	2 or more	3 or more	Vitamins A and C, folate
Milk	2 or more	—	Protein, riboflavin, vitamins D and B-12, and calcium

**This yields about 1600 to 1800 kcalories. Increase the number of servings or add other foods to meet higher energy needs.*
†Base serving size on those listed for the Food Guide Pyramid (see Chapter 2).
‡One serving of vitamin- and mineral-enriched breakfast cereal is recommended.
§A calcium-fortified food, such as orange juice or soy milk, is needed unless a calcium supplement is used. In addition, use of a vitamin B-12 supplement or foods supplemented with vitamin B-12 is a must.
‖Contains about 75 grams of protein in 1650 kcalories.
¶Contains about 79 grams of protein in 1800 kcalories.

needs, protein needs should also be met. A wide variety of protein sources, including the excellent ones just mentioned, should provide all amino acids needed for a complete protein diet. In other words, the essential amino acids deficient from one food protein are supplied by those of another protein in the same meal or in the next.[8]

Table 7-2 lists traditional dishes where vegetable proteins combine to provide high-quality (complete) protein in the meal.

The vegan diet also needs good sources of riboflavin, vitamins D and B-12, calcium, iron, and zinc (Table 7-6).[6] Riboflavin can be obtained by eating green leafy vegetables, whole grains, yeast, and legumes. Most vegans eat these foods. Note that the major source of riboflavin in the American diet is milk, which is omitted from the vegan diet. Vitamin D can be obtained through regular sun exposure. Otherwise, a supplement containing vitamin D should be considered (see Chapter 8).

The vegan should find a reliable source of vitamin B-12, such as fortified soybean milk or special yeast grown on media rich in vitamin B-12 (check the label). Vitamin B-12 occurs naturally only in animal foods; plants can contain soil or microbial contamination that provides at most a trace amount of vitamin B-12. Because the body can store enough vitamin B-12 for up to 4 years, it takes a long time for a deficiency to develop after someone has given up animal foods. If a deficiency develops, nerves can be damaged irreversibly and brain function can decrease. Therefore vegans need to make sure to prevent a vitamin B-12 deficiency (see Chapter 8).

TABLE 7-6

Nutrients Likely to Be Low in the Diet of a Total Vegetarian (Vegan)

Nutrient	Plant Sources
Vitamin D	Fortified margarines, fortified breakfast cereals
Riboflavin	Whole and enriched grains, leafy vegetables, mushrooms, beans, nuts, seeds
Vitamin B-12	Fortified breakfast cereals, fortified yeast, fortified soybean milk
Iron	Whole grains, prune juice, dried fruits, beans, nuts, seeds, leafy vegetables
Calcium	Fortified soybean milk,* tofu, almonds, dry beans, leafy vegetables, some fortified breakfast cereals, flours, certain brands of orange juice (check the label)*
Zinc	Whole grains, wheat germ, beans, nuts, seeds

**Fortified soybean milk and fortified orange juice are the best sources.*

To obtain calcium, the vegan can drink fortified soybean milk or fortified orange juice. Tofu, green leafy vegetables, and nuts also contain calcium, but it is either not well absorbed from them or not very plentiful. Calcium supplements are another option.

For iron the vegan can consume whole grains, dried fruits, and legumes. The iron in these foods is not absorbed as well as that found in animal foods, but a good source of vitamin C taken with these foods can greatly enhance iron absorption. Thus an excellent strategy is to consume vitamin C with every meal that contains adequate iron-rich plant foods.

The vegan can find zinc in whole grains and legumes. Phytic acid in whole grains limits zinc absorption. Grains are most nutritious when leavened, as in bread, because this process reduces the influence of phytic acid.[9]

Of all these nutrients, sufficient calcium is the most difficult to consume. Special diet planning is required (Table 7-6).

Veganism during childhood can pose problems.[8] The sheer bulk of a plant-based diet may make it difficult for a child to eat foods that supply enough energy to permit dietary protein to be used for synthesis of body proteins, rather than used for energy needs. Vegan children need concentrated sources of energy to avoid this problem.[1,12] Examples include fortified soybean milk, nuts, dried fruits, avocados, cookies made with vegetable oils, and fruit juices. Excellent zinc sources need attention in diet planning as well. Overall, both infancy and childhood are life stages in which vegetarianism is appropriate, but it must be implemented with knowledge and professional guidance.

Anyone considering vegetarianism should realize that a healthful diet does not occur automatically. It takes planning and common sense (Figure 7-11). We keep stressing the importance of eating a wide variety of foods. This is especially important for the vegetarian.

FRANK & ERNEST® by Bob Thaves

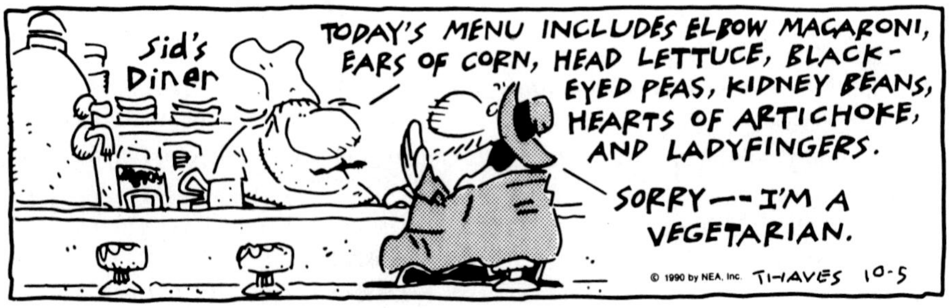

FIGURE 7-11
Frank and Ernest.

Reprinted by permission of NEA, Inc.

chapter

8 VITAMINS

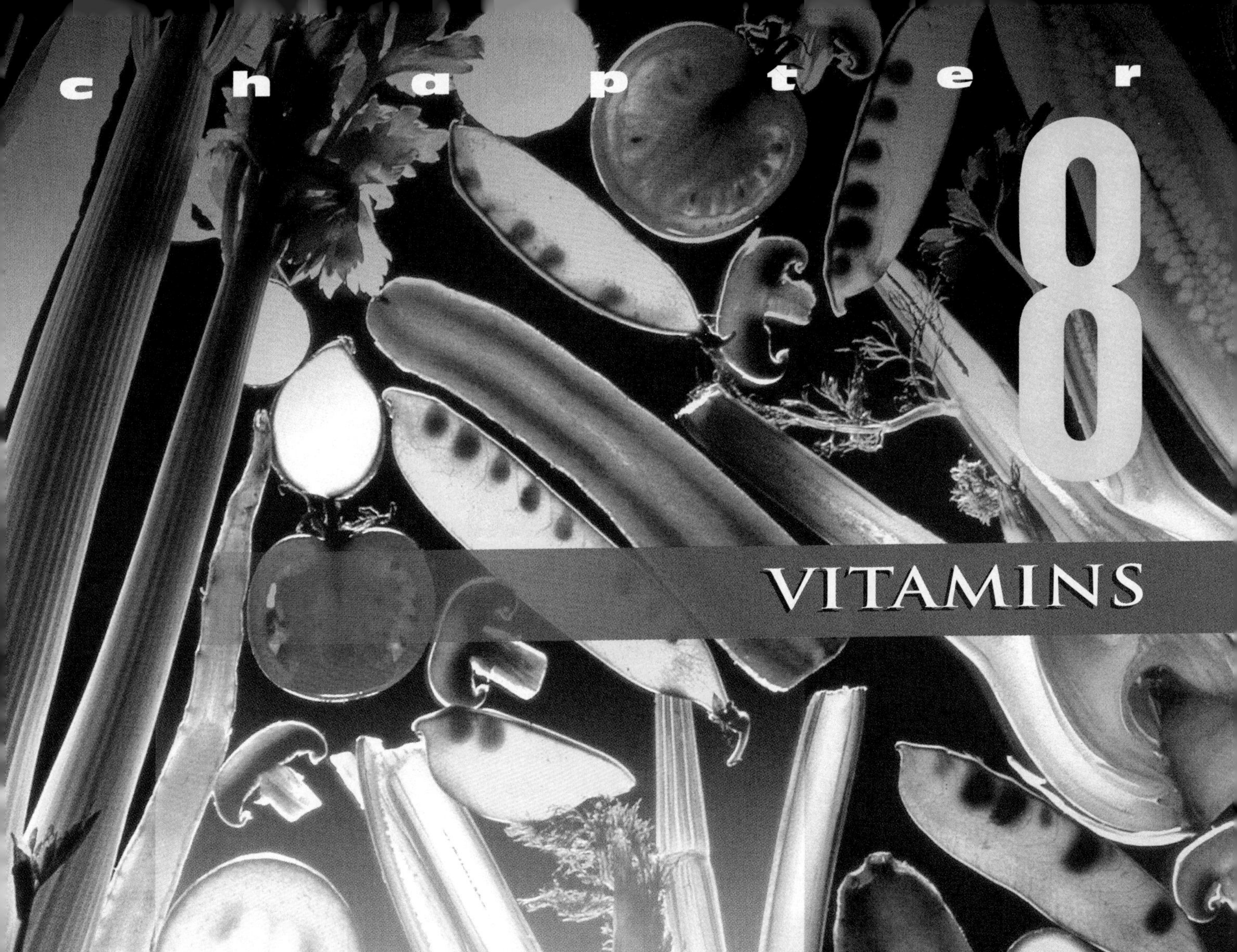

WHEN IT COMES TO VITAMINS AND MINERALS, PEOPLE ARE often told: If a little is good, more is better. This is a popular belief held by some people in their pursuit of better health. Today about 40% of the adults in some areas of the United States take vitamin supplements.[2] This fuels a $3 billion industry. The number of people who take large doses in the belief that vitamins provide extra energy, health, and protection from disease is unknown, but sales suggest the number is enormous.

In stark contrast, our total vitamin needs are really quite small, about 1 ounce (28 grams) for every 150 pounds (70 kilograms) of food we eat. Most plants can synthesize all the vitamins they need. Certain animal species can even synthesize some vitamins; cats and dogs make their own vitamin C. However, human bodies cannot make most vitamins, and so we rely on diet to supply them.

Who should take vitamin supplements and what dosage should be taken? What are the best sources of vitamins? Are there important differences between dietary sources of vitamins and man-made vitamins? How do vitamins work in our bodies? Can vitamins—especially vitamins A, E, and C—help prevent cancer? These are some of the questions we will address.

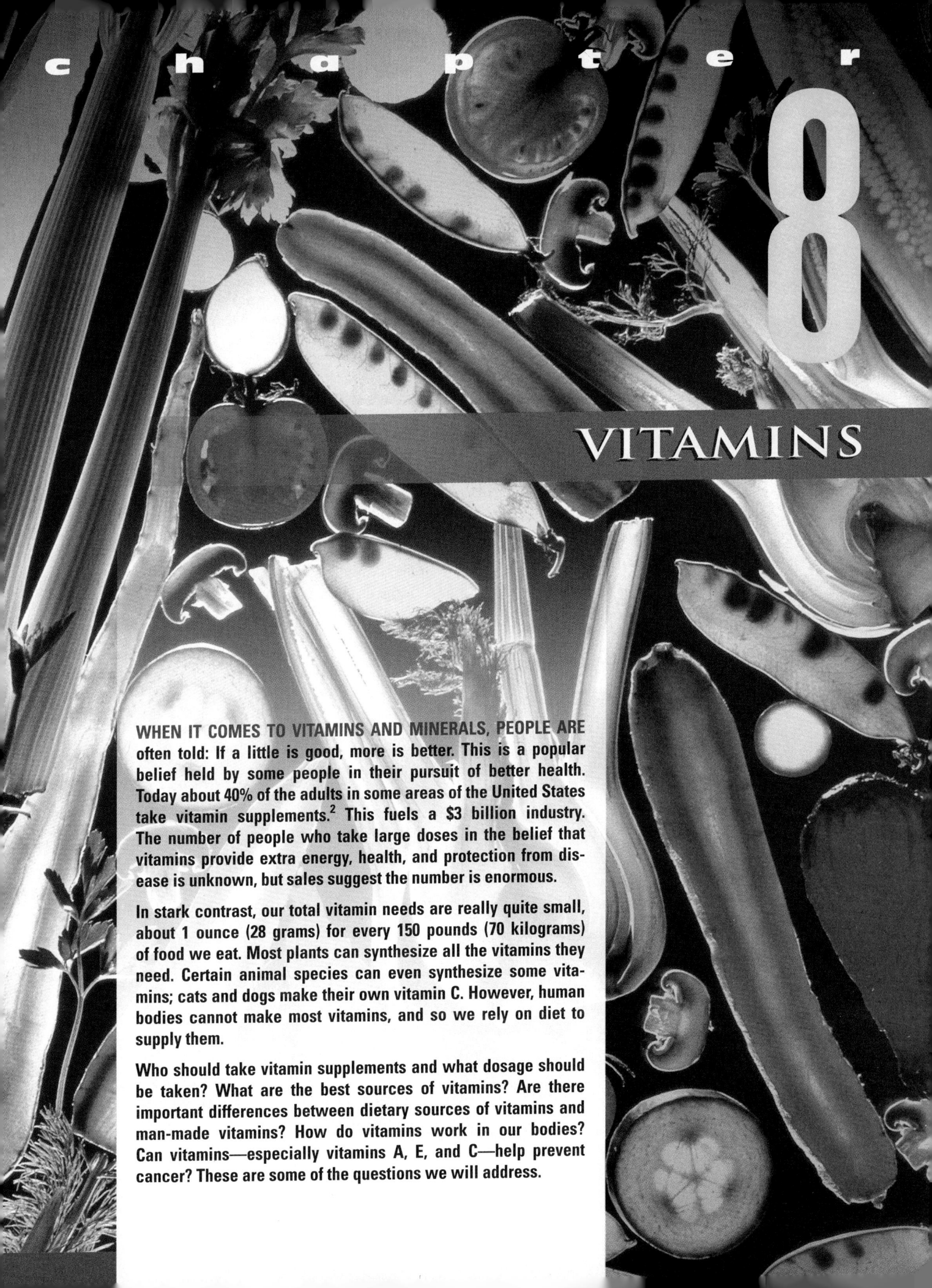

ASSESS

TEST YOUR KNOWLEDGE

yourself

WHAT DO YOU BELIEVE ABOUT VITAMIN SUPPLEMENTS?

Below is a brief article about vitamins, typical of one you might find in a popular health and fitness or women's magazine. As you read it, decide whether you think the claims are true or false. A blank is provided next to each claim to record your answers. Write "T" if you think the statement is true or "F" if you think it is false.

Vitamins: Our Health Promoting Allies by Dr. Wilbert Gruntaloud

Do you take vitamins? If not, you probably aren't doing all you can to promote your health. There are some hidden truths about vitamins that the medical community rarely discloses. Do you suffer from frequent colds and flu? Many people spend their hard-earned dollars for cold medicines and lose a number of workdays because of these ailments. We now know that certain vitamin supplements can prevent colds and flu ._____

Do you eat a relatively poor diet because of all the responsibilities you must handle? Vitamin supplements can completely make up for a poor diet ._____ Do you feel tired and fatigued frequently? You may be one of those people who requires very high intakes of vitamins to be healthy ._____ In addition, vitamin supplements will give you extra energy, especially during times of increased stress ._____ Most of us can't get all the vitamins we need from the food we eat. Plants, potentially rich sources of vitamins, are vitamin deficient today because the soil is so depleted of the nutrients needed for healthy plant growth ._____ Worried about the negative health effects of chemical pollutants in our air and water? Vitamin supplements can protect you ._____

See all the benefits vitamin supplements can bring you? Our Vitablast pack can provide you with all the vitamins you need. These vitamins are from natural sources and therefore safer and much better than synthetic ones ._____ We at Vitablast Distributors can provide you with a regular supply of vitamins and other supplements for a nominal fee.

Can you afford not to take vitamin supplements? Decide for yourself. Vitamin supplements are harmless, so taking extra amounts will just give extra benefits and security. _____ So what do you have to lose?

Check the answers you gave above against Table 8-1. Should you spend your money on vitamin supplements? Read on to find out.

VITAMINS—A TWENTIETH CENTURY PHENOMENON

Based on what we just said, ***vitamins*** can be defined as carbon-containing substances that the body must obtain—although in only small amounts—to maintain health. In this case *obtain* means either ingested or produced by the skin or bacteria in the intestine. The latter occurs, however, in only a few cases. Vitamins are used by the body to help promote and regulate various chemical reactions and processes. Deficiency diseases arise when our bodies are deprived of a vitamin for a prolonged time. Furthermore, to be a *true* vitamin, it must cure the deficiency disease if resupplied in time. While vitamins do not directly yield energy, many water-soluble vitamins do participate in energy-yielding reactions in the body. In contrast, fat-soluble vitamins mainly act to regulate growth and development processes.

Doses of vitamins well above the RDA have also proved useful as medicinal agents in a small number of diseases. For example, high doses of niacin are an accepted part of blood cholesterol–lowering treatment for appropriately selected individuals.[12] Other medical applications of vitamins to prevent or treat nondeficiency diseases need further study. At this time any claims concerning vitamin supplement use—especially if in excess

Vitamins *Carbon-containing compounds that are needed in very small amounts in the diet to help promote and regulate chemical reactions and processes in the body.*

TABLE 8-1

Myths and Facts About Vitamin Supplementation

Most of us view scientific knowledge with awe, and we are quite justified, considering the scientific achievements of our age. Misconceptions about vitamins and their proper functions are understandable. We addressed some misconceptions about vitamins briefly in Chapter 3. Let's spend some more time and clear up other misconceptions.

Myth	Fact
Vitamins give you "pep" and "energy."	Vitamins yield no energy. They, of themselves, provide no extra pep or vitality beyond normal expectations, nor do they provide unusual levels of well-being.
Daily timing of vitamin intake is crucial.	There is no medical or scientific basis for this contention.
Some people need very high intakes of vitamins to be healthy.	A multitude of studies have shown that it is rare for anyone to need amounts higher than the RDA to maintain health.
Vitamin supplements are necessary because today the soil is so depleted.	Crops can't grow in depleted soil. If a nutrient is low, the yield will be low, but the vitamin content will be normal.
Vitamins must be taken in precisely formulated amounts and ratios to each other to have the best effects.	Intake should be adequate, but not excessive, for each. No precise ratios are required.
Organic or natural vitamins are nutritionally superior to synthetic vitamins.	Synthetic vitamins, manufactured in the laboratory, are identical to the natural vitamins found in foods. The body cannot tell the difference and gets the same benefits from either source. Statements to the effect that "nature cannot be imitated" and "natural vitamins have the essence of life" are without meaning.
Vitamin C "protects" against the common cold.	Too bad, but extensive clinical research fails to support this.
The more vitamins, the better.	The opposite is true. In fact, excess amounts of any of several different vitamins can be harmful.
You cannot get enough vitamins from the conventional foods you eat.	Anyone who eats a reasonably varied diet that includes animal products should normally not need supplemental vitamins to maintain health.
Vitamin supplements are needed to protect against harmful chemicals and pollution.	Vitamin supplements do not have special abilities beyond the vitamins that a healthful diet supplies to ward off harmful agents.

of RDA values—should be examined cautiously, because many claims are unproven (Table 8-1).

Vitamins for the human diet come from both the plant and animal kingdoms. Whether isolated from foods or synthesized in a laboratory, vitamins are the same chemical compounds and work equally well in the body. Claims by health food literature that "natural" vitamins isolated from foods are more healthful than are those synthesized in a laboratory are unfounded.

Disorders caused by what we know were vitamin deficiencies are part of written history. The link between foods containing vitamin A and vision has been known since ancient Egyptian times, when topical application of juice extracted from liver was used as a cure for night blindness. Native Americans in the United States used pine needle extracts to cure scurvy, the vitamin C deficiency disease. During the fifteenth and sixteenth centuries, it was observed that scurvy developed during long sea voyages when few fruits and vegetables were eaten. British scientists later discovered that lime juice cured the scurvy. Using this knowledge, the British navy used the lime to develop a healthier work force and went on to dominate seas worldwide.

The twentieth century brought key scientific breakthroughs in the field of vitamins. These began in the early 1900s when Casimir Funk isolated a chemical substance he called "vitamine." This term came from the root phrase "vital amine" (an amine is a compound with a carbon bonded to a nitrogen). This later became the term vitamin we use today.

As scientists began to identify various other substances we call vitamins, such vitamin deficiencies as scurvy, beriberi, pellagra, and rickets were then dramatically cured. For the most part, as the vitamins were discovered, they were named alphabetically—A, B, C, D, E, and so on. Later many substances originally classified as vitamins were found not to

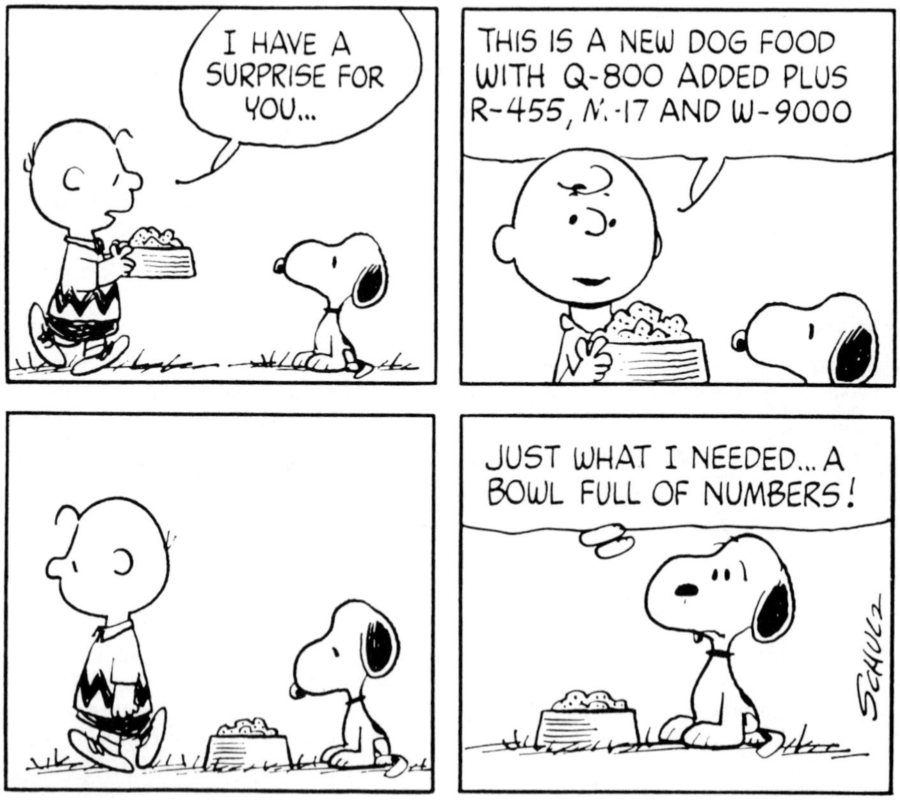

FIGURE 8-1
Peanuts.

be essential for humans and were dropped from the list. This explains the many gaps in the alphabetical listing. Other vitamins, thought at first to have only one chemical form, turned out to take many forms, so the alphabetical name had to be broken down by numbers (B-6, B-12, and so on) (Figure 8-1).

We class vitamins into two types—***fat soluble*** and ***water soluble.*** Based on this difference, they each behave differently in the body. The water in cells dissolves water-soluble vitamins—the B vitamins and vitamin C—and easily flushes them out of the body via the kidneys. Fat-soluble vitamins—vitamins A, D, E, and K—are not readily excreted and rapidly can build up in the body, causing toxic reactions. For that reason, we need to keep track of the amount of fat-soluble vitamins we ingest, especially vitamins A and D.

Fat-Soluble Vitamins
Vitamins that dissolve in such substances as ether and benzene. These vitamins are A, D, E, and K.

Water-Soluble Vitamins
Vitamins that dissolve in water. These vitamins are the B vitamins and vitamin C.

Hemochromatosis
A disorder of iron metabolism characterized by increased iron absorption and deposition in the liver tissue. This eventually poisons the liver cells.

Have We Found All the Vitamins?

You may wonder whether there are still more vitamins lurking in foods that have not been discovered. After all, the first structure and chemical formula of a vitamin (thiamin) were not determined until 1937, and the last structure was characterized in 1948 (vitamin B-12). Though some optimistic researchers hope to discover another vitamin, most scientists are confident that all vitamins needed by humans have been discovered. Evidence supports this assumption. For example, people have lived well for years on intravenous diets that consist of protein, carbohydrate, fat, all the known vitamins, and the essential minerals. With appropriate medical monitoring, these people not only continue to live, but also build new body tissues, have babies, heal wounds, and fight existing diseases. They do not develop deficiency diseases or fail to thrive. Hence, we feel that no essential substance (vitamins included) remains undiscovered. Experiences with intravenous diets have also taught us that some lesser known vitamins, such as biotin, are still very important to health.

SHOULD YOU USE VITAMIN AND MINERAL SUPPLEMENTS?

Almost as soon as vitamins were identified, scientists began to synthesize them in laboratories or isolate them from plant or animal sources. This opened the door for vitamin supplements. Still, consuming vitamin-rich foods on a daily basis is ideal. Even an occasional lapse in the intake of one or more water-soluble vitamins should cause no harm. A typically healthy person takes 10 days to develop the first symptoms of a thiamin deficiency[22] and 20 to 40 days to develop symptoms of a vitamin C deficiency when these vitamins are completely lacking from the diet. Therefore we can infer that we have reserves, although sometimes small, for all vitamins.

To determine whether you need supplements, first look closely at your diet. If it follows the Food Guide Pyramid discussed in Chapter 2—with an emphasis on such nutrient-dense sources as whole grains, low-fat and nonfat dairy products, leafy and dark green vegetables, fruits and vegetables that contain vitamin C, and a serving of vegetable oil—you are probably meeting your nutrient needs. However, some women with heavy menstrual flows may still need more iron to compensate for that lost in the blood. If you are still uncertain whether your diet provides enough vitamins and minerals, take a close look at what you eat for breakfast. Most breakfast cereals have extra vitamins and minerals added, some even matching the adult RDA levels (Figure 8-2).

GOLDEN CRUNCH CEREAL

NUTRITION INFORMATION
SERVING SIZE: 1.2 OZ. (1 OZ. CEREAL WITH 0.2 OZ. NUTS AND FRUIT; 33.1 g, ABOUT 1/2 CUP)
SERVINGS PER PACKAGE: 13

	CEREAL, NUTS & FRUIT	WITH 1/2 CUP VITAMINS A & D SKIM MILK
CALORIES	120	160*
PROTEIN, g	3	7
CARBOHYDRATE, g	25	31
FAT, TOTAL, g	2	2*
UNSATURATED, g	2	
SATURATED, g	0	
CHOLESTEROL, mg	0	0*
SODIUM, mg	170	230
POTASSIUM, mg	115	320

PERCENTAGE OF U.S. RECOMMENDED DAILY ALLOWANCES (U.S. RDA)

PROTEIN	6	15
VITAMIN A	15	20
VITAMIN C	**	2
THIAMIN	25	30
RIBOFLAVIN	25	35
NIACIN	25	25
CALCIUM	2	15
IRON	25	25
VITAMIN D	10	25
VITAMIN E	20	20
VITAMIN B_6	25	25
FOLIC ACID	25	25
VITAMIN B_{12}	20	30
PHOSPHORUS	8	20
MAGNESIUM	8	10
ZINC	20	25
COPPER	4	6
PANTOTHENATE	20	25

*2% MILK SUPPLIES AN ADDITIONAL 20 CALORIES, 2 g FAT, AND 10 mg CHOLESTEROL.
**CONTAINS LESS THAN 2% OF THE U.S. RDA OF THIS NUTRIENT.

FIGURE 8-2
The fortification levels for various vitamins and minerals in a typical breakfast cereal.

What Do the Experts Say?

Nutrition scientists generally agree with us that most people can obtain needed vitamins and minerals from a varied, balanced diet. We think you should start there first. Using the information in this chapter and Chapter 2 can help you improve your diet where needed. If you still think you need a supplement, talk to a registered dietitian and/or your physician. There is some risk from consuming even typical multivitamin and mineral supplements. For example, women in the early months of pregnancy may risk birth defects from ingesting too much vitamin A. People who are genetically prone to a liver disease called ***hemochromatosis*** can easily develop iron toxicity from supplement use.

Recently a panel of scientists from the American Institute of Nutrition and the Ameri-

Only a fraction of our population requires higher-than-normal dietary levels—supplements—of certain nutrients to compensate for impaired use or absorption of them. Examples include greater needs for vitamin D and vitamin B-6 by some individuals.[23] However, a physician must guide therapy, because toxicity is possible.

Lactation
The period after childbirth during which milk is produced in the woman's breasts.

Diuretic
A substance that, when ingested, increases the flow of urine.

can Society for Clinical Nutrition suggested specific cases for which vitamin and mineral supplements should be considered[7]:

- Women who bleed excessively during menstrual periods may need more iron.
- Pregnant or ***lactating*** women may need extra iron, calcium, and the vitamin folate.
- People with low energy intakes (about 1200 kcalories or less) need the range of vitamins and minerals. This can include elderly people who perform little physical activity.
- Some vegetarians may need extra calcium, iron, zinc, and vitamin B-12. Vitamin B-12 is found in reasonable amounts only in animal products.
- Newborns, under the direction of a physician, need a single dose of vitamin K to last until diet and synthesis by intestinal bacteria suffice.
- People with specific illnesses or diseases, and those on certain medications, may need supplementation of specific vitamins and minerals at the direction of a physician. Examples include extra potassium for someone using thiazide ***diuretics*** and possibly extra vitamin D and calcium for someone being treated for osteoporosis.

Supplementation during illness or drug therapy should be directed by a physician because some vitamins and minerals counteract the effect of certain medications. Vitamin B-6 can counteract the action of levodopa, a medication used to treat Parkinson's disease. Similarly, taking too much vitamin E can inhibit vitamin K metabolism and in turn increase the action of drugs designed to reduce blood clotting. By consuming many folate supplements, people with epilepsy who require anticonvulsant medication jeopardize their health; folate decreases the effectiveness of their medication. These examples illustrate the need for professional advice when you take vitamin and mineral supplements that exceed RDA levels. Only with professional advice can you appropriately evaluate whether supplementation is in your best interest.[7]

Which Supplement Should You Choose?

If you do decide to take a vitamin and mineral supplement, the Council on Scientific Affairs of the American Medical Association recommends taking no more than 50% to 150% of the adult U.S. RDA (now called RDI) for vitamins.[12] For minerals, we suggest the same guidelines, especially with regard to iron (see Chapter 9 for details). These are typical supplemental doses, basically a one-a-day type of supplement, but always read the label to be sure. ***Megadoses*** are defined as greater than 10 times one's RDA. A moderate, balanced formulation in a multivitamin and mineral supplement is important because it minimizes the chances of vitamin and mineral competition, which can lead to an imbalance. For instance, a high amount of zinc in a supplement can inhibit copper absorption, and a large amount of the vitamin folate can mask the symptoms of a potentially life-threatening deficiency of vitamin B-12.[17]

Buyer Beware!

Sometimes, what goes into a supplement is mostly a matter of economics. For example, the most expensive vitamin is biotin, and so many supplements contain only a fraction in relation to human needs. Most of the other B vitamins are inexpensive, which explains why it's common to find a supplement with 5000% of our needs for the B vitamins thiamin and niacin. We must keep in mind that FDA does not regulate all vitamin and mineral supplements closely. The Proxmire Amendment to the 1938 Food, Drug, and Cosmetic Act, along with legislation passed in 1992, limits regulation of supplements unless they are known to be inherently dangerous or marketed with illegal claims. Therefore Americans cannot always depend on the federal government to protect them from vitamin and mineral supplement overuse. FDA is working to clamp down on outrageous health claims made for supplements by their manufacturers, but current laws prevent this action. We take our chances when using supplements. For health's sake, people should know what they are ingesting and preferably should seek the advice of physicians and registered dietitians.

Currently, some scientists feel that the concept of the RDA needs to be broadened. One daily recommendation for a nutrient could be designed to prevent known vitamin deficiency diseases. Another higher value would be set to optimize the disease-preventing properties of such nutrients as the antioxidant vitamins C and E.[25] However, the question of benefits for already healthy people by supplementing a balanced diet with vitamin pills remains controversial among knowledgeable scientists. We will point out the pro and con arguments surrounding this issue as we take a look at each vitamin.

CONCEPT CHECK

Vitamins are carbon-containing compounds needed in small amounts by the body. They do not directly yield energy, but many are needed for energy-yielding reactions in the body. Vitamins A, D, E, and K are fat soluble, whereas the B vitamins and vitamin C are water soluble. In general, the fat-soluble vitamins are not readily excreted from the body and have the potential to build up rapidly to toxic levels. Water-soluble vitamins are much more readily excreted. Some people take vitamin supplements believing that they provide health benefits over dietary vitamins, but most nutrition scientists agree that a well-chosen diet that includes some animal products can supply the vitamin needs of almost all people.

THE FAT-SOLUBLE VITAMINS—A, D, E, AND K

First, we will take a look at what we know about the fat-soluble vitamins—vitamins A, D, E, and K (Table 8-2).

Absorption of Fat-Soluble Vitamins

Vitamins A, D, E, and K are absorbed along with dietary fat. These vitamins travel with dietary fats through the bloodstream to reach body cells. Special carriers in the bloodstream help distribute vitamins A and K. Fat-soluble vitamins are stored mostly in the liver and fatty tissues.

When fat absorption is efficient, about 40% to 90% of the fat-soluble vitamins are absorbed. Anything that interferes with normal digestion and absorption of fats also interferes with fat-soluble vitamin absorption. People who use mineral oil as a laxative at mealtimes risk vitamin deficiencies, because the intestine does not absorb mineral oil. Fat-soluble vitamins are simply eliminated with the mineral oil in the stool.

VITAMIN A

The amount of vitamin A you consume is very important. Either too much or too little vitamin A can cause severe problems (Figure 8-3). Vitamin A is found in foods in a variety of forms. Retinol is one example. As a family, the various forms are called preformed vitamin A or ***retinoids.*** Vitamin A activity in the diet also occurs in the form of common plant pigments—***carotenoids***—such as the yellow-orange, beta-carotene pigment in carrots. Carotenoids are also called provitamin A because parts can often be turned into vitamin A. Over 600 carotenoids are found in nature; 50 of them serve as provitamin A. The most potent form is beta-carotene. The preformed vitamin A and the provitamin A carotenoids both make up what is generically referred to as vitamin A. Most vitamin A is stored in the liver in animals, including humans.

Retinoids *Chemical forms of preformed vitamin A; one source is animal foods.*

Carotenoids *Pigment substances in plants that can often form vitamin A. Beta-carotene in the most active form.*

Functions of Vitamin A

Vitamin A performs many important functions in the body. But although researchers have studied vitamin A since its discovery in 1913, its exact roles in the cell are still baffling. Its importance to vision is perhaps its best-known role and the only role clearly under-

TABLE 8-2

Summary of the Fat-Soluble Vitamins, Their Functions, Deficiency Conditions, and Food Sources

Vitamin	Major Functions	Deficiency Symptoms	People Most at Risk	Dietary Sources	RDA	Toxicity Symptoms
Vitamin A (retinoids) and pro-vitamin A (carotenoids)	Vision: light and color Promote growth Prevent drying of skin and eyes Promote resistance to bacterial infection	Night blindness Xerophthalmia Poor growth Dry skin (keratinization)	People in poverty, especially preschool children (still very rare in the United States)	Vitamin A Liver Fortified milk Provitamin A Sweet potatoes Spinach Greens Carrots Cantaloupe Apricots Broccoli	Females: 800 RE* (4000 IU †) Males: 1000 RE* (5000 IU †)	Fetal malformations, hair loss, skin changes, pain in bones
D (chole- and ergo-calciferol)	Facilitates absorption of calcium and phosphorus Maintains optimal calcification of bone	Rickets Osteomalacia	Breastfed infants, elderly shut-ins	Vitamin D–fortified milk Fish oils Tuna fish Salmon	5-10 micrograms (200-400 IU)	Growth retardation, kidney damage, calcium deposits in soft tissue
E (tocopherols, tocotrienols)	Antioxidant: prevents breakdown of vitamin A and unsaturated fatty acids	Hemolysis of red blood cells Nerve destruction	People with poor fat absorption (still very rare)	Vegetable oils Some greens Some fruits	Females: 8 Alpha-tocopherol equivalents Males: 10 Alpha-tocopherol equivalents	Muscle weakness, headaches, fatigue, nausea, inhibition of vitamin K metabolism
K (phyllo- and mena-quinone)	Helps form prothrombin and other factors for blood clotting	Hemorrhage	People taking antibiotics for months at a time	Green vegetables Liver	60-80 micrograms	Anemia and jaundice

**Retinol equivalents*
†International units.

Visual Cycle *A chemical process in the eye that participates in vision. Forms of vitamin A participate in the process.*

stood at the chemical level. Researchers are investigating other ways that vitamin A functions in the body. Body changes that occur when vitamin A is lacking provide clues to its function.

Vision. The link between vitamin A and night vision has been known since ancient Egyptian times, when juice extracted from liver was used as a cure for night blindness. Vitamin A performs important functions in light/dark and color vision. It is a key part of the ***visual cycle.*** For a person to see in dim light, retinal—one form of vitamin A—is needed to start the chemical process that signals the brain that light is striking the eye. This allows the eye to adjust from bright to dim light (such as after seeing the headlights of an oncoming car). Without sufficient dietary vitamin A, eventually the eye cannot quickly readjust to dim light. The condition is known as night blindness. An injection of vitamin A into the bloodstream can cure night blindness in a matter of minutes!

If night blindness is not corrected and vitamin A deficiency progresses, the cells that line the cornea of the eye (the clear window of the eye) also lose their ability to produce mucus.[28] The eye then becomes dry. Eventually, when dirt particles scratch the dry surface of the eye, bacteria infect it. The infection soon spreads to the entire surface of the

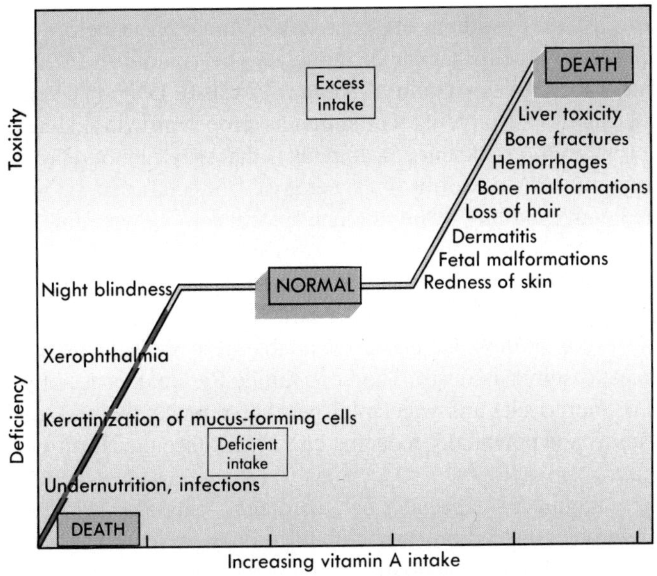

FIGURE 8-3
Consuming the right amount of vitamin A is critical to overall health. A very low (deficient) and a very high (toxic) vitamin A intake can produce damaging symptoms and even lead to death. The severity of effects with regard to levels of intake vary for individuals. Note however, that RDA levels promote health of a variety of body tissues.

eye and leads to blindness. This disease process is called ***xerophthalmia,*** which means dry eye.

Vitamin A deficiency is second only to accidents as a worldwide cause of blindness. Americans are at little risk because of generally good diets. However, people in less-developed nations—especially children—are very susceptible to vitamin A deficiency.[28] Poor dietary intakes and low stores of vitamin A fail to meet the children's high needs during rapid childhood growth. Over 250,000 children in Asia become blind each year because of vitamin A deficiency.

Today, widespread deficiencies of vitamin A constitute one of the most important public health problems in developing countries. Worldwide, attempts to reduce this problem have included giving large doses of vitamin A twice yearly and supplementing sugar and monosodium glutamate with vitamin A. These food vehicles are used because they are commonly consumed by the populations of less-developed nations. In some countries this effort has proven effective.

Health of Cells. Vitamin A maintains the health of cells that line internal and external "skin" surfaces in the lungs, intestines, stomach, vagina, urinary tract, and bladder, as well as the eyes and skin.[28] These cells (called ***epithelial cells***) serve as important barriers to bacterial infection. As we just noted for the eye, some epithelial cells secrete mucus, a needed lubricant. Without vitamin A, mucus-forming cells deteriorate and no longer synthesize mucus. Instead, the cells make a protein, typically found in the hair and nails, called keratin. This causes the cells to harden and crack, disabling them as barriers to invading microorganisms. First affected by this loss of mucus-synthesizing capacity are the eyes.

Vitamin A deficiency also causes insufficient mucus production in the intestines and lung cells and poor health of cells in general, all of which increase the risk of body infections. Vitamin A deficiency also reduces the activity of certain immune cells. Together, these effects leave the vitamin A–deficient person at a great risk for infections.[28]

Growth, Development, and Reproduction. Vitamin A is necessary for cell growth and development. This is most easily demonstrated with laboratory animals, but human

Xerophthalmia
Literally "dry eye." This is a cause of blindness that results from a vitamin A deficiency. The specific cause is linked to a lack of mucus production by the eye, which then leaves it at a greater risk of damage from surface dirt and bacteria.

Epithelial Cells
The surface cells that line the outside of the body and all external passages within it.

BETA-CAROTENE SOURCES FOR YOUR DIET

Vegetables:	Fruits:
Spinach	Cantaloupe
Sweet potatoes	Mango
Pumpkin	Papaya
Carrots	Apricots
Butternut and Hubbard squash	Nectarines
Collard greens	Peaches
Dandelion greens	
Kale	
Turnip greens	
Beet greens	
Red peppers	
Swiss chard	
Bok choy	
Mustard greens	
Tomatoes	
Broccoli	

NOTE: Foods are ranked according to beta-carotene content from highest to lowest.

Fetus *The developing human life form from 8 weeks after conception until birth.*

International Unit (IU) *A crude measure of vitamin activity, often based on the growth rate of animals. Today these units have been replaced by more precise milligram and microgram measures.*

growth is also affected. Resorbing old bone, which must occur before new bone can be deposited, requires bone cells that can be stimulated by vitamin A. Producing some components of bone also requires vitamin A. Vitamin A causes DNA in a cell's nucleus to increase its synthesis of cell proteins that stimulate proper growth and development. One consequence of vitamin A deficiency in animals is that they cannot reproduce.

Cancer Prevention? Most forms of cancer arise from cells that are influenced by vitamin A. Coupled with its ability to aid immune system activity, vitamin A could be a valuable tool in the fight against cancer. This is especially true for skin, lung, bladder, and breast cancers.[36] Scientists have been encouraged by research using animals. Human studies using various forms of vitamin A are now under way in many centers in America. However, until results of these studies are available, it is advisable to avoid personal experimentation, as toxicity can result. The Food Guide Pyramid, especially with its combination of five or more fruits and vegetables per day, remains the best guide for both obtaining all vitamins and potentially reducing cancer risk (see the Nutrition Issue at the end of the chapter).

Forms of provitamin A—especially beta-carotene—may also help prevent cancer because they help protect the carbon-carbon double bonds present in the cells of the body.[21] Free oxygen atoms and other potentially toxic compounds most likely initiate the cancer process in some cells by destroying these bonds. Carotenes appear to limit this destruction. Some evidence shows that regular consumption of vegetables high in carotenes decreases the risk of lung cancer in smokers. However, more investigation is needed in this area before specific recommendations can be made regarding carotenes and cancer prevention. The best advice is still to eat fruits and vegetables regularly and not smoke.

Vitamin A for Acne. The acne medication tretinoin (Retin-A) is made of one form of vitamin A. It has been used as a topical treatment (applied to the skin) for acne for more than 10 years. It appears to work by altering cell activity in the skin. Another derivative of vitamin A, 13-cis retinoic acid (Accutane), is an oral drug used to treat serious acne. We have mentioned that taking high doses of vitamin A itself would not be safe. Even Accutane, a less toxic form, can induce toxicity symptoms. A person using either Retin-A or Accutane must also limit sun exposure, because these drugs cause skin to sunburn easily. Furthermore, Accutane carries a very high risk for ***fetal*** malformations when pregnant women use it. Even the topical use of Retin-A is not recommended during pregnancy.

Vitamin A in Foods

Vitamin A in foods exists in either the animal form (preformed vitamin A) or plant form (provitamin A). Preformed vitamin A is found in liver, fish oils, vitamin A–fortified milk, and eggs. Butter and margarine are also sources, as these are fortified with vitamin A. Provitamin A is found mainly in dark green and orange vegetables and some fruits. Carrots, spinach, squash, broccoli, papayas, and apricots are examples of sources. Beta-carotene contributes to the yellow-orange color of carrots. The yellow-orange color is often masked, however, by dark-green chlorophyll pigments in vegetables, such as in broccoli. Consuming a varied diet rich in green vegetables and carrots ensures sufficient sources for meeting vitamin A needs. About half of the vitamin A in the American diet comes from animal sources, the other half from plants.

Retinol Equivalents (RE)

For vitamin A, the preferred unit of measurement is the ***retinol equivalent (RE).*** In this system, all potential forms of vitamin A are scaled based on their activity. Most nutrient levels in foods, including vitamin A, were formerly expressed in less precise ***international units (IU).*** Some food labels still show the older IU values for nutrients because the U.S. RDA is based on the RDA from 1968, which used the IU system. The current RDA does not. Based on a mixture of preformed and provitamin A, 1 RE of vitamin A is equivalent to 5 IU of vitamin A.

RDA for Vitamin A

The current RDA for vitamin A is 1000 RE for men and 800 RE for women. (Throughout this and the next chapter, refer to the inside cover for nutrient recommendations for other ages and to Appendix B for Canadian recommendations.) The recommendation approximates, but is often slightly above, the average intake for adult men and women in the United States. A higher intake of green vegetables could easily raise intakes to RDA levels.

In America, poor vitamin A status has been noted among preschool children who do not eat enough vegetables. This is especially true in Hispanic communities where typical food choices are not likely to provide adequate vitamin A. The urban poor, the elderly, and people who are alcoholics or who have liver disease (which limits vitamin A storage) can also show poor vitamin A status, especially poor vitamin A storage. Finally, children with severe fat malabsorption, as in cases of cystic fibrosis, may also show a vitamin A deficiency.

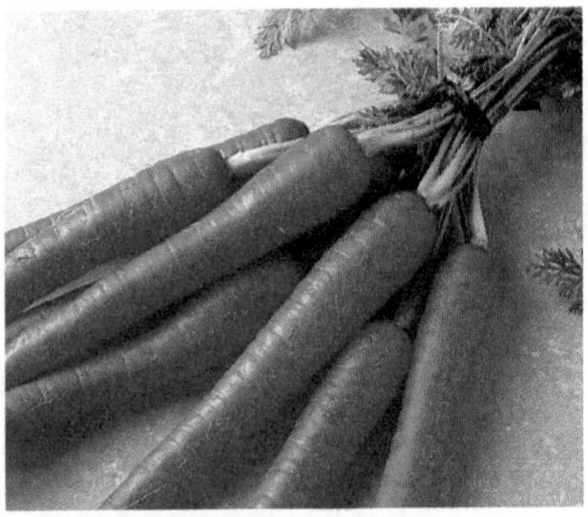

Carrots are a rich source of carotenes and vitamin A activity—good reasons to eat these regularly.

another BITE

Parents often encourage their children to eat vegetables. Besides contributing to good food habits, this practice helps children consume enough vitamin A. Parents provide important role models for children, and they can positively influence their children's eating interests by also eating their vegetables.

Toxicity of Vitamin A

An intake of just 10 times the RDA for vitamin A can cause problems if taken for a prolonged time. Skin, hair, internal organs, and the central nervous system are affected. Most adverse effects disappear after the doses stop. Permanent damage to the liver, bones, and eyes and recurrent joint and muscle pain, however, can occur.

A high vitamin A intake is especially dangerous during pregnancy because it may cause fetal malformations. Birth defects and spontaneous abortions caused by vitamin A toxicity have been clearly demonstrated in experimental animals. In humans, excessive vitamin A intake has been associated with birth defects in infants.

The ingestion of large amounts of vitamin A–yielding carotenoids does not cause vitamin A toxicity. If someone consumes large amounts of carrots or takes pills containing beta-carotene (more than 30 milligrams daily), or if infants eat a great deal of squash, high carotene levels can occur in the bloodstream. This can turn the skin yellow-orange. The palms of the hand and soles of the feet in particular become colored. This condition does not appear to cause harm and disappears when the excess cartotenes decrease. Carotenes do not cause vitamin A toxicity because (1) their rate of conversion into vitamin A is relatively slow and regulated and (2) the efficiency of carotenoid absorption from the small intestine decreases markedly as oral intake increases. Thus nature protects us from serious toxic effects from dietary carotenoids.

VITAMIN D

Vitamin D is not just a vitamin. It is also considered a hormone because cells in the skin can convert a cholesterol-like substance to vitamin D using sunlight, and these cells are different from those cells that mostly respond to vitamin D—bone cells and kidney cells (Figure 8-4).[35]

Recall from Chapter 4 that a hormone is a substance made in the body that travels from the point of synthesis through the bloodstream to act at a different site.

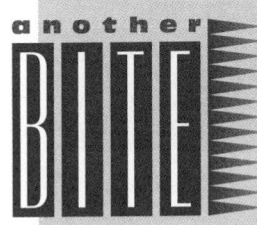

The amount of sun-time needed to produce vitamin D in skin cells depends on the darkness of the skin. Light-skinned people need approximately 15 minutes a day of direct sun exposure on the face and hands. Dark-skinned people need more sun exposure. The process is also more efficient in younger people than in the elderly. The farther you live from the equator and the more smog, fog, and smoke present, the greater the length of exposure needed to produce enough vitamin D. Anyone who does not receive enough sun-

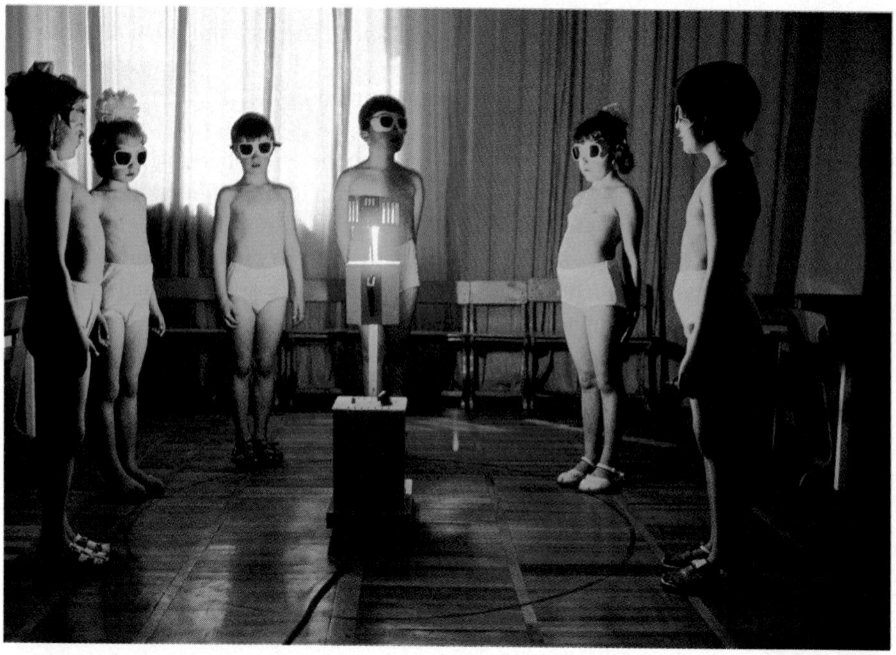

FIGURE 8-4

Who's got the tanning oil? Southern Russia endures a long winter. These Stavropol kids are exposed to a quartz lamp to provide the vitamin D synthesis they would normally experience from playing outdoors.

Calcitriol
The active hormone form of vitamin D (1,25-dihydroxyvitamin D)—not to be confused with calcitonin, a hormone that also affects calcium use.

Parathyroid Hormone (PTH)
A hormone made by the parathyroid glands that increases synthesis of the vitamin D hormone and aids calcium release from bone and calcium uptake by the kidneys, among other functions.

Rickets
A disease characterized by softening of the bones because of poor calcium content. This deficiency disease arises from insufficient vitamin D activity in the body.

light to make sufficient vitamin D must consume vitamin D as well. Most Americans rely on the diet to help supply adequate vitamin D, particularly in winter.

As we noted, the starting product for vitamin D synthesis in the body is a cholesterol-like substance. Ultraviolet light shining on the skin is needed to convert this into vitamin D. Vitamin D toxicity does not result from tanning in the sun too long because the body regulates the amount made in the skin. The same cannot be said for dietary vitamin D sources. Its uptake into the body is not blocked when eaten at high doses.

Function of Vitamin D

To become the active hormone, vitamin D must be metabolized by the liver and then the kidney. The main function of the vitamin D hormone (called ***calcitriol***)—produced by this two-step process—is to help regulate calcium and bone metabolism. In concert with other hormones, especially ***parathyroid hormone (PTH),*** vitamin D closely regulates blood calcium levels to supply appropriate amounts of it to all cells. This overall task entails a variety of processes: the vitamin D hormone helps regulate absorption of calcium and phosphorus from the intestine, it reduces kidney excretion of calcium, and it helps regulate the deposition of calcium in the bones (Figure 8-5).[35] Even tissues in the brain, pancreas, and pituitary gland appear to be influenced by the vitamin D hormone.

Rickets and Osteomalacia

The net result of vitamin D hormone action is to increase calcium and phosphorus deposition in bones. Without adequate calcium and phosphorus, bones weaken and bow under pressure. A child with these symptoms has the disease ***rickets.*** Symptoms also include enlarged head, joints, and rib cage and a deformed pelvis.[35]

To prevent rickets, infant diets, especially those of breast-fed infants in their first 6 months of life, should contain a food or supplement source of vitamin D if sufficient exposure to sunlight is not possible. Keep in mind that supplements should be used very

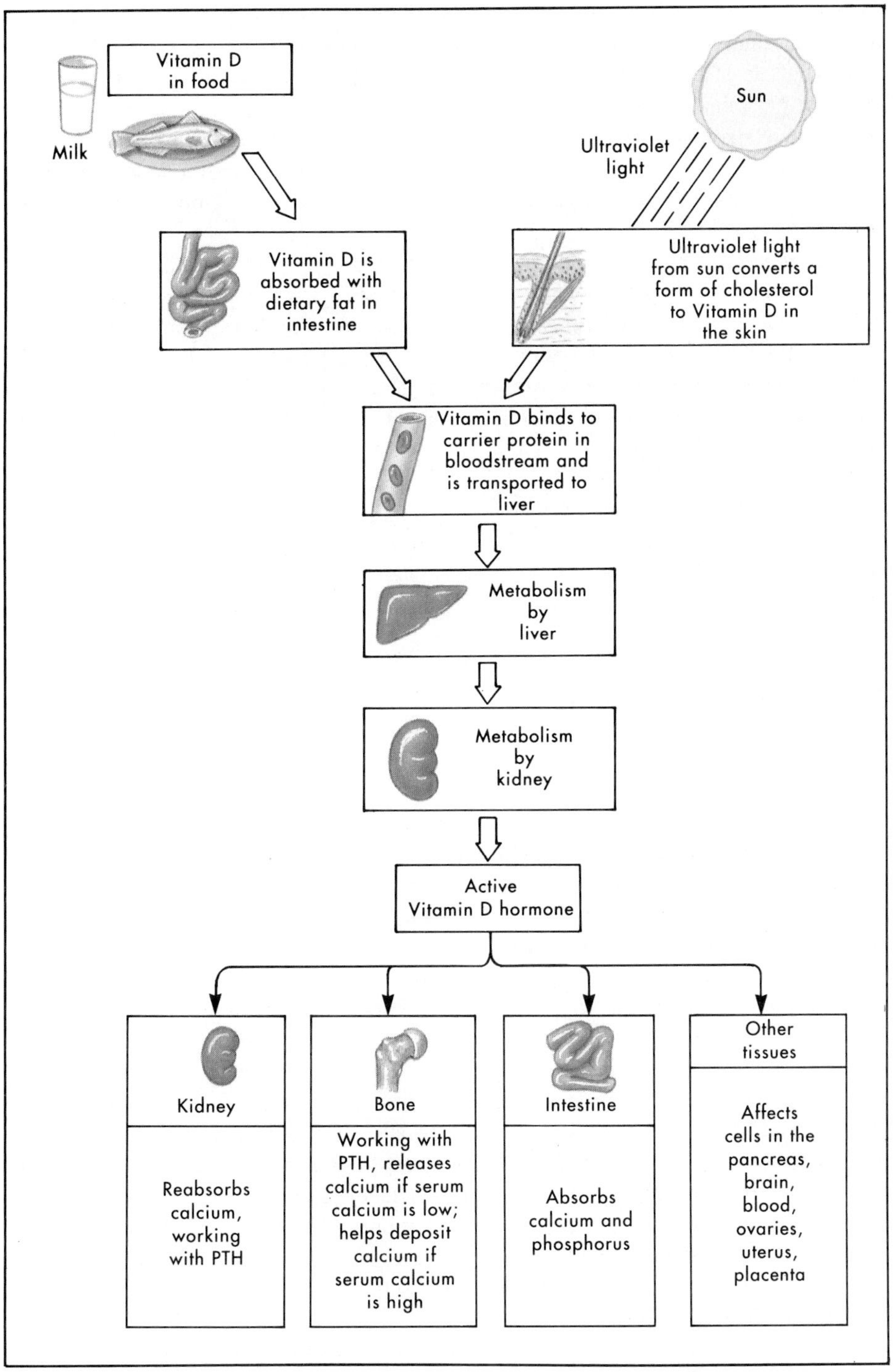

FIGURE 8-5

The many facets of vitamin D metabolism. Note than when made by the body using sunshine, vitamin D is actually a hormone. Recall that a hormone is a substance made in one part of the body that then travels through the bloodstream to act at a distant part of the body.

Osteomalacia Adult form of rickets. The weakening of the bones that is seen in this disease is caused by poor calcium content. A reduction in the amount of the vitamin D hormone activity in the body is the cause.

Be careful not to confuse this with osteoporosis, another type of bone disorder we discuss in Chapter 9.

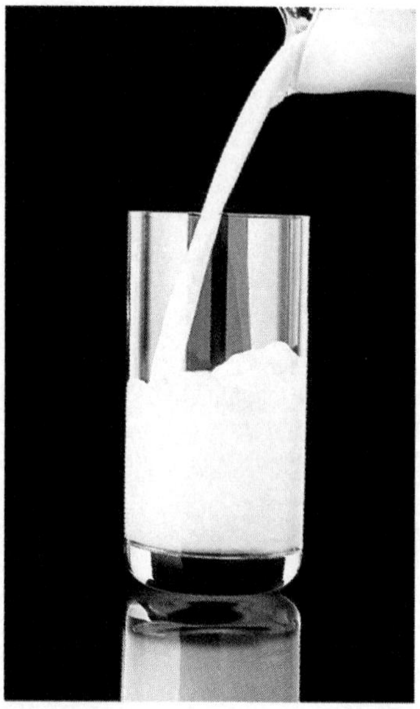

Milk is often fortified with vitamin D, which is important especially for people who receive little sun exposure.

carefully to avoid vitamin D toxicity. Vitamin D fortification of milk has greatly reduced the risk of rickets in children. Today, rickets is most commonly associated with fat malabsorption, such as occurs in children with cystic fibrosis. It is important to maximize the amount of vitamin D these children make using sunlight.

An adult disease comparable to rickets is ***osteomalacia,*** which means soft bones. It results when calcium is withdrawn from the bones to make up for inefficient absorption in the intestine or poor conservation by the kidneys. Both of these calcium-related problems can be caused by vitamin D deficiency. Bones then lose their minerals and become porous and weak and break easily. This leads to fractures in the hip, spine, and other bones.

Osteomalacia in adults occurs most commonly in people with kidney, stomach, gallbladder, or intestinal disease (especially when most of the intestine has been removed) and in people with cirrhosis of the liver. These diseases affect both vitamin D metabolism and calcium absorption. Adults with limited sun exposure may also develop the disease. In fact, current studies show that osteomalacia is common among some elderly people.[6] Combinations of sun exposure and/or vitamin D intake should be used to prevent this problem.

An Even Larger Role for Vitamin D?

The vitamin D hormone influences the development of cells of the intestine, skin, immune system, and bones. More interestingly, vitamin D is capable of influencing the development of some cancer cells, such as skin, bone, and breast cancer cells. However, it is not yet entirely clear how vitamin D regulates these cells or how significant its action may be on tissues other than those associated with its classic roles. In any event, these findings certainly have awakened interest in a vitamin about which we used to think we knew almost everything.

Vitamin D in Foods and the RDA

When exposure to sunshine does not create sufficient vitamin D, fatty fish (and fish oils) and fortified milk serve as the most nutrient-dense sources. Because milk is not a naturally rich source of vitamin D, it is fortified in the United States by adding 10 micrograms (400 IU) of vitamin D to each quart. Milk is a good vehicle for vitamin D supplementation because it is also the main source of calcium for children. Eggs, butter, and liver contain vitamin D but require too great a serving size to be considered significant sources. So few other foods contain vitamin D that food tables do not list sources.

The RDA for adults for vitamin D varies from 5 to 10 micrograms per day (200 to 400 IU per day). Recall that young light-skinned people are able to make this amount of vitamin D in about 15 minutes of sun exposure, and then on just the face and hands. Infants, children, and adolescents have higher RDAs because of their growing bones.

As we noted, anyone who both stays inside most of the day and ingests little or no vitamin D is at risk for developing vitamin D deficiency. This includes infants who are fed only human milk, and elderly people. These groups of people need either a more predictable amount of sun exposure and/or a regular food source of vitamin D.

Toxicity of Vitamin D

As little as four to five times the RDA of vitamin D taken regularly can create an overdose. Anyone who takes a dietary supplement should avoid a dosage higher than 150% of the RDA. Consuming more than 25 micrograms (1000 IU) of vitamin D per day requires close monitoring by a physician—above this level, toxicity problems can occur, particularly overabsorption of calcium and eventual calcium deposits in the kidneys and other organs. The person also suffers the typical symptoms of high blood calcium levels—weakness, loss of appetite, diarrhea, vomiting, mental confusion, and increased urine output. Calcium deposits in organs cause metabolic disturbances and cell death.

CONCEPT CHECK

Vitamin A is found in foods as preformed vitamin A and as provitamin A carotenoids. The most understood function of vitamin A is its importance in vision. Blindness caused by vitamin A deficiency is a major problem in many parts of the world. Vitamin A is also needed to maintain health of many types of cells, to support the immune system, and to promote proper growth and development. Vitamin A may be important in preventing cancer. However, because taking supplements of preformed vitamin A can build up to a toxic level, the best recommendation is to eat plenty of provitamin A–rich foods, such as fruits and vegetables.

Vitamin D is a true vitamin only for people who fail to produce enough from sunlight. Using a cholesterol-like substance, people synthesize vitamin D by the action of sunlight on their skin. The vitamin D is later metabolized by the liver and kidneys to form the active hormone calcitriol. This hormone increases calcium absorption in the intestine and works with other hormones to maintain proper calcium metabolism in bones and other organs in the body. Significant food sources of vitamin D are fish oils and fortified milk. Dietary vitamin D can be quite toxic.

VITAMIN E

Vitamin E has been called the "vitamin in search of a deficiency disease." However, growing evidence suggests it may be a valuable tool in the battle against heart attacks and cancer.[11,26]

Functions of Vitamin E

Vitamin E, a fat-soluble antioxidant, resides mostly in cell membranes. As we discussed in Chapter 6, an antioxidant can form a barrier between a target molecule—an unsaturated fatty acid in a cell membrane, for example—and a compound seeking its electrons (Figure 8-6). The antioxidant donates electrons and/or hydrogens to the electron-seeking compound (called an ***oxidizing compound***) to neutralize it. This protects other molecules

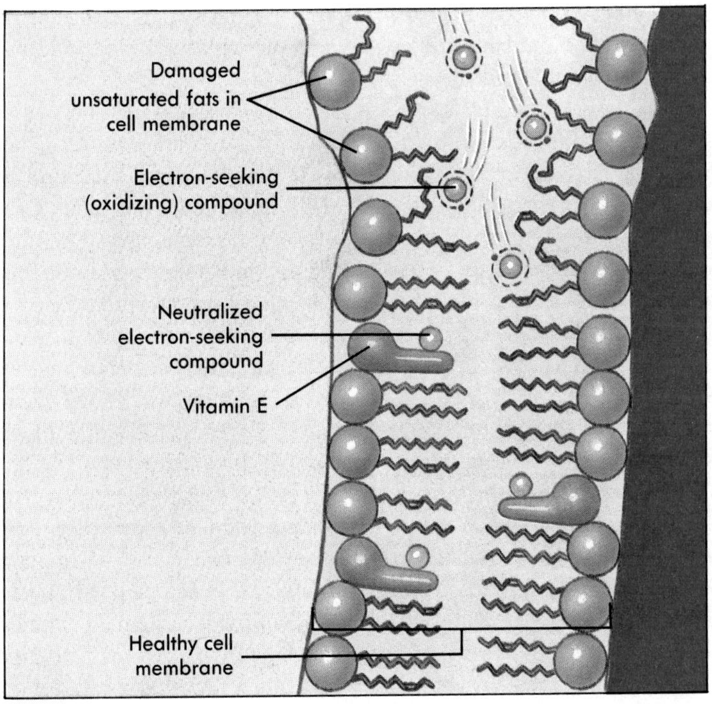

FIGURE 8-6
Vitamin E helps stop cell membrane damage. This needs to happen before much cell damage takes place.

or parts of a cell from having electrons nabbed.[25] Note that vitamin C is a water-soluble antioxidant.

If vitamin E is not present, electron-seeking compounds can oxidize parts of cell membranes, DNA, and other electron-dense cell parts. Oxidization either alters the DNA, which may increase the risk for cancer, or destroys the cell membrane, causing cell death and possibly the speeding of the aging process. After vitamin E donates two electrons, it is broken down and can no longer function. Much of this breakdown product is then excreted in the urine; some is recycled back to an active state using electron donors, such as vitamin C.

another BITE

The mineral selenium can spare some of the body's need for vitamin E. Selenium enables an enzyme in cells to decrease the formation of certain oxidizing compounds. Thus an adequate dietary intake of selenium—from cereals, meats, and seafood—reduces the need for vitamin E, whereas low selenium intake in the diet increases it.

Hemolysis *Destruction of red blood cells. The red blood cell membrane breaks down, allowing cell contents to leak into the fluid portion of the blood.*

A deficiency of vitamin E causes cell membrane breakdown, especially in red blood cells of premature infants. Unsaturated fatty acids in the red blood cell membrane are very sensitive to attack by oxidizing compounds. Because vitamin E neutralizes these agents, it protects the red blood cell membrane from damage. Red blood cell breakage, called ***hemolysis,*** commonly occurs in premature infants because they did not receive sufficient vitamin E from their mothers. The rapid growth of premature infants, coupled with the high oxygen concentration found in infant incubators, greatly increases the stress on red blood cells. This raises the risk of cell damage. Special formulas and supplements for premature infants are used to help compensate for lack of vitamin E.

Vitamin E can help improve vitamin A absorption if the dietary intake of vitamin A is low. In addition, vitamin E is used to metabolize iron in the cell and to help maintain nervous tissues and immune function.[18]

Related to vitamin E's abilities as an antioxidant are its abilities to detoxify compounds, specifically compounds that oxidize cell parts. These compounds include, but are not limited to, lead and mercury and compounds particularly toxic to the liver, such as benzene and carbon tetrachloride.

A Larger Role for Vitamin E?

We noted in Chapter 6 that evidence supports the idea that lipid oxidation products are damaging to coronary arteries and that antioxidants help prevent such damage. Such arterial damage is likely the forerunner to atherosclerosis. It now appears that the lipoprotein LDL must first undergo oxidation before plaque accumulations can occur. Because LDL is the primary carrier of fat-soluble vitamins, it is plausible that antioxidants such as vitamin E can fortify LDLs with antioxidant power to increase resistance to oxidation. Epidemiological evidence has supported the concept that elevated dietary and serum levels of antioxidants are associated with a reduced risk of heart disease.[32] One other key aspect of heart disease involves the function of platelets. These agents create blood clots that trigger a heart attack by lodging in arteries partially blocked by plaque. Vitamin E reduces the tendency of platelets to form clots.

Thus there is mounting evidence that antioxidant vitamins may provide some protection against oxidative stress, which in turn may be one cause of important disease processes. Doses used have been about 66 mg (100 IU) a day. Still, we must learn more before scientifically recommending what, if any, antioxidant supplementation is useful. Until then, most of us would be better served to abide by the proven recommendation of obtaining our vitamin E needs by eating in moderation a variety of healthful foods.[32]

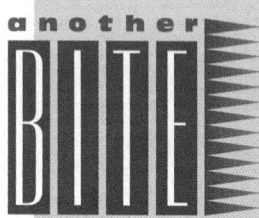

Note that popular health food literature attests to many other benefits of vitamin E. None has been shown to be true for humans. A vitamin E deficiency in laboratory animals can result in muscular dystrophy, fetal death, and impotence. The link between vitamin E deficiency and fetal death in rats—noted in 1922—gave vitamin E its chemical name ***tocopherol,*** which means to bring forth birth. However, vitamin E supplementation in humans is unable to cure any of these conditions. Vitamin E has also been promoted as an antiaging vitamin. Unquestionably, consuming the RDA for vitamin E is important for minimizing cell destruction by oxidizing compounds and maintaining cell health. However, there is no firm evidence that an intake beyond this amount enhances health.

Tocopherols *The chemical name for some forms of vitamin E.*

Prothrombin *A blood protein needed for blood clotting that requires vitamin K for its synthesis.*

Vitamin E in Foods and the RDA

The most nutrient-dense food sources of vitamin E are plant oils; some fruits and vegetables, such as asparagus and green leafy vegetables; and margarine. Animal fats have practically no vitamin E. The actual vitamin E content of a food depends on how it was harvested, processed, stored, and cooked because vitamin E is very susceptible to destruction by oxygen, metals, light, and especially repeated use of oils in deep-fat frying.

Vitamin E content in plant oils is usually high because it is used to protect the unsaturated fats found in plant oils. For healthy people, a varied diet that includes vegetable oils should supply sufficient vitamin E. Selenium in the diet, as mentioned, also spares the need for vitamin E by decreasing the formation of oxidizing compounds.

The RDA for adults for vitamin E is 8 to 10 milligrams per day. This is about the amount we eat each day. To convert from the older IU system, 10 milligrams equals about 15 IU. A variety of forms of vitamin E exist. The RDA is based on the alpha-tocopherol form. Amounts of other forms in foods are adjusted downward to reflect reduced activity when vitamin E content is expressed as alpha-tocopherol equivalents. For example, only one tenth of the amount of gamma-tocopherol is counted.

Toxicity of Vitamin E

Some studies show that an amount in excess of approximately 500 milligrams (800 IU) per day of vitamin E can cause nausea, weakness, headache, diarrhea, and fatigue, as well as interfere with vitamin K metabolism. This is about 50 times the RDA. Antagonizing vitamin K metabolism can be especially dangerous if medications that decrease blood clotting are being used, because vitamin K plays a major role in blood clotting. However, other studies show that intakes up to 2100 milligrams (3200 IU) may be safe for months. People with such diseases as phlebitis, in which blood clots form easily, sometimes benefit from large supplements of vitamin E, but they should follow such a regimen under the careful supervision of a physician. Otherwise, hemorrhages may result.

VITAMIN K

A family of compounds known collectively as vitamin K is found in plants, fish oils, and meats. One form is synthesized by bacteria in the human intestine. These bacteria supply us with about half the vitamin K we absorb every day. The other half comes from diet. The amount in our diets each day alone is generally about five times higher than our daily needs.

Functions of Vitamin K

Vitamin K is vital for blood clotting. The K stands for koagulation, as it is spelled in Denmark. This spelling is used because a Danish researcher first noted the relationship between vitamin K and blood clotting. Vitamin K contributes to the synthesis of several blood-clotting factors, including ***prothrombin.***[33]

Inactive blood-clotting factors

↓ **Action of vitamin K**

Active blood-clotting factors

A newborn's intestinal tract does not yet contain sufficient vitamin K–producing bacteria to allow for blood to clot effectively if the infant is injured. Therefore vitamin K injections are routinely given shortly after birth to bridge the gap until enough bacteria are synthesized. In adults, deficiencies of vitamin K have occurred when a person takes antibiotics for a long period and in the presence of severe long-standing fat malabsorption.

Long-term antibiotic use most likely leads to this problem because it destroys many of the intestinal bacteria that normally account for much of the vitamin K absorbed.[8]

another BITE

Physicians today often treat blood-clotting disorders by using drugs whose structures resemble that of vitamin K. The drugs dicumarol and warfarin antagonize the action of vitamin K because of their resemblance to it. People taking these drugs must be warned against consuming supplements of vitamin K and moderating intake of foods especially rich in vitamin K. This would reduce the action of the drugs.

Vitamin K in Foods and the RDA

The most nutrient-dense food sources of vitamin K are green, leafy vegetables; other vegetables, such as peas and green beans; and liver. Vitamin K provides yet another reason to consume a diet rich in fruits and vegetables. Vitamin K is quite resistant to damage from heat and cooking.

The adult RDA for vitamin K is 60 to 80 micrograms per day. The average U.S. diet contains 300 to 500 micrograms of vitamin K per day, again making a deficiency very unlikely.

Most vitamin K consumed in a day is gone by the next. This limits its toxic potential, even though it is fat soluble. At the same time, vitamin K is so abundant in the diet that there is low risk of suffering a deficiency.

CONCEPT CHECK

Vitamin E functions primarily as an antioxidant. It can donate electrons to electron-seeking (oxidizing) compounds. By neutralizing these compounds, vitamin E helps prevent cell destruction, especially the destruction of red blood cell membranes. The best sources of vitamin E are plant oils, but it occurs in a wide variety of foods.

Vitamin K plays a key role in efficient blood clotting; it contributes to the synthesis of certain blood-clotting proteins, such as prothrombin. About half the vitamin K we absorb every day is synthesized by intestinal bacteria and about half comes from our diets. The amount in the daily diet alone generally greatly exceeds our daily needs. Thus, except for newborns, a deficiency of vitamin K is unlikely, even though it is readily excreted from the body.

THE WATER-SOLUBLE VITAMINS—THE B VITAMINS AND VITAMIN C

Water-soluble vitamins are more readily excreted than are fat-soluble vitamins. Any excess generally ends up in the urine or stool, so it is important to consume the water-soluble vitamins regularly. Because they dissolve in water, large amounts of these vitamins can be lost during food processing and preparation. A summary of much of what we know about water-soluble vitamins is presented in Table 8-3.

The B Vitamins

The B vitamins are thiamin, riboflavin, niacin, pantothenic acid, biotin, vitamin B-6, folate, and vitamin B-12. Because they often occur in the same foods, a lack of one B vitamin may mean other B vitamins are low as well. The B vitamins all are changed into ***coenzymes,*** small molecules that can interact with enzymes to enable enzymes to function. In essence, the coenzymes allow enzymes to take on *active* forms (Figure 8-7).

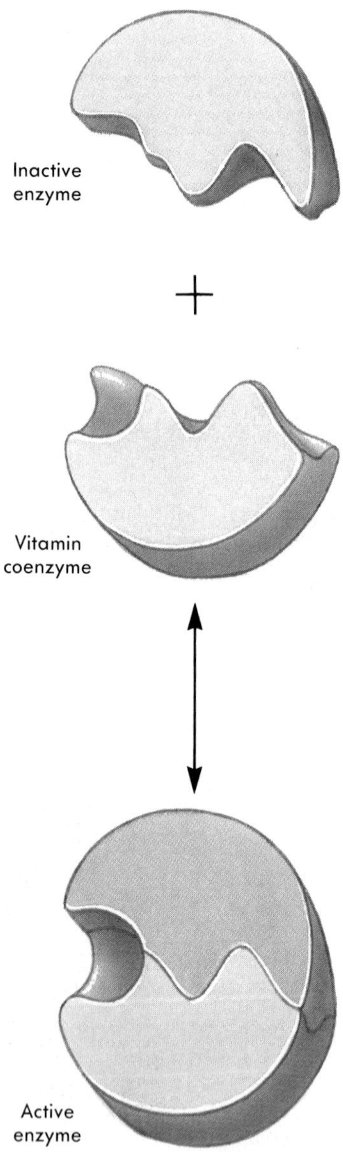

FIGURE 8-7
Coenzymes, such as those formed from B vitamins, aid in the function of certain enzymes.

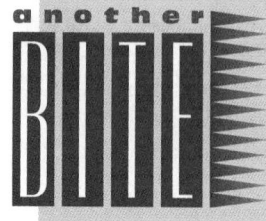

TABLE 8-3

A Summary of the Water-Soluble Vitamins, Their Functions, Deficiency Conditions, and Food Sources

Name	Major Functions	Deficiency Symptoms	People Most at Risk	Dietary Sources	RDA or ESADDI	Toxicity
Thiamin	Coenzyme involved in carbohydrate metabolism; nerve function	Beriberi: nervous tingling, poor coordination, edema, heart changes, weakness	People with alcoholism or in poverty	Sunflower seeds, pork, whole and enriched grains, dried beans, peas, brewer's yeast	1.1-1.5 milligrams	None possible from food
Riboflavin	Coenzyme involved in energy metabolism	Inflammation of mouth and tongue, cracks at corners of the mouth, eye disorders	Possibly people on certain medications if no dairy products consumed	Milk, mushrooms, spinach, liver, enriched grains	1.2-1.7 milligrams	None reported
Niacin	Coenzyme involved in energy metabolism, fat synthesis, fat breakdown	Pellagra: diarrhea, dermatitis, dementia	Severe poverty where corn is the dominant food; alcoholism	Mushrooms, bran, tuna, salmon, chicken, beef, liver, peanuts, enriched grains	15-19 milligrams	Flushing of skin at >100 milligrams
Pantothenic acid	Coenzyme involved in energy metabolism, fat synthesis, fat breakdown	Using an antagonist causes tingling in hands, fatigue, headache, nausea	People with alcoholism	Mushrooms, liver, broccoli, eggs; most foods have some	4-7 milligrams	None
Biotin	Coenzyme involved in glucose production, fat synthesis	Dermatitis, tongue soreness, anemia, depression	People with alcoholism	Cheese, egg yolks, cauliflower, peanut butter, liver	30-100 micrograms	Unknown
Vitamin B-6, pyridoxine, and other forms	Coenzyme involved in protein metabolism, neurotransmitter synthesis, hemoglobin synthesis, many other functions	Headache, anemia, convulsions, nausea, vomiting, flaky skin, sore tongue	Adolescent and adult women; people on certain medications; alcoholism	Animal protein foods, spinach, broccoli, bananas, salmon, sunflower seeds	1.8-2 milligrams	Nerve destruction at doses >500 milligrams
Folate (folic acid)	Coenzyme involved in DNA synthesis	Megaloblastic anemia, inflammation of tongue, diarrhea, poor growth, mental disorders	People with alcoholism, pregnancy, people on certain medications	Green leafy vegetables, orange juice, organ meats, sprouts, sunflower seeds	180-200 micrograms	None; nonprescription vitamin dosage is controlled by FDA
Vitamin B-12 (cobalamins)	Coenzyme involved in folate metabolism, nerve function	Macrocytic anemia, poor nerve function	Elderly people because of poor absorption; vegans	Animal foods, especially organ meats, oysters, clams (not naturally in plant foods)	2 micrograms	None
Vitamin C (ascorbic acid)	Collagen synthesis, hormone synthesis, neurotransmitter synthesis	Scurvy: poor wound healing, pinpoint hemorrhages, bleeding gums, edema	People with alcoholism, elderly men living alone	Citrus fruits, strawberries, broccoli, greens	60 milligrams	Doses >1-2 grams cause diarrhea and can alter some diagnostic tests

Vitamin status can be tested by measuring enzyme activities in red blood cells that require vitamins to function. Such biochemical tests for enzyme activity can be used to determine thiamin, riboflavin, and vitamin B-6 status.

Beriberi *The thiamin deficiency disorder characterized by muscle weakness, loss of appetite, nerve degeneration, and sometimes edema.*

The B vitamins play many key roles in metabolism. The metabolic pathways used by carbohydrates, fats, and amino acids together require input from B vitamins in their coenzyme forms. This makes many B vitamins interdependent, because they participate in the same processes.[22] Their key roles in energy metabolism allow the necessity for some B vitamins to be expressed in terms of energy use, such as 0.5 milligrams of thiamin per 1000 kcalories expended. When setting the RDA, age and gender are factored into the estimate of energy use to yield the final value—for example, 1.1 to 1.5 milligrams of thiamin for adults.

After being ingested, the B vitamins are first broken down from their coenzyme forms into free vitamins in the stomach and small intestine. The vitamins are then absorbed, primarily in the small intestine. Typically, about 50% to 90% of the B vitamins in the diet are absorbed. Once inside cells, the coenzyme forms are resynthesized. Because we make them when needed, we don't need to consume the coenzyme forms themselves.

Thiamin. Thiamin (sometimes called vitamin B-1) is used to release energy from carbohydrate, to transmit nerve impulses, and to metabolize alcohol, among other purposes. Its coenzyme participates in reactions in which a carbon dioxide is lost from a larger molecule—a reaction that is particularly important in metabolizing glucose, the primary nutrient yielded from carbohydrate digestion (Figure 8-8).[22]

Beriberi. The thiamin deficiency disease is called ***beriberi,*** a word which means "I can't, I can't" in the Sri Lankan language of Sinhalese. The symptoms include weakness, loss of appetite, irritability, nervous tingling throughout the body, poor arm and leg coordination, and deep muscle pain in the calves. A person with beriberi often develops an enlarged heart and sometimes severe edema (*wet* beriberi).

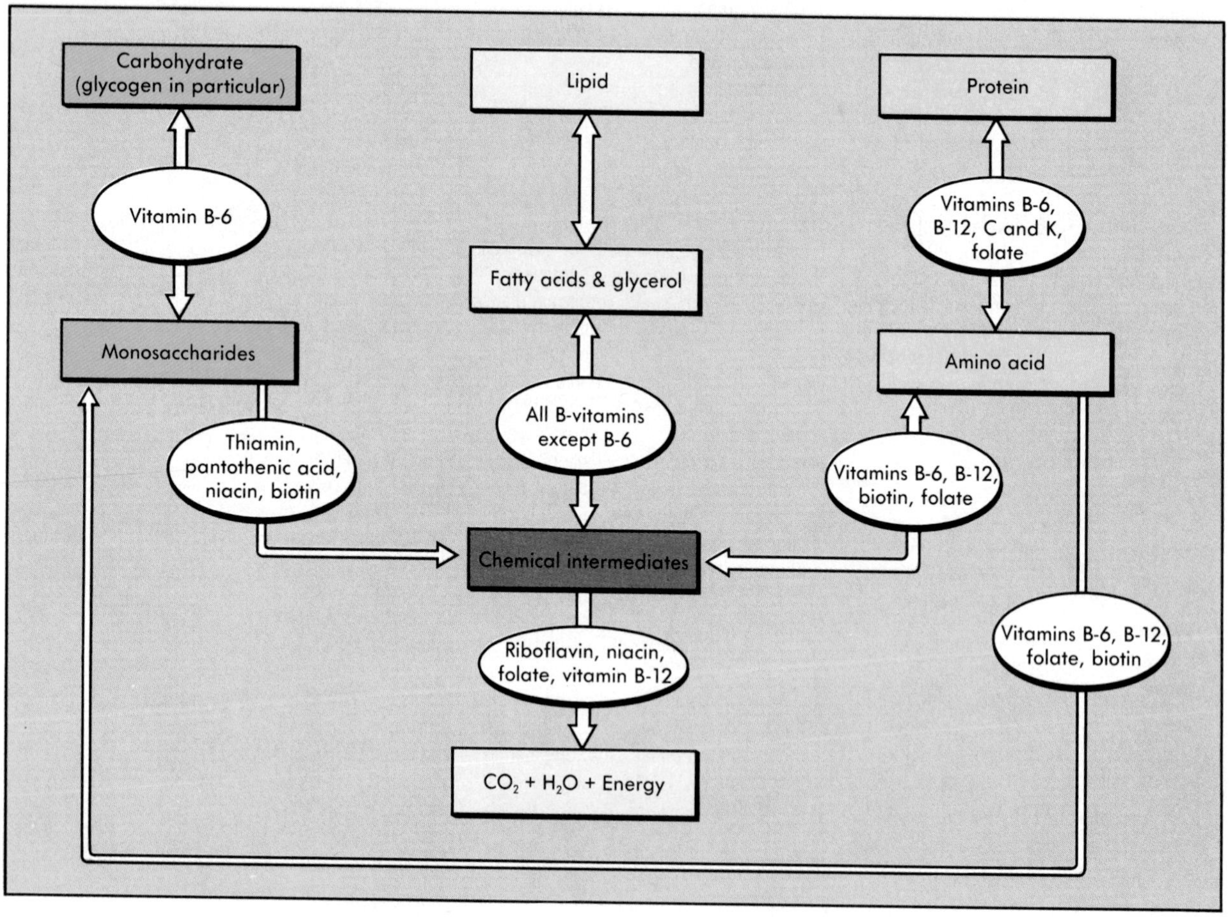

FIGURE 8-8

Examples of metabolic pathways for which vitamins are essential. The metabolism of energy-yielding nutrients requires vitamin input.

Beriberi is seen where rice is a staple and the polished (white) form is consumed rather than the brown (whole grain) form. In most parts of the world, brown rice has had its bran and germ layer removed to make white rice. This makes it a poor source of thiamin. However, thiamin is often replaced during the ***enrichment*** of white rice in the United States (see Chapter 2).

Beriberi results when glucose, the primary fuel for brain and nerve cells, is poorly metabolized. Because the thiamin coenzyme participates in glucose metabolism, body functions associated with brain and nerve action quickly show signs of a thiamin deficiency. Symptoms of depression and weakness can be seen after only 10 days on a thiamin-free diet.[22] This shows how limited the body's stores of thiamin are and how important it is to consume thiamin-rich foods daily.

Thiamin in Foods and the RDA. Foods that contain a very high nutrient density of thiamin include pork products and sunflower seeds. Whole grains (wheat germ), enriched grains, green beans, organ meats, peanuts, dried beans, and other seeds are also good sources.

Major contributors of thiamin to the American diet are white bread and rolls, crackers, pork, hot dogs, luncheon meat, cold cereals, orange juice, and dairy products. White bread, bakery products, and cereals are usually enriched with thiamin. They serve as important sources because many people eat them so often.

Aside from pork products, there is really no one excellent source of thiamin in the American diet. The foods we eat tend to contribute small amounts of thiamin. Eating a wide variety of foods is the best way to obtain enough thiamin.

The adult RDA for thiamin is about 1.5 milligrams per day for men and 1.1 milligrams per day for women. The U.S. food supply yields approximately one-and-a-half times the RDA for thiamin per person per day, but that does not account for the thiamin lost in food preparation and in cooking.

Some groups of people, such as the poor and the elderly, probably barely meet their needs for thiamin. A diet dominated by highly processed and unenriched foods, sugar, fat, and alcohol also creates a potential for thiamin deficiency. Women should be especially careful to consume good sources of thiamin. Their average intake barely meets the RDA. Oral thiamin supplements are essentially nontoxic.

Enriched *Generally refers to the addition of specific nutrients to a food following FDA guidelines. The terms* enriched bread *and* enriched rice *signify that the vitamins thiamin, riboflavin, and niacin and the mineral iron have been added to the product to improve nutritional quality.*

Dermatitis *Inflammation of the skin.*

another BITE

People with alcoholism are at great risk for thiamin deficiency because alcohol profoundly diminishes the ability to absorb and use thiamin. Furthermore, they often eat poorly. An alcohol-related thiamin deficiency can lead to a cluster of symptoms, including mental confusion, memory loss, and poor nervous system control of arms and legs.

Riboflavin. The name riboflavin comes from its yellow color—flavus means yellow in Latin. Riboflavin is sometimes referred to as vitamin B-2.

Functions of Riboflavin. The coenzymes of riboflavin participate in many energy-yielding metabolic pathways. When cells form energy using oxygen or when fats are broken down and burned for energy, the coenzymes of riboflavin are used. Some vitamin metabolism also requires riboflavin.[22]

The symptoms associated with riboflavin deficiency include inflammation of the mouth and tongue, ***dermatitis,*** cracking of tissue around the corners of the mouth (called cheilosis), various eye disorders, sensitivity to the sun, and confusion. The first symptoms of a deficiency are inflammation of the mouth and tongue. All symptoms associated with deficiency develop after approximately 2 months on a riboflavin-poor diet (containing one fourth or less of the RDA).

Clinicians have great difficulty identifying true riboflavin deficiency because it shares symptoms with deficiencies of other B vitamins, such as thiamin, vitamin B-6, and folate.

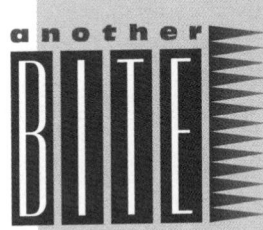

NUTRITION insight

PRESERVING VITAMINS IN FOOD

Substantial amounts of vitamins in foods can be lost from the time a fruit or vegetable is picked until you eat it. The water-soluble vitamins—particularly thiamin, vitamin C, and folate—can be destroyed with improper storage and excessive cooking. Heat, light, exposure to the air, cooking in water, and alkalinity are all factors that can destroy vitamins. The sooner the food is eaten, the less chance of nutrient loss.

In general, if the food is not to be eaten within a few days, freezing is the best method to retain nutrients. In fact, frozen vegetables and fruits are often better than supermarket *fresh* ones. Frozen foods are often processed immediately after harvesting. As part of the freezing process, vegetables are quickly blanched in boiling water. This destroys the enzymes that would otherwise degrade the vitamins. Fresh food often lingers in the grocery store or at home for a while before it is eaten.

Below are some tips to aid in preserving the vitamins in food:

- Keep fruits and vegetables cool. Enzymes in foods begin to degrade vitamins once the fruit or vegetable is picked. Chilling reduces this process, so refrigerating these foods until they are consumed is important.
- Refrigerate foods in moisture-proof containers. Nutrients keep best at temperatures near freezing, at high humidity, and away from exposure to air.
- Avoid trimming and cutting fruits and vegetables into small pieces as much as possible. The greater surface exposed speeds vitamin breakdown by oxygen. Keep in mind the outer leaves of lettuce and other greens have higher values of vitamins and minerals than the inner, tender leaves or stems. In addition, the skins of potatoes and apples and the outer layer of carrots are higher in vitamins and minerals than is the center part.
- To retain the high levels of nutrients in vegetables, microwave cooking, steaming, or using a pan or wok with very small amounts of water and a tight-fitting lid are best. The less contact with water and the shorter the cooking time, the more nutrients retained. Whenever possible, cook fruits or vegetables in their skins.
- Minimize reheating food. This reduces the vitamin content.
- Don't add baking soda to vegetables to enhance the green color. The alkalinity destroys much vitamin C, thiamin, and other vitamins.
- Store canned goods in a cool place. To get maximal nutritive value from the canned goods, serve any liquid packed with the food, whenever possible. Canned foods vary in the amount of nutrients lost, largely because of differences in storage time and temperatures in the canning process.
- Keep milk cold, covered, and away from strong light. Riboflavin may be lost in direct light. Pasteurizing raw milk does not destroy the main nutrients that milk products provide—protein, riboflavin, and calcium, among others.

Microwave cooking provides many advantages as far as preserving nutrients during cooking. When cooking vegetables in a microwave, little water is needed, decreasing the amount of vitamins that can be lost into the surrounding fluid. Also, microwave cooking exposes food to heat for a shorter period than does a conventional oven or stove.

In addition, isolated riboflavin deficiencies probably do not exist. Instead, a riboflavin deficiency would occur with deficiencies of niacin, thiamin, and vitamin B-6 because these nutrients often occur in the same foods.

Riboflavin in Foods and the RDA. Most riboflavin in the U.S. diet comes from one of its most nutrient-dense sources—milk and milk products. Including dairy products in your diet is the best guarantee for a sufficient riboflavin intake. The remainder of the U.S. riboflavin intake comes from enriched white bread, rolls, and crackers; meat; and eggs. For some people, a high meat consumption partially offsets a low intake of dairy products in terms of riboflavin intake.

Riboflavin is very stable at temperatures used to ***pasteurize*** milk and reheat foods in a microwave. However, riboflavin breaks down rapidly when exposed to light. To protect milk products from light, paper and plastic cartons—not glass—work well.

The adult RDA for riboflavin is 1.4 to 1.7 milligrams per day for men and 1.2 to 1.3 milligrams per day for women. On average, people in the United States consume the RDA for riboflavin. Athletes may need extra riboflavin because they use more fat for fuel and because their greater demand for energy taps many chemical pathways that require riboflavin. However, the RDA should still suffice. Overall, riboflavin deficiencies are rare, but some people—especially those who do not regularly consume milk and milk products—may be at risk. Athletic women should particularly take note of this. People with alcoholism risk riboflavin deficiency because they generally eat nutrient-poor diets.

We suggest that if you do not consume much milk or milk products, you should search for another dietary source of riboflavin. Enriched breakfast cereals are a good choice.

Niacin. Niacin is actually composed of a pair of related compounds. Both can function as niacin in the body. Niacin is sometimes referred to as vitamin B-3.

Functions of Niacin. The coenzyme forms of niacin function in many cellular metabolic pathways. In general, when cell energy is being formed, a niacin coenzyme is used. Synthetic pathways in the cell—those that make new compounds—also often use a niacin coenzyme. This is especially true for fat synthesis.[22]

Pellagra. Because almost every cellular metabolic pathway uses a niacin coenzyme, a deficiency causes widespread changes in the body. The entire group of symptoms is known as pellagra, which means rough or painful skin. The symptoms of the disease are known as the *three Ds—**dementia,*** diarrhea, and dermatitis (especially on areas of skin exposed to the sun). Later, death often results. Early symptoms include poor appetite, weight loss, and weakness. Pellagra became epidemic in southern Europe in the early 1700s when corn became a staple food. It became a major problem in the southeastern United States in the late 1800s and persisted until the late 1930s when standards of living and diets improved. The pellagra epidemic in the United States in the early 1900s gave impetus to a federally sponsored program in 1941 to enrich grains. Because pellagra is extremely uncommon today, there is no general need for niacin supplements.

Niacin in Foods and the RDA. The most nutrient-dense sources of niacin are mushrooms, wheat bran, tuna and other fish, chicken, asparagus, and peanuts. Most niacin in the American diet comes from enriched white bread, rolls, crackers, and breakfast cereals (to which niacin is added as part of the enrichment process), beef, chicken, and turkey. Niacin is very heat stable, so little is lost in cooking.

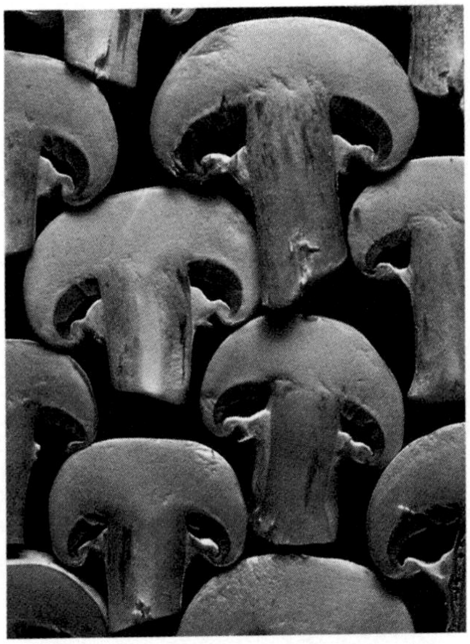

Mushrooms are rich in the B-vitamins: riboflavin, niacin, and pantothenic acid.

Pasteurize
The process of heating food products to kill pathogenic microorganisms. Under one method, milk heated to 161°F for no less than 15 seconds.

Dementia
A general loss or decrease in mental function.

another BITE

Niacin in corn is bound by a protein. This hampers its absorption. Soaking corn in an alkaline solution, such as lime water (water with calcium hydroxide), releases bound niacin and renders it more usable. Hispanic people traditionally soak corn in lime water before making tortillas. This treatment is one reason Hispanic populations never suffered much pellagra.

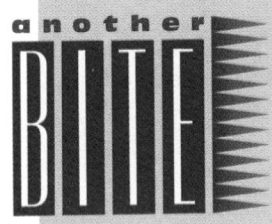

Besides the preformed niacin found in protein foods, each leftover 60 milligrams of the amino acid tryptophan—remaining from intake after protein synthesis—yields about 1 milligram of niacin.

The adult RDA for niacin is 15 to 19 milligrams per day for men and 13 to 15 milligrams per day for women. The difference in muscle mass between genders accounts for the different recommendations. The RDA is expressed as niacin equivalents to account for niacin received intact from the diet, as well as that made from tryptophan.

The average American diet contains 1.4 times the RDA, without considering the contribution from tryptophan. Note that tables of food values also ignore this contribution. Thus it is unlikely that you will develop a niacin deficiency when consuming a wide variety of foods. People with alcoholism are generally the only group to show a niacin deficiency.

Toxicity of Niacin. Intakes of 100 milligrams or more of the nicotinic acid form of niacin can lead to increased blood flow to the skin, causing a general blood vessel dilation or *flushing* in various parts of the body. Headache and itching also may result. This excessive intake is sometimes used, under a physician's guidance, to lower elevated blood cholesterol levels.

CONCEPT CHECK

The B vitamins thiamin, niacin, and riboflavin are all important in the metabolism of carbohydrates, proteins, and fats. Energy metabolism in particular requires adequate amounts of coenzymes of these three vitamins. Enriched grains are adequate sources of all three vitamins. Otherwise, pork is an excellent source of thiamin, milk is an excellent source of riboflavin, and protein foods in general—such as chicken—are excellent sources of niacin. Deficiencies of all three vitamins can occur with alcoholism; a thiamin deficiency is the most likely.

Pantothenic Acid. Like the other B vitamins, pantothenic acid helps release energy from carbohydrates, fats, and protein. By forming its coenzyme, called coenzyme A, pantothenic acid allows many important energy-yielding metabolic reactions to occur. Coenzyme A makes other molecules much more reactive. For example, coenzyme A must activate fatty acids before they can break down to yield energy. It is also used in the beginning steps of fatty acid synthesis.[22]

Pantothenic acid is so widespread in foods that a nutritional deficiency among healthy people who eat varied diets is unlikely. A full-blown deficiency is so rare that it has possibly been observed only during World War II. Prisoners in the Philippines and Japan displayed a "burning foot" syndrome described by numbness and tingling in the toes and burning and shooting pains in the feet, in addition to other mental and neurological symptoms. To study possible consequences of a pantothenic acid deficiency, researchers induce it in subjects by having them consume an antagonist to the vitamin. When antagonists are given, people suffer from such general symptoms as tingling hands, fatigue, headache, sleep disturbances, nausea, and abdominal distress.

Pantothenic Acid in Foods and the ESADDI. Pantothenic acid is present in all foods. Pantothen actually means *from every side* in Greek. Nutrient-dense sources of pantothenic acid are mushrooms, peanuts, and eggs. Other good sources are meat, milk, and many vegetables. Because pantothenic acid is not added to enriched grains, they are not especially good sources of the vitamin.

The ***estimated safe and adequate daily dietary intake (ESADDI)*** for pantothenic acid is 4 to 7 milligrams per day for adults. Not enough is known about this nutrient to set an RDA (see Chapter 2). The average U.S. intake is about 6 milligrams of pantothenic acid

Estimated Safe and Adequate Daily Dietary Intake (ESADDI) *Nutrient intake recommendations made by the Food and Nutrition Board where a range for intake of some nutrients is given, because not enough information is available to set an RDA (see Chapter 2).*

per day.[22] A deficiency of pantothenic acid might occur in alcoholism along with a very nutrient-deficient diet. However, the symptoms would probably be hidden among deficiencies of thiamin, riboflavin, vitamin B-6, and folate, so the pantothenic acid deficiency might be unrecognizable. There is no known toxicity for pantothenic acid.

Biotin. Biotin exists in two active forms in foods. In the ultimate coenzyme form, biotin acts in fat and carbohydrate metabolism. Specifically, biotin assists the addition of carbon dioxide to other compounds. By doing so, it promotes the synthesis of glucose, fatty acids, and DNA, as well as helps break down some amino acids.

No accurate measure is available for assessing biotin status. Symptoms of biotin deficiency include a scaly inflammation of the skin, changes in the tongue and lips, decreased appetite, nausea, vomiting, anemia, depression, muscle pain and weakness, and poor growth.[22]

Biotin in Foods and the ESADDI. Cauliflower, egg yolks, peanuts, and cheese are the most nutrient-dense sources of biotin. Fruits are generally poorer sources. Intestinal bacteria synthesize and supply some biotin, making a biotin deficiency unlikely. We eat even less biotin than we eliminate in the stool. However, we don't know what amount of biotin that is synthesized by bacteria in our intestines is actually absorbed. Still, if the intestinal bacteria are not sufficient, as in people who are missing a large part of the small intestine or who take antibiotics for many months, special attention should be paid to eating good food sources of biotin.

A protein called ***avidin*** in raw egg whites can bind biotin and inhibit its absorption. Feeding many raw egg whites to animals leads to classic *egg white injury* deficiency symptoms, as described previously. An occasional raw egg in eggnog is of no concern, because it would take a regular daily consumption of 12 to 24 raw eggs to produce a biotin deficiency. In cases of alcoholism, however, biotin deficiency symptoms resulting from raw eggs have been reported in people with a regular consumption of just three raw eggs a day. These people probably had very poor diets. Nevertheless, consuming raw eggs is still a concern when you consider the increased risk for *Salmonella* bacteria foodborne illness (see Chapter 17).

The ESADDI for biotin is 30 to 100 micrograms per day for adults. The average American diet is thought to contain 100 to 300 micrograms per day. It is important to avoid a biotin supplement that exceeds the ESADDI, unless a physician recommends it. We know very little about this vitamin, especially its potential for toxicity.

Avidin
A protein found in raw egg whites that can bind biotin and inhibit absorption; cooking destroys avidin.

Neurotransmitter
A compound made by a nerve cell that allows for communication between it and other cells.

Vitamin B-6. Vitamin B-6 is actually a family of three compounds. All can be changed to the active vitamin B-6 coenzyme. The general vitamin name is pyridoxine.

Functions of Vitamin B-6. The coenzymes of vitamin B-6 are needed for the activity of more than 50 enzymes involved in carbohydrate, protein, and fat metabolism. Because vitamin B-6 is needed in so many areas of metabolism, a deficiency results in widespread symptoms, such as depression, vomiting, skin disorders, irritation of the nerves, and impaired immune response.

The most important function of vitamin B-6 concerns protein, because metabolizing any amino acid requires the vitamin B-6 coenzyme. By helping to split the nitrogen group ($—NH_2$) from an amino acid, the coenzyme participates in reactions that allow a cell to either synthesize some amino acids or to break them down for energy.[22] In normal circumstances, our bodies can synthesize about half of the 20 or so types of amino acids we need. If vitamin B-6 were missing, every amino acid would become an essential amino acid—that is, an amino acid that has to be supplied by the diet.

The vitamin B-6 coenzyme is important for the synthesis of hemoglobin, the oxygen-carrying part of the red blood cell. Vitamin B-6 is also necessary for the synthesis of white blood cells, which perform a major role in the immune system.

The syntheses of many ***neurotransmitters*** require the vitamin B-6 coenzyme. Neurotransmitters allow nerve cells to communicate with each other and with other body cells. We noted previously that deficiency of vitamin B-6 results in depression, headaches, confusion, and seizures. These results are predictable, given the importance of vitamin B-6 in the metabolism of key nervous system regulators. In the 1950s, infants fed oversterilized commercial formulas developed vitamin B-6 deficiency symptoms, particularly convulsions. Heat destroyed vitamin B-6 in the formulas, possibly contributing to the infants' decreased ability to synthesize a vital neurotransmitter. Today, manufacturers are more careful to maintain adequate vitamin B-6 levels in formulas.

Premenstrual Syndrome (PMS) *A disorder found in some women in the days surrounding menstrual periods that is characterized by depression, headache, bloating, and mood swings.*

Cirrhosis *A loss of functioning liver cells, which are replaced by nonfunctioning connective tissue. Any substance that poisons liver cells can lead to cirrhosis. The most common cause is a long-standing, excessive alcohol intake.*

The link between vitamin B-6 and neurotransmitters suggested to some researchers that vitamin B-6 might be helpful in the treatment of ***premenstrual syndrome (PMS).*** This disorder appears in some women and is associated with menstrual periods. It is characterized by depression, headache, bloating, and mood swings. Researchers thought that increasing vitamin B-6 intake might increase the synthesis of a neurotransmitter that controls mood and in turn decrease the depression associated with PMS. Until more well-controlled studies are conducted, it is not possible to conclude that vitamin B-6 supplements alleviate the symptoms of PMS.[27] In addition, vitamin B-6 has a great potential for toxicity. Some women have suffered toxic side effects of vitamin B-6 in attempting to treat themselves for PMS. The cause of PMS is not well understood, but a better approach to treatment is to eat a nutrient-rich diet; emphasize starches over fats; decrease alcohol, caffeine, nicotine, and salt to decrease symptoms of nervousness, depression, and bloating; and increase exercise to stimulate relaxation.[27] If nutrition-related therapy is not helpful, women with PMS should seek a physician's advice. They should definitely avoid the PMS "cures" widely available today. These are sold both in drug stores and by mail order.

Similarly, the benefits of using vitamin B-6 to treat carpal tunnel syndrome are open to question. This syndrome is thought to affect people whose jobs involve repetitive motions that have an adverse impact on the carpal tunnel, an opening in the wrist through which tendons, nerves, and blood vessels pass. Of seven studies in which vitamin B-6 was used to treat this syndrome, five showed modest improvement in certain symptoms. The one controlled study showed a variable effect. Several of these studies were not double-blind, placebo-controlled trials, and criteria for improvement of symptoms varied between studies. Thus there is no strong evidence for a benefit of vitamin B-6, but a reduction in pain is possible.[4] Because of potential toxicity, any therapy must be supervised by a physician.

Vitamin B-6 in Foods and the RDA. The most nutrient-dense sources of vitamin B-6 are such fruits and vegetables as bananas, cantaloupe, broccoli, and spinach. But animal foods are the best sources, because the vitamin B-6 present is often more absorbable than that in plant foods.[20] Good animal sources include meat, fish, and poultry (vitamin B-6 is stored in muscles). Because vitamin B-6 is not added to foods as part of an enrichment process, breads, cakes, and cookies are not major sources as they are for some other B vitamins. Food tables listing vitamin B-6 are often incomplete because measuring this vitamin in foods is difficult.

The adult RDA for vitamin B-6 is 2 milligrams per day for men and 1.6 milligrams per day for women. The RDA is set high in response to high protein intakes (which leads to more protein metabolism) of people in the United States. Average consumption of vitamin B-6 in the United States approximately equals the RDA. Athletes may need more vitamin B-6 because they use more glycogen for fuel (glycogen metabolism requires vitamin B-6), use more amino acids for fuel, and eat a lot of protein. However, their usual dietary protein intake should easily supply any extra vitamin B-6 needed.

Numerous studies show that about 35% to 40% of adolescent, adult, and elderly women do not meet their RDA for vitamin B-6.[13] However, because vitamin B-6 values of many foods are not known, they are not counted. True intakes, then, may be greater. Women also often eat less protein than that on which the RDA is based. Today, it is not possible to reliably separate adequate vitamin B-6 status from an abnormal or deficient state. Still, nutritionists are concerned that the vitamin B-6 status of many women needs improvement.

People with alcoholism are susceptible to a vitamin B-6 deficiency, because acetaldehyde—a metabolite formed when ethanol (alcohol) is metabolized—can displace the vitamin B-6 coenzyme from its enzyme. This process increases the tendency for vitamin B-6 to be broken down. In addition, alcoholism decreases both the absorption of vitamin B-6 and its synthesis into the coenzyme form. ***Cirrhosis*** also disables liver tissue from actively metabolizing vitamin B-6. Cirrhosis often accompanies alcoholism (see Chapter 15).

Toxicity of Vitamin B-6. Intakes of 2 to 6 grams of vitamin B-6 per day for 2 to 40 months can lead to irreversible nerve damage. These high doses have usually been used by women with PMS. Symptoms of toxicity include walking difficulties and hand and foot numbness. Some nerve damage is probably reversible, but other nerve damage is probably permanent. There is concern about toxicity from doses of vitamin B-6 as low as 500 milligrams per day. This concern deserves note. Since 500 milligram tablets of vitamin B-6 are available in health food stores, it is quite easy to take a toxic dose.

CONCEPT CHECK

Pantothenic acid and biotin both participate in the metabolism of carbohydrate and fat. A deficiency of either vitamin is unlikely: pantothenic acid is found widely in foods, and our need for biotin is probably partially met by intestinal synthesis from bacteria. Vitamin B-6 is important for protein metabolism, neurotransmitter synthesis, and other key metabolic functions. Headache, anemia, nausea, and vomiting can result from a vitamin B-6 deficiency. Women should take particular care to consume a diet rich in vitamin B-6, emphasizing animal protein foods, broccoli, spinach, and bananas.

Folate. In the past, folate was known as folic acid and folacin. Today, the term folate is preferred, because it encompasses the variety of food forms of the vitamin.

Functions of Folate. Probably the most important role of the folate coenzymes is helping to form DNA.[17] The active coenzymes help in this synthesis by supplying or accepting single carbon compounds. The coenzymes also help metabolize various amino acids and their derivatives. One major result of a folate deficiency is that in the early phases of red blood cell synthesis the immature cells cannot divide because they cannot form new DNA. The cells grow larger and larger, because they can still synthesize enough protein and other cell parts to make new cells. But when it is time for the cells to divide, the amount of DNA is insufficient to form two nuclei. The cells then remain in a large immature form, known as a ***megaloblast.*** Megaloblasts can convert to abnormally large red blood cells, called ***macrocytes,*** but they have a hard time doing so because of difficulty leaving the bone marrow to enter the bloodstream.

Because the bone marrow of a folate-deficient person produces mostly immature megaloblast cells, few mature red blood cells (called erythrocytes) arrive in the bloodstream. When fewer mature red blood cells are present, the blood's capacity to carry oxygen decreases, causing ***anemia.*** In short, a folate deficiency causes megaloblastic anemia.[10]

The changes in red blood cell formation occur after 7 to 16 weeks on a folate-free diet, depending on the person's folate stores. White blood cell formation is also affected but to a lesser degree. In addition, cell division throughout the entire body is disrupted. We focus primarily on red blood cells because they are easy to examine and have a relatively short life span. The need to continually replenish red blood cells leads to a great demand for folate, making anemia the first major symptom of folate deficiency. Other symptoms of folate deficiency are inflammation of the tongue, diarrhea, poor growth, mental confusion, and problems in nerve function.[17]

Some forms of cancer therapy provide a vivid example of the effects of a folate deficiency on DNA metabolism. A cancer drug, methotrexate, closely resembles a form of folate but cannot act in its place. Because of this resemblance, when methotrexate is taken in high doses, it hampers folate metabolism. In essence, methotrexate crowds out folate in the metabolic pathways. The result is less formation of the active folate coenzymes. DNA synthesis, and consequently cell division, then decreases. Because cancer cells are among the most rapidly dividing cells in the body, they are among those affected first. However, other rapidly dividing cells, such as intestinal cells and skin cells, are also

Folate deficiencies also often occur with alcoholism. Symptoms of a folate-related anemia can signal a physician to the possibility of alcoholism.

Megaloblast
A large, immature red blood cell that results from the particular cell's inability to divide when it normally should.

Macrocyte
A greatly enlarged mature red blood cell; it has a short life span.

Anemia
Generally refers to a decreased oxygen-carrying capacity of the blood. This can be caused by many factors.

affected. Not surprisingly, typical side effects of methotrexate therapy are diarrhea, vomiting, and hair loss. These are also typical folate deficiency symptoms.

Folate in Foods and the RDA. Green, leafy vegetables (*folate* is derived from the Latin word *folium,* which means foliage), organ meats, sprouts, other vegetables, and orange juice are the most nutrient-dense sources of folate. In fact, 1 cup of orange juice contains about half of the RDA. While orange juice is promoted for its vitamin C content, an added benefit is its substantial folate contribution. The vitamin C in the juice also reduces folate destruction.

Food processing and preparation destroy 50% to 90% of the folate in food. Folate is very susceptible to destruction by heat. This underscores the importance of regularly eating fresh fruits and raw or lightly cooked vegetables. Vegetables retain their nutrients best when cooked quickly in minimal water—steaming, stir-frying, or microwaving.

The adult RDA for folate is 180 to 200 micrograms per day. These figures approximate the current folate content of the typical American diet without accounting for losses incurred during preparation and cooking. Folate deficiencies are possible during pregnancy. Pregnant women need extra folate to meet the greater cell division rate, and therefore greater DNA synthesis, for themselves and the fetus. The risk of certain types of birth defects is increased if pregnant women underconsume folate (see Chapter 14). One important reason that women need to see their physicians early in pregnancy is to find out whether they need to increase their dietary folate sources (or start folate supplements). The most prudent course is to make sure one's diet is rich in folate when there is a chance of becoming pregnant. Some birth defects take place in the very early stages of pregnancy.[37] Young women, especially those taking oral contraceptives, often register low serum folate values.[1] It is important for all women to seek good sources of folate in foods and eat those foods regularly. FDA is currently examining the need to fortify flour with folate to aid in reaching this goal.

Legal Limits Imposed on Folate Supplements. FDA limits the amount of folate in a vitamin supplement to 400 micrograms. This measure is taken to prevent excess folate from masking a vitamin B-12 deficiency. The metabolisms of folate and vitamin B-12 are linked, as we will soon discuss. For now, note that the major early detectable symptom of a vitamin B-12 deficiency is a change in blood cell formation, which results mainly in a folate-related anemia. However, this symptom does not occur if a large amount of folate is consumed regularly. Hence, the other serious effects of a vitamin B-12 deficiency can exist undetected.[17]

A vitamin B-12 deficiency, for other reasons, can eventually result in paralysis and death. If a vitamin B-12 deficiency is developing in a person, it is important for a physician to diagnose and treat it early. Limiting folate in supplements aids in this goal.

Vitamin B-12. Vitamin B-12 represents a family of compounds that contain the mineral cobalt. All vitamin B-12 compounds are synthesized by bacteria, fungi, and other lower organisms.

Absorption of Vitamin B-12. The body's complex means of absorbing vitamin B-12 is unique among vitamins. Vitamin B-12 in food enters the stomach and is released from other materials by digestion, especially by stomach acid. The free vitamin B-12 then binds with a protein called ***R-protein,*** which is produced by salivary glands in the mouth (Figure 8-9). The R-protein/vitamin B-12 complex travels to the small intestine, where enzyme action removes the R-protein.

Once vitamin B-12 is free again, it binds to the ***intrinsic factor,*** a type of protein made by the stomach's acid-producing cells. The resulting intrinsic factor/vitamin B-12 complex travels to the last portion of the small intestine, called the ***ileum.*** Ileum cells absorb vitamin B-12 and transfer it to a special blood transport protein.[17]

Using this system, approximately 30% to 70% of dietary vitamin B-12 is absorbed, depending on the body's need for it. Any failure in this system results in only 1% to 2% absorption of dietary vitamin B-12.

Vitamin B-12 absorption can be disrupted by such causes as inefficient synthesis of intrinsic factor, a genetic deficiency in R-protein synthesis, absence of the ileum or stom-

R-Protein
A protein produced by the salivary glands that participates in vitamin B-12 absorption.

Intrinsic Factor
A proteinlike compound produced by the stomach that enhances vitamin B-12 absorption.

Ileum
Essentially, the area consisting of the last half of the small intestine.

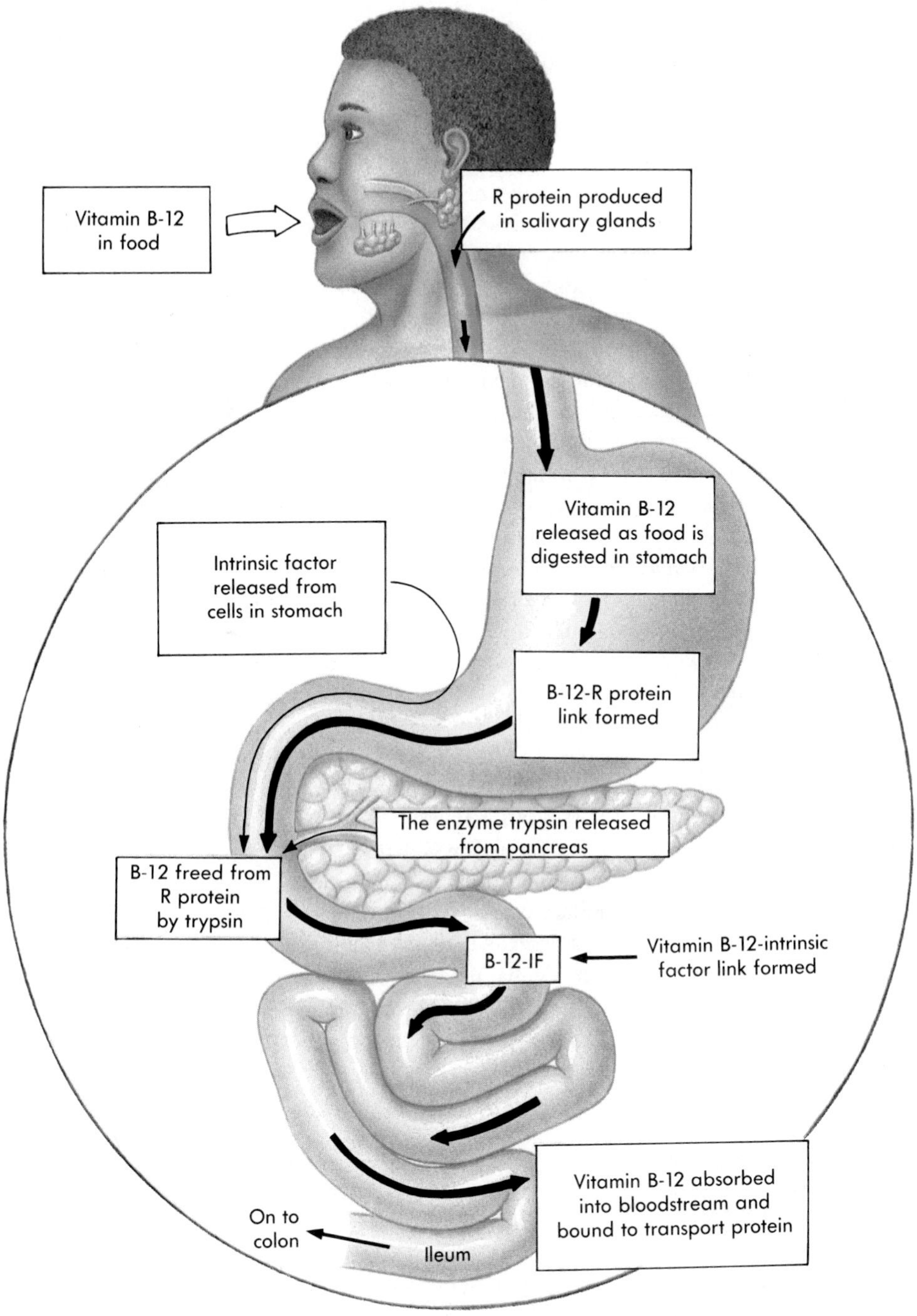

In the 1920s, researchers noted that they could cure a vitamin B-12 deficiency with massive amounts of liver or with concentrated water extracts of liver. In this case, the researchers cured a vitamin B-12 absorption defect by providing enough vitamin to allow simple diffusion across the intestinal tract to suffice. No R-protein/intrinsic factor system was needed.

FIGURE 8-9
Absorption of vitamin B-12. Many factors and sites in the GI tract participate.

ach, or tapeworm infestations. Once a defect in absorption is established, the person usually takes monthly injections of vitamin B-12 to bypass the need for absorption. About 95% of all cases of vitamin B-12 deficiencies in healthy people result from defective vitamin B-12 absorption, rather than from inadequate intakes. This is especially true for elderly people. As we age the stomach loses its ability to synthesize the intrinsic factor needed for vitamin B-12 absorption.[17]

Functions of Vitamin B-12. Vitamin B-12 participates in a variety of cellular reactions. Probably its most important function is in folate metabolism. Vitamin B-12 is required to convert folate coenzymes to the active forms needed for important metabolic reactions, such as DNA synthesis. Without vitamin B-12, reactions that require certain active forms of folate do not take place in the cell. Thus a vitamin B-12 deficiency contributes to what amounts to a folate deficiency. Another vital function of vitamin B-12 is

Pernicious Anemia *The anemia that results from a lack of vitamin B-12 absorption; it is* pernicious *because of associated nerve degeneration that can result in eventual paralysis.*

maintaining the myelin sheaths that insulate nerve fibers from each other.[24] People with vitamin B-12 deficiencies show patchy destruction of the myelin sheaths. This destruction eventually causes paralysis and perhaps death.

Pernicious Anemia. In the past the inability to absorb vitamin B-12 eventually led to death. Researchers in mid-nineteenth century England noted a form of anemia that caused death within 2 to 5 years of the initial illness, mainly because it destroyed the nerves. They called it ***pernicious anemia*** (pernicious literally means *leading to death*). Clinically, the anemia looks much like a folate deficiency anemia.

You can probably guess why the two types of anemia are similar—the folate/vitamin B-12 connection. Without vitamin B-12, folate can't convert to the active coenzymes needed to synthesize red blood cells. Because many macrocytes appear in the bloodstream, the vitamin B-12 anemia is called a macrocytic anemia. In pernicious anemia, symptoms of nerve destruction take about 3 years to appear. When a vitamin B-12 deficiency is caused strictly by a lack of the vitamin in the diet, it would take even longer for significant nerve damage to show up because whenever absorption is possible, tiny amounts suffice. Besides the anemia, symptoms of pernicious anemia include weakness, sore tongue, back pain, apathy, and tingling in the extremities.[17]

Vitamin B-12 in Foods and the RDA. The most nutrient-dense sources of vitamin B-12 are clams, oysters, and hot dogs. Beef, pork, eggs, and milk are also good sources. Vitamin B-12 is present in large amounts only in animal foods. While plants can contain vitamin B-12, they do not make it. Any vitamin B-12 present in plants comes from contamination with organisms that can make it—soil organisms, stray bacteria, or yeast. This contamination can contribute some vitamin B-12 to the vegan's diet. However, these are not reliable sources (see Chapter 7).[17]

The RDA for vitamin B-12 for adults is 2 micrograms per day. The average diet in the United States includes approximately 8 micrograms of vitamin B-12 per day. This high intake provides the average meat-eating person with 2 to 3 years' storage of vitamin B-12 in the liver. Thus if you eat animal foods regularly and can absorb vitamin B-12, a vitamin B-12 deficiency is highly unlikely. It takes approximately 20 years of consuming a diet essentially free of vitamin B-12 for a person to exhibit nerve destruction caused by a diet deficiency. Vegans, who eat no animal products, should find a reliable source of vitamin B-12. As noted earlier, elderly persons are at risk for developing pernicious anemia, and regular physical examinations should test for this possibility.[17] Vitamin B-12 supplements are essentially nontoxic.

CONCEPT CHECK

Folate is needed for cell division mostly because it influences DNA synthesis. A folate deficiency results in anemia, as well as inflammation of the tongue, diarrhea, and poor growth—all signs of poor cell division. Folate is found in fresh vegetables and organ meats. It is important to emphasize fresh and lightly cooked vegetables, because much folate is lost during cooking. Folate needs during pregnancy are especially high.

Vitamin B-12 is necessary for the formation of the active coenzymes of folate. Without dietary vitamin B-12, folate deficiency symptoms—such as macrocytic anemia—develop. In addition, vitamin B-12 is necessary for maintaining the nervous system. Paralysis can develop from a vitamin B-12 deficiency. The absorption of vitamin B-12 requires a number of specific factors. If absorption is inhibited, the resulting deficiency can lead to pernicious anemia and its associated nerve destruction. Concentrated amounts of vitamin B-12 are found only in animal foods; meat eaters generally have a 2- to 3-year supply stored in the liver. Vitamin B-12 absorption may decline as we age. Monthly injections can make up for this.

Vitamin C

Scurvy—the vitamin C deficiency disease—was long ago a constant threat to the health of sailors. Its symptoms include weakness, opening of previously healed wounds, slower wound healing times, bone pain, fractures, bleeding gums, diarrhea, and pinpoint hemorrhages around hair follicles on the back of the arms and legs. On long sea voyages, captains often lost half or more of their crews to scurvy. Epidemics of scurvy occurred in Europe from 1556 to 1857, and soldiers in the U.S. Civil War died of it. In 1740, the Englishman Dr. James Lind first showed that citrus fruits—two oranges and one lemon a day—could cure scurvy. Fifty years after Lind's discovery, rations for British sailors included limes to prevent scurvy. That is how the British earned the nickname *limey*—and one reason for their preeminence at sea during the nineteenth century.

Vitamin C (ascorbic acid) is a puzzling vitamin. It is found in all living tissues, and most animals synthesize their own from the simple sugar glucose. Only guinea pigs, monkeys, some birds, a few fish, and humans need vitamin C in their diets. What is strange is that animals who synthesize vitamin C often make quite a lot of it. For instance, a pig produces 8 grams per day (though we do not benefit from it when we eat pork, because it is lost in processing). This amount is over 130 times our human RDA of 60 milligrams, and even 60 milligrams appears to be quite a generous intake for humans. As little as 10 milligrams daily can prevent scurvy.

Why some animals make so much vitamin C while other animals, including humans, appear to need so little has fueled much controversy. Is the amount of vitamin C that prevents the disease scurvy the same amount that promotes optimal health? This question hasn't been fully answered.

Absorption of Vitamin C. Vitamin C is absorbed in the small intestine. About 80% to 90% of vitamin C is absorbed when a person eats between 30 and 180 milligrams of it per day. If someone ingests 6 grams (6000 milligrams) per day, absorption efficiency drops to about 20%. A common side effect of high vitamin C intakes is diarrhea. The unabsorbed vitamin C stays in the small intestine and attracts water, finally causing diarrhea. Some health food enthusiasts even claim that the ideal dosage of vitamin C is one that produces diarrhea.

Functions of Vitamin C

Promoting Collagen Synthesis. The best understood function of vitamin C is its role in synthesizing the protein ***collagen.*** This protein is highly concentrated in connective tissue, bone, teeth, tendons, and blood vessels. It is very important for wound healing. Vitamin C increases the cross-connections between amino acids in collagen, greatly strengthening the tissues it helps form.

When a person is deficient in vitamin C, widespread changes in tissue metabolism occur. Most symptoms of scurvy are linked to a decrease in collagen synthesis. It takes about 20 to 40 days with no vitamin C intake for the first symptoms of scurvy to appear.

Acting as an Antioxidant. Vitamin C is one of the cell's water-soluble antioxidants. Recall that vitamin E is a fat-soluble antioxidant for the cell membrane. The antioxidant capabilities of vitamin C can reduce the formation of cancer-causing nitrosamines in the stomach and also keep the folate coenzymes intact, preventing their destruction. In addition, risk of cataracts in the eye is reduced by diets rich in vitamin C,[34] as well as the fat-soluble antioxidant vitamin E.[15] If vitamin C is found effective in preventing cancer, its effectiveness will probably be related to its antioxidant capabilities (see the Nutrition Issue at the end of the chapter).[5]

Enhancing Iron Absorption and the Immune System. Vitamin C facilitates iron absorption by keeping iron in the most absorbable (ferrous) form. This renders the iron much more usable in the small intestine's alkaline environment than would be for other forms of iron. Thus iron absorption is enhanced. To produce this effect, about 50 milligrams of vitamin C (about 4 ounces of orange juice) must be consumed at the same meal with the iron. Increasing vitamin C intake is very beneficial if one has poor iron stores. One symptom of vitamin C toxicity—which can occur with doses of 1 to 2 grams per day—can be overabsorption of iron, with the potential for iron toxicity.[16]

Vitamin C is also necessary for the synthesis of a number of hormones, neurotransmitters, and other vital compounds, such as bile acids and DNA. In animal studies, vitamin C deficiency allows cholesterol to accumulate in the liver and leads to high levels in the blood.

Preventing Colds and Other Infections. Vitamin C is vital for the function of the immune system, especially for the activity of certain cells in the immune system. Thus disease states can increase the need for vitamin C, but we don't know what amount above the RDA is needed (if any). Based partly on this observation, Dr. Linus Pauling gained great notoriety by claiming that vitamin C could do battle with the common cold. His 1970 book, *Vitamin C and the Common Cold,* claimed that 1000 milligrams (1 gram) of vitamin C daily (about 15 times the RDA) could reduce the number of colds for most people by nearly half. A 1976 revision recommended still higher doses. Pauling has claimed to take a daily dose of 12,000 milligrams of vitamin C and raises the intake to 40,000 if he feels a cold coming on. As a result of the popularity of his books and the respectability of his scientific credentials, millions of Americans supplement their diets with vitamin C.

But does vitamin C reliably and effectively work against colds and other infections? Most medical and nutrition scientists strongly disagree with Pauling's views of vitamin C.[16] Since the 1930s, medical investigators have rigorously explored the role of vitamin C in preventing infection. Numerous well-designed, double-blind studies have not shown vitamin C to reliably prevent colds, though it seems to slightly reduce cold symptoms. Pauling's conclusions, based on the same studies, dispute the other scientists' results. Nevertheless, most vitamin C consumed in large doses ends up in the stool or the urine. Only a small fraction of such large doses can be used. The body is totally saturated at intakes of 100 to 200 milligrams per day. This means that if more than 100 to 200 milligrams of vitamin C is ingested, it is quickly excreted.

We don't believe that colds are severe enough or last long enough to merit vitamin C therapy. However, that is a personal decision. Consuming vitamin C may alleviate a cold's symptoms somewhat, so we see no reason to discourage people from drinking a few glasses of orange juice when they have a cold. If it doesn't help them physically, it may help them psychologically. Psychological effects often work wonders. In addition, no credible evidence suggests that a dose even as high as 10 grams a day will cure colon cancer.

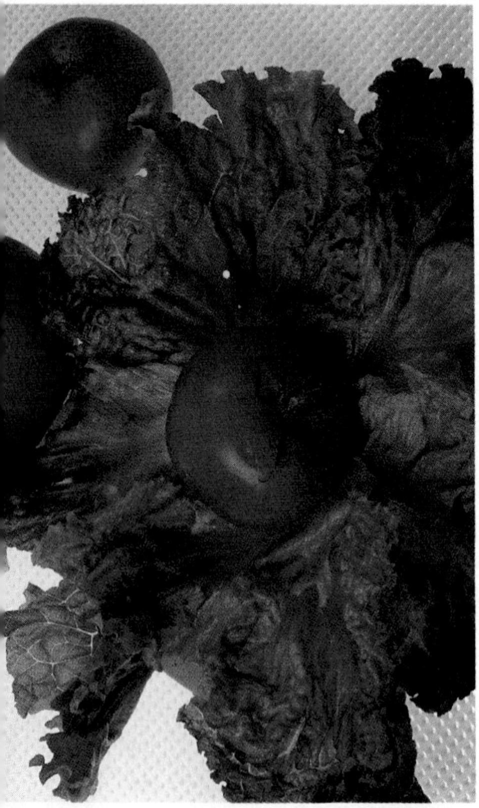

Many vegetables are good sources of vitamin C.

Vitamin C in Foods and the RDA. The most nutrient-dense sources of vitamin C are green peppers, cauliflower, broccoli, cabbage, strawberries, papayas, and romaine lettuce. Citrus fruits, potatoes, and other green vegetables are also good sources of vitamin C. The five to eight servings of fruits and vegetables from the Food Guide Pyramid can easily provide enough vitamin C. The major contributors of vitamin C in the U.S. diet are orange juice, grapefruit and grapefruit juice, tomatoes and tomato juice, fortified fruit drinks, oranges, tangerines, and potatoes.

Vitamin C is easily lost in processing and cooking. Juices are good foods to fortify with vitamin C, because their acidity reduces vitamin C destruction. Vitamin C is very unstable when in contact with heat, iron, copper, or oxygen.

The adult RDA for vitamin C is 60 milligrams per day. The 1989 RDA publication suggests that cigarette smokers consume 100 milligrams per day, because they greatly stress their lungs with oxygen and toxic by-products of cigarette smoke. The average U.S. diet yields about twice the adult RDA (120 milligrams) of vitamin C.

Today vitamin C deficiency appears mostly in alcoholic people who eat nutrient-poor diets and in elderly men who live alone and also eat poorly. Men are more susceptible to vitamin C deficiency than are women because, as a group, they tend to smoke more and are less apt to consume vitamin supplements. Studies show that about 20% of adult and elderly men have low serum vitamin C levels. Overall, a diet with limited fruit and vegetable consumption puts a person at risk of deficiency. Worldwide, scurvy is associated with poverty. It is especially common in infants who are fed boiled milk (all forms of milk are poor sources of vitamin C) and not provided with a good food source of vitamin C or a supplement.

Toxicity of Vitamin C. Vitamin C is probably not toxic when consumed in amounts less than 500 milligrams. Regularly consuming more than that can cause stomach inflammation, diarrhea, and iron toxicity (caused by overabsorption of iron).[16]

NUTRITION insight

BOGUS VITAMINS

Health food enthusiasts promote a variety of compounds as vitamins even though these substances have no importance in human nutrition. Because some of these so-called *vitamins* may cause increased growth in lower organisms, vitamin hucksters try to pass them off as necessary for humans (Figure 8-10). As these pseudovitamins continue to be represented as vitamins, sales profits amount to more and more dollars yearly.

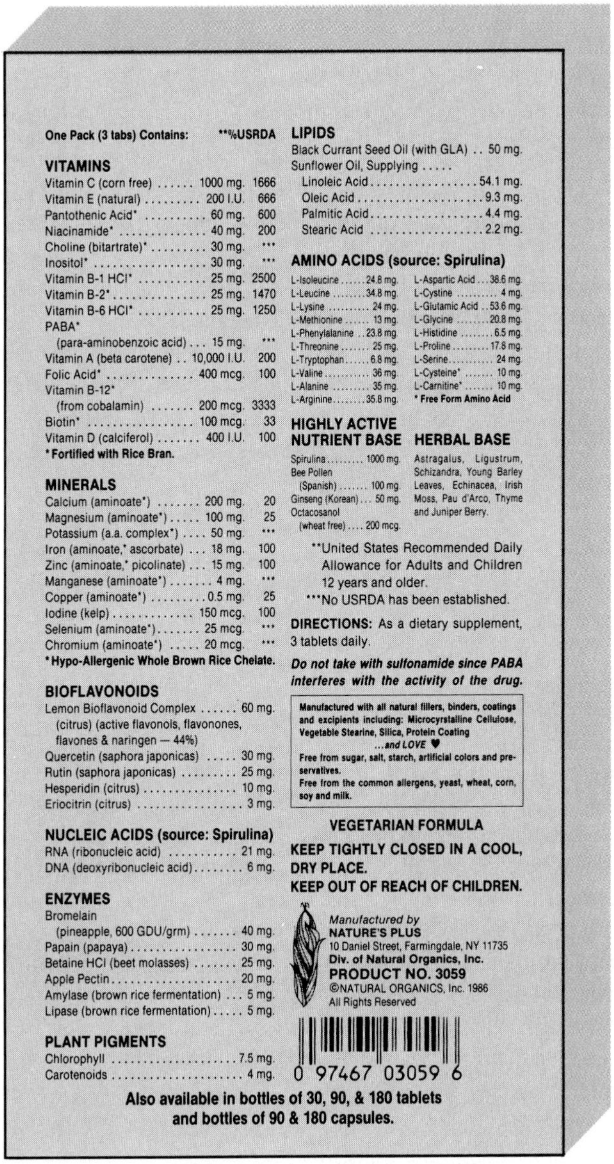

FIGURE 8-10
Health foods *are noted for containing substances the healthy body does not need—vitamin-like compounds, such as inositol, and bogus vitamins, such as bioflavonoids.*

The list of these pseudovitamins changes frequently. The following are some of the more persistent pseudos[17]:

- *Para-aminobenzoic acid (PABA):* Although this compound is part of the vitamin folate, we can't use it to make folate. Entrepreneurs represent PABA as "a member of the B complex family," omitting the words "for bacteria," so that they can sell it as a food supplement. If consumed along with sulfa antibiotics, it can defeat the effect of the antibiotic.
- *Laetrile:* This cyanide-containing compound—wrongly labeled vitamin B-17—is promoted as a cure for cancer. FDA does not recognize it as a legitimate cancer therapy. Chronic cyanide intoxication from laetriles in the diet has produced thousands of cases of slowly progressing nerve damage, resulting in blindness, deafness, and muscle weakness.
- *Bioflavonoids:* These compounds—sometimes incorrectly called "vitamin P"—include rutin and hesperidin. They were originally thought to be more effective than vitamin C alone for treating fragile blood vessels in scurvy. Today there is no recognized nutritional or medical need for bioflavonoids, although they may enhance vitamin C absorption. Most flavonoids are concentrated in the skin, peel, and outer layers of fruits and vegetables. Beverages such as tea, coffee, wine, and beer also contain significant amounts.
- *Pangamic acid:* This bogus compound—wrongly labeled vitamin B-15—has no link to nutrition and deserves no attention from anyone, including athletes. Its roots are quackery, pure and simple.

Other compounds will surely come and go in the next few years. Again, because people have been maintained for years on intravenous feedings that contain all the known essential nutrients without developing deficiency symptoms, it is unlikely that any vitamin remains to be discovered. You can be sure that if a *new* compound has the potential to be a vitamin, the Food and Nutrition Board of the National Academy of Sciences will closely examine it. If it then appears with the rest of the nutrients that have an RDA or ESADDI, you can be confident that the compound can be called a vitamin and is worth your attention.

CONCEPT CHECK

Vitamin C is important in the synthesis of collagen, a major connective tissue protein. A vitamin C deficiency, known as scurvy, causes many changes in the skin and gums, such as small hemorrhages. This is mainly because of poor collagen synthesis. Vitamin C also improves iron absorption, is involved in synthesizing certain hormones and neurotransmitters, and is a general body antioxidant. Citrus fruits, green peppers, cauliflower, broccoli, and strawberries are good sources of vitamin C. As with folate, it is important to eat fresh or lightly cooked foods, because vitamin C loses a lot of its potency in cooking. High doses of vitamin C can lead to diarrhea. These high doses do not prevent the common cold or cure cancer. However, consuming the RDA of vitamin C is part of the overall approach to good health.

Now that we have discussed the vitamins, review the Food Guide Pyramid in Chapter 2 and note how each group makes an important vitamin contribution.

VITAMIN-LIKE COMPOUNDS

A variety of vitamin-like compounds are found in the body. These include the following:

- Choline
- Carnitine
- Inositol
- Taurine
- Lipoic acid

All these vitamin-like compounds are necessary to maintain proper metabolism in the body.[3,14,29] They can be synthesized by cells using common building blocks, such as amino acids and glucose.

In disease states, synthesis of vitamin-like compounds may not meet needs, and so dietary intake can be crucial. The needs for choline, carnitine, and taurine in certain conditions, such as for premature infants, are currently being investigated.[9] Although promoted and sold by health food stores, there is no concern that these vitamin-like compounds are needed by the average healthy adult (Figure 8-10). We make them each day. Some are present only in animal foods, and because vegans—who eat no animal products—show no evidence of deficiencies, body synthesis most likely suffices for us.

SUMMARY

- Vitamins are compounds we generally need daily in small amounts from foods. They yield no energy directly, but many contribute to energy-yielding chemical reactions in the body and promote growth and development. Many vitamins act as coenzymes, which help enzymes function. Vitamins A, D, E, and K are fat soluble, whereas the B vitamins and vitamin C are water soluble.
- Vitamin A consists of a family of compounds that includes several forms of preformed vitamin A. Some carotenoids, such as beta-carotene, function as antioxidants and can also yield vitamin A. Vitamin A functions in vision, immune function, and cell development. Vitamin A is found in liver and fish oils; carotenoids are especially plentiful in dark green and orange vegetables. Vitamin A can be quite toxic, even when taken at just 5 to 10 times the RDA. High vitamin A intakes are especially dangerous during pregnancy, because they can lead to fetal malformations.
- Vitamin D is both a hormone and a vitamin. Human skin synthesizes it using sunshine and a cholesterol-like substance. If we don't spend enough time in the sun, such foods as fish oils and fortified milk must supply the vitamin. The active hormone form of vitamin D helps regulate blood calcium levels by influencing calcium absorption from the intestine. Children who don't get enough vitamin D may develop rickets, and adults with inadequate amounts in the body develop osteomalacia. Vitamin D is a very toxic substance. An intake just 2.5 to 5 times the RDA can cause problems.
- Vitamin E functions primarily as an antioxidant and is found in plant oils. By donating electrons to electron-seeking (oxidizing) compounds, it neutralizes them. This shields cell membranes and red blood cells from breakdown. Claims are made about the curative powers of vitamin E, but few have been scientifically validated.

- Vitamin K helps blood clot. About half the vitamin K absorbed each day comes from bacterial synthesis in the intestine, and the other half comes from foods, primarily green, leafy vegetables. Vitamin K is poorly stored in the body, but our dietary intake alone is usually sufficient. People who can't absorb fat well or who are on antibiotics for long periods may need extra vitamin K.
- Thiamin, riboflavin, and niacin play key roles as coenzymes in energy-yielding reactions. They help metabolize carbohydrates, fats, and proteins. Alcoholism and a poor diet can create deficiencies of these three nutrients. Enriched grain products are common sources of all three of these vitamins.
- Pantothenic acid, which participates in many aspects of cell metabolism, is widely distributed among foods. Biotin—which participates in glucose production, fat synthesis, and DNA synthesis—can be synthesized by bacteria in the intestine. We probably synthesize about half our requirement for biotin. The rest comes from such foods as eggs and cheese.
- Vitamin B-6 performs a vital role in protein metabolism, especially in synthesizing nonessential amino acids. It also helps synthesize neurotransmitters and performs other metabolic roles. Headaches, anemia, nausea, and vomiting result from a B-6 deficiency. Generally, women are more likely to have poor vitamin B-6 stores than do men. Regular consumption of animal protein foods, cauliflower, and broccoli provides needed vitamin B-6. Taking high doses causes malfunction of the nervous system.
- Folate plays an important role in DNA synthesis. Symptoms of a deficiency are generally poor cell division in various areas of the body, anemia, tongue inflammation, diarrhea, and poor growth. Pregnancy puts high demands for folate on the body. A deficiency is most likely to occur in people with alcoholism. Excellent food sources are leafy vegetables, organ meats, and orange juice. Great amounts of folate can be lost in prolonged cooking.
- Vitamin B-12 is needed to metabolize folate and to maintain the insulation surrounding nerves. A deficiency results in anemia (because of its relationship to folate) and nerve degeneration. Elderly people often absorb vitamin B-12 inefficiently. If so, they can benefit from monthly injections of the vitamin. Generally, a deficiency is unlikely because vitamin B-12 is highly concentrated in animal foods, which constitute a major part of the American diet. Vitamin B-12 does not occur naturally in plant foods. Vegans need a supplemental source.
- Vitamin C is used mainly to synthesize collagen, a major protein for building connective tissue. A vitamin C deficiency results in scurvy, which is evidenced by poor wound healing, pinpoint hemorrhages in the skin, and bleeding gums. Vitamin C also enhances iron absorption and is needed for synthesizing some hormones and neurotransmitters. Fresh fruits and vegetables, especially citrus fruits, are generally good sources. Because a great amount of vitamin C is lost in cooking, a good diet should emphasize fresh or lightly cooked vegetables. Deficiencies can occur in people with alcoholism and in those whose diets lack sufficient fruits and vegetables. Smoking makes matters worse for people already at risk.

STUDY QUESTIONS

1. Why do fat-soluble vitamins tend to be much more toxic to the body than the water-soluble vitamins?
2. Name three vitamins whose needs increase during increased energy expenditure and explain why.
3. What three vitamins have a source originating within the body? Describe those sources.
4. Although folate is not known to produce any toxic effects, FDA allows only a limited amount in supplementary forms. Why?
5. Because the deficiency disease of vitamin C is so severe, is it a good idea for Americans to take excess supplementation to avoid such a deficiency? Do the benefits of vitamin C supplementation above and beyond the RDA outweigh negative consequences? Discuss these two questions.
6. What distinguishes the vitamin-like compounds from actual vitamins? Do they warrant any special diet planning?

REFERENCES

1. Bailey LB: Evaluation of a new recommended dietary allowance for folate, *Journal of The American Dietetic Association* 92:463, 1992.
2. Bender MM and others: Trends in prevalence and magnitude of vitamin and mineral supplement usage and correlation with health status, *Journal of The American Dietetic Association* 92:1096, 1992.
3. Berdanier CD: Is inositol an essential nutrient? *Nutrition Today,* p. 22, March/April 1992.
4. Bernstein AL, Dinesen JS: Brief communication: effect of pharmacologic doses of vitamin B-6 on carpal tunnel syndrome, electroencephalographic results, and pain, *Journal of the American College of Nutrition* 12:73, 1993.
5. Block G: The data support a role for antioxidants in reducing cancer risk, *Nutrition Reviews* 50:207, 1992.
6. Burnand B and others: Serum 25-hydroxyvitamin D: distribution and determinants in the Swiss population, *American Journal of Clinical Nutrition* 56:537, 1992.
7. Callaway CW and others: Statement on vitamin and mineral supplements, *Journal of Nutrition* 117:1649, 1987.
8. Carlin A, Walker WA: Rapid development of vitamin K deficiency in an adolescent boy receiving total parenteral nutrition following bone marrow transplantation, *Nutrition Reviews* 49:179, 1991.
9. Carroll JE: Carnitine deficiency revisited, *Journal of Nutrition* 117:1501, 1987.
10. Clark NG and others: Treatment of iron-deficiency anemia complicated by scurvy and folic acid deficiency, *Nutrition Reviews* 50:134, 1992.
11. Comstock GW and others: Prediagnostic serum levels of carotenoids and vitamin E as related to subsequent cancer in Washington County, Maryland, *American Journal of Clinical Nutrition* 53:260S, 1991.
12. Council on Scientific Affairs: Vitamin preparations as dietary supplements and as therapeutic agents, *Journal of the American Medical Association* 257:1929, 1987.
13. Driscoll JA and others: Longitudinal assessment of vitamin B-6 status in Southern adolescent girls, *Journal of The American Dietetic Association* 87:307, 1987.
14. Feller AJ, Redman D: Role of carnitine in human nutrition, *Journal of Nutrition* 118:541, 1988.
15. Hankinson SE and others: Nutrient intake and cataract extraction in women: a prospective study, *British Medical Journal* 305:335, 1992.
16. Herbert V: Viewpoint: does mega-C do more good than harm or more harm than good? *Nutrition Today* p. 28, January/February 1993.
17. Herbert V: "Folic acid" and "vitamin B-12" and "pseudovitamins." In Shils ME, Young VR, editors: *Modern nutrition in health and*

disease, ed 7, Philadelphia, 1988, Lea & Febiger.

18. Howard LJ: The neurologic syndrome of vitamin E deficiency: laboratory and electrophysiologic assessment, *Nutrition Reviews* 48:169, 1990.
19. Jacobs MM: Diet, nutrition and cancer: an overview, *Nutrition Today* p. 19, May/June 1993.
20. Leklem JE: Vitamin B-6: of reservoirs, receptors and requirements, *Nutrition Today,* p. 4, September/October 1988.
21. Malone WF: Studies evaluating antioxidants and β-carotene as chemopreventives, *American Journal of Clinical Nutrition* 53:305S, 1991.
22. McCormick DB: "Thiamin," "riboflavin," "niacin," "vitamin B-6," "pantothenic acid," and "biotin." In Shils ME, Young VR, editors: *Modern nutrition in health and disease,* ed 7, Philadelphia, 1988, Lea & Febiger.
23. Merrill AH, Henderson JM: Diseases associated with defects in vitamin B-6 metabolism or utilization, *Annual Review of Nutrition* 7:137, 1987.
24. Metz J: Pathogenesis of cobalamin neuropathy: deficiency of nervous system s-adenosylmethionine? *Nutrition Reviews* 51:12, 1993.
25. Packer L: Protective role of vitamin E in biological systems, *American Journal of Clinical Nutrition* 53:1050S, 1991.
26. Prasad KN, Edwards-Prasad J: Vitamin E and cancer prevention: recent advances and future potentials, *Journal of the American College of Nutrition* 11:487, 1992.
27. Reid RL: Premenstrual syndrome, *New England Journal of Medicine* 324:1208, 1991.
28. Ross AC: Vitamin A and protective immunity, *Nutrition Today,* p. 18, July/August 1992.
29. Sheard NF, Zeisel SH: Choline: an essential dietary nutrient, *Nutrition* 5:1, 1989.
30. Sherman SS and others: Vitamin D status and related parameters in a healthy population: the effects of age, sex and season, *Journal of Clinical Endocrinology and Metabolism* 71:405, 1990.
31. Smith JR and others: Why are transformed cells immortal? Is the process reversible? *American Journal of Clinical Nutrition* 55:1215S, 1992.
32. Stampfer MJ and others: Vitamin E consumption and the risk of coronary heart disease in women, *New England Journal of Medicine* 328:1444, 1993.
33. Sutie JW: Vitamin K and human nutrition, *Journal of The American Dietetic Association* 92:585, 1992.
34. Taylor A: Cataract: relationships between nutrition and oxidation, *Journal of the American College of Nutrition* 12:138, 1993.
35. Walters MR and others: What is vitamin D deficiency? *Proceedings of the Society for Experimental Biology and Medicine* 199:385, 1992.
36. Weisburger JH: Nutritional approach to cancer prevention and emphasis on vitamins, antioxidants, and carotenoids, *American Journal of Clinical Nutrition* 53:226S, 1991.
37. Werler MM and others: Periconceptional folic acid exposure and risk of occurrent neural tube defects, *Journal of the American Medical Association* 269:1257, 1993.

MEASURING YOUR VITAMIN INTAKE AGAINST THE RDA

This activity requires you to reexamine the nutritional assessment you completed in Chapter 2. You recorded the types, quantities, and amounts of nutrients in the foods and drinks you consumed for one day. Then you assessed your intake by recording the total amounts of nutrient you consumed. You were then asked to compare your intake of nutrients with certain standards. Many of the standards you used were the 1989 RDA found on the inside cover of this book. Using your completed assessment, record your intakes of vitamins A, E, C, B-6, B-12, thiamin, riboflavin, niacin, and folate in the table below. Next, record the RDA for each nutrient from your assessment. Then, record the percentage of the RDA you had for each vitamin. Last, place a +, –, or = in the space provided reflecting an intake higher, lower, or equal to the RDA.

VITAMIN	INTAKE	RDA	% OF RDA	+/–/=
A				
E				
C				
THIAMIN				
RIBOFLAVIN				
NIACIN				
B-6				
FOLATE				
B-12				

Analysis

1. Which of your vitamin intakes equaled or exceeded your RDA? Are any excesses in a possibly toxic range?

____

2. Which of your vitamin intakes were below the RDA?

____

3. What foods could you eat to improve your dietary intake of vitamins? (Review sources of certain vitamins in the text.)

____

____

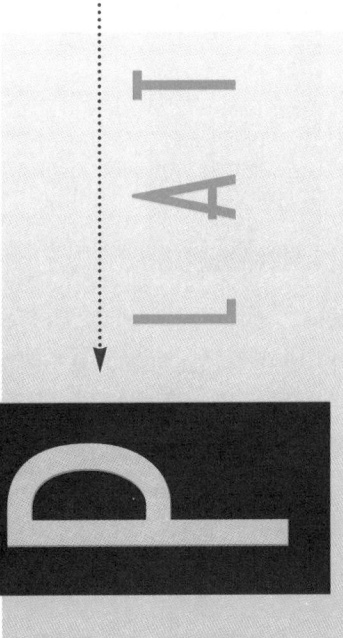

Nutrition ISSUE

NUTRITION AND CANCER

Cancer is the second leading cause of death for adults in the United States. Cancer is actually many diseases; it affects different types of cells and arises from many different causes (Figure 8-11). Causes of skin cancer differ from the causes of breast cancer, and their treatments also differ. We need to look seriously at cancer in general and consider our risk of getting it. As we age, the risk of cancer steadily increases.

Cancer occurs more in some families than in others; genetic background plays a role in the risk for cancer, especially colon cancer. However, lifestyle is also a critical factor. We know this because rates of cancer differ around the world. The Japanese, for example, have more stomach cancer and Americans have more colon cancer. When Japanese people immigrate to the United States, their rates of stomach cancer decrease but their rates for colon cancer increase. In addition, one third of all cancer cases in America are caused by smoking tobacco.

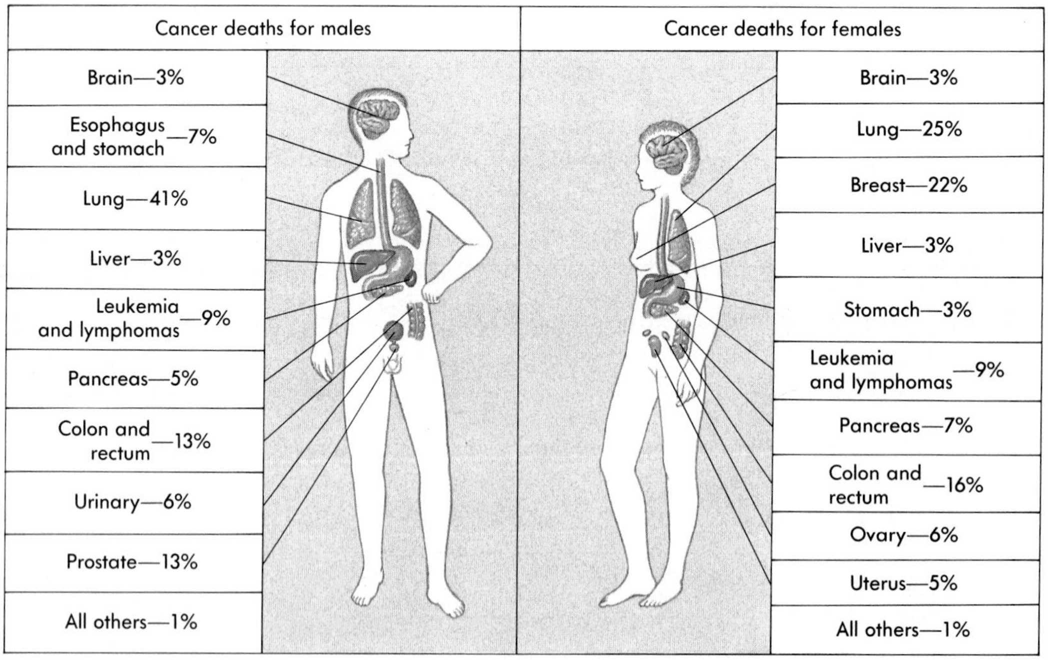

FIGURE 8-11

Approximate cancer deaths by site and gender. Lung cancer is now the number one cancer killer in both men and women.

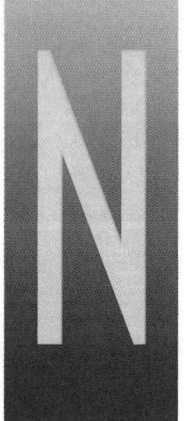

Cancer-Causing Mechanisms

To understand how to prevent cancer we first need to examine how cancer develops in the body. The process begins with an alteration in DNA, the genetic material in our cells. This is called the *initiation phase.* When the DNA is altered, the cell may no longer respond to normal body control signals. The cell can then dictate its own rate of growth. It is not inhibited from growing and may do so at the expense of the cells around it.[31]

Agents That Alter DNA Initiate the Cancer Process. There are many ways to alter DNA and so initiate the cancer process. A substance or phenomenon can either directly alter DNA or lead to processes that in turn alter DNA (Figure 8-12). The timeline for disruption of DNA ranges from less than a second to days. And the longer we live, the more the opportunity exists for this to happen. ***Radiation*** from the sun (ultraviolet rays) can cause DNA to bind itself or break into pieces. This is one way skin cancer begins. The altered skin cells may then begin to grow out of control. Cancer can result. X-rays, another type of radiation, readily damage the genetic material. Certain chemicals, both natural and man-made, can alter DNA. These are often called ***carcinogens.*** Viruses alter DNA by inserting their ***genes*** into human cells. If the genes promote growth, the cell may begin to grow out of control.

Thus three common means of altering DNA are through radiation, certain chemicals, and viruses. However, having a cell with altered DNA does not mean cancer is inevitable. Special enzymes travel up and down the DNA to repair breaks and changes in it. The repair enzymes may fix alterations before the cell begins to grow out of control.

Promotion is Part of the Process That Increases Cancer Risk. Cells in which the cancer process has been initiated must be encouraged to undergo cell division for cancer to occur. This is the second phase of the cancer process, called the *promotion phase.* Compounds that increase cell division are thought to promote cancer by either decreasing the time available for repair enzymes to act or simply encouraging cells with altered DNA to develop and grow (Figure 8-12). Likely candidates are high levels of estrogen in the bloodstream, alcohol intake, and probably dietary fat intake. Once a cell divides, any altered DNA will be reproduced along with the rest of the genetic material. Now the cell will follow its newly altered genetic instructions. Development and growth of these altered cells may take up to 20 years.

Radiation ■
Literally, energy that is emitted from a center in all directions. Various forms of radiation energy include x-rays and ultraviolet rays from the sun.

Carcinogens ■
Compounds that have potential to cause cancer.

Genes ■
The genetic material on chromosomes that make up DNA. Genes provide the blueprints for the production of cell proteins.

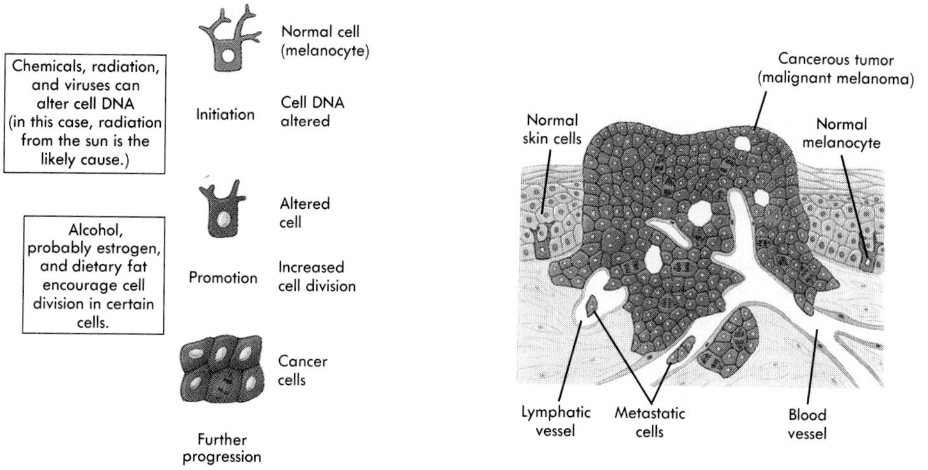

FIGURE 8-12
Progression from a normal skin cell to cancer through the initiation, promotion, and progression phases. The ball of cells is a developing cancer tumor. As the mass of cells grows, it can invade surrounding tissues, eventually penetrating into both lymph and blood vessels. These vessels carry spreading (metastatic) cancer cells throughout the body, where they can form new cancer sites.

Alcohol in large amounts is toxic to cells. The resulting cell death creates a need for new cell division. In this way, alcohol can increase cell division and therefore the risk for cancer especially in the mouth and esophagus.

Once an altered cell has multiplied, there is still a chance that cancer won't result. First, the cell mass must increase until it can significantly affect body metabolism. During this initial stage of growth, called the *progression phase,* the immune system may find the altered cells and destroy them. Or the cancer cells may be so defective that their own DNA limits their ability to grow, and they die anyway.[31]

another BITE

If the cancer is left untreated, it can spread throughout the body. This makes death more likely. For this reason early detection is important. Aids to early detection include the seven warning signals of cancer:

1. A change in bowel or bladder habits
2. A sore that does not heal
3. Unusual bleeding or discharge
4. A thickening or lump in the breast or elsewhere
5. Indigestion or difficulty in swallowing
6. An obvious change in a wart or mole
7. A nagging cough or hoarseness

There are other ways to detect cancer early. Colon and rectum examinations for adults of both genders and pap tests and regular breast examinations for women are recommended by the American Cancer Society.

Diet and Cancer

Besides a generally nutritious diet, other factors related to diet and lifestyle can reduce your risk of cancer (Table 8-4). For example, maintain a desirable body weight and practice regular physical activity. Both obesity and physical inactivity are linked to increased risk of many types of cancer.

In fact, obesity is related to all major forms of cancer except lung cancer. These include breast cancer, colon cancer, endometrial cancer, and prostate cancer. The link probably occurs because adipose tissue synthesizes estrogen from other hormones in the bloodstream. High levels of estrogen in the bloodstream promote cancer. Habitual excessive overeating, especially fatty foods, may also promote cancer. When animals are fed diets high in fat or total energy, they tend to experience more cancer, especially in the colon and breast.

TABLE 8-4

General Dietary Recommendations to Reduce the Risk of Cancer*

1. Avoid obesity.
2. Reduce fat intake to a maximum of 30% of total kcalories as a start. Further reduction to about 20% of kcalories has also been endorsed by some cancer researchers.
3. Eat more high-fiber foods, such as fruits, vegetables, and whole-grain cereals.
4. Include foods rich in vitamins A and C in the daily diet.
5. If alcohol is consumed, do not drink excessively.
6. Use moderation when consuming salt-cured, smoked, and nitrite-cured foods.

**The National Cancer Institute (U.S.) generally endorses the above but warns not to exceed 35 grams of dietary fiber intake.*
The American Cancer Society and The Canadian Dietetic Association generally endorse the above, but the specific language differs.

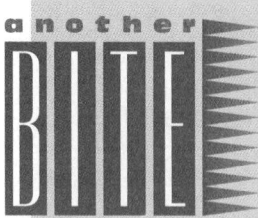

The National Cancer Institute believes that dietary fat is sufficiently linked to cancer, especially colon cancer, to warrant encouraging Americans to eat less fat. It recommends reducing dietary fat consumption to as little as 20% of total kcalories. The Institute is sponsoring a 7-year study of breast cancer risk in 2000 women on a very low fat diet—15% to 20% of total kcalories from fat. Some nutritionists, however, believe that this agency has overreacted to the fat and cancer issue. Epidemiological evidence relates fat intake to cancer, but the evidence is not strong. The question of how much fat can be eaten while minimizing the risk of cancer is not settled. A figure of up to 30% of total kcalories has the widest support, but the lower amounts of 20% of kcalories could be considered by adults.

Total kcalories eaten actually show an even stronger link to cancer than fat intake in animals. Rats with low energy intakes have about a 40% reduction in tumor yield, when compared with rats consuming typical amounts. The amount of fat in the diet is not important, as long as the experimental diet is about 70% of the animal's usual energy intake. An altered hormonal balance probably orchestrates the effect of a lower energy intake.

Can we use this evidence from animals? Americans want to avoid cancer, but very few of us are willing to settle for only 70% of our usual energy intake. While a strong link ties some types of cancer and obesity, this evidence has failed to persuade many of us to slim down to desirable body weights. It is an even bigger task to reduce kcalories to 70% of usual intake. In addition, once cancer is present, energy restriction is no longer helpful. Still, controlling fat intake and balancing energy intake with output is a wise recommendation.

Antioxidants May Be Anticarcinogens

Many single nutrients are promoted as keys to preventing cancer. They are called ***anticarcinogens*** (Table 8-5). The most important ones are beta-carotene (plant form of vitamin A), vitamins E and C, and selenium.[5] All four of these nutrients function as, or contribute to, antioxidant systems in the body. These antioxidant systems help prevent DNA alteration by electron-seeking (oxidizing) substances. Recall that the antioxidant vitamin E also helps protect unsaturated fatty acids from being oxidized. More research on the potential benefits of antioxidants in terms of cancer prevention is needed. There is speculation that substances other than the ones mentioned here are additional key cancer-preventive agents in fruits and vegetables.[19] For now, a diet rich in fruits and vegetables is a good path to take.[36]

Anticarcinogens *Compounds that can potentially inhibit the development of cancer.*

Are Dietary Fiber and Calcium Anticancer Agents?

In Chapter 5 we mentioned a possible role of fiber in preventing colon cancer. Fiber may do this by decreasing transit time so that the feces is in contact with the colon for a shorter period. This would reduce the contact of potential carcinogens with the colon wall. In addition, soluble fibers can bind bile acids. Bile acids are thought to promote cancer by irritating the colon cells, increasing cell division. However, the evidence regarding the importance of fiber in preventing colon cancer is still inconclusive. For now, the recommendation to eat 20 to 35 grams of fiber a day is probably best. Liberal intake of whole grains, fruits, and vegetables should suffice to yield this amount.

A current nationwide study under way in the United States to reduce colon cancer risk employs a diet with fat at 20% of kcalories and five to eight servings of fruits/vegetables per day. This diet also aims for about 30 grams of dietary fiber in the diet.

Dietary calcium is also linked to a decreased risk for developing colon cancer. As with fiber, the evidence is weak. Some studies show that calcium decreases the growth of colon cells. Therefore it probably decreases the risk of altered cells developing into a cancer. Calcium may also bind fatty acids and bile acids in the colon so they are less apt to interact with cells and cause cancer. We need more research before we can claim that calcium acts as a cancer-preventing agent. Nevertheless, there are many important reasons for consuming the RDA for calcium. We will discuss those in Chapter 9.

A Bottom Line?

Table 8-4 lists a variety of dietary changes you can make to reduce the risk of cancer. Start by controlling energy, alcohol, meat, and total fat intake and by increasing intake of

TABLE 8-4

Possible Anticarcinogens in Foods

Substance	Source	Action
Vitamin A	Liver, fortified milk, fruits, vegetables	Encourages normal cell development
Vitamin E	Whole grains; vegetable oil; green, leafy vegetables	Antioxidant
Vitamin C	Fruits, vegetables	Antioxidant; can block conversion of nitrites and nitrates to potent carcinogens
Folate	Fruits, vegetables, whole grains	Encourages normal cell development
Selenium	Meats, whole grains	Part of the glutathione peroxidase antioxidant system
Carotenes	Fruits, vegetables	Many are antioxidants
Indoles, phenols, and other plant substances	Vegetables, especially cabbage, cauliflower, brussels sprouts, garlic, green tea	May reduce carcinogen activation
Dietary fibers	Whole grains, fruits, vegetables, beans	May bind carcinogens in the stool, decrease stool transit time, thus lowering risk of colon and rectal cancer
Calcium	Dairy products, green vegetables	Slows cell division in the colon, binds bile acids and free fatty acids
Omega-3 fatty acids	Cold-water fish	May inhibit tumor growth
Soy compounds	Soybeans	Phytic acid component may bind carcinogens in the intestinal tract; the genistein component may reduce growth of malignant cells.

**Fruits and vegetables contain carotones, many of which are converted to vitamin A.*
†Chemical substances found in many plants.

fruits, vegetables, whole grains, beans, and low-fat or nonfat dairy products. In other words, follow the Food Guide Pyramid. Remember that 35% of all cancer cases are caused by cigarette smoking. Therefore a priority in avoiding cancer is to eliminate tobacco use—even smokeless varieties (chewing tobacco).

In your effort to eat more fruits and vegetables, consider the following suggestions:

- Use fresh or canned fruit as a topping for puddings, yogurt, hot or cold cereal, and frozen desserts.
- Put raisins, grapes, apple chunks, pineapple, grated carrots, zucchini, or cucumber into coleslaw, chicken, or tuna salad.
- Toss raw or steamed vegetables into potato salad, pasta, or rice. Try broccoli or cauliflower florets, mushrooms, peas, carrots, corn, or peppers.
- Be creative at the salad bar; try fresh spinach, leaf lettuce, red cabbage, sprouts, zucchini, yellow squash, cauliflower, peas, mushrooms, or red or yellow peppers.
- Pack fresh or dried fruit for snacks away from home instead of grabbing a candy bar or going hungry.
- On sandwiches, lettuce and tomato are just the beginning. Add slices of cucumber or zucchini, bean sprouts, spinach, carrot slivers, or snow peas.
- Try one or two vegetarian meals per week, such as beans and rice or pasta, or spaghetti squash and tomato sauce.
- When daily protein intake more than meets required amounts, reduce use of the meat, fish, or poultry in casseroles, stews, and soups by one third to one half and add more vegetables.
- In the refrigerator, keep a bowl of fresh vegetables handy for snacks.
- Choose 100% fruit or vegetable juices instead of sodas.
- Have a bowl of fruit on hand.

chapter

9

WATER AND MINERALS

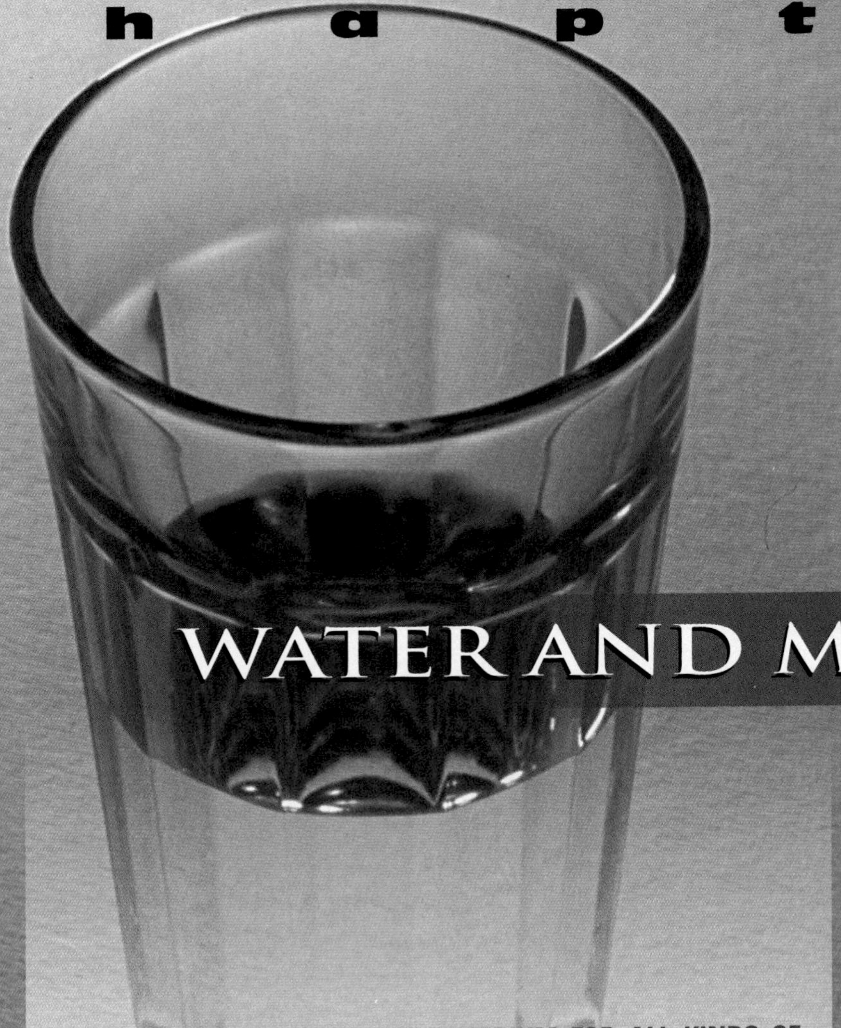

WATER—THE MOST VERSATILE MEDIUM FOR ALL KINDS OF chemical magic—constitutes the major portion of our bodies. Without water, our life processes would cease in a matter of days. We lose about 2 quarts (2 liters) of water daily, and this should be replenished daily because the body does not store water well. We know the resulting constant demand for water as *thirst.*[22]

Minerals, like water, are vital to health. They are key players in body growth and metabolism, muscle movement, and water balance, among other wide-ranging processes. Researchers are still defining what minerals the body requires and the quantities needed for good health. We are not sure that all the minerals found in our bodies—for example, vanadium and tin—are necessary to sustain human life.[18] Some minerals, such as lead, may be found in humans only as a contaminant. The mere presence of a mineral in our bodies is not proof that we need it.

Based on the amount we need each day, minerals are categorized as major (requiring >100 milligrams per day) or trace (requiring $\geq$100 milligrams per day). These categories do not reflect their importance to the body; deficiencies of some trace minerals can cause severe health problems. In this chapter, you will see why the study of water and minerals is critical to understanding human nutrition.

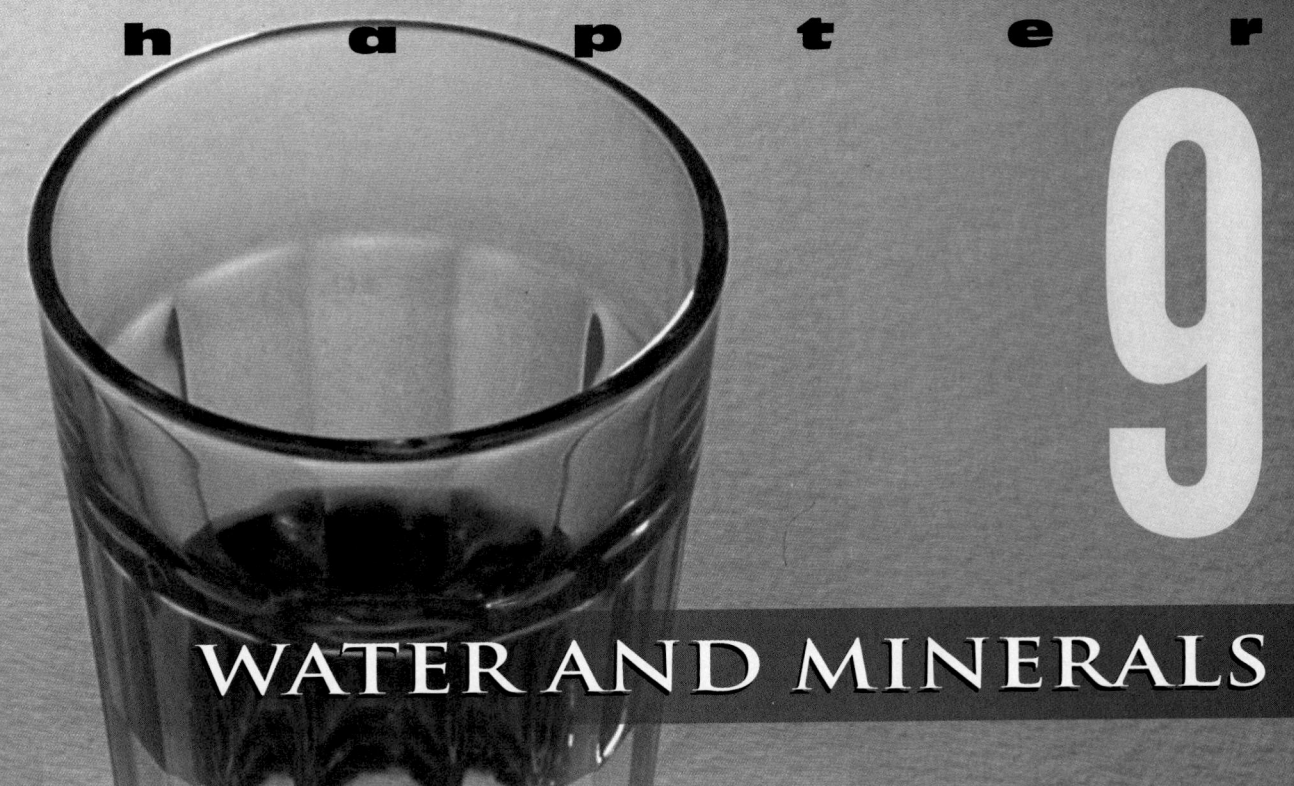

ASSESS

TEST YOUR KNOWLEDGE

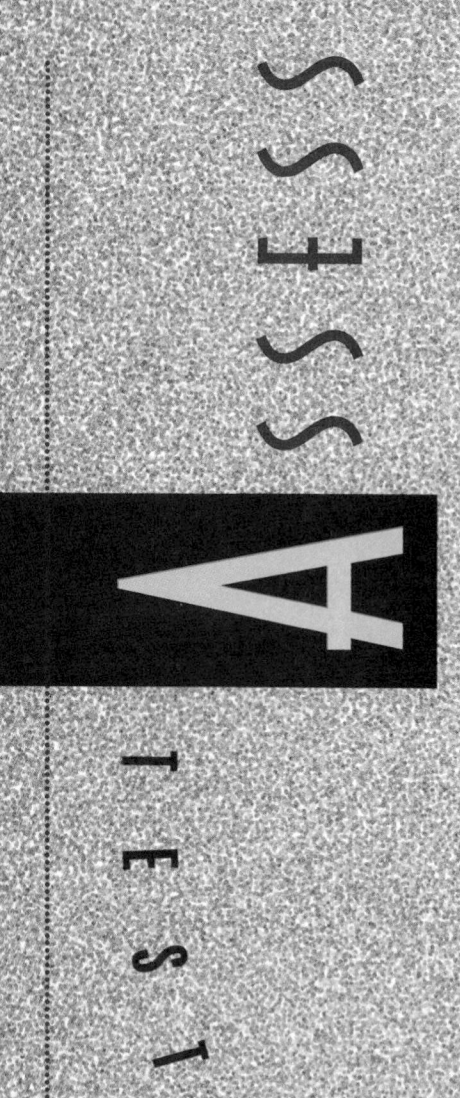

WORKING FOR DENSER BONES

In this chapter you will learn important information about the disease *osteoporosis*, characterized by thinning and brittle bones.

Osteoporosis affects 25 million people in the United States. One third of all women experience fractures because of it, amounting to 1.2 million bone fractures per year. In addition, 12% to 20% of all elderly people who suffer hip fractures die from complications. Given the rise in the number of elderly people in the United States, osteoporosis-related illness and death are anticipated to increase dramatically in coming years.

This is a disease you can do something about. Some risk factors can't be changed, but others can. To what degree are you doing the things that can help prevent this debilitating disease? Answer "yes" or "no" to the following questions by placing an "X" in the appropriate blank:

	YES	NO
1. Do you average at least 30 minutes of sun exposure per day to at least your hands and face to get vitamin D, or drink vitamin D–fortified milk regularly?	_______	_______
2. Do you engage in weight-bearing exercise (jogging, brisk walking, etc.) at least 3 times a week?	_______	_______
3. If you are a woman, do you experience regular menstruation?	_______	_______
4. Do you avoid smoking cigarettes?		
5. Do you avoid regular consumption of large amounts (greater than two drinks) of alcohol?	_______	_______
6. Do you consume milk and cheese regularly, or substitute other foods to meet the RDA for calcium?	_______	_______

The more *yes* answers you have, the more you are actively preserving your bone density for the future. Also, remember that this is not just a consideration for women, because if men plan to live well into their 80s and 90s they are at risk for osteoporosis. In fact, about 14% of all spine fractures and 25% of all hip fractures linked to osteoporosis occur in men.

yourself

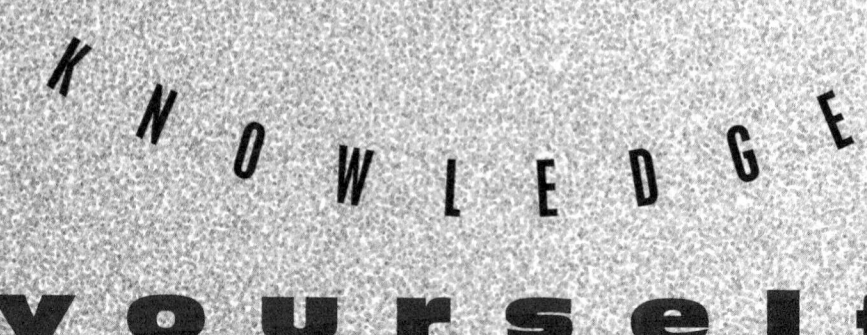

WATER

To appreciate how minerals operate in the body, we must understand the nature and general chemical properties of water, as well as specific nutrient-related functions.

Water—an Overview

Water is the perfect medium for body processes because it enables chemical reactions to occur. Water even participates directly in many of these reactions. It forms the greatest component of the human body, making up 50% to 60% of the body's weight. Lean muscle tissue contains about 73% water. Fat tissue is about 20% water. Thus, as fat content increases (and the percentage of lean tissue decreases) in the body, total body water content declines toward 50%.

Depending on how much fat has been stored, an adult can survive for about 8 weeks without eating food but only a few days without drinking water. This occurs not because water is more important than carbohydrate, fat, protein, vitamins, or minerals, but rather because we can neither store nor conserve water as well as we can the other components of our diet.[22]

Water in the Body—Intracellular and Extracellular Fluid

Water flows in and out of body cells through cell membranes. Water inside cells forms part of the intracellular fluid—the fluid within the cells. When water is outside cells or in the bloodstream, it is part of the extracellular fluid—that outside cells (Figure 9-1). Because cell membranes are permeable to water, water shifts freely in and out of cells. For example, if blood volume decreases, water can move from the areas inside and around cells to the bloodstream to increase blood volume. On the other hand, if blood volume increases, water can shift out of the bloodstream into cells and the surrounding areas.

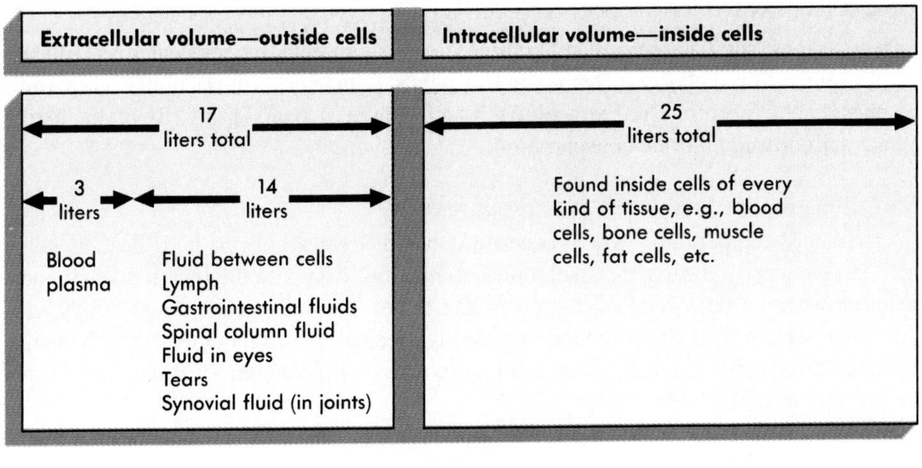

FIGURE 9-1
The body's fluid compartments—both intracellular (within cells) and extracellular (outside cells) spaces.

Osmosis ■ *The passage of solutions through a semipermeable membrane.*

The body controls the amount of water in the intracellular and extracellular compartments mainly by controlling ion concentrations. Ions have electrical charges. Water is attracted to ions, such as sodium, potassium, chloride, phosphate, magnesium, and calcium. By controlling the movements of ions in and out of the cellular compartments, the body maintains the appropriate amount of water in each compartment. Where ions go, water follows.

Examples that demonstrate osmosis are sugar pulling fluid from strawberries and a salty salad dressing wilting lettuce.

Osmosis

Osmosis is the process that regulates and equalizes the proportion of water in cells and in the bloodstream. Osmosis operates when fluids containing different ion concentrations

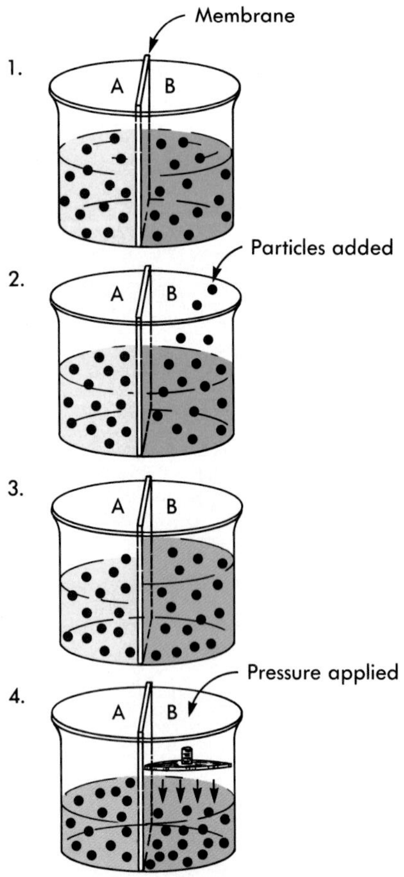

FIGURE 9-2
A graphic representation of osmosis and osmotic pressure. **1.** *Equal number of particles on both sides allows equal amounts of water.* **2.** *Now additional particles are added to side A, but the particles cannot flow across the membrane.* **3.** *Water can flow across the membrane, and so it flows to side B, causing the concentrations on sides A and B to again become equal.* **4.** *If physical pressure (such as a pump) compressed the fluid on side B to restore the original volume, that pressure would equal the osmotic pressure exerted by the added particles.*

are separated by a semipermeable membrane. In the body, for example, a semipermeable cell membrane separates cells from the fluid-filled spaces (compartments) surrounding cells. The semipermeable membrane allows water to pass into cells but controls the flow of ions. If adjoining fluid compartments contain dissimilar concentrations of particles (have different total ion concentrations), it is water that flows through the cell membrane to equalize the particle concentrations in each compartment.

Figure 9-2 illustrates osmosis. Adding particles to the right compartment increases its particle concentration and, in turn, decreases its relative water concentration. This happens in the bloodstream when you eat sodium. Because particles cannot easily pass through the membrane depicted in Figure 9-2, water shifts from the compartment with a low particle concentration (the more diluted compartment) to the more highly concentrated one. To counteract a high sodium concentration in the bloodstream, one body response is to shift fluid from cells into the bloodstream.

Water and Ions in the Body—A Balancing Act

Adding water—instead of particles—to a compartment dilutes its particle concentration, and so the compartment tends to donate water to more concentrated compartments nearby. This happens when you drink water. Some water absorbed by the body moves from the bloodstream into body cells, which in turn equalizes the particle concentrations in the cells with that in the various nearby body compartments. Therefore, because of the action of osmosis, water is forced to move across membranes to balance changes in particle—or ion—concentrations.

Cells have pumping mechanisms that constantly draw potassium ions into the cell and pump sodium ions out. Other ions are exchanged as well. It is this pumping action, in effect, that leaves cell membranes semipermeable—that is, permeable to water but not to many ions. Ions, such as sodium, may cross into the cell, but the cell quickly pumps them back out.

Positive ions, such as sodium and potassium, pair with negative ions, such as chloride and phosphate. Intracellular water volume depends primarily on intracellular potassium and phosphate concentration. Extracellular water volume depends primarily on the extracellular sodium and chloride concentration.

Water Contributes to Temperature Regulation

Water changes temperature slowly because it has a great ability to hold heat. It takes much more energy to heat water than it does to heat fat. Compare the time it takes to melt ice cubes with the time it takes to melt frozen butter in a microwave oven. Foods with high water content heat up and cool down slowly. Because water requires so much energy to change states—for example, from a liquid to a gas—it forms an ideal medium for removing heat from the body.

The body secretes fluids in the form of perspiration, which evaporates through skin pores. To evaporate water, heat energy is required. So, as perspiration evaporates, heat energy is taken from the skin, cooling it in the process.[9] Each quart (liter) of perspiration evaporated represents approximately 600 kcalories of energy lost from the skin and surrounding tissues. For this reason, fever increases one's need for energy.

However, to cool efficiently, perspiration must be allowed to evaporate. If it simply rolls off the skin or soaks into clothing, perspiration doesn't cool us much. Evaporation of perspiration occurs readily when humidity is low. This is why humans often tolerate hot, dry climates far better than they do hot, humid climates.

Water Helps Remove Waste Products

Water is an important vehicle for ridding the body of waste products. Most unusable substances in the body can dissolve in water and leave the body in urine.

A major body waste product is ***urea.*** This by-product of protein metabolism contains nitrogen. The more protein we eat in excess of needs, the more nitrogen we excrete—in the form of urea—in the urine. Likewise, the more sodium we consume, the more sodium

Urea
A by-product of protein metabolism that contains nitrogen.

we excrete in the urine. Overall, the amount of urine a person needs to produce is determined primarily by excess protein and sodium chloride (salt) intake. By limiting excess protein and sodium intakes, it is possible to limit urine output—a useful practice, for example, in space flights. This type of diet is also used to treat some kidney diseases where the ability to produce urine output is hampered.

A typical urine volume is about 1 to 2 liters (1 to 2 quarts) per day, depending mostly on the amount of fluid intake. Somewhat more urine output than that is fine, but less—especially less than 600 milliliters (2½ cups)—forces the kidneys to form a very concentrated urine. The heavy ion concentration increases the risk of kidney stone formation in susceptible people, which includes men in general. Kidney stones are simply minerals and other substances that have precipitated out of the urine and accumulated in kidney tissues.

How Much Water Do We Need?

Adults need roughly 1 milliliter of water per kcalorie expended. We consume about 1 liter (1 quart) of water a day in various liquids (Figure 9-3). Foods supply another liter of fluid; many fruits, vegetables, and beverages are more than 80% water. Water as a by-product of metabolism provides approximately 350 milliliters (1½ cups) of additional water. This yields a total of about 2.4 liters (10 cups) of water for a 2400-kcalorie diet, or about 1 milliliter per kcalorie expended.

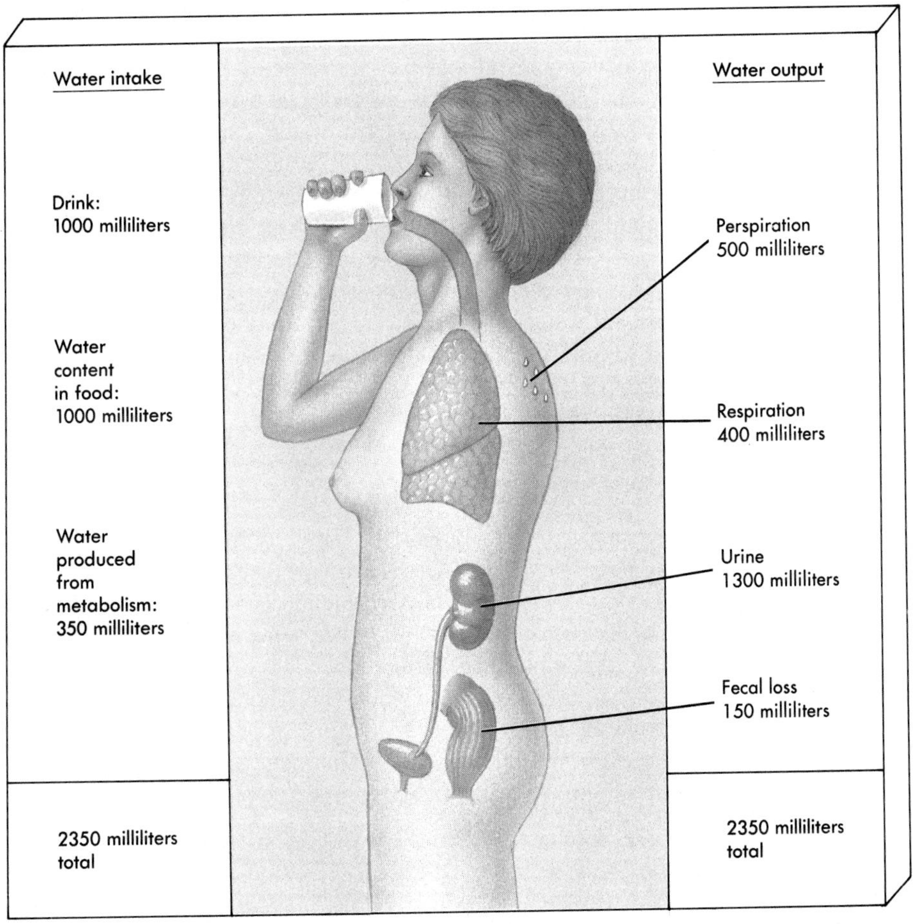

FIGURE 9-3
Water balance—intake versus output. We maintain body fluids at an optimal level by adjusting water intake and output. Most water comes from the liquids we consume. Some water comes from the moisture in more solid foods, and the remainder is manufactured in metabolism. Water output occurs via lungs, kidneys, skin, and bowels.

NUTRITION insight

BOTTLED WATER

These days, it is common to see 5-gallon bottles of water being delivered to homes. Grocery store shelves are now stocked with all kinds of bottled waters—over 700 brands in the United States—ranging from simple plastic jugs containing "pure spring water" to fancier, imported varieties of mineral water in glass bottles.[14] In Europe, bottled water is an institution, as popular as soft drinks are in the United States.

It is quite the fashion to order a bottle of Evian at a restaurant or bar. People are concerned not only with alternatives to alcoholic beverages and soft drinks, but also with the perceived health value or taste of bottled water. The bottled water industry does more than $2 billion a year in business.

Bottled waters vary, depending on the source, use, mineral content, and carbonation. All bottled waters must list the source of the water on the label. This can include wells, spas, springs, geysers, and quite often, the public water supply. Some bottled water companies add minerals—such as calcium, magnesium, and potassium—to give water a better taste. But the term *mineral water* is misleading, because all water (except distilled and specially purified water) contains minerals. In fact, FDA notes there is an increasing number of bottled water products on the market with labels that may be misleading. In response, FDA recently proposed definitions for "artesian water," "distilled water," "purified water," "spring water," "mineral water," and "well water." In essence, the source must be that listed on the label. Thus "spring water" will have to come from an underground spring. When carbon dioxide gas is present in the water source, it results in carbonation. Bottled waters from such sources are said to be *naturally sparkling*. Other carbonated waters have had carbon dioxide added during bottling.

Many people choose bottled water over tap water, because they doubt the safety of public drinking water. Some concern over municipal water supplies is warranted. We need to encourage close vigilance over the purity of our drinking water. The Environmental Protection Agency (EPA) is responsible for tap water quality. Under the Safe Water

Insensible *In this case, not perceived by the person, such as water lost with each breath.*

Of the 2.4 liters of water needed, about 1.4 liters is used to produce urine. The rest, about 1 liter, compensates for typical water losses through the lungs (400 milliliters), feces (150 milliliters), and skin (500 milliliters) (see Figure 9-3). We are not normally aware of these ***insensible*** water losses. Note also that when we consider the large amount of water used to lubricate the gastrointestinal (GI) tract, the loss of only 150 milliliters of water a day through the feces is remarkable. About 8000 milliliters of water enters the GI tract daily via secretions from the mouth, stomach, intestine, pancreas, and other organs. Diet supplies an additional 2000 milliliters or more. The kidneys also greatly conserve water. They reabsorb about 97% of the water filtered from waste products.

another BITE

Too much water—whatever amount the kidneys are unable to excrete—can be toxic. However, an excessive amount would have to approach many quarts (liters) each day. Most people have little risk of drinking too much water, but problems do accompany some disease states and mental disorders. When excessive water overwhelms the kidneys' capacity to excrete, blurred vision is one resulting symptom.

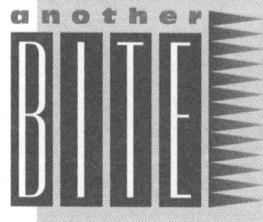

Drinking Act, all public drinking water supplies are monitored for contaminants, such as bacteria, various chemicals, and such toxic metals as lead and mercury. Still, only some bottled water currently meets these same standards—not all. FDA and private inspections of these products are less frequent than are tests done on municipal utilities. The proposed FDA standards will improve these products by also increasing surveillance of them.[14]

another BITE

Water can be classified by whether it is hard or soft. Hard water generally comes from underground wells and characteristically contains calcium, magnesium, and iron. The more minerals it contains the harder the water. Soft water has a low content of these minerals and is often produced by replacing other minerals with sodium. The mineral content of hard water interacts with soap and detergents, inhibiting the chemical processes that cause a soap lather to form.

A recent EPA poll showed that 21 of 50 bottlers surveyed revealed their source as the public water supply. This information, available on the label, indicates that often bottled water is from the same source as the tap water found in many homes. On the other hand, bottled waters derived from springs and wells may lack potentially helpful minerals that many communities have in their drinking water (like fluoride, magnesium, and calcium) and also may be vulnerable to the same groundwater contamination as the public supply. Sometimes bottled water is simply filtered, and minerals are either removed or added for taste.

Keep in mind that, by most standards, bottled water ranges from moderately expensive to expensive. In many cases, you are paying for water that is not much different from tap water. If you are concerned about the safety of your tap water, have it tested. A local testing laboratory or local health department can be of service. Compared with the cost of bottled water, the testing fee will be insignificant. And as we note in Chapter 17, letting cold water run for a minute or so before taking a drink or using it in meal preparation is a good way to limit possible lead exposure, especially if the water has been off for an hour or so.

Thirst

If you don't drink enough water and total body water falls by 1% to 2%, your body often lets you know by signaling thirst. Your brain is communicating to you the need to drink. This thirst mechanism is not always reliable, however, especially during illness, in elderly years, and during vigorous exercise, such as in athletic events.[9] Athletes should weigh themselves before and after training sessions to determine their rate of water loss and thus their water needs. Two cups (½ liter) of water weigh about a pound (about half a kilogram) (see Chapter 11 for details on fluid use in athletics). Ailing children—especially those with fever, vomiting, diarrhea, and increased perspiration—and elderly persons often need to be reminded to drink plenty of fluids. As we cover in Chapter 14, infants easily become dehydrated. Long airplane flights are another situation that demands extra fluid intake: a traveler can lose about 6 cups (1.5 liters) of water during a 3-hour flight. The dehumidified air in an airplane is so dry that it induces excessive insensible perspiration and evaporation.

What If the Thirst Message Is Ignored? Once the body registers a shortage of available water, it increases fluid conservation. The pituitary gland releases ***antidiuretic hormone (ADH)*** to force the kidneys to conserve water. The kidneys respond by reducing

Antidiuretic Hormone (ADH) ■ *A hormone secreted by the pituitary gland that acts on the kidneys to cause a decrease in water excretion.*

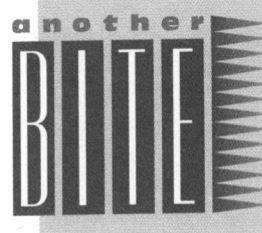

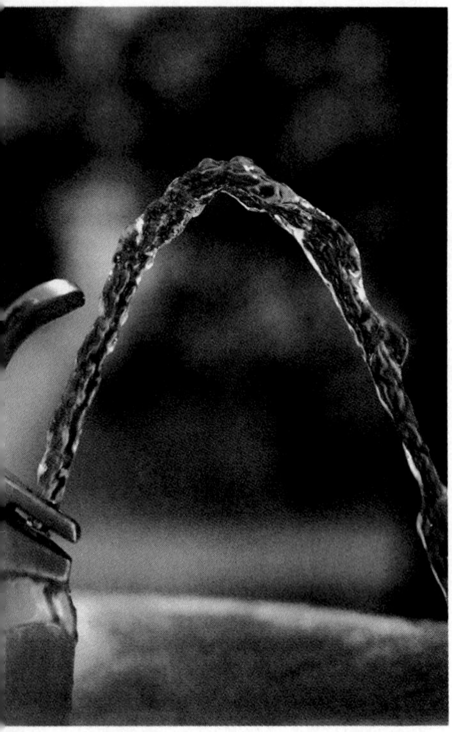

We need water in our diets every day.

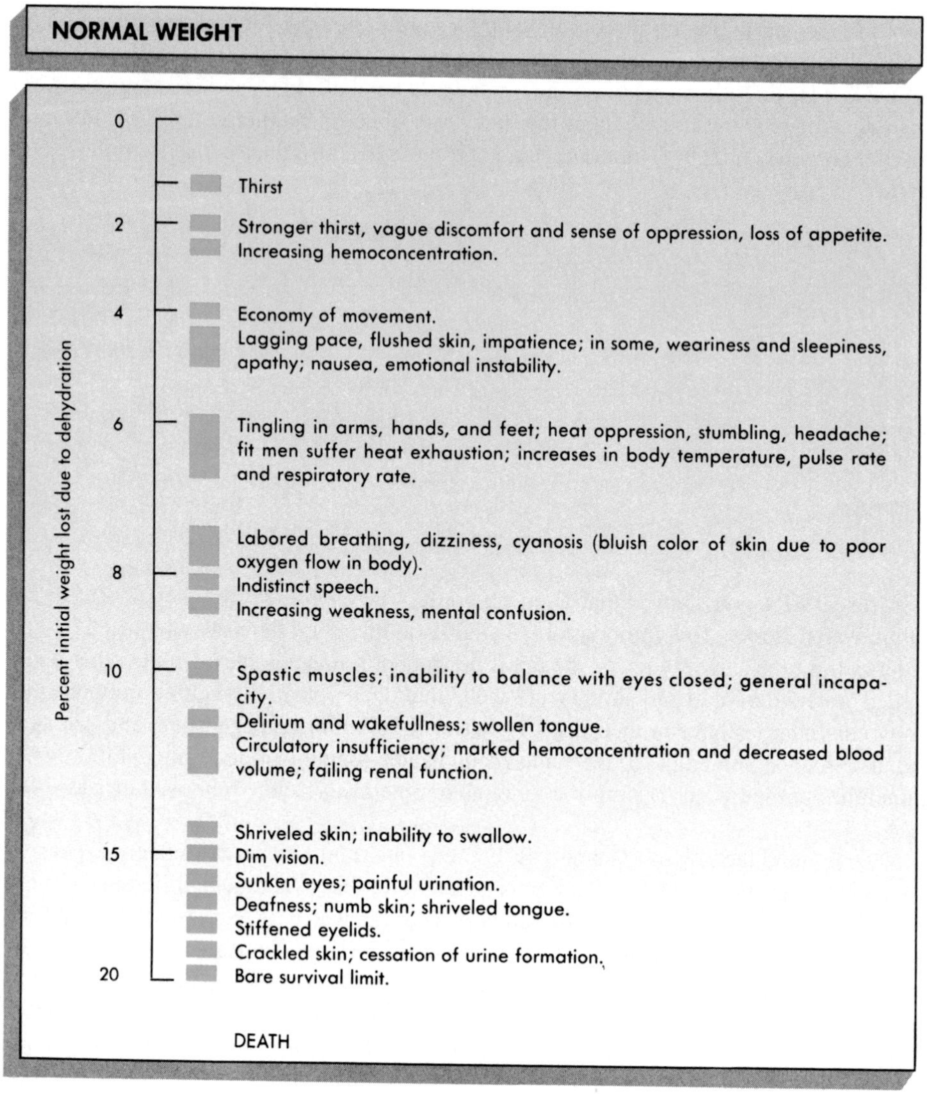
NORMAL WEIGHT
Percent initial weight lost due to dehydration
0
2
4
6
8
10
15
20
Thirst
Stronger thirst, vague discomfort and sense of oppression, loss of appetite.
Increasing hemoconcentration.
Economy of movement.
Lagging pace, flushed skin, impatience; in some, weariness and sleepiness, apathy; nausea, emotional instability.
Tingling in arms, hands, and feet; heat oppression, stumbling, headache; fit men suffer heat exhaustion; increases in body temperature, pulse rate and respiratory rate.
Labored breathing, dizziness, cyanosis (bluish color of skin due to poor oxygen flow in body).
Indistinct speech.
Increasing weakness, mental confusion.
Spastic muscles; inability to balance with eyes closed; general incapacity.
Delirium and wakefullness; swollen tongue.
Circulatory insufficiency; marked hemoconcentration and decreased blood volume; failing renal function.
Shriveled skin; inability to swallow.
Dim vision.
Sunken eyes; painful urination.
Deafness; numb skin; shriveled tongue.
Stiffened eyelids.
Crackled skin; cessation of urine formation.
Bare survival limit.
DEATH

FIGURE 9-4
The effects of dehydration. These range from thirst, as weight initially falls, to death.

Alcohol inhibits the action of antidiuretic hormone (ADH). One reason people feel so bad the day after heavy drinking is that they are very dehydrated. Even though they may have consumed a lot of liquid in their drinks, they have excreted even more liquid because alcohol has inhibited ADH.

urine flow. At the same time, as fluid volume decreases in the bloodstream, blood pressure falls. This eventually signals the kidneys to retain more sodium and, in turn, more water.

However, despite mechanisms that work to conserve water, fluid is constantly lost via the insensible routes—feces, skin, and lungs. Those losses must be replaced. In addition, there is a limit to how concentrated urine can become. Eventually, if fluid is not consumed, the body becomes dehydrated and suffers ill effects.

Again, by the time a person loses 1% to 2% of body weight in fluids, he or she will be thirsty. At a 4% loss of body weight, muscles lose significant strength and endurance. By the time body weight is reduced by 10% to 12%, heat tolerance is decreased and weakness results.[9] At a 20% reduction, coma and death may soon follow (Figure 9-4).

CONCEPT CHECK

Because the body can neither readily store nor entirely conserve water, we can survive only a few days without it. Water functions to dissolve substances, is a medium for chemical reactions and a lubricant, and aids in temperature regulation. Water constitutes 50% to 70% of body weight and distributes itself all over the body: among lean and other tissues (in both intracellular and extracellular fluids) and in urine and other body fluids. Adults need about 1 milliliter of water for each kcalorie expended. Thirst is the body's first sign of dehydration. If this thirst mechanism is faulty, as it may be during illness or vigorous exercise, hormonal mechanisms also help conserve water by reducing urine output.

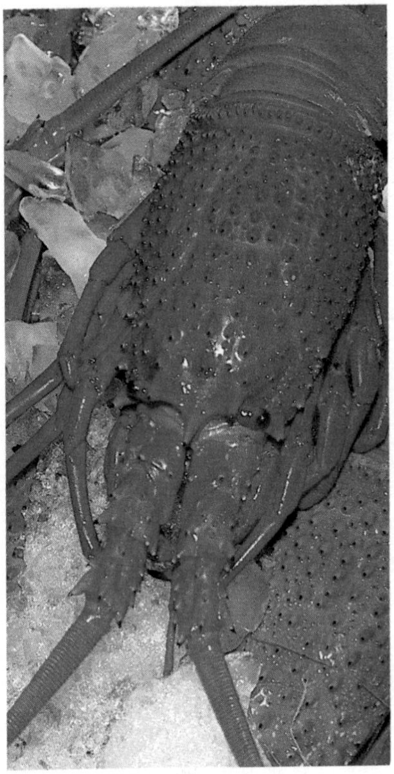

Seafood is a rich source of many trace minerals.

MINERALS

The metabolic roles of minerals vary considerably. Some minerals, such as copper and selenium, work as cofactors, which by definition enable enzymes to function. Minerals also contribute to important body compounds. For example, iodine is a component of the hormone thyroxine that comes from the thyroid gland. Iron is a component of hemoglobin in red blood cells. Sodium, potassium, and calcium aid in the transfer of nerve impulses throughout the body. Calcium is a key participant in muscle contraction. Body growth and development (i.e., bony skeleton) also depend on certain minerals, such as calcium and phosphorus. Water balance requires sodium, potassium, calcium, and phosphorus. At all levels—cellular, tissue, organ, and whole body—minerals clearly play important roles in maintaining body functions.

Mineral Bioavailability

Although foods contain and supply us with many minerals, our bodies vary in their capabilities to absorb and use available minerals. While minerals may be present in foods, they are not ***bioavailable*** unless a body can absorb them. The ability to absorb minerals from a diet depends on many factors. A number listed in a food composition table for the amount of a mineral in a food is just a starting point for estimating the true contribution a food makes to our mineral needs. Spinach is a good example. It contains plenty of calcium, but only about 5% of it can be absorbed because of the vegetable's high concentration of oxalic acid, a calcium-binder. Usually, about 20% to 40% of calcium is absorbed from foods by adults, with the higher figures coming from dairy products.

Bioavailability *The degree to which the amount of an ingested nutrient is absorbed and so available to the body.*

Minerals in the American diet come from both plant and animal sources. Overall, minerals from animal products are absorbed better, because binders and dietary fiber (as we soon will discuss) are not issues. The mineral content of plants depends on mineral concentration in the soil. Animals, however, may consume foods from multiple soil conditions and eat a variety of plant products, because they are often shipped across country during their growth, processing, and finishing in a feed lot. So soil conditions have less of an influence.

Generally the more refined a food—as in the case of white flour—the lower its content of minerals. The enrichment process for grains adds only the mineral iron. The selenium, zinc, copper, and other minerals lost when grains are refined are not replaced.

Fiber-Mineral Interactions

Mineral bioavailability can be greatly affected by nonmineral substances in the diet. Components of fiber, especially phytic acid (phytate) in grain fiber, can limit absorption of some minerals by binding to them.[5] Oxalic acid, mentioned before, is another substance in plants that binds minerals and makes them less available to the body. High-fiber diets can decrease the absorption of iron, zinc, magnesium, and probably other minerals.

An intake above the recommendation of 20 to 35 grams of dietary fiber per day then can cause problems with mineral status of the body.[11]

If grains are leavened with yeast, as they are in bread, enzymes produced by the yeast can break some of the bonds between phytic acid and minerals. This increases mineral absorption. The zinc deficiencies found among some Middle Eastern populations are attributed partly to their consumption of unleavened breads, resulting in low bioavailability of dietary zinc. We discuss this in detail in a later section.

Mineral-Mineral Interactions

Many minerals are of similar sizes and chemical charges, such as magnesium, calcium, iron, and copper. Having similar sizes and the same chemical charge causes these minerals to compete with each other for absorption, and so they affect each other's bioavailability. We caution people against taking individual mineral supplements, unless a medical condition specifically warrants it. This is because an excess of one mineral influences the absorption and metabolism of other minerals. For example, the presence of a large amount of zinc in the diet decreases copper absorption. High doses of calcium supplements can interfere with magnesium and iron absorption.

Mineral Toxicities

Excess mineral intake can lead to toxic results, especially with the trace minerals, such as iron and copper.[10] This potential for toxicity is yet another reason to carefully consider the use of mineral supplements. Every year, people poison themselves using mineral supplements, even though their intent is to maximize health. Many trace minerals are quite toxic at doses not much above the RDA or ESADDI. Mineral supplements exceeding 150% (1.5 times) of nutrient recommendations should be taken only under a physician's supervision, because toxicity and nutrient interactions are possible. We will discuss this concept further as we review each individual mineral.

CONCEPT CHECK

Minerals are vital to the functioning of many body processes. Their bioavailability depends on many factors, including a mineral's interaction with fiber and other minerals. Animal products often yield better mineral absorption than do plants. Still, both animal and plant sources help us meet our mineral needs. Taking an individual mineral supplement can greatly diminish the absorption and metabolism of other minerals. In addition, some minerals are potentially toxic. These are two good reasons to consider carefully any use of mineral supplements.

Major Mineral A mineral vital to health that is required in the diet in amounts greater than 100 mg per day.

MAJOR MINERALS

We have discussed some general characteristics of minerals and how some of them interact with water in the body. Now let us review the individual properties of the ***major minerals*** in the context of the American diet. Recall that these are the minerals we need in excess of 100 milligrams each day (Figure 9-5).

Sodium (Na)

We both crave and fear sodium and its primary dietary source, table salt. Some of this fear is warranted, and some is not.

For your information, the chemical symbols for the minerals we discuss are given next to each mineral heading.

Functions of Sodium. We absorb almost all sodium that we eat. It then becomes the major positive ion in extracellular fluid and a key factor for retaining body water. Fluid balance throughout the body depends partly on varied sodium concentrations among the water-containing compartments in the body. Sodium ions also function in nerve impulse conduction.

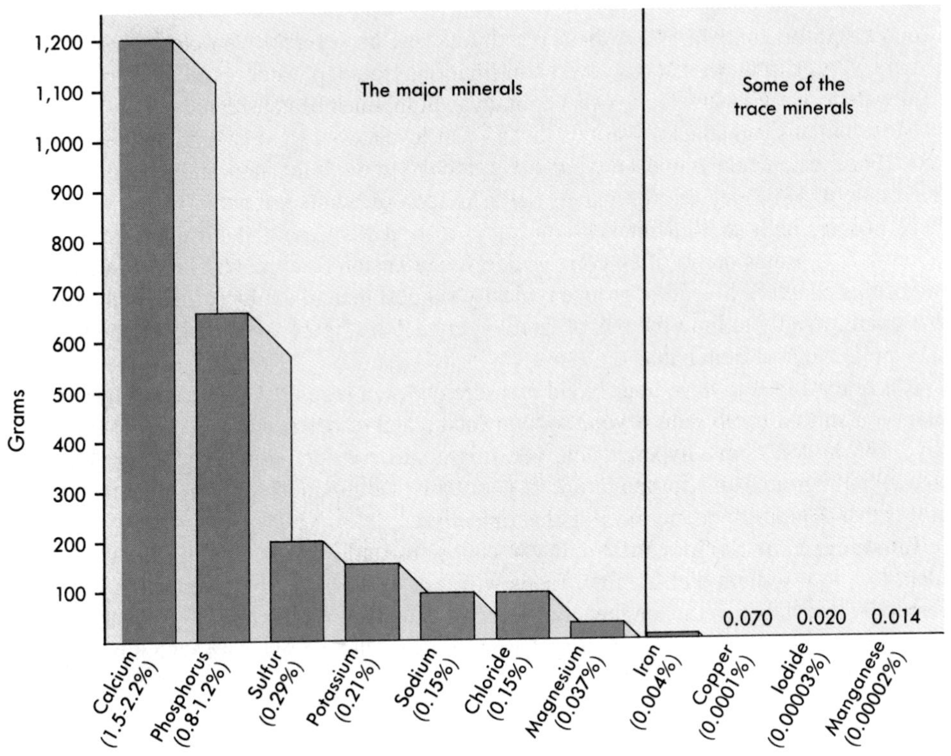

FIGURE 9-5
A list of minerals found in a 130-pound (60-kilogram) person. The percent figures represent percent of body weight. Other trace minerals of nutritional importance include chromium, fluoride, molybdenum, selenium, and zinc.

A low-sodium diet—coupled with high perspiration losses, persistent vomiting, or diarrhea—can deplete the body of sodium. This state can lead to muscle cramps, nausea, vomiting, dizziness, and later to shock and coma. Early kidney responses to a low sodium status, however, eventually trigger the body to conserve sodium. Thus, even in cases of high rates of perspiration, sodium depletion in the body is unlikely, especially since we generally eat a lot of sodium.

Note that although perspiration tastes salty on the skin, sodium is not highly concentrated in perspiration. Rather, water evaporating from the skin leaves concentrated sodium behind. Perspiration contains about two-thirds the sodium concentration found in blood.

Sodium in Foods and the Minimum Requirement for Health. About one third to one half the sodium we consume is added during cooking or at the table. Most of the rest is added during food manufacturing. Many health authorities are calling for manufacturers to use less sodium so that our total sodium intakes fall.[8] Almost all foods naturally contain little sodium; the higher amount found in milk is one exception. The more home cooking one does, the more sodium control one has. Major contributors of sodium in the adult diet are white bread and rolls, hot dogs and lunch meats, cheese, soups, and spaghetti with tomato sauce, partly because these foods are eaten so often.[20] Other foods especially high in sodium are tomato-based products in general, salted snack foods, French fries and potato chips, and sauces and gravies.

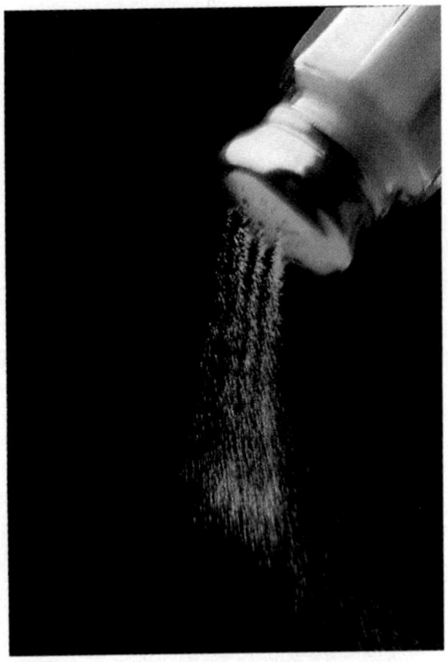

Salt is a major source of sodium for most of us.

If we ate only unprocessed foods and added no salt, we would get about 500 milligrams of sodium per day. This is also the minimum sodium requirement for health in adults set by the current RDA publication (see the inside cover for references to mineral needs for other age-groups). Even this is a generous amount, considering that we really need only about 100 milligrams a day.

If we compare 500 milligrams of sodium from unprocessed food with the 3000 to 7000 milligrams typically eaten by adults, it is clear that food processing and cooking contribute most of our dietary sodium. As we discussed in Chapter 2, nutrition labels list

Commercially prepared condiments, sauces, and seasonings are often high in sodium. Examples include onion, celery, garlic, seasoned, and sea salts; baking powder; salad dressings; pickles; soy, steak, barbecue, chili, and Worcestershire sauces; meat tenderizer; baking soda; salt pork; brine; catsup; mustard; bouillon; monosodium glutamate (MSG); and relish.

a food's sodium content. When dietary sodium must be severely restricted, these labels become very helpful. In that case even contributions from tap water (especially from softened water), as well as medicines that contain sodium, must be considered.

Most humans can adapt to various dietary salt levels, though very high intakes can be toxic. For most people who eat a typical diet, today's sodium intake is simply tomorrow's urine output. However, approximately 10% to 15% of adults are sodium sensitive. For these people, high sodium intakes contribute to hypertension, and lower sodium diets (about 2 to 3 grams daily) often correct their hypertension (see the Nutrition Issue at the end of this chapter). Scientific groups typically suggest that all adults reduce intake to 2.4 to 3 grams, mostly to limit the risk of later hypertension (Figure 9-6). Table 9-1 helps you to examine your sodium habits.

It is a good idea to have your blood pressure checked regularly. If you have hypertension, you should try to reduce your sodium intake and to determine what effect this can have. If you don't have hypertension, you might still consider slowly reducing your intake to build good habits for the future. If your daily sodium intake is already in the range of less than 3 grams, you are meeting that objective.

Lowering Your Sodium Intake. If you choose to eat less sodium, you can eventually adapt to a low-sodium diet. At first, foods will taste quite bland, but eventually you will perceive more flavor as the tongue's salt receptors are triggered by less salt. By slowly reducing dietary sodium and substituting garlic, oregano, lemon juice, and other herbs and

TABLE 9-1

Examining Your Sodium Habits

Examine how the foods you eat and the way you prepare and serve them affect the amount of sodium in your diet.

	Less than Once per Week	1 or 2 times per Week	3 to 5 times per Week	Almost Daily
How often do you:				
1. Eat cured or processed meats, such as ham, bacon, sausage, frankfurters, and other luncheon meats?	☐	☐	☐	☐
2. Choose canned or frozen vegetables with sauce?	☐	☐	☐	☐
3. Use commercially prepared meals, main dishes, or canned or dehydrated soups?	☐	☐	☐	☐
4. Eat cheese?	☐	☐	☐	☐
5. Eat salted nuts, popcorn, pretzels, corn chips, or potato chips?	☐	☐	☐	☐
6. Add salt to cooking water for vegetables, rice, or pasta?	☐	☐	☐	☐
7. Add salt, seasoning mixes, salad dressings, or condiments—such as soy sauce, steak sauce, catsup, and mustard—to foods during preparation or at the table?	☐	☐	☐	☐
8. Salt your food before tasting it?	☐	☐	☐	☐

The more checks you have in the last two columns, the higher your dietary sodium intake. However, not all items listed contribute the same amount of sodium. For example, many natural cheeses are relatively low in sodium. Most processed cheeses and cottage cheese are higher.

To cut back on sodium intake, you can start by eating some items less often, particularly those you checked as "3 to 5 times a week" or more. This does not mean eliminating foods from your diet. You can moderate your sodium intake by choosing lower-sodium foods from each food group more often and by balancing high-sodium foods with low-sodium ones. For example, if you serve ham for dinner, plan to serve it with fresh or plain frozen vegetables cooked without added salt, or use less salt when preparing other foods in the meal. Salt used in food preparation contributes greatly to sodium intake.

From USDA Home and Garden Bulletin No. 232-6, April 1986.

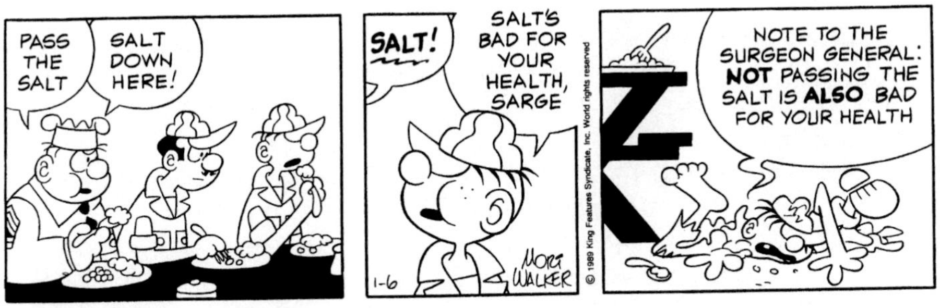

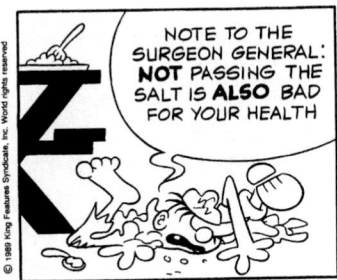

FIGURE 9-6
Beetle Bailey.

spices, you can eventually consume a diet that has only about 3 grams of sodium daily without sacrificing much flavor. Many new cookbooks offer excellent recipes for flavorful foods. Except for yeast breads, omitting salt from food preparation can still yield excellent products.

Table salt is 40% sodium and 60% chloride. The range of sodium intakes seen in adults of 3 to 7 grams per day translates to 7.5 to 18 grams of salt. A teaspoon of salt contains about 2 grams of sodium (2000 milligrams).

CONCEPT CHECK

Sodium is the major positive ion of extracellular fluid. It is important for maintaining fluid balance and conducting nerve impulses. Sodium depletion is unlikely, since the American diet has abundant sources and most sodium consumed is absorbed. The more foods we prepare at home, the more control we have over our sodium intakes. The minimum sodium requirement for health for adults is 500 milligrams per day. The average adult consumes 3000 to 7000 milligrams daily. About 10% to 15% of the population is sensitive to sodium. In these people, hypertension can develop as a result of high-sodium diets. Scientific groups suggest that for all adults sodium intake should be limited to about 3 grams (3000 milligrams) per day.

Potassium (K)

Potassium performs many of the same functions as sodium, such as fluid balance and nerve impulse transmission. However, it operates inside of rather than outside of cells. Intracellular fluids—those inside cells—contain 95% of the potassium in the body. Also, unlike sodium, potassium is associated with lower rather than higher blood pressure values.[8] We absorb about 90% of the potassium we eat.

Results of a Potassium Deficiency. A low blood potassium level is a life-threatening problem. Symptoms often include a loss of appetite, muscle cramps, confusion and apathy, and constipation. Eventually, the heart beats irregularly, decreasing its capacity to pump blood.

Potassium in Foods and the Minimum Requirement for Health. Generally, fruits and vegetables are nutrient-dense sources of potassium. Milk, whole grains, dried beans, and meats are also good sources. Major contributors of potassium to the adult diet include coffee, tea, milk, potatoes, orange juice, and animal products.[20]

The adult minimum potassium requirement for health set by the current RDA is 2000 milligrams (2 grams) per day. A typical adult's diet supplies enough potassium if a variety of foods is eaten. Americans average 2 to 3 grams per day. If kidneys function normally, typical intakes of dietary potassium are not toxic; otherwise, high amounts in the body can lead to heart failure.

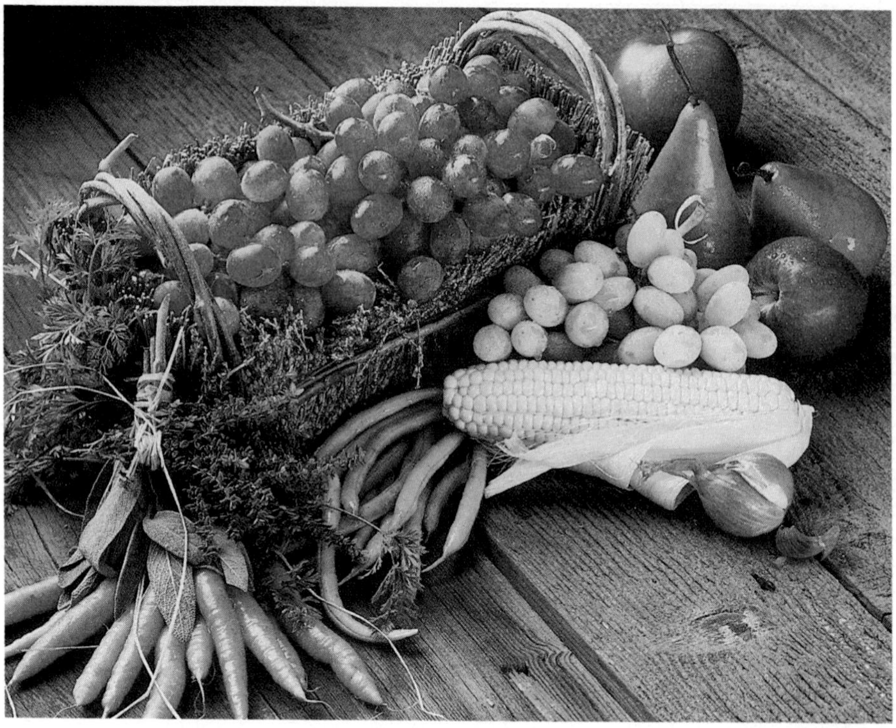

Many fruits and vegetables are good sources of potassium.

Bodies are more likely to be deficient in potassium than sodium, because we generally do not add potassium to foods. Some ***diuretics*** used to treat hypertension, such as thiazides and furosemide, deplete body potassium. Water is excreted along with the potassium, in turn reducing blood volume and blood pressure. People who take such potassium-wasting diuretics need to monitor their potassium intakes carefully. High-potassium foods—such as fruits, fruit juices, and vegetables—are good additions to their diet and perhaps so too are potassium chloride supplements, if recommended by a physician.

A continual poor food intake, as may be the case in alcoholism, can also result in potassium deficiency. People with anorexia nervosa and bulimia, whose diets are poor and whose bodies are nutrient depleted from vomiting, are also at risk for potassium deficiency (see Chapter 12). In addition, people on very low-kcalorie diets are at risk, as well as athletes that exercise heavily. As we will cover in Chapters 10 and 11, all of these people can compensate for potentially low body potassium levels by consuming potassium-rich foods.

Chloride (Cl)

Chlorine is a very poisonous gas. Public water utilities often rely on it to kill bacteria in water supplies. Consequently, many water-borne diseases are rare in America. Health authorities in Columbus, Ohio note that in pre-chlorine days, when cholera and typhoid were common, the cholera rate once was 135 cases per 100,000 people. However, a case hasn't been associated with Columbus water in the last 50 years. Chlorination has probably saved more lives than any other thing we're doing in this country to support health.

In our bodies, chloride—an ion form of chlorine—forms an important negative ion for the extracellular fluid. These ions are a component of the hydrochloric acid produced in the stomach and are also used during immune responses as white blood cells attack foreign cells. In addition, nerve function relies on the presence of chloride. As is the case with sodium, most of the body's chloride is excreted by the kidneys; some is lost in perspiration. It is also implicated in the blood pressure–raising ability of sodium chloride.

A chloride deficiency is unlikely, because our dietary sodium chloride (salt) intake is so high. Frequent and lengthy bouts of vomiting—if coupled with a nutrient-poor diet—can contribute to a deficiency, because stomach secretions contain much chloride. From 1978 to 1979, insufficient chloride added to a brand of infant formula caused severe convulsions and other health problems in the infants who consumed it. This incident shows what can happen when the need for a nutrient normally abundant in our diets is not given adequate attention.

Chloride in Foods and the Minimum Requirement for Health. A few fruits and some vegetables are naturally good sources of chloride. Chlorinated water is also a source. However, we consume most chloride as salt added to foods. If we know a food's salt content, we can predict closely its chloride content; salt is 60% chloride. Naturally occurring sodium or chloride won't significantly affect the prediction.

The minimum chloride requirement for health in adults set by the current RDA is 700 milligrams per day. Assuming that the average adult consumes at least 7.5 grams of salt daily, that yields 4.5 grams (4500 milligrams) of chloride, an abundance of this ion. Some research has revealed an association between certain forms of cancer and by-products of water chlorination. Nevertheless, EPA officials note that the public health benefits of clean water far outweigh the potential health risks of chlorination.

CONCEPT CHECK

Potassium performs functions similar to those of sodium, except that it is the main positive ion found inside, not outside, cells. Potassium is vital to fluid balance and nerve transmission. A potassium deficiency caused by poor intake, persistent vomiting, or use of some diuretics can lead to loss of appetite, muscle cramps, confusion, and heartbeat irregularities. Fruits and vegetables are generally rich sources of potassium. Potassium intake can be toxic if a person's kidneys do not function properly. Chloride is the major negative ion of extracellular fluid. Chloride also functions in digestion as part of hydrochloric acid and in immune and nervous system responses. Deficiencies of chloride are unlikely because we eat so much sodium chloride (salt).

Calcium (Ca)

All cells need calcium, but over 99% of the calcium in the body is used to strengthen bones and teeth. This calcium represents 40% of all the minerals present in the body and equals about 2½ pounds (1200 grams). As calcium circulates in the bloodstream, it supplies the calcium needs of all body cells. Growth and bone development in laboratory animals is closely tied to calcium intake. This link is seen in humans, too, but is not as well established.[1]

Functions of Calcium. Forming and maintaining bones are calcium's major roles in the body, but it is important in many other processes as well. Calcium is essential for blood clotting and for muscle contraction. If the blood calcium level falls below a critical point, muscles cannot relax after contraction; the body stiffens and shows signs of ***tetany.*** In normal nerve transmission, calcium works to release chemical messengers and permits the flow of ions in and out of nerve cells. Without sufficient calcium, nerve transmission fails, opening another path to tetany. Finally, calcium helps regulate cellular metabolism by influencing the activities of various enzymes and hormonal responses. It is the hormonal regulation of blood calcium levels that keeps all these processes going, even if you fail to eat enough calcium on a day-to-day basis.

Tetany *A body condition marked by sharp contraction of muscles and failure to relax afterward; usually caused by abnormal calcium metabolism.*

Absorption of Calcium. Calcium requires an acid environment to be absorbed efficiently. Absorption occurs primarily in the upper part of the small intestine. The area

TABLE 9-2

Absorption of Calcium from the Intestinal Tract Depends on Many Factors

Factors Favoring Absorption	Factors Hindering Absorption
Acid nature of upper intestinal tract	Alkaline state in lower intestinal tract
Normal digestive activity and motility of intestinal tract	Large amounts of dietary fiber
Dietary calcium and phosphorus in about equal amounts	Laxatives or any circumstances that cause diarrhea or rapid flow of the intestine
Vitamin D	*Great* excess of phosphorus or magnesium in proportion to calcium
Need for higher amounts by the body, as during pregnancy	Phytic acid, oxalic acid, and unabsorbed fatty acids: they all bind calcium in the intestine
Low calcium intake	Vitamin D deficiency
Parathyroid hormone (increases active vitamin D synthesis)	Menopause
Lactose	Old age
Glucose	Tannins in tea

tends to remain acidic because it receives the acidic stomach contents. Much calcium absorption in the upper small intestine depends on the active vitamin D hormone.

We absorb about 20% to 40% of calcium in the foods we eat, but during times when the body needs extra calcium—such as in infancy and pregnancy—absorption might reach as high as 50% to 75%. Young people tend to absorb calcium better than do older people, especially those over 70 years of age. Postmenopausal women generally absorb the least calcium, unless they receive supplements of the hormone estrogen. Estrogen therapy increases synthesis of the active vitamin D hormone, which aids calcium absorption. Estrogen also has a direct effect on bones to promote bone health.[21]

Many factors end up enhancing calcium absorption: the acidic environment of the small intestine and the presence of the active vitamin D hormone, mentioned previously; parathyroid hormone, dietary glucose, and lactose; and normal intestinal motility (flow). Factors limiting calcium absorption include large amounts of phytic acid in dietary fiber from grains; great excess of magnesium or phosphorus in the diet; tannins in tea; a vitamin D deficiency; menopause; diarrhea; and old age (Table 9-2).

One problem in setting an RDA for calcium is predicting how much calcium will be absorbed by the body. The RDA is based on an estimated 30% to 40% total calcium absorption. But calcium absorption efficiency varies among people. Those who absorb calcium less efficiently need to consume more.

Because we have excellent hormonal systems to control blood calcium levels, a normal blood calcium level can be maintained despite poor calcium intake. The bones, however, pay the price. Bone loss caused by insufficient calcium intake proceeds slowly. Only after many years are clinical symptoms apparent. By not meeting the RDA for calcium, some people—especially women—are most likely setting the stage for future bone fractures.[1] However, because we don't know how efficiently each individual absorbs calcium, we often cannot predict who is at the highest risk.

Osteoporosis. If bone mass is not maintained sufficiently, ***osteopenia*** (meaning *little bone*) eventually results. There are many contributors to bone loss, including osteomalacia, a condition where bones are poorly calcified (see Chapter 8); the use of certain medications; and cancer tumors (Table 9-3). If all these causes of bone loss are ruled out, the diagnosis is ***osteoporosis.*** Osteoporosis is further classified as Type I (postmenopausal), which appears in the years right after menopause, and Type II (senile), which is found in

Osteopenia
Decreased bone mass caused by cancer, hyperthyroidism, or other reasons.

Osteoporosis
Decreased bone mass where no outward cause can be found. Related to effects of aging, poor diet, and hormonal effects of menopause in women.

TABLE 9-3

Factors Associated With Bone Maintenance Versus Bone Loss

Maintenance	Loss	
Normal menses	Lack of menses	Alcoholism
Estrogen replacement	Early menopause	Cigarette smoking
African-American race	Glucocorticoid use	Slender figure
Thiazide diuretics	Hyperparathyroidism	Bed rest (months)
Physical activity*	Hyperthyroidism	Dietary fiber (large amounts)
Dietary calcium	Thyroid hormone replacement	Anorexia nervosa
Vitamin D nutriture	Factors made by white blood cells	High sodium intakes (pulls calcium into the urine)

**The degree of effect remains to be established.*

people of advanced ages.[21] A long-standing poor calcium intake can contribute to both forms.

Bone composition in osteoporosis is essentially normal; basically there is just less bone mass throughout the body. Because the bones are not as dense as are normal bones, osteoporosis can lead to a decrease in height, hip fractures in old age, and eventual loss of teeth (Figure 9-7).

Other Possible Benefits of Calcium in the Diet. Besides contributing to bone strength, dietary calcium may reduce the risk of colon cancer. It appears that abundant calcium in the feces—from calcium intake of about 2 grams per day—binds with the fats and bile acids there. These compounds, when free, tend to irritate the colon. Such irritation may increase cell turnover there, increasing the risk of cancer. Researchers warn, however, that use of calcium in this manner is still experimental.[27]

Another possible benefit of dietary calcium may be its effect on blood pressure. Consuming the RDA for calcium, when compared with the consumption of about half that amount, has slightly decreased blood pressure in some people in some studies, but the effect has not been consistent[16] (see the Nutrition Issue at the end of this chapter).

Both of these areas of calcium research—colon cancer and high blood pressure—are new. Practical dietary recommendations stemming from this research, aside from meeting the RDA for calcium, are not yet established.

Calcium in Foods. Dairy products—such as milk, yogurt, and cheese—provide most of the calcium in the adult diet. Of these, nonfat milk is the most nutrient-dense source. Cottage cheese, however, is not a good source of calcium, because most of its calcium is lost in production. White bread, rolls, crackers, and other foods made with milk products are also contributors. Although green, leafy vegetables are the most nutrient-dense calcium sources, their oxalic acid content prevents much of their calcium from being absorbed, making them unreliable sources. The new calcium-fortified versions of orange and other fruit drinks are excellent calcium sources and particularly helpful for people who do not drink much milk. Soybean curd (tofu) is also a good source of calcium if it is made with calcium carbonate (check the label).

One reason the Food Guide Pyramid contains a milk, yogurt, and cheese group is to supply calcium to the diet. In addition, this group provides protein, vitamins A and D, riboflavin, potassium, and magnesium. People who do not like milk can use products made

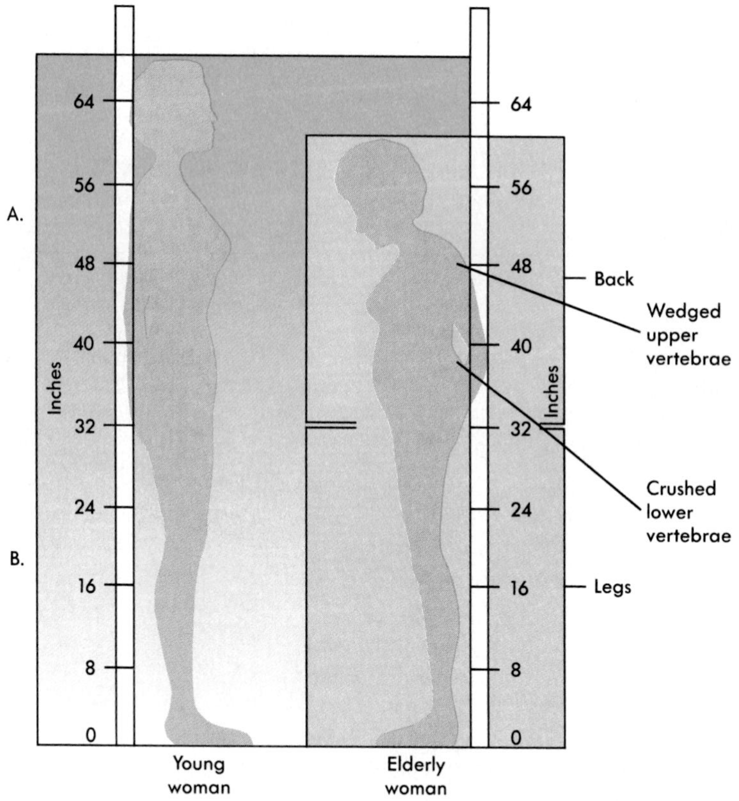

FIGURE 9-7

A loss of height and a misshapen body are common results of osteoporosis. Monitor yourself for these changes in adulthood to detect early signs of osteoporosis.

with milk, such as chocolate milk, yogurt, cheese, and ice cream. All forms of milk, yogurt, and cheese allow about the same degree of calcium absorption. However, we hesitate to recommend a lot of either cheese or ice cream, because they are usually high in saturated fat. Some low-fat cheeses and frozen desserts, such as nonfat frozen yogurt and ice milks, are good calcium sources and have a low saturated-fat content. Bones found in canned fish, such as salmon and sardines, also supply calcium. Calcium supplements are an additional source.

The target for calcium intake for adults over the age of 24 years is 800 milligrams a day. From adolescence through age 24 years, the target is 1200 milligrams a day. To estimate your calcium intake, use the rule of 300s. Give yourself 300 milligrams to start with. This accounts for small amounts of calcium provided by a moderate energy intake from foods scattered throughout a typical diet. Add to that another 300 milligrams for every 1 cup (0.25 liter) of milk or yogurt, 1.5 ounces (45 grams) of cheese, or 1 cup of calcium-fortified juice.

If you eat a lot of tofu, almonds, or sardines, using Appendix A will give you a more accurate account of your calcium intake. Our shortcut method underestimates it, especially for people eating a strictly vegetarian diet. It is important for vegans to focus on eating good plant sources of calcium, as well as on the total amount of calcium ingested.

We hesitate to encourage calcium supplement use, even though most supplements are absorbed about as well as milk calcium. Many people have difficulty adhering to a supplement regimen. Regular food habits can be integrated more easily into a routine than can remembering to take several pills a day. The major risk from taking excess calcium another BITE

Some calcium supplements are poorly digested, because they do not readily dissolve. To test for this, put a supplement in 6 ounces of cider vinegar. Stir every 5 minutes. It should dissolve within 30 minutes.

supplements is poor absorption of other minerals and possibly the development of kidney stones in some people. Moderate use (1000 milligrams per day), however, does not raise the same concerns. Toxic products that are part of dolomite, bone meal, or oyster shell calcium supplements are also of concern if those are used.

RDA for Calcium. As mentioned above, the RDA for calcium is 800 milligrams per day for most adults over age 24 years. For ages 11 through 24 the recommendation increases to 1200 milligrams, with the intent that higher calcium intakes will help build a greater bone mass. We know that youth is the time to accumulate calcium and build strong bones.[11] The greater bone mass can then benefit the person for the rest of his or her life. At 800 milligrams a day, adolescents have enough calcium to maintain bone, but many will not have enough to build their bones to maximal strength.

A recent National Institutes of Health (NIH) committee also recommended that postmenopausal women who do not take estrogen replacements consume 1500 milligrams of calcium daily. Note that an intake up to 2500 milligrams per day is safe for adults. Still, as we will discuss in the Nutrition Insight on preventing osteoporosis, even 1500 milligrams is not enough to prevent bone loss in the spine during the years right after menopause. Estrogen replacement is much more reliable.[21] Women who take estrogen at menopause still need calcium—about 800 to 1000 milligrams a day is recommended.

Unfortunately, the average calcium intake of adult women ranges from approximately 500 to 600 milligrams a day. For men the figure is 800 to 900 milligrams a day.[20] About 25% of women consume less than 300 milligrams per day. This is a major public health concern.[1] So women's diets tend to be deficient in calcium, whereas men's do not. Men eat more food in general to support their higher energy outputs, and that accounts for part of the difference. An easy way for women to consume more calcium is to increase their activity level and, in turn, to eat more in general.

CONCEPT CHECK

About 99% of calcium in the body is found in the bones. Aside from its critical role in bone formation and strength, calcium also functions in blood clotting, muscle contraction, nerve transmission, and cell metabolism. Calcium requires a slightly acid pH and the active vitamin D hormone for efficient absorption. Other factors that reduce calcium absorption include large amounts of dietary fiber, decreased blood estrogen levels, and excess levels of magnesium or phosphorus in the diet. Osteoporosis is bone loss caused by no other obvious condition. Women are particularly prone to osteoporosis because they make less bone than do men, lose it faster, and live longer. Replacing estrogen at menopause for women and following a healthful diet remain the best methods of prevention of osteoporosis. Dairy products and calcium-fortified orange juice are rich sources of calcium. Supplemental forms, such as calcium carbonate, are well absorbed. However, overzealous supplementation may interfere with the absorption of other minerals.

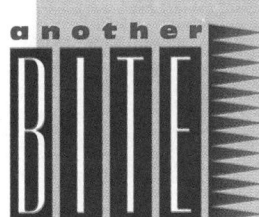

NUTRITION insight

PREVENTING OSTEOPOROSIS

Widespread advertising has made it almost impossible for women to ignore osteoporosis. Its crippling effect on elderly persons is now recognized as a medical emergency. The disease affects 25 million people in the United States, most of them women. About one third of all women experience osteoporosis-related fractures in their lifetimes.

Osteoporosis leads to approximately 1.5 million bone fractures per year, usually in the hip, spine, and wrist. The slender, inactive woman who smokes is most susceptible to osteoporosis, but any person who lives long enough can suffer from the disease. Table 9-3 lists many risk factors for the disease. Both genetic background and lifestyle are implicated. As we age into our 80s and 90s, osteoporosis often becomes the rule—not the exception. This is the case for both women and men. And it is not only debilitating, it can be fatal. Between 12% and 20% of all elderly persons who suffer hip fractures eventually die from fracture-related complications.[21]

Bone Density at Different Ages

Rapid and continual bone growth and calcification occur throughout the adolescent years. Small increases in bone density then continue through the ages of 20 to 30 years. Women make less bone than do men, lose it at a faster rate, and tend to live longer. Thus women start their adult years with less bone and have a longer time in which to lose it. Also, bone density varies among young adult women—some have much denser bone than others, perhaps because they built more bone when they were young. Some women also may more easily adapt to lower-calcium diets. In either case, if a higher bone mass results, this allows a person to sustain greater bone loss in aging without more fractures when compared with women who have less bone density.[1]

For women, bone loss begins around age 30 and proceeds slowly and continuously to menopause (approximately age 50). It often speeds up at menopause and continues at a high rate for the next 5 to 10 years. By age 65, the rate of bone loss falls to about the same rate as before menopause. In men, bone loss is slow and steady from around age 30.[21]

Can Bone Loss Be Prevented?

Hormone replacement therapy with estrogen is widely recommended for women at menopause to prevent osteoporosis, especially if (1) they have no contraindications to use and (2) they fall in the lower third of bone density values for their age.[21] Estrogen is also used to reduce the symptoms of menopause. Studies show that estrogen replacement at menopause virtually stops further bone loss in women. Thus it is reasonable to assume that estrogen replacement therapy will virtually eliminate the risk for significant osteoporosis in women who begin treatment right after menopause and continue to take it for 20 years or so. This therapy is relatively safe for most women but still must be closely supervised by a physician, because a slight increased risk for certain forms of cancer has been observed.[2] Thus close monitoring of the woman is needed. An additional benefit of estrogen replacement therapy is a significant reduction in the risk of heart disease. When the decreased risk for osteoporosis and heart disease are added together, estrogen replacement ends up greatly improving the overall health risk profile for many women.

Is Estrogen Therapy the Only Answer?

Some women cannot take estrogen because they have estrogen-sensitive breasts or uterine tumors. Other therapies, such as taking the active vitamin D hormone or the hormone calcitonin, are available and quite effective. However, will increasing calcium intake substitute for taking estrogen or other medications?

Studies from the United States and Denmark have found that taking as much as 200 milligrams of extra calcium daily (equal to 7.5 glasses of milk) does not prevent bone loss in the spine, hip, or wrist after menopause as successfully as estrogen replacement does. Consuming extra dietary calcium more effectively reduces bone loss in some bony areas better than doing nothing at all. But a high calcium intake may be no better for reducing the often significant bone loss in the spine that occurs in the 5- to 10-year interval after menopause than just meeting the RDA.[21]

Spinal fractures in women cause considerable pain and deformity and decrease physical ability. In addition, no reliable cure exists for osteoporosis. Therefore preventing these fractures is very important. Overall, for most women at high risk for osteoporosis it is not a question of estrogen versus calcium, but estrogen plus calcium that constitutes one of the most effective treatments. Also, as women age 10 years beyond menopause, meeting the RDA for calcium leads to less bone loss throughout the body than does consuming half that amount. This in turn leads to a significant reduction in the risk of hip fracture.[3]

Will a Nutritious Diet in Youth Prevent Osteoporosis Later?

Meeting the RDA for calcium from childhood through adolescence builds a stronger bone structure than does a poor calcium intake. The degree to which this happens is currently under study. Some researchers think that the RDA for ages 11 through 24 for women is even too low. They feel that an additional 300 to 400 milligrams (to a total of 1500 to 1600 milligrams per day) would result in more bone being laid down, as compared with just following the RDA. We will likely have the answer to this controversy by 1996.

A Plan for Fracture Prevention

As women mature, different strategies for preventing osteoporosis are needed, based on risk factors present (Table 9-3). Young women should see a physician at any sign of irregular menstruation and should pursue an active lifestyle that includes sun exposure (to promote synthesis of vitamin D) and weight-bearing exercise (to stimulate bone building). In young women, regular menstruation is the overwhelming key to bone maintenance, as evidenced by poor bone density in nonmenstruating female athletes and other women with irregular menstruation. Exercise cannot prevent the bone loss associated with irregular menstruation. It is also important to at least meet the RDA for calcium. If foods from the milk, yogurt, and cheese group are not usually consumed, it is wise to find other calcium sources.

Smoking and excessive alcohol work against bone strength. Smoking lowers estrogen levels in women, increasing bone loss. Alcohol is toxic to all cells—this includes bone cells. Alcoholism is probably a major undiagnosed and unrecognized cause of osteoporosis today.

At menopause, women should discuss estrogen replacement therapy with a physician.[21] They also need to accurately track their height. A decrease of more than 1 inch from premenopausal values is a sign that significant bone loss is taking place. If a plan to prevent osteoporosis is not being pursued, a loss in height is the signal to see a physician and establish a plan.

Elderly men and women need to stay as physically active as possible and meet their RDA for calcium. As we mentioned, this most likely limits bone loss in some areas of the body, such as the hip. They also need to minimize the risk for falls, especially by limiting their use of medications and alcohol, which might disturb coordination. Getting regular sun exposure and consuming food sources of vitamin D are also good ideas. Securing throw rugs and liberal installation of handrails in the house can help decrease the risk of falls and so fractures.[21]

Phosphorus (P)

Phosphorus plays many important roles in the body. Although no disease is currently associated with a poor phosphorus intake, a deficiency may contribute to bone loss in elderly women. The body absorbs phosphorus quite efficiently and can increase absorption from 60% to 90% as body needs vary. This high absorption rate, plus the wide availability of phosphorus in foods, makes this mineral less important than is calcium in diet planning. The active vitamin D hormone enhances phosphorus absorption, as it does for calcium. Kidney excretion primarily regulates phosphorus levels. This regulating mechanism differs from that of calcium, where changes in the rates of absorption are a more significant factor.

Functions of Phosphorus. Phosphorus is a component of enzymes, other key metabolic compounds, DNA (genetic material), cell membranes, and bone. About 85% of the body's phosphorus is inside bone. The remaining phosphorus circulates freely in the bloodstream and functions inside cells.

Phosphorus in Foods and the RDA. Milk, cheese, bakery products, and meat provide most of the phosphorus in the adult diet. Cereals, bran, eggs, nuts, and fish are also good sources. About 20% to 30% of dietary phosphorus comes from food additives, especially in baked goods, cheeses, processed meats, and many soft drinks (about 75 milligrams per 12-ounce—⅓-liter—serving of soft drinks). Next time you have a soft drink, look for a listing of phosphoric acid on the label.

The same amounts of phosphorus and calcium intake is recommended—800 milligrams per day for adults over age 24. Adults eat about 1400 to 1500 milligrams of phosphorus per day.[20] Thus deficiencies of phosphorus are unlikely in healthy adults, especially because it is so efficiently absorbed.

Marginal phosphorus status can be found in premature infants, vegans, people with alcoholism, elderly people on nutrient-poor diets, people with long-term bouts of diarrhea, and people who use aluminum-containing antacids daily (these bind phosphorus in the small intestine).

Phosphorus does not appear to be toxic for healthy adults, but high amounts can lead to problems in people with certain kidney diseases. Early studies using animals led scientists to believe that a high phosphorus intake, coupled with a low calcium intake, contributed to bone loss. However, recent research casts doubt on the importance of the calcium to phosphorus ratio in a diet, as long as the RDA for calcium is met.[25] If calcium intake is not sufficient, a high phosphorus intake may compound the resulting bone loss.

Magnesium (Mg)

Magnesium is important for nerve and heart function and aids many enzyme reactions. It is found mostly in the plant pigment chlorophyll, where it functions in respiration. We normally absorb about 30% to 40% of the magnesium in our diets, but absorption efficiency can increase up to about 75% if intakes are low. The active vitamin D hormone appears to enhance magnesium absorption.

Functions of Magnesium. Bone contains 60% of the body's magnesium. The rest circulates in the blood and operates inside cells. Over 300 enzymes use magnesium, and many energy-yielding compounds in cells require magnesium to function properly.

Animals deficient in magnesium become very irritable and, with severe deficiency, eventually suffer convulsions and often die. In humans a magnesium deficiency causes an irregular heart beat, sometimes accompanied by weakness, muscle pain, disorientation, and seizures. However, a magnesium deficiency develops very slowly, because our bodies store it readily. A link between magnesium deficiency and sudden heart attacks has been observed, and so now an intravenous dose is commonly administered to people during the early phases of treatment for a heart attack.[24]

Magnesium in Foods and the RDA. The best sources for magnesium are plant, rather than animal, products. Good food sources are whole grains (wheat bran), broccoli, squash, beans, nuts, and seeds. Milk and meats do supply some, however. Whole grains and vegetables are important parts of a diet, partly because they are excellent magnesium sources. Chocolate also contributes magnesium. Hard tap water—that containing a high mineral content—often contains a high concentration of magnesium.

The adult RDA for magnesium is 350 milligrams per day for men and 280 milligrams per day for women. Adult men consume an average of 300 milligrams daily, whereas women consume an average of 200 milligrams daily.[20] The low intake for women creates special concern, because many of them are taking more calcium to offset the possibility of osteoporosis. Because calcium can interfere with magnesium absorption, we suggest women, and men too, find good sources of magnesium and eat them regularly.

Besides being a risk to women in general, poor magnesium status is found among users of certain diuretics; some diuretics increase magnesium excretion in the urine. In addition, perspiring heavily for weeks in hot climates and bouts of long-standing diarrhea or vomiting all cause significant magnesium loss. Alcoholism increases the risk of a deficiency, because dietary intake may be poor and alcohol increases magnesium excretion in the urine. The disorientation and weakness from alcoholism resembles those of people with low blood levels of magnesium. Magnesium toxicity typically occurs only in people with kidney failure.

Sulfur (S)

Sulfur is found in many important compounds in the body, such as some amino acids (like methionine) and the vitamins biotin and thiamin. Sulfur helps in the balance of acids and bases in the body and is an important part of the liver's drug-detoxifying pathways. Because proteins supply the sulfur we need, sulfur is naturally a part of a healthful diet. Sulfur compounds are also used to preserve foods (see Chapter 17).

CONCEPT CHECK

Phosphorus is an important component of bones and cell membranes and contributes to many chemical reactions throughout the body. Good food sources include dairy products, baked goods, and meat. The body absorbs phosphorus quite efficiently, especially in the presence of active vitamin D hormone. No clear deficiency symptoms caused by poor intake have been reported. Toxicity can occur in association with kidney disease. Magnesium is found mostly in the plant pigment chlorophyll, where it functions in respiration. Magnesium is important to humans for nerve and heart function and activates many enzymes. Women in general and people with alcoholism are at risk for a poor intake. Toxicity occurs mainly in people with kidney failure. Sulfur is a component of some vitamins and amino acids. Our diets supply sulfur as part of the protein and vitamins we normally consume.

See Table 9-4 for a review of the major characteristics of water and the minerals we have discussed so far.

TRACE MINERALS

Information about ***trace minerals*** is perhaps the most rapidly expanding area of knowledge in nutrition. With the exceptions of iron and iodine, the importance of trace minerals to humans has been recognized only within the last 30 years. Although we need only about 20 milligrams—or less—of each trace mineral daily, they are just as essential to good health as are major minerals. In some cases, discovering the importance of a trace mineral reads like a detective story. And the dramas are still unfolding.

Trace Mineral *A mineral vital to health that is required in the diet in amounts less than or equal to 100 mg per day.*

As recently as 1961, researchers linked dwarfism in Middle Eastern villagers to a zinc deficiency. Other scientists recognized that a rare form of heart disease in an isolated area

TABLE 9-4

A Summary of Water and the Major Minerals

Name	Major Functions	Deficiency Symptoms	People Most at Risk	RDA or Minimum Requirement	Nutrient-Dense Dietary Sources	Results of Toxicity
Water	Medium for chemical reactions, removal of waste products, perspiration to cool the body	Thirst, muscle weakness, poor endurance	Infants with a fever, elderly persons in nursing homes	1 milliliter per kcalorie expended*	As such and in foods	Probably occurs only in those with mental disorders: headache, blurred vision, convulsions
Sodium	A major ion of the extracellular fluid; nerve impulse transmission	Muscle cramps	People who severely restrict sodium to lower blood pressure (250-500 milligrams/day)	500 milligrams	Table salt, processed foods	High blood pressure in susceptible individuals
Potassium	A major ion of intracellular fluid; nerve impulse transmission	Irregular heart beat, loss of appetite, muscle cramps	People who use potassium-wasting diuretics or have poor diets, as seen in poverty and alcoholism	2000 milligrams	Spinach, squash, bananas, orange juice, other vegetables and fruits, milk	Slowing of the heart beat; seen in kidney failure
Chloride	A major ion of the extracellular fluid; acid production in stomach; nerve transmission	Convulsions in infants	No one, probably, when infant formula manufacturers control product quality adequately	700 milligrams	Table salt, some vegetables	High blood pressure in susceptible people when combined with sodium
Calcium	Bone and tooth strength; blood clotting; nerve impulse transmission; muscle contractions; cell regulation	Poor intake increases the risk for osteoporosis	Women in general, especially those who constantly restrict their energy intake and consume few dairy products	800 milligrams (age greater than 24 years)	Dairy products, canned fish, leafy vegetables, tofu, fortified orange juice	Very high intakes may cause kidney stones in susceptible people, poor mineral absorption in general
Phosphorus	Bone and tooth strength; part of various metabolic compounds; major ion of intracellular fluid	Probably none; poor bone maintenance is a possibility	Elderly persons consuming very nutrient-poor diets; possibly total vegetarians and people with alcoholism	800 milligrams (age greater than 24 years)	Dairy products, processed foods, fish, soft drinks	Hampers bone health in people with kidney failure; poor bone mineralization if calcium intakes are low
Magnesium	Bone strength; enzyme function; nerve and heart function	Weakness, muscle pain, poor heart function	Women in general, people on thiazide diuretics	Men: 350 milligrams Women: 280 milligrams	Wheat bran, green vegetables, nuts, chocolate	Causes weakness in people with kidney failure
Sulfur	Part of vitamins and amino acids; drug detoxification; acid-base balance	None have been described	No one who meets his or her protein needs	None	Protein foods	None likely

**Just an approximation; best to keep urine volume at level greater than 1 liter (4 cups).*

of China was linked to a selenium deficiency. In America, some trace mineral deficiencies were first observed in the late 1960s and early 1970s when the minerals were not added to synthetic formulas used for intravenous feeding.

It is difficult to define precisely our trace mineral needs because we need only minute amounts. Highly sophisticated technology is required to measure such small amounts in both food and body tissues.

Iron (Fe)

The importance of dietary iron has been recognized for centuries. The Persian physician Melampus in 4000 BC gave iron supplements to sailors to make up for iron lost from bleeding wounds during battles. Today, iron deficiency is one of the most common nutrient deficiencies worldwide. Iron is the only nutrient for which adult women have a greater RDA than do adult men. Iron is found in every living cell, adding up to about 5 grams (1 teaspoon) for the entire body.

Absorption and Distribution of Iron. The body uses several mechanisms to regulate iron absorption. Controlling absorption is important, because our bodies cannot easily eliminate excess iron once it is absorbed. Iron absorption from foods varies from about 3% to 40%, depending on its form in the food, the body's need for it, and a variety of other factors (Table 9-5).[4]

The form of iron in foods greatly influences how much is absorbed. About 40% of the total iron in animal flesh is in the form of ***hemoglobin*** (the same form as in red blood cells) and ***myoglobin*** (pigment found in muscle cells). This ***heme iron*** is absorbed more than twice as efficiently as the simple elemental iron, called ***nonheme iron.*** Nonheme iron is also present in animal flesh, as well as in eggs, milk, vegetables, grains, and other plant foods.

About 10% to 15% of iron in the typical adult diet is heme iron, and usually 25% to 35% is absorbed. Nonheme iron makes up the rest, and usually 2% to 20% is absorbed.[4] Therefore animal flesh, especially red meat, is the best source of iron in the adult diet, because of both its iron content and the amount in the heme form. Consuming heme iron and nonheme iron together increases nonheme iron absorption. A protein factor in meats may also aid nonheme absorption.[12] Overall, eating meat with vegetables and grain products enhances the absorption of all nonheme iron present.

Vitamin C can increase nonheme iron absorption. So when taking an iron supplement, consider drinking a glass of orange juice with it. Consuming more foods rich in vitamin C is particularly desirable if dietary iron is inadequate or serum iron levels are low. Iron use in the body is also aided by copper, as we explain in a later section.

Several dietary factors interfere with our ability to absorb iron. Phytic acid and other factors in grain fibers and oxalic acid in vegetables can all bind iron and reduce its absorption.[11] Tannins found in tea also reduce iron absorption. When trying to rebuild iron

Hemoglobin The iron-containing part of the red blood cell that carries oxygen to the cells and some carbon dioxide away from the cells. It is also responsible for the red color of blood.

Myoglobin Iron-containing compound that binds oxygen in muscle tissue.

Heme Iron Iron provided from animal tissues in the forms of hemoglobin and myoglobin. Approximately 40% of the iron in meat is heme iron; it is readily absorbed.

Nonheme Iron Iron provided from plant sources and animal tissues other than in the forms of hemoglobin and myoglobin. Nonheme iron is less efficiently absorbed than heme iron.

TABLE 9-5

Dietary Factors That Affect Iron Absorption, Especially Nonheme Forms

Increase	Decrease
Vitamin C	Phytate fiber
Acid in the stomach	Oxalate
Heme iron	Tannins (in tea)
High body demand for red blood cells (blood loss, high altitude, physical training, pregnancy)	Full body stores
Low body stores	Great excess of other minerals (Zn, Mn, Ca)
Meat protein	Reduced stomach acid production
	Some antacids

stores, it is a good idea to keep dietary fiber under 35 grams a day and to reduce tea consumption, the latter particularly at mealtimes. Zinc also interferes with iron by competing with it for absorption. Finally, high-dose calcium supplements can also bind iron—an important consideration when taking more than 1000 milligrams in supplement form per day.

The most important factor influencing iron absorption is the body's need for it.[4] In a deficiency state, nonheme iron absorption can increase about tenfold and heme iron absorption about twofold. When iron stores are inadequate, the main serum protein that carries iron, transferrin, readily binds more iron, shifting it from intestinal cells into the bloodstream. If iron stores are adequate and transferrin is fully saturated with iron, little will be absorbed from the intestinal cells. It stays bound as a ferritin protein in the intestinal cells.

By this mechanism, in normal circumstances, iron is absorbed only as needed. If not needed, when intestinal cells are shed at the end of their 2- to 5-day life cycle, the iron returns to the lumen of the intestinal tract. This whole process is referred to as a *mucosal block* against excess iron absorption. High doses of iron can still be toxic, but absorption is carefully regulated under typical dietary conditions in most of us (Figure 9-8).

Most iron in the body is contained in the hemoglobin molecules of the red blood cells. Some iron is stored in the bone marrow, and a small portion goes to other body cells, such as the liver, for storage. As iron is needed, it can be mobilized from body stores. If dietary intake is inadequate, these iron stores become depleted. Only then do signs of an iron deficiency appear.

Functions of Iron. We mentioned that iron forms part of the hemoglobin in red blood cells and myoglobin in muscle cells. Hemoglobin molecules in red blood cells transport oxygen (O_2) from the lungs to cells and return with carbon dioxide (CO_2) from cells to the lungs for excretion. In addition, iron is used as part of many enzymes, some proteins, and other important compounds that cells use in energy production. Iron is also needed for immune function and contributes to drug detoxification pathways in the liver.

Iron-Deficiency Anemia. If neither the diet nor body stores can supply the iron needed for hemoglobin synthesis, the number of red blood cells decreases in the bloodstream. The blood hemoglobin concentration also falls. When both the percentage of red blood

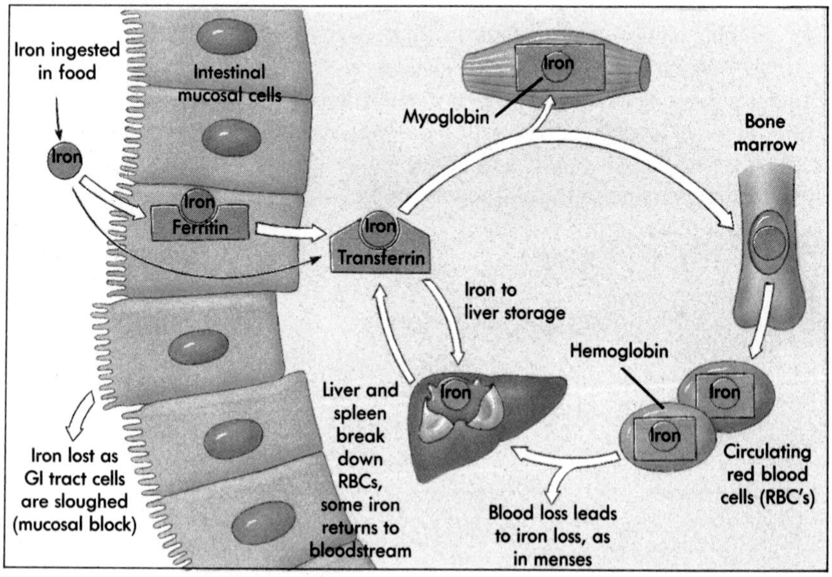

FIGURE 9-8

Iron absorption and distribution. Iron binds with a protein to form a protein called ferritin when stored in cells. If the intestinal absorption cells are shed before iron is absorbed from them, the iron is not absorbed into the bloodstream. This is one way the body can limit overabsorption of iron.

cells (called the ***hematocrit***) and the hemoglobin level fall, a physician would suspect iron deficiency.[19] In severe deficiency, the hemoglobin and hematocrit levels fall so low that the amount of oxygen carried in the bloodstream is decreased. Such a person has anemia, defined as a decreased oxygen-carrying capacity of the blood. While there are many types of anemia, iron-deficiency anemia is the major type worldwide. About 30% of the world's population is anemic, and about half of those cases are caused by an iron deficiency. Probably about 8% of Americans have iron-deficiency anemia.

Iron-deficiency anemia appears most often in infancy, the preschool years, and at puberty for both males and females. Growth, with accompanying expansion of blood volume and muscle mass, increases iron needs, making it difficult to consume enough iron. Women are also very vulnerable during childbearing years when menstruation occurs. In addition, anemia is often found in pregnant women, as we will discuss in Chapter 13. Iron-deficiency anemia in adult men is usually caused by blood loss from ulcers, colon cancer, or hemorrhoids.

Athletes can incur a special type of anemia called ***runner's anemia,*** as we discuss in Chapter 11. Three possible factors contribute to it: additional iron losses via increased perspiration, red blood cell destruction from trauma of the red blood cells being flattened as they pass through the foot when it strikes the ground during exercise, and the increase in blood volume associated with athletic fitness. Runner's anemia can decrease sports performance and so should be avoided. Although actual evidence of anemia is not often seen in athletes, they should have their hemoglobin levels and other iron status indicators monitored and should attempt to meet their iron needs by either dietary means or iron supplementation.

Clinical symptoms of iron-deficiency anemia primarily include pale skin, fatigue, poor temperature regulation, loss of appetite, and apathy. Insufficient iron for the synthesis of red blood cells and key cell compounds may cause the fatigue. Researchers suspect that poor iron stores may also decrease learning ability, attention span, work performance, and immune status even before a person is actually anemic (see Chapter 18).

More people have an iron deficiency than iron-deficiency anemia, especially in America. Probably about 6% of all adults and 30% of women have few or no iron stores.[10] Their blood hemoglobin values are still normal, but they have no stores to draw from in times of pregnancy or illness, and basic functioning may not be up to par. That could mean anything from too little energy to perform everyday tasks in an efficient manner to difficulties staying alert, say, in school or on the job.

To speed the cure of iron-deficiency anemia, a person needs to take iron supplements. A physician should also find the cause—a poor diet or a bleeding ulcer, for example—so that the anemia does not recur. A good diet may prevent iron-deficiency anemia, but supplemental iron is the only reliable cure. Recall that a vitamin C source consumed with an iron supplement enhances absorption.

Iron in Foods. The most nutrient-dense iron sources are spinach, oysters, liver, clams, peas, and legumes. However, total iron content of foods and nutrient density are not the only considerations when choosing dietary iron sources. Serving size and bioavailability are probably more important. For example, although spinach is rich in iron, the body absorbs very little of it. Animal sources contain some heme iron, the most bioavailable form. These then are our best iron sources. Iron present in iron supplements is also absorbed well. The major iron sources in the adult diet are animal and grain products. Most of the iron in bakery products has been added to refined flour in the enrichment process.

The use of iron-fortified formulas and cereals in the Special Supplemental Food Program for Women, Infant, and Children Program (WIC) in the United States is probably a major contributor to decreasing rates of iron-deficiency anemia in preschool children (see Chapter 14).[19] Another possible iron source is cooking utensils. When acidic foods, such as tomato sauce, are cooked for prolonged times in iron pots and cast iron frying pans, some iron from the cookware is taken up by the food.

Milk is a very poor source of iron. A common cause of iron-deficiency anemia in children is an overreliance on milk, coupled with an insufficient meat intake. Total vegetari-

Hematocrit
The percentage of blood that is made up of red blood cells.

Runner's Anemia
Anemia that may be caused by iron loss through perspiration, red blood cell destruction resulting from the impact of exercise, or increased blood volume; found in athletes.

A red blood cell has a life span of approximately 120 days. A rapid cell turnover such as this puts great nutrient demands on the body, and iron is one of those nutrients in great demand.

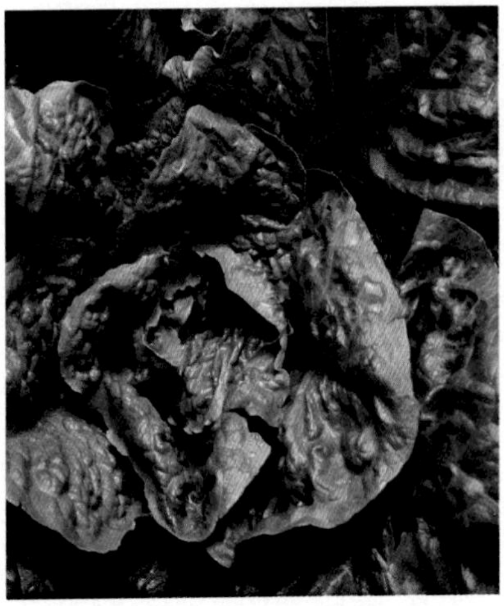

Spinach is rich in iron, but the bioavailability of iron from spinach is low.

ans (vegans) are particularly susceptible to iron-deficiency anemia, because of their lack of dietary heme iron.

Recall that vitamin C enhances iron absorption and so is another nutrient to focus on if an adequate iron status is difficult to maintain.

RDA for Iron. The daily adult RDA for iron is 10 milligrams for men and 15 milligrams for women. The RDA value assumes that about 10% of dietary iron is absorbed. If iron absorption exceeds that, less dietary iron is needed.

The higher RDA for women is primarily because of menstrual blood loss. Women who menstruate more heavily and longer than average may need even more dietary iron, and those who have lighter and shorter flows may need less iron. The variation in menstrual blood loss, and hence, loss of iron, makes it difficult to set an RDA for iron for women.

By recording dietary intakes from a variety of women, we find that most women do not consume 15 milligrams of iron daily. The average daily value is closer to 11 milligrams.[20] Of course, not all women need 15 milligrams of iron daily, because the RDA is set high enough to allow for variations in menstrual flow and absorption rates. Whether male or female, if you are not consuming the RDA for iron, you should be concerned, but not alarmed. Try to consume a diet that meets the RDA for iron. It is difficult to tell whether a lower iron intake is actually harmful. Although we have very sensitive measures of iron stores in the body, we lack the knowledge to reliably predict the resulting effects on health status when people register low values.

another BITE

The adult human body contains about 21 cups (5 liters) of blood. Blood donations are generally 2 cups (500 milliliters). Thus a blood donor gives about a tenth of his or her total supply. Healthy people generally can donate blood four times a year without harmful consequences. As a precaution, blood banks first screen potential donors' blood for the presence of anemia.

The adult diet contains about 5 to 7 milligrams of iron per 1000 kcalories. Thus men generally achieve a good iron status, because a daily energy intake of 2000 to 3000 kcalories meets their RDA for iron. By these criteria, most women would have to eat 3000 kcalories daily to meet the RDA of 15 milligrams of iron. For women with typical activity levels, it would be difficult to maintain desirable weight while eating so much. One way to resolve this problem is to eat nutrient-dense forms of iron, such as those found in fortified breakfast cereals, with an accompanying glass of orange juice to improve absorption of the iron. If that is not sufficient, a supplement can be used. Poor iron stores and iron-deficiency anemia do not develop only in the poor; they cut across all levels of society.

Toxicity of Iron. Although iron deficiency is a common problem, an overabundance of iron can also be a serious problem. Even a large single dose of iron can be life-threatening. Iron pills and vitamin supplements that contain iron poison children each year. Smaller doses (but still greater than what is needed) over a long period can also cause problems. A form of iron toxicity has been observed in an African tribe that brews beer in iron pots and in people of Mediterranean descent who often show a certain type of anemia. And as we noted in Chapter 6, excess iron in blood may speed atherosclerosis and so clogged arteries, because it makes LDL particles more likely to be taken up by cells in the blood vessels.

In America, iron toxicity also accompanies a genetic disease called ***hemochromatosis.***[7] People with this disorder overabsorb iron, and over time the amount of iron in their bodies builds up to high levels, especially in the bloodstream and liver. If not treated, excess iron is deposited in inappropriate tissues, contributing to severe liver and heart damage. About 1 in 250 to 400 adults may have hemochromatosis.

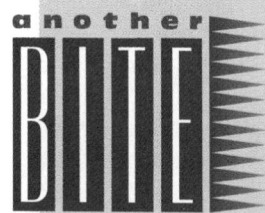

In recent years, geneticists have confirmed that as many as 1 in 10 Americans carry one copy of the hemochromatosis gene. (Sufferers carry two copies, but not everyone with two copies develops the disease.) Evidence is mounting that carrying just one copy can lead to absorption of too much dietary iron, but not as much as for people carrying two genes. The single-gene carriers then could also be prime candidates for iron-related heart disease. Experts now recommend that we all be tested for the possibility of this disease and not consume iron supplements unless prescribed by a physician.[10] Even when iron is prescribed, there should be adequate follow-up so supplementation does not go beyond what is necessary. Diets that are low in iron and frequent blood donation are key parts of the therapy for hemochromatosis.

Many people with hemochromatosis are probably saved from serious effects of the disease by consuming a low amount of iron. For many years, some nutrition interest groups have recommended increasing iron enrichment in grain products to decrease the presence of iron-deficiency anemia. However, for people with hemochromatosis, that would probably increase the numbers who actually develop disease symptoms. How could we balance the interests of both groups?

CONCEPT CHECK

Iron absorption depends on its form (heme iron is best) and the body's need for it. Iron absorption increases in the presence of vitamin C and decreases in the presence of high amounts of calcium and some components of grain fiber, such as phytic acid. Iron is important in forming hemoglobin and myoglobin and in supporting immune function. An iron deficiency can cause decreased red blood cell synthesis, which can lead to anemia. It is particularly important for women of childbearing age to consume adequate iron, primarily to replace that lost in menstrual blood. Good sources include meat, enriched grains and cereals, and seafood. Large doses of iron can lead to toxicity, and so any use of iron supplements should be under the direction of a physician.

Zinc (Zn)

Although zinc has been recognized as an essential nutrient in animals since the early 1900s, zinc deficiency was first recognized in humans in the early 1960s in Egypt and Iran. Zinc deficiencies were determined to cause growth retardation and poor sexual development in some groups of people, even though the zinc content of their diets was fairly high. However, the customary diet contained unleavened bread almost exclusively and little animal protein. Unleavened bread is very high in phytic acid and other factors that decrease zinc bioavailability. Parasite infestation and the practice of eating clay and other parts of soil also probably contributed to the severe zinc deficiency.

In America, zinc deficiencies were first observed in the early 1970s in hospitalized patients fed only intravenously. Zinc was not added to solutions used before this time, but the protein source in the solutions was based on milk protein or a blood protein, which are both naturally rich in zinc. When the solutions were changed in the early 1970s to include mostly individual amino acids as the protein source, deficiency symptoms quickly developed. This source of protein is very low in zinc.

A rare disease, acrodermatitis enteropathica, results from an inherited inability to absorb zinc. Symptoms in infants include rash, hair loss, depressed immune response, decreased sense of taste, lack of appetite, and poor growth. This disease can be treated with supplements of zinc in amounts of about twice the RDA.

Symptoms of adult zinc deficiency include an acnelike rash, diarrhea, lack of appetite, reduced sense of taste and smell, and hair loss. In children and adolescents with zinc deficiency, growth, sexual development, and learning ability may also be poor. When children show poor growth, they should be checked for adequate zinc status. A recent report emphasizes this point.[23] Children recovering from semistarvation gain weight much faster when they consume zinc supplements containing approximately three times the RDA, under a physician's guidance.

Like iron, zinc absorption is influenced by foods ingested. About 25% to 40% of dietary zinc is absorbed; the higher figure is more likely when animal protein sources are used and when the body needs more zinc. Supplementary iron competes with zinc for absorption and vice versa. Toasting cereals also reduces zinc absorption. Most people worldwide rely on cereal grains (low in zinc) for their source of protein, energy, and zinc. This makes consuming adequate zinc a problem.

Functions of Zinc. Over 200 enzymes require zinc for optimal activity. Adequate zinc intake is necessary to support many bodily functions, including the following:

- DNA and protein metabolism, wound healing, and growth
- Proper immune function (taking more than the RDA does not provide extra benefit to immune function)
- Proper development of sexual organs and bone
- Storage and release of the hormone insulin
- Alcohol metabolism
- Taste sensation

Zinc in Foods and the RDA. In general, protein-rich diets are also rich in zinc. Animal foods supply almost half our zinc intake; their cost makes zinc a very expensive nutrient. The most nutrient-dense sources of zinc are oysters, shrimp, crab, lean beef, lamb, turkey, beans, and mushrooms. As with iron, nutrient density is not the only issue; bioavailability is probably more important. Animal foods are again our best sources because zinc from animal sources is not bound by phytic acid.[13] However, good plant sources of zinc—such as whole grains, peanuts, and beans—should not be discounted. Studies show they can deliver substantial amounts of zinc to body cells.

Zinc is not part of the enrichment process, so refined flours are not a good source.

The daily adult RDA for zinc is 15 milligrams for men and 12 milligrams for women. The average daily U.S. adult intake of zinc is 9 to 16 milligrams, with men showing the higher values.[20] This raises concern that many women do not consume enough. Still, there are no indications of moderate or severe zinc deficiencies in an otherwise healthy adult population. Probably many Americans have only marginal zinc status—especially women in general, poor children, vegans, the elderly, and people with alcoholism. However, because we lack a sensitive marker for zinc status, a body must be very zinc-depleted for clinical tests to register a deficiency.

Toxicity of Zinc. A high intake of zinc interferes with iron and copper absorption. Oversupplementation with zinc can cause a copper deficiency. Studies have shown that zinc supplements at approximately three to five times the RDA can reduce HDL—the good—cholesterol levels. This is disturbing for two reasons. First, you know low HDL-cholesterol levels are associated with an increased risk of developing heart disease. Second, it is common for people who take zinc supplements to consume this amount. So some adults, by unwittingly lowering their HDL-cholesterol levels, may be increasing their risk for developing heart disease—even though they think that supplementing zinc in the diet contributes to overall health. Again, this shows why mineral supplements should not be consumed except under a physician's supervision. Otherwise, more harm than good may result. Zinc intakes of over 2 grams daily also result in diarrhea, cramps, nausea, vomiting, and sometimes depression of immune system function.

Selenium (Se)

Selenium exists in many forms that are readily absorbed. Selenium's best understood role is aiding the activity of an enzyme that participates in reducing the damage that electron-seeking (oxidizing) compounds can do to cell membranes.

In Chapter 8 we saw that vitamin E helps prevent attacks on cell membranes by electron-seeking compounds. Thus vitamin E and selenium work together toward the same goal. In Chapter 8 we also discussed how electron-seeking compounds can cause cancer. But although selenium could prove to have a role in cancer prevention, it is premature to recommend selenium supplementation for this purpose. Animal studies in this area are encouraging, and via human studies scientists are presently working to clarify selenium's role—if any—in preventing cancer. Selenium may have yet other metabolic functions, but none has been firmly established.

Selenium deficiency symptoms in farm animals and humans include muscle pain and wasting and a form of heart disease. Farm animals in areas with low selenium soil concentration, such as New Zealand, and humans in some areas of China develop characteristic muscle and heart disorders associated with poor selenium intake. Other factors probably also contribute.

Selenium in Foods and the RDA. Fish, meats (especially organ meats), eggs, and shellfish are good animal sources of selenium. Grains and seeds grown in soils containing selenium are good plant sources. Major selenium contributors to the adult diet are animal and grain products. Because we eat a varied diet of foods supplied from many geographic areas, it is unlikely that low soil levels of selenium in a few locations will mean inadequate selenium in our diets.

The RDA for selenium is 55 to 70 micrograms for adults. In general, adults meet the RDA, consuming on average 60 to 110 micrograms of selenium each day.[20]

Toxicity of Selenium. Selenium at daily intakes as low as 2 to 3 milligrams (35 times the RDA) can cause toxicity symptoms if taken for many months. These symptoms include garlicky breath odor, hair loss, nausea and vomiting, and general weakness. Rashes and cirrhosis of the liver may also develop. Selenium clearly illustrates the saying: "It's the dose that makes the poison." Because of this, FDA has limited supplemental doses in studies using humans to 200 micrograms per day.

CONCEPT CHECK

Zinc functions as a cofactor for many enzymes and is important for growth, immune function, and sense of taste. Beef, seafood, and whole grains are good food sources. As in the case of iron, the intestinal cells regulate zinc absorption according to the body's needs for the mineral. If taken in excess amounts, copper and iron compete with zinc for absorption. Selenium activates an enzyme that helps change electron-seeking (oxidizing) compounds into less toxic compounds, so these do not attack and break down cell membranes. By helping to dismantle the electron-seeking compounds, selenium works toward the same goal as vitamin E. A selenium deficiency results in muscle and heart disorders. Animal products and grains are good selenium sources; however, the selenium content in plants depends on the selenium concentration in the soil. The use of both selenium and zinc supplements can easily lead to toxic results.

Goiter An enlargement of the thyroid gland; this is often caused by insufficient iodide in the diet.

Iodine (I)

Iodine in foods is actually found in the ion form, called iodide. During World War I, a link was discovered between a deficiency of iodide and the production of a ***goiter,*** an enlarged thyroid gland (Figure 9-9). Men drafted from the Pacific Northwest and the Great Lakes Region of the United States had a much higher rate of goiter than did men from other areas of the country. The soils in these areas have very low iodide contents. In the 1920s, researchers in Ohio found that low doses of iodide given to children over a 4-year period could prevent goiter. That finding led to the addition of iodide to salt beginning in the 1920s.

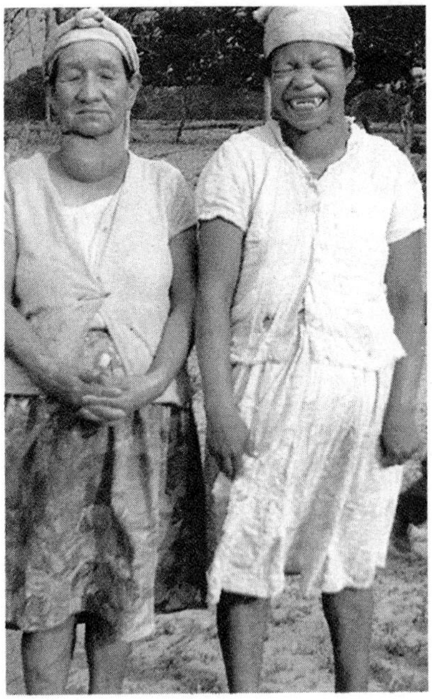

FIGURE 9-9
Iodide deficiency and goiter in Bolivia. The mother (on the left) is goitrous, but otherwise normal. The daughter is goitrous, mentally retarded, and a deaf-mute.

Today, many nations require iodide-fortification of salt. In the United States, salt can be purchased either iodized or plain. Check for this on the label of a package of salt next time you are in a grocery store. Some areas of Europe, such as northern Italy, have very low soil levels of iodide, but have yet to adopt the practice of fortifying salt with iodide. People in these areas, especially women, still suffer from goiter, as do people in areas of Central America, South America, and Africa.[6]

Function of Iodide. The thyroid gland actively accumulates and traps iodide from the bloodstream to support its hormone synthesis. Thyroid hormones, such as thyroxine, are synthesized using iodide. These hormones help regulate metabolic rate, growth, and development; in addition, they promote bone and protein synthesis.[26]

If a person's iodide intake is insufficient, the thyroid gland enlarges as it attempts to take up more iodide from the bloodstream. This eventually leads to goiter. Although iodide can prevent goiter formation, it does not shrink a goiter once it has formed. Goiters have been described in people—usually women—as far back as 3000 BC.

Goitrogens ■ *Substances in food that interfere with the absorption and use of iodide. They therefore may cause goiter if consumed in large amounts.*

Cretinism ■ *Stunting of body growth and poor mental development that result from inadequate maternal intake of iodide during pregnancy.*

another BITE

Goiters are sometimes found in people who consume large amounts of raw turnips and rutabagas. These vegetables contain compounds called ***goitrogens,*** which inhibit the function of the thyroid gland and, in turn, thyroid hormone synthesis. However, goitrogens are generally not an important cause of goiter because the cooking process destroys them, and turnips and rutabagas are not typically staples in human diets.

If a woman consumes an iodide-deficient diet during the early months of her pregnancy, the fetus suffers iodide deficiency because the mother's body uses up the available iodide. The infant then may be born with short stature and develop mental retardation. This stunted growth that results is part of what is known as ***cretinism.*** Cretinism appeared in America before iodide fortification of table salt began. Today, cretinism still appears in Europe, Africa, Latin America, and Asia.[6]

Food Sources of Iodide and the RDA. Saltwater fish, seafood, iodized salt, dairy products, and grain products contain various forms of iodide. Sea salt found in health food stores, however, is not a good source because the iodide is lost during processing.

The RDA for iodide for adults is 150 micrograms. A half teaspoon of iodide-fortified salt (about 2 grams) supplies that amount. Most adults consume much more iodide than the RDA—an estimated 240 to 400 micrograms daily.[20] This extra amount adds up because dairies and quick-service restaurants use it as a sterilizing agent, bakeries use it as a dough conditioner, food producers use it as part of food colorants, and it is added to salt.

Toxicity of Iodide. Reports in scientific literature raise concern about a high iodide intake. Levels of up to 1 milligram (6.6 times the RDA) per day appear to be safe. However, when very high amounts of iodide are consumed, thyroid gland function is hampered. This can occur in people who eat a lot of seaweed, because some seaweeds contain much iodide; total iodide intake can then add up to 60 to 130 times the RDA. Because it is potentially toxic, manufacturers are currently working to reduce unnecessary iodide use in dairies, restaurants, and bakeries.

Copper (Cu)

Copper is a critical element in the metabolism of iron; it operates in processes that form hemoglobin and transport iron. A copper-containing enzyme, ceruloplasmin, appears to aid in the release of iron from storage.[13]

Copper is needed by enzymes that create cross-connections in collagen and elastin, connective tissue proteins. In laboratory animals with copper deficiencies, blood vessels rupture because collagen is unavailable to form the important connective tissue network that strengthens blood vessels.

Copper is also needed by other enzymes, such as those that defend the body against electron-seeking (oxidizing) compounds and those that act in the brain and central nervous system. In addition, copper also performs in immune system function, blood clotting, and blood lipoprotein metabolism. Symptoms of copper deficiency include anemia, low white blood cell count, bone loss, poor growth, and some forms of heart disease.

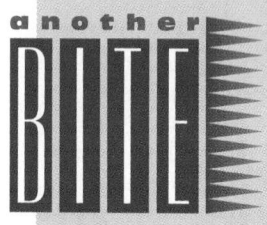

Copper in Foods and the ESADDI. Copper is found primarily in liver, cocoa, legumes, nuts, dried fruits, and whole-grain breads and cereals. It is not added to breakfast cereals because it speeds fat breakdown in the product. Milk is also a very poor source of copper. Overall, we need whole grains, nuts, and legumes to supply our copper needs. We absorb about 25% to 40% of dietary copper.

The estimated safe and adequate daily dietary intake (ESADDI) for copper is 1.5 to 3 milligrams daily for adults. The average adult intake is about 0.9 to 1.2 milligrams per day.[20] Women generally consume the lesser amount. Even so, the copper status of adults appears to be good, though we lack sensitive measures for copper status. We suggest that you regularly eat good sources of copper.

The groups most likely to develop copper deficiencies are premature infants, infants recovering from semistarvation on a milk-dominated diet (which is a poor source of copper), and people recovering from intestinal surgery (during which time copper absorption decreases). Recall that a copper deficiency can also result from overzealous supplementation of zinc, because zinc and copper compete with each other for absorption.

An inherited condition known as Menkes' kinky hair syndrome is characterized by slow growth, brain degeneration, kinky white hair, and low serum copper levels. This condition results from a defect of copper absorption and incorporation into proteins, such as ceruloplasmin. Supplemental copper is given in an attempt to partially reverse this condition.

Toxicity of Copper. Copper can cause vomiting at single doses of greater than 10 to 30 milligrams. When copper is used to treat a deficiency, it must be given in divided doses to limit this effect. An inherited condition called Wilson's disease results in accumulation of copper in the liver, brain, kidneys, and cornea of the eye. If recognized early, treatment that binds copper in the bloodstream and increases its excretion in the urine can prevent damage to these tissues and reduce the mental degeneration commonly seen in active cases.

Fluoride (F)

Dentists in the early 1900s noticed a lower rate of dental caries (cavities) in the southwestern United States. These areas contained high amounts of fluoride in the water. The levels were sometimes so high that small spots on the teeth, called mottling, appeared. Even though mottled teeth were quite discolored, they contained very few dental caries. After experiments showed that fluoride in the water did indeed decrease the rate of dental caries, controlled fluoridation of water in parts of the United States began in 1945.

Those of us who grew up drinking fluoridated water generally have 50% to 70% fewer dental caries than people who did not drink fluoridated water as children. Dentists can provide fluoride treatments, and schools can provide fluoride tablets, but it is much less expensive and more reliable to simply add fluoride to a community's drinking water. State and private water sources do not always contain enough fluoride, however. When in doubt, contact your local water plant or have the water in your home analyzed for fluoride content. If it is less than 1 part fluoride per million parts of water (1 ppm), talk to your dentist about the best means for your children to obtain the needed fluoride.

Functions of Fluoride. Dietary fluoride consumed during childhood, when bones and teeth are developing, aids the synthesis of tooth crystals that strongly resist acid. Therefore teeth become very resistant to dental caries. Fluoride also inhibits the growth of bacteria that cause dental caries (Chapter 5 reviews the development of dental caries).

Dietary fluoride has also been shown to improve growth rate in mice, but scientists are not sure whether fluoride is actually necessary for growth in humans. High doses also stimulate bone formation, and so fluoride is used experimentally to treat severe cases of osteoporosis. Results to date have been poor, but ongoing refinement in dosing schedules holds some hope for the use of fluoride as a therapeutic agent.[21]

Fluoride in Foods and the ESADDI. Tea, seafood, seaweed, and some natural water sources are the only good food sources of fluoride. Most fluoride consumed in America comes from water-fortification, toothpaste, and fluoride treatments performed by dentists. No evidence shows that water fluoridation is harmful at levels currently used in the United States.

The estimated safe and adequate daily dietary intake (ESADDI) of fluoride for adults is 1.5 to 4 milligrams. This amount provides resistance to dental caries without causing mottling of the teeth or other toxicity symptoms. Adults generally meet this level of intake.

Toxicity of Fluoride. A fluoride intake of greater than 6 milligrams daily can ***mottle*** (stain) teeth during their development. High-fluoride intake in adults does not cause mottling. When fluoride intakes reach 20 milligrams daily during tooth development, the tooth structure is weakened and can crumble. This is called *fluorosis* and appears in humans and other animals. High doses of fluoride (20 or more milligrams per day) can also cause other side effects, such as stomach upset and bone pain.

CONCEPT CHECK

Iodide is vital for the synthesis of thyroid hormones. A prolonged insufficient intake causes the thyroid gland to enlarge, resulting in a goiter. The use of iodized salt in America has virtually eliminated this condition. Copper functions mainly in iron metabolism and in the cross-bonding of collagen. A deficiency can result in an iron-deficiency type of anemia. Good food sources of copper are seafoods, legumes, nuts, dried fruits, and whole grains. Fluoride aids in tooth and bone development. When incorporated into the diet during development, fluoride makes teeth resistant to acid and bacterial growth, in turn reducing development of dental caries. Most adults get adequate amounts of fluoride via water fortification and in toothpaste. All three minerals can lead to toxic effects when consumed in excess of recommended levels.

Chromium (Cr)

The importance of chromium in human diets has been recognized only in the past 20 years. There is much we do not understand about this mineral, but chromium deficiency may be related to both diabetes and heart disease.

Functions of Chromium. Chromium helps with glucose entry into cells, but the mechanism by which it works continues to puzzle researchers.[17] In both laboratory animals and humans, a chromium deficiency results in impaired glucose clearance from the bloodstream and elevated blood cholesterol levels. We don't know how chromium influences cholesterol metabolism either, but the mechanism may involve enzymes that control cholesterol synthesis. Chromium deficiency appears in people maintained on intravenous feedings not supplemented with chromium and in children during semistarvation. Some people with diabetes have shown improvement when taking chromium supplements under a physician's scrutiny.[17] Because sensitive measures of chromium status are not available, marginal chromium deficiencies can go undetected.

Food Sources of Chromium and the ESADDI. Overall, we have little information about chromium values of foods. Egg yolks, whole grains, and meats are good sources. Poor sources are fruits, vegetables, many seafoods, highly processed foods, and drinking water. The ultimate chromium level in foods is closely tied to soil content, which varies with locality. To provide yourself with good chromium sources, eat mostly whole—not refined—forms of grains.

The estimated safe and adequate daily dietary intake (ESADDI) of chromium is 50 to 200 micrograms. We eat about 25 to 90 micrograms per day. Marginal to low chromium intakes in elderly persons may contribute to an increased risk for developing diabetes. Chromium toxicity has been reported in people exposed to industrial waste and in painters using art supplies with a very high chromium content. Liver damage and lung cancer can result.

Manganese (Mn)

It is easy to confuse the mineral manganese with magnesium. Not only are their names similar, but they also often substitute for each other in metabolic processes. Manganese is needed by some enzymes, such as those used in carbohydrate metabolism. Manganese is also important in bone formation.

TABLE 9-6

A Summary of Key Trace Minerals

Mineral	Major Functions	Deficiency Symptoms	People Most at Risk	RDA or ESADDI	Nutrient-Dense Dietary Sources	Results of Toxicity
Iron	Part of hemoglobin and other key compounds used in respiration; used for immune function	Low serum iron levels; small, pale red blood cells; low blood hemoglobin values	Infants, preschool children, adolescents, women in childbearing years	Men: 10 milligrams Women: 15 milligrams	Meats, spinach, seafood, broccoli, peas, bran, enriched breads	Toxicity is seen when children consume 200-400 milligrams in iron pills and in people with hemochromatosis
Zinc	Over 200 enzymes need zinc, including enzymes involved in growth, immunity, alcohol metabolism, sexual development, and reproduction	Skin rash, diarrhea, decreased appetite and sense of taste, hair loss, poor growth and development, poor wound healing	Vegetarians, women in general, elderly persons	Men: 15 milligrams Women: 12 milligrams	Seafoods, meats, greens, whole grains	Reduces iron and copper absorption; can cause diarrhea, cramps, and depressed immune function
Selenium	Part of antioxidant system	Muscle pain, muscle weakness, heart disease	Unknown	55-70 micrograms	Meats, eggs, fish, seafoods, whole grains	Nausea, vomiting, hair loss, weakness, liver disease
Iodide	Part of thyroid hormone	Goiter; poor growth in infancy when mother is deficient during pregnancy	None in America, because salt is usually fortified	150 micrograms	Iodized salt, white bread, saltwater fish, dairy products	Inhibition of function of the thyroid gland
Copper	Aids in iron metabolism; works with many enzymes, such as those involved in protein metabolism and hormone synthesis	Anemia, low white blood cell count, poor growth	Infants recovering from semistarvation, people who use overzealous supplementation of zinc	1.5-3 milligrams	Liver, cocoa, beans, nuts, whole grains, dried fruits	Vomiting; nervous system disorders
Fluoride	Increases resistance of tooth crystal to dental caries	Increased risk of dental caries	Areas where water is not fluoridated and dental teatments do not make up for a lack of fluoride.	1.5-4 milligrams	Fluoridated water, toothpaste, dental treatments, tea, seaweed	Stomach upset; mottling (staining) of teeth during development; bone pain
Chromium	Enhances blood glucose control	High blood glucose levels after eating	People on total parenteral nutrition, and perhaps elderly people with non–insulin-dependent diabetes	50-200 micrograms	Egg yolks, whole grains, pork	Due to industrial contamination, not dietary excess
Manganese	Aids action of some enzymes, such as those involved in carbohydrate metabolism	None in humans	Unknown	2-5 milligrams	Nuts, rice, oats, beans	Unknown in humans
Molybdenum	Aids action of some enzymes	None in humans	Unknown	75-250 micrograms	Beans, grains, nuts	Unknown in humans

No human deficiency symptom is associated with a low manganese intake. Animals on manganese-deficient diets suffer alterations in brain function, bone formation, reproduction, and blood glucose regulation. If human diets were low in manganese, these symptoms would probably appear as well. As it happens, our need for manganese is very low, and our diets tend to include a lot of manganese.

Good food sources of manganese are nuts, rice, oats and other whole grains, beans, and leafy vegetables. The estimated safe and adequate daily dietary intake (ESADDI) of manganese is 2 to 5 milligrams. Manganese is toxic at high doses, so be cautious with supplement use that exceeds your needs.

Molybdenum (Mo)

Molybdenum interacts with iron and copper, especially to inhibit copper absorption. Several human enzymes use molybdenum. No molybdenum deficiency has been noted in people who consume normal diets, though deficiency symptoms have appeared in people maintained on intravenous feedings. These symptoms include increased heart and respiration rates, night blindness, mental confusion, edema, and weakness.

Good food sources of molybdenum include beans, whole grains, and nuts. The estimated safe and adequate daily dietary intake (ESADDI) for molybdenum is 75 to 250 micrograms. When consumed in high doses, symptoms of molybdenum toxicity in laboratory animals include weight loss and decreased growth.

OTHER TRACE MINERALS

Although a variety of other trace minerals is found in humans, many of them have not yet been shown to be required. The list of minerals in this category includes boron, nickel, vanadium, arsenic, lithium, silicon, tin, and cadmium.[18] Widespread deficiency symptoms in humans have never been noted, probably because typical diets provide adequate amounts and they are needed by very few enzymes and metabolic systems. Their potential for toxicity should make one question any supplementation not supervised by a physician. These trace minerals may achieve more importance as more research is reported.

See Table 9-6 to review what we have discussed about the trace minerals.

CONCEPT CHECK

Chromium acts to maintain normal glucose uptake into cells. The amount of chromium found in food depends on soil content. Meats, whole grains, and egg yolks are some good sources. Manganese is a component of bone and used by many enzymes, including those involved in glucose production. Because our need for manganese is low, deficiencies are rare. Nuts, rice, oats, and beans are good food sources. Molybdenum is another trace mineral required by a few enzymes. Deficiencies appear only with intravenous diets. The needs for some other trace minerals—such as boron, nickel, arsenic, and vanadium—have not been fully established in humans. If required, they are needed in such small amounts that our current diets are probably adequate sources of them.

SUMMARY

- Water constitutes 50% to 70% of the human body. Its unique chemical properties enable it to dissolve substances, as well as serve as a medium for chemical reactions, temperature regulation, and lubrication. Water also helps regulate the acid-base balance in the body. For adults, daily water needs are estimated at 1 milliliter per kcalorie expended.
- Many minerals are vital for sustaining life. For humans, animal products are the most bioavailable sources of most minerals. Supplements of minerals exceeding 150% of recommended amounts should be taken only under a physician's supervision, because toxicity and nutrient interactions are a likely possibility.
- Sodium, the major positive ion found outside cells, is vital in fluid balance and nerve impulse transmission. The American diet provides abundant sodium through processed foods and table salt. About 10% to 15% of the adult population is sodium-sensitive and is at risk for developing hypertension from consuming excessive sodium.
- Potassium, the major positive ion found inside cells, functions similarly to sodium. Milk, fruits, and vegetables are good sources. Chloride is the major negative ion found outside cells. It is important in digestion as part of gastric hydrochloric acid and in immune and nerve functions. Table salt supplies most of the chloride in our diets.
- Calcium forms a vital part of bone structure and is also very important in blood clotting, muscle contraction, nerve transmission, and cell metabolism. Calcium absorption is enhanced by stomach acid and the active vitamin D hormone. Dairy products are important calcium sources. Bone loss in osteoporosis is linked to low calcium intake. Women are particularly at risk for this condition and should get plenty of calcium and exercise regularly. Estrogen replacement at menopause is currently the most accepted way to stop significant adult bone loss in women after menopause.
- Phosphorus aids enzyme function and forms part of key metabolic compounds, cell membranes, and bone. It is efficiently absorbed, and deficiencies are rare, although there is concern about possibly poor intake by some elderly women. Good food sources are dairy products, bakery products, and meats. Sulfur is incorporated into certain vitamins and amino acids. Magnesium is a mineral found mostly in plants. It is important for nerve and heart function and as an activator for many enzymes. Whole grains (bran portion), vegetables, nuts, seeds, milk, and meats are good food sources.
- Iron absorption depends mainly on the form of iron present and the body's need for it. Heme iron from animal sources is better absorbed than the nonheme iron obtained primarily from plant sources. Consuming vitamin C simultaneously with iron will increase nonheme absorption. Iron operates mainly in synthesizing hemoglobin and myoglobin and in the action of the immune system. Women are at great risk for developing iron deficiency, which decreases blood hemoglobin level and red blood cell number. When this condition is severe enough to decrease the amount of oxygen carried in the blood, iron-deficiency anemia develops. Iron toxicity usually results from a genetic disorder called hemochromatosis. This disease causes overabsorption and accumulation of iron, which can result in severe liver and heart damage.
- Zinc aids in the action of over 200 enzymes that are important for growth, development, immune function, wound healing, and taste. A zinc deficiency results in poor growth, loss of appetite, reduced sense of taste and smell, hair loss, and a persistent rash. Zinc is best absorbed from animal sources. The most nutrient-dense sources of zinc are oysters, shrimp, crab, and beef. Good plant sources are whole grains, peanuts, and beans. Copper is important for iron metabolism, collagen cross-linking, and other functions. A copper deficiency can result in an iron-deficiency–type anemia. Copper is found mainly in liver, cocoa, legumes, and whole grains. Milk is a poor source.

- An important role of selenium is decreasing the action of electron-seeking (oxidizing) compounds. In this way, selenium acts along with vitamin E. Muscle pain, muscle wasting, and a form of heart disease may result from a selenium deficiency. Meats—especially organ meats—eggs, fish, and shellfish are good animal sources of selenium. Good plant sources include grains and seeds.
- Iodide forms part of the thyroid hormones. A lack of dietary iodide results in the development of an enlarged thyroid gland or goiter. Iodized salt is a good food source.
- Fluoride incorporated into dietary intake during development makes teeth resistant to dental caries. Most Americans receive the bulk of their fluoride from fluoridated water and toothpaste.
- Chromium appears to help regulate glucose uptake by cells. Egg yolks, meats, and whole grains are good sources of chromium. Manganese and molybdenum are used by various enzymes. Deficiencies are rarely seen for any of these three nutrients. Human needs for other trace minerals are so low that deficiencies are uncommon.

STUDY QUESTIONS

1. Minerals in the diet are likely to interact with each other. Provide two examples of this for trace minerals.
2. What is the relationship between sodium and water, and how is that relationship monitored and maintained in the body?
3. What might you need to tell a 12-year-old child about the importance of consuming enough calcium?
4. Phosphorus is second only to calcium in terms of mineral content within the body. Name two ways in which phosphorus and calcium are alike, and then name two ways in which they differ.
5. Outline the histories of iodide and fluoride in human nutrition—from epidemiological observations to dietary intervention.
6. Describe what is meant by a marginal deficiency state with respect to trace minerals. What two factors make studying this state of health difficult?

REFERENCES

1. Anderson JJB: The role of nutrition in the functioning of skeletal tissue, *Nutrition Reviews* 50:388, 1992.
2. Barrett-Connor E: Risks and benefits of replacement estrogen, *Annual Review of Medicine* 43:239, 1992.
3. Chapuy MC and others: Vitamin D_3 and calcium to prevent hip fractures in elderly women, *New England Journal of Medicine* 327:1637, 1992.
4. Cook JD: Adaptation in iron metabolism, *American Journal of Clinical Nutrition* 51:301, 1990.
5. Davis CD and others: Interactions among dietary manganese, heme iron, and nonheme iron in women, *American Journal of Clinical Nutrition* 56:926, 1992.
6. Dunn JT: Iodine deficiency—the next target for elimination? *New England Journal of Medicine* 326:267, 1992.
7. Edwards CQ, Jushner JP: Screening for hemochromatosis, *New England Journal of Medicine* 328:1616, 1991.
8. Fifth Joint National Committee Report of High Blood Pressure, *American Family Physician* 45:526, 1993.
9. Greenleaf JE: Problem: thirst, drinking behavior, and involuntary dehydration, *Medicine and Science in Sports and Exercise* 24:645, 1993.
10. Herbert V: Everyone should be tested for iron disorders, *Journal of the American Dietetic Association* 91:1502, 1992.
11. Hurrell RF and others: Soy protein, phytate, and iron absorption in humans, *American Journal of Clinical Nutrition* 56:573, 1992.
12. Johnson JM, Walker PM: Zinc and iron utilization in young women consuming a beef-based diet, *Journal of the American Dietetic Association* 92:1474, 1992.
13. Johnson MA, Kays SE: Copper: its role in human nutrition, *Nutrition Today,* p. 6, January/February 1990.
14. Lambert V: Bottled water, *FDA Consumer,* p. 9, June 1993.
15. McGovern PG and others: Trends in mortality, morbidity, and risk factor levels for stroke from 1960 through 1990, *Journal of the American Medical Association* 3:1475, 1990.
16. Mikami H and others: Blood pressure response to dietary calcium intervention in humans, *American Journal of Hypertension* 3:147S, 1990.
17. Morris BW and others: The trace element chromium—a role in glucose homeostasis, *American Journal of Clinical Nutrition* 55:989, 1992.
18. Nielsen FH: Nutritional requirements for boron, silicon, vanadium, nickel, and arsenic: current knowledge and speculation, *FASEB Journal* 5:2661, 1991.
19. Oski FA: Iron deficiency in infancy and childhood, *New England Journal of Medicine* 329:190, 1993.
20. Pennington JAT, Young FE: Total diet study nutritional elements, *Journal of the American Dietetic Association* 91:179, 1991.
21. Riggs BL, Melton LJ: The prevention and treatment of osteoporosis, *The New England Journal of Medicine* 327:620, 1992.
22. Rolls BJ, Phillips PA: Aging and disturbance of thirst and fluid balance, *Nutrition Reviews* 48:137, 1990.
23. Sandstead HH: Zinc deficiency: a public health problem? *Journal of Diseases in Children (AJDC)* 145:853, 1991.
24. Seelig MS: Interrelationship of magnesium and estrogen in cardiovascular and bone disorders, eclampsia, migraine, and premenstrual syndrome, *Journal of the American College of Nutrition* 12:442, 1993.
25. Spencer H and others: Do protein and phosphorus cause calcium loss? *Journal of Nutrition* 118:657, 1988.
26. Zamula E: Thyroid disorders often unsuspected, *FDA Consumer,* p. 34, December 1992.
27. Zimmerman J: Does dietary calcium supplementation reduce risk of colon cancer? *Nutrition Reviews* 51:109, 1993.

RATE

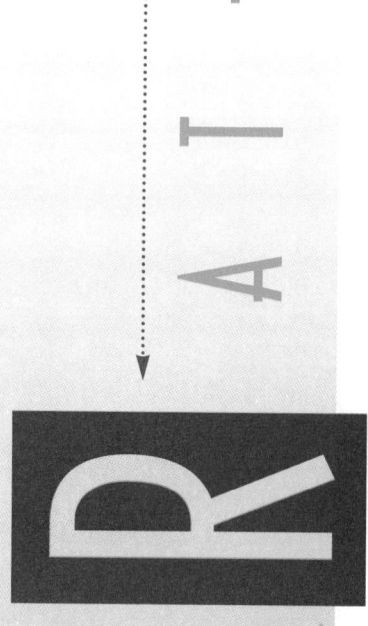

HOW DOES YOUR MINERAL INTAKE MEASURE UP AGAINST VALUES FROM THE CURRENT RDA?

To complete this activity, you must reexamine your nutritional assessment from Chapter 2. Compare your intake of selective minerals with the RDA (or other standards given). Use your completed nutritional assessment to complete the table below. For each mineral, record your intake, the RDA, the percentage of the RDA you consumed, and a +, –, or = to indicate an intake higher, lower, or equal to the RDA. Note that for sodium and potassium, minimum requirements of health are designated and are already recorded in the table (these can also be found on the inside front cover of the book). RDAs have not been established for these two minerals.

Mineral	Intake	RDA	% of RDA	+/–/=
Calcium				
Phosphorus				
Sodium		500 mg		
Potassium		2000 mg		
Iron				
Zinc				

Analysis

1. Which of your mineral intakes equaled or exceeded the RDA (or other standard given)? Do the nutrients for which you exceeded the RDA pose a likely risk for toxicity, as noted in the chapter?

____

2. Which of your intakes were below the RDA (or other standard given)?

____

3. What foods or cooking practices could be emphasized or deemphasized to modify your weaknesses?

____

____

____

____

____

Nutrition ISSUE

MINERALS AND HYPERTENSION

Blood pressure is expressed by two different numbers. The higher number represents systolic blood pressure, the pressure in the arteries when the heart actively pumps blood. The second value is diastolic pressure, the pressure in the arteries when the heart is relaxed. Normal systolic blood pressure values vary from 100 to 130 millimeters of mercury (mm Hg). Normal diastolic blood pressure values vary from 60 to 85 mm Hg.

Hypertension is defined as sustained high blood pressure, with systolic pressure exceeding 140 mm Hg or diastolic blood pressure exceeding 90 mm Hg on at least two occasions after the original detection. Most hypertension (90% to 95%) has no apparent cause. It is called primary or ***essential*** hypertension. Kidney disease often causes the other 5% to 10% of cases.

About 20% of American adults have essential hypertension. This is called a *silent* disease, because—unless blood pressure is measured periodically—no one knows it is developing. A physician usually does not treat hypertension with medication until the diastolic blood pressure measures at least 90 mm Hg on three or more occasions. But any value over about 85 mm Hg is actually too high and deserves dietary and lifestyle interventions.[8]

Why Control Hypertension?

Hypertension needs to be controlled mainly to prevent heart disease, kidney disease, and strokes. All three diseases are much more likely to be found in people with hypertension than in those with normal blood pressure. People with hypertension should be diagnosed and treated as soon as possible. We now know the value of aggressively treating hypertension; in the last 20 years, blood pressure values have fallen, along with the incidence of strokes and heart attacks.[15]

Causes of High Blood Pressure

A variety of factors affect blood pressure. Blood pressure usually increases as a person ages. Atherosclerosis causes some increase (see Chapter 6). As plaque builds up, arteries become less flexible and cannot expand as the heart pumps. When vessels remain rigid, blood pressure remains high. Eventually the plaque begins to choke off blood supply to the kidneys, decreasing their ability to control blood volume and, in turn, blood pressure.

Obesity is associated with high blood pressure, especially in men. Inactivity also increases the risk for high blood pressure. If an obese person can lose weight and become more physically active by exercising three or four times a week, blood pressure often returns to normal values.[8] A weight loss of as little as 10 to 20 pounds can help, especially in men. Often a minor change in lifestyle can greatly reduce, or even eliminate, the need for medications.

African-Americans are more likely to have high blood pressure than are Caucasians. In addition, alcohol has a greater tendency to raise blood pressure in African-Americans than it does in Caucasians. However, both races should moderate alcohol intake, especially men, to control blood pressure. Various blood enzymes and hormonelike compounds also affect blood pressure.

Sodium and Blood Pressure

Sodium tends to increase blood pressure in some people. The average adult intake of 3 to 7 grams can elevate blood pressure, particularly in those who are sensitive to its effects. However, not all of the 20% of Americans with hypertension are very sensitive to sodium. Therefore sodium in the diet is not a problem for everyone, even among people with hypertension. Nevertheless, in populations that eat 1.5 grams or less of sodium daily, hypertension is rare. A decrease in blood pressure usually appears when sodium is restricted to a level of approximately 2 to 3 grams a day. When medications are used to treat hypertension, a sodium restriction of 4 grams per day is generally employed. This restriction aids the function of the medications typically used, such as diuretics. These reduce blood volume by increasing urination and, in turn, lead to a fall in blood pressure. Although some experts recommend that all people with hypertension reduce sodium intake, we feel dietary advice should be given on an individual basis once a response to treatment is verified.

Calcium and Blood Pressure

Since 1983 there has been debate concerning whether calcium intake can affect blood pressure. Careful studies show that some people register slightly lower blood pressures when they consume the RDA for calcium, compared with about half of the RDA. Systolic blood pressure is affected more than diastolic blood pressure. It is reasonable for a person with hypertension to experiment, in consultation with a physician, by increasing calcium intake to see whether that produces a benefit.[16]

Preventing Hypertension

Hypertension develops in many adults, especially in those with family histories of hypertension. To prevent hypertension, we recommend maintaining an active lifestyle and a desirable body weight. Regular exercise is a key component. Limiting alcohol use is also very important (Table 9-7). A reduction in stress adds to the list of preventive measures.

Population studies suggest that a low-sodium diet may lead to less hypertension later in life. But many people never develop hypertension, regardless of their sodium intake. Sodium appears to be a villain only for some of us. If you have hypertension or a family history of hypertension, it is a good idea to reduce sodium intake. The American Heart Association suggests that you keep your sodium intake under 3 grams per day. Some people may choose to limit their sodium only if hypertension develops. As we said before, most of us need to be prudent—not paranoid—about dietary sodium.

In addition, we suggest consuming a diet rich in dairy products, fruits, and vegetables. This provides ample potassium, calcium, and magnesium—all of which may contribute to a lower blood pressure.[8] Even if drugs are needed, a proper diet and lifestyle approach can often reduce the necessary dosage and, in turn, reduce the expense and side effects of medications. Nutritional therapy is a key to treating hypertension.

TABLE 9-7

A Nutritional Plan to Minimize Hypertension Risk and Aid in Therapy

1. Lose weight, and try to attain a desirable body weight.
2. Incorporate regular physical activity into your lifestyle.
3. Meet the RDA for calcium, potassium, and magnesium.
4. Consume alcoholic beverages in moderation, if at all.
5. Consume moderate to scant amounts of sodium.

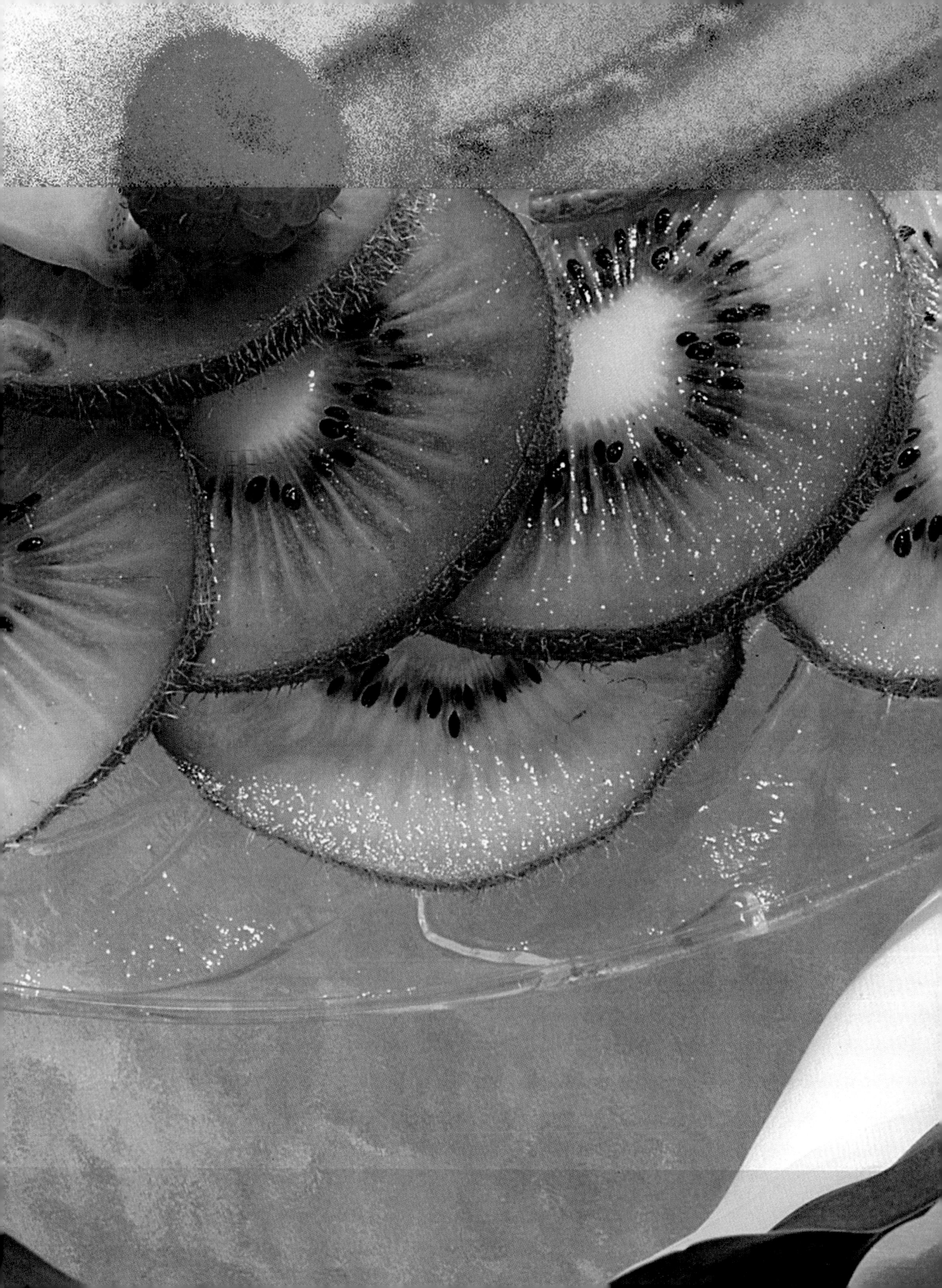

ENERGY: BALANCE AND IMBALANCE

3

c h a p t e r

10

WEIGHT CONTROL

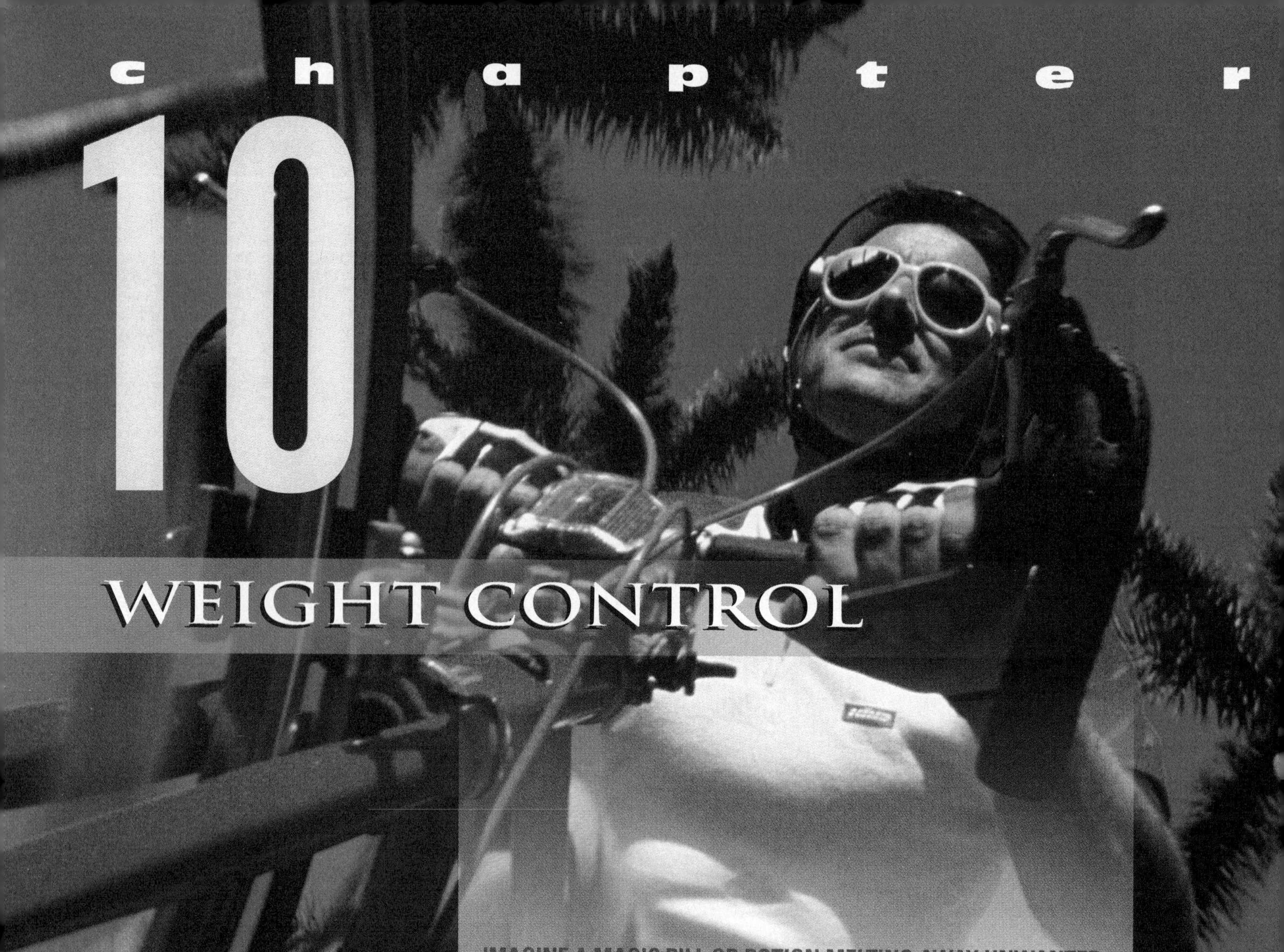

IMAGINE A MAGIC PILL OR POTION MELTING AWAY UNWANTED pounds. No sweat or starvation, just a sleek body in a few quick swallows. Many proponents of *magical* drinks and diet programs erroneously claim they eliminate excess fat forever. Consumers presently pour $30 billion into the diet industry, a business predicted to increase by $20 billion within 5 years. The diet industry digests dollars, and consumers lose not only pounds. They often lose cash—and sometimes good health— needlessly.

Of people you see on the street, one fourth of the men and nearly half the women will be struggling to control weight.[17] But for all the struggles, the ranks of the obese in America are still bulging. Most diets fizzle before bodies become slim. Monotonous, ineffective, and confusing, fad diets even endanger some populations, such as children, teenagers, pregnant women, and people with various health disorders.

The secret to weight loss is actually very straightforward: (1) eat less, especially fat, (2) exercise more, and (3) change problem eating behaviors.[27] This chapter discusses these recommendations to help you understand obesity's causes, treatments, and effects. You will learn how to take charge of a weight problem by replacing fad diets with the three key actions recommended above.

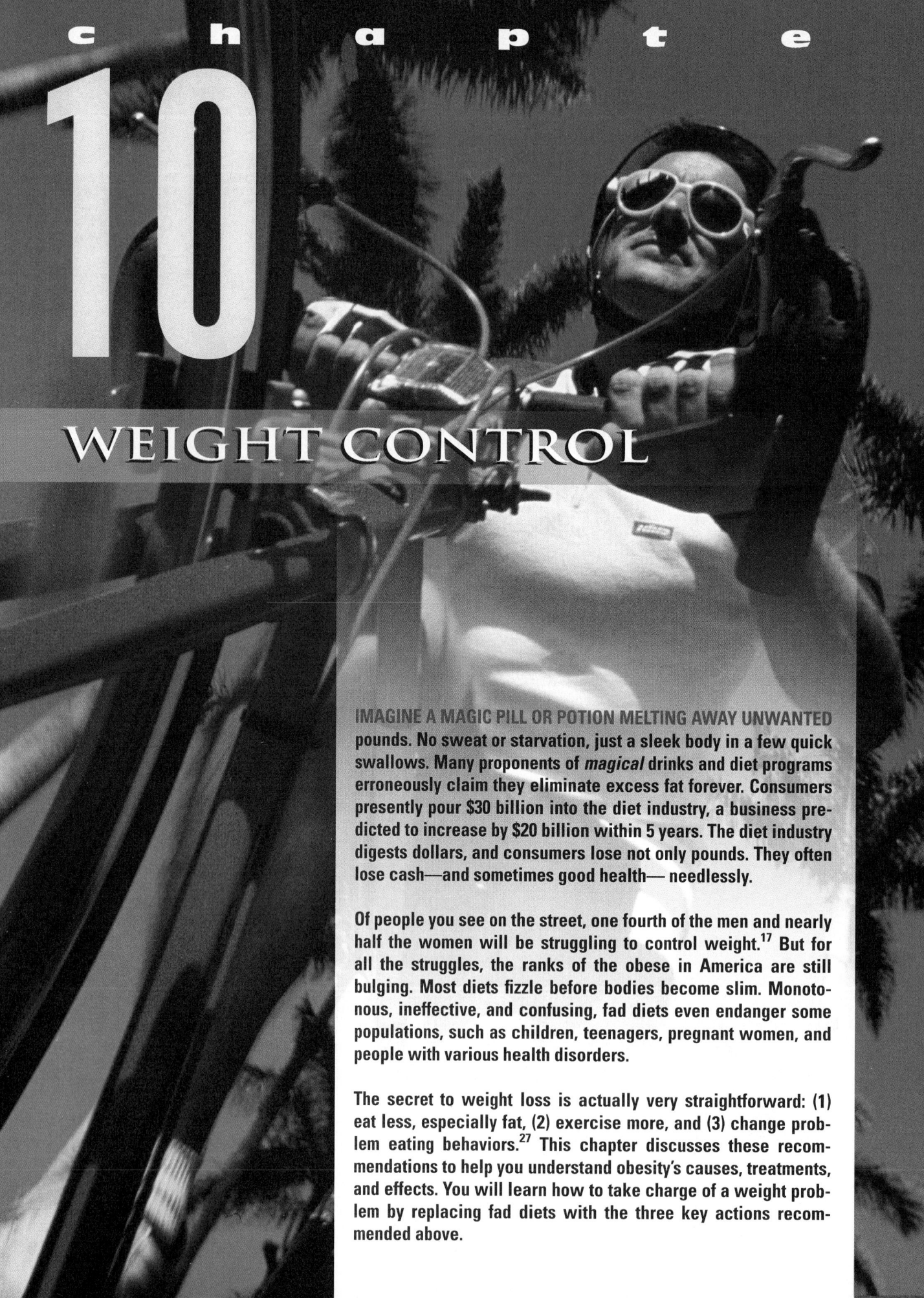

ASSESS YOUR KNOWLEDGE

IS THE TTFV LIPOLOSS WEIGHT LOSS PLAN FOR YOU?

Read the following discussion of the TTFV Lipoloss Weight Loss Plan. See whether it is one you would want to follow.

Do you want to turn your body into a high-powered fat burner? Try the TTFV Lipoloss Weight Loss Plan, scientifically proven to be the quickest and most permanent fat loss miracle in America. The nutritional part of the TTFV Plan consists of eating 800 kcalories of delicious tuna, turkey, fruits, and vegetables. Combine the fruits with the turkey and the vegetables with the tuna to achieve the greatest lipoloss effect (remember, *lipo* means fat).

We encourage at least 30 minutes of aerobic exercise—brisk walking, jogging, swimming, or biking—three to five times per week. And we haven't forgotten those diet-wrecking urges and cravings. Fight them with our high-fiber Urge-Smasher Wafers. These wafers fill you up, fighting the gnaw of hunger.

If you have any health problems, see your physician for approval and clearance for regular exercise. Overall, with the TTFV LipoLoss Plan you can lose 3 to 5 pounds each week and enjoy a variety of tasty food.

Now rate this diet based on the following questions; a perfect score of 100 points indicates a good weight loss plan. Start at 100 points.

1. Will the diet meet all nutritional needs with a wide variety of foods? IF NOT, SUBTRACT 10 POINTS.
2. Does the program stress slow and steady weight loss of about 1 to 2 pounds per week rather than rapid loss? IF NOT, SUBTRACT 10 POINTS.
3. Is the diet tailored to individual habits and tastes, diminishing feelings of deprivation? IF NOT, SUBTRACT 10 POINTS.
4. Does the plan avoid rigid rituals, such as eating fruits only in the morning or not eating meat after milk products? IF NOT, SUBTRACT 10 POINTS.
5. Does the diet minimize hunger and fatigue by containing at least 1000 kcalories per day? IF NOT, SUBTRACT 10 POINTS.
6. Does the diet include readily obtainable foods, with no special products to buy to speed weight loss? IF NOT, SUBTRACT 10 POINTS.
7. Is the diet socially acceptable, allowing the dieter to attend parties, eat at restaurants, and participate in normal daily activity? IF NOT, SUBTRACT 10 POINTS.
8. Does the plan promote changes in eating habits and lifestyle so that weight maintenance will be possible? IF NOT, SUBTRACT 10 POINTS.
9. Does the plan emphasize regular physical activity? IF NOT, SUBTRACT 10 POINTS.
10. Does the plan encourage the dieter to see a physician before starting if the person has existing health problems, wants quick weight loss, is over 35 years of age, or plans to perform vigorous physical activity? IF NOT, SUBTRACT 10 POINTS.

Now, having assessed the TTFV Lipoloss Weight Loss Plan, how many points would you give it? SCORE ______________________

Would you choose this weight loss plan if you were attempting to lose fat and keep it off?
YES ______ NO ______

To assess the legitimacy of any weight loss plan, ask yourself questions like those above. With so many competing diet plans available, you can save yourself money, disappointment, effort, and time by asking the right questions.

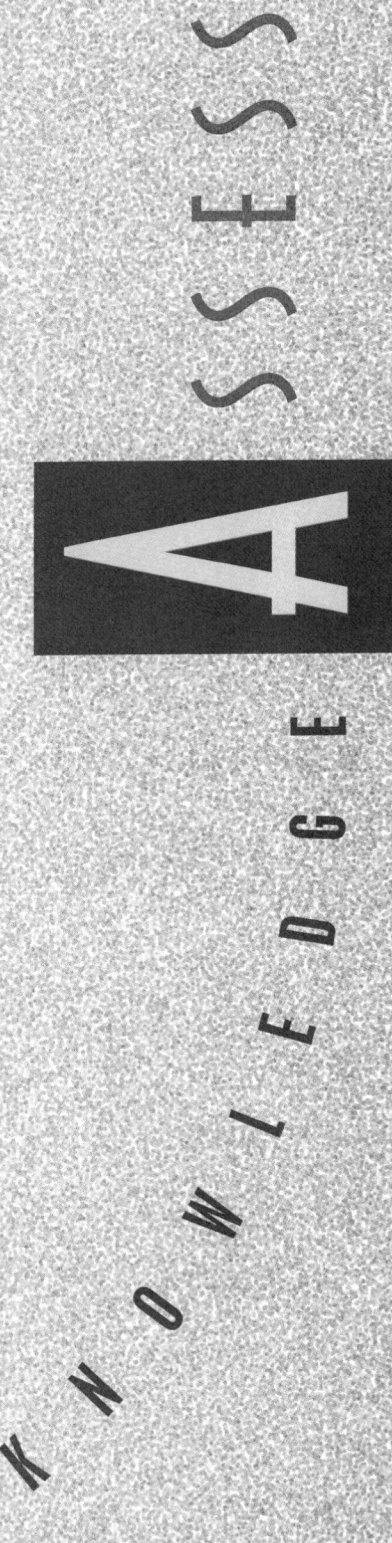

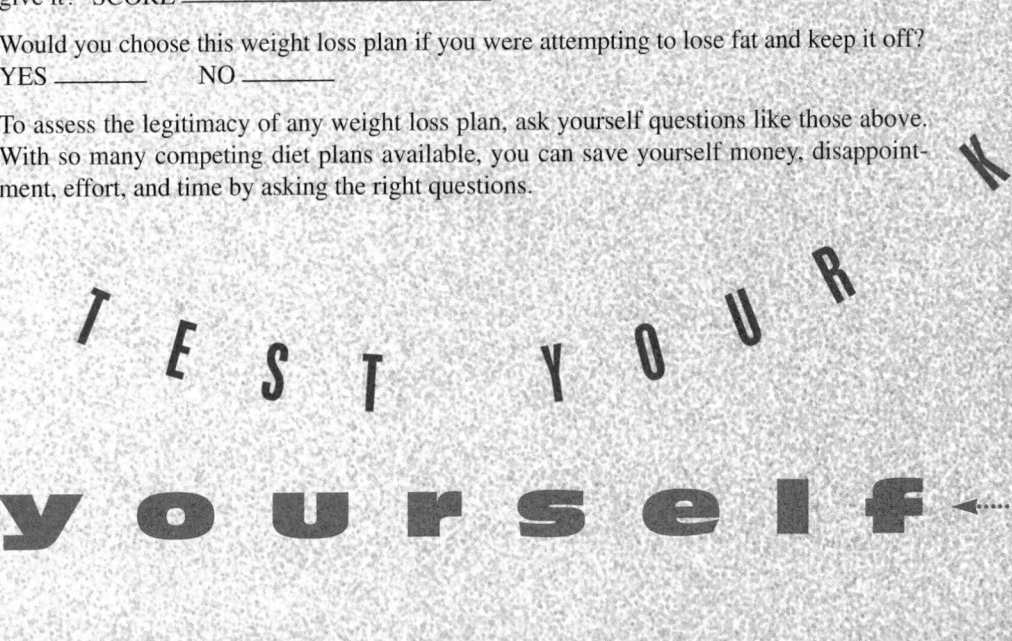

TEST YOUR yourself

ENERGY INTAKE: THE FIRST HALF OF ENERGY BALANCE

Does your weight yo-yo up and down while you aim for your ideal? If the scales keep you emotionally off balance, consider another scale—that of energy balance. This balance depends on energy input and energy output (Figure 10-1). Excesses or deficits in this balance go on to influence energy stores, primarily in adipose (fat) tissue[9] (Figure 10-2). Let's look at the factors affecting this balance.

Two drives influence our desire to eat, ***hunger*** and ***appetite.*** These differ dramatically. Hunger is our physiological drive to eat and is controlled by internal body mechanisms. Appetite can be seen as our psychological drive to eat and is affected by external food choice mechanisms, such as seeing a tempting dessert. Fulfilling either or both drives normally brings a state of ***satiety,*** temporarily halting the desire to eat.[23]

Hunger *The physiological or internal drive to find and eat food.*

Appetite *The psychological or external drive to find and eat food, often in the absence of hunger.*

Satiety *A state in which there is no longer a desire to eat.*

Hypothalamus *A grouping of cells at the base of the brain. These cells participate in many body functions, such as in the regulation of hunger.*

The Hypothalamus: A Satiety Regulator

The ***hypothalamus,*** a portion of the brain stem, helps regulate satiety. When stimulated, cells in the *feeding center* of the hypothalamus signal us to eat. Then as we eat, hunger decreases. Eventually, we stop eating as cells in the *satiety center* of the hypothalamus are stimulated.[23] Blood glucose levels probably stimulate both centers. When glucose levels drop, we eat. Other cues to eat probably come from amino acids and fatty acids in the bloodstream and from various hormones and other substances.[14] Such internal signals both inhibit and encourage food intake.

Chemicals, surgery, and some cancers can destroy the feeding and satiety centers in the hypothalamus. Without satiety center activity, laboratory animals (and humans) eat their way to obesity. Without feeding-center activity, animals eat little and eventually lose weight.

Satiety Is Regulated at Other Body Sites

Satiety is actually controlled by a complex network of mechanisms spread throughout the body that regulate the desire to either eat or avoid food. The satiety and feeding centers in the hypothalamus especially communicate and interact with other decision points in the brain and in the liver.[7]

Hormones Regulate Satiety

Endorphins, the body's natural painkillers, and hormones, such as high amounts of cortisol, can prod us to eat. On the other hand, other hormones, hormone-related compounds, and still other chemical factors in the body can contribute to the feeling of satiety.[23] With eating, blood concentrations of some digestive hormones—cholecystokinin (CCK), secretin, gastrin, and others—increase. This increase, combined with stomach distention, helps shut off hunger. Certain arms of the nervous system also contribute to this satiety.[4]

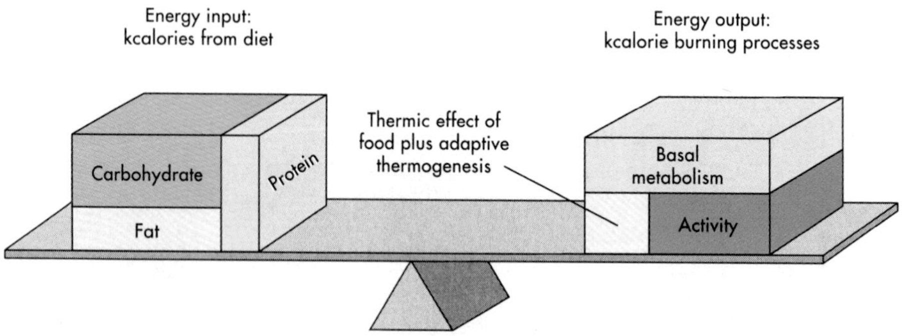

FIGURE 10-1
A model for energy balance. This model incorporates the major variables that influence energy balance.

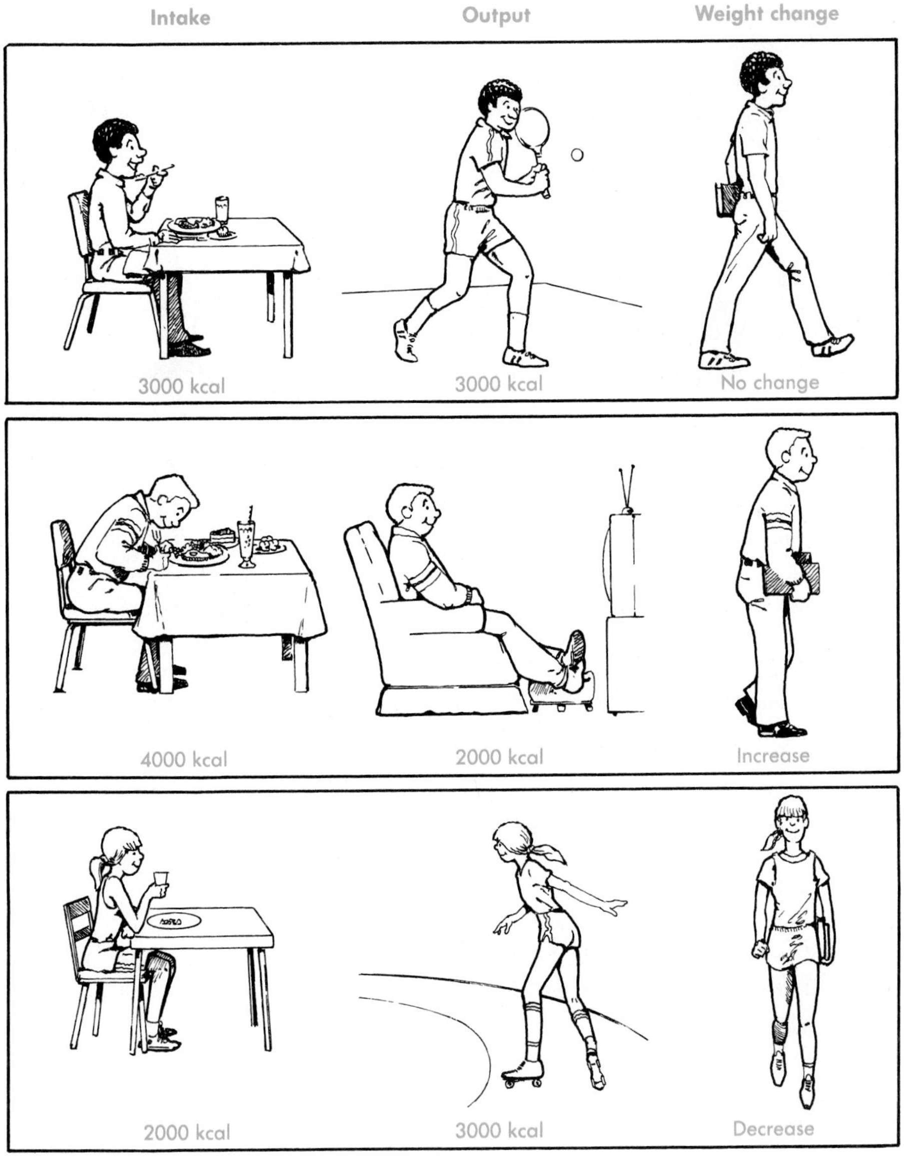

FIGURE 10-2
The energy equation. Overall, to maintain weight we need to use roughly the same number of kcalories we consume. It's a simple equation, but an unforgiving one if we deviate either way.

Does Appetite Regulate What We Eat?

Various feeding and satiety messages from body cells do not singlehandedly determine what we eat. Almost everyone has encountered a mouthwatering dessert and devoured it, even on a full stomach (Figure 10-3). Appetite can be affected by a great variety of external forces, such as environmental and psychological factors and social customs.

We often eat because food confronts us. It smells good, tastes good, and looks good. We might eat because it is the right time of day, we are celebrating, or we are trying to overcome the blues. Appetite may not be a biological process, but it does influence food intake.[8] After a meal, memories of pleasant tastes and feelings reinforce appetite. If stress or depression sends you to the refrigerator, you are mostly seeking comfort, not energy.

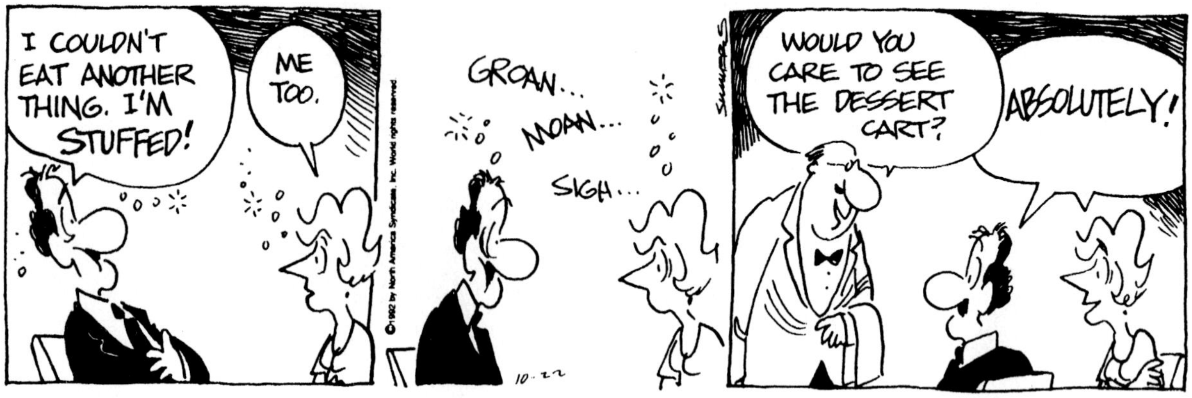

Reprinted with permission of North America Syndicate, Inc.

FIGURE 10-3
The Middletons.

Internal and external signals—driving hunger and appetite—generally operate simultaneously and combine into a momentary decision whether to reject or eat a food item. Often we don't think about why or what we eat, but a simple reconsideration of what motivates your food choices may show you whether you respond to hunger or to external factors linked to appetite, such as what you feel like eating. American prosperity and ample food supply set the stage for a population that eats primarily from appetite and habit, not hunger. If you rarely feel real hunger, you probably reach for food mostly as a reflex.[11]

Putting Hunger and Appetite into Perspective

The next time you pick up a candy bar or ask for second helpings, remember the physiological and psychological influences on eating behavior (Figure 10-4). Body cells (brain, mouth, stomach, intestine, liver, and other organs), hormones (like cortisol), and social customs all influence food intake.[7] Where food is ample, appetite—not hunger—mostly triggers eating. Keep track of what triggers your eating for a few days. Is it primarily hunger or appetite?

CONCEPT CHECK

Hunger is the physiological drive to find and eat food and is regulated by internal mechanisms, such as the brain, adipose tissue, liver, and hormones. Appetite is the psychological drive to find and eat food and is affected mostly by external factors, such as social custom, time of day, and food palatability. Internal and external factors influence decisions about food intake. Appeasing both hunger and appetite typically leaves us in a state of satiety. Americans probably respond more to external appetite-related forces than to hunger-related ones in choosing when and what to eat.

ENERGY USE: THE OTHER SIDE OF ENERGY BALANCE

We have examined some factors that encourage energy intake. Now let's look at the other side of the relationship—energy output.

Energy Use by the Body

The body uses energy for three general purposes: basal metabolism, physical activity, and the thermic effect of food (see Figure 10-1). Shivering, the body's reflex to cold, demon-

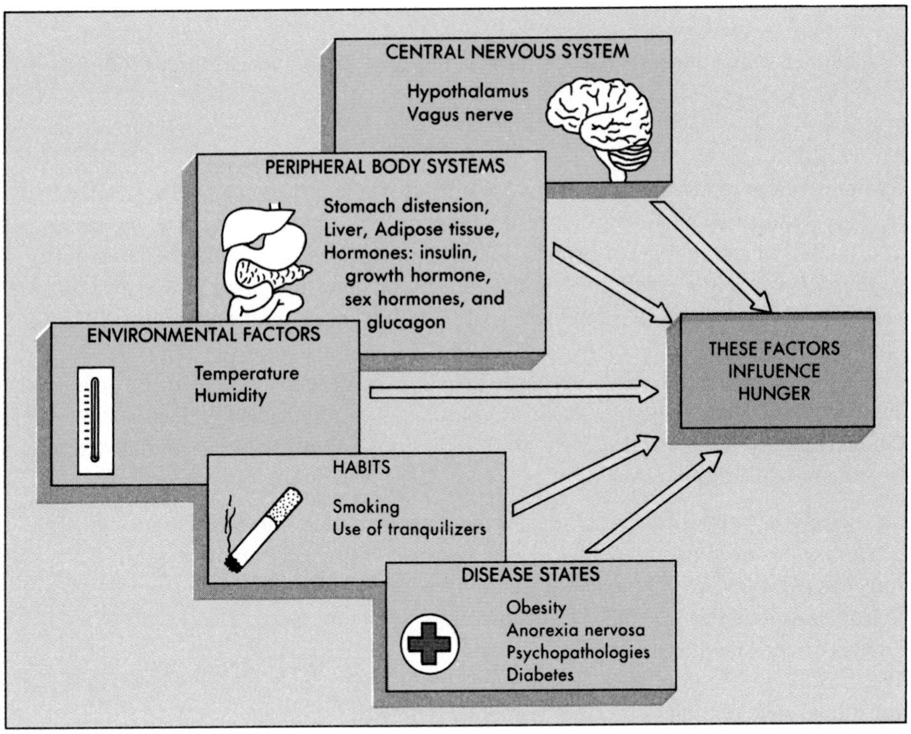

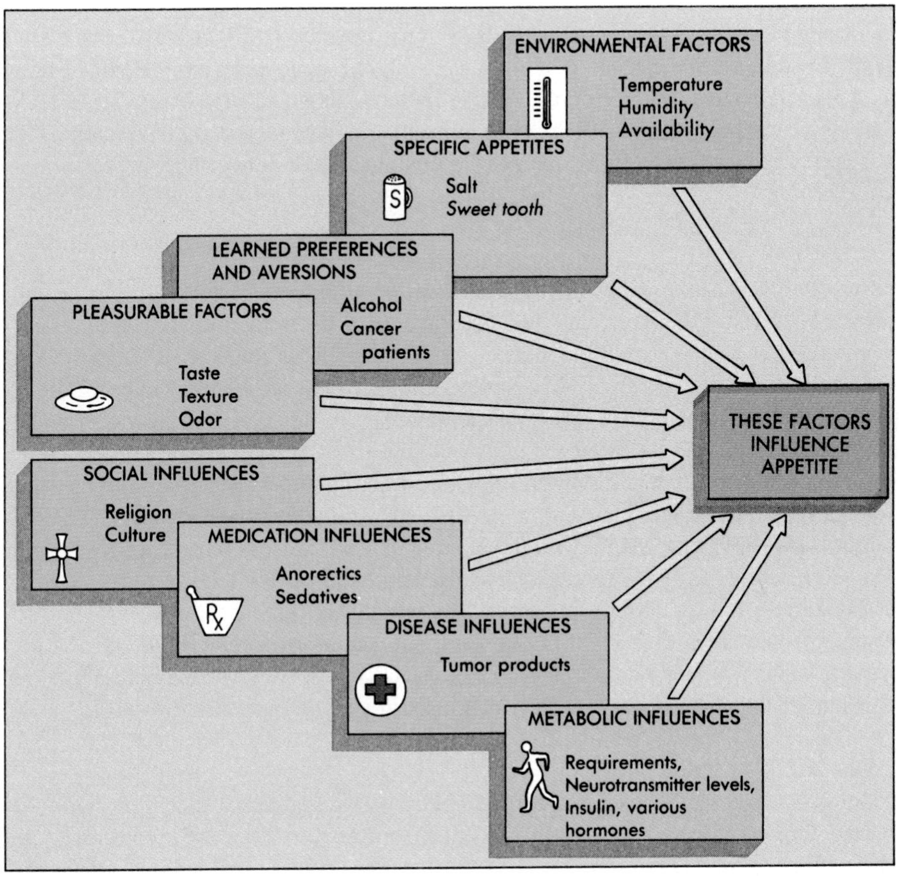

FIGURE 10-4
A model incorporating many factors that influence hunger and appetite. Together these influences regulate satiety.

strates another minor form of energy turned into heat production, often called *adaptive thermogenesis.*

Basal Metabolism *The minimal energy the body requires to support itself when resting and awake. It amounts to roughly 1 kcalorie per minute, or about 1400 kcalories per day.*

Thermic Effect of Food *The increase in metabolism occurring during the digestion, absorption, and metabolism of energy-yielding nutrients. This represents 5% to 10% of kcalories consumed.*

While a person is resting, percent of total energy use by various organs is about as follows:

Liver	26%
Muscle	26%
Brain	18%
Heart	9%
Kidney	7%
Other	14%

Basal Metabolism

Basal metabolism represents the minimal energy expended to keep a resting, awake body alive. This requires about 60% to 70% of total energy use by the body. The processes involved include maintaining a heartbeat, respiration, temperature, and other functions. It does not include energy used for physical activity or digesting foods. Basal metabolism accounts for about 1 kcalorie per kilogram of body weight per hour, or about 1400 kcalories per day.

The amount of energy used for basal metabolism depends primarily on lean body mass. The participating tissues—such as muscle, liver, brain, and kidney—show high metabolic activity at rest and have high energy needs. Other influences that determine basal metabolism are the following:

- The amount of body surface (the greater the area, the greater the heat loss)
- Gender (males average higher energy use, because of greater lean body mass)
- Body temperature (fever increases metabolic rate)
- Thyroid hormone levels (higher levels increase metabolic rate)
- Aspects of nervous system activity
- Age (metabolic rate falls as we age through adulthood)
- Nutritional state (eating less slows metabolic rate in the short term)
- Pregnancy (increases metabolic rate)
- Caffeine and tobacco use (increases metabolic rate)

A low-kcalorie intake decreases the basal metabolic rate (BMR) by about 10% to 20%, or about 150 to 300 kcalories per day.[18] This lowered BMR makes losing weight difficult. In addition, the effects of aging make weight maintenance hard. BMR declines about 2% each decade past age 30 as actively metabolizing cells slowly and steadily decrease. However, because physical activity helps maintain lean body mass, remaining active as one ages helps maintain a high basal metabolism and, in turn, aids in weight control.

Energy for Physical Activity

Basal metabolism uses roughly the same proportion of energy in most people (usually varies ± 25% to 30% between individuals). Physical activity then increases our energy expenditure above and beyond our basal energy needs by as much as 25% to 40%. In choosing to be inactive or active, we determine much of our total energy expenditure for a day. Unlike basal metabolism, energy expenditure from physical activity varies widely among people.

Climbing stairs rather than riding the elevator, walking rather than driving to the store, and standing in a bus rather than sitting increase physical activity and, hence, energy use. Recent studies show that people who fidget and can't sit still use more energy (an extra 100 to 800 kcalories daily in one study) than do those who readily relax.

The alarming rate of obesity in America is caused by our inactivity.[10] We eat little more than people did at the turn of this century, but we are less active (Figure 10-5). Jobs demand less physical activity, and leisure time usually is spent slouched before a television. What are the alternatives to obesity and inactivity? One answer is *movement!*

Thermic Effect of Food

In addition to basal metabolism and physical activity, the body uses energy to digest, absorb, and further process food nutrients.[21] Energy used for these tasks contributes the ***thermic effect of food.*** The energy cost of this thermic effect is analogous to a sales tax. It is like being taxed about 5% to 10% for the total energy you eat. The charge covers the cost of processing that energy. To supply the body with 100 kcalories for basal metabolism and physical activity, a person must eat between 105 and 110 kcalories. The process-

NUTRITION insight

THE TRUE ENERGY VALUE OF FAT

In the bomb calorimeter, fats produce about 9 kcalories per gram. However, when stored for energy, fats function very efficiently. Dietary fats induce little thermic effect of food, because most fat consumed bypasses the liver on its way to the bloodstream and ultimately to body cells. Thus because no energy is used to metabolize it in the liver, very little energy in fat is lost when it transfers from food directly to fat storage.

In contrast, all carbohydrate and protein eaten must pass through the liver, the latter as amino acids. We have an especially limited ability to store carbohydrate.[25] Excess amounts generally are metabolized into various fats once liver glycogen stores are full. The fats then enter the bloodstream. This applies to excess protein intake as well. Metabolic processing demands about a quarter of the energy content of carbohydrates or proteins eaten.

Scientists note that when fed equal amounts of energy, growing rats on high-fat diets gain more weight than do rats on low-fat diets. If fats use fewer kcalories per gram during their initial distribution in the body, it follows that high-fat diets will cause greater weight gain. We also have an essentially limitless ability to store this fat. As well, fat intake does not stimulate fat use for energy, whereas carbohydrate and protein intake stimulate use of these fuels.[25] Overall, high-fat foods tend to make us fat, whereas high-carbohydrate foods may not necessarily do so.[7,22] In cutting kcalories, eliminating fat first is the best policy.

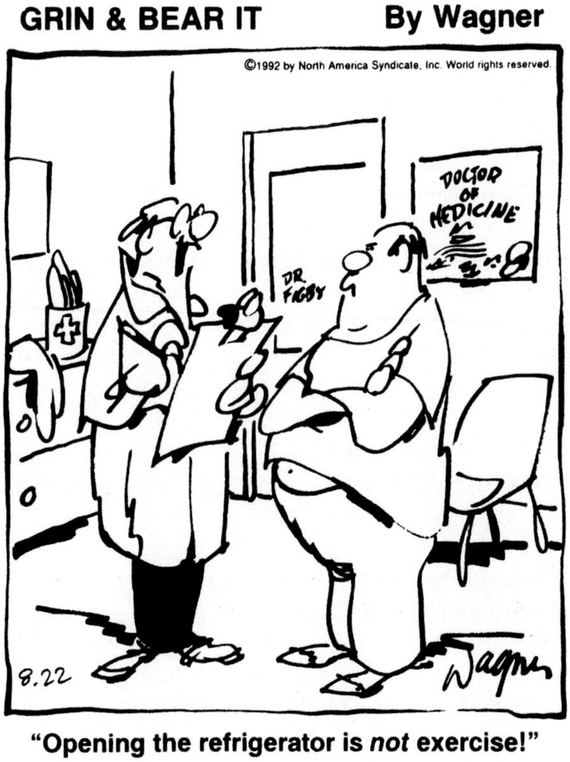

FIGURE 10-5
Grin and Bear It.

es of digestion, absorption, and metabolism use the extra 5 to 10 kcalories to modify the energy-yielding nutrients for use. Given a daily kcalorie intake of 3000, the thermic effect of food would use 180 to 300 kcalories. However, the total amount can vary somewhat among individuals.

Adaptive Thermogenesis

The body expends some energy to produce heat in response to a cold environment and as a result of overfeeding. This process is known as *adaptive thermogenesis.* Some studies of overfeeding show that heat is produced without work being done. This subject has produced much controversy and interest. Some studies show that people who were overfed did not gain the amount of weight that might be expected. Though adaptive thermogenesis probably does not play a major role in weight regulation, it appears to represent a small portion of energy use.[9]

In many animals, including humans to an undetermined extent, adaptive thermogenesis is linked to the presence of brown adipose tissue. Most fat is stored in white adipose tissue. Brown adipose tissue, so named because of its appearance, is less than 1% of body weight in humans. This tissue represents a specialized form of fat storage found primarily in the shoulder area. For hibernating animals, it is a main source of heat during their long winter sleep. Brown adipose tissue fails to use energy in the same method as white adipose tissue does. Most brown adipose cell energy is lost in the form of heat; little is used to perform useful work beyond simply warming the body. So these cells can produce a lot of heat and, in turn, "waste" a lot of potentially useful energy. If you touch an infant's back, you can feel the heat produced by brown adipose tissue. The extent to which brown adipose tissue is both present and operative in humans has not been clearly determined.

Decreased activity of brown adipose tissue during overfeeding and cold adaptation is associated with obesity in rats. Researchers are not in agreement, but some evidence suggests that impaired adaptive thermogenesis resulting from abnormalities in the functioning of brown adipose tissue may contribute to human obesity.[19]

In sum, a sedentary person uses about 80% of energy for basal metabolism and the thermic effect of food. The remainder is used for physical activity and adaptive thermogenesis.

CONCEPT CHECK

The body uses energy for four main purposes.

- Basal metabolism represents the minimal amount of energy needed to maintain a body in a resting state. The rate of a person's basal metabolism depends greatly on the amount of lean body mass, the amount of body surface, thyroid hormone levels, and other hormone levels.
- Physical activity expenditure represents energy use for total body cell metabolism above what is needed during rest (i.e., basal metabolism).
- The thermic effect of food represents the energy needed to digest, absorb, and process absorbed nutrients. This corresponds to about 5% to 10% of energy used for basal metabolism and physical activity.
- Adaptive thermogenesis is heat production in response to cold or overfeeding. This phenomenon may be linked to the presence of brown adipose tissue.

In a sedentary person, about 80% of energy is used for basal metabolism and the thermic effect of food; the remainder is used for physical activity and adaptive thermogenesis.

MEASURING ENERGY USE BY THE BODY

Direct and Indirect Calorimetry

The amount of energy a body uses can be measured by both direct and indirect calorimetry. To understand ***direct calorimetry,*** imagine a science fiction film in which a creature is submerged in ice water. The creature gradually raises the water temperature to a tropic warmth simply by releasing body heat. Direct calorimetry uses this concept to measure the body heat released by a person. The subject is put into an insulated chamber, often the size of a small bedroom, and body heat released raises the temperature of a layer of water surrounding the chamber. A kcalorie, recall, is the amount of heat required to raise the temperature of 1 liter of water 1 degree Celsius. By measuring the water temperature in the direct calorimeter before and after the body releases heat, scientists can determine the number of kcalories expended. This method resembles the bomb calorimeter method for measuring the energy content in food (see Figure 1-2).

Direct Calorimetry *A method to determine energy use by the body by measuring heat that emanates from the body.*

Indirect Calorimetry *A method to estimate the energy use by the body by measuring oxygen uptake and then using formulas to convert that gas usage into energy use.*

another BITE

Today, scientific journals often express energy intake and output in kjoules, rather than kcalories. A kjoule is a measure of work, not heat. It is the amount of work involved in moving 1 kilogram for 1 meter with the force of 1 newton. Heat and work are just two forms of energy. Energy expressions in the form of either heat or work can be exchanged for each other; 4.18 kjoules equals 1 kcalorie.

Direct calorimetry works because all the energy used by the body eventually leaves as heat. However, few studies use direct calorimetry, mostly because of its expense and complexity.

In ***indirect calorimetry,*** instead of measuring heat output, a technician measures the amount of oxygen a person uses (Figure 10-6). A predictable relationship exists between the body's use of energy and oxygen. For example, when burning a mixed diet of carbohydrate, fat, and protein—a typical blend of nutrients we use—the human body needs 1 liter of oxygen to burn about 4.85 kcalories.

Instruments used to measure oxygen consumption for indirect calorimetry have great versatility. They can be mounted on carts and rolled up to a hospital bed or carried in backpacks while a person plays tennis or jogs. Tables showing energy demands of various exercises rely on information gained from indirect calorimetry studies (see Appendix K).

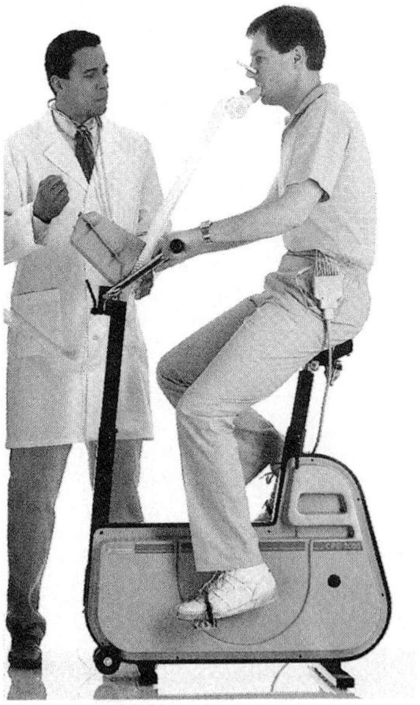

FIGURE 10-6
Indirect calorimetry. This method can be used to measure energy output during daily activities.

Estimating Energy Needs

The RDA provides rough estimates of total energy needs for healthy people who perform light activity (see inside cover). Another rough estimate uses a person's weight and activity level. Total energy needs for a sedentary person are set at 9 kcalories per pound (20 kcalories per kilogram). The value is then decreased by 100 kcalories for every 10 years of age over age 30. People performing light activity, such as routine walking, start with 13 kcalories per pound (30 kcalories per kilogram); those regularly performing heavy activity, as required in some sports play, start at 20 kcalories per pound (45 kcalories per kilogram). These values are then adjusted for age, as mentioned previously. For example, a 150-pound, 40-year-old woman performing light activity needs to eat about 1850 ([13 × 150] – 100) kcalories to meet total energy needs.

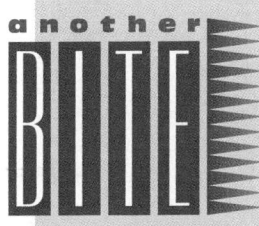

CONCEPT CHECK

Energy use by the body is measured by direct calorimetry as heat given off and by indirect calorimetry as oxygen used. Total energy needs can be estimated based on the RDA or by using a person's weight, age, and activity level.

TABLE 10-1

Health Problems Associated with Excess Body Fat

Health Problem	Partially Attributed To:
Adult-onset diabetes (NIDDM)	Enlarged fat cells, which then poorly bind insulin and also poorly respond to the message insulin sends to the cell
Surgical risk	Increased anesthesic needs and greater risk of wound infections
Pulmonary disease	Excess weight over lungs
Hypertension	Increased miles of blood vessels found in the fat tissue; however, no validated cause is yet known
Coronary heart disease	Increases in serum cholesterol and triglyceride levels, as well as a decrease in physical activity
Bone and joint disorders	Excess pressure put on knee, ankle, and hip joints
Gallbladder stones	An increase in cholesterol content of bile
Skin disorders	The trapping of moisture and microbes in fat folds
Various cancers	Estrogen production by fat cells; animal studies suggest excess energy intake encourages tumor development
Shorter stature (in some forms of obesity)	An earlier onset of puberty
Pregnancy risk	More difficult delivery and increased anesthetic needs (if the latter is used)
Early death	A variety of risk factors for diseases listed above

The greater the degree of obesity, the more likely and the more serious these health problems generally become. They are much more likely to appear in people who are greater than twice their desirable body weight.

Obesity *A condition characterized by excess body fat. In clinical settings, this is often defined as weighing 20% above desirable weight. Many scientists encourage defining obesity in terms of body mass index (BMI) instead, with a cutoff of 25 to 27 to indicate when obesity-related health risks begin.*

ENERGY IMBALANCE

Problems associated with ***obesity***—the major type of energy imbalance in America—go far beyond any social stigma (Table 10-1). Since 1948 the Framingham Heart Study has medically tracked several thousand residents of Framingham, a small Massachusetts town. The study has observed that carrying an excess of 20% or more above one's desirable weight poses health risks. And the greater the degree of obesity, (1) the more likely one is to develop health problems and (2) the more serious these problems generally become. The Framingham study supports other studies that show excess weight raises the risks for the following[5]:

- Adult-onset (non-insulin dependent) diabetes
- Surgical complications
- Hypertension
- Heart disease
- Arthritis
- Gallstones
- Various forms of cancer—colon, rectal, and prostate cancer in men and breast, uterine, and ovarian cancer in women
- Pregnancy risks
- Sleep disturbances
- Early death

Numerous studies indicate that a significant number of people with hypertension, non-insulin dependent diabetes, and osteoarthritis can reverse the conditions through weight loss. Table 10-1 lists possible explanations of how obesity causes some of these disorders.

Defining Obesity

Obesity can be defined in terms of percent of weight as body fat, body weight itself, and body fat distribution (Figure 10-7). Age of onset is an additional consideration.

Using Body Fat. Risks of being overweight apply mostly to people who are overfat. Men with over 25% body fat and women with over 30% to 35% body fat run health risks and are considered obese. Dropping body fat to about 15% for men and about 25% fat for women also drops risk. Women need more body fat than do men because some gender-specific fat is needed for reproductive functions. Because this extra fat in women is needed, it is factored into calculations of body composition.

DEGREE OF CONFIDENCE	METHOD	CUT OFF VALUE
Rough estimate	% of desirable weight (Current wt. − desirable wt.) x 100 / Desirable weight	Mild: >20% Moderate: >40% Severe: >100% (morbid)
↓	Body mass index (wt (kg)/ht² (m))	Mild: 25-30 through age 35; 27-30 after age 35 Moderate: 30-35 Severe: 35-40
↓	Total body fat from skinfold thicknesses/bioelectrical impedance/infrared measurements or Loss of weight while underwater (hydrostatic weighing)	Men: >25% of body weight Women: >30%-35% of body weight
More sensitive estimates of obesity—related health risk	Upper body distribution of fat stores	Ratio of waist to hip circumference: Men: >0.95 Women: >0.8

FIGURE 10-7

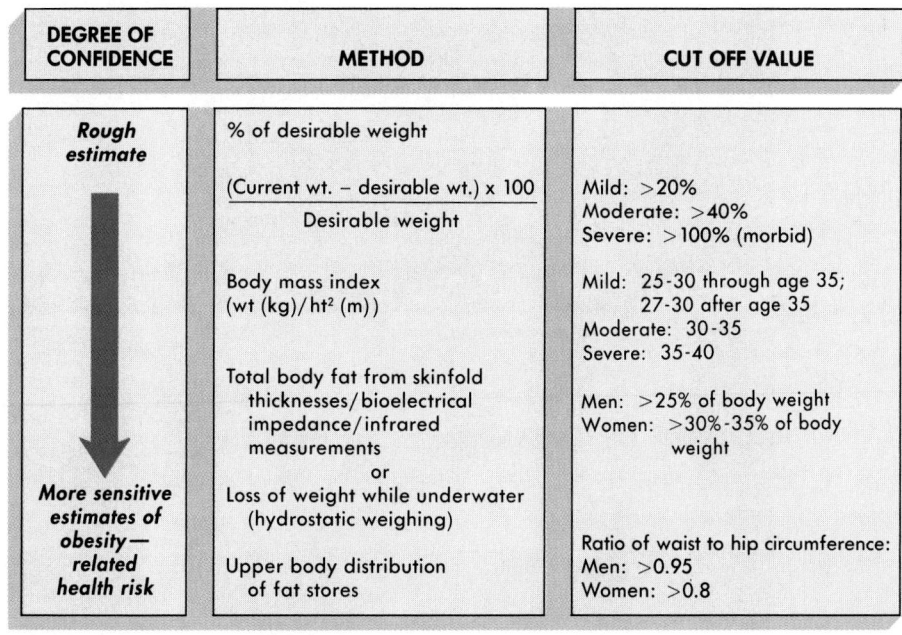

Establishing the extent of obesity to predict health risk. If one is obese by any of these measures and has an upper-body distribution of fat stores, the risk of complications is more likely than if the fat distribution is primarily in the lower body.

Various methods are used to estimate body fat levels. Underwater weighing, the most accurate method, works because fat tissue is less dense than lean tissue; because fat floats, the more fat tissue present, the less a person weighs when submerged. This procedure requires a trained technician and forces the subject to be submerged, and so it is used primarily as a research tool.

Though there are some limits to its accuracy, skinfold thickness is the method most widely used to estimate total body fat. Clinicians use special calipers to measure the fat layer directly under the skin. This 20-minute test works because more than half of all body fat lies directly under the skin (Figure 10-8).

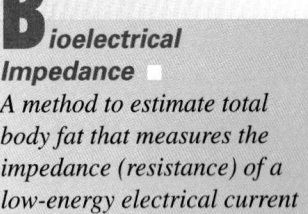

Bioelectrical Impedance ■ *A method to estimate total body fat that measures the impedance (resistance) of a low-energy electrical current by the body.*

Clinicians have recently begun measuring total body fat using ***bioelectrical impedance.*** This technique sends a painless, low-energy electrical current to and from the body via wires and electrode patches. Because fat resists electrical flow, more fat proportionately means greater electrical resistance. Within a few minutes, bioelectrical impedance analyzers convert body electrical resistance into an estimate of total body fat.

Another new method for estimating total body fat exposes the biceps to infrared light, assessing the interactions with the fat and protein in arm muscle. After only 2 seconds, this flashlight-size device can give an estimate.

A further advance in determining body fat is use of x-ray photon absorptiometry. This x-ray system allows the clinician or investigator to separate body weight into three com-

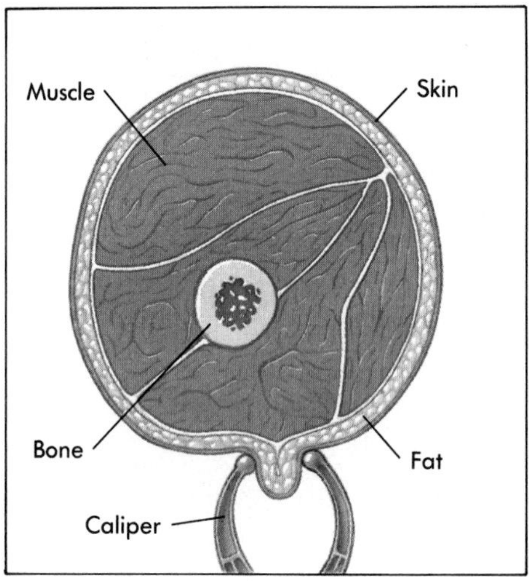

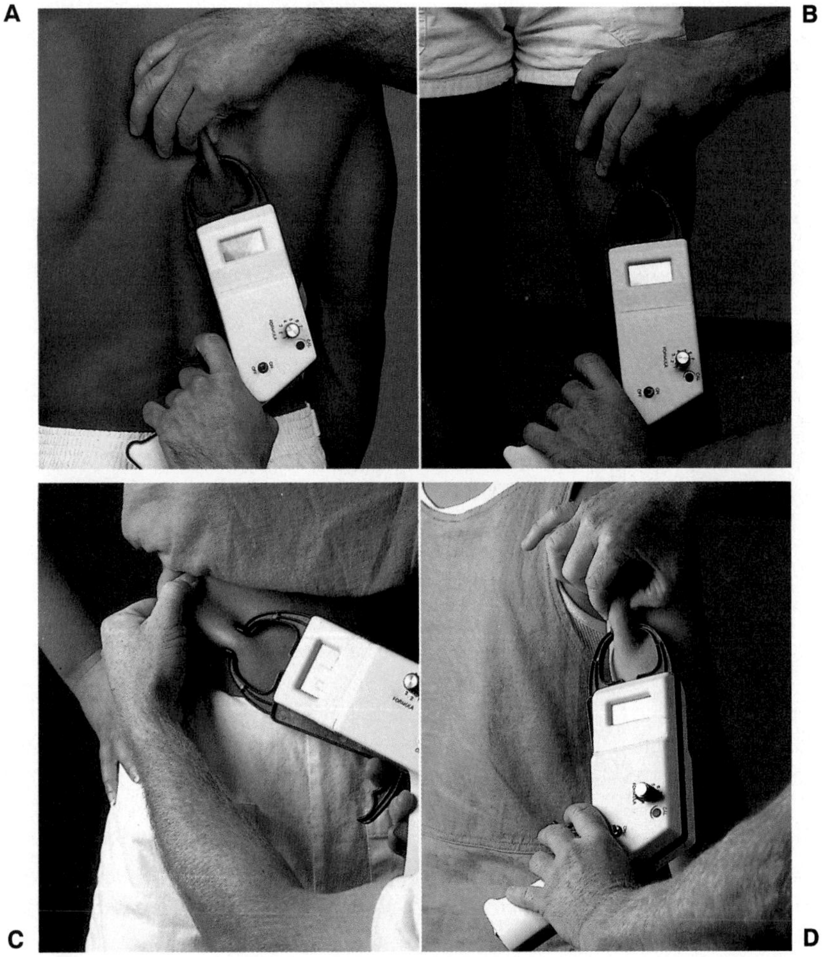

FIGURE 10-8
Skinfold measurements. Using a proper technique, calibrated equipment, and standards, skinfold measurements can be used to accurately predict body fat content in about 20 minutes. Commonly measured skinfolds are, **A,** *subscapular;* **B,** *thigh;* **C,** *suprailiac; and* **D,** *triceps.*

TABLE 10-2

Body Weights in Pounds According to Height and Body Mass Index (BMI)

	BMI (kg/m^2)													
	19	20	21	22	23	24	25	26	27	28	29	30	35	40
Height (Inches)	Body Weight (Pounds)													
58	91	96	100	105	110	115	119	124	129	134	138	143	167	191
59	94	99	104	109	114	119	124	128	133	138	143	148	173	198
60	97	102	107	112	118	123	128	133	138	143	148	153	179	204
61	100	106	111	116	122	127	132	137	143	148	153	158	185	211
62	104	109	115	120	126	131	136	142	147	153	158	164	191	218
63	107	113	118	124	130	135	141	146	152	158	163	169	197	225
64	110	116	122	128	134	140	145	151	157	163	169	174	204	232
65	114	120	126	132	138	144	150	156	162	168	174	180	210	240
66	118	124	130	136	142	148	155	161	167	173	179	186	216	247
67	121	127	134	140	146	153	159	166	172	178	185	191	223	255
68	125	131	138	144	151	158	164	171	177	184	190	197	230	262
69	128	135	142	149	155	162	169	176	182	189	196	203	236	270
70	132	139	146	153	160	167	174	181	188	195	202	207	243	278
71	136	143	150	157	165	172	179	186	193	200	208	215	230	286
72	140	147	154	162	169	177	184	191	199	206	213	221	258	294
73	144	151	159	166	174	182	189	197	204	212	219	227	265	302
74	148	155	163	171	179	186	194	202	210	218	225	233	272	311
75	152	160	168	176	184	192	200	208	216	224	232	240	279	319
76	156	164	172	180	189	197	205	213	221	230	238	246	287	328

From Bray GA, Gray DS: Western Journal of Medicine 148:429, 1988.
Each entry gives the body weight in pounds for a person of a given height and BMI. Pounds have been rounded off. To use the table, find the appropriate height in the far left column. Move across the row to a given weight. The number at the top of the column is the BMI for the height and weight.

ponents—fat, fat-free soft tissue, and bone mineral. The usual whole-body scan requires 15 to 20 minutes and delivers a minimal radiation dose. Obesity, osteoporosis, and other aspects of nutritional health can be investigated using this method.

Using Body Mass Index. ***Body mass index (BMI)*** offers an alternative way to define obesity.[5] This measure is highly predictive of the degree of body fatness. To calculate BMI, divide a person's weight in kilograms by height in meters squared. Table 10-2 does this calculation for you. A 70-kilogram (154-pound) man who is 1.78 meters (70 inches) tall has a BMI of 22 ($70/[1.78]^2$). An optimal BMI is about 19 to 25 through age 35 and about 21 to 27 after age 35, although specific cutoff values are still being debated.[13]

When BMI begins to exceed 25 to 27, obesity-related health risks often begin for men and women and the person is said to be overweight. At a BMI of about 27, the risk for diabetes and hypertension is three times greater than normal and the risk for a high serum cholesterol level (greater than 240 milligrams per deciliter) is two times normal. A BMI above 30 poses even greater health risks and is typically defined as obesity. A value this high suggests that a treatment program should be considered, especially if obesity-related health problems are present.[5] About 10% of Americans exceed this value. A BMI above 40 represents a severe health risk. These BMIs for health risks are the same for both men and women.

Body Mass Index (BMI) *Weight (in kilograms) divided by height (in meters) squared; a value greater than 25 to 27 indicates a higher risk for obesity-related health disorders.*

Desirable body mass index (BMI) range in relation to age[5]

Age-Group (yr)	BMI
19-24	19-24
25-34	20-25
35-44	21-26
45-54	22-27
55-64	23-28
65+	24-29

Upper-Body Obesity The type of obesity, also called android, in which fat is stored primarily in the abdominal area; defined as a waist to hip circumference ratio of greater than 0.95 in men and 0.8 in women; closely associated with a high risk of heart disease, hypertension, and diabetes.

Lower-Body Obesity The type of obesity, also called gynoid, in which fat storage is primarily located in the buttocks and thigh area.

Using Body Fat Distribution. Where we store fat, as well as how much, can predict health risks.[3] Some people store fat in upper body areas. Others hold fat low. Each storage space has risks. Fat deposited in the lower body often resists being shed.[29] However, ***upper-body obesity*** is related to more heart disease, hypertension, and diabetes. While other fat cells empty fat directly into general circulation, the fat contents of abdominal fat cells go straight to the liver, by way of the portal vein, before being circulated to the muscles. This process likely interferes with the liver's ability to clear insulin and alters lipoprotein metabolism by the liver as well. Both changes spell trouble for the body.

High testosterone (a male hormone) levels apparently encourage upper-body obesity. This characteristic male pattern of fat storage appears in the "apple-on-a-stick" shape (large abdomen [pot belly] and small buttocks and thighs). A ratio of waist circumference (at the level of the umbilicus) to hip circumference more than 0.95 in men and 0.8 in women indicates upper body fat storage (Figure 10-9).

Progesterone (a female hormone) encourages lower body fat storage and so ***lower-body obesity***—the typical female pattern. The familiar small abdomen and much larger buttocks and thighs give a pear-shape appearance.

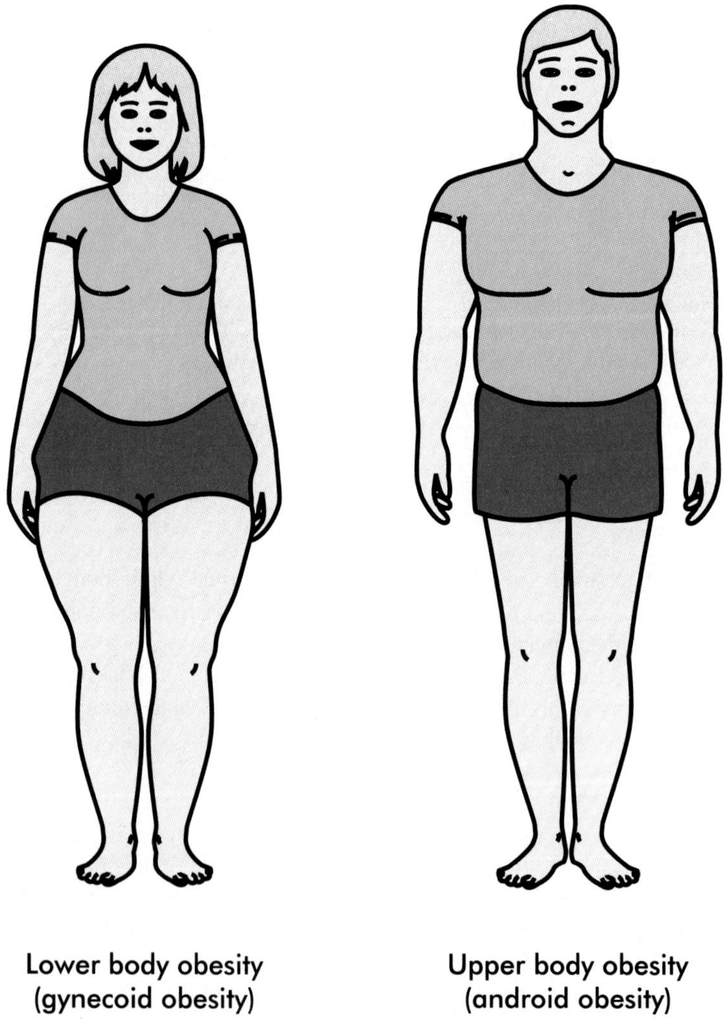

FIGURE 10-9

Body fat distribution. Gynecoid and android obesity. The android form brings higher risks for ill health associated with obesity.

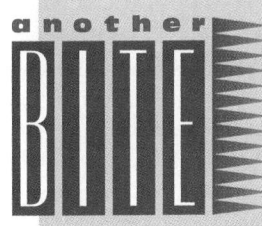

another BITE

In the future we may have obesity standards that apply more strictly to upper-body fat distribution and more leniently to lower-body fat distribution. Excess abdominal fat is more harmful to health than excess fat in the buttocks and thighs. For now it is best to consider one's BMI and pattern of fat distribution when assessing possible health risks from obesity.

Using Body Weight. Body weight is actually a crude measure of obesity, because it can miss the critical factor—being overfat. However, with the exception of the husky athlete, overfat and overweight (obese) conditions generally appear together. The focus in a clinical setting is on body weight because it is easier to measure.

Overweight can be defined as weighing at least 10% more than desirable body weight. Obesity weighs in at 20% more than desired weight. As the following chapter shows, obesity comes in degrees. While mild obesity carries little risk, severe (morbid) obesity raises overall health risk twelvefold.[5]

Degrees of obesity

% Over desirable body weight	% Of cases	Form of obesity
20%-40%	90%	MILD
41%-99%	9.8%	MODERATE
100% +	0.2%	SEVERE (MORBID)

To determine desirable body weight, many clinicians and research scientists use the current (1983) Metropolitan Life Insurance Table (see the inside cover of the textbook). This tool estimates weights that have enabled people to lead a long life. The weight range is based on height, age, and frame size. Methods of estimating frame size use measurements of wrist width or elbow breadth (see Appendix I).

Medical literature currently uses the term *desirable* or *healthy,* rather than *ideal,* when referring to body weight.

The table, however, has its limitations. Because the table's data are derived only from purchasers of life insurance, poor people and minorities may be underrepresented. In addition, height and weight were determined only at the time the insurance policy was purchased and included shoes and clothes. A positive point is that the table does not include insured persons with significant diseases, such as heart disease, cancer, and diabetes. The weight range listed does not, however, necessarily tell which weight offers optimal health. If you have good health and weigh slightly more than the chart range indicates you should, you need not be concerned.

The *pounds per inch of height* method for estimating desirable body weight offers another measurement. For women allow 100 pounds for the first 5 feet, and add 5 pounds for every inch thereafter. To estimate a man's desirable body weight, allow 105 pounds for the first 5 feet and then add 6 pounds for each inch thereafter. A 6-foot-tall man then should weigh about 177 pounds ($105 + [12 \times 6]$) based on this system.

another BITE

The Metropolitan Life Insurance Table does not offer weight estimates for people over 60 years of age. It is not clear whether the condition of overweight or obesity in elderly people follows the same pattern of association with disease as it does in younger people. The height-weight table published with the *Dietary Guidelines for Americans* does allow for some weight gain in the adult years. This table is included in Chapter 15. Currently there is debate as to whether this weight gain is desirable or just adds to the chances of developing health problems.[13]

Using Age of Onset. Obesity can be classified as juvenile-onset or adult-onset. When obesity develops in infancy or childhood, numerous adipose (fat) cells develop, each with the ability to grow larger. In adult obesity, fewer fat cells are usually present, but these contain an excess amount of fat.

Juvenile-onset obesity presents concern, because the greater number of fat cells may increase the body's resistance to cutting down fat stores. Fat cells have a long life span. In addition, fat cells appear to need to store some fat. If more fat cells automatically require more fat storage, reducing total body fat becomes a tough task. Though still a puzzle, it appears long-term obesity makes losing weight more difficult.

THE MULTIPLE CAUSES OF OBESITY

Obesity is a very personal disorder. It may be measured in many ways, but statistics aside, each person has unique characteristics and problems. Treatment needs to consider current energy expenditure, fasting blood glucose levels, family history of obesity, number of years the person has been obese, and the extent of erroneous nutrition practices. Each individual faces possible complications requiring individual treatment plans.[17]

A history of yo-yo dieting, the repeated loss and regain of weight, also bears consideration. Recent studies suggest this pattern can predispose a person to subsequent heart disease.

Achieving body weights and shapes presented in the media often is not a reasonable, appropriate, or achievable goal, and the failure to do so does not represent a weakness of willpower or character. For example, consider a person who is 5 feet 2 inches and has weighed 250 pounds for 25 years. Theoretically she should weigh around 110 pounds according to height and weight charts, but that is not a realistic weight goal for that person. Unreasonably low weight goals invariably result in rapid weight regain. The most important factor in determining the weight goal is the amount of weight loss necessary for weight not to be an impediment to health, employment, or normal life activities.[27]

Before we go on, let's look at one other important concept. Most Americans with obesity show relatively low health risks, because these people have mild forms of obesity. On a population-wide basis, the two typical cutoffs for an increase in obesity-related health risks—(1) a BMI of greater than 25 to 27 or (2) greater than 20% of desirable body weight—are relevant to disease prevention in our society. On an individual basis, however, some people with this amount or somewhat more body weight may not necessarily show negative health effects. The extra body fat can set the stage for future disease, but even that is not guaranteed for a specific person. This suggests that the individual, in conjunction with a physician, is best equipped to establish whether a need for weight reduction exists, based on fat distribution patterns, family history of obesity-related disease, and current health status—not on population-based mathematical models.[17]

CONCEPT CHECK

Obesity refers to a state of excessive body fat storage. The risk of health problems related to obesity increases under the following conditions:

- A man's percent of body fat exceeds 25%; a woman's exceeds 30% to 35%.
- Body mass index (BMI) is over 25 to 27 (calculated as weight in kilograms divided by height in meters squared).
- Scale weight is 20% above desirable body weight as predicted by the 1983 Metropolitan Life Insurance Table.

Body fat storage is estimated clinically using skinfold thickness or bioelectrical impedance. Fat storage distribution further specifies an obese state as either upper body or lower body. Obesity leads to an increased risk for heart disease, some types of cancer, hypertension, adult-onset diabetes, bone and joint disorders, and some digestive disorders. The risks for some of these diseases are especially high with upper-body fat storage.

WHY SOME PEOPLE ARE OBESE—NATURE VERSUS NURTURE

Both genetic traits and psychological factors can increase the risk for obesity. These diverse influences spark controversies concerning which factor yields the greater influence.

How Does Nature Contribute to Obesity?

Identical twins raised apart tend to show similar weight gain patterns, whether lean or obese. It appears that nurture—what we learn about eating habits and nutrition, which varies with twins who are raised apart—has less to do with obesity than do one's genes.[21] In fact, research suggests genetic background accounts for about 70% of weight differences between people. Twins even tend to accumulate fat in the same body sites. Our genes help determine rates of metabolism and differences in brain chemistry. Both affect weight.

We also inherit specific body types, such as pencil-thin or muscular. The specific body types—known as endomorphs, mesomorphs, and ectomorphs—greatly determine human size and shape. Endomorphs, with their stocky builds, have short, stubby bones, short trunks, round heads, wide chest and hips, and very short fingers. Ectomorphs, like Abraham Lincoln, are tall and slender with long, thin bones, and narrow chests, hips, heads, and fingers. Mesomorphs exhibit a medium, muscular build.

Ectomorphs appear to have an inherently easier time maintaining desirable body weight. Basal metabolism increases as body surface increases. Tall people have more body surface (based on body weight comparisons) than do short, stocky people. Therefore, even when resting, taller people use more energy than do shorter ones.

You've heard of fat cats, but have you heard of fat rats? Some rats and mice have a genetic predisposition to obesity. They inherit a ***thrifty metabolism,*** one that uses energy frugally.[21] This enables them to store fat more readily than does the typical animal. Some people probably inherit a thrifty metabolism as well. Farmers once bred cows and hogs based on their ability to acquire fat. Today, because we know that eating too much animal fat can increase the risk for heart disease, farmers breed leaner animals.

A thrifty human metabolism requires less energy to get through the day. In earlier times, when food supplies were scarce, a thrifty metabolism helped protect against starvation. With today's general abundance of food, operating in this low gear requires a high-energy output and wise food choices to prevent obesity.

We cannot measure small differences in energy efficiency among humans. In the long run, however, even a 1% or 2% difference in metabolic rate may be a decisive factor between massive weight gain and healthy weight maintenance. Resting metabolic rates among family members tend to be more similar than a comparison with those of the general population. Families with lower resting metabolic rates have higher rates for obesity. Even after adjusting for the amount of body fat, research shows that resting metabolic rate varies as much as 30% between leaner and more obese families. Some Native American tribes also show a high rate of obesity, linked in part to lower metabolic rates.[21]

If you think your metabolism promotes weight gain, you may have inherited a thrifty metabolism to some extent. A child with no obese parent has only a 10% chance of becoming obese. A child with one obese parent has a 40% risk, and one with two obese parents an 80% risk. It can be argued that these probabilities are related, in part, to the eating behaviors a child learns. ***Fraternal twins*** vary less in weight than do two unrelated people. That pattern supports the theory that environment, or nurture, affects obesity. Still the close association of body weights between identical twins strongly supports the genetic explanations. This varied evidence shows how complicated it is to separate nature from nurture when searching for the causes of obesity.

Does Nurture Have a Role?

Genetic factors determine some differences in energy metabolism and explain certain weight gain variations among people. However, environmental factors, such as high-fat diets and inactivity, can literally shape us as well. Family members often have similar eating habits and choose similar foods. Even husbands and wives—who have no genetic

Identical Twins
Two offspring that develop from a single ovum and sperm and consequently have the same genetic makeup.

Thrifty Metabolism
A metabolism that characteristically conserves more energy than normal, such that it increases the risk of weight gain and obesity.

Fraternal Twins
Offspring that develop from two separate ova and sperm and therefore have separate genetic identities, although they develop simultaneously in the mother.

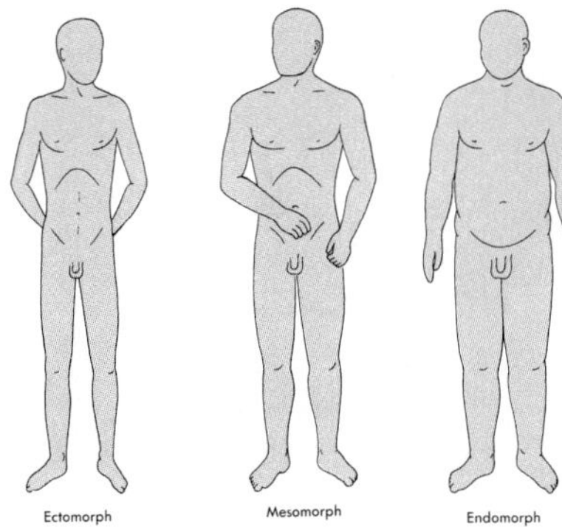

Ectomorph, mesomorph, and endomorph body shapes.

Nature or nurture—what causes these twins to have similar body weights?

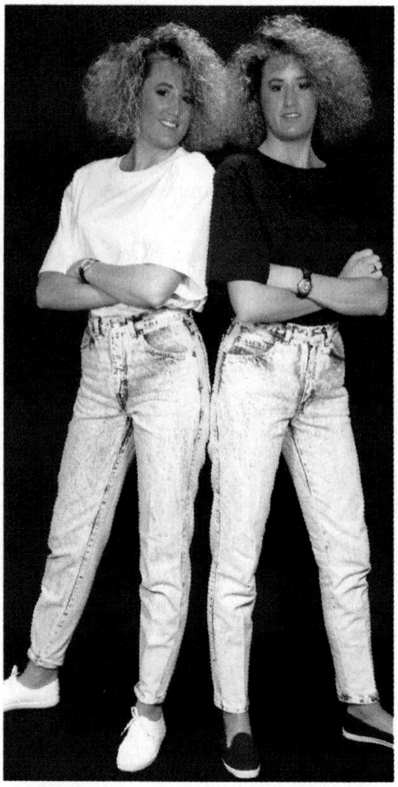

link—may behave similarly toward food and eventually assume similar degrees of leanness or chunkiness. Therefore the family that bonds at the quick-service restaurant counter can influence each other's eating habits and, ultimately, fatness.

Is poverty associated with obesity? By a peculiar twist of irony, the answer is often yes. In America, people of lower socioeconomic status, especially females, are more likely to be obese than those in upper socioeconomic groups. Are cultural expectations or socioeconomic stress the cause of this?

Adult obesity in women is often rooted in childhood obesity. In addition, periods of stress and boredom and excess weight gain in pregnancy contribute to female obesity. Relative inactivity further adds to the problem.[10] These patterns suggest both social and genetic links. Male obesity, however, is not strongly linked to childhood obesity and instead tends to appear after age 30. In part, a working life encourages a sedentary life for men. This powerful and prevalent pattern suggests a primary role of nurture in obesity, with less genetic influence.

another BITE

Early research suggested that infant feeding practices, such as introducing solid foods and bottle feeding before age 6 months, encourage infant weight gain and higher risk of obesity later in life. However, many recent studies reexamining this issue show very little relationship between how an infant was fed or how much weight was gained in the first year of life and the presence or absence of obesity in later childhood. The exception could be the infant who gains weight very rapidly in the first 6 weeks of life. Most overweight or obese infants become normal-weight schoolchildren. However, if a child has become obese by 5 years of age, immediate attention is necessary. Obesity in childhood is strongly related to obesity in adulthood.

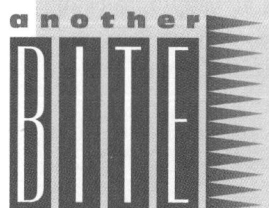

TABLE 10-3

What Encourages Some of Us to Develop Excess Body Fat Stores?

Factor	Reason for Increase
Age	Excess body fat is more common in adults and middle-aged individuals.
Gender	Females have more fat.
Positive energy balance	Excess energy intake is especially important over a relatively long period.
Composition of intake	High-fat intake and preference for sugary, fat-rich foods may be contributing factors.
Physical activity level	Low or decreasing level of activity affects body fat stores.
Resting metabolic rate	A low value with respect to lean body mass is linked to weight gain.
Thermic effect of food	Low for some obesity cases.
Use of fat for energy	Poor fat use is linked with body fat gain.
Ratio of fat to lean tissue	A high fat-mass–to–fat-free-mass ratio is correlated with weight gain.
Adipose-tissue lipoprotein lipase activity	High in obese individuals and remains high (perhaps even increases) with weight loss.
Variety of social and behavioral factors	Obesity is associated with socioeconomic status, familial conditions, network of friends, pattern of leisure activities, television time, smoking habits, alcohol intake, and so on.
Undetermined genetic characteristics	These affect energy balance, particularly via the energy expenditure components, the deposition of surplus kcalories as fat or as lean tissue, and the relative proportion of fat and carbohydrate use by the body.
Certain medications	Food intake increases.

From Bouchard C: American Journal of Clinical Nutrition *53:1561S, 1991.*

Nature and Nurture Together

Evidence suggests that both nature and nurture influence the tendency toward obesity (Table 10-3). Consider the possibility that obesity is nurture allowing nature to express itself, like an accident waiting to happen. Some people begin with a slower metabolism. Put these people into an inactive environment, feed them high-kcalorie foods, and praise them for eating. They, like any of us, can be nurtured into gaining weight, allowing their natural tendency for obesity to blossom, with the eventual location of fat storage strongly influenced by genetics.[5] Weight gain in adulthood often alternates with periods of weight maintenance. This suggests that for some of us a natural tendency to gain weight persists and that changes in our nurturing environment cause spurts of weight gain.

If your parents are obese, you're likely to be at risk for obesity all your life.[17] To avoid it will require eternal vigilance. Eat the right foods at the right times for the right reasons. Remember as well, genes are not destiny. With increased exercise and decreased food consumption, even those of us with a genetic tendency toward obesity can maintain a healthy body weight.

CONCEPT CHECK

Genetic background plays a role in obesity via body shape, sites of fat deposition, and rate of basal metabolism. The role of nurture is exhibited in similar eating habits, activity levels, and degrees of fatness in families. Men's tendency to develop obesity after age 30 and women's pattern of having both childhood and adult roots for obesity suggest an especially important influence of nurture in men. Because both factors have an impact, we speculate that nurture may serve as a catalyst for expressing or denying a genetic tendency toward obesity.

NUTRITION insight

A SET POINT FOR BODY WEIGHT?

Set Point ■
The close and essentially automatic regulation of body weight. It is not known what cells control set point or how it actually functions in weight regulation. There is no doubt, however, that there are mechanisms that help regulate weight.

Adipsin ■
A protein that appears to be made by fat cells and acts as a communication link between these cells and the brain.

Some scientists suggest that in humans and laboratory animals, cells in the brain continually monitor the amount of body fat. This self-regulating fat level or ***set point*** supposedly reacts when weight shoots up or edges down. A protein produced by fat cells, called ***adipsin,*** may form the regulating (communication) link between fat cells and the brain.

Researchers compare set point with the tight regulation of blood pressure and body temperature. One researcher described the set point as a coiled spring: the further you stray from your set weight, the stronger the force pulls you back.

Sound evidence suggests that the body tends to maintain a set weight. After an illness, most people regain the lost weight. Conversely, if you just eat less, the blood level of a thyroid hormone falls, decreasing metabolic rate.[16] Your body begins to resist further weight loss. These findings suggest that adjustments in energy output are important in regulating body weight. They present evidence for the set-point theory of body-weight regulation. In addition, weighing less results in burning less energy during activity. And because total lean tissue decreases, total energy use decreases. Furthermore, the enzyme used by fat cells and muscle cells to pull in fat from the bloodstream can turn more active as one tries to lose weight, and as fat cells shrink, they become more responsive to the action of insulin and do not release their contents as readily.

Arguments against the set-point theory cite the fact that during pregnancy women slowly increase body weight and fat with little fight to maintain this trend. Also, an average person's weight does not remain constant throughout adulthood; it usually increases slowly, at least until old age. This means that one must be able to shift one's set point. If an individual is placed in a different social, emotional, or physical environment, weight can become markedly higher or lower and will be maintained. These arguments would

TREATMENT OF OBESITY

If a *successful formula* to weight loss or weight control exists, it is—as we said before—to practice eating a moderate amount of total kcalories, minimizing fat kcalories, and staying physically active.[17,27] Unfortunately, this simple formula hasn't the glamour or hype of the latest fad diet nor does it promise effortless slimness. If only kcalories didn't count or a beautifully proportioned body could be had with just moments of exercise. Then the continuing assault of diet books, special programs, dietary supplements, and medical procedures for weight loss might disappear. Obesity would vanish as a public health problem and a common cause of great personal agony. Don't hold your breath.

Basic Premises for a Weight-Loss Program

Let's focus on three other important principles concerning weight loss for adults: (1) the body naturally resists weight loss, (2) preventing obesity is key, and (3) weight should mostly be lost from fat storage.

First, the body resists weight loss. Thyroid hormone levels, and consequently basal metabolism, drop during weight loss. The basal metabolic rate (BMR) returns to predictable values when the diet stops.[26] But the BMR stays lower if the person has lost lean body mass, making it difficult to keep losing weight or maintain a lower weight. Recent studies show that a fat storage enzyme increases its activity in fat cells after weight loss.[17] So after dieting, the body takes up and stores fat from the bloodstream more efficiently.

say that humans, rather than having a set point determined by genetics or number of adipose cells, actually settle into a particular stable weight based on an interaction between nature and nurture influences.

Putting Some Numbers on Set Point

You will eat about 35 tons of food in about as many adult years. Daily energy intake varies from about 20% below to 20% above a monthly average (about ± 400 kcalories). But a 2% (40-kcalorie) overconsumption of energy per day, if continued for 20 years, adds up to an 82-pound weight gain. Still, people tend to gain only 15 to 20 pounds between the ages of 18 and 54 years. The significant gain possible from such a small error—far in excess of what we usually see—suggests some degree of set point exists. Considering that 35 tons of food equals about 30 million kcalories, your body's regulation of that tonnage, though imperfect, is still quite impressive.

Will exercise or a low-fat diet lower your set point? Popular books and magazines suggest so. Science hasn't decided. Whether a set point exists is even immaterial. With or without it, you need to consider that (1) exercise is important for weight maintenance, (2) a high-fat diet is often very high in kcalories, and (3) dieting is very difficult. If these phenomena are easier to understand using the concept of set point, use it. However, very little valid evidence shows how set point operates. We must remember to eat moderately, stay active, and face the fact that—even with a set point helping us—we must stay vigilant against creeping weight gain in adulthood.[17]

Beyond Set Point

Perhaps it's time for a radical idea. Instead of focusing on what we should weigh, we could let our lifestyles guide us. Shift focus from a particular weight or set point. Focus instead on moderate intake of healthful foods, plenty of exercise, positive thinking, and learning to cope with stress. Let the pounds fall where they may. For most people, the result will be close to the recommended weight ranges discussed earlier. For some people, weight will be somewhat higher than societal norms—but right for them (and their set point?). By focusing on a healthful lifestyle for weight control, we might shift our fixation (and that of the nation) away from dieting hysteria.

This is a good reason to stay on a low-fat diet for weight maintenance. Insulin action on fat cells also improves with weight loss, and this reduces fat release by fat cells.

Second, prevent obesity. Reversing it is a demanding battle. Only about 5% of those who diet actually lose weight and keep it off.[17] A weight-loss program should be considered successful only when participants remain at their lower weight for 3 to 5 years. The overall statistics for maintaining this degree of weight loss are grim.

From ages 25 to 44 a weight gain danger zone exists, especially for women. If weight gain has plagued you, practice particular prudence in this decade. Childhood and adolescent years also deserve special focus. Rapid weight gainers should closely monitor food intake and activity level. In addition, we need to avoid the trap of today's crash diet, setting the stage for next month's weight gain.

Third, the goal is to drop weight from fat storage, with little coming from muscle and other lean tissues. Quick weight loss fools those who follow fad diets. Weight drops, but little of it is fat loss. Rapid, initial weight loss often represents fluid lost because of decreased salt intake and glycogen lost from the liver and muscles. Muscle tissue in the body drops as well.[16] As the diet continues, weight loss slows down. As a result, dieters often believe their efforts have failed. They give up, not realizing that smaller losses later in a diet are actually better because, unlike the initial big losses, these represent mostly fat losses.

Wishful Shrinking—Why Can't We Lose Mostly Fat?

Because losing fat tissue demands such a severe energy deficit, rapid weight loss must necessarily be caused by depletion of other tissues. Fat storage—adipose tissue plus lean support tissues, such as connective tissue—represents approximately 2700 kcalories per pound.[19] The fat itself holds about 3500 kcalories per pound. To lose 1 pound of fat storage each week, energy intake must be cut by about 400 to 500 kcalories a day. Cutting about 1000 kcalories a day for 6 weeks, while keeping activity the same, would then yield about a 12-pound fat loss. Diets that promise a 10- to 15-pound weight loss every week cannot promise weight loss from fat storage alone. One would have to cut about 5000 kcalories a day for that 10-pound loss of fat, a feat neither practical nor healthy.

A SOUND WEIGHT-LOSS PLAN—WHAT TO LOOK FOR

A sound weight-loss program addresses the three key issues we have stressed: controlling energy intake, changing problem food habits, and increasing physical activity. Cutting back on kcalories is important. Unfortunately, 100 kcalories represents a trivial amount of food compared with the minutes of exercise required to burn it off. We need also to look for the following characteristics in a weight-loss program:

1. The plan should meet nutritional needs, except for kcalories. This means following the Food Guide Pyramid, emphasizing lower fat choices among a wide variety of foods. Conscious eating should replace unconscious eating.
2. The plan should stress realistic goals, especially gradual—not rapid—weight loss. Look for a fat storage loss of 1 to 2 pounds per week.
3. The plan should adapt to habits and tastes. This will diminish discouraging feelings of deprivation, food binges, and rebound weight gain—all hallmarks of relapse. We should avoid plans that support such practices as eating fruits only in the morning or not eating meat after milk products. No rigid rituals should be required.
4. The plan should minimize hunger and fatigue while ideally supplying at least 1500 kcalories per day. With a daily intake of only 1200 to 1500 kcalories, young women especially may become iron deficient. These lower-kcalorie regimens should recommend either fortified foods (breakfast cereals, for example) or a vitamin and mineral supplement (see Chapter 8 for advice on using supplements).
5. The plan should include a range of readily obtainable foods. No magical food speeds weight loss. If a plan promotes a particular food's *extraordinary* properties—whether ginseng, tofu, or garlic—look elsewhere for advice.
6. The plan should be socially acceptable, allowing the dieter to attend parties, eat at restaurants, and participate in normal daily activities. There is also no need for it to be expensive to follow.
7. The plan should help reshape lifestyle and problem eating habits to make weight loss and later maintenance possible. Positive coping skills are a must. Building a strong social support network is also important.
8. The plan should improve overall health. It should emphasize regular physical activity, proper rest, stress reduction, and other healthful changes in lifestyle.
9. The plan should require physician approval if the dieter
   - Has existing health problems
   - Intends to lose weight as quickly as possible
   - Is over 35 years of age and intends to perform substantially greater-than-usual physical activity

CONTROLLING ENERGY INTAKE

Women often need to reduce kcalories to about 1200 per day and men to about 1500 to lose 1 to 2 pounds of fat storage per week. We need to eat at least 1000 kcalories to keep hunger at bay. When weight loss slows, a person should increase activity level, which allows one to consume enough energy to satisfy nutrient needs.

High-carbohydrate foods—such as spaghetti, rice, and whole-wheat bread (minus the butter)—fill us up with few kcalories and reduce our intake of high-fat foods. We can replace pepperoni, sausage, and extra cheese on pizza with vegetables. Carbohydrates provide less than half as many kcalories as fat. Eating at least 150 grams (600 kcalories) of carbohydrate daily promotes normal metabolism and reduces the risk of eating binges, particularly on sweets, because of intense hunger.

Avoiding hunger is crucial. A regular meal pattern decreases extreme hunger, one roadblock to weight control. Eating breakfast is one excellent suggestion. Sticking with a diet is easier when we make small, daily changes and include a variety of foods.

A person should not reduce the fat content of a diet below 20% of kcalorie intake. A diet very low in fat produces little satiety, so hunger returns quickly after eating. A diet

A good idea is to keep low-fat snack foods close at hand, especially during peak snacking periods. Reaching for fruit by the refrigerator may prevent snacking on fat-laden foods. While it would be desirable to have the willpower to not eat high-fat foods, most people find that the best alternative is to avoid the temptation.

TABLE 10-4

Choosing "Thin" Foods

The chart below can help you plan your meals while following the simple guidelines for healthful eating. When you select a variety of foods from those listed in the far left column, you'll be eating foods that are low in fats and/or high in dietary fiber.

Types of Food	Select Most Often	Select Moderately	Select Least Often
Animal protein	Lean cuts of beef/pork Salmon, halibut (broiled) Canned tuna in water Poultry (without skin) Egg Crab	Untrimmed beef and pork Canned tuna in oil Poultry (with skin) Lobster, shrimp Canadian bacon	Fatty beef, lamb, pork Luncheon meats/hot dogs Fried chicken Fried fish Liver, kidneys Bacon
Dairy	Nonfat yogurt Nonfat milk (or ½%) Nonfat dry milk Nonfat frozen yogurt	Reduced fat and part-skim cheeses Low-fat cottage cheese Low-fat milk Low-fat yogurt 95% Fat-free frozen yogurt	Whole milk cheese (cheddar, muenster) Whole milk Sour cream, ice cream Cream, half-and-half
Vegetable proteins	Dried beans and peas (kidney, lima, and soy beans; lentils; split peas) Tofu (bean curd)	Raw or dry-roasted nuts and seeds Peanut and other nut butters (moderate amounts)	Oil-processed nuts and seeds
Vegetables	Raw, fresh vegetables Fresh or frozen, slightly cooked vegetables	Canned vegetables Canned tomato or vegetable juice	Vegetables in cream or butter sauces Fried vegetables
Fruits	Fresh, raw fruit Dried fruit Frozen and fresh fruit juices	Canned fruit packed in juice Canned fruit juices Frozen fruit	Fruit-flavored beverages Canned fruit packed in syrup Avocados Olives
Grain products	Shredded wheat, oats Whole-grain cereals Whole-grain breads Brown rice Wheat bran, oat bran Bagels Fig bars	Refined cereals Enriched white breads Refined pastas White rice Granolas Toast with margarine Plain cookies	Cookies, cakes, pies Sweetened cereals Tortilla chips Donuts Oil-processed crackers Cream-filled cookies Croissants, doughnuts
Other (still limit quantity)	Popcorn (air popped)	Low-fat salad dressings Low-fat mayonnaise Pretzels	Fat-rich salad dressings Mayonnaise Gravies, cream sauce Potato chips

with 30% kcalories as fat permits most commonly eaten foods. To lose weight and keep it off, dietary changes must fit daily life for years to come.

Many other appealing foods can keep us lean. Healthful, low-fat substitutes can replace the worst high-fat offenders (Table 10-4). Tomato sauce on pasta instead of a creamy Alfredo sauce is one idea; substituting fresh fruit or frozen yogurt for ice cream and pie is another. In some cases, minor switches help, like leaving the cheese off a hamburger.

Most people need to lose fewer than 50 pounds. By consuming a lower-kcalorie diet, that goal can be reached within 1 year or less. Weight is gained slowly and should come off at the same steady pace. This helps make the overall weight loss attempt a long-term success.

One suggested reason for failure with restrictive diets is the sense of restraint people feel. They feel limited in the amount and types of food they can eat. Often a trade-off is constructed, classifying some foods as "good" and others as "bad." One violation of the diet will be considered a failure. This exerts considerable pressure on the dieter. All it takes is one small emotionally disturbing event or environmental change to "release" the individual trying to lose weight. The person eats a little of the forbidden food, feels a sense of relief from restraint, and binges. This leads the dieter to classify himself or herself as a failure and abandon the weight-loss attempt. We recommend substituting a more "healthful" view of eating and self, stressing the positive aspects we see in ourselves and in the nutritious foods that surround us.

CONCEPT CHECK

Dieting deserves consideration of these points:

1. The body resists weight loss.
2. Prevent obesity; reversing the condition is much harder.
3. Lose weight from fat stores, not from lean tissues.

Good weight-loss diets

1. Meet nutritional needs (you can evaluate this by referring to the Food Guide Pyramid).
2. Accommodate the dieter's habits and tastes.
3. Include a range of readily obtainable foods, preferably low in fat.
4. Promote changing habits that lead to overeating.
5. Encourage an increase in physical activity.

Chain-Breaking Breaking the link between two or more behaviors that encourage overeating, such as snacking while watching television.

Contingency Management Forming a plan of action to respond to an environment where overeating is likely, such as when snacks are within arm's reach at a party.

BEHAVIOR MODIFICATION—WHAT MAKES US TICK?

Does dieting test your self-control? Do you know what habits sabotage your good intentions? Controlling food intake, so important to weight loss, means modifying *problem* behaviors. Only you can decide what behaviors keep you from reaching for the wrong foods at the wrong times for the wrong reasons. Overall, there is no good or bad treatment; there is only the appropriate treatment for you. And only you can modify those behaviors. What events start (or stop) your eating? What factors influence food choices? Psychologists often use terms like ***chain-breaking, stimulus control, cognitive restructuring, contingency management,*** and ***self-monitoring*** when discussing behavior modification[11] (Table 10-5). This terminology, as we will cover in detail in Chapter 16, helps place the problem in perspective and organize the intervention strategy into manageable steps.

TABLE 10-5

Behavioral Principles of Weight Loss

Stimulus Control

Shopping
1. Shop for food after eating—buy nutritious foods.
2. Shop from a list; do not buy irresistible "problem" foods.
3. Avoid ready-to-eat foods; let others who want them buy them and store them.
4. Put off shopping until absolutely necessary.

Plans
1. Plan to limit food intake as needed.
2. Substitute exercise for snacking.
3. Eat meals and snacks at scheduled times; don't skip meals.

Activities
1. Store food out of sight, preferably in the freezer, so that impulsive eating is discouraged.
2. Eat all food in the same place.
3. Keep serving dishes off the table, especially sauces and gravies.
4. Use smaller dishes and utensils.

Holidays and Parties
1. Drink fewer alcoholic beverages.
2. Plan eating behaviors before parties.
3. Eat a low-kcalorie snack before parties.
4. Practice polite ways to decline food.
5. Don't get discouraged by an occasional setback.

Eating Behavior
1. Put fork down between mouthfuls.
2. Chew thoroughly before taking the next bite.
3. Leave some food on the plate.
4. Pause in the middle of the meal.
5. Do nothing else while eating (e.g., reading, watching television).

Reward
1. Solicit help from family and friends and suggest how they can help you.
2. Help family and friends provide this help in the form of praise and material rewards.
3. Use self-monitoring records as basis for rewards.
4. Plan specific rewards for specific behaviors (behavioral contracts).

Self-Monitoring

Diet Diary
1. Note time and place of eating.
2. List type and amount of food eaten.
3. Record who is present and how you feel.
4. Use diet diary to identify problem areas.

Cognitive Restructuring
1. Avoid setting unreasonable goals.
2. Think about progress, not shortcomings.
3. Avoid imperatives like "always" and "never."
4. Counter negative thoughts with positive restatements.

From Frankle RT, Yang M: Obesity and weight control, *Rockville, MD, 1988, Aspen Publishers.*
See Chapter 6 for low-fat methods of cooking.

Cognitive Restructuring
Changing one's frame of mind regarding eating—for example, instead of using a difficult day as an excuse to overeat, substituting other pleasures for rewards, such as a relaxing walk with a friend.

Stimulus Control
Altering the environment to minimize the stimuli for eating—for example, removing foods from sight and storing them in kitchen cabinets.

Self-Monitoring
A process of tracking foods eaten and conditions affecting eating; actions are usually recorded in a diary, along with location, time, and state of mind. This is a tool to help a person understand more about his or her eating habits.

Chain-breaking separates behaviors that tend to occur together—for example, snacking on chips while watching television. While these activities do not have to occur together, they often do. Dieters may need to break the chain reaction.

Stimulus control puts us in charge of temptations. You might want to push tempting food to the back of the refrigerator, remove fat-laden snacks from the kitchen counter, or avoid the path by the vending machines. Provide a positive stimulus by keeping low-kcalorie snacks ready to satisfy hunger/appetite. Note that alcohol and foods offer quick, easy stress relief. We need to plan healthful alternatives.[11]

Cognitive restructuring changes our frame of mind. For example, after a hard day, a person should respond with a walk or satisfying talk with a friend instead of a binge. Replace eating reactions to stress with healthful, relaxing alternatives.

Decreeing some food off limits sets up an internal struggle to vigilantly resist the urge to eat that food. This hopeless battle can keep us feeling deprived. We lose the fight. It is best to manage food choices with the principle of moderation. If a favorite food becomes troublesome, place it off limits only temporarily, until you can face it frugally.

Contingency management prepares us for potential pitfalls and high-risk situations. We might rehearse ahead responses to pressure—like food being passed at a party.

Did you keep a record of what you ate and what catalysts urged you to pick up the fork or put it down as we suggested in Chapter 1? If so, you already know one key tool in modifying behavior—self-monitoring. A self-monitoring record can reveal patterns—such as unconscious overeating—that may explain problem eating habits. This record can encourage new habits to counteract unwanted behaviors.

New habits often need to replace defeating ones. For example, limiting eating to a single room in the house might eliminate television snacking. Eating rapidly, holding an ever-ready forkful of food while chewing, outpaces the natural satiety response. It takes about 20 minutes for the brain to register satiety. Put the fork down! Because appetite, not physical hunger, often opens the mouth, one may need to simply stop purchasing irresistible foods.

Studies show that people inaccurately estimate portion sizes.[15] During the first week of self-monitoring, it is best to measure food as precisely as possible. Including estimated amounts of toppings, gravies, and garnishes is important. If an eating plan allows only 3 ounces of skinless chicken breast, we need to know what a 3-ounce portion looks like on the plate. It's not much bigger than a pack of playing cards, or the palm of your hand. Investing in a kitchen scale may serve us as well as the one in the bathroom.

Overall, we need to analyze shortcomings that make dieting difficult. Address specific problems, such as snacking, compulsive eating, or mealtime overeating. In all, consult Chapter 16 for a more detailed discussion of how to develop a plan to change behavior.

another BITE

People carry on an internal dialogue—self-talk—to sort out their own truth, beliefs and attitudes, and responses to events around them. Positive self-talk leads us kindly through changes, like choosing to lose weight. We praise ourselves for success. Negative self-talk is different. Praise is replaced with self-deprecating remarks; self-blame; and angry, guilt-producing put-downs. Negative self-talk undermines efforts at self-control—dieting included—and leads to anxiety and depression. Beliefs and self-talk influence how we interpret events of today and expectations of the future, as well as how we feel and react. Positive self-talk and problem-solving efforts and realistic beliefs and goals lead us to a healthful, self-caring lifestyle.

A dieter can tolerate an occasional lapse but needs to plan for lapses. Encourage calm when you slip, but take charge immediately. Change responses like "I ate that cookie; I'm a failure," to "I ate that cookie, but I did well to stop after only one!" An occasional cookie is fine; a pound of cookies in an afternoon deserves reconsideration. When a dieter lapses from the diet plan, newly learned food habits should steer one back toward the plan. This should enable the dieter to avoid the lapse-relapse-collapse trap. Without a strong behavioral plan, a lapse frequently turns into a relapse.[28] Once a pattern of poor food choices begins, the dieter feels like a failure and strays further from the plan. As the relapse lengthens, the diet plan collapses, and the person falls short of the weight-loss goal. Even with a good behavioral plan, a person may fail at a diet. Losing weight is difficult.

CONCEPT CHECK

We should consider the following changes when dieting: (1) Modify behavior to improve conditions for losing weight. (2) Break habit chains that encourage overeating, such as snacking while watching television. (3) Reduce temptations by not buying irresistible foods and by storing foods out of sight. (4) Preplan how to refuse food temptations at a party. (5) Rethink the role of food, replacing food with relaxing activities as a reward for coping with stress. (6) Carefully observe and record eating habits to reveal subtle behaviors that lead to overeating.

PHYSICAL ACTIVITY—ANOTHER KEY TO WEIGHT LOSS

Exercising—until recently a relatively neglected strategy in weight control—causes us to expend far more energy than when we rest (Figure 10-10). Burning only 200 to 300 extra kcalories a day—above and beyond the normal activity level—can eliminate about a half pound of fat storage per week: that's about 25 pounds of fat in a year. Fat burning is greatest during moderate activity—when you can exercise and carry on a conversation at the same time.

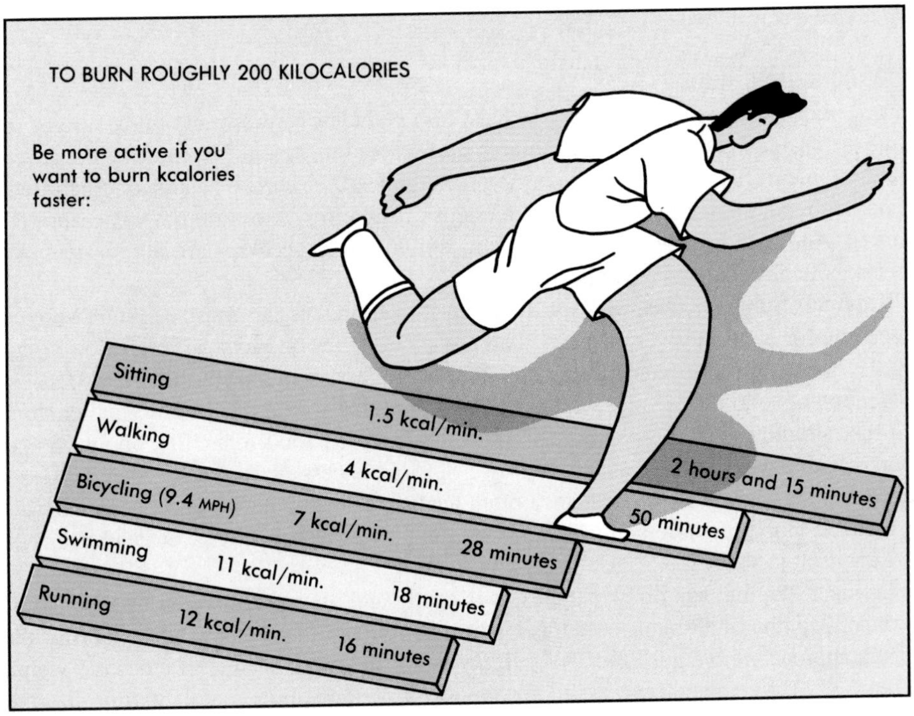

FIGURE 10-10
Exercise improves any diet. Weight loss will occur because we burn more kcalories when in motion than at rest.

Walking and riding bicycles, transportation for much of the world, offer an easy way to increase daily physical activity. Experts recommend an hour or so of brisk walking every day as one option.

Exercise also reduces the stress and boredom of a diet. A walk takes the dieter out of the house and away from temptations. Regular exercise gradually increases muscle mass as well. More lean tissue raises basal metabolism so that we burn more energy, even while we are sitting still. A higher ratio of lean tissue to fat gives us a "losing" advantage.

Becoming even lighter may require more exercise. As the body responds to exercise, weight loss usually slows; the lighter body weight reduces the energy cost of activity. The metabolic rate also slows as the body loses lean tissue along with fat tissue during dieting. Walking 15 minutes more each day to help receive the same exercise benefit during efficient energy use is one response. The goal is to keep exercising.[10] A lifelong commitment to exercise promises leaner bodies and better health for all.

PROFESSIONAL HELP FOR WEIGHT LOSS

The dieter needs to see the family physician or student health service professionals for advice about a weight-loss program. Doctors, trained to assess overall health and the appropriateness of weight loss, can refer dieters to a registered dietitian. With their knowledge of food composition and how people use foods to cope with psychological challenges, registered dietitians can answer diet-related questions and design a specific weight-loss plan.

Self-help weight-loss organizations, such as Take Off Pounds Sensibly (TOPS) and Weight Watchers, offer sensible guidance and support. The classes offer the opportunity to discuss problems with a group and possibly gain new coping mechanisms. Other programs—such as Jenny Craig, Diet Center, and Physician's Weight Loss Center, among others—are often less helpful for the average dieter. These are generally expensive, because of the intense counseling and/or mandatory diet foods and supplements required.

Many programs unfortunately pay only lip service to maintenance. Weight Watchers, an exception, offers free meetings as long as one stays within the goal weight range. People generally need 18 to 24 months in an organized maintenance program to incorporate the lifestyle changes that keep weight off. If the program doesn't encourage exercise, take our advice—stay active.

Treating Severe Obesity

Severe (morbid) obesity—weighing at least 100 pounds over desirable body weight (or twice the desirable body weight)—requires professional treatment.[5] Because of the severe health problems related to morbid obesity, drastic measures can be necessary. Such treatments are recommended, though only for those people for whom no other measure has worked. And it should be noted that drastic weight-loss procedures are not without side effects, both physical and psychological.

Gastroplasty
Surgery on the stomach to limit its volume to approximately 50 milliliters, which is the size of a shot glass.

Stomach Surgery. ***Gastroplasty,*** or stomach stapling, is the most common surgical procedure for treating severe obesity. The procedure relies on physical restriction of eating. By reducing the stomach to the size of a shot glass, about 50 milliliters (2 ounces), overeating of solid foods is less likely.[12] Rapid vomiting would result. The smaller stomach also promotes more rapid satiety. With the enforced food reduction, about 75% of people with severe obesity eventually lose 50% of excess body weight. The surgery's success at long-term loss maintenance often leads to dramatic health improvements, such as reduced blood pressure and correction of adult-onset diabetes. Risk of death from the surgery itself is about 1%.

Stomach stapling has disadvantages. It is costly and often not covered by medical insurance. Months of difficult emotional adjustments face the dieter while enduring this drastic approach to weight loss. This surgery is not reversed, even after a desired weight is reached. Thus, though successful for weight loss, it requires major lifetime lifestyle changes.

NUTRITION insight

DIET PILLS

Over-the-counter medications that claim to help weight loss sell briskly. Though some can be effective, none matches diet moderation and physical activity for long-term weight loss. Diet aids include caffeine, fiber pills, phenylpropanolamine, and benzocaine. Caffeine tends to blunt appetite. Benzocaine numbs the tongue and affects the sense of taste, so a person tends to eat less. Fiber pills can increase bulk in the stomach and ideally lead to satiety. A typical side effect is significant intestinal gas. Can you guess why? (See Chapter 5.)

Phenylpropanolamine is an epinephrine-like drug that can cause a slight decrease in food intake.[17] At a typical dose of 75 milligrams per day, the degree of appetite suppression varies among people. FDA recommends that phenylpropanolamine be used with caution in people with hyperthyroidism, cardiovascular disorders (including hypertension), and diabetes. Adverse reactions may also occur among those taking various other medications at the same time.

Phenylpropanolamine *An over-the-counter stimulant that has a mild appetite-reducing effect.*

Prescription Medications

Physicians sometimes prescribe amphetamines for weight loss.[6] Amphetamines decrease appetite, but they can have a hook: addiction. In addition, amphetamines can increase heart rate and nervousness and lead to insomnia. Thyroid hormone preparations, once popular, cause significant loss of lean tissue.

Fenfluramine and fluoxetine have been prescribed by physicians to promote weight loss. By increasing the action of a neurotransmitter in the brain, they may lead to less food craving, especially for high-carbohydrate foods. Note that some people complain of rapid weight gain after discontinuing the drug, and fenfluramine worsens depression in those people who already show signs of this disorder.

The experimental medications naloxone and naltrexone significantly decrease food intake in laboratory animals. Results from human studies, however, have proved discouraging. Development of related drugs is continuing.

Overall, in skilled hands, prescription medications can aid weight loss when coupled with diet control[6]; however, they do not substitute for the more conservative approaches of reducing energy intake, modifying problem behaviors, and increasing physical activity.

Useless Medications

The hormone cholecystokinin (CCK) may regulate food intake within the body, but bought in a bottle, it wastes money. It is widely available in health-food stores in the form of ground-up animal intestines (recall CCK is produced in the small intestine). However, the amount of CCK in each pill is almost too small to detect, let alone suppress appetite. In addition, CCK is a protein and so is destroyed by digestion in the stomach; little is absorbed as such from an oral dose. It must be injected to be effective, and you can't buy a form that is safe to inject.

Another class of useless and potentially harmful diet aids is diuretics or "water pills." They have a legitimate medical use in the treatment of hypertension, but they cannot control body fatness. Obesity is not primarily caused by excess water accumulation in healthy people.

another BITE

Lipectomy, surgically removing localized fat deposits from humans, is a cosmetic choice for diet-resistant areas of the body. A pencil-thin tube inserted through an incision in the skin suctions off fat tissue from the buttocks, thighs, and other areas. Risks include infection; large, lasting skin depressions; and blood clots that can lead to kidney failure. This often painful surgery requires an experienced physician but can help reshape body areas. Over 100,000 procedures were performed in 1990, with women receiving 85% of them. Cost is about $1500 per site.

Lipectomy
Surgical removal of body fat; also known as liposuction.

Very Low-Calorie Diet (VLCD)
Also known as a protein-sparing modified fast (PSMF), this diet allows the consumption of 400 to 800 kcalories per day in liquid form. Of this, about 30 to 120 grams are made up of carbohydrate; the rest is mostly protein.

Very low-calorie diets. Physician-supervised ***very low-calorie diets (VLCD)*** offer an alternative for severely obese people who prefer no temptations from conventional food.[20] These 400- to 800-kcalorie-per-day diets, usually in liquid form, were earlier called protein-sparing modified fasts. They provide about 30 to 120 grams of carbohydrates. The remainder, about 50 to 100 grams, is high-quality protein, such as is found in egg whites, chicken, turkey, and lean beef. The diets include vitamin and mineral supplements. The minimal energy and absence of food choice can usually produce about a 3- to 5-pound loss per week. On these diets, men tend to lose weight faster than women.

Some researchers support the use of VLCD therapy with people who have body weights of greater than 30% to 40% above desirable weight. However, recent studies show few people can maintain the weight loss after following a VLCD alone. Changing behavior and exercising regularly still are key parts of long-term therapy. These concepts are given greater attention in the latest commercial VLCD programs.[2] In addition, losing weight too rapidly on a VLCD can cause gallstones, as well as a significant loss of heart tissue, which has occasionally led to sudden death from heart attack. These risks demand that a person use careful, physician-guided consideration when choosing and while following VLCD therapy.

VLCD therapy has other less serious side effects, such as cold intolerance, fatigue, light-headedness, nervousness, euphoria, constipation, diarrhea, dry skin, thinning reddened hair, anemia, and menstrual irregularities.[1]

Very low-calorie diets (VLCDs) should not be used by infants, children, teenagers, pregnant women, or elderly persons.

CONCEPT CHECK

Severe (morbid) obesity's high failure rate with conservative weight loss strategies suggests a need for other interventions. Two options include surgery to reduce stomach volume to about 50 milliliters or a very low-calorie diet consisting of 400 to 800 kcalories per day. Both require careful monitoring by a physician to evaluate health risks. Behavior modification and exercise should be included to maintain weight loss and overall health.

PUTTING WEIGHT LOSS INTO PERSPECTIVE

Have you known anyone who has lost and regained the same 10 pounds—plus more—many times? It appears that dieting actually promotes obesity. Can you imagine the time and trouble that went along with each lost pound? The emotional demands of dieting require strong motivation and strong social support to sustain the loss. We need to put supports in place first. Weight loss and subsequent weight maintenance demand ongoing attention. This essentially boils down to a lifelong commitment. Any treatment program should continue until the dieter feels the sense of control needed to take this lifelong step. Then extensive follow-up is needed, much like what is done when people with diabetes are treated.

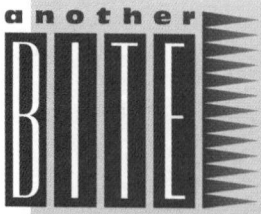

If this lifelong commitment will be a struggle for you, make dieting choices wisely so that each pound is lost forever. You deserve not to repeat your struggling steps. If you have healthy, acceptable body weight, simple maintenance is a positive step.

Otherwise healthy people who do not exceed a BMI of 25-27 do not necessarily need weight loss for health's sake. These people would be better served if our culture simply rethought its obsession with slimness.[5] For people who have heart disease, hypertension, diabetes, arthritis, or another disorder that is often worsened by obesity, weight loss is recommended.

Our own strengths and weaknesses will determine which weight loss techniques work. A true measure of diet success is improved health and self-esteem as weight is lost.

TREATING THE UNDERWEIGHT PERSON

Sometimes being underweight requires medical intervention. A physician should be consulted to rule out hormonal imbalances, depression, cancer, infectious diseases, digestive tract disorders, excessive physical exercise, and other hidden disease, such as anorexia nervosa or bulimia. Risks associated with being underweight include complications in surgery and slow recovery after illness. Underweight women may have menstrual irregularities, stop menstruating altogether (which is associated with bone loss—see Chapter 9), risk infertility, and deliver low-birth-weight newborns. Underweight is also associated with increased death rates, especially when associated with cigarette smoking. This surprises some people, because we hear about the risks of obesity, but not underweight. In our society, being underweight is much more socially acceptable than being obese.

The causes of underweight are not altogether different from the causes of obesity. Internal and external satiety signal irregularities, metabolism, hereditary tendencies, and psychological traits can all contribute to being underweight.

For growing children, the demand for energy to support physical activity and growth can cause underweight. During growth spurts in adolescence, an active child may not take the time to consume enough energy to support his or her high energy needs. And gaining weight can be a formidable task for an underweight person. More than 500 extra kcalories per day may be required to gain weight, even at a slow pace. This is due in part to the expenditure of energy in adaptive thermogenesis. In contrast to the weight loser, the person who wants to gain weight may need to increase portion sizes and learn to like new energy-dense foods.

When underweight requires medical intervention, one approach for treating adults is to gradually increase their consumption of energy-dense foods (foods that provide many kcalories in a small volume), especially those higher in vegetable fat. Italian cheeses, nuts, and granola are good kcalorie sources with low saturated fat content (read the label to see whether the product is high in mostly unsaturated fat). Dried fruit and bananas provide energy-dense fruit choices. If eaten at the end of a meal, they don't cause early satiety. Underweight people should replace such foods as diet soft drinks with good energy sources, like fruit juices. Keeping a daily food record for weekly review can help point one toward wise high-kcalorie food choices (the right side of Table 10-4 lists some possible choices). In addition, encouraging a regular meal and snack schedule aids in weight gain and maintenance. Sometimes people who are underweight have experienced stress at work or have been too busy to eat. Making regular meals a priority can not only aid with attaining an appropriate weight, but can also help with digestive disorders—such as constipation—which are sometimes associated with irregular eating times.

A physically active person could reduce activity. If weight still stays low, a weight-lifting or exercise program might be used to add muscle mass, but energy intake must be increased to support that exercise. Otherwise, weight gain will be hindered.

If these efforts fail to achieve the desired weight, they should at least prevent health problems associated with being underweight. After achieving that, the person may have to accept his or her very lean frame.

SUMMARY

- Hunger is the internal physiological drive to find and eat food. It is triggered partly by cells that form satiety and feeding centers in the hypothalamus. Destroy the satiety center in animals or humans, and overeating with eventual obesity results. Destroy the feeding centers, and semistarvation results. These centers monitor and respond to blood glucose and other nutrients. Hormones and other compounds made by cells also help regulate satiety.
- Appetite is the psychological desire to find and eat food. It is affected by external factors, such as time of day, food availability and palatability, and social custom. Because food is so readily available in America, appetite—not hunger—is often the catalyst for food intake.
- Basal metabolism, the thermic effect of food, and physical activity account for most of the body's energy use. Basal metabolism, the minimal energy needed to keep the resting body alive, is primarily determined by lean body mass, amount of body surface, and thyroid hormone levels. The thermic effect of food is energy the body uses to digest, absorb, and process nutrients recently consumed.
- We measure the body's energy use directly from heat output or indirectly from oxygen uptake. Formulas based on various combinations of body weight, height, and age estimate the body's energy needs.
- The existence of obesity and risk for related disease can be defined along several dimensions:
  - A total body fat exceeding 25% in men and 30% to 35% in women; body fat is most often measured by skinfold thickness and bioelectrical impedance.
  - A body mass index (BMI) (weight in kilograms divided by height in meters squared) over 25 to 27.
  - Weighing 20% more than desirable body weight (based on the Metropolitan Life Insurance Table, published in 1983).
- Fat distribution predicts health risks linked to obesity. Upper-body obesity (characterized by a large abdomen and small buttocks and thighs) means higher risks of hypertension, heart disease, and diabetes than lower-body obesity (characterized by small abdomen and larger buttocks and thighs).
- Genetic factors influence basal metabolism and body shape, and so influence the tendency to obesity. How one is raised (or nurtured) also influences obesity. Family members often develop similar eating habits and activity patterns. Obesity may essentially be nurture allowing nature to express itself.
- To some extent, body weight tends to regulate itself naturally. Does a set point for weight level exist? Trusting a set point to maintain a desirable weight isn't reliable; adults tend to gain 15 to 20 pounds between the ages of 18 and 54.
- When considering a treatment for obesity, remember (1) the body resists weight loss, (2) because obesity is difficult to reverse, the goal is prevention, and (3) losing weight mostly from fat storage, not from muscle and other lean tissues is the goal.

- A sound weight-loss diet should meet a dieter's nutritional needs by following the Food Guide Pyramid. A good plan should adapt to the person's habits, encourage readily obtainable foods, strive to change poor eating habits, promote regular physical activity, and foster a lifelong commitment to treatment. It should also insist that the dieter see a physician if weight is to be lost rapidly or if the person is over 35 years of age and plans to perform substantially greater physical activity than usual.
- A pound of fat stores—gained or lost—represents approximately 2700 kcalories. If energy output exceeds energy intake by 400 to 500 kcalories per day, one can lose a pound of fat storage in a week. We can best cut kcalories by decreasing intake of high-fat foods.
- Behavior modification helps weight-loss programs because current habits may encourage overeating and discourage weight maintenance. Specific behavior modification techniques, such as stimulus control and self-monitoring, help change problem behaviors.
- Increasing physical activity sheds pounds. A good goal is to expend an extra 200 to 300 kcalories in activity each day.
- Severe (morbid) obesity, defined as weighing at least 100 pounds over desirable body weight or twice the desirable body weight, may require (1) stomach surgery to reduce stomach volume to approximately 50 milliliters or (2) very low-calorie diets (VLCDs) containing 400 to 800 kcalories per day. Only people who fail at more conservative approaches to weight loss should use these procedures.
- Over-the-counter weight-loss medications include caffeine and other mild stimulants and fiber pills. None of these, however, replaces a good diet, behavior changes, and increased physical activity, which are essential to long-term weight loss.

STUDY QUESTIONS

1. John walked into his physician's office and his body status was assessed using the 1983 Metropolitan Life Insurance Table. Provide one advantage and one disadvantage of using this method.
2. What are the two most convincing pieces of evidence that both genetic and environment factors play significant roles in the development of obesity?
3. What are the major psychological and physiological problems associated with rapid weight loss?
4. When searching for a sound weight-loss program, what six characteristics would you look for? Give four characteristics of fad diets for weight loss.
5. You are following a nutritional plan for weight loss. What are five specific ways you could save kcalories?
6. Describe the term *behavior modification.* Relate it to the terms *stimulus control, self-monitoring, chain-breaking, relapse prevention,* and *cognitive restructuring.* Give examples of each in the latter group.

REFERENCES

1. Anderson JW and others: Benefits and risks of an intensive very-low-calorie diet program for severe obesity, *The American Journal of Gastroenterology* 87:6, 1992.
2. Atkinson RL and others: Combination of very-low-calorie diet and behavior modification in the treatment of obesity, *American Journal of Clinical Nutrition* 56:199S, 1992.
3. Bjorntorp P: Metabolic implications of body fat distribution, *Diabetes Care* 14:1132, 1991.
4. Booth DA: Integration of internal and external signals in intake control, *Proceedings of the Nutrition Society* 51:21, 1992.
5. Bray GA: An approach to the classification and evaluation of obesity. In Bjorntorp B, Brodoff BN, editors: *Obesity,* Philadelphia, 1992, JB Lippincott.
6. Bray GA: Drug treatment for obesity, *American Journal of Clinical Nutrition* 55:538S, 1992.
7. Bray GA: The nutrient balance approach to obesity, *Nutrition Today* p. 13, May/June 1993.
8. Castonguay TW, Stern JS: Hunger and appetite. In Brown ML, editor: *Present knowledge in nutrition,* Washington, DC, 1990, International Life Sciences Institute.
9. Diaz EO and others: Metabolic response to experimental overfeeding in lean and overweight healthy volunteers, *American Journal of Clinical Nutrition* 56:641, 1992.
10. Forbes GB: Exercise and lean weight: the influence of body weight, *Nutrition Reviews* 50:157, 1992.
11. Foreyt JP, Goodrick GK: Weight management without dieting, *Nutrition Today* p. 4, March/April 1993.
12. Gastrointestinal surgery for severe obesity: National Institutes of Health Consensus Development Conference Statement, *American Journal of Clinical Nutrition* 55:615S, 1992.
13. Kushner RF: Body weight and mortality, *Nutrition Reviews* 51:127, 1993.
14. Leibel RL: Fat as fuel and metabolic signal, *Nutrition Reviews* 50:12, 1992.
15. Lichtman SW and others: Discrepancy between self-reported and actual caloric intake and exercise in obese subjects, *The New England Journal of Medicine* 327:1893, 1992.
16. Luke A, Schoeller DA: Basal metabolic rate, fat-free mass, and body cell mass during energy restriction, *Metabolism* 41:450, 1992.
17. National Institutes of Health Technology Assessment Conference Statement: Methods for voluntary weight loss and control, *Nutrition Reviews* 50:340, 1992.
18. Nelson KM and others: Effect of weight reduction on resting energy expenditure, substrate utilization, and the thermic effect of food in moderately obese women, *American Journal of Clinical Nutrition* 55:924, 1992.
19. Owen OE: Regulation of energy and metabolism. In Kinney JM and others, editors: *Nutrition and metabolism in patient care,* Philadelphia, 1988, WB Saunders.
20. Pi-Sunyer FX: The role of very-low-calorie diets in obesity, *American Journal of Clinical Nutrition* 56:240S, 1992.
21. Ravussin E, Bogardus C: A brief overview of human energy metabolism and its relationship to essential obesity, *American Journal of Clinical Nutrition* 55:242S, 1992.
22. Rolls BJ, Shide DJ: The influence of dietary fat on food intake and body weight, *Nutrition Reviews* 50:283, 1992.
23. Stricker EM, Verbalis JG: Control of appetite and satiety: insights from biologic and behavioral studies, *Nutrition Reviews* 48:49, 1990.
24. Sweeney ME and others: Severe vs moderate energy restriction with and without exercise in the treatment of obesity: efficiency of weight loss, *American Journal of Clinical Nutrition* 57:127, 1993.
25. Swinburn B, Ravussin E: Energy balance or fat balance? *American Journal of Clinical Nutrition* 57:766S, 1993.
26. Wadden TA and others: Relationship of dieting history to resting metabolic rate, body composition, eating behavior, and subsequent weight loss, *American Journal of Clinical Nutrition* 56:203S, 1992.
27. Willard MD: Obesity: types and treatments, *American Family Physician* 43(6):2009, 1991.
28. Wing R: Behavioral treatment of severe obesity, *American Journal of Clinical Nutrition* 55:545S, 1992.
29. Zamboni M and others: Effect of weight loss on regional body fat distribution in premenopausal women, *American Journal of Clinical Nutrition* 58:29, 1993.

AM I A CANDIDATE FOR WEIGHT LOSS?

Determine the following two indices of your body status: body mass index and waist to hip ratio.

Body Mass Index (BMI)

Record your weight in pounds: ________________ lbs.
Divide your weight in pounds by 2.2 to determine your weight in kilograms: ________________ kg.
Record your height in inches: ________________ in.
Divide your height in inches by 39.3 to determine your height in meters: ________________ m.
Calculate your BMI using the following formula:

BMI = Weight (kg)/height $(m)^2$

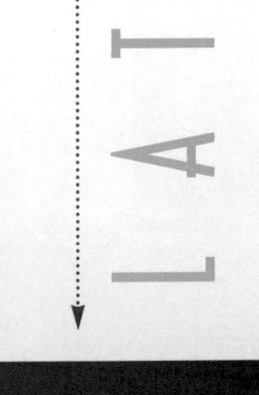

BMI = ____________ kg/____________ m^2 = ________________.

Waist to Hip Ratio

Take a tape measure and measure the circumferences of your waist (at the belly button) and hips (widest point).

Circumference of waist (umbilicus) = ________________ in.

Circumference of hips = ________________ in.

Calculate your waist to hip ratio using the following formula:

Circumference of waist/circumference of hips

Waist to hip ratio = ____________ in/____________ in = ____________.

Interpretation

1. When BMI is greater than 25 to 27, health risks from obesity begin. It would be especially advisable to attempt weight loss if your BMI exceeds 30.
   Does yours exceed 25 to 27? Yes ____________ No ____________
2. When a person is greater than 20% above desirable weight, a waist to hip ratio exceeding 0.95 in men and 0.8 in women indicates upper-body obesity. This is associated with an increased risk of heart disease, hypertension, and diabetes.
   If appropriate, does your ratio exceed the standard appropriate for your gender?
   Yes ____________ No ____________
3. Do you feel you need to pursue a program of weight loss?
   Yes ____________ No ____________

Application

From what you've learned in this chapter, what habits could you change in eating and exercise to lose weight and help ensure you maintain the loss?

____

____

____

____

FAD DIETS—WHY ALL THE COMMOTION?

Bowker's *Books in Print* lists an astounding 455 titles under diet books. Quacks probably make more unreasonable, unproven, and dangerous claims for fat loss treatments than for any other products. So-called cures show up everywhere—television, magazines, newspapers. In fact, dieting quackery has existed for years, as we mentioned in Chapter 3. Today, advertisers push pills, hypnosis, and wonder diets, all promising fewer fat cells, just like magic. But any dieter should know magic can't do the trick.

Still, many overweight people attempt to turn fad diet books into self-treatment. As you will see, most of these diets provide no special help, and some can do harm (Table 10-6).

Why do fad diet books still exist? Why doesn't the government ban them? Many contain obvious misinformation. FDA gets tough only when products threaten serious harm. FDA's heavy demands prevent it from pursuing every new fad diet. So the ancient advice still applies: *Let the buyer beware.* Authors and publishers seeking success may shirk their responsibility to the reader with little risk. Outrageous claims sell more books than does telling people to eat less fat and exercise more.

How to Recognize a Fad Diet

Fad diets typically share some common characteristics. We list a few here:

1. They promote quick weight loss, but it is primarily through glycogen, sodium, and muscle mass depletion. All lead to a loss of body water. Little fat is lost.
2. They limit food selections and dictate specific rituals, such as eating only fruit for breakfast.
3. They use testimonials from famous people and tie the diet to celebrity cities, such as Beverly Hills and New York.
4. They bill themselves as cure-alls. Whatever the type of obesity or whatever a reader's specific strengths and weaknesses, these diets claim to work for everyone.
5. They often recommend expensive supplements. Some supplements can be harmful, such as high doses of vitamin A, vitamin D, niacin, or vitamin B-6.
6. No attempts are made to change eating habits permanently. The dieter follows the diet until reaching the desired weight, then reverts to old eating habits. Eat rice for a month, lose weight, and then return to old habits.
7. The authors generally criticize the scientific community, suggesting that physicians and registered dietitians do not really want people to lose weight. They encourage dieters to seek advice outside the medical and scientific establishment.

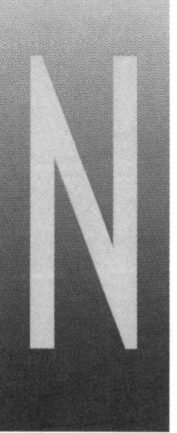

TABLE 10-6

Summary of Popular Diet Approaches to Weight Control

Approach and Examples	Characteristics and Possible Negative Health Consequences
Moderate Kcalorie Restriction	
The Setpoint Diet Slim Chance in a Fat World Weight Watcher's Diet The American Heart Association Diet Mary Ellen's Help Yourself Diet Plan The Beyond Diet Nutripoints	Usually 1000-1800 kcalories per day Reasonable balance of macronutrients Encourages exercise May employ behavioral approach None Weaknesses: none if vitamin and mineral supplement used and permission of family physician is granted
Macronutrient Restriction	
Low carbohydrate Atkins' Diet Revolution Calories Don't Count Wild Weekend Diet Miracle Diet for Fast Weight Loss Drinking Man's Diet Woman Doctor's Diet for Women The Doctor's Quick Weight Loss Diet (Stillman's) The Complete Scarsdale Medical Diet Four Day Wonder Diet	Less than 100 grams of carbohydrate per day Weaknesses: ketosis; poor exercise capacity due to poor glycogen stores in the muscles; excessive animal fat intake
Low-Fat The Rice Diet Report The Macrobiotic Diet (some versions) The Pritikin Diet The Tokyo Diet The Palm Beach Lifelong Diet The James Coco Diet The 35+ Diet 7-Week Victory Diet Fat to Muscle Diet T-Factor Diet Fit or Fat Two Day Diet Complete Hip and Thigh Diet The Maximum Metabolism Diet The Pasta Diet The McDougall Plan	Less than 20% of energy from fat Limited (or elimination of) animal protein sources; also all fats, nuts, seeds Weaknesses: little satiety; flatulence; possibly poor mineral absorption from excess fiber; limited food choices → deprivation
Novelty Diets	
Dr. Abravanel's Body Type and Lifetime Nutrition Plan (or his other books) Dr. Berger's Immune Power Diet Fit for Life The Rotation Diet The Hilton Head Metabolism Diet The Junk Food Diet The Beverly Hills Diet Dr. Debetz Champagne Diet Sun Sign Diet F-Plan Diet Fat Attack Plan	Promote certain nutrients, foods, or combination of foods as having unique, magical, or previously undiscovered qualities Weaknesses: malnutrition; no change in habits → relapse; unrealistic food choices → leading to possible bingeing

Diets may be listed in more than one category if multiple characteristics apply.

TABLE 10-6 CONT'D

Summary of Popular Diet Approaches to Weight Control

Approach and Examples	Characteristics and Possible Negative Health Consequences
Novelty Diets—cont'd	
The Ultrafit Diet The Princeton Plan The Diet Bible Bloomingdale's Diet The Love Diet Eat to Succeed The Underburner's Diet Eat to Win	
Very Low-Calorie Diets (VLCDs)	
Optifast Cambridge Diet The Last Chance Diet Genesis Medifast New Direction HMR Ultrafast	Less than 800 kcalories per day Also known as protein-sparing modified fasts Weaknesses: organ tissue loss—especially from the heart; low serum potassium level → heart failure; expense → must be under close physician scrutiny; kidney stones; gout
Formula Diets	
U.S.A. (United States of America), Inc. Optifast Genesis Cambridge Diet Herbalife The Last Chance Diet Slimfast	Can help people who find it easier not to eat whole foods while dieting to lose weight Based on formulated or packaged products Weaknesses: many are very low-kcalorie diet regimens (see above); no change in habits → increased chance of relapse; expensive; constipation
Premeasured Diets	
Jenny Craig	Most food supplied in premeasured servings to take much of the decision making out of the process of eating Weaknesses: expensive; may not allow for easy sound eating later

Fad diets fail. Most cruelly, dieters are left to assume the guilt and burden, believing they are failures. Fad diets are built for the quick fix. They often don't address problem eating habits (Figure 10-11). They can severely limit food selection, dooming the dieter to quit within a few weeks. But the hook comes with quickly vanishing pounds. Although dieters assume they have lost fat, they actually lose much water and lean tissue mass as well.[24]

An important principle to remember is that weight loss does not always equate with fat loss. Rapid weight loss signifies lean tissue and water loss and suggests that foods have been restricted to less-than-minimal nutrient needs.[17] When normal eating resumes, the lost water and tissue return. In a matter of weeks, most of the lost weight returns, too. This whole scenario sets up an emotionally damaging cycle of hope, discipline, failure, and guilt. Professional help, which fad diets rarely offer, is preferable.

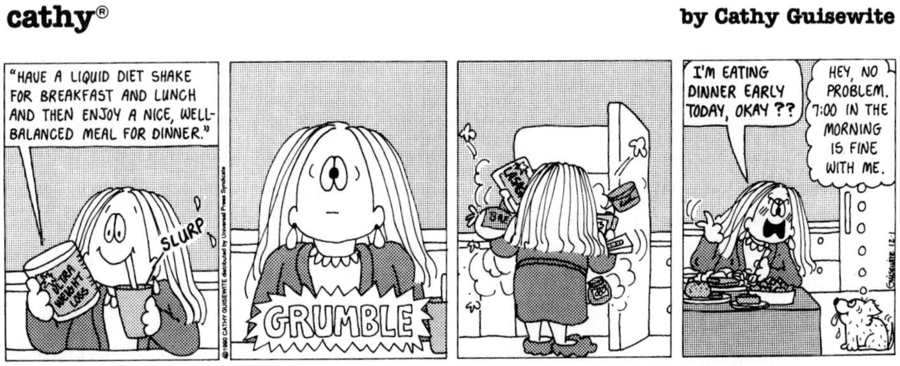

FIGURE 10-11
Cathy.

Types of Fad Diets

Low-Carbohydrate Approaches. The most common form of fad diet, the low-carbohydrate diet, forces the body to provide the glucose vital to such cells as red blood cells. Muscle and other lean tissue generate the carbons used to make new glucose. Thus a low-carbohydrate diet depletes muscle tissue. Because muscle tissue is mostly water, the person loses weight rapidly. When a normal diet is resumed, the muscle tissue is rebuilt and weight quickly returns.

Low-carbohydrate dieting does not guarantee weight loss. Restricting energy intake is what helps. A low-carbohydrate diet by itself results in no more weight loss than other diets. Low-carbohydrate diets include Dr. Atkins' Diet Revolution, Dr. Stillman's Calories Don't Count Diet, the Scarsdale Diet, the Drinking Man's Diet, Four Day Wonder Diet, and the Air Force Diet. Check new fad diets for carbohydrate levels. Extremely limited amounts of breads, cereals, fruits, and vegetables indicate a low-carbohydrate diet.

Low-Fat Approaches. Very low-fat diets—though not harmful—generally fail because fat restrictions (as low as 5% to 10% of kcalories) generate eventual cravings for foods rich in fat. Overall, the very low-fat diet—the Pritikin Diet, for example—turns out to be a very high-carbohydrate diet. The dieter primarily eats grains, fruits, and vegetables. The rigid restrictions lead dieters to a lapse, then a relapse, and probably a collapse. These diets are too far removed from our usual diets for most of us to follow consistently.

Novelty Diets. Gimmicks sell many diets. The Rotation Diet, for example, rotates the total amount of energy intake every few days, attempting to prevent dieting's usual drop in metabolic rate. No scientific data show that this diet works or even how it might work.

Some novelty diets suggest gorging on particular foods or food groups. An egg diet suggests swallowing all the eggs you can eat. The Beverly Hills Diet promotes dining almost exclusively on fresh fruit. A rice diet, designed in the 1940s to lower blood pressure, recently resurfaced for weight loss: more fruit, lots of rice. It is useless in the long run, and most often not nutritionally sound.

The rationale behind these diets is that you can eat only eggs, or fruit, or rice for so long. You will soon become bored and, in theory, reduce your energy intake. These diets are based on fake science. And chances are that you will abandon the diet entirely before you lose much weight.

In the 1960s, diet aids were introduced. For appeal, the popular grapefruit diet enlisted help from some aids: lecithin to help release fat from the tissues, vitamin B-6 to act as a diuretic, vinegar to provide potassium, and kelp to stimulate the thyroid gland. These aids don't deliver what they promise. In the 1980s we had an entirely new product, Herbalife. The aid in Herbalife is herbs high in caffeine; caffeine stimulates the metabolic rate. None of these diet aids can substitute for moderating food intake, modifying behavior, and increasing activity.

The most bizarre of the novelty diets propose that "food gets stuck in your body." Fit for Life and the Beverly Hills Diet suggest that food gets stuck in the intestine, putrifies, and creates toxins that invade the bloodstream and cause disease. This is utter nonsense. Nevertheless, health food books have proposed this chain of events since the 1800s. Today, Fit for Life suggests meat eaten with potatoes will not be digested and that only fresh fruit should be consumed before noon. These recommendations are absurd. These supposedly controversial gimmicks are really designed to sell books. If weight loss does occur, it is because the books combine such complicated rules and rituals that, by the time the dieter has figured out what to eat, it is the wrong time to eat it!

Does your food make you sick? One scheme suggests 30% of us have food allergies that in turn cause most current disease. Find the food allergy, treat it, and, like magic, disease will be waved away; obesity as well. This theory of the early 1980s was made popular by Dr. Berger's Immune Power Diet Book. However, we know of no research that supports Dr. Berger's claim that 30% of people have food allergies.

Now in the nineties there are diets to hook everyone: if astrology guides you, follow the Sun Sign Diet; if you need a drink, celebrate with the Champagne Diet; or match your "dominant" gland with the Body Type and Lifetime Nutrition Diet. Quackery never sleeps, so keep on your toes.

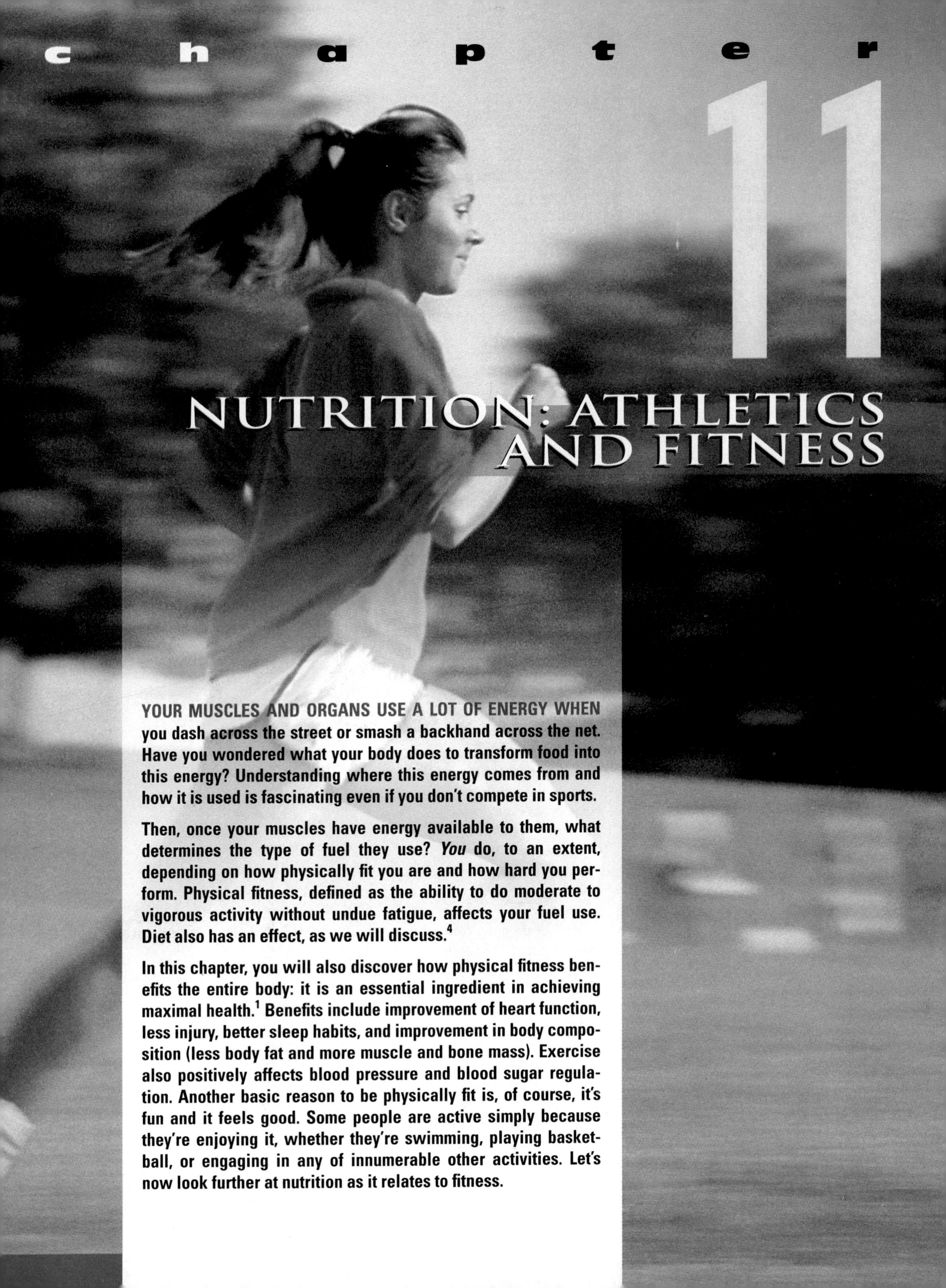

c h a p t e r

11

NUTRITION: ATHLETICS AND FITNESS

YOUR MUSCLES AND ORGANS USE A LOT OF ENERGY WHEN you dash across the street or smash a backhand across the net. Have you wondered what your body does to transform food into this energy? Understanding where this energy comes from and how it is used is fascinating even if you don't compete in sports.

Then, once your muscles have energy available to them, what determines the type of fuel they use? *You* do, to an extent, depending on how physically fit you are and how hard you perform. Physical fitness, defined as the ability to do moderate to vigorous activity without undue fatigue, affects your fuel use. Diet also has an effect, as we will discuss.[4]

In this chapter, you will also discover how physical fitness benefits the entire body: it is an essential ingredient in achieving maximal health.[1] Benefits include improvement of heart function, less injury, better sleep habits, and improvement in body composition (less body fat and more muscle and bone mass). Exercise also positively affects blood pressure and blood sugar regulation. Another basic reason to be physically fit is, of course, it's fun and it feels good. Some people are active simply because they're enjoying it, whether they're swimming, playing basketball, or engaging in any of innumerable other activities. Let's now look further at nutrition as it relates to fitness.

ASSESS

TEST YOUR KNOWLEDGE

HOW PHYSICALLY ACTIVE ARE YOU?

How physically active are you really? Here are five activity levels: (1) sedentary, (2) mostly inactive, (3) moderately active, (4) active, and (5) superactive. Each category is defined below. Your task is to track your activities for the next 3 weeks (even if this class ends before 3 weeks). Assign yourself an activity level each week. Then average the three values and place yourself (X) in the appropriate place on the ladder. Note that you may end up halfway between two classifications.

(5) **Superactive**—One hour of vigorous activity at least 5 days per week. Examples are full-court basketball, mountain climbing, treadmill work, soccer, and other similar activities.

(4) **Active**—Twenty minutes of sustained activity at least 5 days per week. Examples are swimming, tennis singles, cycling, jogging, cross-country skiing, or walking briskly for 45 minutes.

(3) **Moderately Active**—Twenty minutes of sustained activity at least 3 days per week or 10 to 15 minutes of sustained activity at least 4 days a week. Examples include tennis doubles, downhill skiing, skating, aerobic dancing, golf, or similar activities.

(2) **Mostly Inactive**—Sustained activity fewer than 3 days per week that usually involves mostly walking. Examples including fishing, bowling, or sporadic jogging.

(1) **Sedentary**—Most activities are limited to sitting or minimal walking.

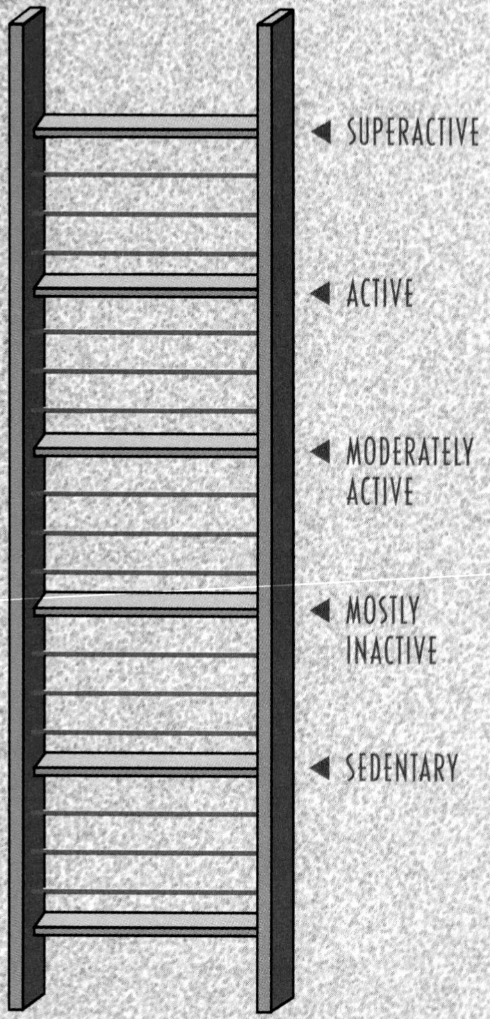

What kind of program of regular physical activity would allow you to move up the ladder, if appropriate?

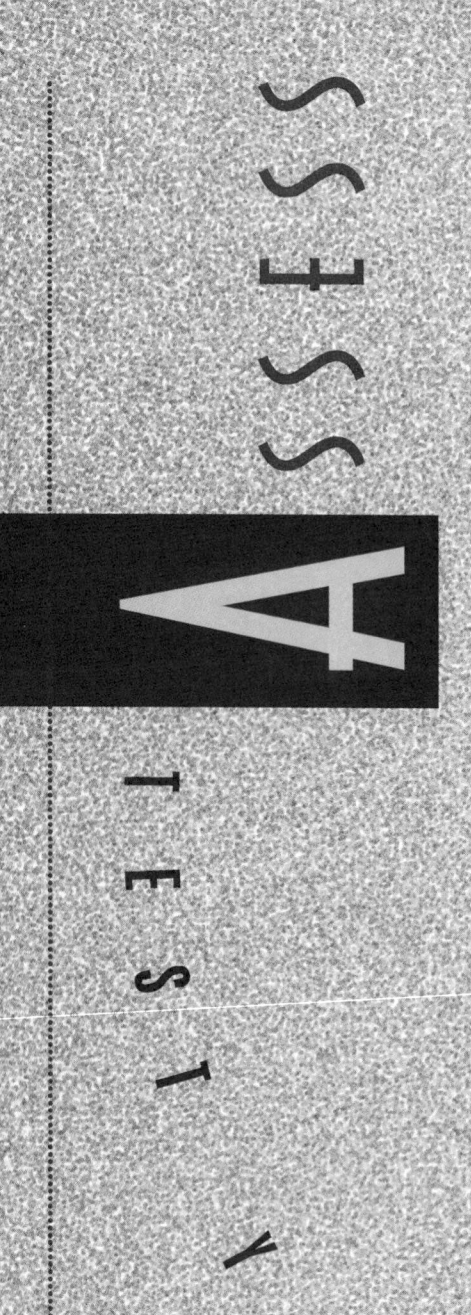

yourself

METABOLISM

Muscle cells, like all cells, need energy to perform. Cells need to capture this energy and then release it to do work.

Our discussion of this process—energy ***metabolism***—must start with the definition of metabolism. This term refers to all chemical processes that take place in the body. Any sequence of a chemical process from beginning to end—for example, burning glucose for fuel—is called a ***pathway.***

Metabolic pathways can produce both ***anabolic*** and ***catabolic*** results. Anabolic pathways build compounds. In these pathways the typical building blocks—oxygen (O_2), water (H_2O), and carbon dioxide (CO_2)—are used to form new, larger compounds. These parts can be combined to form a fatty acid, glucose, or even the complex cholesterol molecule. The process of building requires energy input to make it go.[20]

Conversely, catabolic pathways—which break down compounds into smaller units—often release energy. Glucose and fatty acids, for example, are catabolized when broken down into carbon dioxide and water. Energy is released as a by-product. Anabolic and catabolic pathways take place simultaneously in cells.

Overall, the catabolism needed for energy production from foodstuffs occurs in two stages. In the first stage, large compounds in food—proteins, starches, and triglycerides—are broken down during digestion into smaller units, such as amino acids, simple sugars, and fatty acids. These units are then delivered to working cells, such as muscle cells, via the bloodstream. In this second stage these compounds are eventually broken down into carbon dioxide and water inside the cell. During this second process, large amounts of energy are released to power the cell.[20]

Metabolism *Chemical reactions occur in the body, enabling cells to release energy from foods, convert one substance into another, and prepare end products for excretion.*

Pathway *A metabolic progression of individual steps from starting materials to ending products, such as glucose* $\rightarrow\rightarrow\rightarrow CO_2 + H_2O$

Anabolism *The process of building compounds.*

Catabolism *The process of breaking down compounds.*

Energy a Cell Can Use

The energy that runs the body originates as solar energy. Plants capture this energy through the process of ***photosynthesis.*** As we discussed in Chapter 5, plants use the energy to produce carbohydrates, proteins, and fats. In essence, plants trap solar energy and store it as chemical energy in these nutrients. Every amino acid, glucose, and fatty acid molecule contains a specific amount of chemical energy stored within chemical bonds used to hold the molecule together. When these bonds are broken, the energy that is released can be used to perform cellular work.

One key function of metabolism is to convert energy stored in foodstuffs to a form human cells can use. Overall, each cell must first break down glucose or other energy-rich sources to release stored energy and then convert that energy into usable and smaller energy packets.[20]

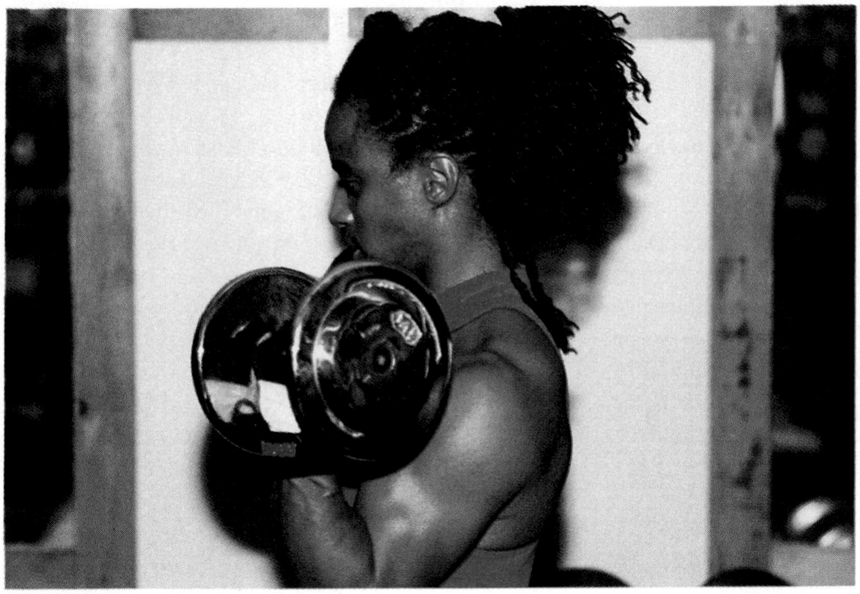

Bursts of muscle activity utilize a variety of fuel sources.

Almost every step in any metabolic pathway depends on input from an enzyme to allow the step to take place.

Photosynthesis
The process by which plants use energy from the sun to produce energy-yielding compounds, such as glucose.

Adenosine Triphosphate (ATP)
The main energy currency for cells. ATP energy is used to promote ion pumping, enzyme activity, and muscular contraction.

Phosphocreatine (PCr)
A high-energy compound that can be used to reform ATP.

Anaerobic
Not requiring oxygen.

Adenosine Triphosphate (ATP). As you may have guessed from our previous discussion, cells can't directly use the energy released from breaking down glucose or fat. Rather, the energy must first be stored in a special form known as ***adenosine triphosphate (ATP).*** To store chemical energy, our cells make ATP. Again, the cells are using the energy obtained from foodstuffs. Conversely, to release energy from ATP, cells partially break down ATP. This releases usable energy for cell functions.

Essentially, ATP is the immediate source of energy for body functions. This includes locomotion.[20] The overall goal of any fuel use—carbohydrate, fat, or protein—is to make ATP. A resting muscle cell has only a small amount of ATP that can be used. If no resupply of ATP were possible, this stored ATP could keep the muscle working maximally for only about 2 to 4 seconds. Fortunately, there are several types of chemical compounds—***phosphocreatine (PCr),*** carbohydrates, fats, and proteins—that can be broken down to release enough energy to make more ATP. Cells actually must constantly use and then reform ATP, over and over again.

another BITE

Think about ATP the next time you race after a bus. When you finally sit down, you are exhausted, you breathe hard, and your heart races. Your muscle cells have used up most of their ATP and other high-energy compounds. While you rest, muscle cells begin to resynthesize the ATP used up during your run. Reforming ATP requires energy. Again, cells can get this energy from foodstuffs. If you sit long enough, you can then race off to class using some of the newly formed ATP.

Phosphocreatine Is the First Line of Defense for Resupplying ATP in Muscles. The instant that breakdown products of ATP begin to accumulate in the contracting muscle, an enzyme is activated to split PCr. This releases the energy needed to reform ATP from its breakdown product adenosine diphosphate (ADP). If no other source of energy for ATP resupply were available, PCr could probably maintain maximal muscle contractions for about 10 seconds. But because other ATP resupply sources kick in, PCr ends up the major source of energy for all events lasting up to about 1 minute (Figure 11-1).

The main advantage of PCr is that it can be activated instantly and can replenish ATP at rates fast enough to meet the energy demands of the fastest and most powerful sports events, including jumping, lifting, throwing, and sprinting actions. The disadvantage of PCr is that there is not enough of it made and stored in the muscles to sustain a high rate of ATP resupply for more than a few minutes. Many attempts have been made over the years to improve the muscle ATP and PCr stores by dietary means, but none has been effective.

Releasing the Energy in Carbohydrate Begins with Glycolysis. Carbohydrates are a valuable fuel for muscles. The most useful form of carbohydrate fuel is the simple sugar glucose. This is available to all cells from the bloodstream. The breakdown of liver glycogen (a storage form of glucose) helps maintain blood glucose levels. In muscles, breakdown of glycogen stored there helps meet carbohydrate demand of that particular muscle. In the catabolic pathway that breaks down glucose, the six-carbon glucose splits into two three-carbon compounds. The net energy released equals two ATPs. This is about 5% of the total number of ATPs that can be made from one glucose.[20] But although this phase of glucose metabolism does not extract much energy from a single glucose molecule, a muscle cell can break down thousands of glucose molecules per second. Therefore this form of glucose metabolism resupplies ATP at a very high rate for a brief period.

When glucose breaks down, the resulting three-carbon compound follows either of two main routes. When oxygen supply in the muscle is limited (***anaerobic*** conditions)

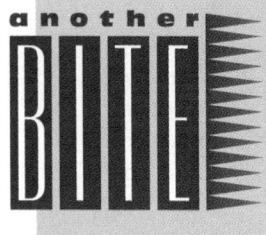

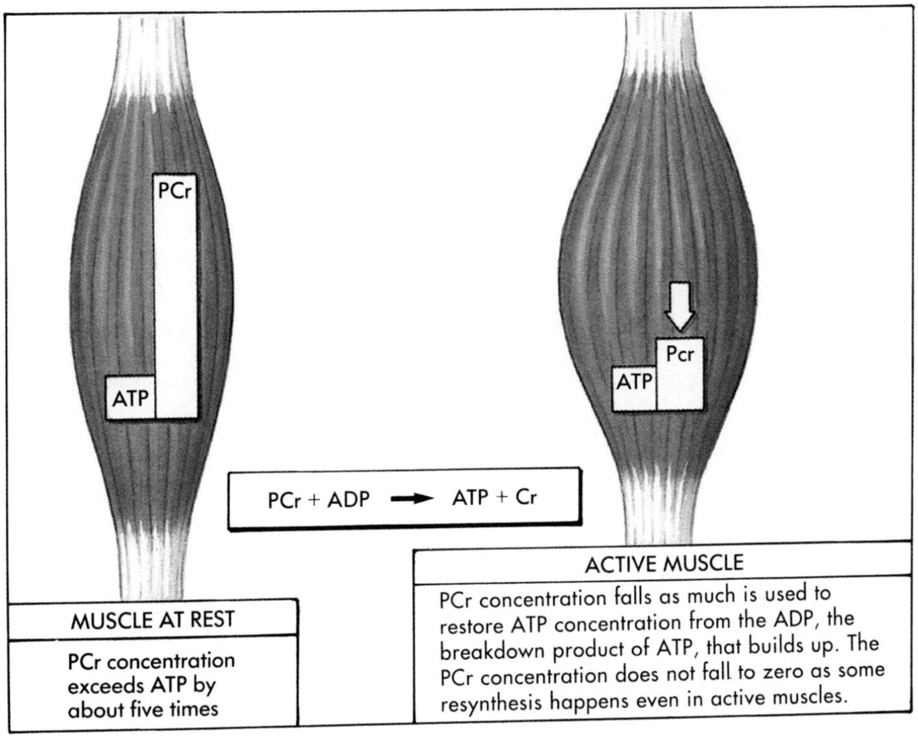
PCr
ATP
Pcr
ATP
PCr + ADP → ATP + Cr
ACTIVE MUSCLE
PCr concentration falls as much is used to restore ATP concentration from the ADP, the breakdown product of ATP, that builds up. The PCr concentration does not fall to zero as some resynthesis happens even in active muscles.
MUSCLE AT REST
PCr concentration exceeds ATP by about five times

FIGURE 11-1
Quick energy for muscle use includes a supply of phosphocreatine (PCr). This can rapidly replenish adenosine triphosphate (ATP) stores as activity begins. PCr can be almost totally depleted in maximally contracting human forearm muscles in less than 60 seconds. It then takes 4 minutes of rest to replenish 95% of the PCr. Similarly, it takes about 7 minutes of rest to replenish 95% of the PCr depleted with repeated knee extensions against resistance.

and when the exercise is intense (e.g., running 400 meters or swimming 100 meters), the three-carbon compound accumulates in the muscle and is converted to ***lactic acid.*** No further ATP is directly formed. This conversion of glucose to lactic acid is called anaerobic ***glycolysis*** (*glyco* means sugar, and *lysis* means breakdown). Carbohydrate is the only fuel that can be used for this process (Table 11-1).

If there is plenty of oxygen available in the muscle (***aerobic*** conditions) and the exercise activity is of moderate to low intensity (e.g., jogging or distance swimming), the bulk of the three-carbon compound is shuttled to the ***mitochondria*** of the cell, where it is further metabolized into carbon dioxide (CO_2) and water (H_2O). This is known as aerobic glycolysis, because the breakdown of glucose in this manner uses oxygen. This aerobic stage of glycolysis forms about 95% of the ATP made from complete glucose metabolism to carbon dioxide and water (Figure 11-2).[20]

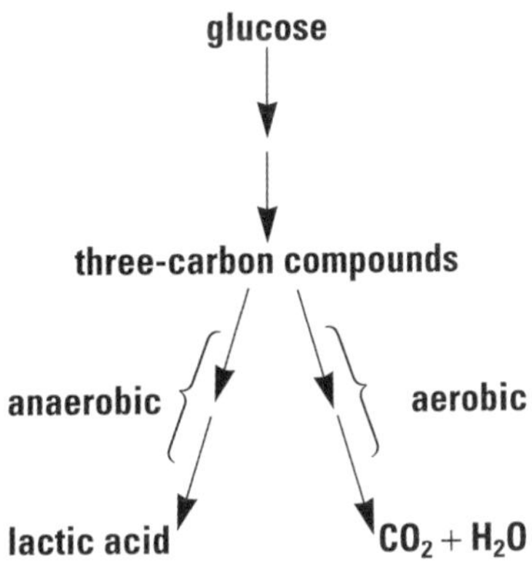

Lactic Acid A three-carbon acid formed during anaerobic cell metabolism; a partial breakdown product of glucose; also called lactate.

Glycolysis The pathway that results in the breakdown of glucose into two three-carbon compounds.

Aerobic Requiring oxygen.

Mitochondria The main sites of energy production in a cell. Structure inside most cells, including muscle cells. Mitochondria also contain the pathway for burning fat for fuel, among other metabolic pathways.

TABLE 11-1

Energy Systems for Muscle Cell Use

System*	When in Use	Example of an Exercise
Adenosine triphosphate (ATP)	At all times	All types
Phosphocreatine (PCr)	All exercise initially; extreme exercise thereafter	Shotput, jumping
Anaerobic glycolysis (carbohydrate)	High-intensity exercise, especially lasting 30 seconds to 2 minutes	200-yard (200-meter) run for time
Aerobic glycolysis (carbohydrate)	Exercise lasting 2 minutes to 4 to 5 hours; the higher the intensity (such as running a 6-minute mile), the greater the use	Basketball, swimming, jogging
Aerobic fat use	Exercise lasting more than a few minutes; greater amounts are used at lower levels of exercise intensity	Long-distance running, long-distance cycling; 70%-90% of fuel use in a brisk walk is fat
Aerobic protein use	Low levels during all exercise; moderate levels in endurance exercise, especially when carbohydrate fuel is lacking	Long-distance running

**Note that at any time more than one system is operating.*

Anaerobic Glycolysis. The advantage of anaerobic glycolysis is that, other than PCr breakdown, it is the fastest way to resupply ATP. Anaerobic glycolysis provides most of the energy for events ranging from about 30 seconds to 2 minutes. The two major disadvantages of anaerobic glycolysis are that (1) the high rate of ATP production cannot be sustained for long events and (2) the rapid accumulation of lactic acid greatly increases the acidity of the muscle. This acid inhibits the activities of key enzymes in the glycolysis pathway. That slows anaerobic ATP production and, in turn, causes fatigue.

For the most part, lactic acid accumulates in active muscle cells until it is released into the bloodstream. The liver picks up the lactic acid and resynthesizes it into glucose. Glucose then can reenter the bloodstream where it is available for cell uptake and breakdown. The heart also can use the lactic acid directly for its energy needs, as can less active muscle cells situated near active ones.[20]

Aerobic Glycolysis. Aerobic glycolysis supplies ATP more slowly than does anaerobic glycolysis but releases more energy. Furthermore, the slower rate of aerobic energy supply can be sustained for hours. Accordingly, aerobic glycolysis makes a major energy contribution to sports events that last anywhere from 2 minutes to 4 or 5 hours (see Table 11-1).[18]

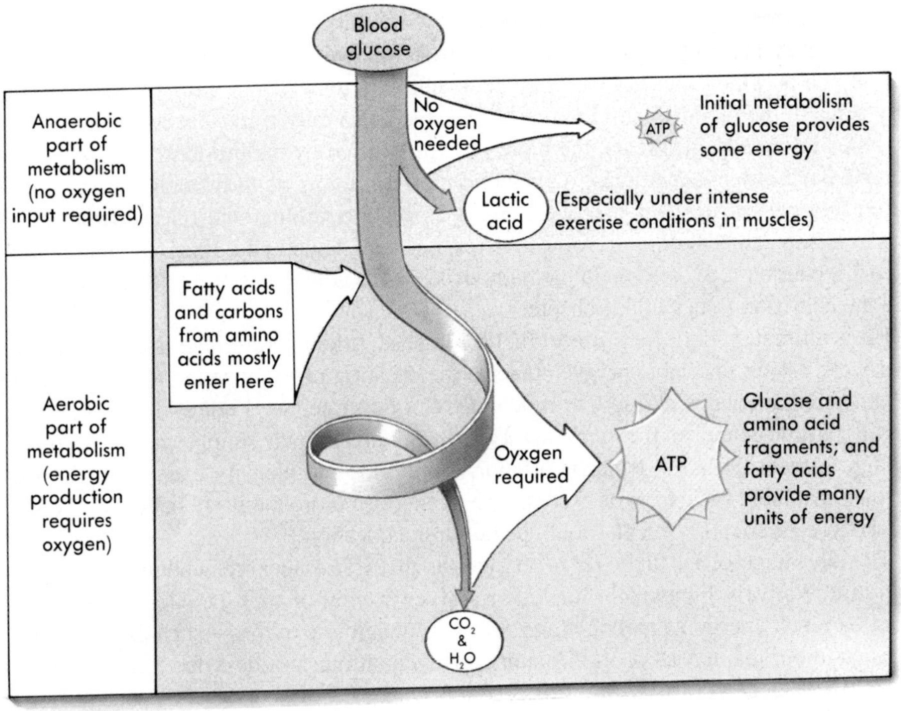

FIGURE 11-2
Carbohydrate, fat, and protein fuels can all supply ATP energy for a muscle cell. Carbohydrate can follow both aerobic and anaerobic pathways, whereas fat and protein are limited for the most part to the aerobic pathway.

Importance of Glycogen Versus Blood Glucose for Carbohydrate Fuel. It is important to note that muscle glycogen is the preferred fuel for both anaerobic and aerobic glycolysis in fairly intense muscular activities that last for less than about 2 hours. For these activities, the depletion of glycogen fuel in the muscle can cause fatigue. Diets high in carbohydrate can be used to build up muscle glycogen stores before athletic competition, thereby forestalling fatigue and improving endurance.[18] We discuss this technique—carbohydrate loading—in a later section.

As exercise duration increases beyond 20 to 30 minutes, blood glucose becomes increasingly important, along with glycogen, as a fuel for glycolysis.[4] The use of glucose from the bloodstream can spare some glycogen use, saving it in the muscle for sudden bursts of effort that may be required—for example, for a sprint to the finish in a marathon race. Because it is important to maintain normal concentrations of glucose in the bloodstream for prolonged exercise, many researchers have studied various types of carbohydrate feedings before and during exercise to maximize glucose supply to muscles. Overall, the techniques have succeeded.[4,17] Carbohydrate feedings during strenuous endurance exercise like cycling can aid in maintaining adequate blood glucose levels and in turn result in a delay of fatigue by 30 to 60 minutes. We discuss this issue further in a later section as well.

Fueling Muscles Using Fat. When fat stores in body tissues are broken down for energy, one triglyceride molecule first yields three fatty acids and a glycerol. The majority of the stored energy is found in the fatty acids. During physical activity, the fatty acids are released from various fat depots into the bloodstream and travel to the muscles, where they are taken into each cell and aerobically broken down to carbon dioxide and water.[20]

The rate at which muscles use fatty acids is partly dependent on the concentration of fatty acids in the bloodstream. In other words, the more fatty acids that are released from fat stores into the bloodstream, the more fat will be used by the muscles. Recently, some athletes have attempted to raise their blood concentrations of fatty acids by consuming caffeinated beverages. This practice actually can increase fatty acid release from the fat depots and so can be helpful to some athletes, but it is illegal under International Olympic rules if the amount of caffeine in the body exceeds the equivalent of 6 to 8 cups of coffee (see the Nutrition Issues in this chapter).

Fat is ultimately not a very useful fuel for intense, brief exercise, but it becomes a progressively more important energy source as the duration of exercise increases, especially when exercise remains at a low or moderate (aerobic) rate (see Figure 11-2). The reason for this is that some of the steps involved in fat breakdown simply cannot occur fast enough to meet the ATP demands of short-duration, high-intensity exercise. If fat were the only available fuel, we would be unable to exercise more intensely than a fast walk or jog. High-caliber sports events would be out of the question.[12]

The advantage of fat fuel over other types is that it provides tremendous stores of energy in a relatively lightweight form. For a given weight of fuel, fat supplies more than twice as much energy as carbohydrate. For very lengthy activities—such as a triathalon, ultramarathon, manual labor in a foundry, or even sitting at a desk for 8 hours a day—fat supplies about 70% to 90% of the energy required. For short events, such as a 100-meter sprint or even a 1500-meter race, the contribution of fat used to resupply ATP is minimal. Keep in mind that the only fast-paced (anaerobic) fuel we eat is carbohydrate; slow and steady (aerobic) activity uses carbohydrate, fat, and protein energy sources (Figure 11-3).[20]

Does This Mean We Use Protein to Fuel Activity? Protein, actually amino acids, can be used for fueling muscles, but in most circumstances protein contributes only about 2% to 5% of the body's general energy needs.[10] This is also true for the typical energy needs of exercising muscles. However, proteins can contribute somewhat more to energy needs in endurance exercise, perhaps as much as 10% to 15%, especially as carbohydrate stores in the muscles are exhausted. We easily eat enough to supply this amount of fuel.[14] Protein or amino acid supplements are not needed. Contrary to what many athletes believe, protein is used less for fuel in resistance types of exercise, such as weight lifting, than for endurance exercise, such as running. The primary fuels for the actual act of weight lifting are PCr and carbohydrate.

CONCEPT CHECK

Adenosine triphosphate (ATP) is the main form of energy that cells use. Metabolic pathways use food energy to form ATP. Phosphocreatine (PCr) can rapidly reform ATP from adenosine diphosphate (ADP), but PCr supplies are quite limited. Carbohydrate metabolism to form ATP begins as glucose becomes available from the bloodstream or from glycogen breakdown. In a muscle cell, each glucose is broken down through a series of steps to yield either lactic acid or carbon dioxide (CO_2) plus water (H_2O). The process that occurs when glucose is broken down into carbon dioxide and water is called *aerobic glycolysis,* because oxygen is used. The conversion of glucose to lactic acid is called *anaerobic glycolysis,* because no oxygen is used. This latter process allows the cell to quickly reform ATP and supports the demand for energy during intense exercise. Fat is a key aerobic fuel for muscle cells, especially at low exercise intensities. At rest, muscles primarily burn fat for energy needs. On the other hand, little protein is used to fuel muscles. It supplies about 2% to 5% of energy needs and, at most, 10% to 15% of energy needs during endurance events.

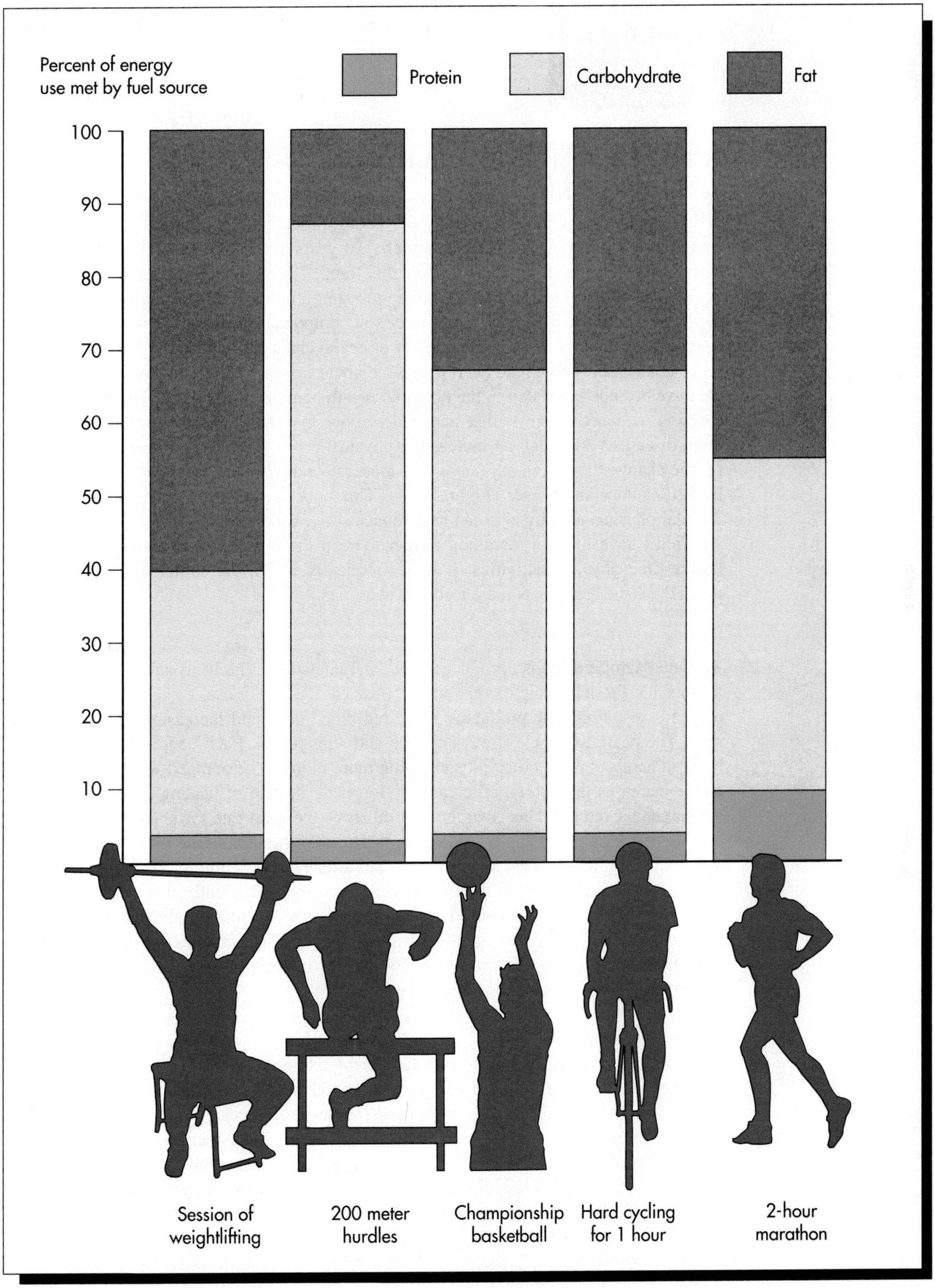

FIGURE 11-3
Rough estimates of food fuel use during various forms of physical activity.

NUTRITION insight

WHAT CAN A PHYSICALLY ACTIVE LIFESTYLE PROMISE?

Was your New Year's resolution to start exercising? Do you often wish that you could be healthier and more physically fit? Today, the interest in physical fitness that blossomed into a full-fledged movement nearly 20 years ago shows no signs of fading. Experts in medicine and nutrition support this trend.[16] More people than ever engage in a wide range of activities, from mall walking to stair climbing and triathalons. This interest in physical activity, particularly as an integral component of overall health and wellness, is evident by the explosion in the number of health clubs nationwide.

To counteract widespread heart disease, diabetes, obesity, and osteoporosis, many people have become interested in the potential health benefits of regular physical activity. Increasing evidence suggests that physical activity may delay the onset and/or help treat these diseases.[1] Although an increase in physical activity is hardly a magic bullet, many people change their habits in hopes that moderate exercise will improve their chances of living healthier and longer (Figure 11-4). This hope is not without scientific support.[16] Regular physical activity also can help reduce stress and increase self-esteem. Best of all, you don't have to be a marathon runner to reap the benefits of exercise. Moderate or leisure-time physical activities, if done frequently and for a sufficient duration, offer much the same benefits as more rigorous activities.

Overall Exercise Fitness

Repeated aerobic exercise produces beneficial changes in the heart and in blood vessels responsible for delivering oxygen to the muscles. Because it uses more oxygen, the body responds to training by producing more red blood cells and increasing total blood volume. The heart, a muscle itself, enlarges and strengthens. Each contraction empties the heart's chambers more efficiently, enabling more blood to be pumped with each beat. Exercise increases the heart's efficiency by lowering its rate of beating at rest and during submaximal exercise. This is an index of fitness—the heart rate lowers as fitness increases. In addition, oxygen can be delivered more easily throughout the muscles because the number of capillaries in the muscles increases after exercise training.

After a period of aerobic training, muscles can more efficiently fuel themselves from fatty acid stores. Changes caused by aerobic exercise eventually allow muscle cells to produce more ATP using oxygen-requiring pathways. This includes the pathway used to burn fat for fuel. This in turn allows for greater intensity during aerobic exercise and harder and longer training at an aerobic pace.

Heart Disease

Cardiovascular *Pertaining to the heart and blood vessels.*

How can a physically active lifestyle reduce the risk of coronary heart disease? Exercise can improve ***cardiovascular*** fitness, help maintain weight, regulate blood pressure, and often modestly boost HDL cholesterol (good cholesterol) levels.

Based on a review of many studies on heart health, the American College of Sports Medicine recommends at least 20 to 60 minutes of vigorous, aerobic exercise, 3 to 5 days per week, with a heart rate elevation of 60% to 90% of one's age-dependent maximal heart rate (220 minus current age).[8] Other researchers suggest adding to that about 60 minutes of more moderate or leisure-time physical activity, such as walking or stair climbing. This can benefit the body even further.[1] And, significantly, we are more likely to perservere in the more moderate—rather than more rigorous—physical activities. Daily, routine stair climbing is one easy way to get moderate aerobic stimulation. For sedentary and middle-aged people who have not maintained a physically active lifestyle, brisk walking and other such moderate activities are preferable at the start to jogging and more rigorous types of activities.

Diabetes

Exercise contributes to weight loss in obesity, which in turn enhances the action of the hormone insulin. Poor insulin action is characteristic of adult-onset (non-insulin dependent) diabetes, the most predominant form of diabetes in the United States. Interestingly, the majority of individuals with this insulin-resistant type of diabetes are also obese. Enhancing insulin sensitivity also improves glucose removal from the bloodstream and potentially allows the insulin dosage to be reduced for those who use it. A person with diabetes must work with a physician to make the correct alterations in diet and medications to perform exercise safely. This is because physical activity can adversely affect some people with diabetes (by inducing low blood sugar, for example). These people need to be aware of their blood glucose response to exercise. To determine this response, they can self-monitor their blood glucose levels before, during (if exercise is prolonged), and after physical activity. The benefits of exercise on insulin action are short-lived, so regular moderate physical activity is encouraged.

Obesity

As a means of losing or controlling weight, a physically active lifestyle offers several benefits, as noted in Chapter 10. In review, first, by increasing energy use, exercise may allow a person to lose weight while eating more than normal. More food and greater variety can then allow better overall nutrient intake. Losing weight by dieting usually entails losing lean tissue, as well as body fat. Performing regular physical activity along with dieting spares some of this lean tissue loss, while promoting the loss of fat tissue. Furthermore, physical activity, especially if it helps someone lose fat, may also help reverse some risk factors associated with obesity, such as diabetes, hypertension, and premature cardiovascular disease.[1]

At moderate levels of activity, exercise increases one's resting metabolic rate, but only for a short time after exercise ceases. Therefore, to get a regular boost in kcalorie burning, exercise should be a daily routine for an obese person, and for that matter, any of us. Note that little bursts of activity can mount up to a lot of daily activity.

Chapter 16 lists many guidelines for setting goals and sticking to them. These suggestions are quite applicable to a goal of performing regular exercise.

Osteoporosis

Osteoporosis is a disease that leads to a high risk for bone fracture caused by bone loss. Each year, osteoporosis leads to over 1 million bone fractures in people over 45 years of age, most of whom are women. Both genetic and environmental factors are implicated as causes. Estrogen deficiency at menopause is a major factor. Regularly getting too little calcium is another contributor. Physical activity, particularly moderate weight-bearing exercise, can help to prevent osteoporosis.[1]

An extremely sedentary lifestyle causes bone loss. Bone loss occurs under extreme conditions of prolonged bed rest or weightlessness, as astronauts experience in space. Experts agree that regular moderate exercise is important for bone health. Regular physical activity may offer even more benefits for elderly persons, who in general are at great risk of osteoporosis. The agility and strength from activity can reduce both the likelihood of falls and/or injuries caused by falls.

Maintaining One's Drive

Even a minimal amount of exercise—a brisk half-hour walk a few times a week—is important for promoting cardiovascular fitness, as well as forestalling disease from a wide range of other causes. Overall, exercise should be a regular part of one's life. Note that adults in the United States have an average of 41 hours of free time each week. There **is** time to exercise.

FRANK & ERNEST® by Bob Thaves

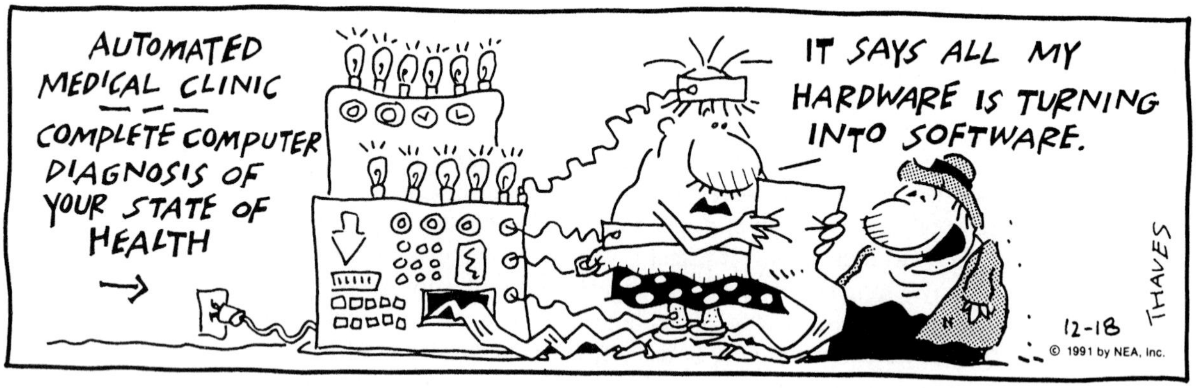

FIGURE 11-4
Frank and Ernest.

POWER FOOD: WHAT SHOULD AN ATHLETE EAT?

Athletic training and genetic makeup are two very important determinants of athletic performance. A good diet won't substitute for either, but as we have mentioned, diet can further enhance and maximize an athlete's potential. More important, a poor diet certainly can harm performance.[3]

How Much Food Energy Does an Athlete Need?

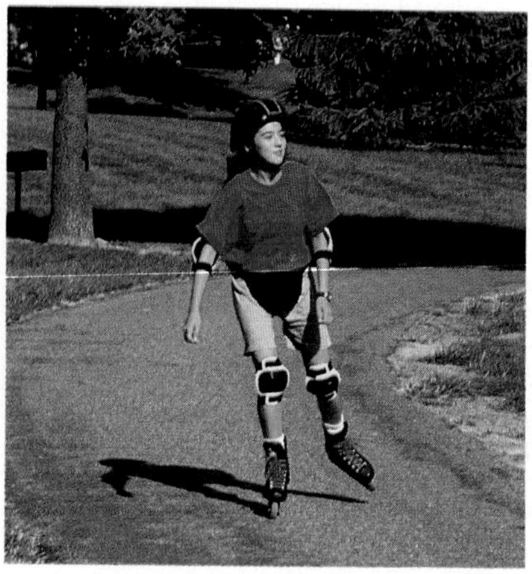

A goal should be to stay physically active throughout one's life.

Athletes need varying amounts of food energy, depending on the athlete's body size and the type of training or competition being considered. A small person may need only 1700 kcalories daily to sustain normal daily activities without losing body weight. A large muscular man may need 3000 kcalories. These are only estimates and need to be individualized based on the experience of each athlete. Kcalories required for sports training or competition have to be added to energy needed for normal activities (see Table 11-2). An hour of bowling, for example, requires few kcalories in addition to those required to sustain normal daily living. On the other extreme, 12-hour endurance bicycle races over mountains can require an additional 4000 kcalories per day. Therefore some athletes may need as much as 7000 kcalories daily just to maintain body weight while training, whereas others may need 1700 kcalories or less.[3]

How can we determine whether an athlete is getting enough energy from food? The first step is to estimate the athlete's body fat percentage by measuring skinfold thickness, estimating bioelectrical impedance, or using the underwater weighing technique (see Chapter 10). Body fat should be in the desirable range—about 6% to 12% for most male athletes and 15% to 25% (but sometimes less) for most female athletes. The next step is to monitor body-weight changes on a daily or weekly basis. If body weight starts to fall, food energy should be increased; if weight rises because of increases in body fat, the athlete should be encouraged to eat less, especially if performance suffers.

If the body composition test shows that the athlete carries too much body fat, the athlete should eat about 200 to 500 fewer kcalories per day until the desirable fat percentage is achieved while maintaining a regular exercise program. Reducing fat intake is the best nutrient-related approach. On the other hand, if the athlete needs to gain weight, an additional 500 to 700 kcalories per day will eventually lead to the needed weight gain. A mix of carbohydrate and fat is advised, coupled again with exercise to ensure the gain is mostly from lean tissue and not just added fat stores.

Rapid Weight Loss by Dehydration. Wrestlers, boxers, and oarsmen often try to lose weight so that they can be certified to compete in a lower weight class. This helps them gain a mechanical advantage over an opponent of smaller stature. Most of the time, this weight is lost a few hours before the athlete steps on the scale for weight certification. Athletes can lose up to 22 pounds (10 kilograms) of body water in 1 day by sitting in a sauna, exercising in a plastic sweat suit, and/or taking diuretic drugs that speed water loss via urine. Losing as little as 3% of body weight by dehydration can sometimes adversely affect endurance performance.[6] A pattern of repeated weight loss and weight gain of

TABLE 11-2

Approximate Energy Costs of Various Activities for a 150-Pound (68-Kilogram) Person

Activity	Kcalories/Hour
Aerobics—heavy	544
Aerobics—light	204
Aerobics—medium	340
Backpacking	612
Basketball—vigorous	680
Bicycling (5.5 MPH)	204
Bowling	265
Calisthenics—heavy	544
Calisthenics—light	272
Canoeing (2.5 MPH)	224
Cleaning (female)	253
Cleaning (male)	236
Cooking	190
Cycling (13 MPH)	659
Dressing/showering	106
Driving	117
Eating (sitting)	93
Food shopping	245
Football—touch	476
Golf	244
Horseback trotting	346
Ice skating (10 MPH)	394
Jogging—medium	612
Jogging—slow	476
Lying—at ease	89
Racquetball—social	544
Roller-skating	346
Running or jogging (10 MPH)	897
Skiing (10 MPH)	598
Sleeping	80
Swimming (.25 MPH)	299
Tennis	414
Volleyball	346
Walking (2.5 MPH)	204
Walking (3.75 MPH)	299
Water skiing	476
Weight lifting—heavy	612
Weight lifting—light	272
Window cleaning	240
Writing (sitting)	118

From Mosby Diet Simple, *N-Squared Computing, Salem, Oregon 97302.*

more than 5% of body weight by dehydration carries some risk of kidney malfunction or heat illness. Dehydration also causes a reduction in blood volume, increases body temperature, and may result in heat cramps or heat exhaustion.

This practice of losing weight by dehydration is common in such sports as interscholastic and intercollegiate wrestling. Most competitors in wrestling face opponents who have gone through the same misery to gain an "advantage." If an athlete wishes to compete in a lower body-weight class and has enough extra fat stores, that athlete should begin a gradual, sustained reduction in food energy intake long before the competitive season starts. In so doing, the athlete will have a presumably healthier body composition (less fat) and can avoid the potentially harmful and certainly misery-creating effects of severe dehydration. An athlete who has no extra body fat should be discouraged from attempting to compete at a lower body-weight class. It is important for coaches and trainers to be aware of the decreased performance and other potentially serious side effects of severe dehydration in athletic events (see Table 9-4).[2]

General Principles for Meeting Nutrient Needs in the Training Diet

Anyone who exercises regularly, including the dieter, needs to consume a diet that includes moderate to high amounts of carbohydrates.[3] This should be about 55% to 70% of total kcalories, rather than our typical 46%. Endurance athletes should meet the higher value. Fat intake should then fall from our typical 38% of total kcalories to 30% or less. Protein should make up the rest of the energy—about 12% to 15% of the total.[10] This creates a plate with about two thirds carbohydrate-rich foods and one third protein-rich foods.

All athletes should consume a variety of foods and adhere to the Food Guide Pyramid (see Chapter 2). Numerous selections of starches and fruits will help maintain adequate muscle glycogen stores and replace glycogen losses from the previous day.[18] Triathletes and marathon participants should consider eating close to 10 grams of carbohydrate per kilogram of body weight per day. This recommendation is designed to (1) prevent chronic fatigue and (2) load the muscles and liver with glycogen. A diet rich in carbohydrate is especially important when performing multiple training bouts in 1 day, such as swim practices, or heavy training on successive days, such as in cross-country running.[9] Table 11-3 can help plan a high carbohydrate intake. Table 11-4 provides an example of such a diet. One does not have to give up any specific food. The diet focus just must turn to more of the best—high carbohydrate foods—and away from the rest—concentrated fat sources.

A Further Look at Carbohydrate—Carbohydrate Loading

Carbohydrate-loading *A process in which a very high carbohydrate diet is consumed for about 3 days before an athletic event in an attempt to increase muscle glycogen stores.*

For athletes who compete in events lasting 90 to 120 minutes or longer or in shorter events repeated in a 24-hour period, it is often advantageous to undertake a ***carbohydrate-loading*** regimen to maximize muscle glycogen stores.[18] One possible regimen includes a gradual reduction or tapering of exercise intensity and duration, coupled with a gradual increase in dietary carbohydrate as a percentage of energy intake, to about 70% of total kcalories. For example, 7 days before a competition, an athlete consumes about 350 grams of carbohydrate per day. Then during the 72 hours before the competition, 525 to 650 grams of carbohydrate per day is recommended. Avoiding moderate to heavy exertion 2 to 3 days before competition is also recommended. This carbohydrate-loading technique usually increases muscle glycogen storage by 50% to 85% over usual conditions—that is, when a typical amount of carbohydrate is consumed (46% of kcalories). The greater carbohydrate stores then often contribute to improved athletic endurance.[18]

A potential disadvantage of carbohydrate loading is that, along with the glycogen, some water is also stored in the muscles. The water adds body weight and may cause muscle stiffness. For some people, this makes carbohydrate loading an unfeasible practice. Athletes considering carbohydrate loading should try it once during training (and well before an important event) to experience its effects on performance. They can then determine whether it is worth the effort.

TABLE 11-3

Grams of Carbohydrate in Typical Foods

Starchy Vegetables, Breads, and Cereals—15 Grams Carbohydrate Per Serving

One serving:
Breakfast cereals,* dry, ½ cup
Breakfast cereals, cooked, ½ cup
Grits, cooked, ½ cup
Rice, cooked, ⅓ cup
Pasta, cooked, ½ cup
Baked beans, ¼ cup
Corn, ½ cup
Beans, ½ cup
Potato, baked, small
Bagel, ½
English muffin, ½
Bread, 1 slice
Pretzels, ¾ oz
Saltine crackers, 6
Pancakes, 4-inch-diameter, 2
Taco shells, 2

Vegetables—5 Grams Carbohydrate Per Serving

One serving:
Vegetables, cooked, ½ cup
Vegetables, raw, 1 cup
Vegetable juice, ½ cup
EXAMPLES : Carrots, green beans, broccoli, cauliflower, onions, spinach, tomatoes, vegetable juice

Fruits—15 Grams Carbohydrate Per Serving

One serving:
Fruit, fresh, ½ cup
Fruit juice, ½ cup
Fruit, dried, ¼ cup
Apple, small
Apricots, 4
Banana, ½
Cherries or grapes, 12
Grapefruit, ½
Nectarine
Orange
Peach
Watermelon, 1¼ cup

Milk—12 Grams Carbohydrate Per Serving

One serving:
Milk, 1 cup
Yogurt, plain, low-fat, 8 oz

Sweets—15 Grams Carbohydrate Per Serving

One serving:
Cake, ½ slice
Cookies, small, 2
Ginger snaps, 3
Ice cream, ½ cup
Sherbet, ¼ cup

From: Exchange lists for meal planning, *the American Diabetes Association and American Dietetic Association: 1986, Chicago, American Dietetic Association.*

**Note that the carbohydrate content of ½ cup of dry cereal varies widely. Check the label of the ones you choose and adjust serving size accordingly.*

another BITE

Appropriate Activities for Carbohydrate Loading	Inappropriate Activities for Carbohydrate Loading
Marathons	Football games
Long-distance swimming	10-kilometer runs
Cross-country skiing	Walking and hiking
30-kilometer runs	Most swimming events
Triathalons	Basketball games
Cycling time trials	Weight lifting
Long-distance canoe racing	Most track and field events

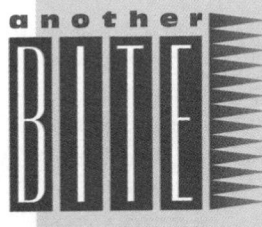

TABLE 11-4

Example of a High-Carbohydrate Diet to Support Daily Vigorous Activity

4000 kcalories:
- 623 grams of carbohydrates (61% of kcalories)*
- 139 grams of protein (14% of kcalories)*
- 118 grams of fat (26% of kcalories)*

Menu	Carbohydrate (Grams)
Breakfast	
Orange	14
Oatmeal, 2 cups	50
Skim milk, 1 cup	12
Bran muffins, 2	48
Snack	
Dates, chopped, 3/4 cup	98
Lunch	
Lettuce salad:	
Romaine lettuce, 1 cup	2
Garbanzo beans, 1 cup	45
Alfalfa sprouts, 1/2 cup	5.5
French dressing, 2 Tbsp	2
Macaroni and cheese, 3 cups	80
Apple juice, 1 cup	28
Snack	
Whole-wheat toast, 2 slices	26
Margarine, 1 tsp	—
Jam, 2 Tbsp	14
Dinner	
Turkey breast (no skin), 2 oz	—
Potatoes, mashed, 2 cups	74
Peas and onions, 1 cup	23
Banana	27
Skim milk, 1 cup	12
Snack	
Pasta, 1 cup, with	33
margarine, 2 tsp, and	—
parmesan cheese, 2 Tbsp	—
Cranberry juice, 1 cup	36
Total	628 grams

**A carbohydrate:protein:fat ratio of 60:15:25 is a good general goal when planning a diet to aid athletic performance.*

Carbohydrate loading is safe for adolescents, but the activities this technique is useful for, like marathon runs, may not be. A physician's approval should be sought for the latter.

Sports nutritionists emphasize the difference between a high-carbohydrate meal and a high-carbohydrate/high-fat meal.[3] Before endurance events, such as marathons or triathalons, some athletes attempt carbohydrate loading by eating potato chips, French fries, banana cream pie, and pastries. These foods do contain carbohydrate, but they also contain a lot of fat. Better food choices are pasta, rice, potatoes, bread, and many breakfast cereals. Sports drinks appropriate for carbohydrate loading, such as GatorLode, can also help. Eating only a moderate amount of dietary fiber during the final day is a good precaution to reduce the chances of bloating and intestinal gas during the next day's event.

Muscle-Bulking Diets

Muscles contain protein, but eating protein alone does not build muscles. Exercise that provides overload work for the muscles of interest is what is needed. During muscle-building regimens, athletes should be sure to consume enough protein, about 1 to 1.5 grams of protein per kilogram (0.5 to 0.7 grams per pound) of body weight daily.[14] This amount ranges from slightly above to about double the protein RDA (0.8 grams per kilogram of desirable body weight). Anyone eating a variety of foods can easily meet the higher intake. Extra protein supplements, such as protein pills, are not needed.[10] For example, a 123-pound (53-kilogram) woman can consume close to her upper range of 80 grams of protein by eating 4 ounces of chicken (one chicken breast) and 3 ounces of beef (a small lean hamburger) and drinking three glasses of milk during a single day. And this does not even include the protein in the grains or vegetables she will also eat. A 180-pound (77-kilogram) man needs to consume only 6 ounces of chicken (a large chicken breast), a 6-ounce can of tuna, and three glasses of milk during a day to obtain close to his upper range of 115 grams of protein. Many athletes eat many more protein-rich foods than this as they meet their energy needs (see Table 11-4).

Athletes who either feel they must significantly limit their energy intake or are vegetarians should determine how much protein they eat; they should make sure it equals at least 1 gram per kilogram of desirable body weight. Skimping on protein is not a good idea.[3]

Vitamins and Minerals

Athletes usually consume many kcalories, and so they tend to consume plenty of vitamins and minerals. The B vitamins and the minerals iron and copper are especially needed to support energy metabolism, but needs barely exceed, if at all, RDA levels.[5] Some researchers are examining whether more antioxidant nutrients, such as vitamins C and E and the provitamin beta-carotene, are needed because of the stress muscles undergo during exercise. We advise waiting for proof before undertaking supplementation of these nutrients beyond what a well-balanced diet supplies (Table 11-5). If a low energy intake—less than 1200 to 1600 kcalories—is needed, athletes should pay very close attention to their vitamin and mineral intake. A focus on nutrient-dense foods—such as low-fat milk, broccoli, tomatoes, oranges, strawberries, whole grains, lean beef, kidney beans, turkey, fish, and chicken—is a good idea. Vitamin- and mineral-fortified foods (e.g., many breakfast cereals) or a balanced multivitamin supplement also can be used. Note that vitamin and mineral supplements supply no known ***ergogenic*** (work-producing) benefit[19] (see the Nutrition Issue in this chapter). They benefit the body only when a medically diagnosed deficiency exists.[14]

Ergogenic *Work-producing.*

Iron. Athletes, especially females and adolescents, should pay special attention to iron intake. In all athletes, iron stores can be depleted by iron losses in sweat, enhanced red blood cell production associated with athletic fitness, and foot-strike destruction of red blood cells (red cells are broken by trauma as they pass through the foot during exercise). Young women are at special risk because of the additional iron loss during menstruation. If iron stores are not replenished, iron-deficiency anemia and markedly impaired endurance performance can result.[11] Although true anemia (noted as a depressed blood hemoglobin concentration) is quite rare among athletes, it is a good idea—especially for adult women athletes—to have blood hemoglobin levels checked regularly by a physician and to monitor dietary iron intake. Vegetarian female athletes should be especially careful to watch iron status. If blood iron levels are consistently low, the use of extra lean meats and iron supplements is advisable.[13] Extra iron can improve athletic performance if the athlete is truly anemic, but it appears to have no effect on endurance when the athlete simply has low blood levels of iron that have not resulted in anemia.[11]

Calcium. Athletes, especially women who are attempting to lose weight by restricting their intake of dairy products, can have marginal or low dietary intakes of calcium. This practice jeopardizes optimal bone health. Of still greater concern are women athletes who

TABLE 11-5

Vitamins and Minerals: Function and Usage with Regard to Exercise

Vitamins and Minerals	Exercise-Related Function	Proposed Benefit to Performance	Effects of Supplementation in Excess of RDA/ESADDI
Thiamin	Carbohydrate metabolism	Enhances endurance performance	Does not enhance performance
Riboflavin	Energy metabolism	Enhances aerobic performance	Does not enhance performance
Niacin	Energy metabolism	Enhances energy metabolism	May impair performance by reducing fatty acid release
Vitamin B-6	Formation of hemoglobin	Enhances exercise performance	Does not enhance performance
Pantothenic acid	Energy metabolism	Enhances aerobic performance	Unclear research results to date
Vitamin B-12	Red blood cell development	Enhances endurance performance	Does not enhance performance
Folate	Cell synthesis; red blood cell formation		No studies available
Biotin	Fat and glycogen synthesis		No studies available
Vitamin C	Antioxidant	Prevents tissue damage; speeds repair	Well-controlled studies show no effect on performance, but some researchers think extra amounts may reduce muscle damage from exercise
Vitamin A and beta-carotene	Antioxidant	Prevents tissue damage; speeds repair	Enhanced performance unlikely, but some researchers think extra amounts may reduce muscle damage from exercise
Vitamin D	Bone mineral metabolism	Bone formation during muscle building	Does not affect work performance; may affect muscle building (one study), but needs likely do not exceed the RDA. Note that excess intakes can be toxic
Vitamin E	Antioxidant	Prevents tissue damage; speeds repair	Does not enhance performance; may reduce exercise damage caused by breakdown in fat structure in cell membranes; research is ongoing
Zinc	Carbohydrate, fat, and protein metabolism; tissue repair	Repair of exercise damage	Enhances some measures of muscle performance after 2 weeks (one study), but the dose was too high to be safely consumed on a regular basis (nine times the male RDA)
Copper	Red blood cell synthesis; energy metabolism	Enhances aerobic performance	No studies available
Chromium	Carbohydrate metabolism; increases effects of insulin	Delays fatigue	No studies available
Selenium	Antioxidant	Protects against exercise damage; delays fatigue	No studies available
Iron	Oxygen transport and delivery	Reduces fatigue; enhances endurance	No effect on performance in nonanemic or non–iron-deficient subjects

Primarily taken from Clarkson PM: Vitamins and trace minerals. In Lamb DR, Williams M, editors: Perspectives in exercise science and sports medicine, *vol 4, Ergogenics: enhancement of exercise and sport performance, Indianapolis, 1991, Benchmark Press.*

stop menstruating because of arduous exercise training and often low-energy diets that have interfered with the normal secretion of the reproductive hormones. Disturbing reports show that female athletes who do not menstruate regularly have far less dense spinal bones than both nonathletes and female athletes who menstruate regularly.[15]

Researchers have just begun to understand the importance of regular menstruation in promoting bone maintenance. Current studies imply that a woman runner who does not menstruate regularly may also have a higher risk of developing a ***stress fracture.***[14] Female athletes whose menstrual cycles become irregular should consult a physician to ascertain the cause. Decreasing the level of training and/or increasing body weight often restores regular menstrual cycles. If irregular menstrual cycles persist, severe bone loss and osteoporosis may result. Extra calcium in the diet does not necessarily compensate for this loss of menstruation, but inadequate dietary calcium can make matters worse.

Stress Fracture *A fracture that occurs from repeated jarring of a bone. Common sites include bones of the foot.*

Pre-Event Meal

A light meal (300 or more kcalories) can be eaten 2 hours before an endurance event to top off muscle and liver glycogen stores and prevent hunger during the event. Extra fluid intake is also advised. The foods in the overall meal should consist primarily of carbohydrate, contain little fat or dietary fiber, and include a moderate amount of protein.[3] Good choices are pasta, bagels, muffins, bread, and breakfast cereals with low-fat milk. Liquid meal replacement formulas can also be used. Fiber-rich foods should be consumed the previous day to help clear the bowels before the event, but not the night before. Foods that are fatty or fried—such as sausage, bacon, sauces, and gravies—should be avoided. A meal high in carbohydrate is quickly digested, promotes normal blood glucose levels, and avoids the need to dip right away into glycogen stores. If an athlete feels a pre-event meal harms performance, eating a high-carbohydrate diet the day and night before can help meet the same goal.

Consuming carbohydrate 15 to 45 minutes before competition was previously thought to adversely affect performance because it increases insulin release, and insulin causes blood glucose to fall. However, such feedings do not cause premature fatigue or decrease endurance for most people. In fact, recent studies show positive benefits of this type of pre-event feeding.[4] However, some athletes are extremely sensitive to an insulin surge. Thus athletes should experiment with pre-event carbohydrate feedings to see whether their performance is adversely or positively affected.

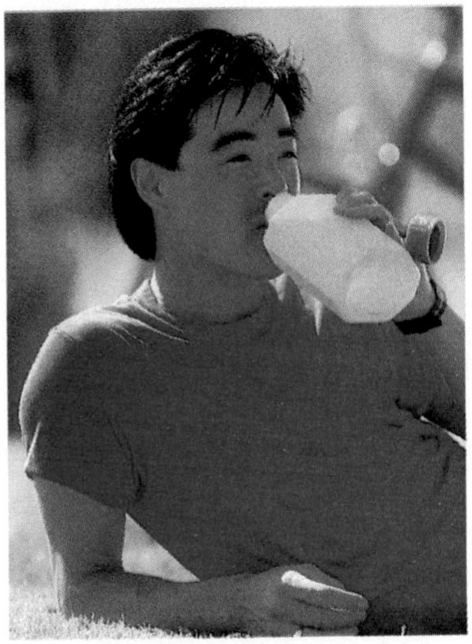

Attention to fluid consumption is one key for the person seeking peak athletic performance, or anyone who exercises, for that matter.

Maximizing Body Fluids and Energy Stores During Exercise

Athletes need enough water to maintain the body's ability to regulate its internal temperature and so keep itself cool, even in winter months when perspiration is not that noticeable.[6] Most energy released during metabolism appears immediately as heat. Unless this heat is quickly dissipated, heat cramps, heat exhaustion, or deadly heat stroke may ensue (see Figure 9-4). As we noted in Chapter 9, sweat evaporating from the skin helps remove this heat from the body. Sweat rates during prolonged exercise range from 3 to 8 cups (750 to 2000 milliliters) per hour. To keep the body from becoming dehydrated, fluid intake during exercise, when possible, should be adequate to minimize body weight loss. However, most athletes find it very uncomfortable to replace more than about 75% to 80% of this sweat loss during exercise.

By experimenting, athletes can determine how much fluid they require to maintain weight and how much fluid intake they can tolerate without experiencing stomach cramps. This determination will be most accurate if the athlete is weighed before and after a typical workout. For every 1 pound (½ kilogram) lost, 2 cups (0.5 liter) of water should be consumed during exercise or immediately afterward. For example, an athlete who loses 5 pounds during a 3-hour practice should drink 10 cups of water—that is, perhaps 6 to 8 cups during practice and 2 to 3 cups after practice.

Thirst is not a reliable indicator of fluid need; exercise blunts this sensation.[6] By relying on thirst alone, an athlete might take 48 hours to replenish fluid loss. After several days of practice, the increasing fluid debt can begin to impair performance. By the time thirst registers, the person may have lost 3% of body weight through sweat.

NUTRITION insight

SPORTS DRINKS: ARE THEY NECESSARY?

Electrolytes Compounds that break down into ions in water and, in turn, are able to conduct an electrical current. These include sodium, chloride, and potassium.

A question that often arises is whether to drink water or a sports-type carbohydrate-***electrolyte*** drink—such as Bodyfuel, Exceed, Gatorade, or 10-K—during competition. For sports that require less than 30 minutes of exertion, replacing the water lost in sweat is of greater concern than are the losses of body carbohydrate stores and electrolytes (sodium, chloride, potassium, and other minerals), which are not usually too great in such activities.[6] Electrolytes are lost in sweat, but the quantities lost in exercise of brief to moderate duration can be easily replaced later by consuming normal foods, such as orange juice, potatoes, or tomato juice.

Water is certainly cheaper than a sports drink. But sports-type drinks can taste better than water, and that may make one drink more often—a clear benefit for fluid replenishment. In addition, the carbohydrate in these drinks quickly replaces carbohydrate used up during practice or competition. The sodium also aids glucose absorption.

For endurance athletes—those whose sports demand exertion for longer than 30 minutes—the issue of sports drinks becomes more critical.[4] Beverages for the endurance athlete must provide water for hydration, electrolytes to both enhance water absorption from the intestine and help retain blood volume, and carbohydrate to provide energy. Beyond 60 to 90 minutes of exercise, electrolyte replacement becomes increasingly important.

Prolonged exercise results in large sweat losses, and some of the fluid for sweat comes from the bloodstream. If only water is used to replace the fluid losses in the blood, the concentration of essential electrolytes in the bloodstream may become too diluted. Small amounts of sodium and potassium are included in sports drinks to help maintain blood volume.[8]

A good rule of thumb is to drink beverages freely for up to 2 hours before an event. Don't worry about thirst. Then consume 1 to 2 cups (0.25 to 0.5 liter) of fluids (water, diluted fruit juice, or sports drinks) about 15 minutes before a sports event. This is called *hyperhydration.* The extra fluid in the body can replace sweat losses as needed. Next, consume approximately 1 to 1.5 cups of fluid (preferably at refrigeration temperature on hot days to help cool the body) each 15 to 20 minutes for events that last longer than 30 minutes. If the weather is hot and/or humid, even more fluids may be required.[6] The athlete need not worry that gradual consumption of fluids will cause bloating or impair performance. But skipping fluids will almost certainly cause problems!

Carbohydrate Intake During Recovery from Exercise

A large portion of the day's carbohydrate-rich foods should be eaten within 2 hours of a training exercise bout, and the sooner the better. During this period, glycogen synthesis is the greatest.[12] Athletes who are training hard can consume a simple sugar candy, sugared soft drink, fruit juice, or a sports-type carbohydrate supplement right after training as they attempt to reload their muscles with glycogen. At quick-service restaurants, the athlete can order extra crust on pizza, load up at the salad bar, and have extra rolls and muffins.

Fluid and electrolyte intake is also an essential component of the athlete's recovery diet.[2] This helps reestablish normal levels of body fluids as quickly as possible. Again, a return to preexercise weight is a good goal. This is especially true if the athlete works out twice a day and if the environment is hot and humid.

Including carbohydrates in sports drinks has also been found to delay fatigue in endurance exercise.[4] In exercise at intensities of a 3-hour marathon pace, ingesting carbohydrate improved endurance, presumably by either preventing great drops in blood glucose levels or providing an outside source of glucose for muscle use, thereby sparing glycogen use somewhat. Athletes should experiment to see whether the use of glucose in fluids agrees with them and is worth the trouble.[2]

If practiced, the amount of carbohydrate recommended for consumption about 15 minutes before endurance exercise is 1 to 2 cups of a 10% to 20% solution of carbohydrate (10 to 20 grams of carbohydrate per 100 milliliters of water), such as in GatorLode or Exceed High Carbohydrate Source. Once exercise begins, 1 cup or so of a 5% to 8% carbohydrate solution (5 to 8 grams per 100 milliliters of fluid) should be consumed every 15 to 20 minutes, depending on the athlete's sweat rate. This is the carbohydrate concentration of typical sports drinks (check the label to be sure). Athletes who compete longer than 6 to 8 hours should consume adequate electrolytes, particularly sodium (approximately 1 gram/hour), through either sports drinks or foods.[9]

Some beverage labels mention ***glucose polymers*** (glucoses linked together in short chains). Solutions containing glucose polymers were initially thought to empty from the stomach faster than did solutions containing glucose, and so to be advantageous for the athlete during exercise. We now know, however, that there's little difference in stomach-emptying times between sports drinks containing glucose polymers and those containing simple sugars, such as glucose or sucrose. Thus glucose polymers offer no important advantage to the athlete. Furthermore, comparisons of drinks containing glucose polymers (more properly known as *maltodextrins*), glucose, or sucrose show that all these carbohydrates have similar positive effects on exercise performance and physiological function, as long as the concentrations of carbohydrate are in the 5% to 8% range. The exceptions to this rule are drinks whose only carbohydrate source is fructose. Fructose is absorbed from the intestine more slowly than is glucose and often causes bloating or diarrhea.

Overall, the decision to use a sports drink hinges primarily on the duration of the activity. As the duration of continuous activity begins to total 30 minutes or longer, the advantages of using a sports drink over plain water begin to emerge.

Glucose Polymer *Carbohydrate sources used in some sports drinks that consist of a grouping of a few glucose molecules.*

Alcohol and caffeine both have a dehydrating effect on the body, so fluids containing them should not be part of any hydration plan for exercise.

another BITE

It cannot be emphasized enough that any nutrition strategies, including fluid replacement, should be tested during practice and trial runs. An athlete should never try a new food or beverage on the day of competition. Some food items or beverages may not be tolerated well, and the day of competition is not the time to find that out.

CONCEPT CHECK

All athletes would do well to plan a diet that follows the Food Guide Pyramid. High-carbohydrate foods should be emphasized, and these should dominate the pre-event meal. Additional protein intake above a usual American intake is not necessary. Nutrient supplements should be taken only to correct actual nutrient deficiencies or to compensate for a low nutrient intake. Fluid should be consumed as liberally as possible before, during, and after an event. A sports-type drink can be helpful for endurance athletes.

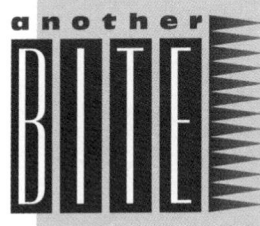

SUMMARY

- All energy available to humans comes from solar energy. Adenosine triphosphate (ATP) is the major form of energy used for cellular metabolism. Plants capture solar energy using photosynthesis. Human metabolic pathways are able to extract that energy from foodstuffs and convert it into ATP energy. Phosphocreatine (PCr) also can provide the energy to form ATP in a human cell.
- In glycolysis, glucose is broken down into three-carbon compounds, yielding some ATP. The three-carbon compounds can then proceed to an aerobic pathway to form carbon dioxide (CO_2) and water (H_2O) or to an anaerobic pathway to form lactic acid.
- At low workloads, muscle cells mainly use fat for fuel. For intense exercise of short duration, muscles use PCr for energy. For more sustained intense activity, muscle glycogen breaks down into lactic acid. For endurance exercise, fat and carbohydrate are used as fuels; carbohydrate is used increasingly as activity intensifies. Little protein is used to fuel muscles.
- Exercise is a vital part of a healthy lifestyle. Aerobic stimulation of the heart should constitute a goal of the exercise plan. Physically active people show lower risks for premature heart disease, diabetes, and other common chronic diseases.
- Anyone who exercises regularly needs to consume a diet that is moderate to high in carbohydrates and that follows the Food Guide Pyramid. Vitamin and mineral supplements are indicated if a low energy intake makes it difficult to meet nutrient needs or a nutrient deficiency exists.
- Carbohydrate loading can increase usual stores of muscle glycogen by 50% to 85%. Participants in endurance events that last more than 2 hours benefit most from carbohydrate loading. This basically involves eating a diet very high in carbohydrate for about 3 days before the event.
- Athletes should consume enough fluid to both minimize loss of body weight from fluid loss and ultimately restore preexercise weight. A sports-type drink can be helpful for endurance athletes.

STUDY QUESTIONS

1. How does greater physical fitness contribute to greater use of aerobic metabolism in exercise? Explain the process.
2. ATP is a continuously supplied fuel source. Describe how ATP is maintained in the muscle, from immediately after initiation of exercise to long-distance endurance exercise.
3. Based on your knowledge of protein, why is it unnecessary to supplement the diet of an athlete with specific amino acids, although they are often touted as beneficial to exercise?
4. Your roommate is running a 20-kilometer race tomorrow and asks your advice on fluid recommendations for before and during the event. What will you tell him?
5. Your neighbor asks, "Why exercise?" Give convincing and factual reasoning in your answer.

REFERENCES

1. Blair SN and others: How much physical activity is good for health? *Annual Review of Public Health* 13:99, 1992.
2. Clark N and others: Feeding the ultraendurance athlete: practical tips and a case study, *Journal of the American Dietetic Association* 92:1258, 1992.
3. Clark N: *Nancy Clark's sports nutrition guidebook: eating to fuel your active lifestyle,* Champaign, Ill, 1990, Leisure Press.
4. Coyle EF: Carbohydrate supplementation during exercise, *Journal of Nutrition* 122:788, 1992.
5. Fogelholm GM and others: Dietary and biochemical indices of nutritional status in male athletes and controls, *Journal of the American College of Nutrition* 11:181, 1992.
6. Gisolfi CV, Duchman SM: Guidelines for optimal replacement beverages for different athletic events, *Medicine and Science in Sports and Exercise* 24:679, 1992.
7. Hallagan JB and others: Anabolic-androgenic steroid use by athletes, *The New England Journal of Medicine* 321:1042, 1989.
8. Holt WS: Nutrition and athletes, *American Family Physician* 47:1757, 1993.
9. Hoffman CJ, Coleman E: An eating plan and update on recommended dietary practices for the endurance athlete, *Journal of the American Dietetic Association* 91:325, 1991.
10. Houston ME: Protein and amino acid needs of athletes, *Nutrition Today,* p. 36, September/October 1992.
11. Klingshirn LA and others: Effect of iron supplementation on endurance capacity in iron-depleted female runners, *Medicine and Science in Sports and Exercise* 24:819, 1992.
12. Kris-Etherton PM: Nutrition and athletic performance, *Nutrition Today,* p. 35, September/October 1990.
13. Lyle RM and others: Iron status in exercising women: the effect of oral iron therapy vs increased consumption of muscle foods, *American Journal of Clinical Nutrition* 56:1049, 1992.
14. Position of the American Dietetic Association and the Canadian Dietetic Association: Nutrition for physical fitness and athletic performance for adults, *Journal of the American Dietetic Association* 93:691, 1993.
15. Ropp KL: Steroid substitutes: no-win situation for athletes, *FDA Consumer,* p. 8, December 1992.
16. Sandvik L and others: Physical fitness as a predictor of mortality among healthy, middle-aged Norwegian men, *The New England Journal of Medicine* 328:533, 1993.
17. Sherman WM and others: Dietary carbohydrate, muscle glycogen, and exercise performance during 7 days of training, *American Journal of Clinical Nutrition* 57:27, 1993.
18. Simopoulos AP: Nutrition and fitness: a conference report, *Nutrition Today,* p. 24, November/December 1992.
19. Singh A and others: Chronic multivitamin-mineral supplementation does not enhance physical performance, *Medicine and Science in Sports and Exercise* 24:726, 1992.
20. Stryer L: *Biochemistry,* ed 3, New York, 1988, WH Freeman.
21. Williams MH: Ergogenic and ergolytic substances, *Medicine and Science in Sports and Exercise,* 24:S344, 1992.

RATE

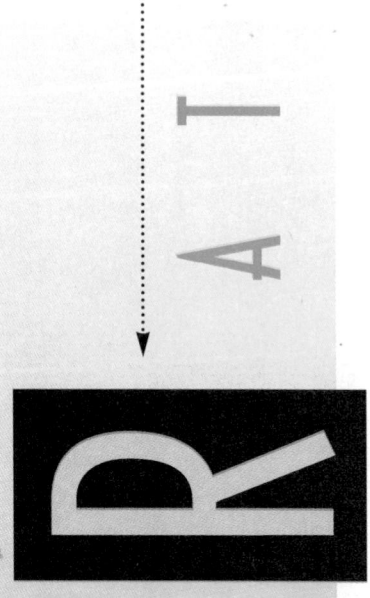

ARE YOU MEASURING UP TO THE NUMBERS?

In this chapter, several key nutrients were discussed in relation to exercise performance. The following guidelines were mentioned, not only for athletes, but for everyone maintaining generally good fitness:

- Eat a moderate to high amount of carbohydrates (55% or more of total kcalories).
- Athletes should eat about 1 gram of protein per kilogram of body weight.
- Consume the RDA for vitamins and minerals.
- Make sure iron and calcium intake is at RDA levels (especially in women).
- Consume enough fluid to maintain weight during exercise.

Review the results of the dietary assessment you completed in Chapter 2. Remember that you assessed 1 day's food intake. Now answer the following questions whether or not you consider yourself an athlete:

1. What percentage of your kcalories came from carbohydrate? Was your intake 55% of your total kcalories or greater?

___

2. Did you eat at least 0.8 grams of protein per kilogram of body weight? If you are an athlete, did you consume about 1 gram per kilogram of body weight?

___

___

3. Did you consume at least the RDA for all vitamins and minerals assessed, especially iron and calcium? Which ones were below the RDA?

___

___

___

4. Did you consume enough fluid—about 6 to 8 cups for a good starting point?

___

___

5. What can you do to improve your dietary intake to aid general fitness, and if you are an athlete, to promote maximal performance in your chosen event(s)?

___

___

___

___

your plate

Nutrition ISSUE

ERGOGENIC AIDS: SOME SUBSTANCES CAN ENHANCE ATHLETIC PERFORMANCE

Manipulating one's diet for better performance has a long history. As long as 30 years ago, American football players were encouraged on hot practice days to "toughen up" for competition by consuming salt tablets before and during practice and by not drinking water. Now it is recognized that this practice can be fatal. Today's athletes are also likely to experiment—bee pollen, seaweed, freeze-dried liver flakes, gelatin, ginseng, freeze-dried adrenal glands from cattle, and artichoke hearts are just some of the worthless substances known today as ergogenic aids.[21]

Still, modern-day athletes can benefit from recently documented scientific evidence that some dietary substances do have ergogenic properties. These include sufficient water, lots of carbohydrate, and a balanced and varied diet that follows the Food Guide Pyramid.[3] Protein and amino acid supplements are not in the list. The average American athlete eats plenty of protein.

Clearly, it is not possible to change average athletes into champions simply by altering diet. This means nutrient supplements require careful evaluation. Use should be designed to meet a specific dietary weakness, such as a poor iron intake. These and other aids, whose benefit is often dubious and which can pose health risks, must be given close scrutiny before use. The cost-benefit ratio of these ergogenic aids especially needs to be examined, keeping in mind the expense, health risks, and potential illegality. Athletes must stay on guard against false promises.

Carnitine

The majority of the energy stored in the body for muscle use is found in fat. During physical activity, fatty acids are released into the bloodstream from the fat depots and travel to the muscles, where they are taken into each cell and aerobically broken down to carbon dioxide and water. These fatty acids must enter the cell's mitochondria before they can be broken down. The fatty acids are transported mostly from the fluid portion of the cell into the mitochondria using a transport system that contains a compound called ***carnitine.*** Athletes sometimes take carnitine pills hoping it will help them burn fat faster in exercise. But because our cells can make carnitine quite easily, carnitine supplements provide no reliable benefit.[21]

Carnitine
A compound used to shuttle fatty acids into the cell mitochondria. This allows for the fatty acids to be burned for energy.

Sodium Bicarbonate
An alkaline substance made of basically sodium and carbon dioxide ($NaHCO_3$).

Bicarbonate Loading

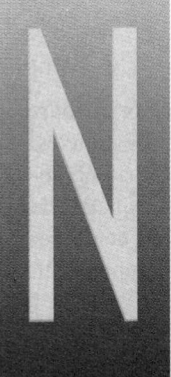

We have noted that muscles that contract vigorously during athletic performance produce lactic acid. Lactic acid buildup inhibits the activity of enzymes involved in energy metabolism and leads to early fatigue. In the 1930s, athletes attempted to counter lactic acid accumulation by ingesting small doses of ***sodium bicarbonate,*** a base. However, this failed to improve their athletic performances. On the other hand, more recent experiments using large doses of bicarbonate (30 milligrams per kilogram of body weight) demonstrate performance improvement. Athletes who consume large doses of bicarbonate 1 or 2 hours before exercise generally have improved strenuous performance lasting 2 to 10 minutes. About 20 minutes of warm-up typically precedes the event. The bicarbonate loading apparently speeds the removal of lactic acid from contracting muscle cells. Unfortunate side effects of large doses of sodium bicarbonate are nausea and diarrhea, often at unpredictable times.[21] For this reason, bicarbonate loading has so far not become popular with athletes.

Caffeine

Drinking three to four cups of coffee (4 to 5 milligrams of caffeine per kilogram of body weight) or using caffeine suppositories about 1 hour before an endurance competition (lasting more than 2 hours) enhances performance in some athletes. The effect is less apparent in athletes who have ample stores of glycogen. The reason for the overall effect is not well established: increased use of fatty acids for muscle fuel, psychological effects, and enhancement of glycolysis in muscle all deserve consideration. However, some athletes experience changes in heart rhythm, nausea, or lightheadedness that can actually impair performance.

Athletes are permitted small amounts of caffeine before competition, but intake of about 800 milligrams (the amount in 6 to 8 cups of coffee) will elicit a urine level that would be grounds for disqualification according to standards set by the International Olympic Committee.[21]

Alcohol

Alcohol is thought to enhance endurance performance by altering a person's perception of fatigue and by providing additional energy. Alcohol's ergogenic value is not borne out by research findings, however, and it appears more likely that alcohol may impair rather than enhance physical performance. Alcohol decreases glucose release from the liver, which reduces blood glucose availability and can lead to hypoglycemia and possible premature fatigue. In cold environments, this hypoglycemia can also contribute to hypothermia.[21]

Anabolic Steroids

Steroids ■ *A group of hormones and related compounds that are derivatives of cholesterol.*

Androgen ■ *A general term for hormones that stimulate development in male sex organs and such male characteristics as facial hair—for example, testosterone.*

Public attention focused on the use of anabolic ***steroids*** when Ben Johnson, winner of the gold medal for the 100-meter dash in the 1988 Olympic Games, was disqualified. Johnson acknowledged that he took anabolic steroids regularly as part of his training regimen. These steroids are used by athletes to enhance performance in a variety of sports but most commonly in strength sports, such as football, wrestling, weight lifting, and certain track-and-field events.[7] Steroids have also been used by swimmers and cyclists and are often used by male and female body builders and even nonathletic high school students in an attempt to "get big."

Steroids are synthetic versions of sex hormones that promote two types of effects: masculinization and growth. Athletes have taken various forms of these drugs, often in doses 10 to 30 times normal ***androgen*** output, to increase muscle size, strength, and performance. No cardiovascular benefit has been found.

Although they can increase muscle mass in some people, steroid use is unsafe and, in athletics, illegal. The consequences of steroid use also can occasionally be devastating. For example, steroids can cause growth plates in bones to close prematurely (thus limiting the adult height of a teenage athlete); produce bloody cysts in the liver; accelerate the development of heart disease; and cause high blood pressure, sterility, and many other detrimental physical effects. Psychological consequences vary from increasing aggressiveness, drug dependence, and mood swings to decreased sex drive, depression, and even roid-rage—violence attributed to steroid use. Some football players consider the increased aggressiveness an additional benefit.

Athletes may begin to use steroids during high school, and perhaps as early as junior high school.[7] Many serious athletes must make a hard choice—to not use steroids and

TABLE 11-6

Suggestions for the Athlete Making Choices About Steroid Use

1. Know the facts about steroids.
2. View your body as something to keep safe from harm and free from contamination.
3. Think about your plans for the future and your health.
4. Go for natural methods that allow you to look good and perform well.
5. Enjoy and appreciate your uniqueness; don't ever try to be somebody else.
6. When in doubt, check out the recommendation with somebody who really cares.
7. After considering all possible consequences, have the courage to make a good decision based on healthy practices.

From American Family Physician *41:1163, 1990.*

face a large field of artificially endowed opponents or to use the drugs and risk side effects and legal sanctions (Table 11-6).

Growth Hormone

There is too little scientific information available regarding the effects of ***growth hormone*** on muscle mass and strength to allow firm conclusions to be made about this drug. However, it is known that the skin, tongue, and bones may grow abnormally under growth hormone stimulation. Abusing growth hormone may increase height if consumed at critical ages, but uncontrolled growth of the heart and other internal organs and even death are also potential consequences. All in all, use of growth hormone is dangerous—it requires careful monitoring by a physician. Arginine and ornithine supplements (basically amino acids), a new rage among body builders, are promoted as growth hormone boosters. Current evidence suggests that any increase in growth hormone after consuming amino acids is rather modest and probably of little physiological consequence.[10]

Growth Hormone *A pituitary hormone that produces body growth and release of fat from storage, among other effects.*

Blood Doping *A technique by which an athlete's red blood cell count is increased. Blood is taken from the athlete. The red blood cells are concentrated by removing fluid from that blood sample and then later reintroduced into the athlete.*

Blood Doping

Injecting red blood cells into the bloodstream—known as ***blood doping***—is a technique that may enhance aerobic capacity. In this procedure, an athlete donates at least 2 pints of blood at least 6 weeks before the event and freezes the cells while the body makes more blood to replace it. Then, 1 or 2 days before competition, the frozen red cells are thawed and reinfused into the veins; the added cells elevate the total red blood cell count and hemoglobin concentration above normal.

A simpler, faster, but more dangerous way to blood dope is to inject a synthetic form of the hormone *erythropoietin.*[15] The kidney secretes erythropoietin to stimulate red blood cell production by the bone marrow; it is also available commercially. Erythropoietin can increase the concentration of red blood cells so greatly that blood clots develop in the lungs or brain, leading to strokes that can paralyze or kill. It is widely speculated in the medical community that erythropoietin abuse is responsible for a sudden dramatic increase in deaths of young competitive cyclists in Europe over the last few years.

Studies of blood doping show that it is a means to improve endurance performance. Admissions by world-class athletes—including members of the victorious United States cycling team in the 1984 Olympics—that they used blood doping to reduce race times continue to stimulate questions about both sports ethics and how well the procedure actually works. Several studies confirm an aerobic benefit to the athlete as a result of blood doping, but the possible negative health consequences remain. It is also an illegal practice under Olympic guidelines.

Diphosphoglycerate (DPG)
A compound in the red blood cell that is involved in oxygen release from hemoglobin.

Phosphate Loading

Contrary to beliefs of many athletes and coaches, phosphate pills do not always improve performance or efficiency of heart function during endurance events. Some studies have suggested that loading phosphate for 4 days increases the levels of a metabolically important phosphate compound, ***diphosphoglycerate (DPG),*** in red blood cells. These studies also showed that increased levels of DPG potentially improved the delivery of oxygen to muscles and reduced work by the heart during vigorous exercise. We now know that rigorously trained athletes already have high levels of DPG in their red blood cells. Thus although a single dose of phosphate can induce blood chemistry changes, it does not reliably improve the ability to perform endurance exercise, nor does it necessarily increase the efficiency of aerobic metabolism. In addition, some people may suffer gastrointestinal distress, such as abdominal distention and diarrhea, which could inhibit their performance.[21]

Inosine

Inosine is a compound with a variety of metabolic roles, many of which are species-specific. Inosine has been marketed for endurance athletes because it might reduce glycogen breakdown, promote blood flow, and improve oxygen release to the muscles by increasing red blood cell levels of DPG (mentioned earlier). However, an investigation of the ergogenic potential of inosine found no effect on DPG levels, metabolic changes during exercise, endurance, or overall treadmill performance.[21]

Summing Up

Although many claims of ergogenic effects in athletes are unfounded, the few exceptions we've described are based on systematic scientific investigations. This is not to say that there are no other potentially ergogenic substances, but just that such aids are not scientifically verified.[21]

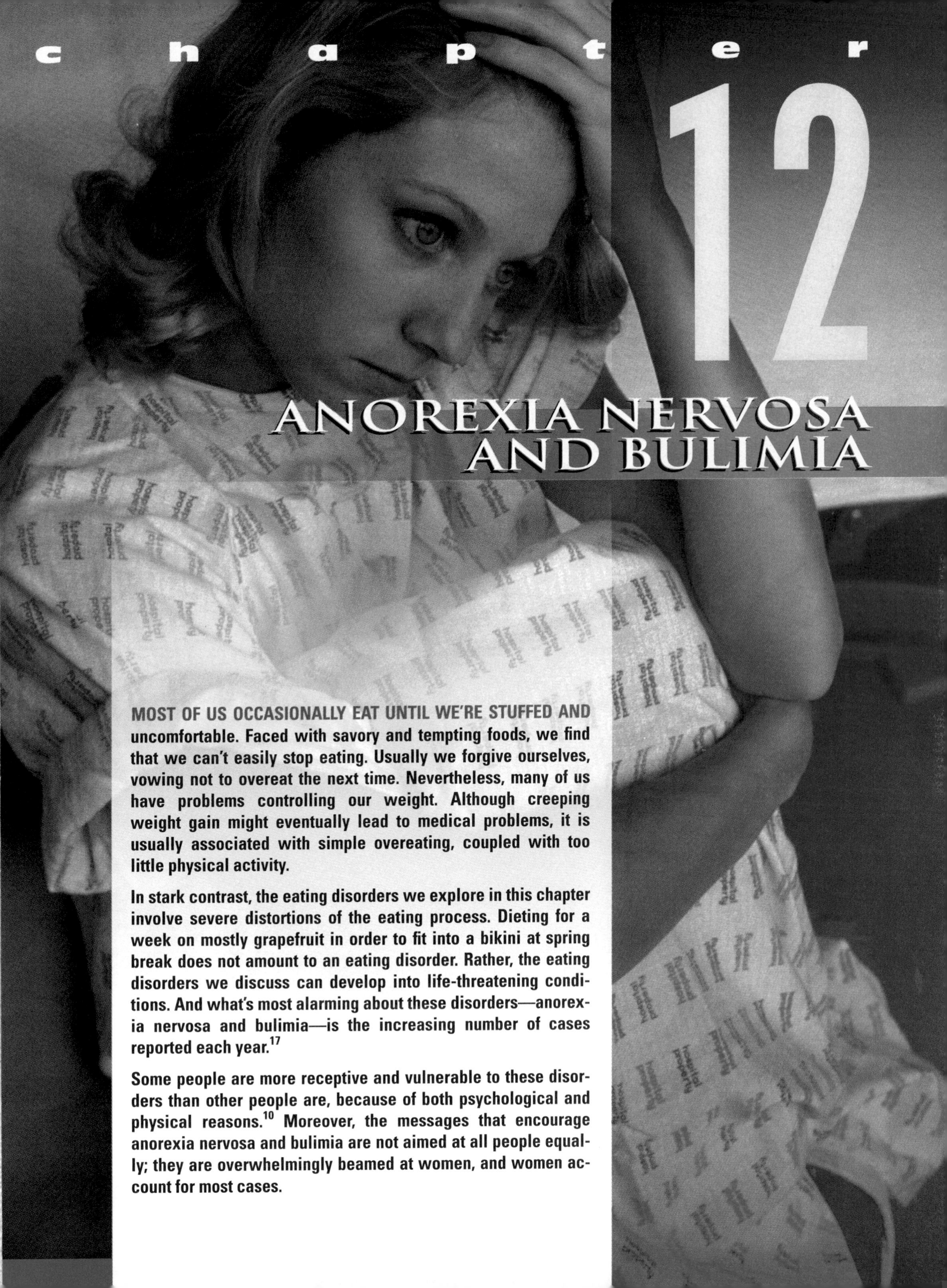

chapter 12

ANOREXIA NERVOSA AND BULIMIA

MOST OF US OCCASIONALLY EAT UNTIL WE'RE STUFFED AND uncomfortable. Faced with savory and tempting foods, we find that we can't easily stop eating. Usually we forgive ourselves, vowing not to overeat the next time. Nevertheless, many of us have problems controlling our weight. Although creeping weight gain might eventually lead to medical problems, it is usually associated with simple overeating, coupled with too little physical activity.

In stark contrast, the eating disorders we explore in this chapter involve severe distortions of the eating process. Dieting for a week on mostly grapefruit in order to fit into a bikini at spring break does not amount to an eating disorder. Rather, the eating disorders we discuss can develop into life-threatening conditions. And what's most alarming about these disorders—anorexia nervosa and bulimia—is the increasing number of cases reported each year.[17]

Some people are more receptive and vulnerable to these disorders than other people are, because of both psychological and physical reasons.[10] Moreover, the messages that encourage anorexia nervosa and bulimia are not aimed at all people equally; they are overwhelmingly beamed at women, and women account for most cases.

Progression of eating habits—from ordered to disordered

Attention to hunger and satiety signals; limitation of energy intake to restore weight to a healthful level

↓

Some "disordered" eating habits begin as weight loss is attempted

↓

Clinically evident eating disorder can be recognized

WE ALL NEED TO EAT

Eating—a completely instinctive behavior for animals—serves an extraordinary number of psychological, social, and cultural purposes for humans. As we mentioned in Chapter 1, eating practices may take on religious meanings; identify bonds among cultural, ethnic, and family groups; and be a means of expressing hostility and affection, prestige, and class values. Similarly, providing, preparing, and distributing food may be a means of expressing love or hatred, or even power in family relationships. Given these possibilities, it is not surprising that some eating behaviors take on unusual and strange rituals, progressing from (1) normal responses to hunger and satiety cues to (2) obsessive weight loss to (3) a full-blown eating disorder.

Food Can Represent Much More Than Nutrients

From birth we link food with personal emotional experiences. An infant associates milk with security and warmth, and so the bottle or breast becomes a source of comfort as well as food. We are further exposed to the use of foods as rewards. Here are some typical statements heard at the dinner table:

"You can't play until you clean up your plate."
"I'll eat the broccoli if you let me watch TV."
"If you love me, you'll eat what I fixed for dinner."

On the surface, this practice appears harmless enough, but, eventually, both caregivers and children can build behavior patterns that use foods to achieve unstated goals. Food, then, can take on a much larger role. At the extreme—when food is regularly used as a bargaining chip rather than simply as a source of nutrients—it can contribute to abnormal eating patterns. At worst, these patterns can lead to disordered eating behavior.[20]

Anorexia Nervosa
An eating disorder involving a psychological loss or denial of appetite and self-starvation, related in part to a distorted body image and various social pressures commonly associated with puberty.

Bulimia
An eating disorder in which large quantities of food are eaten at one time (binge eating) and then purged from the body by vomiting, use of laxatives, or other means.

TWO COMMON TYPES OF EATING DISORDERS

Anorexia nervosa and ***bulimia*** (sometimes called bulimia nervosa) have been written about for centuries, at least as far back as the Middle Ages. Anorexia nervosa is characterized by extreme weight loss, poor and distorted body image, and an irrational, almost morbid, fear of obesity and weight gain. The term ***anorexia*** implies a loss of appetite; however, denying one's appetite more accurately describes anorectic behavior. By rough estimate, approximately 1 of every 100 girls (1%) between the ages of 12 and 18 years suffers from anorexia nervosa.[9] It occurs less commonly among adults. Few men are affected, partly because the ideal image for men is big and bulky. Men in weight-control sports, such as wrestling or judo, may practice bulimia,[23] but poor self-esteem and other psychological problems don't seem to be related to this behavior as they are to anorexia nervosa. Most of these athletes vomit and dehydrate so that they can compete in lower weight classes. On the other hand, people with anorexia nervosa typically see themselves as fat even though they are extremely thin.

Bulimia means "ox hunger," or being as hungry as an ox. It is characterized by episodes of binge eating followed by attempts to purge the food from the body, usually by vomiting, fasting, taking diuretics, exercising, or using laxatives. People with this disorder may be difficult to identify because they keep their binge-purge behaviors secret and their symptoms are not obvious. Researchers think that approximately 4% or more of adolescent and college-age women suffer from this disorder.[9] A growing number of male athletes also report these practices, especially swimmers, wrestlers, and track participants. "Get thin and win" is a slogan heard around gyms.[21]

The Diagnostic and Statistical Manual of Mental Disorders (3rd edition, revised) of the American Psychiatric Association lists specific criteria for diagnosing eating disorders (Table 12-1).[19] People may exhibit some symptoms of an eating disorder but not sufficiently enough to enable a medical worker to diagnose it. People may also show characteristics of both anorexia nervosa and bulimia. The diseases overlap considerably (Figure 12-1). Studies suggest that 20% to 50% of women diagnosed as having anorexia nervosa eventually develop bulimic symptoms.[13] Anorexia nervosa and bulimia nervosa are both

TABLE 12-1

Criteria for Eating Disorder

Criteria for the diagnoses of anorexia nervosa and bulimia. Milder habits and symptoms that point in these directions are still troubling, since they suggest the person is developing the ultimate disease patterns.

Anorexia nervosa

A. Refusal to maintain body weight over a minimal normal weight for age and height, for example, weight loss leading to maintenance of body weight 15% below that expected; or failure to make expected weight gain during period of growth, leading to body weight 15% below that expected.
B. Intense fear of gaining weight or becoming fat, even though underweight.
C. Disturbance in the way in which one's body weight, size, or shape is experienced. The person claims to "feel fat" even when emaciated, believes that one area of the body is "too fat" even when obviously underweight.
D. In females, absence of at least three consecutive menstrual cycles when otherwise expected to occur (primary or secondary amenorrhea). (A woman is considered to have amenorrhea if her periods occur only after administration of a hormone, such as estrogen.)

Bulimia nervosa

A. Recurrent episodes of binge eating (rapid consumption of a large amount of food in a discrete period of time).
B. A feeling of lack of control over eating behavior during the eating binges.
C. Regularly engaging in either self-induced vomiting, use of laxatives or diuretics, strict dieting or fasting, or vigorous exercise to prevent weight gain.
D. A minimum average of two binge eating episodes a week for at least 3 months.
E. Persistent overconcern with body shape and weight.

Source: Diagnostic and Statistical Manual for Mental Disorders, DSM IIIR.[19]

Groups of people with long-standing histories of anorexia nervosa include models, ballet dancers, and gymnasts. Earning their living often depends on maintaining ultra-slim bodies.

potentially serious diseases. When practiced, both conditions can harm one's physical and mental health and lead to long-term health problems.

Table 12-2 lists some characteristics of people with anorexia nervosa and bulimia. Do you know someone who is at risk? If so, a professional diagnosis, coupled with professional help, is needed. The sooner help begins, the better. The first step is to rule out other diseases, such as cancer, gastrointestinal disease, schizophrenia, and depression. If an eating disorder is diagnosed, the person should consider immediate treatment. The best a friend can do is to lead the person to treatment. Professional help is often available at student health centers and student guidance/counseling facilities on college campuses. We need to be cautious of diagnosing eating disorders in friends and family members. A number of diagnostic criteria must be met before this is possible, and only a professional is equipped to diagnose a disorder.

There are no simple causes or solutions to eating disorders. They are rooted in multiple causes—biological, psychological, and social.[10] In the Nutrition Issue we review some sociological aspects of these disorders. From this perspective you might see how the disorders develop and why some people are more susceptible than others.

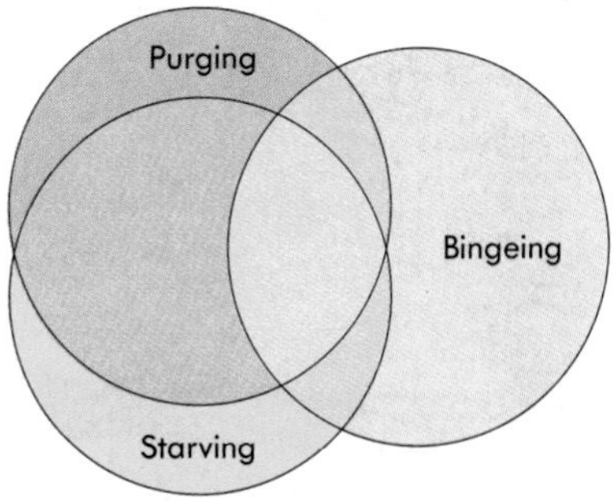

FIGURE 12-1
The overlap of eating disorders. A combination of binge eating, purging, and/or starving can be found in both anorexia nervosa and bulimia.

ANOREXIA NERVOSA

Anorexia nervosa evolves from a dangerous mental state to an extremely dangerous physical condition. People suffering from this disorder think they are fat and intensely fear obesity and weight gain. They lose much more weight than is healthful. Recent studies indicate that 3% to 8% of people with anorexia die prematurely—from suicide, heart ailments, and infections.[20] About half those who survive it recover within 6 years; the rest

TABLE 12-2

Are You at Risk for an Eating Disorder?

Some characteristics of eating disorders. This can be used as a tool for group discussion to help people discover their risks. Having some of these characteristics does not diagnose the disease but should cause a person to reflect on eating habits and related concerns.

Characteristics of anorexia nervosa

- Rigid dieting causing dramatic weight loss
- False body perception—thinking "I'm too fat," even when emaciated; relentless pursuit of thinness
- Rituals involving food, excessive exercise, and other aspects of life
- Maintenance of rigid control in lifestyle; security found in control and order
- Feeling of panic after a small weight gain; intense fear of gaining weight
- Feelings of purity, power, and superiority through maintenance of strict discipline and self-denial
- Preoccupation with food, its preparation, and observing another person eat
- Helplessness in the presence of food
- Lack of menses after what should be the age of puberty

Characteristics of bulimia

- Secretive binge eating; never overeating in front of others
- Eating when depressed
- Bingeing followed by fasting, laxative abuse, self-induced vomiting, or excessive exercise
- Shame, embarrassment, deceit, and depression; low self-esteem and guilt (especially after a binge)
- Fluctuating weight resulting from alternate bingeing and fasting
- Loss of control; fear of not being able to stop eating
- Food is the only comfort/escape in an otherwise carefully controlled and regulated life
- Erosion of teeth, swollen glands

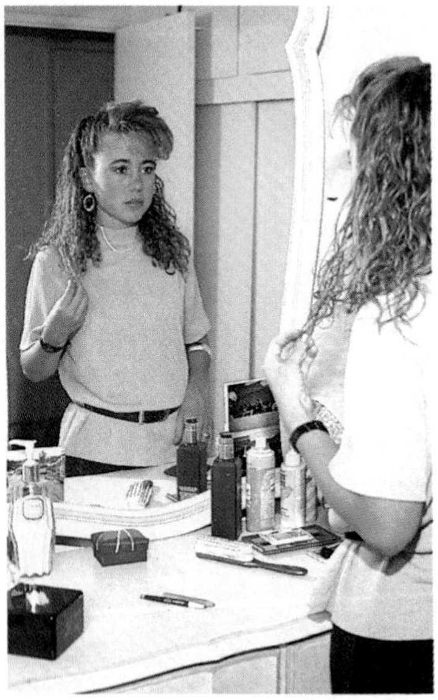

FIGURE 12-2
Self-image can be ever changing. For people with eating disorders, the difference between the real and desired body image may be too difficult to accept.

simply exist with the disease. The longer one suffers from anorexia nervosa, the poorer the chances for complete recovery. A young patient with a short episode and a cooperative family has a better outlook. Prompt and vigorous treatment with close follow-up improves the chances.[9]

Anorexia nervosa may begin as a simple attempt to lose weight. A comment from a well-meaning friend or relative suggesting that the person seems to be gaining weight or is too fat may be all that is needed. The stress of having to maintain a certain weight to look attractive or competent on a job can set off a problem. Physical changes associated with puberty, the stress of leaving childhood, or losing a friend may also trigger extreme dieting (Figure 12-2). Leaving home for boarding school or college or starting a job can reinforce the desire to make oneself more "socially acceptable."[9]

Adolescence is a period of turbulent sexual and social tensions. Teenagers seek—and are often expected—to establish separate and independent lives. While declaring independence they seek acceptance and support from peers and parents, and react intensely to how they think others perceive them.[12] At the same time, their bodies are changing, and much of the change is beyond their control. Adolescents often lack appropriate coping mechanisms for the stresses of teen years. The attempt to take charge of their lives sometimes results in their maintaining extreme control over their bodies. Genetic factors also appear to increase the risk for anorexia nervosa: usually both identical twins—rather than only one—develop the disorder.

Once dieting begins, a person developing anorexia nervosa does not stop. The results are long periods of semistarvation practiced rigidly, almost with a vengeance, in a relent-

less pursuit of thinness.[20] Anorexia may eventually lead to bingeing on large amounts of food in a short time, then purging. Purging occurs primarily through vomiting, but laxatives, diuretics, fasting, and exercise are also used. Thus a person with anorexia nervosa may exist in a state of semistarvation, or may alternate periods of starvation with periods of bingeing and purging.[4]

Once a person drops 15% below normal body weight, there is great risk for lifelong suffering from anorexia nervosa. After a person falls 25% below normal body weight, a cure becomes very difficult, hospitalization is almost always necessary, and premature death is more likely.[20]

Profile of a Person with Anorexia Nervosa

A person with anorexia nervosa refuses to eat. This refusal is the hallmark of the disease, whether or not other practices, such as binge-purge cycles, appear. The person is usually a girl from the middle or upper socioeconomic class. Perhaps her mother also has distorted views of a desirable body shape and acceptable food habits. The girl is often described by parents and teachers as "the best little girl in the world." She is competitive and often obsessive.[9] Her parents set high standards for her. At home, she may not allow clutter in her bedroom. Physicians note that after a physical examination, she may fold her examination gown very carefully and clean up the examination room before leaving. Even though such behaviors may be apparent, it takes a skilled professional to tell the difference between anorexia nervosa and other common adolescent complaints, such as delayed puberty, fatigue, and depression.[7]

A common thread underlying many—but not all—cases of anorexia nervosa is conflict within the family structure, especially rooted in an overbearing mother. When family expectations are always too high, resulting frustration leads to fighting. Overinvolvement, rigidity, overprotection, and denial also typically appear in the daily transactions of such families.[10] Often the eating disorder allows the person to exercise control over an otherwise powerless existence.

A person with anorexia nervosa may use the disorder to gain attention from the family, sometimes in hopes of holding the family together.

Early Warning Signs

A person developing anorexia nervosa will exhibit important warning signs. At first, dieting becomes the life focus. The person may feel, "The only thing I am good at is dieting. I can't do anything else." This innocent beginning often leads to very abnormal self-perceptions and eating habits (Figure 12-3). Cutting a pea in half before eating it may be

For Better or For Worse® **by Lynn Johnston**

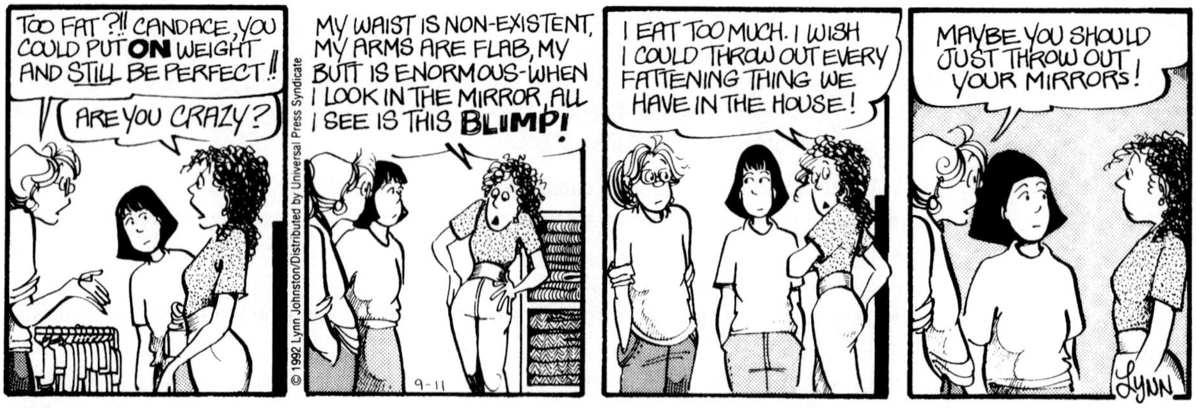

FIGURE 12-3
For Better or For Worse.

seen. An anorectic woman may cook a large meal and watch others eat it while refusing to eat any herself. As the disease progresses, she narrows her own food choices considerably. For someone developing anorexia nervosa, these practices say "I am in control." The anorectic person may be hungry but denies it. She is driven by the belief that good things will happen for her if she just becomes thin enough. It becomes a question of willpower.

another BITE

Some Americans feel that a thin body might make life perfect. This whirlwind hope especially appeals to young people. Most vulnerable are young women who feel alienated from or suffocated by their parents. Parents may not consider a teenager mature enough to make decisions, for instance. She disagrees, and if the situation is very tense, may turn to purging or starving as a way to show her power. "You may try to control my life, but I can do anything I want with my body."

In the words of one young woman: "I couldn't get angry, because it would be like destroying someone else, like my mother. It felt like she would hate me forever. I got angry through anorexia nervosa. It was my last hope. It's my own body and this was my last-ditch effort."

Soon the anorectic person becomes irritable and hostile and begins to withdraw from family and friends. School performance generally crumbles. The person refuses to eat out with family and friends, thinking, "I won't be able to have the foods I want to eat," or "I won't be able to throw up afterward." The person also tends to be excessively critical of herself and others. Nothing is good enough. Because it cannot be perfect, life appears meaningless and hopeless. A sense of joylessness colors everything.

As stress increases in an anorectic person's life, sleep disturbances and depression are common. For a female, these problems—coupled with lower and lower body weight and fat stores—cause menstrual periods to stop.[7] This may be the first sign of the disease a mother notices. Parents, teachers, friends, and coaches need to be aware of the early warning signs of anorexia nervosa. As we stated earlier, this disease is much easier to treat when caught at an early stage. If not treated right away, it quickly leads to self-destruction.

Ultimately, an anorectic person eats very little food; 300 to 600 kcalories daily is not unusual. In place of food the person may consume up to 20 cans of diet soft drinks each day.

Physical Signs and Symptoms

Rooted in the emotional state of the victim, anorexia nervosa produces profound physical effects. A typical medical description reveals a reluctant young woman and a frantic family.[10] The anorectic person is often 20% to 40% below desirable body weight and appears to be skin and bones. This state of semistarvation disturbs many body systems as it forces the body to conserve as much energy as possible. Hormonal responses to semistarvation then cause an array of predictable effects[7,16]:

- Lowered body temperature caused by loss of fat insulation.
- Slower basal metabolism caused by decreased synthesis of active thyroid hormone.[5]
- Decreased heart rate as metabolism slows, leading to easy fatigue, easy fainting, and an overwhelming need for sleep.
- Iron-deficiency anemia from poor nutrient intake, which leads to further weakness.
- Rough, dry, scaly, and cold skin from a poor nutrient intake and anemia.
- Low white blood cell count caused by poor nutrient intake, especially protein and zinc. This condition increases the risk of infection, a cause of death in anorectic people.
- Loss of hair caused by a poor nutrient intake.

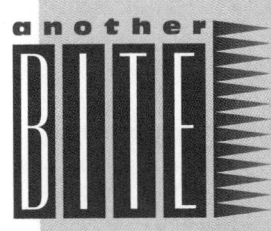

NUTRITION insight

ANOREXIA NERVOSA: A CASE STUDY

At fifteen Alma had been healthy and well-developed; she had menstruated at age 12, was 5 feet 6 inches tall, and weighed 120 pounds. At that time her mother urged her to change to a school with a higher academic standing, a change she resisted; her father suggested that she should watch her weight, an idea that she took up with great eagerness, and she began a rigid diet. She lost weight rapidly, and her menses ceased. That she could be thin gave her a sense of pride, power, and accomplishment. She also began a frantic exercise program, would swim by the mile, play tennis for hours, or do calisthenics to the point of exhaustion. Whatever low point her weight reached, Alma feared that she might become too fat if she regained as little as an ounce.

At age 20 when she came for a consultation with her physician, she looked like a walking skeleton, scantily dressed in shorts and a halter, with her legs sticking out like broomsticks, every rib showing, and her shoulder blades standing up like little wings. Alma insisted that she looked fine and that there was nothing wrong with being so skinny.

- Appearance of ***lanugo,*** downy hairs on the body that trap air, insulating against heat loss and in turn replacing some insulation lost with the fat layer.
- Constipation from semistarvation and laxative abuse.
- Low blood potassium because of a poor nutrient intake, possible vomiting, and the use of some types of diuretics. This increases the risk of heart rhythm disturbances, another leading cause of death in anorectic people.
- Loss of menstrual periods because of low body weight, low body fat content, and the stress of the disease. Periods cease when body weight drops to around 100 pounds or less in many women. Accompanying hormonal changes cause a loss of bone mass and increase the risk of osteoporosis.
- Eventual loss of teeth caused by frequent vomiting. Loss of teeth and bone mass can be lasting signs of the disease, even if the other physical and mental problems are resolved.

A person with anorexia nervosa is psychologically and physically ill and needs help.

Lanugo *Downlike hair that appears after a person has lost much body fat through semistarvation. The hair stands erect and traps air, acting as insulation for the body to compensate for the relative lack of insulation usually supplied by body fat.*

CONCEPT CHECK

Anorexia nervosa is an eating disorder characterized by semistarvation. It is found primarily—but not only—in adolescent girls, starting at or around puberty. An anorectic person dwindles essentially to "skin and bones," but often thinks she is fat. Semistarvation produces hormonal and other changes that lower body temperature, slow the heart rate, decrease immune response, stop menstrual periods, and contribute to hair loss. It is a very serious disease that often produces lifelong consequences. It can end with death.

Treatment of Anorexia Nervosa

Anorectic persons often sink into shells of isolation and fear. They deny that a problem exists. Frequently, friends and family members meet in a group with the person to confront the problem in a loving way. They present evidence of the problem and encourage entrance into treatment immediately. Treatment then requires a team of physicians, registered dietitians, psychologists, and other health professionals working together. An ideal setting is an eating disorders clinic in a medical center.[10]

Once the medical team has gained the cooperation of the anorectic person, they work together to restore a sense of balance, purpose, and future.[4] As we said, anorexia nervosa usually is rooted in psychological conflict. However, a person who has been barely existing in a state of semistarvation cannot focus on much besides food. A psychiatrist cannot counsel a starving person. Dreams and even morbid thoughts about food will interfere with therapy until sufficient weight is regained.

Nutrition Therapy. The first goal of therapy then must be to have a person increase food intake. Weight gained must be enough to raise the metabolic rate to normal and to reverse as many physical signs of the disease as possible. Food intake is designed to first minimize or stop any further weight loss. Then the focus shifts to restoring regular food habits. After this is accomplished, the expectation can be switched to slow weight gain, from 1 to 4 pounds (0.5 to 2 kilograms) each week until weight exceeds 90% of body weight seen before the disorder began. Weight gain is not the sole goal of treatment but rather a prelude to fuller engagement in psychological issues.[3] The medical team should stress that patients will not be abandoned after they gain weight.

One critical goal at early stages of treatment is to allow the person a feeling of control over life. Only when the patient knows exactly what to expect can this be achieved. Unanticipated weight gain at this stage of treatment—even when caused by fluctuating menstrual fluids after periods resume—can easily set up a feeling of being completely out of control.

Health professionals should measure and compare weight and height to standards—not merely rely on appearance—because our assessments of "thin" are distorted by the very thin models in advertisements.

Experienced, professional help is the key. An anorectic person may be on the verge of suicide and near starvation. Today suicide is the most common cause of death in people with anorexia nervosa.[20] In addition, anorectic people are often very clever and resistant. They may try to hide weight loss by wearing many layers of clothes, putting coins in their pockets, and drinking numerous glasses of water.

Psychological Therapy. Once the physical problems are addressed, the therapist tries to determine how dieting became such a dominant force, knowing that it usually signals a deeper emotional illness. To heal, the anorectic person must reject the sense of accomplishment associated with an emaciated body. If therapists can discover reasons for the disorder, they can develop strategies to restore normal weight and eating habits by resolving psychological conflicts.

A key aspect of psychological treatment is showing the person how to regain control of some facets of his or her life and how to cope with tough situations. As eating evolves into a normal routine, the person can turn to previously neglected activities.

Family therapy is important in treating anorexia nervosa.[4] It focuses on the role of the illness among family members, how individual family members react, and how through their behavior they might unknowingly contribute to the abnormal eating patterns. Therapy involves all family members relevant to the behavior problem. Frequently, a therapist finds family struggles at the heart of the problem. As the disorder resolves, the person has to relate to family members in new ways in order to gain the attention previously tied to the disease. The family needs to help the young person ease into adulthood and to accept its responsibilities as well as its advantages.

Self-help groups for anorectic and bulimic persons, as well as their families and friends, represent nonthreatening first steps into treatment. People also can attend to get a sense of whether they really do have an eating disorder.

With professional help, many people with anorexia nervosa can again lead normal lives. They then do not have to depend on unusual eating habits to cope with daily problems. Although they may not be totally cured, they do recover a sense of normalcy in

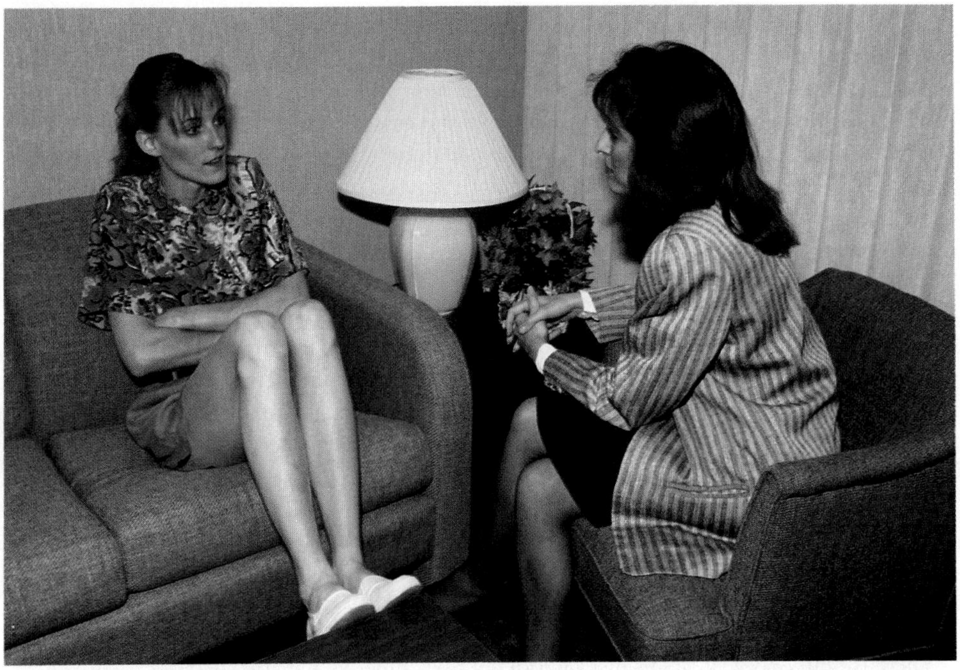

A psychologist cannot counsel a starving person—issues surrounding food intake must be addressed early in therapy.

their lives. There are no set answers or approaches; each case is different. Medications are useful mainly when depression accompanies the disorder. Still, establishing a strong relationship with either a therapist or another supportive person is a key to recovery. Once the anorectic person feels understood and accepted by another person, he or she can begin to build a sense of self and exercise some autonomy.[4]

These words are from a young woman on recovering from anorexia nervosa: "I have lost a specialness that I thought it gave me. I was different from everyone else. Now I know that I'm somebody who's overcome it, which not everybody does."

CONCEPT CHECK

Treatment of anorexia nervosa first requires a person to be brought back from a semistarvation state. Once weight gain allows normal basal metabolism to be maintained, psychotherapy can begin to uncover the causes of the disease and to help the person develop skills needed to return to a healthy life. Family therapy is an important tool in treatment.

BULIMIA

One of your best friends may practice bulimia without your knowing it. The person may feel desperate, yet goes to great lengths to keep it secret. This eating disorder involves episodes of binge eating followed by attempts to purge the food. College-age students practice it most commonly. However, high school students also are at risk.[8] Susceptible people may have both biological factors and life-style patterns that predispose them to becoming overweight. As teenagers, these people probably tried many weight-reduction diets. Now as young adults, their fear of gaining weight is overwhelmed by periods of real hunger.

Bulimia was first characterized in 1979 in college students. Like people with anorexia nervosa, those with bulimia are usually female and successful. But they are usually at or slightly above a normal weight. Females with bulimia are more likely to be sexually active than those with anorexia nervosa. The person with bulimia may think of food constantly. The major difference from anorexia nervosa is actually that the bulimic person turns to food during a crisis or problem, not away from it. Also, unlike those with anorexia nervosa, people practicing bulimia know their behavior is abnormal.[12] These people often have very low self-esteem and are depressed. Lingering effects of child abuse may be one reason for these feelings. The world sees their competence, while inside they feel out of control, ashamed, and frustrated.

Bulimic people tend to be impulsive. It has been suggested that part of the problem may actually arise from an inability to control responses to impulse and desire. Some studies have demonstrated that bulimic people tend to come from disengaged families, ones that are loosely organized. Roles for family members are not clearly defined. Too little protection is given for family members, and rules are very loose. This is in contrast to homes of anorectic people whose families may be so actively engaged that roles may be too well defined.

Men, especially athletes, are increasingly likely targets of bulimia as they attempt to maintain a certain weight.[23]

Pinpointing the number of people who practice bulimia is difficult if the strictest medical guidelines are followed. These guidelines specify that to be diagnosed as bulimic a person must vomit at least twice a week for 3 months. Approximately 2% to 4% of college-age women fit this description.[9] However, people with bulimia lead secret lives. There is really no way to tell just by looking that someone has this disorder. Estimates of cases come largely from self-report and may therefore be unreliable. The problem, especially of milder cases, may be much more widespread than we think.

Among sufferers of bulimia, binges often alternate with attempts to rigidly restrict food intake.[11] Elaborate "food rules" are common. One frequently practiced rule is to avoid eating sweets. Thus if they eat even one cookie or donut, they may feel they have broken a rule and must get rid of the objectionable food. Usually this leads to further overeating, both because it is easier to regurgitate a large amount of food than a small amount, and because "having blown it," a decision is made to "go all the way" and start over tomorrow.

Binge-purge cycles may be practiced daily, weekly, or at other intervals. A special time is often set aside. Most binge eating occurs at night when other people are less likely to interrupt, and usually lasts from a half-hour to 2 hours. A binge can be triggered by a combination of stress, boredom, loneliness, and depression. It often follows a period of strict dieting, and so can be linked to intense hunger. The binge is not at all like normal eating and, once begun, seems to propel itself. The person loses control. Bulimic people often report that they do not taste or enjoy the food once the binge has started (Figure 12-4).

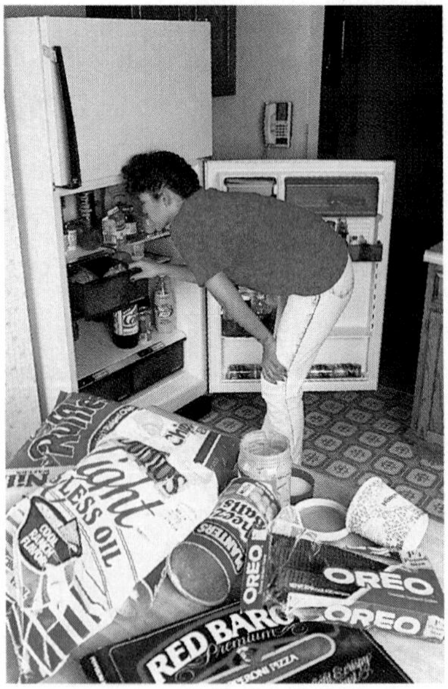

FIGURE 12-4
The binge-purge cycle. It can lead to a sense of helplessness.

Foods chosen for a binge are usually convenience foods—cakes, cookies, pies, ice cream, donuts, and pastries. Even 15,000 or more kcalories might be eaten in a binge.[9] Purging follows in hopes that no weight will be gained. But even when vomiting follows the binge very quickly, 20% to 33% of the food energy taken in is still absorbed. Even more energy is absorbed when laxatives are used for purging. People are mistaken in thinking that there will be little or no energy uptake as long as they purge soon after a binge.

Since people beginning to practice bulimia often use their fingers to induce vomiting, bite marks around the knuckles are a characteristic sign of this disorder. Therefore, it is important for physicians to routinely examine the hands of young people. Once the disease is established, however, a person often can vomit simply by contracting the abdominal muscles. Vomiting may also occur spontaneously.

People practicing bulimia are not proud of these behaviors. After a binge, they usually feel guilty and depressed.[9] Over time they feel hopeless about their situations. Compulsive lying and drug abuse can further intensify these feelings. All this just makes things worse (Figure 12-5). If a person has just started a binge when somebody comes to visit, the response may be, "Get out of my house." The person distances herself from friends and family, becoming more preoccupied with bingeing and purging, an activity that takes up a lot of time.

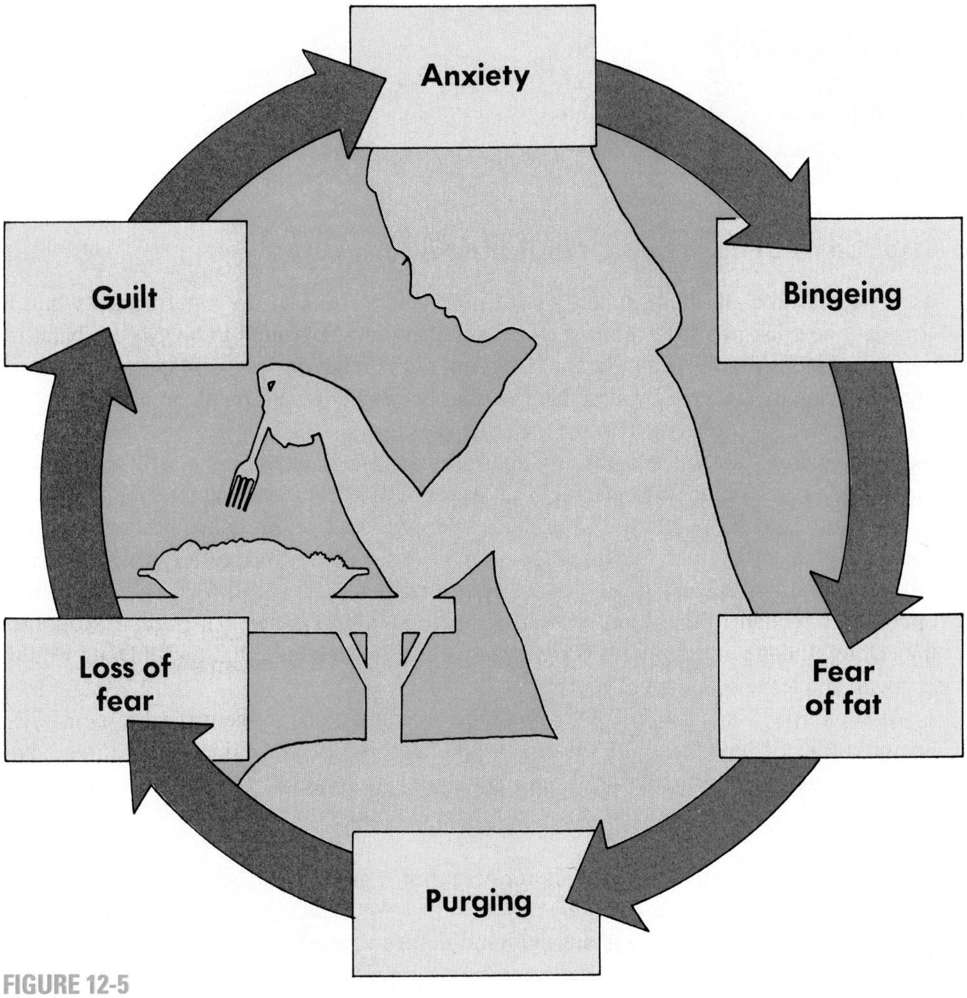

FIGURE 12-5
Bulimia's vicious cycle of obsession.

Health Problems Stemming from Bulimia

Most health problems in bulimia arise from vomiting. While vomiting is the most effective way of purging, it is also the most physically destructive. Dental professionals are sometimes the first health practitioners to notice signs of bulimia.[22] Repeated exposure to the acid in vomit demineralizes teeth. The person complains of painful teeth that are sensitive to heat, cold, and acids. Eventually, the teeth may severely decay, erode away from fillings, and finally fall out.

Blood potassium levels can drop significantly with regular vomiting or use of certain diuretics. This can disturb the heart's rhythm and even produce sudden death. Salivary glands may swell because of infection and irritation from the vomit. The person may even suffer from stomach ulcers and bleeding and tears in the esophagus. Constipation may result from frequent laxative use.[7] Body immune function also has been found to decline.[15]

Ipecac syrup, also used to induce vomiting, is poisonous to the heart, liver, and kidneys. It has caused accidental poisoning when taken repeatedly.

Treatment of Bulimia

Therapy for bulimia, as for anorexia nervosa, requires a team approach. Treatment should last at least 15 to 20 weeks. Clinicians have yet to agree on the best method. Generally, psychotherapy aims primarily to help a person accept herself and to be less concerned

NUTRITION insight

THOUGHTS OF A PERSON WITH BULIMIA

I am wide awake and immediately out of bed. I think back to the night before when I made a new list of what I wanted to get done and how I wanted to be. My husband is not far behind me on his way into the bathroom to get ready for work. Maybe I can sneak onto the scale to see what I weigh this morning before he notices me. I am already in my private world. I feel overjoyed when the scale says that I stayed the same weight as I was the night before, and I can feel that slightly hungry feeling. Maybe *it* will stop today; maybe today everything will change. What were the projects I was going to get done?

We eat the same breakfast, except that I take no butter on my toast, no cream in my coffee, and never take seconds (until Doug gets out the door). Today I am going to be really good and that means eating certain predetermined portions of food and not taking one more bite than I think I am allowed. I am very careful to see that I don't take more than Doug. I judge myself by his body. I can feel the tension building. I wish Doug would hurry up and leave so I can get going!

As soon as he shuts the door, I try to get involved with one of the myriad responsibilities on my list. I hate them all! I just want to crawl into a hole. I don't want to do anything. I'd rather eat. I am alone; I am nervous; I am no good; I always do everything wrong anyway; I am not in control; I can't make it through the day, I know it. It has been the same for so long.

I remember the starchy cereal I ate for breakfast. I am into the bathroom and onto the scale. It measures the same, *but I don't want to stay the same!* I want to be thinner! I look in the mirror. I think my thighs are ugly and deformed looking. I see a lumpy, clumsy, pear-shaped wimp. There is always something wrong with what I see. I feel frustrated, trapped in this body, and I don't know what to do about it.

I float to the refrigerator knowing exactly what is there. I begin with last night's brownies. I always begin with the sweets. At first I try to make it look like nothing is missing, but my appetite is huge and I resolve to make another batch of brownies. I know there is half of a bag of cookies in the bathroom, thrown out the night before, and I polish them off immediately. I take some milk so my vomiting will be smoother. I like the full feeling I get after downing a big glass. I get out six pieces of bread and toast one side of each in the broiler, turn them over and load them with pats of butter, and put them under the broiler again until they are bubbling. I take all six pieces on a plate to the television and go back for a bowl of cereal and a banana to have along with them. Before the last piece of toast is finished, I am already preparing the next batch of six more pieces. Maybe another brownie or five, and a couple of large bowls full of ice cream, yogurt, or cottage cheese.

My stomach is stretched into a huge ball below my rib cage. I know I'll have to go into the bathroom soon, but I want to postpone it. I am in never-never land. I am waiting, feeling the pressure, pacing the floor in and out of the rooms. Time is passing. Time is passing. It is getting to be time.

I wander aimlessly through each of the rooms again, tidying, making the whole house neat and put back together. I finally make the turn into the bathroom. I brace my feet, pull my hair back and stick my finger down my throat, stroking twice, and get up a huge pile of food. Three times, four times, and another pile of food. I can see everything come back. I am so glad to see those brownies because they are *so* fattening. The rhythm of the emptying is broken and my head is beginning to hurt. I stand up feeling dizzy, empty, and weak. The whole episode has taken about an hour.

From Hall L, Cohn L: Bulimia—a guide to recovery, Carlsbad, Calif, 1992, Gurze Books.

with body weight. Therapy focuses on correcting typical bulimic behaviors, such as the "all or none" thinking: if I'm not perfect, I'm a failure, so one slip-up—one cookie—justifies a binge. The person might be asked to role play a scientist testing assumptions and beliefs about food and weight. Patient and therapist together examine the validity of such beliefs. The premise for this therapy is that if abnormal attitudes and beliefs can be altered, normal eating will follow.[10] In addition, the therapist guides the person to establish behaviors that will minimize bingeing. Examples of these behaviors are eating regular meals and using alternate methods—other than food—to cope with stressful situations.[2] Group therapy is often useful. As in cases of anorexia nervosa, if a person enters treatment in a state of starvation, psychotherapy is delayed.

One goal of therapy is to help a bulimic person accept as normal some depression and self-doubt. Therapists may prescribe antidepressant medications to combat some depression associated with bulimia.[1] That often also works to reduce binge eating in early phases of treatment.

Nutritional counseling can help correct misconceptions about food. This entails teaching the person about bulimia and its consequences, focusing on its extreme means of weight control. In early stages it may be best for the person with bulimia to avoid eating binge foods or stepping on a scale. The primary goal, however, is to develop a normal eating pattern.[3] Some nutrition specialists achieve this goal by encouraging daily meal planning.

Nutritional counseling emphasizes setting up regular eating habits rather than stopping the bingeing and purging. Usually a food diary is kept throughout treatment. This helps the person monitor food intake as well as feelings that accompany binge-purge cycles. Alternate coping strategies can then be tried. A therapist might use such information to identify events that seem to trigger binge episodes.

Once regular eating habits are established, the binge-purge cycle should stop by itself. The person should be discouraged from following strict food rules. Stressing the maintenance of healthful eating habits is a key to helping a person regain nutritional perspective.

Bulimia is a serious health problem. If it is not treated, grave medical complications can result. Since relapse is likely, therapy should be long term as mentioned before. People with bulimia can be very depressed and are at a high risk for suicide. For this reason they need professional help.

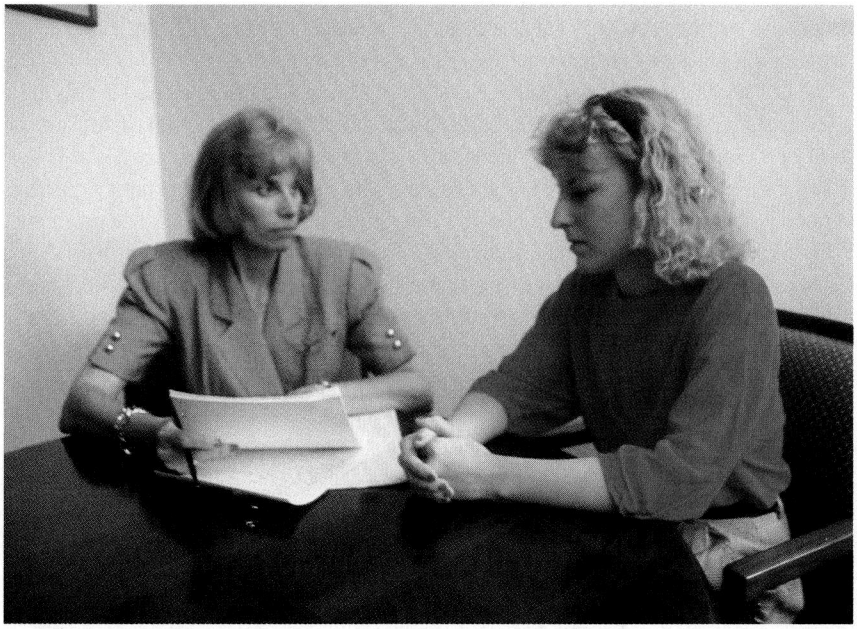

A person practicing bulimia should seek professional advice to help stop the process.

OTHER CASES OF DISORDERED EATING BEHAVIORS

Anorexia nervosa and bulimia affect many people; however, there are abnormal eating patterns that affect others and also require professional treatment. These disordered eating behaviors share some similar characteristics with anorexia nervosa and bulimia, but still differ. Two conditions that have been recognized fairly recently that require treatment are compulsive overeating and baryophobia.

Compulsive Overeating

Compulsive Overeating ■ *A practice in which an abundant amount of food is eaten, generally in response to stress or frustration. Eating then is used as an emotional outlet.*

New criteria for diagnosing eating disorders are set to come out soon. They may define a new category, "compulsive overeating," as a distinct eating disorder, identifying it as frequent binge eating behavior not accompanied by purging, as typifies bulimia. Until now the term *compulsive overeating* has served as a catchall phrase to describe a range of habitual excessive eating. But now health care professionals recognize this condition as a separate, unique eating disorder, as complex and serious a problem as anorexia nervosa or bulimia.[18]

Typical behavior for people with a compulsive overeating disorder is to isolate themselves with a favorite food and to eat large quantities of it. Stressful events or feelings of depression or anxiety can trigger this behavior. They might binge on whatever is easy to eat in large portions—noodles, rice, bread, leftovers. But characteristically they eat foods that carry the social stigma of "junk" or "bad" foods. Among those would be ice cream, cookies, sweets, and snack foods like chips.

In general, people overeat compulsively to induce a sense of well-being and perhaps even numbness, usually in an attempt to avoid feeling and dealing with emotional pain and anxiety.[18] They eat without regard to biological need for nutrients and often repeat the eating behaviors in ritualized fashion. Some people graze—eat food continually over an extended period. Others cycle episodes of bingeing with normal eating. For example, a person who works at a stressful or frustrating job might come home every night and graze until bedtime. Another person might eat normally most of the time but find comfort in consuming large quantities of food when an emotional setback occurs.

While the disorders of anorexia nervosa and bulimia entail persistent preoccupation with body shape, weight, and thinness, compulsive eating behaviors do not necessarily build on those concerns. Compulsive overeating doesn't necessarily involve eating the large quantities of food bulimic people might eat, nor the purging and periods of starvation. In addition, obesity and compulsive overeating are not necessarily linked. Not all obese people overeat compulsively, and though obesity may result from trying to numb emotional pain with food, it is not necessarily an outcome.

Some physicians classify compulsive overeating as an addiction to food involving psychological dependence. The person becomes attached to the behavior itself and has a drive to continue it, senses only limited control over it, and needs to persist at it despite negative consequences. Food is the means used to reduce stress, produce feelings of power and well-being, avoid feelings of intimacy with others, and avoid life problems.

Compulsive overeaters often come from alcoholic families and have suffered sexual abuse. These dysfunctional families do not know how to deal effectively with emotions. They cope by turning to substances. Family members learn to cover up dysfunctional patterns for the alcoholic person and to nurture him or her at the expense of each other and their own needs.

Why does compulsive overeating develop? This behavior frequently evolves in people who never learn to appropriately express and deal with their feelings. Rather than face their problems, they turn to food instead. They continue to do the things that perpetuate the experiences of frustration, anger, and pain. A person, for example, who regularly becomes frustrated because he doesn't assert himself when he needs to, may eat to forget his frustration rather than learn to deal with his lack of courage and to practice assertiveness. The frustration will continue because he never deals with the basic problem. The compulsive behavior forces the person to feel he cannot control the behavior pattern and therefore cannot control his life. Worse, the compulsive overeating usually increases negative self-feelings. Bingeing on a couple of pizzas and half a cake leads to feelings of guilt, embarrassment, and shame.

People who compulsively overeat often have been shaped by families who do not address and express feelings in healthful ways. The parents nurture and comfort their children with food rather than engage in healthful exchanges of self-disclosure of feelings and potential solutions. Members learn to eat in response to emotional needs and pain rather than to eat when hungry. Those who become compulsive overeaters grow up nurturing others instead of themselves, avoiding their own feelings, and taking little time for themselves. Not knowing how to satisfy their personal and emotional needs in healthful ways, they turn to food.

How can compulsive overeaters overcome this disorder? These people must learn to respond to biological signals—hunger—rather than to emotions and external factors like time of day or sensing the presence of food. Experts often direct compulsive overeaters to record their level of physical hunger throughout the day and at the beginning and end of every meal. These people learn to eat just to a prescribed level of fullness at each meal. They must avoid slimming diets because feelings of food deprivation can lead to more disruptive emotions and a greater sense of unmet needs. Diets are likely to encourage more intense problems with compulsive overeating.

Compulsive overeaters must learn to identify their personal needs that require attention. They must find healthful ways to satisfy these needs and to express their emotions. Often they need to be shown how to identify their own buried emotions in anxiety-producing situations and then learn how to have the courage to share them.[18] Learning simple but appropriate phrases to say to oneself can help stop overeating when the desire is strong.

Self-help groups such as Overeaters Anonymous aim to help overeaters recover. Their treatment philosophy parallels that of Alcoholics Anonymous. Overeaters Anonymous attempts to create an environment of encouragement and accountability to overcome this eating disorder. Dietary goals typically range from avoiding restraint in eating to limiting binge foods. Some nutrition experts feel that learning to eat all foods—but in moderation—is a healthful goal for compulsive overeaters. That practice can head off the feelings of desperation and deprivation from limiting particular foods. There is no set answer, but diet extremism is not needed.

Baryophobia

Baryophobia, literally "the fear of becoming heavy," is a relatively new disorder. The term applies to children or young adults who grow slower and less than normal.[14] Decreased growth in a child usually reflects disease. If no hormonal or other abnormality can be found, the possibility of baryophobia should be investigated.

Baryophobia *A disorder associated with a poor growth rate in a child because of parents' underfeeding the child or young adult in an attempt to prevent development of obesity and heart disease.*

This disorder occurs when parents put their children on the same low-fat, high-carbohydrate diet that adults follow. Adults do this in an attempt to prevent their children from developing obesity or heart disease later in life. Today's parents or caregivers, themselves frequently harassed by weight problems, are determined to free their children from that ordeal. Well-intended efforts to prevent obesity in their children can lead parents or caregivers to severely restrict their children's diets. The child doesn't consume enough energy to maintain an adequate growth rate. In young adults, the low-kcalorie diet may be self-imposed to avoid a perceived risk of obesity.

In these cases, counseling is needed. The caregivers and the young adult need to be informed of the nutrient requirements and weight gain patterns for the age group involved. The caregivers will learn that including some sweets and higher-fat foods in a young person's diet is appropriate (see Chapter 14). The diet can still minimize saturated fat, a more important focus in a diet designed to reduce the risk of heart disease. Supplying adequate energy and protein and other nutrients is the key to promoting growth—height and weight—in childhood and young adult years, and it can be done in a healthful manner.

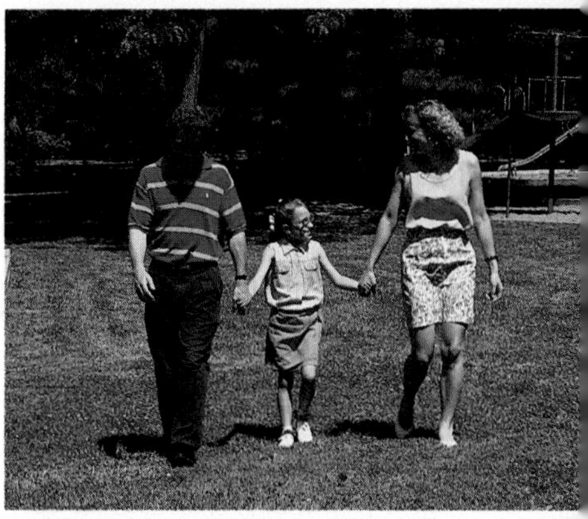

Adults need to be cautious when making weight-related comments to children.

PREVENTING EATING DISORDERS

A key to developing and maintaining healthful eating behaviors is to realize that some concern about diet, health, and weight is normal. It is normal to experience variation in what we eat, how we feel, and even how much we weigh. For example, it is not abnormal to experience some minimal weight change (up to 2 to 3 pounds) throughout the day, and even more over the course of a week. A large weight fluctuation or ongoing weight gain or weight loss is a more likely indicator of a problem. If you identify a large change in your diet, how you feel, or your body weight, it is worth your while to have a check-up with your physician. Treating physical and emotional problems early on helps lead to peace of mind and good health.

We begin to form our opinions about food, nutrition, health, our weight, and our body image especially during puberty. Parents, friends, and professionals working with young adults should consider the following advice for preventing eating disorders:

1. Discourage restrictive dieting, meal skipping, and fasting.
2. Provide information about normal changes that occur during puberty.
3. Correct misconceptions about nutrition, normal body weight, and approaches to weight loss.
4. Carefully phrase weight-related recommendations and comments.

Our society as a whole can benefit from a fresh focus on healthful food practices and a healthful outlook toward food and weight.

another BITE

Along with the references we list at the end of the chapter, these sources can give you more insight into eating disorders:

HOT LINE

Bulimia Anorexia Self Help/Behavior Adaptation Support and Healing (BASH) 1(800)888-4680—Available 24 hours, this is a treatment and research center for eating (anorexia, bulimia, overweight) and mood (depression, anxiety, phobias, panic attacks) disorders. It will provide assistance and information.

BOOKS

Arenson S: *A substitute called food,* ed 2, Blue Ridge Summit, PA, 1989, Tab Books.

Eades MD: *Freeing someone you love from eating disorders,* New York, 1993, Perigee Books/Putnam Publishing Group.

Hall L, Cohn L: *Bulimia: a guide to recovery,* Carlsbad, Calif, 1992, Gurze Books.

Kano S: *Making peace with food,* New York, 1989, Harper & Row.

Tannehaus N: *What you can do about eating disorders,* New York, 1992, Lynn Sonberg Book Services.

NEWSLETTER

National Anorexic Aid Society (NAAS) Quarterly Newsletter, 1925 Dublin Granville Rd., Columbus, Ohio 43229 (phone [614] 436-1112)—Material is appropriate for professional and personal use. Ten back issues and "Overview of Eating Disorders" can be ordered for $10.00. A current subscription also is available through NAAS membership.

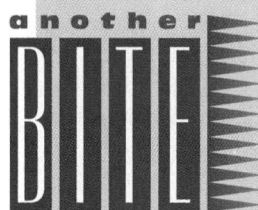

CONCEPT CHECK

Bulimia is characterized by episodes of binge eating followed by purging, usually by vomiting. Vomiting is very destructive to the body, often causing severe dental decay, stomach ulcers, irritation of the esophagus, and blood potassium imbalances. Treatment using nutrition counseling and psychotherapy attempts to restore normal eating habits, help the person correct distorted beliefs about diet and lifestyle, and find tools to cope with the stresses of life. As well, baryophobia and compulsive overeating are now recognized as two conditions that significantly affect people's eating behaviors. In all cases of eating disorders, the underlying causes must first be determined, diagnosed, and treated before eating behaviors can change.

SUMMARY

- The person with anorexia nervosa is usually a girl around the age of puberty who begins to diet but then finds it difficult to stop. She is generally a perfectionist and a high achiever, often described as the "best little girl in the world." Few cases are seen in men.
- Warning signs for anorexia nervosa include abnormal food habits, such as cutting a pea in half before eating it or cooking a large meal and watching others eat. Later, school performance crumbles, and the person often refuses to eat out with family and friends and develops a very critical and joyless nature.
- Physical effects of anorexia nervosa include a decrease in body temperature and heart rate, iron-deficiency anemia, a low white blood cell count, hair loss, constipation, low blood potassium level, and the loss of menstrual periods. A person with anorexia nervosa is physically very ill.
- Treatment of anorexia nervosa includes increasing food intake to at least support basal metabolism and then to allow for gradual weight gain. Psychological counseling attempts to help the person establish regular food habits and to find means of coping with the life stresses that led to the disorder. Hospitalization may be necessary.
- Bulimia is characterized by bingeing on up to 15,000 kcalories at one sitting and then purging by vomiting, laxative use, exercise, or other means. Both men and women are at risk. Vomiting as a means of purging is especially destructive to the body; it can cause severe tooth decay, stomach ulcers, irritation of the esophagus, low blood potassium levels, and other problems. Bulimia poses a serious health problem and is associated with significant risk of suicide.
- Treatment of bulimia includes psychological as well as nutritional counseling. During treatment, the person learns to accept him/herself and to cope with problems in ways that do not involve food. Regular eating patterns are developed as the bulimic person begins to plan meals in an informed, healthful manner.
- Grazing and food bingeing without purging are two behaviors characteristic of compulsive overeating. Emotional disturbances are often at the root of this disordered form of eating. Treatment addresses deeper emotional issues, and endorses avoiding food deprivation and restrictive diets and restoring normal eating behaviors.
- Baryophobia describes a condition in which children are underfed by parents in an attempt to limit risk of future disease, such as obesity or heart disease. Growth failure—weight and height gains—can result if nutrient intake is not increased to appropriate levels.

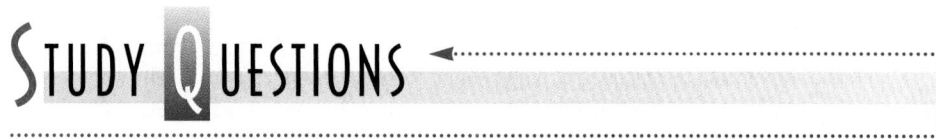

STUDY QUESTIONS

1. What, in your opinion, is a healthful attitude toward food and eating?
2. What are the typical characteristics of a person with anorexia nervosa? What may influence a person to begin rigid, self-imposed dietary patterns? List the long-term health effects of this condition.
3. List the detrimental physical and psychological side effects of bulimia. Describe important goals of psychological and nutrition therapy in treatment of bulimia.
4. How might parents significantly contribute to the development of an eating disorder? Share an attitude that a parent or adult friend of yours displayed that may not have been conducive to developing a normal relationship to food.
5. Based on your knowledge of good nutrition and sound dietary habits, answer the following questions:
   a. How could poor eating habits, such as those exhibited in a binge/purge cycle, cause significant nutrient deficiencies?
   b. How can significant nutrient deficits contribute to major health problems in later life?
   c. A friend asks you, the nutrition expert, if it is OK to "cleanse" his or her body by eating only grapefruit for a week. What is your response?
6. How, in your opinion, has society contributed to the development of disordered eating behaviors? Provide an example.

REFERENCES

1. Alger and others: Effect of a tricyclic antidepressant and opiate antagonist on binge-eating behavior in normal weight bulimic and obese binge-eating subjects, *American Journal of Clinical Nutrition* 53:865, 1991.
2. Anonymous: Orderly dieting and disordered eating: a case report, *Nutrition Reviews* 49:16, 1991.
3. APA issues guidelines for eating disorders, *American Family Physician* 47:1290, 1993.
4. Beresin EV and others: The process of recovering from anorexia nervosa, *Journal of The American Academy of Psychoanalysis* 17:103, 1989.
5. Casper RC and others: Total daily energy expenditure and activity level in anorexia nervosa, *American Journal of Clinical Nutrition* 53:1143, 1991.
6. Collier SW and others: Assessment of attitudes about weight and dieting among college-aged individuals, *Journal of The American Dietetic Association* 90:276, 1990.
7. Comerci GD: Medical complications of anorexia nervosa and bulimia nervosa, *Medical Clinics of North America* 74:1293, 1990.
8. Emmons L: Dieting and purging behavior in black and white high school students, *Journal of The American Dietetic Association* 92:306, 1992.
9. Farley: Eating disorders require medical attention, *FDA Consumer,* March 1992, p. 27.
10. Field, HL: Eating disorders, *Comprehensive Therapy* 15:3, 1989.
11. Greene GW and others: Dietary intake and dieting practices of bulimic and nonbulimic female college students, *Journal of the American Dietetic Association* 90:576, 1990.
12. Grodner M: Forever dieting: chronic dieting syndrome, *Journal of Nutrition Education* 24:207, 1992.
13. Kreipe RE and others: Long-term outcome of adolescents with anorexia nervosa, *American Journal of Diseases of Children* 143:1322, 1989.
14. Lifshitz F: Children on adult diets: Is it harmful? Is it helpful? *Journal of the American College of Nutrition* 11:84S, 1992.
15. Marcos A and others: Evaluation of immunocompetence and nutrition in patients with bulimia nervosa, *American Journal of Clinical Nutrition* 57:65, 1993.
16. McClain CJ and others: Gastrointestinal and nutritional aspects of eating disorders, *Journal of the American College of Nutrition* 12:466, 1993.
17. Mellin LM and others: Prevalence of disordered eating in girls: A survey of middle-class children, *Journal of the American Dietetic Association* 92:851, 1992.
18. Miller KD: Compulsive overeating, *Nursing Clinics of North America* 26:699, 1991.
19. Nicholi AM, editor: *The new Harvard guide to psychiatry,* Cambridge, Mass, 1988, Harvard University Press.
20. Patton G: The course of anorexia nervosa, *British Medical Journal* 299:139, 1989.
21. Roberts WO, Elliot DL: Malnutrition in a compulsive runner: a case study, *Medicine and Science in Sports and Nutrition* 23:513, 1991.
22. Ruff JC and others: Bulimia: dentomedical complication, *General Dentistry,* p. 22, January/February 1992.
23. Thornton JS: Feast or famine: eating disorders in athletes, *The Physician and Sportsmedicine* 18:116, 1990.

RATE your plate

ASSESSING THE RISK OF HAVING AN EATING DISORDER

Figure 12-1 of this chapter lists the criteria for the eating disorders anorexia nervosa and bulimia. These criteria are repeated below. Put an "X" in the space before statements that describe your characteristics and lifestyle. Respond as honestly as possible.

_____ 1. You refuse to keep your body weight over a minimal normal weight for age and height.

_____ 2. You intensely fear gaining weight or becoming fat, even though you are underweight.

_____ 3. You feel fat even though you are quite thin.

_____ 4. If you are female, you have missed at least three consecutive menstrual cycles.

_____ 5. You have recurrent episodes of binge eating.

_____ 6. You feel out of control over eating behavior during the eating binges.

_____ 7. You regularly self-induce vomiting, use laxatives or diuretics, diet strictly or fast, or vigorously exercise to prevent weight gain.

_____ 8. You engage in a minimum average of two binge eating episodes a week.

_____ 9. You have a persistent overconcern with body shape and weight.

Questions 1 through 4 pertain to anorexia nervosa and 5 through 9 to bulimia.

Complete This Activity by Answering the Following Questions:

1. After having completed this checklist, do you feel that you might have an eating disorder or the potential to develop one?

____

____

2. Do you think some of your friends might have an eating disorder?

____

____

3. What counseling and education resources exist in your area or on your campus to help with a potential eating disorder?

____

____

____

____

____

4. If a friend had an eating disorder, what do you think would be the best way to assist him or her in getting help?

____

____

____

If you would like more information, in addition to the sources listed on p. 396, you can contact the following national self-help groups:

American Anorexia/Bulimia Association, Inc.
418 East 76th Street
New York, New York 10021
(212)734-1114

Anorexia Nervosa and Associated Disorders, Inc.
P.O. Box 7
Highland Park, IL 60035
(708)831-3438

Anorexia Nervosa and Related Eating Disorders, Inc.
P.O. Box 5102
Eugene, OR 97405
(503)344-1144

N u t r i t i o n ISSUE

EATING DISORDERS: A SOCIOLOGICAL PERSPECTIVE

We evaluate ourselves in many ways. One way is based on body image. We identify our body with our self and judge it as we think others see us, knowing that our appearance affects their opinions of us.

Early in life, we develop images of "acceptable" and "unacceptable" body types. Of all attributes that constitute attractiveness, body weight is probably perceived as the most important, partly because it is an aspect we feel we can control somewhat.

Yet body weight is probably the aspect of image that dissatisfies us most. Fatness has been ranked as the most dreaded deviation from our cultural ideals of body image, the one most derided and shunned, even among schoolchildren.[17]

Women, in particular, are likely to diet because they feel strongly about what is acceptable size and weight. In general, though, most dieting women aren't technically obese. Rather, they diet to correct some perceived flaw or because they simply feel they should weigh less than they do now.

A *Glamour* magazine survey with 30,000 respondents indicated that 80% were ashamed of their bodies. This dissatisfaction focuses primarily on the desire for lower weight and smaller thighs, hips, buttocks, and waists, typical sites of greatest fat deposition in sexually mature women.

Changing Times

The "full-bodied" woman as a cultural ideal did not survive into the twentieth century. Over the course of this century, a woman's "ideal" body form has become thinner and thinner. Our passion for thinness may have its roots in the Victorian era, which specialized in denying "unpleasant" physical realities, such as appetite and sexual desire. Flappers of the 1920s cemented a trend for thinness (Figure 12-6). Over the past 20 years, the ideal has gradually moved toward a thinner, more angular body shape. Female models for women's magazines are taller and thinner, and more "tubular" in that bust and body circumferences have decreased compared to waist size. At the same time, the population as a whole has gained weight. The same holds true for men in general: a lean, slightly muscular physique characterizes men in advertisements and movies.

Researchers have linked this preference for a lean body type to the recent surge in eating disorders. As the more full-figured woman (earth mother) is displaced by the ultrathin woman, the number of eating disorders increases, along with our society's preoccupation with obesity.[12] It appears that the cultural pressures toward thinness are stretching the physiological capabilities of many women and men. Given the natural variability in human basal metabolism, genetic makeup, our easy access to food, and increasingly sedentary lifestyles, it is no surprise that some of us gain weight. People predisposed to eating disorders for either biological or emotional reasons may be nudged "over the edge" by this change in social values.

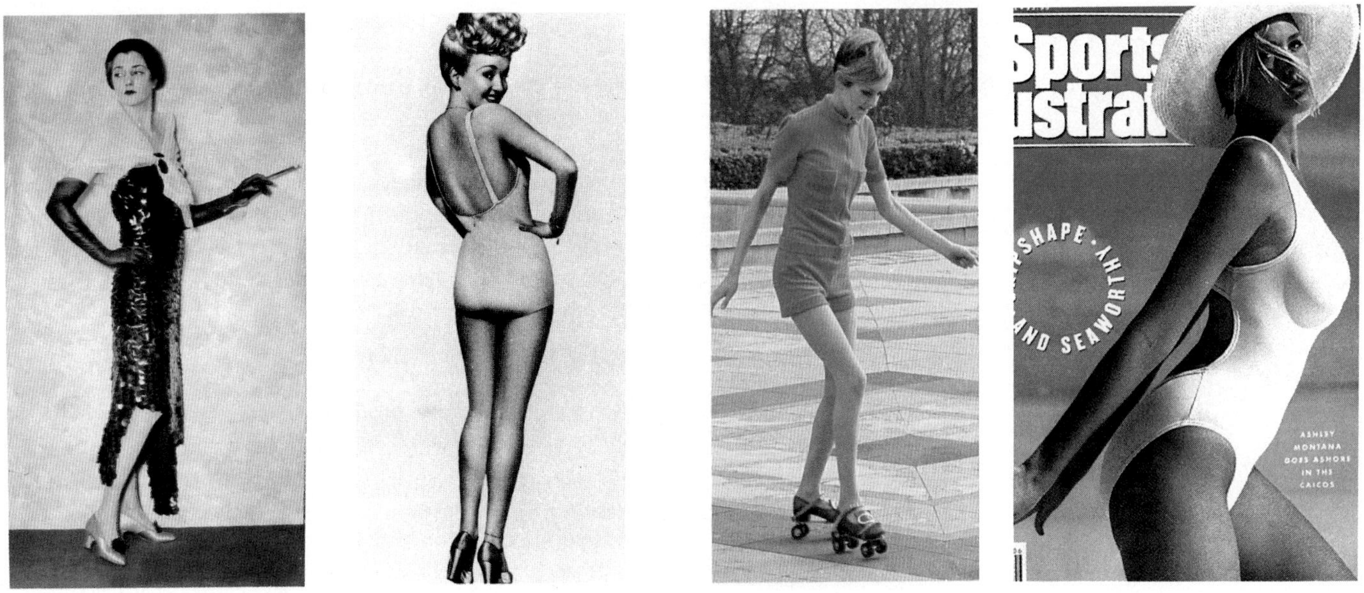

A B C D

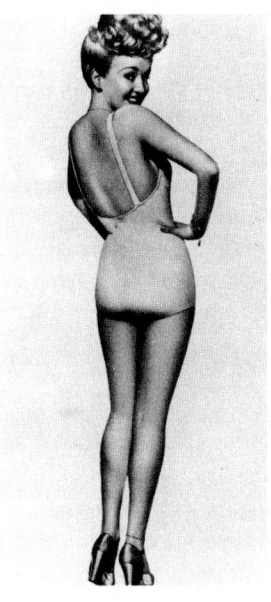

FIGURE 12-6
The changing views of desirable body weight. American society has imposed varying stereotypes for desirable body weight, especially for women. ***A,*** *The svelte flapper of the 1920s.* ***B,*** *The "thin but curvaceous" look of the 1940s.* ***C,*** *Ultra-thin was in during the 1960s.* ***D,*** *Lean and well-toned physiques grace magazine covers of the 1980s and 1990s.*

The Pursuit of Power

Unfortunately, many in society today view obesity as a failure of control, willpower, competence, and productivity. At stake are social acceptance and even access to scarce resources, such as good jobs or an attractive spouse. Whether we like it or not, in today's society our appearance says a lot about us, even though the way we were raised and our genetic background is beyond our control. Some of us were much more likely to become obese in the first place. The question implicit in our society's values is this: if a person cannot control himself enough to stay slim, can he supervise employees, organize the work day, and reliably bear heavy responsibilities?

Mixed Messages

On top of the pressure for thinness, we receive mixed messages. Half the advertisements in women's magazines may be for diets, and the other half for tasty foods. Movie and television stars are almost always perfect physical specimens. Yet television advertisements encourage us to visit our local quick-service restaurant. There you can buy a hamburger, French fries, and milk shake, totaling about 1200 kcalories—about the amount of energy our daily basal metabolism uses—without even leaving the car.

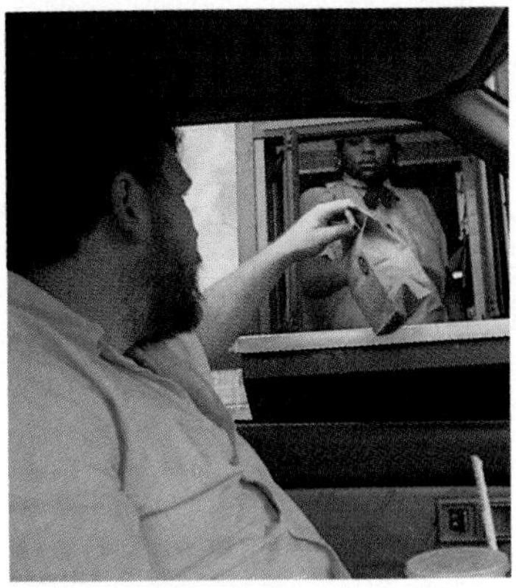

The easy availability of quick-service food has made weight control even harder for many people.

New Pressures

Divorce now ends about one half of all marriages. This increases the stress on children and adolescents, who, like adults, may turn to food. Considering other prevalent stresses—alcoholism in the family, child abuse, school and work pressures, and crowded urban conditions—many of us face family and social environments that encourage us to find a pressure release valve. That valve may be food.

Thin Is In!

All in all, fat has lost favor in our society. Today's myth is that thin people are better than obese people—more competent, healthier, and more strong-willed.

Eating disorders are usually only a symptom of greater emotional trauma in a person's life. When psychiatrists are able to dig deeper, they find that eating disorders mask serious questions of self-worth, family struggles, and sometimes fears of puberty and the future.[9] The real illnesses are not the eating disorders—though they eventually contribute to poor health—but rather, the way people feel about themselves. And negative self-images are reinforced by current social values.

another BITE

By severely restricting energy intake for long periods, people with anorexia nervosa greatly compromise their nutritional status, impair their reproductive systems, retard growth, and put themselves at risk for osteoporosis and even death.[7] The harm produced by milder, shorter periods of diet restriction is not clear. Evidence, however, suggests that even moderate diet restriction, if continued, contributes to the risks for various anemias, pregnancy complications, low-birth-weight infants, and permanently reduced bone density. As we mentioned, it can also impair growth in children and very young adolescents. The percentage of adolescents and young adults who significantly restrict food intake is not known. But at least two problems, iron-deficiency anemia and pregnancy complications, are significant problems in this age-group.

Glimmers of Hope

For women there are some glimmers of hope. Feminists are beginning to point out that true liberation means being free to find one's natural weight. Women who combine careers and motherhood are saying that they have more important things to worry about; fashion leaders are tolerating more curves; exercise programs are encouraging walking, rather than jogging and working out, to feel good. Writers, therapists, and some registered dietitians are working to help women accept and love their bodies.

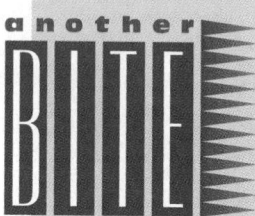

What is the difference between people who can accept themselves—even with a few more pounds than the glamorous people have—and those who chronically diet and feel dissatisfied? Perhaps it is the willingness to recognize that satisfaction with appearance comes from within, not from what they see in the mirror or what someone else tells them (Figure 12-7). The challenge facing Americans today is achieving a healthy body weight without excessive dieting. This means adopting and maintaining sensible eating habits, a physically active lifestyle, and realistic and positive attitudes and emotions, while practicing creative ways to handle stress.

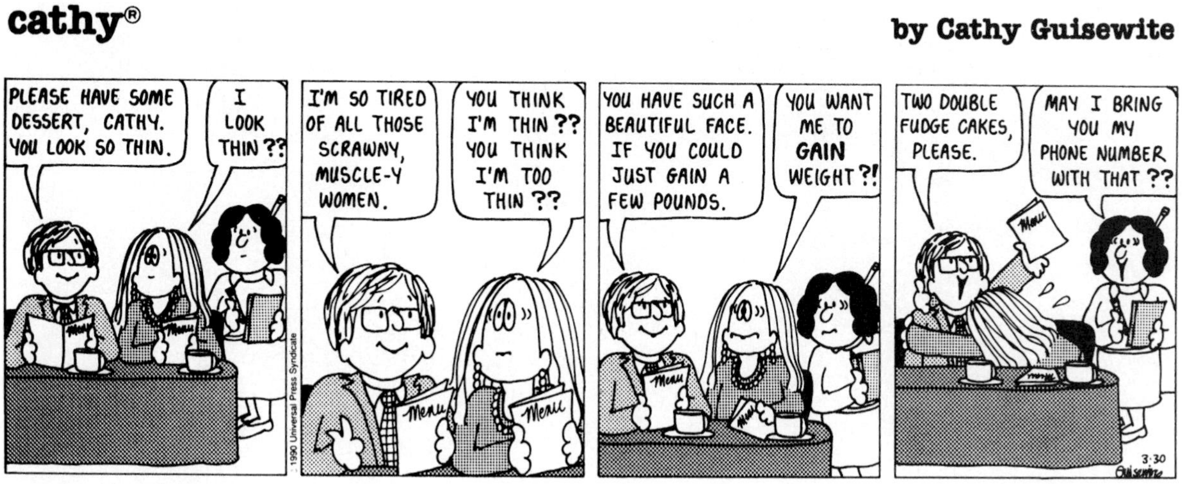

FIGURE 12-7
Cathy.

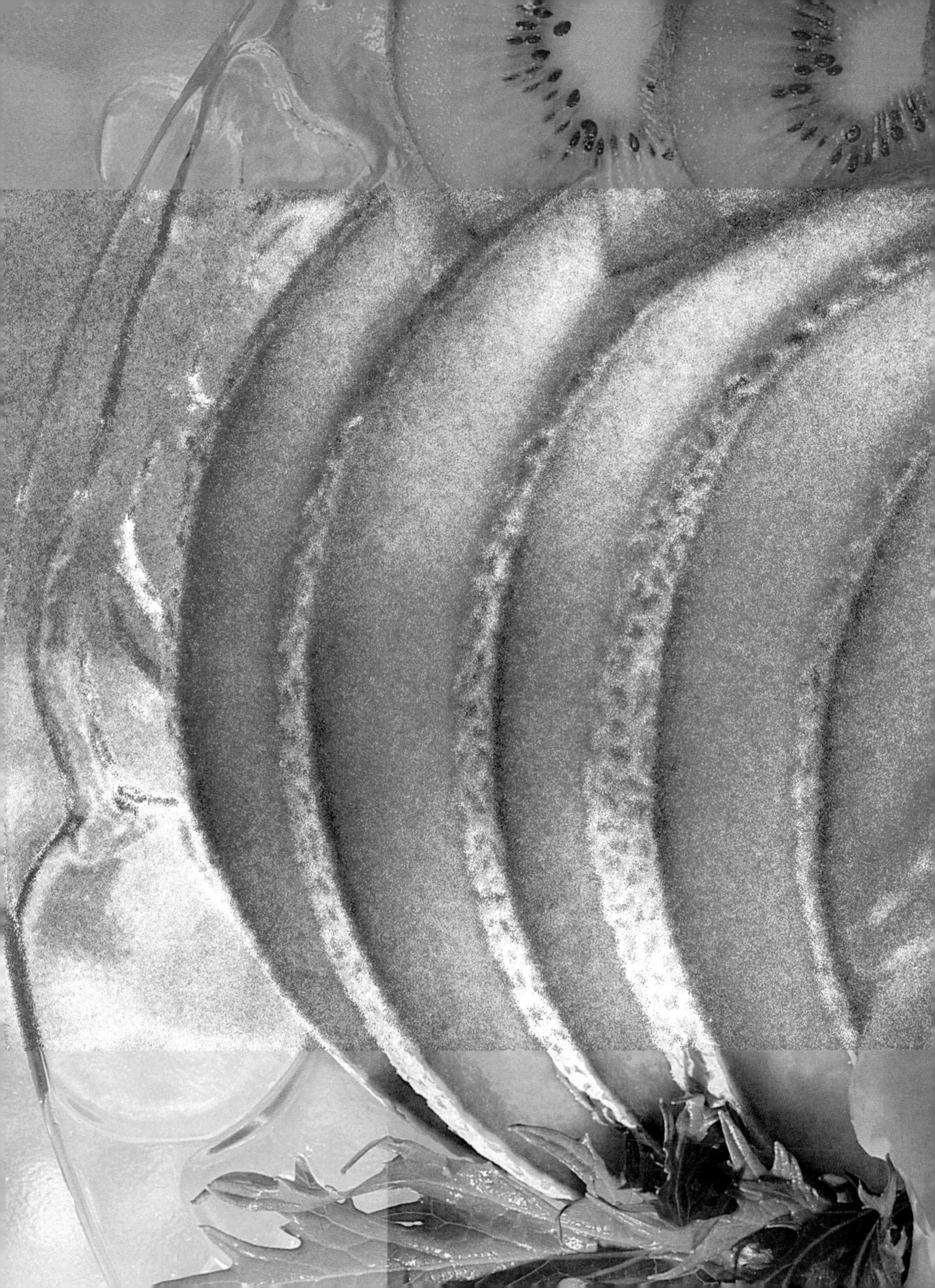

NUTRITION: A FOCUS ON LIFE STAGES

4

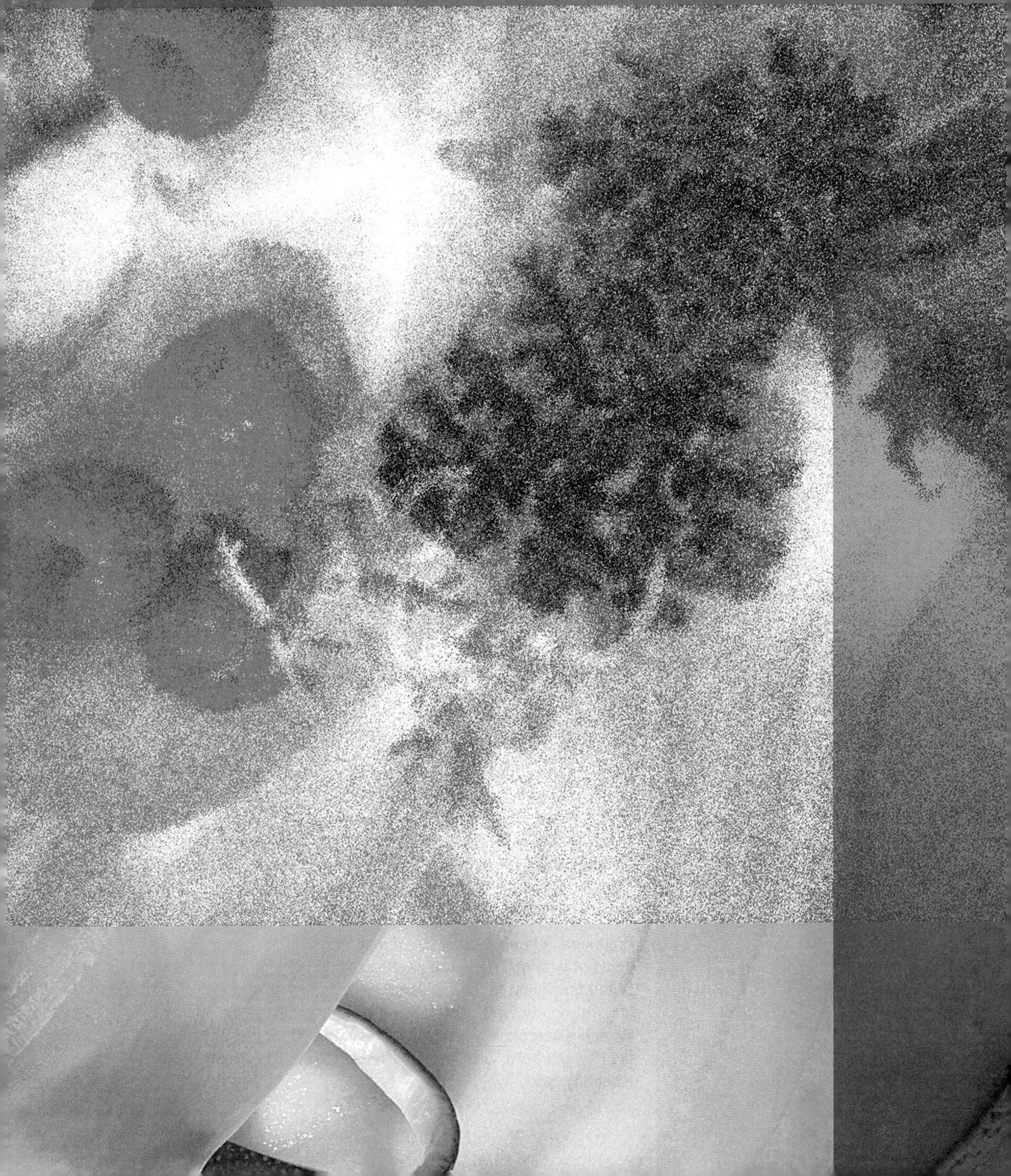

chapter

13 PREGNANCY AND BREAST-FEEDING

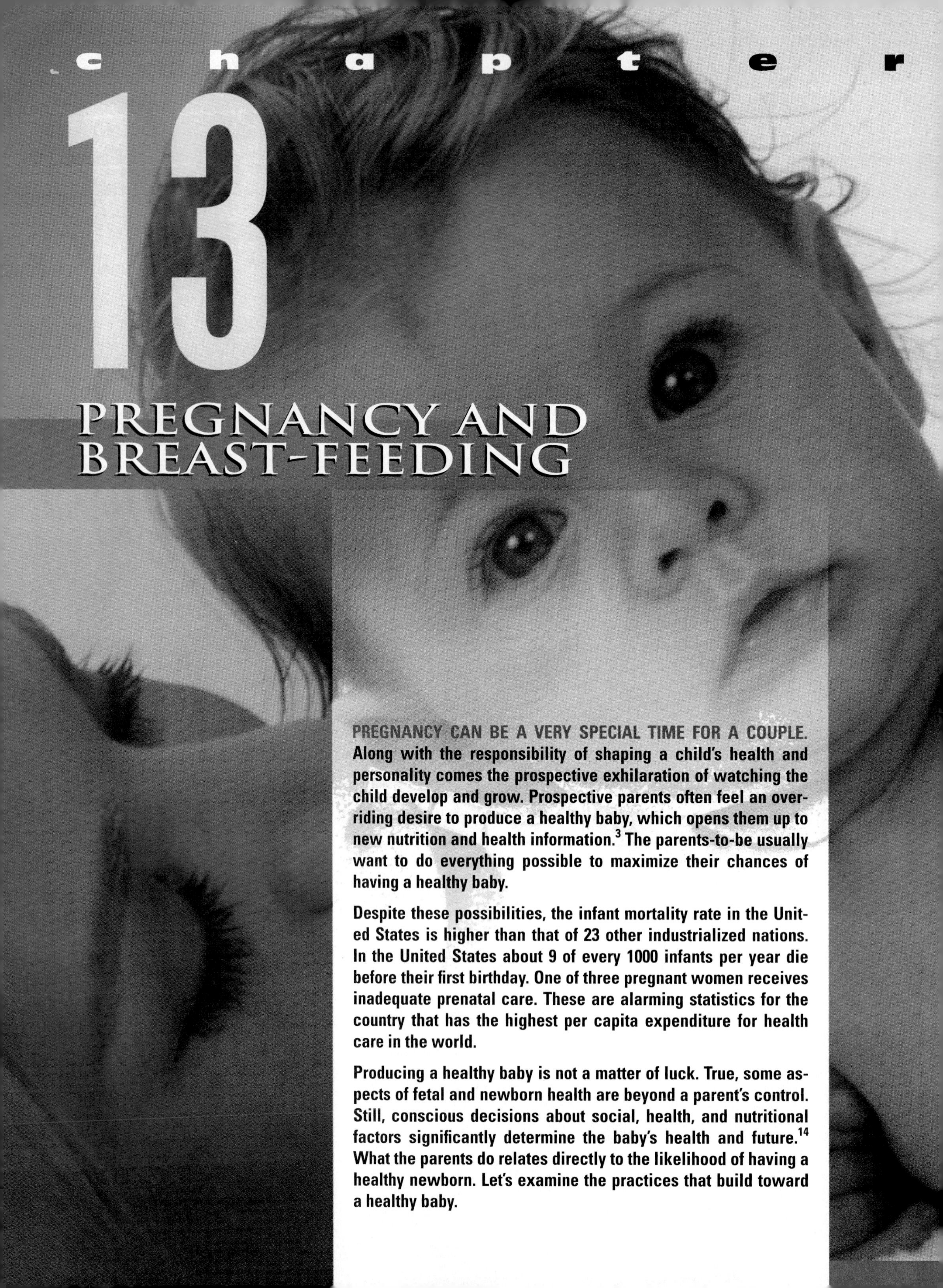

PREGNANCY CAN BE A VERY SPECIAL TIME FOR A COUPLE. Along with the responsibility of shaping a child's health and personality comes the prospective exhilaration of watching the child develop and grow. Prospective parents often feel an overriding desire to produce a healthy baby, which opens them up to new nutrition and health information.[3] The parents-to-be usually want to do everything possible to maximize their chances of having a healthy baby.

Despite these possibilities, the infant mortality rate in the United States is higher than that of 23 other industrialized nations. In the United States about 9 of every 1000 infants per year die before their first birthday. One of three pregnant women receives inadequate prenatal care. These are alarming statistics for the country that has the highest per capita expenditure for health care in the world.

Producing a healthy baby is not a matter of luck. True, some aspects of fetal and newborn health are beyond a parent's control. Still, conscious decisions about social, health, and nutritional factors significantly determine the baby's health and future.[14] What the parents do relates directly to the likelihood of having a healthy newborn. Let's examine the practices that build toward a healthy baby.

THE RIGHT START FOR A HEALTHY LIFE

Premature and low-birth-weight babies are commonplace in the United States today. Do you know the risk factors for these outcomes of pregnancy?

Find out by indicating whether the following statements are true or false.

T F 1. A pregnancy duration of less than 37 weeks does not cause concern with respect to an infant's birth weight.

T F 2. Women younger than 18 years of age have an increased risk of having a low-birth-weight infant.

T F 3. Weight gain during pregnancy is an important factor in determining the infant's birth weight.

T F 4. The greater the number of previous offspring, the less the risk of a premature infant.

T F 5. Risk of having a low-birth-weight infant increases as time between pregnancies decreases.

T F 6. Prenatal education and prenatal care do not significantly increase the chances of having a healthy infant.

T F 7. Financial situation and education level generally affect the outcome of pregnancy.

T F 8. Extreme food faddisms or crash diets can have a detrimental effect on the infant's birth weight.

T F 9. Drug and alcohol use during pregnancy is a major risk factor in delivering a premature or underweight infant.

T F 10. A woman carrying more than one fetus does not run a greater risk for having a low-birth-weight infant than does a woman carrying a single fetus.

Answers: True: 2, 3, 5, 7, 8, 9.
False: 1, 4, 6, 10.

How Did You Do?

Perhaps you would like to learn more about nutrition and pregnancy. In this chapter, we review the guidelines to maximize the chances of having a healthy infant. Knowing the risk factors to avoid and the health habits to foster is vital information for all parents-to-be.

ASSESS

TEST YOUR KNOWLEDGE

yourself

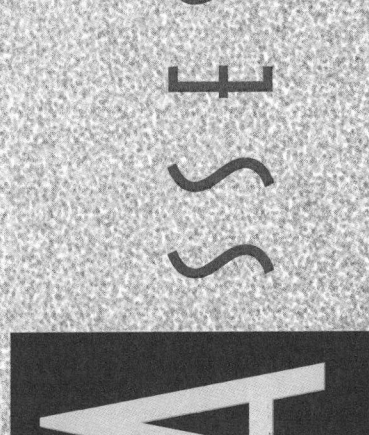

Embryo ■
The developing human life form from the second to eighth week after conception.

Ovum ■
The egg cell from which a fetus eventually develops if the egg is fertilized by a sperm cell.

Trimester ■
The normal pregnancy of 38 to 42 weeks is divided into three 13- to 14-week periods called trimesters.

PRENATAL GROWTH AND DEVELOPMENT

For 8 weeks after its conception, a human ***embryo*** develops from an ***ovum*** into a fetus. For another 30 weeks the incomplete fetus continues to develop. When its body finally matures enough, the infant is born, about 38 weeks after it was conceived. Until birth, the mother nourishes it via a placenta, an organ that forms in her uterus to accommodate the growth and development of the fetus (Figure 13-1).[23]

Women often do not suspect they are pregnant during the first few weeks. They may not even seek medical attention during the first ***trimester.*** Nevertheless, without fanfare, the embryo grows and develops daily. For that reason, a woman's health and nutritional habits are particularly important for several years before pregnancy. Note that a history of anorexia nervosa or bulimia does not set the stage for a healthy pregnancy (as we discussed in Chapter 12). Recent research suggests that an inadequate vitamin and mineral intake, especially of the vitamin folate, in the months before conceiving and during the first months of pregnancy may lead to birth defects.[5] Parents-to-be need to be aware of this kind of information.

During childbearing years, good nutrition practices have a double significance—to the woman and her future fetus. The time to focus on good nutritional and other health habits, then, is before pregnancy. Maternal nutrition should be a focus during all phases of reproductive life. Such practices as smoking and using certain medications (even aspirin), drugs (like cocaine), and alcohol can harm a fetus during its development. On the other hand, once started, healthful habits can be carried into pregnancy, providing optimal health and nutrition from conception until birth.[14]

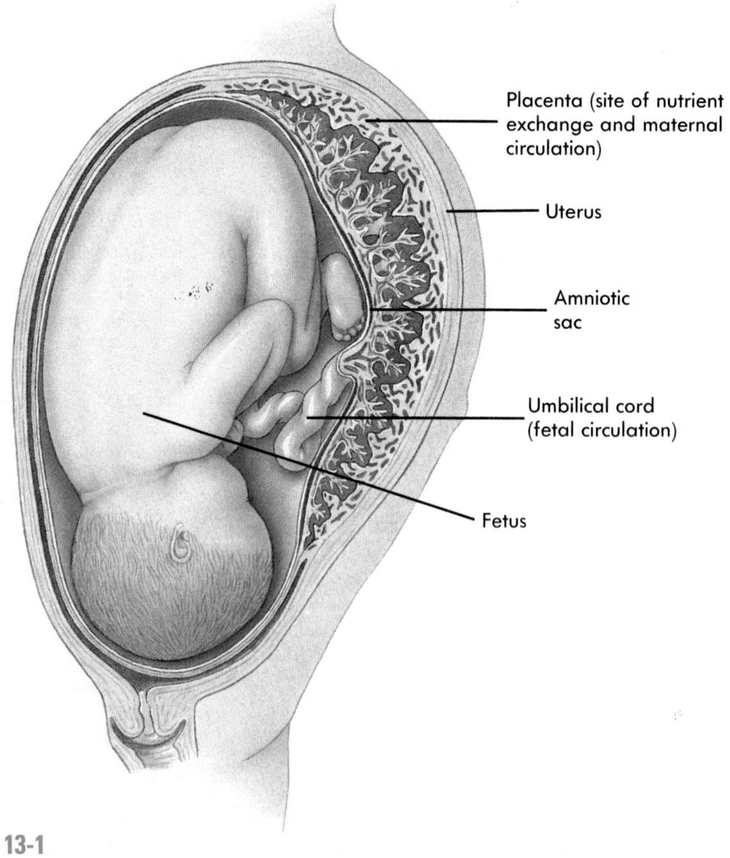

FIGURE 13-1
The fetus in relationship to the placenta. The placenta is the organ through which nourishment flows to the fetus.

Early Growth—The First Trimester

Embryo growth begins with a rapid increase in cell number (called *hyperplasia*). This type of growth also dominates fetal development. Newly formed cells then proceed to grow larger (called *hypertrophy*). Further growth and development combine, increasing cell number and size.[23] At about 3 weeks, cells begin to form specialized organs and body parts. By the end of 13 weeks, the heart is complete and beating, most organs have formed, and the fetus can move (Figure 13-2).[23]

Nutritional deficiencies and other insults transmitted through the mother to a fetus—for example, injuries caused by medications and other drugs, high intakes of vitamin A, radiation, or trauma—can alter or arrest the progressing phase of development. The effects may last a lifetime. The most critical time for fetal development is during the first trimester. Most ***spontaneous abortions***—premature termination of a pregnancy—occur at this time. Currently, about one third of all pregnancies miscarry, often so early that a woman does not realize she was indeed pregnant. Early miscarriages usually result from a genetic defect or fatal error in fetal development.[14]

Spontaneous Abortion
Loss of pregnancy, also called miscarriage, that occurs within 28 weeks of conception.

A woman must avoid substances that may harm the developing fetus, especially during the first trimester. This holds true for the time when a woman is trying to become pregnant. As we mentioned above, she likely will not know of her pregnancy for at least a few weeks. In addition, the fetus develops so rapidly during the first trimester that if an essential nutrient is not available, the fetus may be affected even before the deficiency appears in the mother. Though some women lose their appetite and feel nausea during the first trimester, adequate nutrition is extremely important (Figure 13-3).[23]

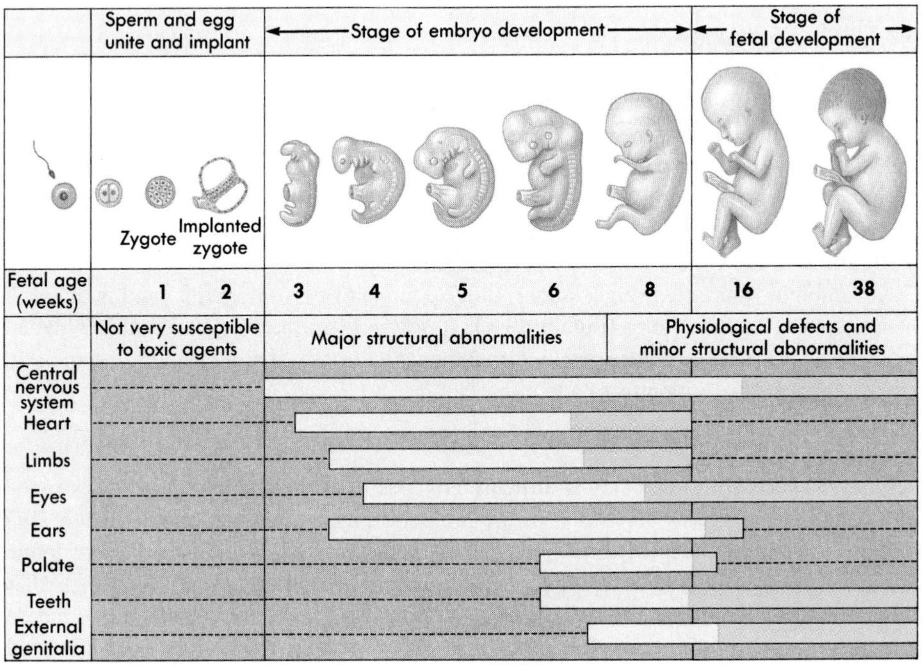

FIGURE 13-2
Vulnerable periods of development. The most serious damage from fetal exposure to toxins is likely to occur during the first 8 weeks after conception (yellow bars). *As the chart shows, however, damage to vital parts of the body—including the eyes, brain, and genitals—can also occur during the last months of pregnancy* (purple bars).

For Better or For Worse® **by Lynn Johnston**

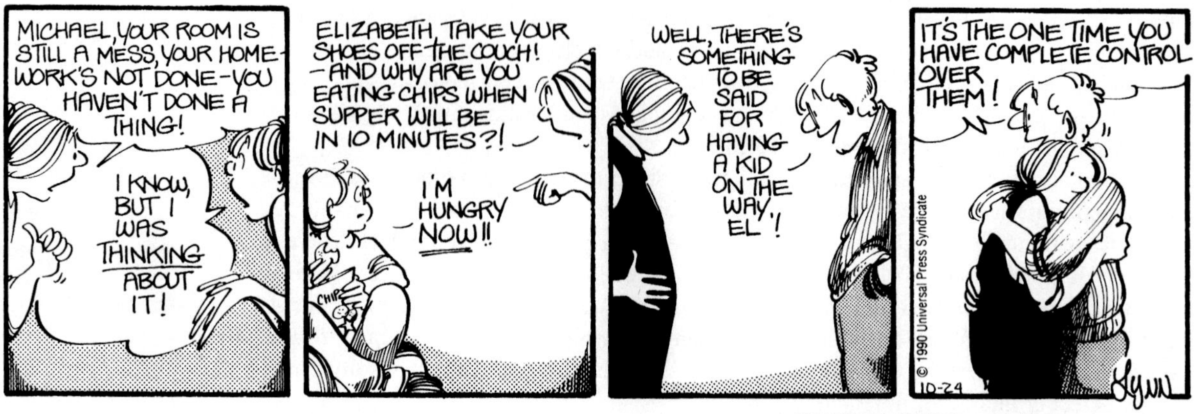

FIGURE 13-3
For Better or For Worse.

Gestation *The time of fetal growth from conception to birth; a period of about 40 weeks after the woman's last menstrual period.*

Premature *An infant born before 37 weeks of gestation.*

Small for Gestational Age (SGA) *Infants born after normal gestational time (38 weeks) who weigh less than about 5.5 pounds (2.5 kilograms).*

The Second Trimester

By the beginning of the second trimester, a fetus weighs about 1 ounce. Soon its movements can be detected by the mother. Arms, hands, fingers, legs, feet, and toes are fully formed. The fetus has ears and begins to form tooth sockets in its jawbone. Organs continue to grow and mature, and with a stethoscope, physicians can detect the fetus' heart beat. Eventually, the fetus begins to look more like a baby (see Figure 13-2). Most bones are distinctly evident throughout the body.[23]

The Third Trimester

By the beginning of the third trimester, a fetus weighs about 2 to 3 pounds. After about 28 to 30 weeks of gestation, an infant born ***prematurely*** (before 37 weeks of gestation) has a good chance of survival if it is cared for in a nursery for high-risk newborns. However, the infant will not contain the mineral and fat stores normally accumulated during the last month of gestation. This and other medical problems, such as a poor ability to suck and swallow, complicate nutritional care for prematurely born infants. More than 1 in 10 infants in the United States are born prematurely.[23]

At 9 months, the fetus weighs about 7 to 9 pounds (3 to 4 kilograms) and is about 20 inches (50 centimeters) long (Figure 13-4). A soft spot in the forehead indicates where the skull bones (fontanels) are growing together. The bones finally close by the time the baby is about 12 to 18 months of age.

What Is a Successful Pregnancy?

Defining a successful pregnancy is difficult. No specific standards have been determined. One dimension concerns protection of the mother's physical and emotional health. Two goals are commonly suggested for health of the infant: (1) a gestational period of longer than 37 weeks and (2) a birth weight of greater than 5.5 pounds (2500 grams).[3] The longer the gestational age, the more time fetal lungs have to develop. Adequate lung development is critical for the infant's survival. By 37 weeks, fetal lungs are well developed, and other medical problems associated with premature birth occur less often.

Infants born after 37 weeks in the uterus who weigh less than 5.5 pounds are considered ***small for gestational age (SGA).***[23] About 1 in 14 infants is born SGA in the United States. These infants are more likely than normal-weight infants to have problems regulating blood sugar and temperature, and they show reduced growth and development in the early weeks after birth.

In 1990 the hospital-related costs of caring for low-birth-weight newborns totaled more than $2 billion, an average of $21,000 per child. Compare this with an average hospital-related cost of $2842 per normal delivery and an average of $500 for preventive prenatal care.

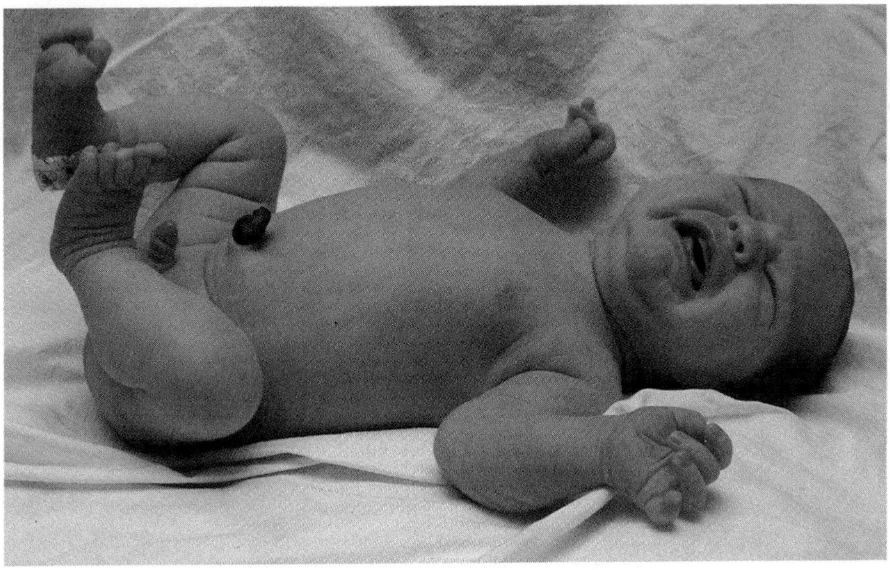

FIGURE 13-4
A healthy one-week-old baby. At birth the baby usually weighs about 7 ½ pounds and is 20 inches long.

In rating the success of a pregnancy, the newborn's quality of life must also be considered. This dimension involves the newborn's ability to grow, develop, learn, and eventually reproduce. Parents should strive toward producing a baby who is born healthy, on time, and with the mental, physical, and physiological capabilities to take advantage of whatever life offers, while also protecting the mother's health.

Nutrition is one key to a successful pregnancy.[14] Eating healthfully is vital during pregnancy to ensure the health of both the fetus and the mother. Fetal organs and body parts begin to develop very soon after conception. The first trimester (13 weeks) is an especially critical period when poor nutrition or drug use can result in birth defects.

CONCEPT CHECK

Infants born after 37 weeks of gestation who weigh more than 5.5 pounds (2.5 kilograms) have the fewest medical problems at birth. To reduce infant and maternal medical problems or death, a mother should strive to carry her baby in the uterus for the entire 9 months and to have a large enough baby. Good nutrition and health practices aid in this goal.

MEETING INCREASED NUTRIENT NEEDS POSED BY PREGNANCY

Over the past century the medical community has changed nutritional advice to pregnant women. In the 1950s, doctors commonly recommended that women restrict weight gain to between 15 and 18 pounds. At times they also recommended severe kcalorie and sodium restrictions to keep the baby small, in hopes of easing labor and avoiding complications. Few of these practices were based on sound scientific information. We know now that many of these recommendations can actually harm the mother and fetus.

The first comprehensive scientific report about nutrition and pregnancy was issued in 1970 by The National Academy of Sciences and updated in 1990.[14] The document emphasizes an increase in nutritional requirements during pregnancy (not restrictions) and the importance of individually assessing and counseling mothers-to-be.

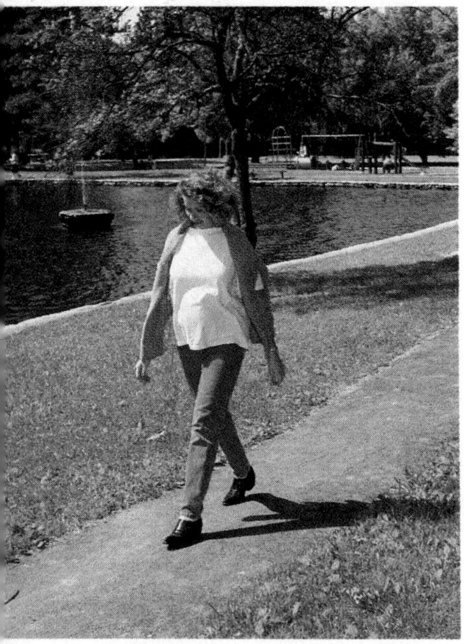

Walking, cycling, swimming, and light aerobics are all suitable exercises during pregnancy.

Increased Energy Needs

An average pregnancy requires approximately 300 extra kcalories daily during the second and third trimesters. Energy needs during the first trimester are essentially the same as for the nonpregnant woman.[14] Just 2 cups of low-fat milk and a piece of bread, for example, can provide 300 kcalories. Though she may "eat for two," the pregnant woman must not double her normal energy intake. She cannot afford a cheeseburger for herself and another for the fetus. She will want to seek the best quality foods to create the best possible health for her child. Many vitamin and mineral needs increase, but the mother can meet those requirements by eating nutrient-dense foods—ones that don't contribute many extra kcalories (Figure 13-5).

If a woman is active during pregnancy, she can add the extra energy she uses to the energy allowance for pregnancy. Her greater body weight requires more energy for activity. Physicians strongly encourage women to continue most activities during pregnancy, except scuba diving, downhill skiing, weight lifting, and contact sports like hockey. Walking, cycling, swimming, and light aerobics are generally advised.[22] However, many women find that they are inactive during the later months, partly because of their increased size, and so an extra 300 kcalories daily is usually enough.

another BITE

The American College of Obstetrics and Gynecology suggests the following guidelines for exercise during pregnancy[22]:

1. Do not allow heart rate to exceed 140 beats per minute.
2. Regular exercise three times per week is recommended, not occasional bursts of activity.
3. Strenuous activities should not exceed 15 minutes.
4. Avoid exercising in hot, humid weather.
5. Avoid contact and jarring sports.
6. Discontinue exercise that causes discomfort of overheating.
7. Drink plenty of liquids to avoid dehydration and becoming overheated.
8. Avoid abrupt decreases in exertion (don't stop and stand around after a hard workout; women should continue exercising, but with less and less vigor, gradually reducing pulse rate).
9. After about the fourth month, don't exercise while lying on your back.

Recommended Weight Gain

Adequate weight gain for a mother is one of the best predictors of pregnancy outcome. Her diet should allow for approximately 2 to 4 pounds (0.9 to 1.8 kilograms) of weight gain during the first trimester, and then a subsequent weight gain of 3/4 to 1 pound (0.3 to 0.5 kilogram) weekly during the second and third trimesters. Total weight gain goal normally averages about 25 to 35 pounds (11.5 to 16 kilograms).[14] Adolescents and black women, who often have smaller babies, are strongly advised to aim for the greater amount (Table 13-1).

For underweight women the goal increases to 28 to 40 pounds (12.5 to 18 kilograms). Body mass index (BMI) currently is the preferred means of establishing this weight status (Table 13-1). The goal decreases to 15 to 25 pounds (7 to 11.5 kilograms) for obese

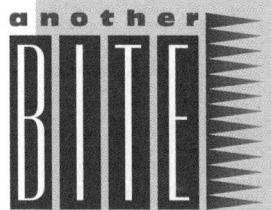

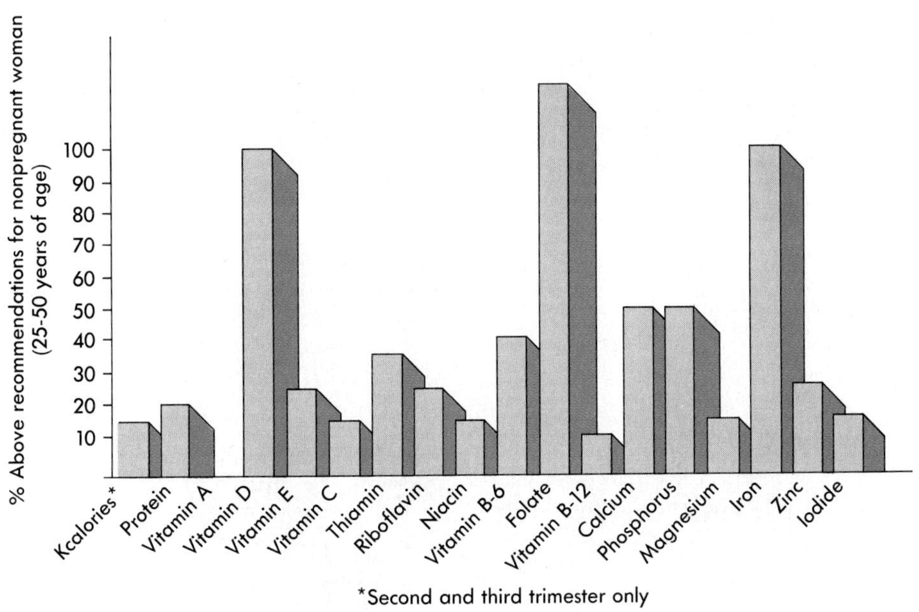

FIGURE 13-5

Changes in the RDA for pregnancy. During pregnancy, many nutrients are needed in greater amounts than at other times. These include vitamin D, folate, and iron. Note, however, that kcalorie needs do not change very much.

TABLE 13-1

Recommended Weight Gain in Pregnancy Based on Prepregnancy Body Mass Index (BMI)

Pre-Pregnancy Weight-for-Height Category	Recommended Total Gain,*† (pounds)
Low (BMI of <19.8)‡	28-40
Normal (BMI of 19.8 to 26)	25-35
High (BMI of >26.0 to 29.0)	15-25
Obese (BMI of >29.0)	≤15

**From National Academy of Sciences—Institute of Medicine:* Nutrition during pregnancy, *Washington, DC, 1990, National Academy of Sciences Press.*

†For singleton pregnancies. The range for women carrying twins is 35 to 45 pounds (16 to 20 kilograms). Young adolescents (<2 years after menarche) and African-American women should strive for gains at the upper end of the range. Short women (<62 inches) should strive for gains at the lower end of the range.

‡See Chapter 10 to review the concept of BMI.

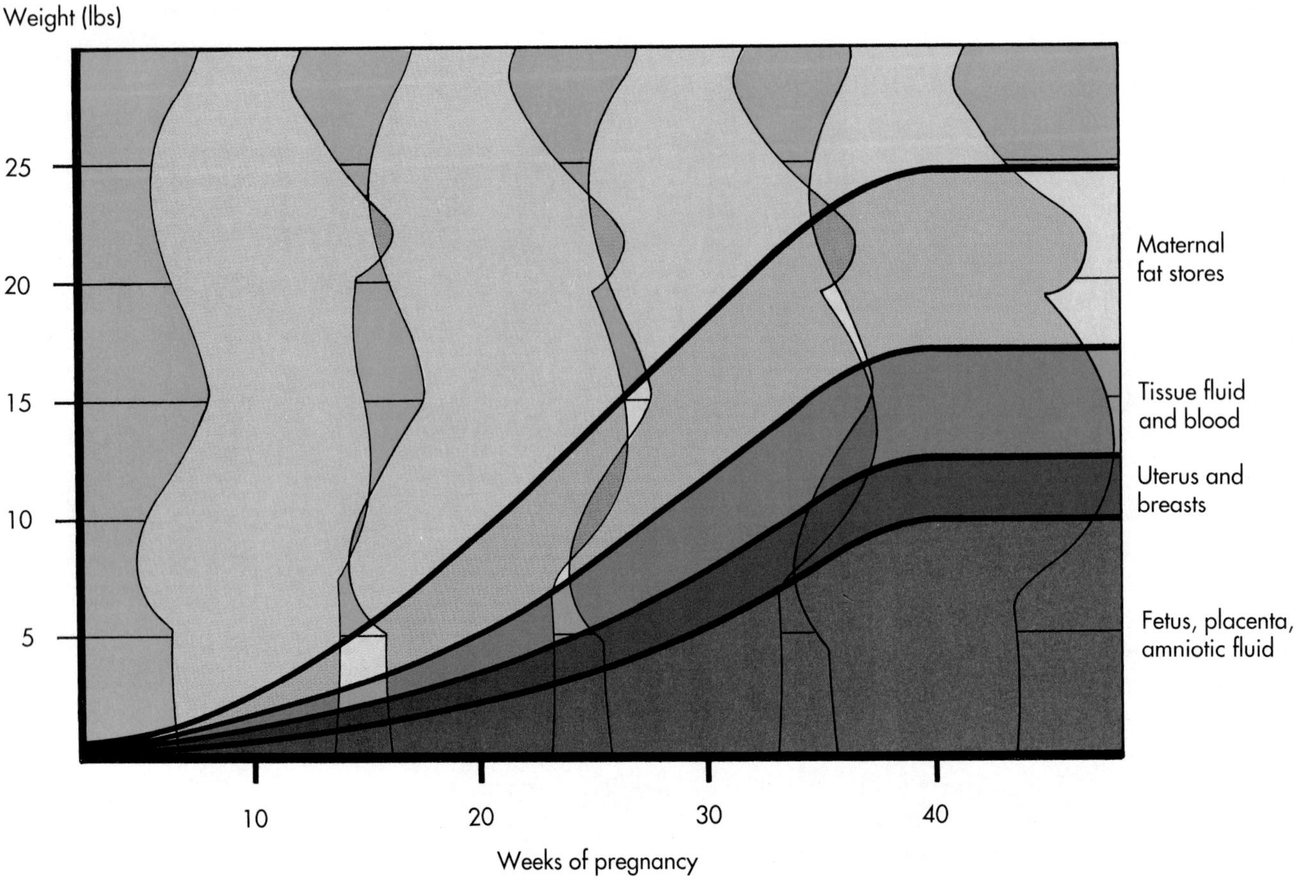

FIGURE 13-6

The components of weight gain in pregnancy. A weight gain of 25 to 35 pounds is recommended. Note that the various components total about 25 pounds.

Low Birth Weight (LBW) *Infant weight at birth of less than 5.5 pounds (2.5 kilograms), usually because of premature birth; these infants are at higher risk for health problems.*

women. Figure 13-6 shows why the typical recommendation begins at 25 pounds. It accounts for the total weight of the baby (8 pounds), placenta (1 pound), amniotic fluid (2 pounds), and the mother's increases in breast tissue (3 pounds), blood supply (4 pounds), fat (2 to 8 pounds), and muscle tissue (2 pounds), which are needed to support pregnancy and lactation.

A weight gain of between 25 to 35 pounds has repeatedly been shown to yield optimal health for both mother and fetus.[14] The poundage especially reduces the risk for delivering an infant of ***low birth weight*** and should yield a birth weight of 8 to 9 pounds (3.6 to 4 kilograms). While some extra weight gain during pregnancy is usually not harmful, it can set the stage for creeping obesity during the childbearing years if the mother does not return to about her prepregnancy weight. This is especially true if the woman intends to have more than one child.

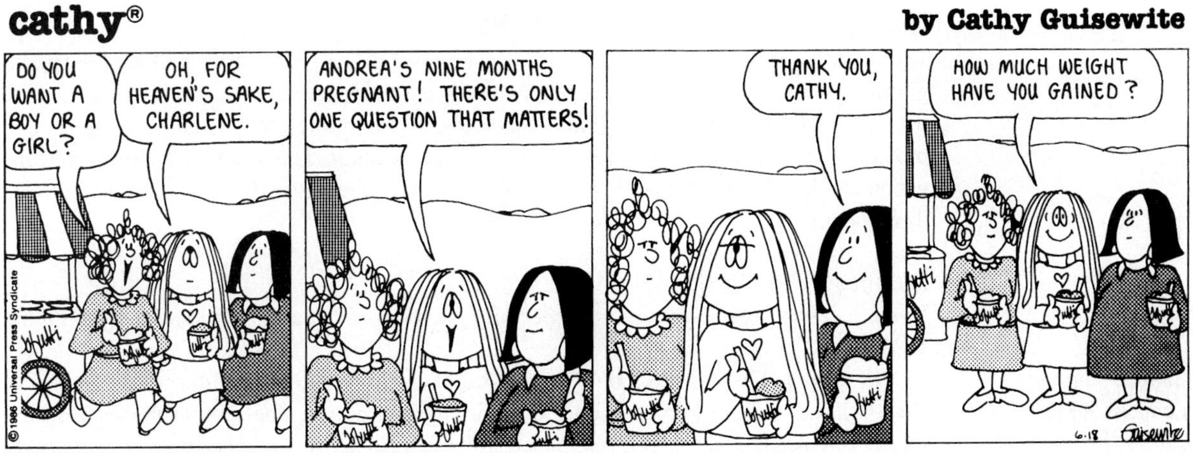

FIGURE 13-7
Weight gain in pregnancy is a concern of more than just the mother.

Weight gain during pregnancy needs regular monitoring, especially in the teenage years.[12] Infant birth weights improve if the mother's weight gain meets the ranges previously mentioned. Keeping weekly records of a pregnant woman's weight gain can help assess how much to adjust her food intake. Weight gain is a key issue in prenatal care and a concern of many mothers (Figure 13-7). Inadequate weight gain can cause many problems. If a woman deviates from the desirable weight gain pattern, she should be warned of this.[11]

If a woman begins to gain too much weight during her pregnancy, she should not be encouraged to lose weight to get back on track. She should simply slow the increase in weight to parallel the rise on the prenatal weight gain chart. If a woman has not gained the desired weight by a given point in pregnancy, she shouldn't be encouraged to gain the needed weight rapidly. Instead, she should slowly gain a little more weight than the typical pattern to meet the goal by the end of pregnancy.[14]

another BITE

During pregnancy, women in America are more likely to gain excess weight and make poor food choices than to eat too few kcalories. The problem is more often how to limit weight gain, so that they don't have many extra pounds to shed after pregnancy. Excessive weight gain increases risk for complications during pregnancy and encourages excess fetal growth, which makes birth trauma more likely. Loose, accommodating maternity clothes designed for comfort do not provide the usual feedback about weight gain, and fluid retention can likewise mask true weight gain during pregnancy. The woman and her physician should work together to monitor weight gain.

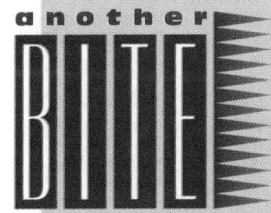

Increased Protein and Carbohydrate Needs

The RDA for protein increases by 10 to 15 grams daily. A glass of milk alone contains 8 grams. Still, many nonpregnant women already eat the recommended 60 grams of protein per day. However, all women should check to make sure they are actually eating enough protein. Carbohydrate needs are at least 100 grams daily. This amount prevents ketosis, which can harm the fetus (see later section). Most women already consume almost twice this amount.

Increased Vitamin Needs

Vitamin needs generally increase, especially the need for vitamin D and folate (see Figure 13-5).

Some recent research suggests that fathers can contribute to a successful pregnancy by consuming adequate amounts of vitamin C. Sperm show inferior development in vitamin C–deficient men.

Vitamin D. The woman's body increases its calcium metabolism during pregnancy to absorb and distribute extra calcium for forming fetal bones. The mother's need for vitamin D doubles to aid the calcium absorption. To provide it, pregnant women should get regular sunlight exposure. If exposure is impossible or insufficient, they can drink vitamin D–fortified milk to make up the difference. A quart (liter) suffices. Pregnant women can also consider a vitamin D supplement that contains 5 to 10 micrograms (200 to 400 IU). The typical prenatal supplement contains this extra amount of vitamin D.

Folate. The synthesis of DNA requires folate. This means both fetal and maternal growth in pregnancy depends on an ample supply of folate. Red blood cell formation increases in pregnancy, and that also requires folate. Serious anemia (the megaloblastic type; see Chapter 8) can result if folate intake is inadequate. The RDA for folate doubles during pregnancy. As mentioned before, folate deficiency in pregnancy has been associated with birth defects, and more recently with ***neural tube defects,*** such as spina bifida.[6]

Neural Tube Defect
Birth defect resulting from failure of the neural tube to close during early fetal developments. Outcomes include spina bifida.

Some women have difficulty consuming sufficient folate through diet alone to satisfy their pregnancy needs. Recent studies show that some pregnant women consume only about the RDA for nonpregnant women. However, by choosing foods wisely—for example, folate-rich fruits and vegetables as outlined in the Food Guide Pyramid—a woman can meet her needs (Table 13-2). Most breakfast cereals also provide folate via the fortification process. A prenatal vitamin supplement may also be used to meet the RDA for folate, especially for women with histories of inadequate folate intake, frequent or multiple births, folate-related anemia, or use of medications that increase folate needs. But normally, wise diet choices alone suffice. Women who have birthed an infant with a neural tube defect should consult a physician about the need for folate supplementation.

There are additional concerns for women who have taken oral contraceptives for extended periods. Oral contraceptives inhibit folate absorption. Taking them necessitates careful attention to folate status during pregnancy. Ideally, one would begin folate-rich foods (or take folate supplements) 4 to 5 weeks before conception.

Increased Mineral Needs

Mineral needs generally increase during pregnancy, especially the need for iron, calcium, zinc, and fluoride (see Figure 13-5).

Iron. Pregnant women need extra iron (twice the RDA for nonpregnant women) to synthesize the greater amount of hemoglobin needed during pregnancy and to provide iron stores for the fetus. The greatest need occurs mostly during the last two trimesters. A supplement is often needed to provide that much iron, especially if iron-fortified foods—such as breakfast cereals—are not eaten. Because iron supplements decrease appetite and can cause nausea and constipation, taking them along with food helps. Combining foods rich in vitamin C with an iron supplement increases iron absorption. Severe iron-deficiency anemia in pregnancy may lead to premature delivery, low birth weight, and increased risk for fetal death in the first weeks after birth.[14]

Calcium. Calcium is needed during pregnancy to promote adequate mineralization of the fetal skeleton and teeth. Most calcium is required during the third trimester, when skeletal bones are growing most rapidly and teeth are forming. However, extra calcium

TABLE 13-2

A Food Plan for Pregnancy and Breast-Feeding

Food Group	Key Nutrients Supplied	Number of Servings
Milk, yogurt, and cheese: 1 cup; 1½ ounces for cheese	Protein Riboflavin Calcium	3*
Meat, poultry, fish, dry beans, eggs, and nuts: 2-3 ounces meat; 1 cup beans; 2 eggs; ½ cup nuts	Protein Thiamin Vitamin B-6 Iron Zinc	3
Vegetables: ½ cup or ¾ cup raw	Vitamin A Vitamin C Folate Dietary fiber	3 (to 5)
Fruits: 1 piece generally	Vitamin C Folate Dietary fiber	2 (to 3)
Breads, cereals, rice, and pasta: 1 slice or ½-¾ cup cooked	B vitamins Iron Dietary fiber	6 (to 11)

**Four servings if a teenager.*

intake should start immediately after conception. The RDA for calcium in pregnancy is the same as for women ages 11 to 24 years and one and a half times the RDA for women over age 24 years. The only practical food sources for calcium are the milk, yogurt, and cheese group and calcium-fortified orange juice. Calcium supplements are needed if these options are not utilized.

Zinc. Zinc is a mineral important for supporting growth and development. The RDA increases 25% for pregnant women. The extra protein foods in the diet of a pregnant woman should supply this much zinc. A poor zinc status in pregnancy increases the risk for having a low-birth-weight infant.

Fluoride. Fluoride may improve fetal tooth development, but this is still a research question. Women should ask their dentists whether extra fluoride is needed.

Is There an Instinctive Drive in Pregnancy to Eat More Nutrients?

Extra needs in pregnancy for folate, iron, calcium, and zinc are the most difficult for women to satisfy. These, then, should be the focus of diet planning for pregnant women. Before we discuss diet planning, however, one important misconception about pregnancy needs to be dispelled. You may have heard that mothers instinctively know what to eat, and that their craving for pickles and ice cream is dictated by a natural desire to consume needed nutrients. These cravings are most common during the last two trimesters and could be related to hormonal changes in the mother. Still, it remains a mystery why some women experience pica, a craving for nonfood items during pregnancy (see p. 424).[10] Is this a natural drive or a learned behavior? We think the latter is the primary reason.

If a woman finds herself with no desire at all for pickles and ice cream or frijoles and hot fudge, there is no need to panic: about a third of pregnant women experience no strong food cravings.

There may be a natural instinct to consume the right foods during pregnancy, but we are so far removed from surviving by instinct that relying on our desires is risky. Good nutritional counseling and the Food Guide Pyramid can focus food choices more reliably.

A FOOD PLAN FOR PREGNANCY

As stated earlier, the Food Guide Pyramid provides a good diet approach during pregnancy (see Table 13-2). It includes three servings from the milk, yogurt, and cheese group (four servings for teens who are pregnant or breast-feeding); three servings from the meat, poultry, fish, dry beans, eggs, and nuts group; three to five servings from the vegetable group; two to three servings from the fruit group; and six to eleven servings from the breads, cereals, rice, and pasta group. More specifically, most of the servings from the milk, yogurt, and cheese group should be portions of low-fat milk, yogurt, or cheese. These supply needed protein, calcium, and riboflavin. Servings from the meat, poultry, fish, dry beans, eggs, and nuts group should include some animal sources and some vegetable sources. Besides protein, these provide some of the extra iron and zinc needed.

The servings of vegetables provide mostly vitamins and minerals. A good vitamin C source should be among the vegetable and fruit servings, as well as a rich source of folate, such as orange juice or a green, leafy vegetable. For the breads, cereals, rice, and pasta group, the servings should be whole grains or enriched grains. Recall that whole grains are good sources of dietary fiber. This basic diet plan can contain as little as 1800 kcalories and still meet the extra needs of pregnancy (Table 13-3).

When Are Prenatal Vitamin and Mineral Supplements Needed?

As outlined previously, maternal dietary changes during pregnancy enable the typical woman to meet all increased nutrient needs, except perhaps for iron. For most pregnancies, the National Academy of Sciences supports only the use of iron supplements.[14]

TABLE 13-3

A Sample Diet Based on the Minimal Recommendations in Table 13-2

Breakfast
Egg, 1
Raisin bran, ¾ cup
Orange juice, 4 oz
1% milk, ½ cup

Snack
Peanut butter, 2 Tbsp
Whole-wheat toast, 1 slice
Plain low-fat yogurt, ½ cup
Strawberries, ½ cup

Lunch
Spinach salad with
oil and vinegar dressing, 2 Tbsp
Tomato, sliced, ½
Whole-wheat toast, 2 slices
Provolone cheese, 1 ½ oz

Snack
Whole-wheat crackers, 4
1% milk, 1 cup

Dinner
Lean hamburger, broiled, 3 oz
Baked beans, ½ cup
Hamburger bun, 1
Broccoli, cooked, ¾ cup
Corn oil margarine, 1 tsp
Iced tea or milk (the latter if a teenager)

This diet meets the RDA for pregnancy and lactation for only 1800 kcalories (including 34 milligrams of iron).

However, physicians routinely prescribe a specially formulated prenatal supplement. They may do this because it is easier to prescribe supplements than to discuss diet changes. Also, some women are just not willing to improve their diets to meet their increased nutrient needs. The supplements typically include the critical nutrients for pregnancy—iron, folate, vitamin D, and calcium—and many others, as well.

Pregnancy, in particular, is not a time to self-prescribe vitamin and mineral pills.

There is no evidence that prenatal supplements cause problems, aside perhaps from the combined amounts of supplementary and dietary vitamin A (mainly during the first trimester). Under some conditions—such as poverty, teenage pregnancy, poor maternal diet, multiple fetuses, and vegetarianism—the necessity for use of supplements deserves a close look.

The Pregnant Vegetarian

The vegetarian woman who becomes pregnant should not necessarily face special nutritional hurdles if she practices either lacto-ovo vegetarianism or lacto vegetarianism. Meeting iron needs is still the major problem. A total vegetarian (vegan), on the other hand, must carefully plan a diet that includes sufficient protein, vitamin B-6, iron, calcium, zinc, and a vitamin B-12 supplement. The basic vegan diet listed in Chapter 7 should be supplemented in the grain group, as well as in the beans, nuts, and seeds group to supply more needed nutrients. Because iron and calcium are poorly absorbed from most plant foods, iron and calcium supplements are probably necessary. The levels provided by a typical prenatal supplement should suffice for iron needs but not for calcium needs.

CONCEPT CHECK

Women need an average of about 300 extra kcalories daily during pregnancy, especially during their second and third trimesters. They should gain weight slowly and steadily. Women starting at normal weight should gain up to a total of 25 to 35 pounds. Protein, vitamin, and mineral needs all increase during pregnancy. Vitamin D, iron, calcium, and zinc are nutrients of particular concern. In addition, because folate status has recently been linked to neural tube defects, folate-rich foods are especially recommended as part of a diet for pregnancy. A pregnant woman's diet should be varied and generally include more milk products than does a nonpregnant woman's diet. Prenatal supplemental vitamins and minerals are commonly prescribed, but taking too many supplements—especially of vitamins A and D—can be hazardous to the fetus.

THE EFFECT OF NUTRITION ON THE SUCCESS OF PREGNANCY

Do we have evidence that all this attention to nutrition is worth the effort? Yes, the effort is justified. Extra nutrients and energy are used for fetal growth, as well as the changes in the mother's body to accommodate the fetus. Her uterus and breasts grow, the placenta develops, her total blood volume increases, the heart and kidneys work harder, and stores of body fat increase. All these changes prepare a woman's body for birth and for producing milk. The nutrients needed for these support-system changes are added to the nutrient needs of both the growing fetus and the mother's own normal body functions.[23]

It is difficult to pinpoint the specific harm to fetal development if a mother either gets too little energy and nutrients during pregnancy or begins pregnancy with only minimal nutritional stores. A daily diet containing only 1000 kcalories has been shown to greatly retard fetal growth and development. Increased maternal and infant death rates recently seen in famine-stricken areas of Africa add further evidence (see Chapter 18). For some nutrients, however, such as iron and calcium, the fetus may also use—and deplete—the mother's stores if she doesn't get enough in her diet.

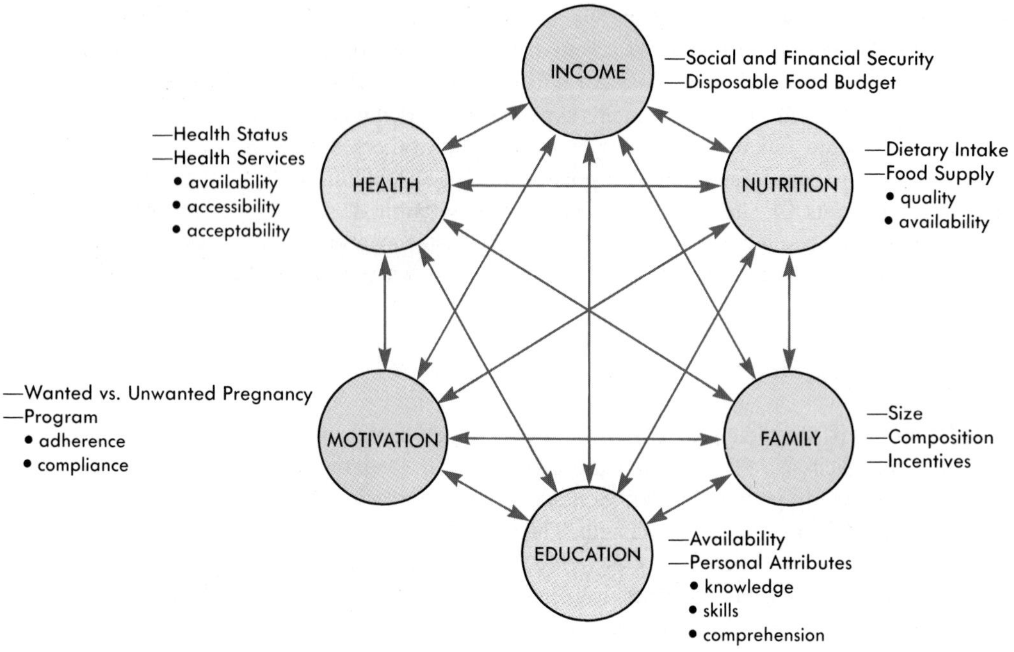

FIGURE 13-8
The seamless web of influences that can affect the outcome of pregnancy. Choices concerning a number of factors influence the chances of having a healthy baby.

The mother's body can adapt to the demands of pregnancy in a variety of ways; it may, for example, absorb more nutrients from foods. However, the success of this adaptation is unpredictable. Both environmental and nutritional factors, such as a mother's prepregnancy weight and weight gain during pregnancy, turn out to be much more important.[3] Figure 13-8 depicts many factors that influence the quality of pregnancy.

Early Research Supports the Importance of Good Nutrition in Pregnancy

During World War II, parts of Russia and much of Holland were blockaded. Food supplies were quickly exhausted. The resulting undernutrition greatly affected birth weights of infants developing in the second or third trimester. Birth defects also occurred more commonly, and the number of new pregnancies fell. After the blockades were lifted, birth weights, subsequent infant health, and the numbers of new pregnancies quickly returned to prewar statistics.[23]

At the same time, researchers working in Boston noticed that a good protein intake was associated with a greater success of pregnancy. It appeared that the mother's diet—not only during pregnancy, but also preceding conception—affected the health of both mother and infant. Studies in Toronto then showed that dietary supplements and nutritional counseling improved the health of the pregnant mother and yielded a healthier baby. Complication rates also dwindled.[23] In addition, researchers in Great Britain showed that height and social class could better predict the outcome of pregnancy than dietary intake during pregnancy. Supporting this is a recent study of middle-class African-American women in Chicago. Their risk of having low-birth-weight babies still exceeded that of middle-class Caucasians, possibly reflecting the effects of poverty on previous generations. This finding again suggests that long-term nutritional intake may be critical to pregnancy outcome.

Laboratory animal studies have supported the importance of diet during pregnancy. Food deprivation during animal pregnancy led to smaller organ size in the offspring, even in the brain, which usually resists nutritional insults. In addition, placentas weighed less and fewer healthy offspring survived the first weeks of life.

Maternal and Infant Mortality—Common Consequences of Poor Nutrition

In the United States, approximately 12 of every 100,000 live births end in the mother's death. In comparison, 920 infant deaths occur for each 100,000 live births. Such grim statistics can be attributed mostly to high-risk teenage pregnancies and inadequate prenatal care for the poor.[14] Compared with other industrial nations worldwide, these U.S. death rates currently rank 23rd—a poor showing. And for African-Americans in the United States, infant deaths are double those of Caucasians or Hispanics. Health professionals are expending considerable effort to reduce both infant and maternal deaths. Good health care and nutritional practices are two key factors in reducing these deaths (Table 13-4). The same principles hold true for pregnant women over 35 years, when age becomes a concern as well.[18]

TABLE 13-4

Women Generally Defined as Nutritionally "at Risk" During Pregnancy

- Women who do not ordinarily consume an adequate diet
- Women carrying more than one fetus
- Women who use cigarettes, alcohol, illegal drugs
- Women whose children are closely spaced together
- Women with lactose intolerance
- Women who are underweight or overweight at conception or who gain inadequate or excessive weight during pregnancy
- Adolescents
- Women with poor knowledge about nutrition, who follow faddish food patterns, or who have insufficient financial resources to purchase adequate food

Beyond the Nutrients

Many nutrition-related factors also affect the health of both the mother and the fetus (infant).[23]

Low socioeconomic status that leads to poverty, inadequate health care, poor health practices, lack of education, and unmarried status is associated with problems in pregnancy.[12] Currently in the United States about 25% of births are to unwed mothers, with a range of 17% to 67% for various racial groups.

Poor, absent, or delayed prenatal care can allow maternal nutritional deficiencies to deprive a fetus of needed nutrients. Chronic diseases, such as hypertension or diabetes, increase the risk of fetal damage. Without prenatal care, a woman is three times more likely to give birth to a low-birth-weight baby—one that will be 40 times more likely to die during the first 4 weeks of life than a normal-birth-weight infant. Ideally, prenatal care should start before conception.[14] Still, about 25% of women in the United States receive no prenatal care in the first trimester—a critical time to change habits.

Smoking, alcohol consumption, use of some medications, and illicit drug use in pregnancy all lead to harmful effects. The Nutrition Issue in this chapter reviews one effect of alcohol—fetal alcohol syndrome. Smoking is linked to premature birth and low infant birth weight and appears to increase the risk of birth defects, sudden infant death, and childhood cancer. These problems are associated with the effect of nicotine, which constricts arteries and may then reduce fetal oxygen flow; carbon monoxide; and other compounds in cigarette smoke. Problem drugs include aspirin, hormone ointments, nose drops, rectal suppositories, weight-control pills, and medications that were prescribed for previous illnesses.

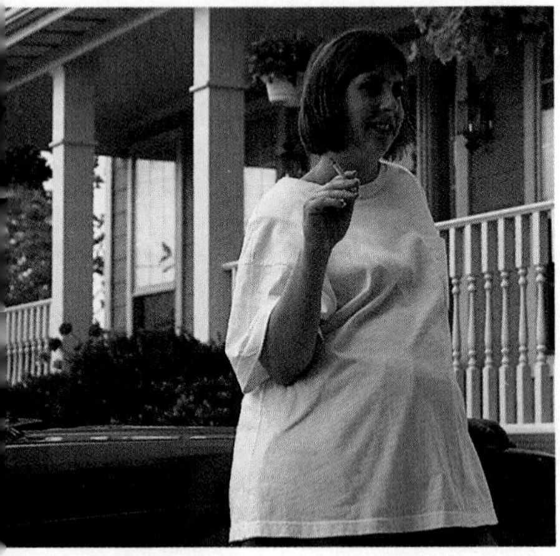

Smoking during pregnancy can lead to lower birth weight in the infant.

A recent survey of 36 hospitals throughout the United States found that overall 11% of women used illicit drugs during pregnancy. The actual range for individual hospitals was 0.4% to 27%. In 1989, research at a major hospital in Philadelphia revealed that 15% of 852 women tested had positive blood studies for cocaine or combinations of cocaine, marijuana, and narcotics. This percentage was equally distributed among private and medical-assistance patients. Clearly, this is not an issue for poor minorities alone: infants in all socioeconomic and ethnic groups are adversely affected.

Fetal exposure to cocaine is of special concern.[20] Its use has become more prevalent in recent years, as has the incidence of infants born to cocaine-abusing women. Prenatal use of cocaine has been linked to premature birth, small body and head size, and several physical malformations. Using cocaine also appears to disrupt brain and nervous system development and may reduce both interactive behaviors and organizational responses to environment stimuli in the infant. Further studies and improved testing procedures are needed to determine long-term developmental abnormalities in infants exposed to cocaine in utero.

Prenatal ketosis is not desirable for the growing fetus. Ketone bodies are thought to be poorly used by the fetal brain. This suggests that they could slow fetal brain development. Researchers stress the need for a pregnant woman not to "crash" diet or fast for more than 12 hours. A pregnant woman can develop significant ketosis after only 20 hours of fasting. Eating about 100 grams of carbohydrate every day prevents ketosis.[14] We noted earlier even nonpregnant women usually eat twice this amount.

Obesity leads to an increased rate of high blood pressure and diabetes during pregnancy.[8] The need for surgery and other complications during delivery likewise increase,[23] especially because the baby can be very large. These pregnancies require intense monitoring.

Inadequate weight gain, especially among underweight women, often produces infants of low birth weight.[23] Undernourished women often have borderline vitamin and mineral intakes and need to build up body stores. They should try to reach desired weight by the end of the first trimester. As mentioned previously, the recommendation for underweight women is to gain more weight (28 to 40 pounds total) than a woman at a more healthy weight. Overweight women who try to avoid weight gain during pregnancy may rob both themselves and their infants of essential nutrients. Also, to efficiently metabolize protein during pregnancy, enough kcalories from carbohydrate and fat are needed to meet energy needs.

In the United States, 7% to 10% of infants have a low birth weight—that is, they weigh less than 5.5 pounds (2.5 kilograms). Low-birth-weight infants are more susceptible to infections, illnesses, and disabilities and are more likely to die than normal weight infants. Premature birth, poor diet during pregnancy, some medical conditions in the mother, and the factors highlighted previously influence an infant's birth weight. Reducing the number of low-birth-weight infants will help reduce infant deaths.[14]

There are still other nutrition-related factors to consider during a pregnancy. *Caffeine* consumption during pregnancy has been investigated, resulting in some provocative findings. Caffeine decreases iron absorption, an important nutrient discussed earlier in this chapter. The risk of spontaneous abortion has been shown to increase in the first trimester and early in the second trimester with moderate to heavy caffeine consumption (moderate use equals 1 to 5 cups of coffee per day). Also, as caffeine intake increases, so does the risk of delivering a low-birth-weight baby. Although more research is needed, it is advisable to limit intake to no more than 2 cups of coffee and no more than 4 cups of caffeinated soft drinks per day.[13]

Phenylalanine, a component of aspartame (Nutrasweet and Equal) causes concern for some pregnant women. High levels of phenylalanine in maternal blood disrupt fetal brain development if the mother has a disease known as *phenylketonuria* (see Chapter 5). Without this condition, however, it is unlikely that the baby will be affected by aspartame use. Some experts still recommend cautious use of aspartame, but total abstinence is hardly warranted, based on our current knowledge.[23]

Pica is the craving for and eating nonfood items, such as starch, ice, or clay, especially during pregnancy. Pica occurs more frequently among African-American women in the United States. [10] As we mentioned before, this practice probably results more from cultural influences than from a need for specific nutrients like iron and zinc. Eating soil raises the risk of infections from parasites and can cause anemia as well as life-threatening blockages of the intestinal tract. Eating laundry starch should be discouraged because it contains toxic compounds. Eating ice can break teeth.

• • • •

Education, an adequate diet, and early and consistent prenatal medical care maximize the chances of producing a healthy baby. The woman should be counseled to avoid x-ray exposure, smoking, vitamin A supplements, medicines, illicit drugs, and alcohol use. If diabetes is present or developing, it must be carefully controlled to minimize complications in the pregnancy.

Given close monitoring, women over the age of 35 have an excellent chance of producing healthy babies. Physicians once considered this a high-risk group. They now feel this age-group has typical problems that are usually manageable.

Again, it is best to begin these examinations and counseling strategies before a woman becomes pregnant, but certainly they should begin early in pregnancy. Many potential problems that develop during pregnancy can be diagnosed and quickly treated medically.[14]

Almost all women need prenatal nutritional counseling, because nutrition needs are unique during pregnancy.[3] Food habits cannot be predicted from income, education, or lifestyle. While some women already have good nutritional habits, most can benefit from nutritional advice. All should be reminded of habits that may harm the growing fetus, such as severe dieting or fasting. By focusing on appropriate prenatal care, good nutritional intake, and proper health habits, as well as using common sense, parents give their fetus—and later infant—its best chance of thriving.

Several U.S. government programs exist to reduce infant mortality by providing high-quality health care and foods. These are designed to alleviate the effects of poverty and insufficient education. An example of such a program is the Special Supplemental Food Program for Women, Infants, and Children (WIC). This program offers health assessments and foods (or vouchers for foods) that supply high-quality protein, calcium, iron, and vitamins A and C to pregnant women, infants, and children (to age 5 years) from low-income populations.

On the WIC program, participants' diets have improved markedly, as has the likelihood that women will have a healthy baby. This program is credited with decreasing the cases of iron-deficiency anemia and low-birth-weight infants within the population it serves. Studies have estimated that every dollar spent on the prenatal component of WIC saves up to three dollars in public health expenditures for the care of low-birth-weight babies.[4]

The WIC program is provided to all areas throughout the United States and has a trained staff ready to help all who need it in providing a healthful diet in pursuit of a healthy baby. Pregnant women are a priority for this program. Budget constraints force some programs to discontinue serving children to make more money available for serving pregnant women.

CONCEPT CHECK

Successful pregnancy depends in part on the mother's healthful diet. It must provide the nutrients necessary for building the new fetus, maintaining the mother's body, and developing the mother's physical support system in the uterus and breasts. A minimal nutrient intake can retard fetal development. Besides nutrient intake, other factors that contribute to poor pregnancy outcome are low socioeconomic status; obesity; poor, absent, or delayed prenatal care; smoking; imprudent medicine use; alcohol consumption; drug use; pica; teenage pregnancy; inadequate prenatal weight gain; and prenatal ketosis.

NUTRITION insight

TEENAGE PREGNANCY

About half a million teenagers birth babies in the United States each year. This is about 13% of all births. Teenage pregnancy poses special health problems for both the mother and child. To accommodate their normal growth even when not pregnant, teenagers need an extraordinary nutrient supply. Women normally continue to grow taller for 2 years after they begin menstruating. Teen pregnancy adds the needs of the growing fetus to those of the growing mother. They both need considerable amounts of nutrients for their growing bodies.[14]

Teen diets—pregnant teens included—vary greatly in nutritional adequacy. Many teens eat irregularly, skip meals, snack on low-nutrient foods, and frequently diet. Many of them eat less than two thirds of the RDA for many vitamins and minerals. Table 13-5 lists some of these problems.

TABLE 13-5

Nutrition-Related Risk Factors in Teenage Pregnancy

- Low pregnancy weight gain
- Low prepregnancy weight for height (or other evidence of poor nutrition)
- Smoking (mothers 18 to 19 years of age smoke more than do any other group of mothers)
- Excessive prepregnancy weight for height
- Anemia

Other risk factors suggested by health histories

- Unhealthful lifestyle (e.g., the use of drugs or alcohol)
- Unfavorable reproductive history
- Chronic diseases
- History of an eating disorder or excessive worry about maintaining a thin appearance

From ADA Reports: Journal of The American Dietetic Association *89:106, 1989.*

PHYSIOLOGICAL CHANGES CAN CAUSE DISCOMFORT IN PREGNANCY

During pregnancy, the fetus' needs for oxygen, nutrients, and excretion increase the burden on the mother's lungs, heart, and kidneys. Although a mother's digestive and metabolic systems work very efficiently, some discomfort accompanies the changes her body undergoes to accommodate the fetus.

Heartburn, Constipation, and Hemorrhoids

Hormones produced by the placenta relax muscles in both the uterus and the intestinal tract. This often causes heartburn as stomach acid slips up into the esophagus (see Chapter 4).[23] When this occurs, the woman should avoid lying down after eating, eat less fat so that foods pass more quickly from the stomach into the small intestine, and avoid spicy foods she can't tolerate. She should also consume liquids between meals to decrease stomach volume and pressure.

Teenagers are more likely than most mothers to be underweight at the beginning of pregnancy and to gain fewer than 16 pounds during pregnancy. Consequently, teens frequently produce low-birth-weight infants.[17] Additional complications, such as infant illness or even death, appear to be closely tied to the teenage mother's day-to-day health practices. If the mother leads a healthful life, she will be healthier and so likely will her baby.[12]

The specific needs of pregnant adolescents vary according to their own growth patterns, body build, and exercise habits. This makes it difficult to predict their nutrient needs. But health workers can evaluate the adequacy of their diet by checking for appropriate weight gain during pregnancy and appropriate food choices. To improve pregnancy outcomes and the health of pregnant teenagers, their eating practices should be routinely examined and they should be counseled concerning nutrition during their prenatal care.[12] They need information about basic nutrition guidelines: the relationship between food and health, issues that affect adequate nutrition and food resources (for example, the WIC program), the kind and amount of food energy needed to support appropriate weight gain, how to select nutrient-rich foods, regular use of prenatal vitamin/mineral supplements, and preparation for breast-feeding or for using infant formulas. They also need to be made aware of the risks involved with smoking, drinking alcohol, and using drugs and medications not approved by their physicians.

The other major problem related to teenage pregnancy and parenthood is their impact on the mother's education and economic future. Young mothers are often deprived of the education that would help them qualify for better jobs, leading to better means of looking after themselves and their children. Few teenagers can successfully care for and support themselves and their children. Thus, ultimately, prevention of teenage pregnancy is generally the best approach.

Constipation often results as the intestinal muscles relax during pregnancy. It especially develops late in pregnancy as the fetus competes with the GI tract for space in the abdominal cavity. To offset these discomforts, a woman should typically perform regular exercise and consume more water, dietary fiber, and dried fruits. These practices can help prevent constipation and an often accompanying problem, hemorrhoids. Straining during elimination can lead to hemorrhoids, which are more likely to occur during pregnancy anyway because of other bodily changes.

Edema

Placental hormones cause various body tissues to retain fluid during pregnancy.[23] Blood volume also greatly expands during pregnancy. The extra fluid normally contributes some swelling (edema). There is no reason to severely restrict salt or use diuretics to limit mild edema. However, the edema may limit physical activity late in pregnancy and occasional-

Physiological Anemia *The normal increase in plasma volume that dilutes the concentration of red blood cells, resulting in anemia; also called hemodilution.*

Pregnancy-Induced Hypertension *A serious disorder that can include high blood pressure, kidney failure, convulsions, and even death of the mother and fetus. Although the exact cause is not known, good nutrition and prenatal care can prevent or limit its severity.*

Today, folate-related anemias do not occur often during pregnancy. Widespread use of prenatal supplements, which supply folate, is probably the major reason.

ly require the woman to elevate her feet to control the effects. Retaining fluid spells trouble only if hypertension and the appearance of protein in the urine accompany it. (We discuss this in a later section.)

Morning Sickness

Women commonly feel nauseated during the early stages of pregnancy, which is possibly a reaction to pregnancy-related hormones circulating in the bloodstream.[23] Although known as "morning sickness," nausea may occur at any time and persist all day. It is often the first signal to a woman that she is pregnant. Some women partially control mild nausea by eating soda crackers or dry cereal before getting out of bed; cooking with open windows to dissipate nauseating smells; eating smaller, more frequent meals; and avoiding foods that increase nausea. Usually, nausea stops after the first trimester, but it can continue throughout the entire pregnancy. In cases of serious nausea, the preceding practices offer little relief. When appetite is severely reduced or vomiting persists, medical therapy is needed.

Anemia

To supply fetal needs, the mother's blood volume expands up to approximately 150% of normal. The red cell mass expands only 20% to 30% above normal and occurs more gradually. This leaves proportionately fewer red blood cells in a pregnant woman's bloodstream. The lower ratio of red blood cells to total blood volume is a condition known as ***physiological anemia.***[23] It is a normal response to pregnancy, rather than the result of poor nutrient intake. If during pregnancy, however, iron stores and/or dietary iron intake is inadequate, any resulting iron-deficiency anemia requires medical evaluation.

Pregnancy-Induced Hypertension

Pregnancy-induced hypertension is a high-risk disorder. In its mild forms it is known as preeclampsia and in severe forms as eclampsia. The problem resolves once the pregnancy ends. Early symptoms include a rise in blood pressure, excess protein in the urine, edema, changes in blood clotting, and nervous system disorders. Very severe effects, including convulsions, can occur in the second and third trimesters. Good nutrition, especially an adequate calcium intake, may prevent or lessen the symptoms.[2] Mild effects can be lessened by bed rest. If not controlled, eclampsia eventually damages the liver and kidneys, and mother and fetus may both die. Careful medical attention is needed.

• • • •

Although pregnancy brings with it some physical discomforts for the mother, the inconvenience is temporary and many potential discomforts can be diffused through generally good eating and health habits. More than that, the good habits bring double benefits, because they are the basis of good health for both mother and infant.

CONCEPT CHECK

Heartburn, constipation, nausea, and vomiting from morning sickness, edema, and anemia are possible discomforts and complications of pregnancy. Changes in food habits can often ease these problems. Pregnancy-induced hypertension, with high blood pressure and kidney failure, can lead to severe complications, and if not treated, can lead to death of both the mother and fetus.

BREAST-FEEDING

Before the 1900s, if a mother didn't breast-feed, a substitute "wet-nurse" was hired to do it. Formula-feeding was fraught with complications, primarily because people did not know the importance of sterilizing formulas against bacteria. Nor did people know much about the nutritional needs of infants. During the early 1900s, the technology of formulas and feeding improved. From the 1920s and especially in the 1940s when women worked in armament factories during World War II, more and more babies were fed formula. Throughout the 1950s and early 1960s, interest in breast-feeding further waned. In the 1970s, breast-feeding enjoyed a resurgence, which has since leveled off.

Recent statistics show that about 60% of Caucasian women nurse their babies in the hospital, and 25% of African-American women do so. The same approximate ratio of Caucasian to African-American women who breast-feed holds after 4 months. The women who choose to breast-feed usually find it an enjoyable and special time in their lives and in the relationship with their new babies.[8]

Bottle-feeding a formula to an infant is also a nutritious choice. We discuss the how-to's in the next chapter.

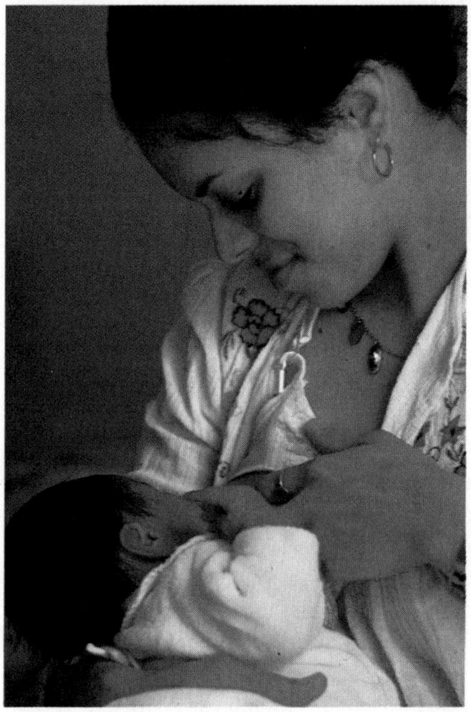

Breast-feeding fosters a closeness and bonding between the mother and the infant.

Physiology of Lactation

Almost all women can breast-feed their children.[1] Major problems are usually caused by a lack of information. Problems such as inverted nipples can be corrected during pregnancy. Breast size does not affect successful breast-feeding: breasts of all sizes normally contain adequate numbers of milk-producing cells. First-time mothers who plan to breast-feed should learn as much as they can about the process before delivering the baby. Interested women should learn the proper technique, as well as what problems to expect and how to respond to them. Familiarity with the process builds the confidence and knowledge necessary for success.

Producing Human Milk

During pregnancy, cells in the breast form milk-producing ***lobules*** (Figure 13-9). Hormones from the placenta stimulate these changes in the breast. After birth, the mother produces more ***prolactin*** hormone to maintain the changes in the breast, and therefore the ability to produce milk.[23] During pregnancy, breast weight increases by 1 to 2 pounds.

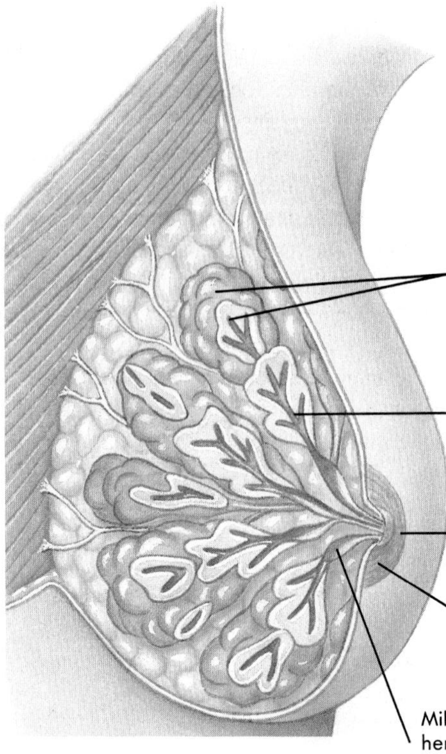

FIGURE 13-9

The breast automatically prepares itself for nourishing the infant. Many structures in the breast contribute to the production and release of human milk.

The hormone prolactin also stimulates the synthesis of milk. Suckling stimulates prolactin release. Milk synthesis then occurs as an infant nurses. The more the infant suckles, the more milk is produced. Milk production closely parallels infant demand.[15] In this way, even twins can be nursed. Demand is the driving force for milk production.

Most protein found in human milk is synthesized by breast tissue. Some proteins also enter the milk directly from the mother's bloodstream. These proteins include immune factors and enzymes. Fats in human milk come from the mother's diet, and some are also synthesized by breast tissue. The simple sugar galactose is synthesized in the breast, while glucose enters from the mother's bloodstream. Together these sugars form lactose, the main carbohydrate in human milk.

The Let-Down Reflex

An important brain-breast connection—the ***let-down reflex***—is necessary for breast-feeding (Figure 13-10).[1] The brain releases the hormone oxytocin to allow the breast tissues to let down (release) the milk from storage sites. It travels to the nipple area. A tingling sensation signals the let-down reflex shortly before milk flow begins. If the let-down reflex doesn't operate, little milk is available to the infant. The infant then gets frustrated, and this can frustrate the mother.

The let-down reflex is easily inhibited by nervous tension, a lack of confidence, and fatigue. First-time mothers should be especially aware of the link between tension and a weak let-down reflex. They need to find a relaxed and supportive environment where they can breast-feed.

After a few weeks, the let-down reflex becomes almost automatic. The mother's response can be triggered just by thoughts about the baby or by seeing or hearing another baby. But at first, the reflex can be a bit bewildering. Because she cannot measure the

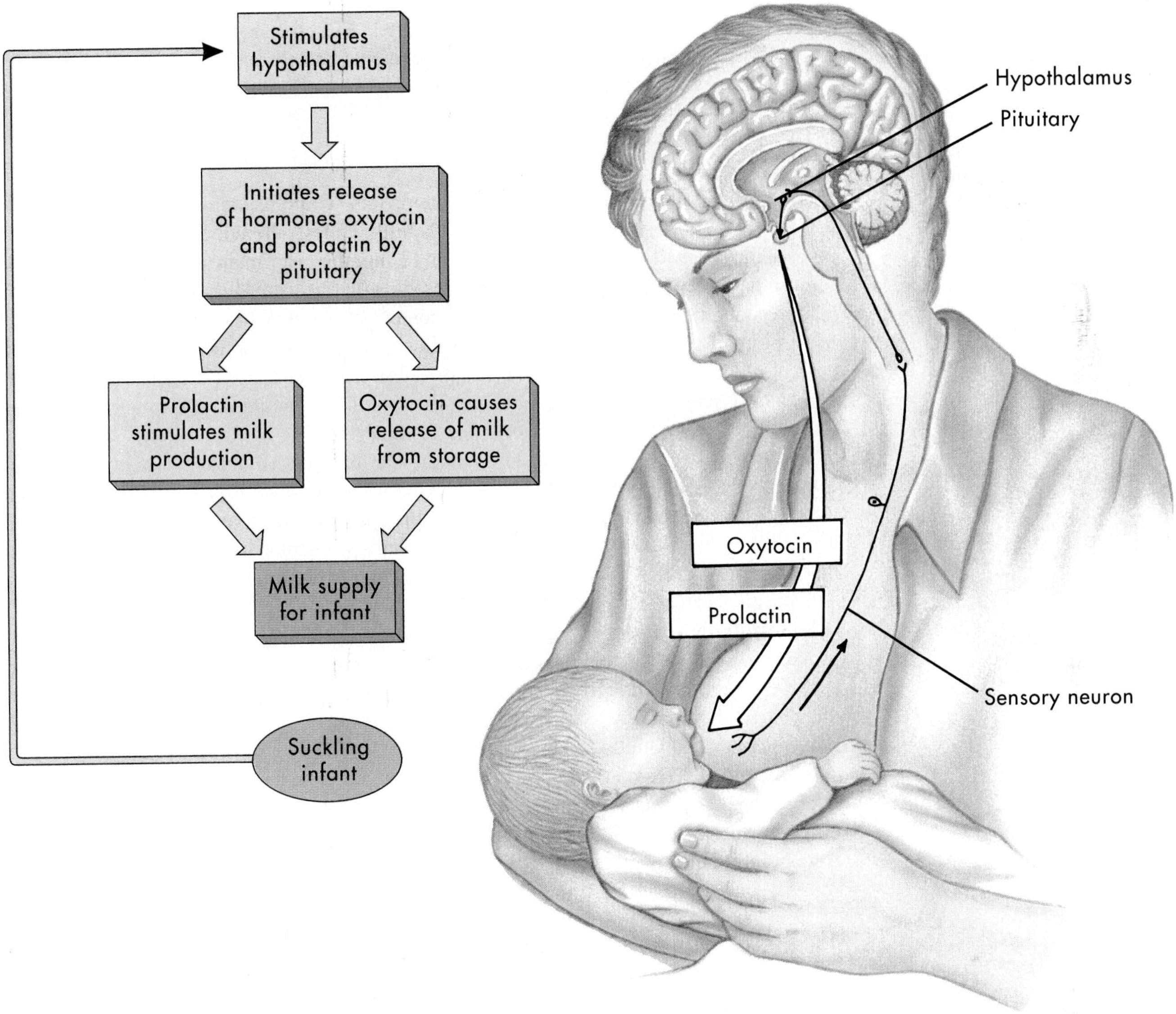

FIGURE 13-10
The let-down reflex. Suckling by the infant initiates hormonal changes in the mother—notably, prolactin and oxytocin release from the pituitary. This leads to milk production and the let-down reflex. This reflex releases the milk from storage cells in the breast.

amount of milk the infant takes in, a mother may fear that she is not adequately nourishing the baby. A good standard of comparison for a breast-fed baby is (1) it should have six or more wet diapers every day and show normal growth, (2) the stool should look like mustard (one to two stools every day is typical), and (3) the breast should soften during the feeding. If so, enough milk is being consumed.[23]

The parents need not be concerned that breast-fed infants grow a bit more slowly after about 3 months of age than do formula-fed infants. Weight gain is more affected than height gain.[9] The infant's physician is the best judge of whether the rate of growth of the breast-fed infant is satisfactory. Growth will likely catch up to that of formula-fed babies by 2 years of age.

It generally takes 2 to 3 weeks to fully establish a feeding routine.[15] By then infant and mother should both feel comfortable, the milk supply should meet infant demand, and

Disposable diapers can absorb so much urine that is difficult to judge when they are wet. A strip of paper towel laid inside a disposable diaper makes a good wetness indicator. Or, cloth diapers may be used for a day or two to assess whether nursing is supplying sufficient milk.

initial nipple soreness should have disappeared. Establishing the routine requires patience, but the rewards are great. The adjustments are easier if supplemental formula feedings are not introduced until breast-feeding is well-established. That occurs after about 2 to 3 months.

Human Milk is for Humans

Human milk is composed of lactose, protein, fats, vitamins, minerals, and other constituents. Its composition differs from cow's milk. Unless altered, cow's milk should not be used in infant feeding for the first 6 to 12 months. The main protein in cow's milk forms a hard curd that is hard to digest unless it is first heat-treated. Infant kidneys are not mature enough to handle the high mineral content of the milk (see Chapter 14). For those reasons, pediatric authorities advise against using cow's milk until the infant is at least 1 year old unless it is processed into a baby formula. In addition, certain compounds in human milk presently under study show other possible benefits for the infant. These factors are not present in cow's milk or infant formulas.[7]

Colostrum. The first milk made by the human breast is ***colostrum.*** This type of milk is produced a few days before birth through the week or so after birth. It is yellowish and thick. Colostrum contains immune factors that protect the infant from some diseases. These immune factors compensate for the infant's immature immune system in its first few months of life.[15] They are one reason that breast-fed infants have fewer respiratory and intestinal infections than formula-fed infants.

Colostrum has potent laxative properties that help the baby pass ***meconium,*** a stool produced during fetal life. One compound in colostrum, the ***Lactobacillus bifidus factor,*** encourages the growth of beneficial *Lactobacillus bifidus* bacteria. These bacteria limit the growth of potentially toxic bacteria in the intestine, such as *Escherichia coli,* and promote the intestinal health of the breast-fed infant.[23]

Mature Milk. Human milk composition gradually changes until several days after delivery, when it achieves the normal composition of mature milk. Human milk looks very different from cow's milk. (Table 14-1 in the next chapter provides a direct comparison.) Human milk is thin and almost watery in appearance and often has a slight bluish tinge. Its nutritional qualities are impressive, especially the quality of protein.

Human milk's main protein, lactalbumin, forms a soft, light curd in the infant's stomach, easing digestion.[23] The other proteins bind iron, reducing the growth of iron-requiring bacteria. Many of these types of bacteria cause diarrhea. Still other proteins offer the important immune protection already noted.

Human milk changes in fat composition during each feeding. The consistency of milk released initially (about 60% of the volume) resembles that of skim milk. The next amount (about 35% of the total volume) has a greater fat proportion, similar to whole milk. Finally, the hindmilk (about 5% of the total) is essentially like cream and is usually released 10 to 20 minutes into the feeding. Babies need to nurse long enough to get the kcalories in the rich hindmilk to be satisfied between feedings and grow well.

Human milk also allows for adequate hydration of the infant, provided the baby is exclusively breast-fed. A question commonly asked is whether the infant needs additional water, if stressed by diarrhea, vomiting, or fever. Extra water given with a physician's guidance may be required to prevent dehydration. Otherwise, breast-feeding should suffice.

A FOOD PLAN FOR WOMEN WHO BREAST-FEED

Nutrient needs for a breast-feeding mother change slightly, if at all, from those of the pregnant woman. Exceptions are decreases in folate and iron needs, and an increase in the need for energy, vitamins A and C, niacin, and zinc. The diet for breast-feeding women can be the same as that for pregnant women, except teenagers should add an additional serving from the milk, yogurt, and cheese group (see Table 13-2). Some researchers recommend eating fish at least twice a week, since the omega-3 fatty acids present in fish are thought to be important for brain development.[16] It is also important for the woman to drink fluids every time the baby nurses. A high fluid intake encourages ample milk production. If a woman restricts her energy intake too severely, the quantity of milk also decreases. This is not a time to crash diet.[15]

Milk production requires approximately 800 kcalories every day. The RDA for energy during lactation is an extra 500 kcalories daily above prepregnancy recommendations. The difference between kcalorie needs and intake should allow for gradual loss of the extra body fat accumulated during pregnancy, especially if breast-feeding is continued for 6 months or more. This shows how practical the link is between pregnancy and breast-feeding.[3] If the mother is physically active, she will need more kcalories.

another BITE

Most substances the mother ingests are secreted into her milk. For this reason, she should limit intake of or avoid all alcohol and caffeine and check all medications with a pediatrician. Some mothers believe that some foods, such as garlic and chocolate, flavor the breastmilk and upset the infant. If a woman notices a connection between a food she eats and the infant's later fussiness, she could consider avoiding that food. However, she might want to experiment again with it later. Infants become fussy for many reasons, and the suspected ingredient may not be the cause.

CONCEPT CHECK

Recognition of the importance of breast-feeding has contributed to its greater popularity during the last 20 years. Almost all women have the ability to breast-feed. The hormone prolactin stimulates breast tissue to synthesize milk. Some components of human milk come directly from the mother's bloodstream. Infant suckling triggers a let-down reflex that releases the milk. The more an infant nurses, the more milk is synthesized. The nutrient composition of human milk is very different from that of cow's milk and changes as the infant matures. The first milk, colostrum, is rich in immune factors. The diet for breast-feeding is generally similar to that for pregnancy, except for additional fluids, as well as an extra serving from the milk, yogurt, and cheese group for a teenage pregnancy.

DECIDING TO BREAST-FEED

Advantages of Breast-Feeding

Human milk is tailored to meet infant nutrient needs for the first 4 to 6 months of life. The possible exceptions are the relative lack of fluoride, iron, and vitamin D. Infant supplements, given under the guidance of a pediatrician, can supply these. Fluoride may be found in the household water supply. If it is not present in adequate amounts or the child is not receiving tap water, a fluoride supplement should be considered. A dentist should be consulted. Regular sun exposure for the infant can supply needed vitamin D. Vitamin B-12 supplements are recommended for the breast-fed infant if the mother is a complete vegetarian (vegan). Although formula feeding can satisfy the infant, mother, and the rest of the family (see Chapter 14), breast-feeding offers many physiological and practical advantages.[1,23]

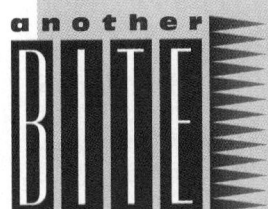

Fewer Infections. Breast-feeding reduces the general risk of infections to the infant. This is partially because of the immune bodies in human milk that an infant can use. As already mentioned, these reduce the risk of respiratory and intestinal infections. Breastfed infants also have fewer ear infections, because they do not sleep with a bottle in the mouth. We strongly discourage allowing any infant to sleep with a bottle in its mouth, because when that happens, milk pools there, backs up through the throat, and eventually settles in the ears, creating a growth medium for bacteria. Infant ear infections are a common problem. By avoiding them, parents can decrease discomfort for the infant and trips to the doctor and prevent possible hearing loss. Tooth decay from nighttime bottles is also likely (see Chapter 14).

Fewer Allergies and Intolerances. Breast-feeding reduces the chances of allergies, especially in allergy-prone infants (see the Nutrition Issue in Chapter 14). Cow's milk contains a number of potential allergy-causing proteins that are missing from human milk. Infants tolerate human milk better than they do formulas. Formulas must sometimes be switched several times until caregivers find one the infant thrives on.

Convenience. Breast-feeding frees the mother from the time and expense involved in buying and preparing formula and washing bottles. Breast milk is ready to go and sterile. This allows the mother to spend more time with her baby. On the other hand, if the child is bottle-fed, the mother may be freed to do other things while others feed the baby. This trade-off needs to be considered.

Barriers to Breast-Feeding

A lack of role models, widespread misinformation, fear of appearing immodest, and working away from the children all serve as barriers to breast-feeding.[8]

Misinformation. Probably the major barriers to breast-feeding are misinformation and lack of role models. If a woman is interested in breast-feeding, she should talk to women who have done it successfully. Experienced mothers can be an enormous help to the first-time mother. She should find a friend she can call on to ask questions. In almost every community, a group called La Leche League offers classes in breast-feeding and advises women who have problems with it.

Returning to an Outside Job. Working outside the home can complicate plans to breast-feed. One possibility after a month or two of breast-feeding is for the mother to regularly express and save her own milk. She can express milk using a breast pump or by hand into a sterile plastic bottle or nursing bag (used in a disposable bottle system). Saving breastmilk requires careful sanitation and rapid chilling. It can be stored in the refrigerator for 1 day and be frozen for 1 month. There is a knack to learning how to express milk, but the freedom can be worth it. Then others can feed the mother's milk to the infant.

Frozen human milk should not be thawed in a microwave. The heat can destroy immune factors in the milk and create hot spots that can scald the infant's tongue.

Some women can juggle both a job and breast-feeding, but others find it too cumbersome and decide instead to formula-feed. A compromise—balancing some breast-feedings, say early morning and night, with formula-feedings during the day—is possible. However, too many supplemental feedings decrease milk production.

another BITE

A schedule of expressing milk and using supplemental formula-feedings is most successful if begun after 1 to 2 months of exclusive breast-feeding. After 2 months, the baby is well adapted to breast-feeding and probably feels enough emotional security and other benefits from nursing that it is willing to drink both ways.

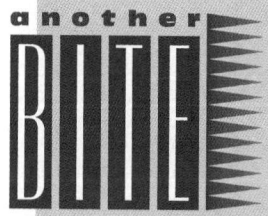

The key months for breast-feeding are the first 2 to 3 months of an infant's life. A longer commitment is even better. The American Academy of Pediatrics recommends it exclusively for the first 4 to 6 months, and as a supplement with solid food for the second 6 months of life. But the first few months are critically important ones. During that time, human milk provides the antiinfective properties needed until the infant begins to synthesize his or her own immune factors in high concentrations.

Social Reticence. Another barrier for some women is embarrassment when nursing a child in public. Our society historically has stressed modesty and frowned on baring breasts in public—even in so good a cause as nourishing babies. With appropriate clothing, it is possible to nurse quite discreetly.

When Is Breast-Feeding Not a Good Idea?

Mothers should not breast-feed their infants if they don't want to do so. There are distinct advantages to breast-feeding, but none so great that a woman who decides to bottle-feed should feel she is penalizing her infant.

Because human milk contains much phenylalanine, it often cannot be fed to infants with the disease phenylketonuria. Infants with galactosemia cannot be fed human milk because of the great amount of galactose in it (see Chapter 7). Mothers who take medications that pass into the milk and adversely affect the child also should not breast-feed. In addition, a woman who has a serious chronic disease, such as tuberculosis or hepatitis, or is being treated for cancer should not breast-feed.

What About Environmental Contaminants in Human Milk?

Some women wonder whether breast-feeding is safe. There is some legitimate concern over the levels of various environmental contaminants in human milk. But the benefits from human milk are very well established, and the risks from environmental contaminants are still largely theoretical. Thus it is probably best to operate with what we know works until sufficiently strong research data dissuade us.

A few measures a woman could take to counteract some known contaminants are to (1) avoid freshwater fish from polluted waters, (2) carefully wash and peel fruits and vegetables, and (3) remove the fatty edges of meat. In addition, a woman should not try to lose weight rapidly while nursing, because contaminants stored in fat tissue then enter her bloodstream and, in turn, her milk. If a woman questions whether her milk is safe, especially if she has lived in an area known to have a high concentration of toxic wastes or environmental pollution, she should consult her local health department.

Can a Premature Infant Be Breast-Fed?

There is no clear-cut answer to whether a woman can breast-feed a premature infant.[23] In some cases, human milk is the most desirable form of nourishment. If so, it must usually be expressed from the breast and fed through a tube. This type of feeding demands great maternal dedication. Fortification of the milk with such nutrients as calcium, phosphorus, sodium, and protein is often needed to match an infant's rapid growth. In other cases, special feeding problems may prevent using human milk or necessitate supplementing it with formula. Sometimes intravenous nutrition is the only option. Working as a team, the pediatrician, neonatal nurses, and registered dietitian guide the parents in this decision.

CONCEPT CHECK

Human milk provides most of an infant's nutritional needs for the first 6 months. Vitamin D, iron, and fluoride may be supplemented. The advantages of breast-feeding over formula-feeding include fewer intestinal, respiratory, and ear infections; fewer allergies and food intolerances; and convenience. Lack of role models, misinformation, and social reticence may dissuade a mother from breast-feeding. A combination of breast-feeding and formula-feeding is possible when a mother is regularly away from her infant. Breast-feeding is not desirable if a mother has certain diseases or must take medication potentially harmful to the infant. The premature infant, depending on its condition, may benefit from consuming human milk.

SUMMARY

- Adequate nutrition is vital during pregnancy to ensure the well-being of both the infant and the mother. Insults from poor nutrition and some medications can cause birth defects, especially if they occur in the first trimester. Growth retardation and altered development are possible if insults occur later in pregnancy.
- Infants born prematurely (before 37 weeks of gestation) or with low birth weight (less than 5.5 pounds or 2.5 kilograms) usually have more medical problems at birth than do full-term infants.
- Daily energy needs increase by an average of 300 kcalories during the last two trimesters of a pregnancy. Weight gain should be gradual to a total of 25 to 35 pounds in a normal-weight mother.
- Protein, vitamin, and mineral requirements increase during pregnancy. Iron and folate status deserve a careful evaluation. Three servings from the milk, yogurt, and cheese group (four if a teenager), in addition to the other recommendations of the Food Guide Pyramid, are recommended. Supplements of iron and folate, in particular, may be needed.
- Teenage pregnancy requires very careful prenatal and nutritional care. Complications are more common in teenage pregnancies because of the very high physiological demands and often poor social and economic support.
- Pregnancy-induced hypertension, heartburn, constipation, nausea, vomiting, edema, and anemia are all possible discomforts and complications of pregnancy. Nutritional therapy can often help minimize these problems.
- The popularity of breast-feeding has increased in the past 20 years. Almost all women have the ability to nurse their infants. The nutrient composition of human milk is very different from that of cow's milk. Colostrum, the first milk produced by humans, is very rich in immune factors. Mature milk is rich in important proteins.
- For the infant, advantages of breast-feeding over formula-feeding include fewer intestinal, respiratory, and ear infections; fewer allergies and food intolerances; and convenience. An infant can be adequately nourished with formula if the mother chooses not to breast-feed. Breast-feeding is not desirable if the mother has certain diseases or must take medication potentially harmful to the infant.

STUDY QUESTIONS

1. What historical evidence establishes the importance of nutrition in pregnancy outcome?
2. Provide three key pieces of advice for a couple who are seeking to maximize their chances of having a healthy baby. Why did you single out those specific factors?
3. What health problems can a woman possibly expect to develop during pregnancy? What nutrition-related advice can you provide to help prevent these problems from developing into serious conditions?
4. Give three reasons why a woman should give serious consideration to breast-feeding her infant.
5. Describe the physiological links between milk production and release. How does knowing about these help you provide more informed advice to nursing mothers?

REFERENCES

1. ADA Reports: Position of the American Dietetic Association: Promotion and support of breast-feeding, *Journal of the American Dietetic Association* 93:467, 1993.
2. Belizan JM and others: Calcium supplementation to prevent hypertensive disorders of pregnancy, *The New England Journal of Medicine* 325:1399, 1991.
3. Boyne L: Nutrition in pregnancy, *Nutri-News* 5:10, 1992.
4. Buescher PA and others: Prenatal WIC participation can reduce low birth weight and newborn medical costs, *Journal of the American Dietetic Association* 93:163, 1993.
5. Butterworth CE: Folate status, women's health, pregnancy outcome, and cancer, *Journal of the American College of Nutrition* 12:438, 1993.
6. Czeizel AE, Dudas I: Prevention of the first occurrence of neural-tube defects by periconceptional vitamin supplementation, *The New England Journal of Medicine* 327:1832, 1992.
7. Ellis LA, Picciano MF: Milk-borne hormones: regulators of development in neonates, *Nutrition Today,* p. 6, September/October 1992.
8. Freed GL: Breast-feeding: Time to teach what we preach, *Journal of the American Medical Association* 269:243, 1993.
9. Heinig MJ and others: Energy and protein intakes of breast-fed and formula-fed infants during their first year of life and their association with growth velocity: the DARLING Study, *American Journal of Clinical Nutrition,* 58:152, 1993.
10. Horner RD and others: Pica practices of pregnant women, *Journal of the American Dietetic Association* 91:34, 1991.
11. Lederman SA: Recent issues related to nutrition during pregnancy, *Journal of the American College of Nutrition* 12:101, 1993.
12. McGrew MC, Shore WB: The problem of teenage pregnancy, *The Journal of Family Practice* 32:17, 1991.
13. Mills JL and others: Moderate caffeine use and the risk of spontaneous abortion and interuterine growth retardation, *Journal of the American Medical Association* 269:593, 1993.
14. National Academy of Sciences—Institute of Medicine: *Nutrition during pregnancy,* Washington, DC, 1990, National Academy of Sciences Press.
15. National Academy of Sciences—Institute of Medicine: *Nutrition during lactation,* Washington, DC, 1991, National Academy of Sciences Press.
16. Nettleton, JE: Are n-3 fatty acids essential nutrients for fetal and infant development? *Journal of the American Dietetic Association* 93:58, 1993.
17. Rees JM and others: Weight gain in adolescents during pregnancy: rate related to birth-weight outcome, *American Journal of Clinical Nutrition* 56:868, 1992.
18. Resnick R: The "elderly primigravida" in 1990, *The New England Journal of Medicine* 322:693, 1990.
19. Streissguth AP and others: Fetal alcohol syndrome in adolescents and adults, *Journal of the American Medical Association* 265:1961, 1991.
20. Volpe JJ: Effect of cocaine use on the fetus, *The New England Journal of Medicine* 327:399, 1992.
21. Werler MM and others: Maternal alcohol use in relation to selected birth defects, *American Journal of Epidemiology* 134:691, 1991.
22. White J: Exercising for two—what's safe for the active pregnant woman? *The Physician and Sportsmedicine* 20:179, 1992.
23. Worthington-Roberts B and others: *Nutrition in pregnancy and lactation,* St Louis, 1993, Mosby–Year Book.

RATE your plate

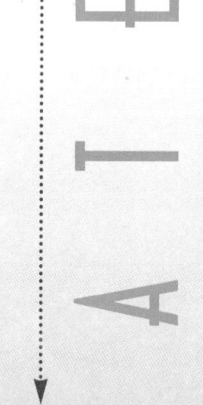

TARGETING NECESSARY NUTRIENTS FOR A PREGNANT WOMAN

In this chapter, we mentioned that the nutrient needs hardest to meet during pregnancy are *folate, vitamin D, iron, calcium,* and *zinc.* Refer to Chapters 9 and 10 to find five foods rich in each nutrient. List them next to the appropriate heading below.

Nutrient	**Foods**	
Folate	1	4
	2	5
	3	
Vitamin D	1	4
	2	5
	3	
Iron	1	4
	2	5
	3	
Calcium	1	4
	2	5
	3	
Zinc	1	4
	2	5
	3	

Did you list any foods next to more than one nutrient? What are they?

____

____

Foods rich in more than one of these nutrients would be doubly useful and valuable. Those foods would be ones to focus on when pregnant.

Are there any reasons that it might be hard for a person to get the needed amount of these nutrients?

____

____

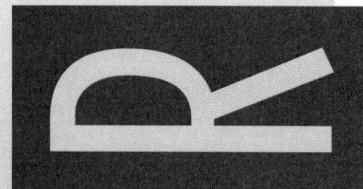

Nutrition ISSUE

FETAL ALCOHOL SYNDROME

Although we know a great deal about diagnosing and treating some learning problems in children, many causes remain elusive. One particular question haunts many mothers: Did something happen while I was pregnant that created a learning disability for my child? This puzzle makes alcohol use during pregnancy a very important issue, especially because alcohol is the most common damaging substance fetuses are exposed to.

Scientists do not know whether alcohol must be totally eliminated from the diet, but there is no question that large amounts of alcohol harm the fetus. Until a safe level can be established, it is recommended that women not drink alcohol at all during pregnancy. When the mother drinks more alcohol than she can metabolize, the excess reaches the fetus, which has no means for detoxifying it. Women suffering from chronic alcoholism produce children with a recognizable pattern of malformations called ***fetal alcohol syndrome (FAS).***[19] A diagnosis of FAS is based mainly on poor prenatal and infant growth, physical deformities (especially of facial features), and mental retardation (Figure 13-11). The infant is frequently irritable and proceeds to develop hyperactivity and a short attention span. Poor hand-eye coordination is not uncommon.

The range of abnormalities varies from severe FAS to reduced birth weight, behavioral effects, growth retardation, and poor learning ability in infants born to women who report only social drinking. The latter category is termed *fetal alcohol effects (FAE).*[19] Without

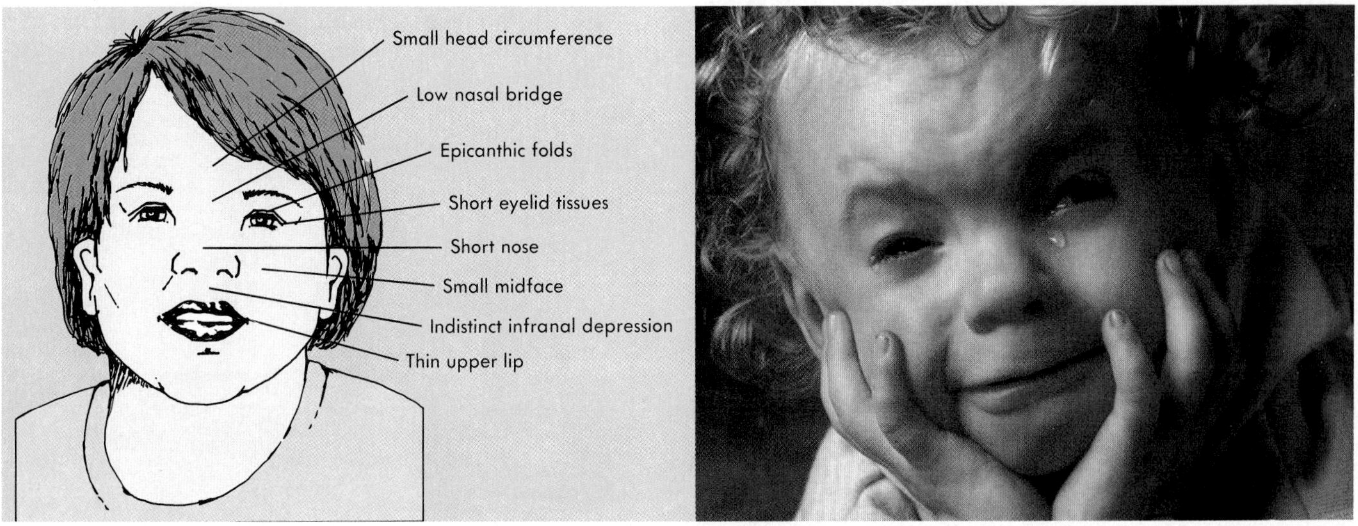

FIGURE 13-11
Fetal alcohol syndrome. Milder forms of alcohol-induced changes on the fetus and the infant are known as fetal alcohol effects.

the clue from the classic facial abnormalities to alert them to the condition's presence, parents may not suspect the presence of subtle defects caused by alcohol. Yet they may exist and can devastate learning potential. Annually, about 4000 to 7000 infants are born in the United States with FAS, and about 30,000 are born with FAE. This makes alcohol the leading cause of preventable birth defects and mental retardation in the United States.[21] Binge drinking is perilous, especially during the first 12 weeks of pregnancy since the signs of pregnancy are few and key aspects of fetal development take place.

Exactly how alcohol causes these defects is not known. One line of research shows faulty cell migration in the brain during early stages of development in the presence of alcohol. Most likely, other factors—such as poor nutrition, cigarette smoking (nicotine intake), and other drug use—also contribute to the overall result. We further do not know how much alcohol it takes to produce the effects. Again, for this reason many authorities—including the U.S. Surgeon General and the American Medical Association—believe it is best that mothers-to-be avoid alcohol altogether. Abstinence is especially important during the first trimester when key growth and development occur. Alcohol reaches the fetal blood at the same concentration as the mother's blood within 15 minutes of her drinking. However, the effect on the fetus may be up to 10 times greater.

Just one bout of binge drinking can arrest and alter cell division occurring during a critical phase of fetal development. The fetus then may develop with an irreversible defect. Physical damage to the fetus results more from first-trimester drinking, because tissues and organs are being developed; emotional and learning problems stem more from third-trimester drinking, because the brain is in a critical stage of development. And throughout the pregnancy, alcohol interferes with growth.[21]

Because alcohol has the capacity to adversely affect each stage of fetal development, the earlier in pregnancy that heavy drinking ceases, the greater the potential for improved outcome. The best course is to consider alcohol an indulgence that can be eliminated until after pregnancy. It is important for pregnant women to abstain from alcohol not only during pregnancy, but also when trying to conceive and any time conception is possible. One step in the right direction is the new congressionally mandated warnings about drinking during pregnancy that appear on all alcoholic beverage containers. Recall that many women are not aware they are pregnant until 2 to 3 months after conception. Pregnancy lasts only 9 months. Parents may spend a lifetime caring for their needlessly handicapped offspring.

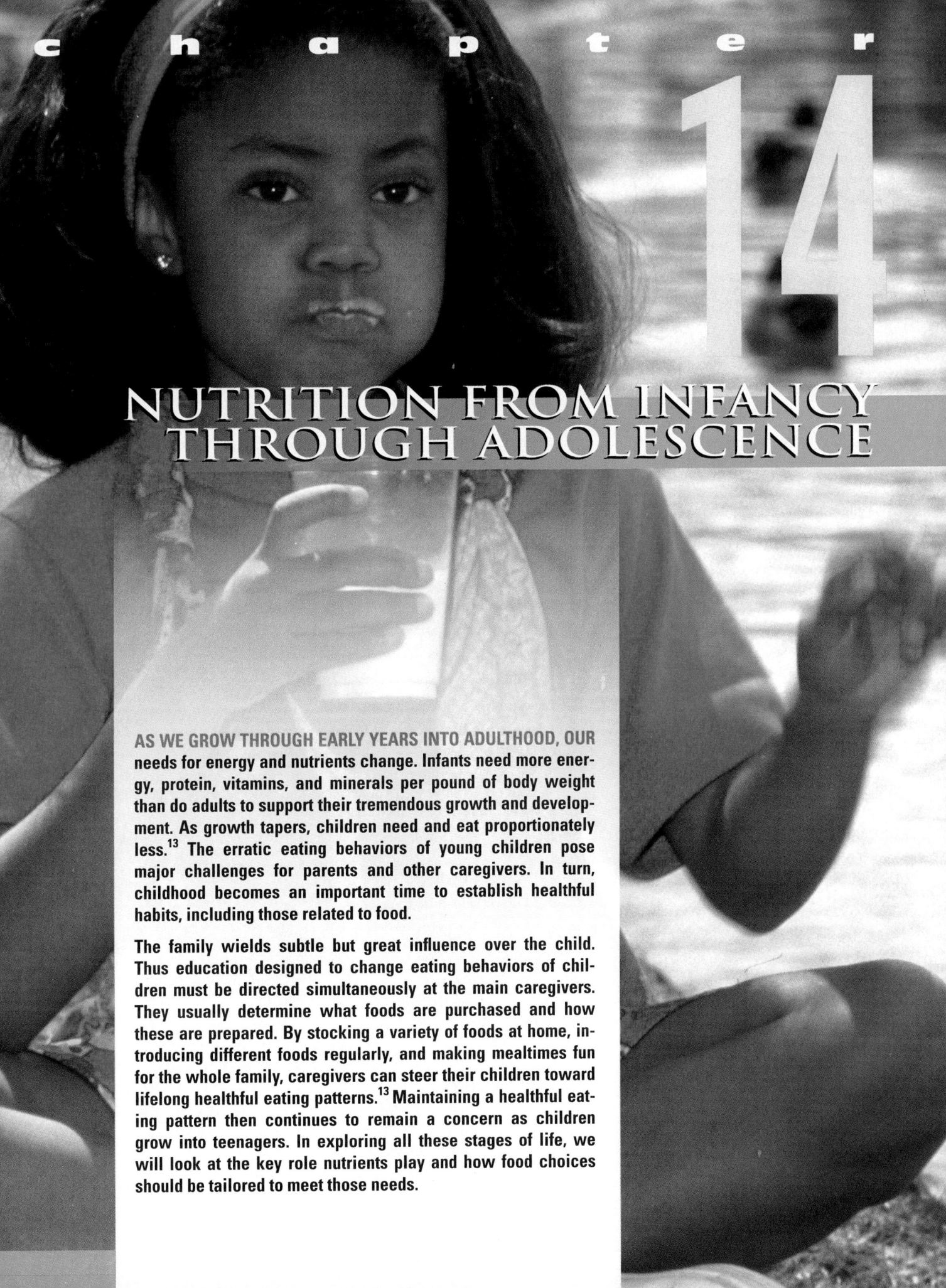

chapter 14

NUTRITION FROM INFANCY THROUGH ADOLESCENCE

AS WE GROW THROUGH EARLY YEARS INTO ADULTHOOD, OUR needs for energy and nutrients change. Infants need more energy, protein, vitamins, and minerals per pound of body weight than do adults to support their tremendous growth and development. As growth tapers, children need and eat proportionately less.[13] The erratic eating behaviors of young children pose major challenges for parents and other caregivers. In turn, childhood becomes an important time to establish healthful habits, including those related to food.

The family wields subtle but great influence over the child. Thus education designed to change eating behaviors of children must be directed simultaneously at the main caregivers. They usually determine what foods are purchased and how these are prepared. By stocking a variety of foods at home, introducing different foods regularly, and making mealtimes fun for the whole family, caregivers can steer their children toward lifelong healthful eating patterns.[13] Maintaining a healthful eating pattern then continues to remain a concern as children grow into teenagers. In exploring all these stages of life, we will look at the key role nutrients play and how food choices should be tailored to meet those needs.

ASSESS YOURSELF

TEST YOUR KNOWLEDGE

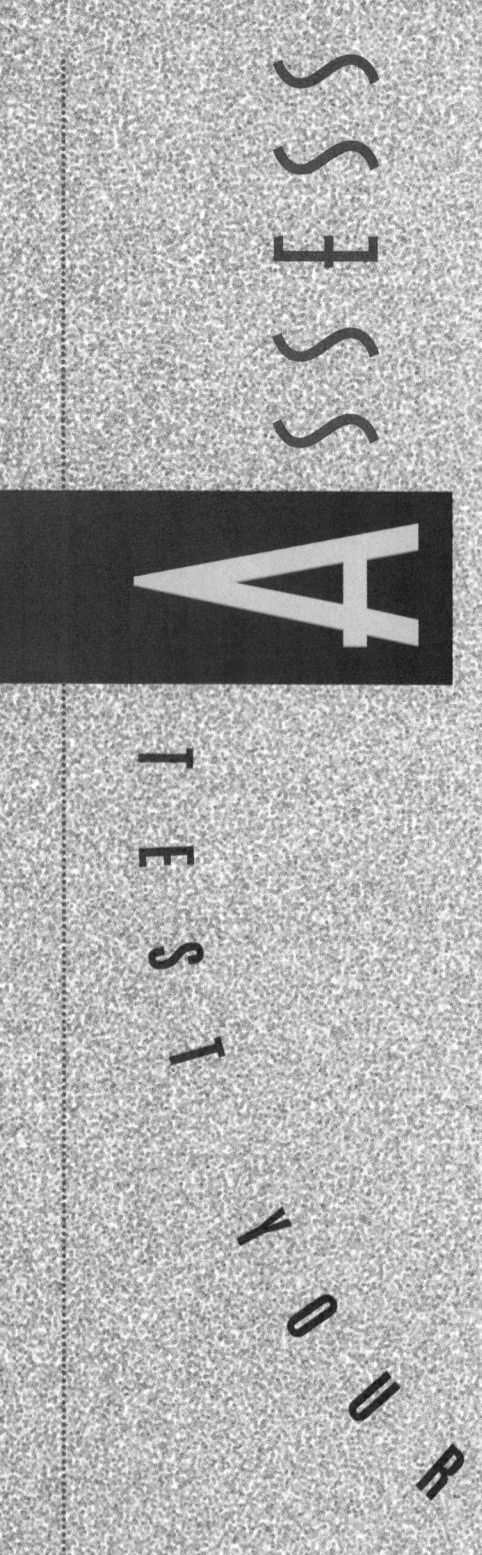

AVOIDING TABLE WARS

If you have children or have ever worked as a babysitter, you probably know how difficult it can be to get kids to eat on command. The problem doesn't go away—caregivers also worry later about the eating habits of their teenagers. During adolescence, teenagers establish their own identities and their busy lifestyles leave little time for structured eating.

How can household wars about eating be avoided? Listed below are some statements about children and adolescents and their eating habits. Which are true? Place a "T" in the blank to the left if you think the statement is true, or an "F" if false. If caregivers know the truths, they possibly can avoid table wars.

____ **1.** Around 9 to 10 months of age, infants explore, test, and play with food. Unless they are disciplined to eat neatly and treat food seriously, they will be undisciplined eaters in the future.

____ **2.** Expect babies to take only two or three bites of solid food at first meals.

____ **3.** Infants enjoy bland foods much more than do adults.

____ **4.** Infants should be encouraged to consume a lot of apple juice, because it's rich in so many nutrients.

____ **5.** Honey is a good sweetener for infants because it has a high nutrient content.

____ **6.** Toddlers typically have less appetite than they had during the first year of life.

____ **7.** You can normally expect children to avoid vegetables and whole grains.

____ **8.** Adult modeling of good eating habits influences a child's behavior.

____ **9.** A good policy is the one-bite rule, which asks children to take at least one bite of the foods presented to them.

____ **10.** Children like foods with soft textures and strong flavors.

____ **11.** Children should be made to eat three meals a day, rather than many small meals.

____ **12.** Children often object to having foods mixed, as in stews and casseroles.

____ **13.** Children should be forced to eat.

____ **14.** Infants and children of all ages should eat low-fat diets to decrease their risk of future heart disease.

____ **15.** Teenagers are more likely to try healthful foods when immediate positive outcomes are emphasized—such as their contributions to a better appearance and physique—as opposed to when potential future health hazards from a poor diet are stressed.

____ **16.** Involving teenagers in cooking and purchasing food helps promote good eating habits.

True: 2, 3, 6, 8, 9, 12, 15, 16
False: 1, 4, 5, 7, 10, 11, 13, 14

INFANT GROWTH AND PHYSIOLOGICAL DEVELOPMENT

During infancy a child's attitudes toward foods and the whole eating process begin to take shape. If parents and other caregivers practice good nutrition and are flexible, they can lead a child into lifelong beneficial food habits. Such an infant has a good chance of starting life with the nutrients needed to support brain and body growth spurts and to develop a willingness to try new foods. However, these physical and psychological advantages alone do not guarantee that a child will thrive. Children additionally need specific attention focused on them; they need to grow in a stimulating environment, and they need a sense of security.[17] Children hospitalized for growth failure tend to gain weight more quickly when tender loving care accompanies needed nutrients.

We use the term *parents* in this chapter, realizing that some infants and children are raised by caregivers other than their true biological parents.

The Growing Infant

It seems that all babies do is eat and sleep. There is a good reason for this. An infant's birth weight doubles in the first 4 to 6 months and triples within the first year. Such rapid growth requires a lot of both nourishment and sleep. Beyond the first year, growth is slower; it takes 5 more years to double the weight seen at 1 year. An infant also increases in length in the first year by 50% and then continues to gain height throughout preschool and teen years.[13] These gains are not necessarily continuous—spurts of growth alternate with plateaus. Height is essentially complete by age 19, though increases of several inches may occur in the early 20s (Figure 14-1). Head size in proportion to total height shrinks from one fourth to one eighth during the climb from infancy to adulthood.

The human body needs a lot more food to support growth and development than to merely maintain itself once growth ceases. In some populations, food is not regularly available. When nutrients are missing at critical phases of growth and development, growth slows and may even stop. From observations of Egyptian mummies, we see that infants were about the same size in 300 BC as they are today. However, adult mummies are much smaller than adults today. Also, the small suits of armor in museum collections

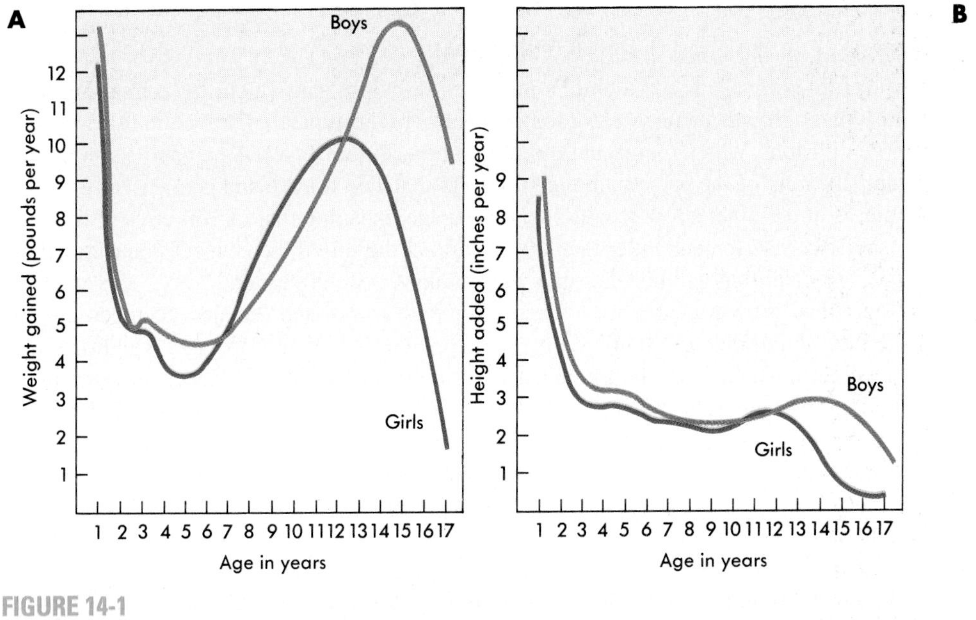

FIGURE 14-1

*Growth rates. **A,** Average gains in weight for girls and boys. **B,** Average additions to height for girls and boys. The higher the line in any one year, the greater the amount of gain compared to other years. Note the great degree of length gained in infancy. Large gains in weight occur in infancy and at puberty. Note also that if parceled into smaller time segments, graphs such as these would show growth spurts spiking from the smooth lines. Growth takes place in spurts, rather than in a steady manner.*

of the Middle Ages indicate that people of that time generally ate nutrient-poor diets that did not support the growth we typically experience today.

In Third World countries today, about half the children are short and underweight for their ages. Poor nutrition—called undernutrition—is at the heart of the problem. This occurs to a lesser extent in America. The undernourished children are simply smaller versions of nutritionally fit children. In poorer countries, when breast-feeding ceases, children are often fed a high-carbohydrate, low-protein diet. This diet supports some growth but does not allow children to attain their genetic potential. To grow, children must consume adequate amounts of protein and other nutrients.

Weight primarily reflects current nutrient intake. Height is a measure of long-term nutrient intake.

Infant development follows a pattern in which body water reduces from about 75% at birth to 60% at 1 year. The latter is also the proportion typical in adults. By 1 year of age an infant's body nitrogen content (and so, protein content) has increased from 2% of body weight at birth to 3%, indicating the infant has synthesized much new lean tissue.[13]

In Utero *In the uterus; in other words, during pregnancy.*

The Effect of Undernutrition on Growth

As with the fetus *in utero,* the long-term effects of nutritional problems in infancy and childhood depend on the severity, timing, and duration of the nutritional insult to cell processes.

Probably the single best indicator of a child's nutritional status is growth.[17] Mild zinc deficiencies in children in the United States have been linked to poor growth. Improving the diets of these children then leads to improved growth. Overall, eating a poor diet as an infant or child hampers cell division that occurs at that critical stage. Getting an adequate diet later usually won't compensate for lost growth, because high levels of key hormones are then missing from the bloodstream, though they were present during the critical time when cells should have been divided. For example, a 15-year-old Central-American girl who is 4 feet 8 inches tall cannot attain the adult height of a typical American simply by now eating better. Girls experience their peak rate of growth before the onset of the menses. Once the time for growth ceases (in women this is about 2 years after they start menstruating), a good nutrient intake will help maintain health and weight but will not make up for all lost growth.

Assessing Infant Growth and Development

Health professionals assess a child's increases in height and weight by comparing these with typical growth patterns recorded on charts.[13] The typical charts contain seven percentile divisions, which represent 90% of children (Figure 14-2). A percentile simply represents the rank of the person among 100 peers matched for age and gender. Tony, for example, is at the ninetieth percentile height for age, meaning that of 100 boys of that age, he is shorter than ten and taller than 89. A child at the fiftieth percentile is considered average. Fifty children will be taller than this child; 49 will be shorter.

Individual growth charts are available for both males and females, for ages ranging from 0 to 36 months or 2 to 18 years (see Appendix L). Height-for-age, weight-for-age, and weight-for-height can be plotted. Infants and children should have their growth assessed during regular health checkups. It takes 1 to 3 years for an infant to establish his or her own genetic percentile. Once this figure is established, such as length-(height)-for-age, the child's measurement should then track along that percentile. If the child's growth does not keep up with its length-for-age percentile, a physician needs to investigate whether a medical or nutritional problem is impeding the predicted growth. Inappropriate weight gain—too little or too much—should also be investigated.

Children under 2 to 3 years of age are measured with knees unflexed and while lying on their backs, and so the term length is used rather than height.

Infants born prematurely may catch up in growth in 2 to 3 years. This requires that the child jump up in the percentiles. If this occurs—especially in length-for-age—it is usually no cause for alarm. On the other hand, jumping percentiles in weight-for-height can be disturbing if the child approaches the eightieth to ninetieth percentiles. Generally a child at the ninetieth percentile for weight-for-height is considered overweight. Above the ninety-fifth percentile, the child is considered obese.[14]

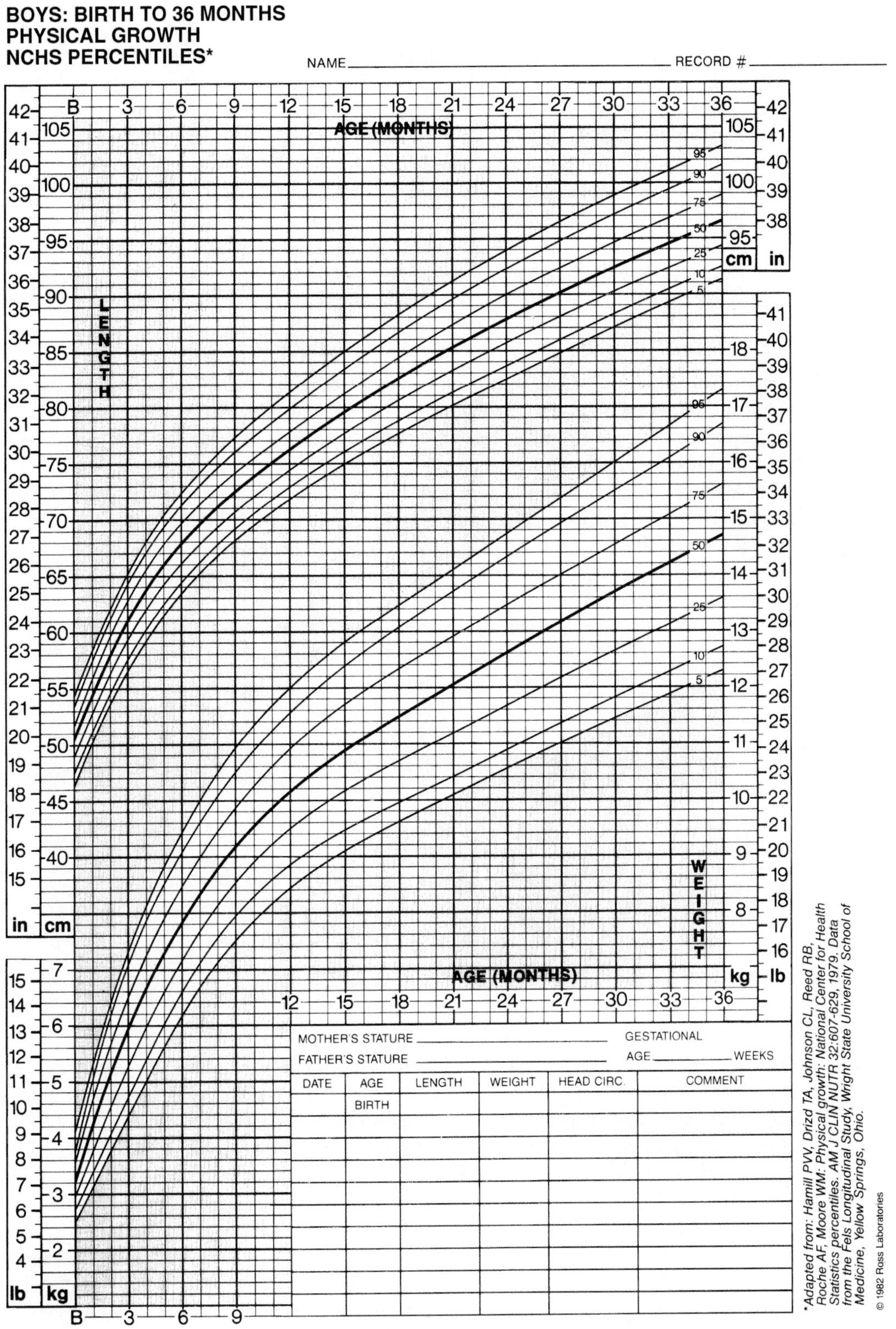

FIGURE 14-2

Growth charts used to assess height (length) and weight in young boys. A certain weight and height (length) corresponds to a percentile value, which is a ranking of the person among 100 peers. See Appendix L for charts that apply to young girls and older children.

Brain Growth

The brain grows faster around the time of birth than at any other time of life. To accommodate the growth, an infant's head must be very large in proportion to the rest of the body. The rapid growth stops between 12 and 15 months of age. The rest of the body eventually grows to fit the head. In early physical checkups, a health professional usually measures the head circumference as another means of assessing growth, especially brain growth. How nutritional status affects brain development and intelligence quotient (IQ) is difficult to measure, because we haven't figured out how to separate the effects of nature from nurture. However, studies from Central America suggest that IQ after age 5 years relates more closely to the amount of schooling a child receives than to nutritional intake during childhood.

Adipose (Fat) Tissue Growth

Since 1970, researchers have speculated that overfeeding during infancy may increase fat tissue cell numbers. Today, we know that fat cells can also increase as adulthood obesity develops (see Chapter 10). Still, if energy intake is limited during infancy to keep down fat cell number, the growth of other organ systems may also be severely retarded. Special concern revolves especially around proper brain and nervous system development. In addition, most obese infants become normal-weight preschoolers. So it is unwise to restrict diet, and especially fat intake, before 2 years of age. About 40% of kcalories from fat is recommended.[13] As mentioned earlier, without adequate nutrients, infants are unlikely to eventually attain their potential adult height.

CONCEPT CHECK

Growth occurs rapidly during infancy: birth weight doubles in 4 to 6 months and triples within the first year. Lean tissue increases, and the percentage of body water falls during infancy. Undernutrition can irreversibly inhibit growth and maturation. Infant and child growth is assessed by tracking body weight, height (or length), and head circumference over time. It is undesirable for infants to become obese, although no evidence strongly indicates that obese infants become obese adults.

Failure to Thrive

Occasionally an infant does not grow much in the first few months. Physical problems that may contribute to retarded growth range from poor oral cavity development, infections, and heart irregularities to constant diarrhea associated with intestinal problems. However, more than half the infants who fail to thrive have no apparent disease. Poor infant-parent interaction is the typical cause.[2] This stems from misinformation, no parent role model, or apathy about the child's welfare. Overall, the problems often arise from the parents' inexperience, rather than intentional negligence.

Infants need cuddling, and they respond to voices and eye contact, especially at feeding times. New parents need to appreciate the importance of these practices to their infant's well-being. Some parents are also overcommitted to maintaining a lean child in hopes of preventing future obesity, as we discussed in Chapter 12. The result, even though well-meaning, can be a child's failure to thrive.

When clinicians encounter an infant who is failing to thrive, they must first determine whether the child is consuming enough energy. For infants, approximately 45 kcalories per pound (95 kcalories per kilogram) of body weight daily is adequate in early infancy. By 6 months of age, closer to 40 kcalories per pound (85 kcalories per kilogram) is recommended. For a breast-fed infant, the clinician needs to make sure that sufficient milk is being consumed. The child should be nursing about six to eight times a day for about 20 minutes a session and have six to eight wet diapers each day. The mother should consume adequate food and fluid (see Chapter 13). Children older than 2 years are less likely to experience failure to thrive because they can often get food for themselves. Younger children are limited to what the caregivers provide.

INFANT NUTRITIONAL NEEDS

Infants' nutrient needs vary as they grow, and these differ from adult needs in both amount and proportion (Figure 14-3). Initially, human milk or formula supplies needed nutrients. Solid foods are usually not needed until after 4 to 6 months.[13] Even after solid foods are added, the basis of an infant's diet for the first year is still human milk or formula.

Energy

As mentioned earlier, infants need about 40 to 45 kcalories per pound of body weight daily (85 to 95 kcalories per kilogram) to supply them adequate energy. At 6 months of age this amounts to about 750 kcalories daily. Based on body weight, this amounts to two

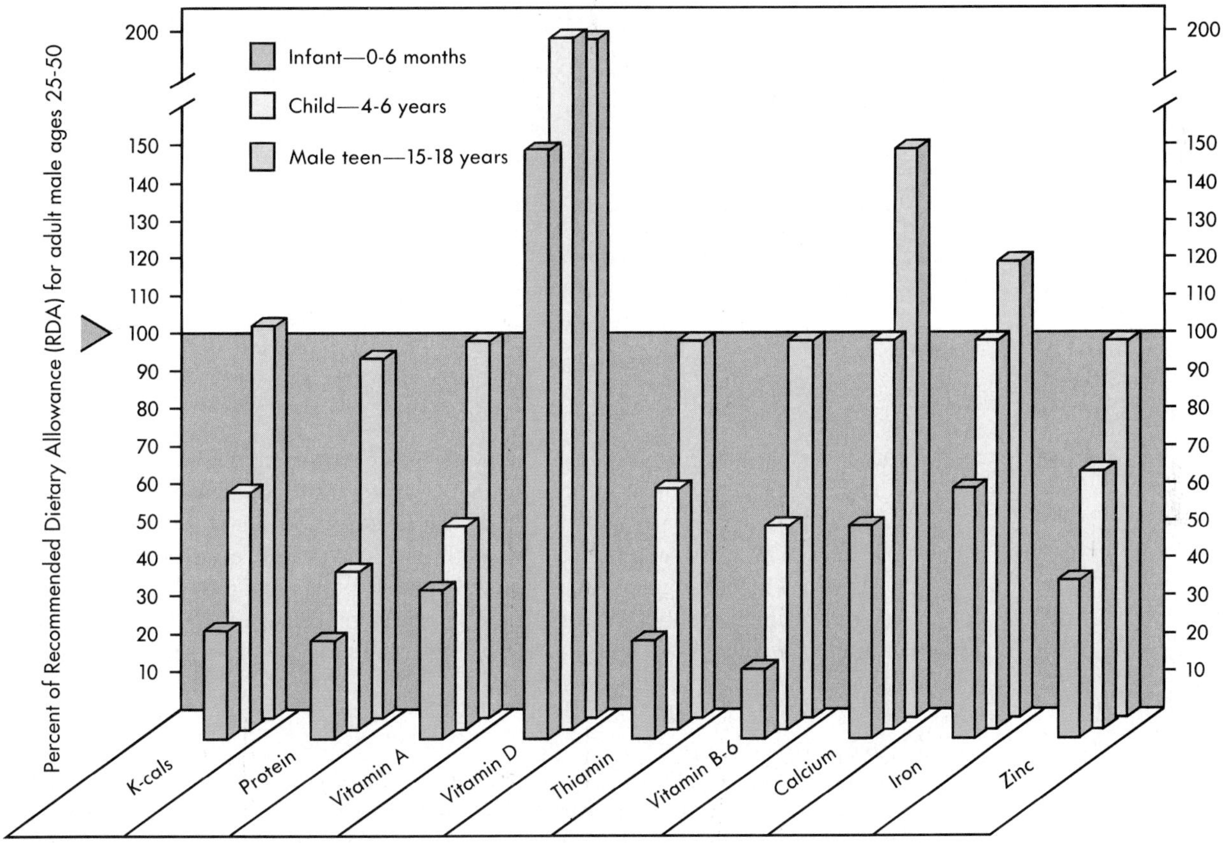

FIGURE 14-3

Compared with energy needs, infants need greater quantities of some nutrients than adults. This is illustrated by comparing the height of the kcalorie bar for infants (in green) with all other bars for infants (again in green). The kcalorie bar is often lower than are the bars for other nutrient needs. Therefore infants need many nutrients from relatively few kcalories in their diet, when compared with adults. This is also true for children, but to a lesser extent. Notice the vitamin D need of an infant is almost as high as that of an adult. However, infants need to fulfill their need for vitamin D within a much lower energy allowance. In other words, adults can more easily fulfill their nutrient needs, because they can eat proportionally more energy and therefore more foods.

TABLE 14-1

Composition of Infant Formulas, Human Milk, and Cow's Milk (Per Liter*)

Milk or Formula	Kcalories	Protein (grams)	Fat (grams)	Carbohydrate (grams)	Minerals† (grams)
Human milk	750	11	45	70	2
Casein-Based Formulas					
Similac	680	16	36	72	3
Enfamil	670	15	38	69	3
SMA	670	15	36	72	3
Gerber	670	15	36	72	2
Cow's Milk					
Whole	670	36	36	49	7
Skim	360	36	1	51	7
Soybean Protein-Based Formulas					
ProSobee	670	20	36	68	4
Isomil	570	20	36	68	4
Nursoy	670	20	36	68	4
Predigested Protein					
Nutramigen	670	19	26	90	1
Alimentum	670	19	38	70	1

**1 liter equals about 30 fluid ounces.*
†Calcium, phosphorus, and other minerals.

to four times more than adults need. Infants need an easy way to get these kcalories. Either human milk or formula is ideal for the first few months. Both are high in fat and supply about 650 kcalories per quart of fluid (700 kcalories per liter; Table 14-1). Later, human milk or formula, supplemented by solid foods, can provide even more energy.

The infant's high energy needs are primarily driven by its rapid growth and high metabolic rate. The high metabolic rate is caused in part by the ratio of the infant's great body surface to its weight. More body surface allows more heat loss from the skin; the body must use extra energy to replace that heat.[13]

Protein

Daily protein needs vary in infancy from 0.7 to 1 gram of protein for each pound of body weight (1.6 to 2.2 grams per kilogram). About 40% of total protein intake should come from essential amino acids. Both goals are satisfied by either human milk or formula. Total protein intake should not exceed 20% of kcalorie needs. Excess nitrogen and minerals supplied by high-protein diets would exceed the ability of an infant's kidneys to excrete the resulting metabolic waste products.

In America, infant protein deficiency is unlikely, except in cases of mistaken feeding practices, such as when an infant's formula is watered down too much. Protein deficiency may also be induced by elimination diets used to detect food allergies. As foods are eliminated from the diet, infants may not be offered enough protein to compensate for the high-protein sources no longer present (see the Nutrition Issue on food allergies and intolerances at the end of the chapter).

Fat

Infants and children up to 2 years of age should get about 40% of their energy from fat. More than 50% may lead to poor fat digestion. About half the energy supplied by both human milk and formula comes from fat. Essential fatty acids should make up 3% of total energy. Fats are an important part of the infant's diet because they are energy-dense and vital to the development of the nervous system. As a concentrated energy source, fat helps resolve the potential problem of the infant's high energy needs and small stomach capacity.[13]

Vitamins of Special Interest

Vitamin K is routinely given (injected) to all infants at birth. This dose lasts until the infant's intestinal bacteria are established and begin to synthesize vitamin K. Formula-fed infants receive the rest of the vitamins they need from the formula. Breast-fed infants, especially dark-skinned ones, may require a vitamin D supplement if they are not exposed to much sunlight. (Sunlight exposure on human skin activates synthesis of vitamin D; see Chapter 8.) The time needed in the sun is approximately 15 to 30 minutes daily on hands and face for white infants and longer for dark-skinned babies. Breast-fed infants whose mothers are total vegetarians (vegans) should receive a vitamin B-12 supplement. Infants who drink goat's milk need a dietary supplement of folate, because the milk doesn't supply a sufficient amount of this essential nutrient.

Minerals of Special Interest

The iron stores a child is born with are generally depleted by the time its birth weight doubles, in 4 to 6 months.[11] The American Academy of Pediatrics recommends that to maintain a good iron status, formula-fed infants be given an iron-fortified formula from birth. Breast-fed infants need solid foods to supply extra iron at about 6 months of age. The need for iron is a major consideration in deciding when to introduce solid foods. Some researchers recommend liquid iron supplements from birth or by 1 month of age for breast-fed infants.

Infants need adequate amounts of iodide and zinc to support growth. Human milk and formula adequately supply these needs when the infant's energy needs are met. In addition, some clinicians recommend fluoride supplements to aid tooth development for breast-fed infants and for bottle-fed infants if the water supply used in home formula preparation—tap or bottled water—does not contain fluoride. Note that formula manufacturers use fluoride-free water in formula preparation. Parents should consult their dentist for advice on the need for fluoride for the infant.

Water

An infant needs about 2 ounces of water and other fluids combined per pound of body weight (about 150 milliliters per kilogram). Infants typically consume enough human milk or formula to supply this amount. In hot climates, supplemental water may be necessary. And any conditions that lead to water loss—diarrhea, vomiting, fever, and too much sun—often call for supplemental water. Infants are easily dehydrated, a condition that has serious effects if not remedied. Dehydration can result in rapidly decreasing kidney function, and the infant may then require hospitalization for rehydration. Special fluid replacement formulas are available to treat dehydration.[13] A physician needs to guide any use of these products. It is important to remember that excessive fluid can also be harmful, especially to the brain. It is best to limit supplemental fluids to about 4 ounces per day, unless the physician feels a greater need exists because of disease or other conditions. Overall, extremes in fluid intake—either too little or too much—can lead to health problems.

CONCEPT CHECK

When an infant does not grow properly, its failure to thrive may stem from physical problems or inappropriate feeding practices. Most nutrient needs in the first 6 months are met by human milk or formula. Breast-fed infants may need vitamin D, fluoride, and iron supplements, and formula-fed infants may need fluoride supplements. Infants usually get enough water from the human milk or formula they drink.

Formula-Feeding for Infants

We discussed breast-feeding in detail in Chapter 13. Let's now focus on formula-feeding. Recall that a major advantage of breast-feeding is provision of immune bodies that impart immune protection to the infant. That advantage is very important in the context of poverty and poor hygiene. It is less important in America, where high standards for water purity and cleanliness make formula-feeding a safe alternative for infants.

Formula Composition. Infants cannot adequately tolerate cow's milk, because of its high protein and mineral content. Cow's milk reflects the greater growth needs of calves. Thus cow's milk must be altered to be safe for infant feeding. The altered forms, known as infant formulas, were first available commercially in 1931. Since 1980 they have been required to conform to strict guidelines for nutrient composition and quality set by federal law. Formulas generally contain lactose or sucrose for carbohydrate, heat-treated proteins from cow's milk, and vegetable oils for fat (see Table 14-1). Soy protein–based formulas are available for infants who can't tolerate lactose or types of proteins found in cow's milk. If the soybean-based formula is not tolerated, the next step is to try a predigested (hydrolyzed) protein formula, such as Nutramigen or Alimentum.[13] Formulas contain vitamins and minerals in amounts suggested by the guidelines of the American Academy of Pediatrics. A variety of specialized formulas also are available.

another BITE

A severely malnourished 5-month-old infant was recently admitted to Arkansas Children's Hospital in Little Rock. Symptoms included heart failure, rickets, inflamed blood vessels, and possible nerve damage. According to the hospital, the baby girl had been fed nothing but a soy beverage sold in health food stores. This kind of soy beverage is not a soy-based infant formula. Unlike true infant formulas, which are nutritionally complete and appropriate for infants, other soy beverages lack some nutrients infants need. Because of cases such as this one, parents should consult their physician when choosing an appropriate infant formula.

Formula and baby foods should not be heated in a microwave oven. Hot spots can develop that may burn the infant's mouth. Bottles are best warmed in a pot of water on the stove or under hot running water.

Formula Preparation. In the 1950s, it was common to prepare a day's supply of bottles and then sterilize them in boiling water for about 30 minutes. Today, it is often more convenient to prepare bottles one at a time. All utensils should be washed before preparing the formula. Powdered formulas are measured into a bottle to which clean water is added (follow label directions). The formula is mixed and fed immediately to the infant. Either warm or cold water can be added, depending on preference. Most people preparing concentrated formula make up the whole can (13 ounces of formula plus 13 ounces of water) and store it in the refrigerator in a clean, covered jar or pitcher until needed. Ready-to-feed formulas are also available. These are poured into a bottle and fed immediately.[13]

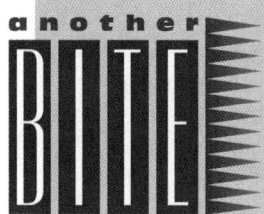

It is safe to refrigerate diluted formula for a day. However, formula left over from a feeding should be discarded, because it will be contaminated by bacteria and enzymes in the infant's saliva. If well water is used, it should be boiled before making formula and should also be analyzed for excessive concentration of naturally occurring nitrates, which can lead to a severe form of anemia.

Because babies swallow a lot of air along with either formula or human milk, it is important to burp a baby after either 10 minutes of feeding or 1 to 2 ounces (30 to 60 milliliters) from a bottle, and again at the end of feeding. Spitting up a bit of milk is normal at this time. Once fed, the child should be placed on its side, with a rolled-up blanket placed behind its back to support that position. In this position the infant has the least chance of choking on any milk it spits up.

It is important to stop a bottle feeding when the infant indicates that it is full. Pay attention to cues that signal the infant has had enough, such as turning its head away, inattention, falling asleep, and becoming playful (Figure 14-4). Trust the infant's appetite rather than a standardized serving recommendation, and allow the infant to refuse some milk in the bottle. It is difficult to tell how much milk a breast-fed baby gets. New mothers who breast-feed often worry whether the baby has had enough milk. Again, watch for signs from the baby. After about 20 minutes, the baby has probably had enough.

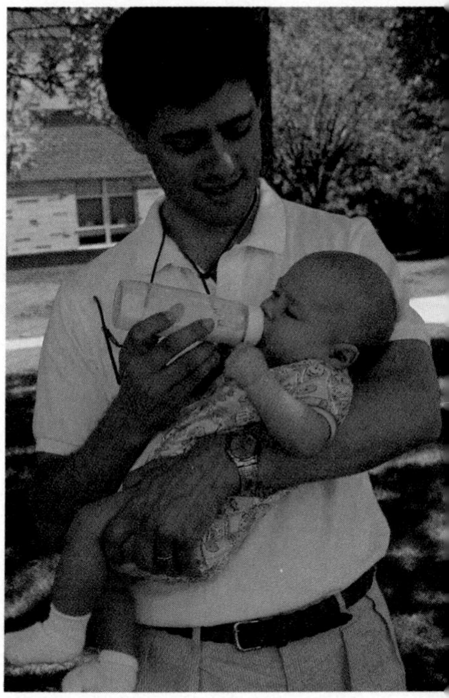

FIGURE 14-4
Careful attention during feeding allows the infant to signal the caregiver when the feeding should cease. In addition, stopping the feeding before putting the infant to bed is important. This helps prevent nursing bottle syndrome, because the infant will not fall asleep with the bottle. Thus carbohydrate-laden fluid, which can lead to severe dental decay, will not pool in the oral cavity as the child sleeps.

SOLID FOODS

Development of Feeding Skills

By 6 to 7 months, the infant has learned to grab and transfer objects from one hand to the other (Table 14-2). At about this time, teeth begin to appear, and the infant begins to handle finger foods with some dexterity. Dry toast, sliced in strips, offers hours of enjoyment.

By age 7 to 8 months, the infant can push food around on a plate and play with a drinking cup. He or she can hold a bottle and self-feed a cracker or piece of toast.[13] In mastering these manipulations the infant develops self-confidence and self-esteem. It is important that parents be patient and support these early feeding attempts, even though they appear inefficient.

At around 10 months of age, the infant practices in earnest self-feeding finger foods and drinking from a cup. Feeding time is often very messy. Food is used as a means to explore the environment. By the infant's first birthday, his or her body has developed sufficiently to accommodate crawling, probably walking, and self-feeding. While attempts at feeding are still erratic, the developing child takes great pride in doing more things independently. As the child drinks from a cup more frequently, fewer bottle-feedings and/or breast-feedings are necessary. The added mobility of walking should naturally lead to gradual weaning from the bottle or breast.[13]

Introducing Solid Foods

The time to introduce solid foods into an infant's diet hinges on a few important factors[8]:

Nutritional need—As noted, iron stores are exhausted by about 6 months of age. Either solid foods or iron supplements are then needed to supply iron if the child is breast-fed or fed a formula not supplemented with iron. Iron, however, is not the only nutrient missing from human milk and unfortified formulas. Vitamin D and fluoride may also deserve attention. Still, adding solid foods is unnecessary for any nutrients other than iron before 4 to 6 months.

Physiological capabilities—Infants cannot readily digest starch before 3 months. As they age, their digestive capabilities increase. Kidney function likewise is quite limited until about 4 to 6 weeks of age. Until then, waste products from high levels of dietary protein or minerals are difficult to excrete.[13]

Physical ability—Three markers indicate that a child is ready for solid foods: (1) the disappearance of the extrusion reflex (thrusting the tongue forward and pushing food out), (2) head and neck control, and (3) the ability to sit up with support. These usually occur around 4 to 6 months of age, but they vary with each infant.

Preventing allergies—An infant's intestinal tract can readily absorb whole proteins from birth until 4 to 5 months of age. Early exposure to many types of proteins—par-

TABLE 14-2

Guidelines for Progression of Solid Foods

Age	Feeding Skills	Oral Motor Skills	Types of Food	Suggested Activities
Birth-4 months		Rooting reflex Sucking reflex Swallowing reflex Extrusion reflex	Breast milk Infant formula	Breast-feed or bottle-feed
5 months	Able to grasp objects voluntarily Learning to reach mouth with hands	Disappearance of extrusion reflex		Possible introduction of thinned cereal
6 months	Sits with balance while using hands	Transfers food from front of tongue to back	Infant cereal Strained fruit Strained vegetables Egg yolk (if no family history of egg allergy)	Prepare cereal with formula or breastmilk to a semiliquid texture Use spoon Feed from a dish Advance to ⅓-½ cup cereal before adding fruits or vegetables
7 months	Improved grasp Can transfer objects from hand to hand	Mashes food with lateral movements of jaw Learns side-to-side or "rotary" chewing Tooth eruption	Infant cereal Strained to junior texture of fruits, vegetables, and meats	Thicken cereal to lumpier texture Sit in highchair with feet supported Introduce cup
8-10 months	Holds bottle without help Drinks from cup without spilling Decreases fluid intake and increases solids Coordinates hand-to-mouth movement		Juices Soft, mashed, or minced table foods	Begin finger foods like toast or crackers Do not add salt, sugar, or fats to food Present soft foods in chunks ready for finger-feeding
10-12 months	Feeds self Holds cup without help	Improved ability to bite and chew	Soft, chopped table foods Whole egg (at 1 year of age)	Provide meals in pattern similar to rest of family Use cup at meals

From Queen P, Lang C: Handbook of pediatric nutrition, *Rockville, Md, 1993, Aspen Publishers.*
This timeline is just an estimate. Infants vary. A pediatrician should be consulted if caregivers are concerned about an infant's developmental progress. In general, there is no nutritional reason to begin solid food introduction before 4-6 months of age.

ticularly proteins in cow's milk—may predispose a child to future allergies, including food allergies, because some types of these proteins may be absorbed intact. For this reason, it is best to minimize the number of different types of proteins in a child's diet during the first 3 months.

With these considerations in mind—nutritional need, physiological and physical readiness, and allergy prevention—the American Academy of Pediatrics recommends that solid foods not be introduced until about 6 months of age (see Table 14-2). In general, a child starting solid foods should weigh at least 13 pounds (6 kilograms) and should be drinking more than 32 ounces (1 liter) of formula daily or breast-feeding more than 8 to 10 times within 24 hours. This description generally applies to 6-month-old infants and to some 4-month-old infants.

Before 4 to 6 months, infants are not physically mature enough to consume much solid food. Attempts to push down solid foods have sometimes led to force-feeding with a feeder (a giant syringe) or to mixing infant cereal with milk and putting it in a bottle.

Even if these are traditional alternatives in your family, there is no reason to carry on these practices. The inconvenience alone should make one consider whether all the effort is worth it. This practice is unnecessary nutritionally, tedious, and possibly dangerous for the infant because it increases the risk of allergies and choking or inhaling food when crying. Even so, many children are already eating solids by 2 months of age.[8] Only occasionally does a rapidly growing infant—one who consumes more than 32 ounces (1 liter) of formula daily—need solid foods at 4 months to meet high energy needs.

A common reason offered for introducing solid foods early—before 4 to 6 months of age—is the belief that it helps the infant sleep through the night. However, many studies show that sleeping through the night is a developmental milestone for the infant. It has nothing to do with how much food the infant eats. Infants naturally begin sleeping through the night between the ages of 1 to 3 months. Girls reach this stage before boys. Filling them with cereal is not going to influence that process.

Which Solid Foods Should Be Fed First?

Before 6 months of age, the first solid foods should be iron-fortified cereals. A good idea is to offer foods after some breast-feeding or formula-feeding when the edge has been taken off the infant's hunger. This practice aids in early spoon-feeding. Rice cereal is the best cereal to begin with, because it is least likely to cause allergies. After the age of 6 months, the first food is not such an important issue. Some pediatricians may recommend lean ground (strained) meats for more absorbable forms of iron. Although yogurt and cottage cheese are also well tolerated and their consistencies make them good candidates for early foods, they are not good sources of iron.

Start with teaspoon amounts and increase the serving size gradually. Once a new food has been fed for several days without ill effects, another food can be added to the infant's diet. At first, this can be another type of cereal or perhaps a cooked and strained (blended) vegetable, meat, fruit, or egg yolk. Each feeding step builds on the last (see Table 14-2).

Waiting several days between each new food is important, because it can take that long for signs of an allergy or intolerance to develop. Symptoms to look for are diarrhea, vomiting, a rash, or wheezing. If one or more of these symptoms appear, the suspected problem food should be avoided for several weeks and then reintroduced in a small quantity. If the problem continues, a doctor should be consulted. It is important not to introduce mixed foods until each component of the mixed food has been given separately. Otherwise, if an allergy or intolerance develops, it will not be easy to identify the offending food. Note that many babies outgrow food sensitivities in childhood.

Some foods that commonly cause an allergic response in infants are egg whites, chocolate, nuts, and cow's milk.[15] It is best not to introduce these foods early in infancy. The American Academy of Pediatrics recommends against the use of cow's milk during the first year of life.

A variety of strained foods is available for infant feeding. Check this out next time you are in a supermarket. Single-food items are more desirable than mixed dinners and desserts, which are less nutrient-dense. Most brands have no added salt, but some fruit desserts contain a lot of added sugar.

As an alternative, plain foods from the table—vegetables, fruits, and meats (no seasoning added)—can be ground up in an inexpensive plastic baby food grinder/mill. Another option is to puree a larger amount of food in a blender, freeze it in ice-cube portions, store in plastic bags, and defrost and warm as needed. Careful attention to cleanliness is necessary. Infant foods made at home should be ground before seasonings are added to please the rest of the family. The infant does not notice the difference if salt, sugar, or spices are omitted. It is best to introduce infants to a variety of foods, so that by the end of the first year the infant is consuming many foods—milk, meats, fruits, vegetables, and grains.

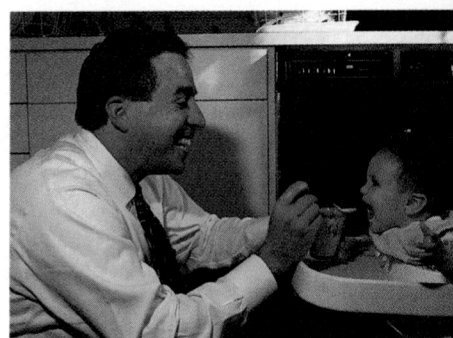

By 6 months of age, a baby is ready for more than just formula or human milk.

As early as possible, juices and formula should be offered in a cup. A heavy cup with a wide, flat bottom aids success. Drinking from a cup helps prevent "nursing bottle syndrome." As an infant plays with a bottle, the carbohydrate-rich fluid bathes the teeth, providing an ideal growth medium for bacteria. Bacteria on the teeth then make acids that

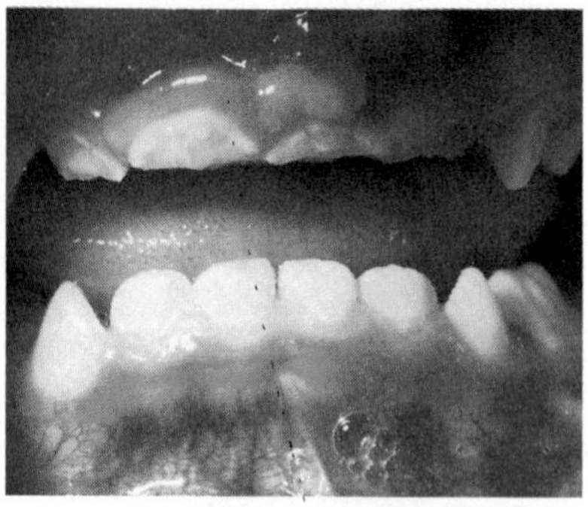

Nursing bottle syndrome—an extreme example of tooth decay. This child was probably often put to bed with a bottle. The upper teeth have decayed almost all the way to the gum line.

dissolve tooth enamel. An infant should never be put to bed with a bottle or placed in an infant seat with a bottle propped up. As the child lies in bed, fluid (even milk) pools around the teeth, increasing the likelihood of dental caries. Again, infants need careful attention when being fed. Propping bottles does not constitute careful attention.

Getting a baby out of the bedtime-bottle habit is difficult. But determined caregivers can either wince through a few nights of their baby's crying or can slowly wean the baby away from the bottle with either a pacifier or water (for a week or so).

In the first attempts to introduce solid foods, just getting the food into the infant, instead of all over him or her, proves to be a challenge. The caregiver must proceed slowly. Initially, table foods supplement—rather than replace—formula or human milk. The infant controls the situation by signaling when he or she is hungry and when he or she has had enough to eat. Self-feeding skills require coordination and can develop only if the infant is allowed to practice and experiment. By 9 to 10 months, the infant's desire to explore, experience, and play with food can also hinder feeding. Caregivers need to relax and take this phase of infant development in stride. Sloppy, friendly mealtimes actually make for good memories.

To ease efforts in feeding solid foods, consider the following tips:

- Use a baby-sized spoon; a small spoon with a long handle is best.
- Hold the infant comfortably on the lap, as for breast-feeding or bottle-feeding, but a little more upright to ease swallowing. In this position, the infant expects food.
- Put a small dab of food on the spoon tip and gently place it on the infant's tongue.
- Convey a calm and casual approach to the infant. The infant needs time to get used to food.
- Expect the infant to take only two or three bites of the first meals. Anything more than that is real success.

By the end of the first year, finger-feeding becomes more efficient, drinking from a cup improves, and chewing is easier as more teeth erupt.[13] Still, experimentation and unpredictability are to be expected.

another BITE

A summary of infant feeding recommendations

Breast-Fed Infants

- Breast-feed for 6 months or more.
- Consider fluoride, iron, and vitamin D supplements.
- Add iron-fortified cereal at about 6 months of age.
- Provide a variety of basic, soft foods after 6 months of age.

Formula-Fed Infants

- Use infant formula for at least 6 months, preferably an iron-fortified type.
- Give a fluoride supplement if water supply is not fluoridated.
- Add iron-fortified cereal at about 6 months of age.
- Provide a variety of basic, soft foods after 6 months.

What Not to Feed an Infant

Following are several foods and practices to avoid when feeding an infant:

- *Honey and corn syrup*—These products may contain spores of *Clostridium botulinum.* The spores can eventually develop into bacteria in the stomach and lead to a food poisoning known as botulism. This is often fatal in children under 1 year old (see Chapter 17).
- *Very salty and very sweet foods*—Infants do not need a lot of sugar or salt added to their foods. They enjoy bland foods much more than do adults.[13]

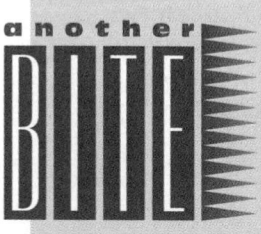

- *Excessive formula or milk (more than 40 ounces [1.2 liters] of formula or 32 ounces [1 liter] of milk daily)*—Solid foods should play a greater role in satisfying an infant's increasing appetite after 6 to 8 months. The switch needs to occur mainly because foods can contain much iron, whereas human milk, cow's milk, and low-iron formulas don't contain much. About 24 to 32 ounces (¾ to 1 liter) of human milk or formula daily is ideal after 6 months, with food supplying the rest of energy needs.
- *Foods that tend to cause choking*—These foods include hot dogs (unless finely cut into sticks, not coin shapes), candy, whole nuts, grapes, coarsely cut meats, raw carrots, and popcorn. Hot dogs, grapes, chunks of meat, carrots, peanuts, popcorn and peanut butter cause the most choking deaths. Caregivers should discourage the practice of allowing younger children to gobble snack foods during playtime and should supervise all meals.
- *Low-fat or nonfat cow's milk*—Beyond 2 years, children can drink 1% or 2% milk, because by then they are consuming enough solid foods to supply energy and fat needs. Before that age, the amount of low-fat milk needed for energy needs would supply too many minerals. That could overwhelm the kidneys' ability to excrete the excess. The lower fat intake might also harm nervous system development. The American Academy of Pediatrics strongly urges parents not to give children under the age of 2 low-fat or nonfat milk.
- *Feeding excessive amounts of apple or pear juice*—The simple carbohydrate sorbitol contained in these juices can lead to diarrhea, because sorbitol is poorly absorbed. Diluting juices with an equal part of water is a good idea, but it should be begun early, before the infant becomes accustomed to full-strength juices.

CONCEPT CHECK

Infant formulas generally contain lactose or sucrose, heat-treated proteins from cow's milk, and vegetable oil. Formulas may or may not be fortified with iron. Sanitation is very important in preparing and storing formula. Solid food should not be added to an infant's diet until the child is both ready for and needs solid food, usually at about 6 months of age. The first solid food given can be iron-fortified infant cereals with very gradual additions of other foods—one at a time each week. Some foods to avoid giving infants in the first year include honey, low-fat cow's milk, very salty or sweet foods, and foods that may cause the child to choke.

NUTRITION-RELATED PROBLEMS IN INFANCY

Parents, other caregivers, and clinicians should be aware of a variety of potential problems related to infant nutrition.

Possible Feeding Problems

Feeding problems to watch out for in infancy include the following:

- Getting insufficient iron in the diet.
- Excluding from the diet an entire food group of the Food Guide Pyramid during introduction and later regular use of solid foods.
- Drinking raw milk from either cows or goats. This raw milk raises the possibility of viral and bacterial contamination (see Chapter 17). Goat's milk, as noted, is low in folate.
- Not progressing from the bottle to a cup by 1 year of age.
- Feeding from a bottle past 18 months of age.
- Getting supplemental vitamins or minerals beyond 150% of an infant's or child's RDA.

All these problems require attention. Parents and other caregivers should consult with a physician.

NUTRITION insight

DIETARY GUIDELINES FOR INFANT FEEDING

In response to various controversies surrounding infant feeding, experts have written the following dietary guidelines for infants:

- Build up to a variety of foods.
- Be sensitive to the infant's appetite to avoid overfeeding or underfeeding.
- Don't restrict fat and cholesterol too much.
- Don't overdo high-fiber foods.
- Sugar is fine in moderation.
- Sodium is fine in moderation.
- Infants need more iron per pound of body weight than do adults.

These guidelines have been accepted by the American Academy of Pediatrics and the American Dietetic Association. The recommendations in this chapter are also consistent with these guidelines. In essence, there is no evidence of positive effects of very restrictive diets during infancy, although their hazards are well documented.[13]

Colic ■ *Periodic crying in a healthy infant; apparently caused by gas buildup or allergies to proteins.*

Colic

The first time an infant has a lengthy, unexplained crying spell, most parents panic. Crying episodes of about 3 or more hours that do not respond to typical remedies—such as feeding, holding, or diaper changes—are characteristic of infants who develop ***colic.***[5] Colic affects about one third of all infants, and so it is neither uncommon nor abnormal. Late afternoon and early evening can be the most common times for crying. Nighttime sleeping is almost always disturbed by crying spells. The only good news is that colic usually goes away after a few intense months.

Colic is thought to be caused by either (1) allergy-causing proteins in formula or human milk or (2) excess gas buildup in the gastrointestinal (GI) tract because of sluggish peristalsis.[5] The infant commonly tucks into a ball in response to colic. Painful accumulation of gas in the GI tract may be the reason for this response. The crying is not usually related to feeding, but positioning a colicky baby upright during feeding allows him or her to expel trapped air more easily by burping. In addition, the infant should be burped regularly during feeding and fed for no longer than 30 minutes. The longer a child suckles at the bottle or breast, the more air he or she takes in.

Changing the infant's diet from a cow's milk protein–based formula to a predigested protein formula sometimes helps in severe cases (see Table 14-1).[4] A recent study suggests that it is helpful for the breast-feeding mother to temporarily avoid dairy products. In addition, the physician may prescribe medications to calm the child and reduce gas buildup.

Overall, parents need the counsel and support of other adults to ease their distress during this trying period, which often lasts for the first 3 to 4 months. Because it is so unnerving to feel powerless to calm an infant in pain, hearing from other parents who have experienced having a colicky child is especially helpful.

Diarrhea

Diarrhea results from various causes in infancy, including bacterial and viral infections. In the United States, about 500 infants die each year of simple dehydration resulting from diarrhea. To prevent dehydration, infants with diarrhea should be given plenty of fluids—

although not milk or full-strength fruit juices. Specialized fluids, such as Pedialyte, are available. These contain glucose, sodium, potassium, chloride, and water.[13] It is best to have a pediatrician's recommendations concerning fluid replacement.

Once diarrhea subsides, a bottle-fed infant may be switched to a soy-based, lactose-free formula for a few weeks. This allows time for the intestine to produce sufficient lactase enzyme to digest the large amount of lactose typically found in formulas. The breast-fed infant should continue at the breast throughout the duration.

Milk Allergy

Over 25 proteins in milk can lead to allergies.[15] Some of these are inactivated by heating (scalding) milk. However, some proteins are very heat stable. A "true" milk allergy is actually quite rare and develops in less than 1% of formula-fed infants. However, infants may be switched to soy-based formulas in an attempt to decrease crying and spitting up. Just because a child thrives better on a soy-based formula does not mean he or she has a true milk allergy. If it is a true milk allergy, the soy formula is not likely to help in the long run. A special formula with predigested protein will be needed (see Table 14-1).

Iron-Deficiency Anemia

Iron-deficiency anemia typically occurs in infants who consume few solid foods and whose diets are dominated by cow's milk, which has little iron.[11] Iron stores are then quickly depleted by the daily demand for new red blood cells to be synthesized. To prevent iron-deficiency anemia, it is best to start an infant at about 6 months on iron-fortified cereals and meats and to limit formula to 16 to 25 ounces (500 to 750 milliliters) daily. The infant should also not consume cow's milk for the first year, and especially before 3 months of age, because cow's milk tends to cause intestinal bleeding. If anemia does develop, medicinal iron supplements are advised with a physician's guidance.

The Premature Infant

The premature infant is fed either human milk or a specially designed formula. As noted in Chapter 13, nutrients may be added to human milk to increase its protein, mineral, and energy content. The premature infant must be fed immediately, because little fat or carbohydrate storage is present.[2] The body composition of a full-term infant includes about 12% fat, whereas the composition of a very premature infant can include as little as 2% fat.

CONCEPT CHECK

Colic is commonly associated with GI tract discomfort. Switching to a formula with predigested proteins may help treat colic. It may also be helpful for breast-feeding mothers to avoid dairy products, under a physician's guidance. Diarrhea requires additional fluids to prevent dehydration. Allergy to milk proteins is rare and may require switching to a formula with predigested proteins. Introducing iron-containing solid foods at an appropriate time and avoiding early use of cow's milk can generally prevent iron-deficiency anemia in infancy.

CHILDHOOD

The rapid growth rate that characterizes infancy tapers quickly during the subsequent few years. The average weight gain is only 5 pounds per year and the average height gain is only 3 inches per year during the second through about the eighth years of life (see Figure 14-1). As a toddler's growth rate tapers, eating behaviors change.[17] Feeding problems can stem from the decreasing appetite that characterizes the preschool years. Adapting food

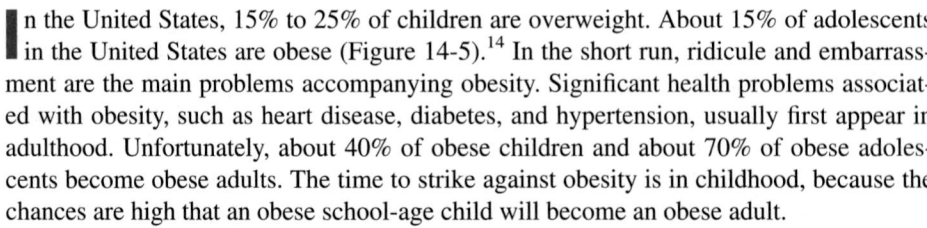

NUTRITION insight

OBESITY IN THE GROWING YEARS

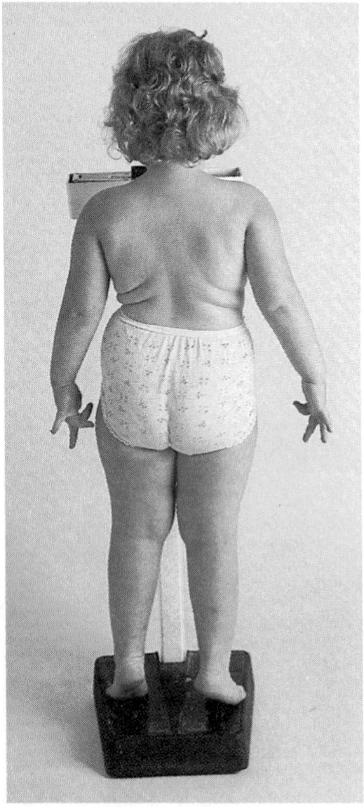

FIGURE 14-5
Childhood obesity. A female child like this one who is still obese after 5 years of age often faces a battle against obesity for the rest of her life.

In the United States, 15% to 25% of children are overweight. About 15% of adolescents in the United States are obese (Figure 14-5).[14] In the short run, ridicule and embarrassment are the main problems accompanying obesity. Significant health problems associated with obesity, such as heart disease, diabetes, and hypertension, usually first appear in adulthood. Unfortunately, about 40% of obese children and about 70% of obese adolescents become obese adults. The time to strike against obesity is in childhood, because the chances are high that an obese school-age child will become an obese adult.

The easiest way to evaluate obesity in childhood is to plot weight-for-height on a growth chart. Children over the ninetieth percentile are considered overweight, and those over the ninety-fifth percentile are considered obese. Skinfold thickness can also be measured to assess obesity (see Chapter 10).

What Causes Childhood Obesity?

Current research indicates that there are many potential causes for childhood obesity.[19] Recall the nature versus nurture discussion in Chapter 10. Some infants are born with lower metabolic rates; they use energy more efficiently and, in turn, have an easier time saving energy intake for fat storage. Some infants are less active than others and so use fewer kcalories each day. Research shows a moderate relationship between the number of hours a child spends watching television and obesity. Obesity is also linked to heredity. We can also expect further environmental influences—such as snacking, decreased physical activity, and high-fat/high-kcalorie food choices—to contribute to childhood obesity.[13]

Treating Childhood Obesity

A first approach to treating childhood obesity is assessing the child's activity level. If a child spends much free time in sedentary activities (such as watching television), more physical activities should be encouraged.[19] At the beginning of the week, a plan for a reasonable allotment of television time and video games for each family member could be set. The television generation now glues itself to the tube for an average of 22 hours a week. Activities to replace television viewing and video games do not necessarily have to be competitive sports. Children should be given opportunities to enjoy activities that they like—such as walking, cycling, swimming, and jazz dancing—and then encouraged to do

choices to the slower growth rate and reduced hunger becomes a challenge. When the child consumes few foods, the nutrient density of each food choice is important. This is a good time to emphasize whole grains and vegetables without increasing fat intake. Choosing a whole-grain breakfast cereal with limited fat is an excellent choice. There is no need to decrease fat intake severely, but fatty food choices should not overwhelm more nutritious ones.

The preschool years are the best time for a child to start a healthful pattern of living and eating, focusing on regular physical activity and nutritious foods. Self-esteem and successful eating are closely tied. Parents and other caregivers are role models: if they eat a variety of foods, the children will eat a variety of foods. One possible policy is the one-bite rule: within reason, children take at least one bite or taste of the foods presented to these often. Getting the family together for a brisk walk after dinner and finding an after-school sport the child enjoys are two good ideas.

Moderation in kcalorie intake is important, especially in limiting high-fat/high-kcalorie food choices and sugar-laden carbonated beverages. More nutrient-dense foods should be the primary focus. A diet containing 30% of kcalories as fat can support normal growth and development during childhood, provided that foods are carefully selected from the Food Guide Pyramid. Resorting to a weight-loss diet is usually unnecessary. Changing habits should be the emphasis in the short run.[14] Children have an advantage over adults in losing weight—some stored energy can be used for growth. If weight gain can be moderated, height gain may soon catch up. This is one reason treating obesity in childhood is so desirable. Further growth can contribute to success.

Sometimes weight loss is necessary if a child will still be obese after attaining ultimate adult height. Then weight loss should be gradual, perhaps ½ pound per week. The child should be watched closely to ensure that during this weight loss the rate of growth is normal. It is important that the child's energy intake not be so low that gains in height diminish.

Behavior modification adds a third important component to treating childhood obesity. One underlying environmental cause of obesity can be parents' attitudes and behaviors toward the child's weight. Struggles around feeding may interfere with a child's ability to eat sensibly. Children often need to find a new way to relate to foods, especially snack foods. An important family rule could be that children are allowed to eat only while sitting at the meal table. This could stop endless hours of snacking in front of the television. It might also help to put portions on plates rather than allow snacking to go on indefinitely, as often happens when children eat directly from a full box of crackers.

Parents play a key role in treating childhood obesity.[19] After all, they select and bring the food home. Overweight children have greater long-term success controlling their weight if their parents provide early support for exercising and eating right. One goal is to keep healthful, nutrient-rich but kcalorie-light snacks on hand. The parents must also help a child turn his or her interest from eating toward other interests, such as sports, hobbies, and school. Any management plan for treating childhood obesity must involve the parents.

The self-esteem of a child is quite fragile. Obesity itself already affects the child's psyche. Humiliation does not work: it only makes the child feel worse. Support, admiration, and encouragement—these are offerings to be emphasized.

Parents should also realize that by denying a child favorite foods, they do not necessarily deny love. The child can have treats, such as candy, in small amounts—not a whole bag. Often parents and children need to develop new ways of relating—ways that do not involve food and obesity.

another BITE

Surprisingly, children eat what they are exposed to. Children can eat a well-rounded and healthful diet if one is served to them. If offered whole-grain breakfast cereals, whole-wheat bread, vegetables, salad, and fresh fruits regularly, young children accept most of these foods and eat them. Only a lack of imagination limits—and possibly deprives—a child's diet. If caregivers don't like a particular food, they should still offer it to the child.

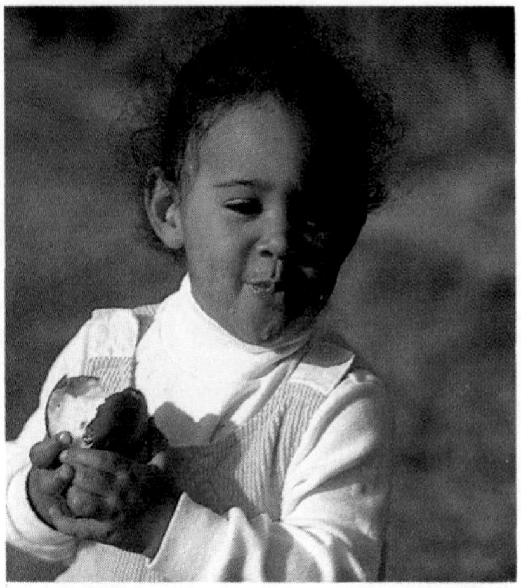

Childhood is the ideal time to begin to enjoy healthy foods.

them. For snacks, parents should decide the options. Children should then be allowed to choose one; responsibility for food choice ideally should start early.[16]

In the early school years, regular meals—especially breakfast—become an important focus. Some research suggests that eating breakfast helps children learn better in the subsequent hours they spend in school. The energy and nutrients consumed can stimulate attention, energy level, and motivation, yielding better test scores. Sports performance can be improved as well. This makes sense, because breakfast can replenish depleted carbohydrate stores in the liver. Still, some researchers dispute the importance of breakfast as it relates to learning. They claim that it is the more motivated students who eat breakfast, rather than eating breakfast that motivates students. In our opinion it is a good idea to give breakfast to all students, especially to otherwise sluggish ones since it can give a nutrient-rich start to the day's intake.

Breakfasts can be imaginative. Instead of conventional breakfast foods, caregivers can offer pizza, spaghetti, soups, yogurt with trail mix on top, chili, sandwiches, or shish kabob for starters.

How to Help a Child Choose Nutritious Foods

One way adults can encourage young children to eat nutritious, well-balanced meals is to serve new foods and repeat exposure to them. If a child observes adults and older children eating and enjoying a food, there is a good chance he or she will eventually accept it.[17] The dinner hour is a good time for children to experience new foods and to develop their own likes and dislikes. Preschool children tend to be wary of new foods. One reason is that their taste buds are more sensitive than those of adults. In addition, they have a general distrust of unfamiliar foods. If adults can be patient and persevere, children will build good food habits. Above all, the dinner table should not become a battleground.

Perseverance with children is critical, because it takes effort and commitment to guide them into liking a variety of foods. Be ready for some surprises (Figure 14-6). Note also that if left to their own devices, preschool children would find a few foods they like and eat them every day. But by constantly being introduced to new foods, children at this age

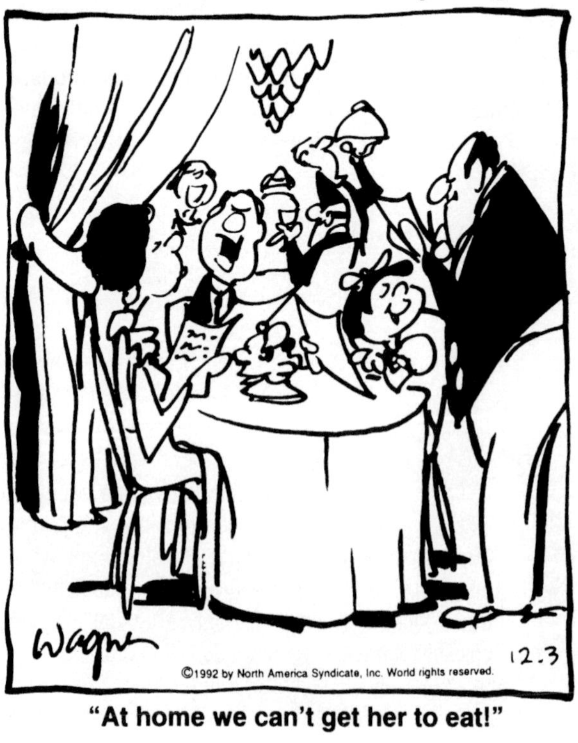
GRIN & BEAR IT
By Wagner
Wagner
12.3
©1992 by North America Syndicate, Inc. World rights reserved.
Reprinted with permission of North America Syndicate, Inc.
"At home we can't get her to eat!"

FIGURE 14-6
Grin and Bear It.

TABLE 14-3

Observed Emotional, Eating, and Food-Related Behaviors of Preschoolers

Age (years)	Emotional Behaviors	Eating Behaviors	Food-Related Behaviors
1-2	• Fears new things • Sharing is difficult • Requires constant supervision • Enjoys helping but can't be left alone • Curious • Often defiant • Eager for attention	• "Finicky" eater • Holds food in mouth without swallowing • May insist on eating the same food at meal after meal (called a food jag)	• Uses spoon with some skill (especially if hungry) • Can begin to tear, break, snap, and dip foods • Has good control of cup—lifts, drinks, sets it down, holds with one hand • Helps self-feed
3	• The "me too" age—wants to be included in everything • Responds well to options rather than demands • Sharing is still difficult • Somewhat rigid about the "right" way to do things	• Eats most foods, except for certain vegetables • Dawdles over food when not hungry • Comments on how foods are served	• Uses spoon in semiadult fashion; may spear with fork • Medium hand muscle development • Feeds self independently, especially if hungry • Can pour milk and juice and serve individual portions from a serving dish if given instructions
4	• Shares well • Needs adult approval and attention—shows off • Understands; needs limits • Follows rules most of the time • Still rigid about the "right" way to do things	• Eating and talking get in the way—prefers to talk • Strong food likes and dislikes • Refuses to eat to the point of tears	• Uses all eating utensils • Small finger muscle development • Can wipe, wash, set table, and pour premeasured ingredients • Can peel, spread, cut, roll, and mash foods; cracks eggs
5	• Helpful and cooperative with family chores and routines • Still somewhat rigid about the "right" way to do things • Very attached to mother, home, and family	• Likes familiar foods; prefers most vegetables raw • Latches on to food dislikes of family members and declares these as own	• Fine coordination in fingers and hands • Makes simple breakfast and lunch • Can measure, cut, grind, and grate

From Sigman-Grant M: Nutrition Today, *p. 13, July/August 1992.*

can expand their nutritional choices, develop an experimental approach, and learn to appreciate a variety of foods. It may take 10 to 15 exposures, but eventually most foods will be accepted. A positive outlook by the caregivers helps a lot.

Research shows that children like certain foods—especially those with crisp textures and mild flavors—and familiar foods. Young children are especially sensitive to and reject hot-temperature foods.

Parents and other caregivers play a central role in teaching by example. Children more readily learn good table manners along with others who practice them. The harmony that comes from working at being polite creates a positive environment for learning good nutrition habits. Preschoolers eventually develop skill with spoons and forks and can even use dull knives (Table 14-3). But finger foods are also a good idea. A goal should be to make mealtime a happy, social time. Share enjoyment of healthful foods. A regular family meal daily—whether breakfast, lunch, or dinner—is an appropriate setting for children to learn about healthful eating and to build good eating habits.

Childhood Feeding Problems

Tensions between parents, or between parents and children, often contribute to eating problems. Getting to the root of family problems and creating a more harmonious family atmosphere are an important part of resolving many childhood feeding problems. In addition, parents must often be educated as to what to expect of a preschool child and what goals to set. Some typical problems, their causes, and suggestions for correcting them follow.

"My Child Won't Eat as Much or as Regularly as He Did as an Infant." This is to be expected. The growth rate slows after infancy, and a child does not need as much food. Parents must often be reminded that they shouldn't expect a 3-year-old to eat as voraciously as an infant or to eat adult-sized portions. Reducing serving size to two thirds of an adult's portion for servings from the Food Guide Pyramid is a good approach for young children aged 2 years and older. Normal-weight children have a built-in feeding mechanism that adjusts hunger to regulate food intake at each stage of growth.[6] If a child is developing and growing normally and the caregiver is providing a variety of healthful foods, all can be confident the child isn't starving. One should avoid nagging, forcing, and bribing.

Appetite also varies with activity level and general health. An initial symptom of a sick child is poor appetite. Picky eating is also just another indication of a child's striving toward independence and his or her strong desire to establish routines. Asserting himself or herself about food preferences is a relatively easy way for the child to do this.

Parents should also be reminded that food likes and dislikes change rapidly in childhood and are influenced by food temperature, appearance, texture, and taste. Sometimes children object to having foods mixed, as in stews or casseroles, even if they normally like the ingredients separately.

Battling to get a child to eat more is rarely worth the effort. Parents should present nutritious food choices, eat some themselves, and let the child decide the serving size. It all boils down to a division of responsibility in feeding. The parents are responsible for what their child is offered to eat and for setting up a pleasant eating environment. The child is responsible for deciding how much or even whether he or she eats.[16] In addition, parents should recognize that this is an important age for children to explore the world around them. Even good eaters are sometimes more interested in exploring than eating. There's room for occasional indulgences, a skipped meal or two, or once-in-a-while poor choices. It's eating and lifestyle habits over the course of a month and lifetime that matter. Children master their eating when adults provide opportunities to learn, give support for exploration, and limit inappropriate behavior.

"My Child Is Always Snacking, yet She Never Finishes Her Meal." Children have small stomachs. Offering them six or so small meals succeeds better than limiting them to three meals each day. Sticking to three meals a day offers no special nutritional advantages; it is just a social custom. Snacking is fine, as long as good dental care is practiced. When we eat isn't nearly so important as what we eat. If nutritious snacks are readily available, these would be good to offer at midmorning or midafternoon when the child becomes hungry (Table 14-4). Fruits and vegetables (fresh, frozen, or juice) are always good snack accompaniments. Working parents should make sure their children are provided with nutritional snacks to tide them over until dinnertime.

Caregivers can use snacks to fill in the foods missing from meals. Fresh fruit, fruit or vegetable juices, ice milk or pudding, a sandwich or burrito, and a bowl of cereal are all good choices.

When a child refuses to eat, it is best not to overreact.[16] Doing so may give the child the idea that eating is a means of getting attention or manipulating a scene. Most children do not starve themselves to any point approaching physical harm. When a child refuses to eat, have him or her sit at the table for a while, and if he or she still isn't interested in eating, remove the food and wait until the next scheduled meal or snack.

"My Child Never Eats His Vegetables." Everyone dislikes certain foods. Again, the one-bite policy can be encouraged, and guidelines can be set to discourage fussing over unfamiliar foods. Children eventually learn that they can eat some of a food they don't particularly like without first gagging, choking, and yelling, "Oh gross!" It takes time for a child to become enthusiastic about a new food, but with continual exposure and a positive role model, chances are the child may even grow to like it.

Children cannot and should not be forced to eat. They need to develop independence and identities separate from their parents. In other words, children have to choose for

TABLE 14-4

Serving Nutritious Snacks and Beverages for School-Age Children

Snack suggestions:	
Fresh raw vegetables	Serve with a dip of cottage cheese or yogurt blended with dried buttermilk dressing
Celery	Spread with peanut butter and sprinkle on raisins, shredded carrots, or finely chopped nuts
Bananas	Dip in sweetened yogurt or spread with peanut butter and roll in coconut, chopped nuts, or granola
Sliced apples or crackers	Serve with a dip of peanut butter, honey, nuts, raisins, and coconut mixed together
Bagels	Spread with cream cheese or peanut butter and top with chopped bananas, crushed pineapple, or shredded carrots
Quick bread or muffins	Make with carrots, zucchini, pumpkin, bananas, nuts, dates, raisins, lemons, squash, or berries
Flour tortillas	Spread with refried beans or canned chili, sprinkle with grated cheese and broil; top with chili sauce
Ready-to-eat cereals	Use brands low in sugar and containing fiber; serve with raisins
Pita bread	Place sliced meat, cheese, lettuce, and tomato in open pocket
English muffins or pita bread	Top with spaghetti sauce, grated cheese, and meats; broil or bake and cut in fourths
Potato skins	Sprinkle with shredded cheese, broil, and top with yogurt and bacon bits
Canned chili	Heat and top with onions, lettuce, and tomato; use as dip for Italian or French bread, biscuits, or corn bread
Kabobs	Make with any combination of the following: fruit, vegetables, and sliced or cubed cooked meat (remove toothpicks before serving)
Popcorn	Serve plain or make three quarts and sprinkle with 1/4 cup grated cheese and 1/2 tsp garlic or onion salt
Parfait	Make with yogurt, fruit, and granola
Gelatin	Add fruit or vegetable juice, vegetables, fruits, or cottage cheese
Frozen fruit cubes	Freeze pureed applesauce or fruit juice into cubes
Fruit fizz	Add club soda to juice instead of serving soft drinks
Fruit shake	Blend milk with fresh fruit (bananas, berries, or a peach) and a dash of cinnamon or nutmeg
Yogurt frost	Combine fruit juice and yogurt; add fresh fruit if desired
Hot chocolate	Make hot chocolate or cocoa with milk chocolate and a dash of cinnamon
Seeds	Shelled sunflower seeds
Fish	Tuna fish
Canned soup	Vegetable or minestrone; nice on a cold winter's day

From A food guide for the first five years, *National Meat and Livestock Board, 444 North Michigan Avenue, Chicago, IL 60611.*

themselves—a practice that should be encouraged. No one food is an essential part of a diet. Hunger is still the best means for getting a child to eat. It may work to feed children vegetables at the start of a meal, when they are hungriest. Offer new foods with familiar ones. A platter of raw or lightly cooked carrots, broccoli, green and red peppers, cabbage, and mushrooms eaten as a snack with friends can do a lot to remedy a vegetable problem. Recall that children often are more sensitive to strong flavors and odors than are adults. Nutritious dips sell vegetables to many children. Using heroes as role models may work. Vegetables may acquire more appeal when children help prepare them. A 4- or 5-year-old child can safely eat raw vegetables without fear of choking.

"How Do I Know Whether My Child Is Eating Healthfully?" The Food Guide Pyramid in Chapter 2 forms the basis for a healthful diet in children aged 2 years and older (Figure 14-7). A child who eats from these food groups and regularly gains height and weight is eating a good diet. In childhood, 1 tablespoon of each food per year of age is a good starting point. Then serving size can increase to full adult portions as energy needs and appetite increase with age. Some nutrients that deserve special attention during childhood are calcium, iron, and vitamins A, B-6, and C.[1] These nutrients should be readily supplied if a child's diet includes choices from all the food groups—milk, yogurt, and cheese group; meat, poultry, fish, dry beans, eggs, and nuts group; fruit group; vegetable group; and breads, cereals, rice, and pasta group.

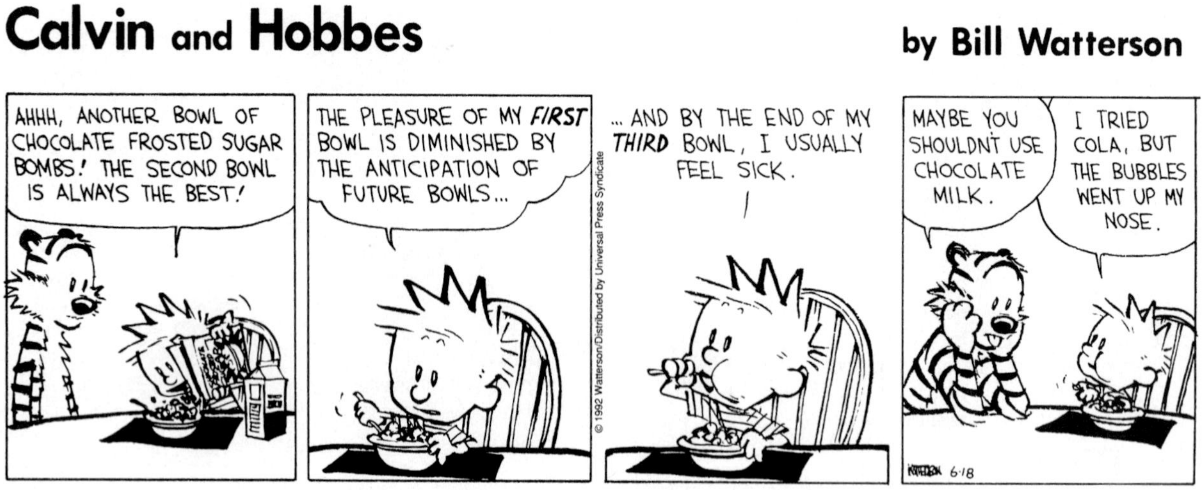

FIGURE 14-7
Calvin & Hobbes.

Two-year-olds commonly prefer peculiar foods, and parents need not worry about this. A child may switch from one specific food focus (often called a jag) to another with equal intensity. If the caregiver continues to offer choices, the child will soon begin to eat a wider variety of foods again, and the specific food focus will disappear as suddenly as it appeared.

Major scientific groups, such as the American Dietetic Association and the American Society for Clinical Nutrition, believe that vitamin and mineral supplements are unnecessary for healthy children. It is better to emphasize good foods. However, a nutrient supplement at the RDA level may be needed when a child is ill, especially if the illness persists. Diets for children who eat totally vegetarian fare should especially focus on protein, vitamin B-12, iron, and zinc. Studies show that many parents offer children conservative amounts of vitamins, so toxicity is unlikely. Still, the practice of giving supplements is often unnecessary, especially given today's typically highly fortified breakfast cereals, which children often eat.

Dental Health Tips for Children
- **Begin oral hygiene when an infant receives his or her first tooth.**
- **Seek early pediatric dental care.**
- **Drink fluoridated water.**
- **Use fluoridated toothpaste twice daily.**
- **Snack in moderation.**
- **Have your dentist apply tooth sealants if needed.**

If current childhood feeding practices aim to follow the most healthful dietary plans, they should gradually shift away from high-fat diets to diets containing more complex carbohydrates.[18] Low-fat, nutritious foods can form the base of a healthful diet for children. Opportunities to learn to enjoy these types of foods need to be provided. After 2 years of age, many authorities recommend eating patterns for children that contain no more than 30% of kcalories as fat and no more than 10% of kcalories as saturated fat. The Food Guide Pyramid, with its emphasis on starches, allows for such a pattern. Children are exposed to high-fat foods in quick-service restaurants. These foods are often sweet and high in salt as well. Caregivers can teach and model healthful ways to eat at quick-service restaurants by ordering from the salad bar. Children aren't born with a preference for high-fat foods; they develop this preference through repeated exposure.[3]

Many of us should consider a diet higher in carbohydrate and lower in fat. For children, the idea is not to force them to follow severely restricted diets, such as adults with weight or cholesterol problems might follow. Instead, children can simply limit the amount of high-fat, nutritionally empty foods they eat each day. Some easy diet changes to begin with are bagels instead of doughnuts, nonfat frozen yogurt instead of ice cream, low-fat milk instead of whole milk, fruit instead of crackers and cheese for snacks, and air-popped popcorn instead of chips.

Nutritional Problems in Childhood

The two most common nutritional problems in childhood are obesity, which we discuss in Nutrition Insight 14-2, and iron-deficiency anemia.

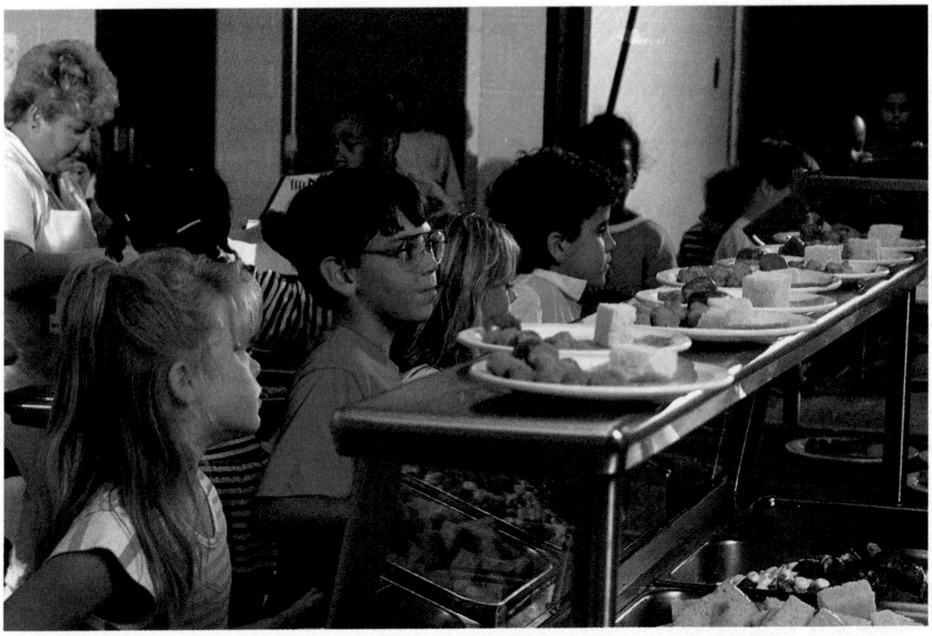

School lunch menus follow federal guidelines in the United States. What is eaten is up to the student.

Iron-Deficiency Anemia

Childhood iron-deficiency anemia is most likely to appear in children between the ages of 6 and 24 months.[11] It can lead to poor stamina and decrease in learning ability, because the oxygen supply to cells decreases. Less resistance to disease is also likely. Fortunately, the incidence of childhood anemia currently is quite low. This is probably because of the use of iron fortified breakfast cereals by children. In addition, the Special Supplemental Food Program for Women, Infants, and Children (WIC), sponsored by the federal government, deserves credit. This program emphasizes the importance of iron-fortified formulas and cereals and distributes them—along with nutrition education—to low-income parents of infants and preschool children considered to be at nutritional risk.

The best way to prevent iron-deficiency anemia in children is to regularly feed them foods that are adequate sources of iron.[15] Iron-fortified breakfast cereals and a few ounces of lean meat are convenient means of getting more iron into a child's diet. The high proportion of heme iron in many animal foods allows the iron to be more readily absorbed than is iron from plant foods. Consuming a vitamin C source along with the less readily absorbed iron in plants and supplements will aid absorption (see Chapter 9).

Is Childhood the Time to Start a Diet Designed to Limit the Risk for Heart Disease?

The American Academy of Pediatrics does not recommend low-fat diets (below 30% of total kcalories) for young children. It does recommend screening for blood cholesterol levels in children from families with histories of early heart disease and then treating children with high blood cholesterol levels with appropriate diet and drug therapy when needed, as discussed in Chapter 6. Currently, children get about 35% of their kcalories from fat, with about half of that from saturated fat.[1]

Heart disease starts in childhood. Autopsies of young military men who died in Korea and Vietnam showed the early signs of plaque buildup in their blood vessels.[18] The same holds for teens killed in auto accidents. As we said before, there is ample evidence to encourage the consumption of foods that have less overall fat and a higher proportion of monounsaturated and polyunsaturated fat. Moderation is the best strategy; very restrictive diets can be detrimental to overall nutrient intake.[13] A child needs to consume adequate energy and to build good habits that can be practiced into the teen years. One strategy to add to previous recommendations is to have children drink 1% or 2% milk after the age of 2 and to limit the intake of fatty meats, high-fat cheese, stick margarine, ice cream, and butter. Lean meats, fruits, vegetables, and breads and cereals form a better diet and generally provide little saturated fat.[10]

Are Low-Sodium Diets Appropriate for Children?

Scientific data neither confirm nor refute the notion that eating less sodium will reduce the risk of future high blood pressure. Moderation in sodium consumption does help build good health habits for the future—especially if the person later develops hypertension and needs to eat even less sodium. If children become accustomed to less salt, they will be less inclined to eat very salty foods as adults.

CONCEPT CHECK

The rapid growth rate of an infant's first year slows during the toddler and preschool years (about ages 1 to 5). As a child's appetite decreases, adults need to serve nutrient-dense foods and allow the child to decide how much to eat. Sudden shifts in food preferences are to be expected. Snacking is fine if there is attention given to the selection of healthful foods and good dental hygiene. Vitamin and mineral supplements are usually not needed—a plan following the Food Guide Pyramid should meet nutrient needs. Children should have plenty of iron-rich foods available to prevent iron-deficiency anemia. Developing heart-healthy habits after the age of 2 years is good health insurance.

THE TEENAGE YEARS

Most girls begin a rapid growth spurt between the ages of 10 and 13 years, and most boys grow more between the ages of 12 and 15 years. Nearly every organ in the body grows during these periods of faster growth, which last about 3 years. Most noticeable are increases in height and weight and development of secondary sexual characteristics. Girls usually begin menstruating (reach menarche) during this growth spurt, and they grow very little—if at all—beyond 2 years after menarche. Early maturing girls may begin their growth spurt as early as ages 7 to 8, whereas early maturing boys may begin growing by ages 9 to 10.

During the growth spurt, girls gain about 10 inches (25 centimeters) in height and boys gain about 12 inches (30 centimeters). Girls also tend to accumulate both lean and fat tissue, whereas boys tend to gain mostly lean tissue. This growth spurt provides about 42% to 51% of ultimate adult weight and 15% to 25% of ultimate adult height (see Figure 14-1).

Fortunately, as the growth spurt begins, teenagers begin to eat more. If teens choose nutritious food, they can take advantage of their increased hunger and easily satisfy their nutrient needs. As with older age-groups, the Food Guide Pyramid provides the basis for meeting these nutrient needs (Table 14-5).

Nutritional Problems and Concerns of Teens

Alcoholism, a significant health problem that may have its roots in the teen years, is covered in detail in Chapter 15.

We discussed anorexia nervosa and bulimia in Chapter 12. Other nutritional problems are more common during the teen years. A major concern is that many teenage girls stop drinking milk, and so they may not consume enough calcium to allow for maximal mineralization of bones through their early twenties. Many investigators are concerned that

TABLE 14-5

Food Guide for Adolescents and Teens*

	Include at Least This Many Servings Daily
Milk, yogurt, and cheese (preferably low-fat or nonfat)	3
Meats, poultry, fish, dry beans, eggs, and nuts	2-3
Vegetables	3-5
Fruits	2-4
Breads, cereals, rice, and pasta (preferably whole grain; otherwise, enriched or fortified)	6-11
Fats, oils, and sweets	Use sparingly

**Use serving sizes from adult Food Guide Pyramid.*
Here we define "teen" as a person who has added height in the past year and is at least 12 years old. This guide should be used through age 24 years.

young women who do not consume enough calcium are sowing the seeds for future osteoporosis.[9] Again, three servings from the milk, yogurt, and cheese group per day are recommended. The RDA for calcium increases between ages 11 and 24 years from 800 to 1200 milligrams for both males and females. This is the equivalent of three or four glasses of milk per day. Only about one in six teenage girls consumes that much calcium.

Another concern is iron deficiency. Iron-deficiency anemia sometimes appears in girls after they start menstruating and in boys during their growth spurt. About 12% of teenagers have low iron stores.[11] Teens who strive to forge an identity by adopting dietary patterns unfamiliar to their families—vegetarianism, for example—may not know enough about the alternate diet pattern to keep from developing health problems, such as iron-deficiency anemia. Overall, it is important that teenagers choose good food sources of iron, such as lean meats, whole grains, and enriched cereals. In addition, it is always a good idea to consume vitamin C with plant or supplemental sources of iron to increase iron absorption. Teenage girls especially need to eat good sources of iron (or regularly consume an iron supplement), particularly those with heavy menstrual flows. Iron-deficiency anemia is not a desirable state for a teen. It can produce increased fatigue and decreased ability to concentrate and learn. School performance may suffer.

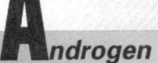

Androgen *A general term for hormones that stimulate development in male sex organs; testosterone is one example.*

Acne is a common teen concern—about 80% of teens experience it.[12] Though one hears that eating nuts, chocolate, and pizza can make acne worse, scientific studies have been unable to show a strong link between any dietary factor and acne. Teens are simply warned to avoid "trigger foods," assuming that planning a well-balanced diet is still possible. Acne naturally waxes and wanes, and so teens fall easy prey to notions about relationships to dietary factors. Acne may be more dormant in summer, because sunlight appears to improve this condition. The effect of artificial ultraviolet light on acne is not so pronounced. The main culprit of acne is overactivity by the sebaceous glands in the skin.[12] They respond to testosterone, which is mainly a male hormone. This is why men tend to have more serious cases of acne and to a greater extent than do women. Women also secrete testosterone and other **androgen** (testosterone-like) compounds. If these compounds are produced in large amounts, a woman also may experience serious acne.

The sebaceous glands surround hair follicles on the face, ears, back, chest, eyelids, and other areas. If substances block a duct in the gland, this can lead to an infection and local pressure, resulting in an acne lesion.

One drug dermatologists sometimes prescribe for acne is tretinoin, which is sold under trade names, such as Retin-A. A derivative of vitamin A, tretinoin is rubbed onto the skin once nightly. It is highly effective for treating blackheads and modestly effective for treating pimples. Scientists do not know exactly how tretinoin works, but research suggests that it both pushes out the plugs in the ducts beneath the skin and helps prevent their reformation. The most exciting news for serious acne is the introduction of Accutane (13-cis retinoic acid or isotretinoin). This prescription oral medication, another derivative of vitamin A, appears to change the nature of sebaceous gland development. It decreases the production of ***sebum*** and in turn reduces the number of acne lesions. The medication is especially helpful in treating cases resistant to antibiotic therapy (see Chapter 8 for more information about Accutane). Teens should not self-medicate with vitamin A itself in hopes of curtailing acne. Instead they should rely on advice from their physician. It is the derivatives of vitamin A—not the vitamin itself—that are helpful, and these are available only by prescription.[12] Recall as well that excess dosages of vitamin A can cause toxicity, so this would also likely be a hazardous choice.

Sebum *Secretion of the sebaceous glands consisting of waxes, and other lipids.*

A Closer Look at the Diets of Teenage Girls

Teenagers in general are apt to adopt fad diets, eat away from home or miss meals completely, and snack a lot. Teenage girls, especially, are very concerned with weight gain, appearance, and acceptability. Recent government statistics revealed that female students were significantly more likely to report currently trying to lose weight (44%) than were male students (15%). Moreover, 27% of female students who considered themselves the right weight reported they were currently trying to lose weight. In an attempt to reach personal goals, they may eat dangerously little, select just a few items, and frequently skip meals altogether. If their limited food choices then consist of French fries, soft drinks, and pastries, little room is left for foods that are good nutrient sources. It's not only calcium and iron that teenage girls need to be concerned about—they often don't get enough folate, zinc, and vitamins A, B-6, and C as well. Common use of diet pills and the increasing number of bulimia cases further add to these nutritional problems.

Helping Teens Eat More Nutritious Foods

Teenagers face a variety of upheavals in their lives. They pursue their independence, experience identity crises, seek peer acceptance, and worry about physical appearance. Advertisers take advantage of this by pushing a vast array of products—candy, gum, soda pop, and snacks—targeted toward the teenage market. All these factors affect food choice.

Teens often do not think of the long-term benefits of good health. They have a hard time relating today's actions to tomorrow's health outcomes. The future is far away. Many teenagers tend to think they can just change habits later; there is no hurry.

Still, healthful teen food habits do not have to include giving up favorite foods. Small portions of fatty foods can complement larger portions of low-fat dairy products, lean meats, vegetable proteins, fruits, vegetables, and grain products. A plain hamburger with a garden salad (minimize the amount of regular dressing or use a low-fat variety) and small order of French fries incorporates these goals.

Overcoming the Teenage Mindset

One strategy for working with teenage boys is to stress the importance of nutrition for physical development—especially muscular development—and for fitness, vigor, and health. With teenage girls, one approach is to help them understand how to choose nutrient-dense foods that lead to better health while maintaining appropriate weight. It can be explained that beauty is based on the glow of health, something that sick people often do not have. For teenagers, it is more effective to focus on the benefits of healthful foods they can reap right now than to talk about health hazards that may or may not happen at some later time if they eat a less than healthful diet.

Are Teenage Snacking Practices Harmful?

As with children, the major focus with snacks should be what one eats. Teens often obtain one fourth to one third of all their energy and major nutrients from snacks (Figure 14-8). Teenagers can obtain many nutrients from snacking. Key reasons for snacking include an opportunity to get out and socialize with friends, accessibility, hunger, and celebrating a special event. Even quick-service restaurants offer some good food choices. By choosing wisely and eating in moderation, teens can eat at quick-service restaurants and still consume a very good diet. Snacks and quick-service restaurants in and of themselves are not the problem; poor food choices are. Unfortunately, a recent Gallup poll has found just what you might expect—that teens snack mostly on potato and corn chips, cookies, candies, and ice cream.

Poor dietary habits formed during teenage years often continue into adulthood, giving rise to an increased risk of chronic diseases, such as heart disease, osteoporosis, and some types of cancer. Getting this message across to teenagers is an important and challenging task for parents and health professionals.

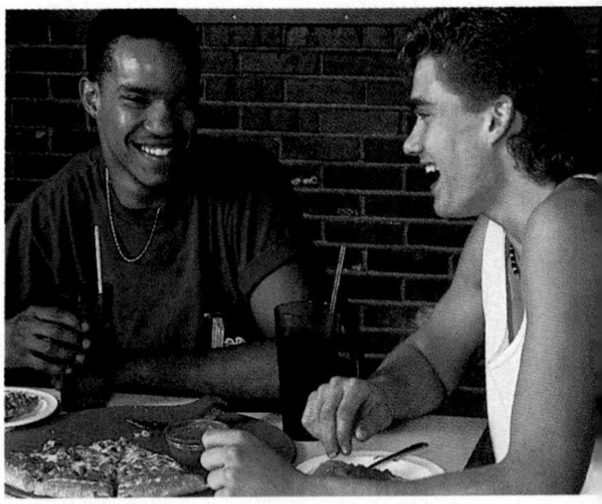

FIGURE 14-8
The teen years are noted for snacking. Still, nutritional problems associated with teenagers' eating at quick-service restaurants are caused more by food choice than by the foods available.

CONCEPT CHECK

Another period of rapid growth occurs during the teen years. Girls generally start this earlier than boys. The Food Guide Pyramid should guide meal planning. Common nutritional problems in these years arise from poor food choices and include inadequate calcium intake in girls, iron-deficiency anemia, and sometimes excessive saturated fat intake. Because changes occur so rapidly during these years, and in so many areas—psychological, social, and physical—it may be difficult to stress the importance of nutrition to teenagers. Moderation in fat intake is one goal to consider when choosing snacks.

SUMMARY

- Growth is very rapid during infancy; birth weight doubles in 4 to 6 months, and length increases by 50% in the first year. An adequate diet, especially protein intake, is very important to support normal growth. Undernutrition can cause irreversible changes in growth and development. Growth in infants and children can be assessed by measuring body weight, height (or length), and head circumference over time.
- Nutrient needs in the first 6 months can be met by human milk or formula. Supplementary vitamin D and iron may be needed in the first 6 months for breast-fed infants, and many infants may need supplemental fluoride.
- Infant formulas generally contain lactose or sucrose, heat-treated proteins from cow's milk, and vegetable oil. Formulas may or may not be fortified with iron. Sanitation is very important when preparing and storing formula.
- Most infants do not need solid foods before about 6 months of age. Solid food should not be added to an infant's diet until the nutrients are needed, the GI tract can digest complex foods, the infant has the physical ability to control tongue thrusting, and the risk of developing food allergies decreases.
- The first solid food given should be iron-fortified infant cereals or ground meats. Other single foods can be added gradually, at the rate of about one each week. Some foods to avoid giving infants in the first year include honey, low-fat cow's milk, very salty or sweet foods, or foods that may cause choking.

- Introducing iron-containing solid food at the appropriate time and not offering cow's milk until appropriate can generally prevent iron-deficiency anemia in late infancy.
- Obese children and adolescents are more likely to become obese adults and so incur greater health risks. Parents can provide healthful food choices, while children should control portion sizes. When controlled early, a problem of obesity may correct itself as the child continues to grow in height. Obese infants, on the other hand, do not necessarily go on to become obese children.
- A slower growth rate in preschool years underlies the importance of children eating nutrient-dense foods and reducing their food serving sizes. Choosing iron-rich foods, such as lean red meats, is important at this age. Portion sizes at meals of 1 tablespoon of each food for each year of life is a good rule of thumb. Teens and young adults particularly need adequate iron and calcium in the diet, especially girls, and should generally strive to moderate high-fat food choices.

Study Questions

1. Describe how you would assess whether an 8-month-old infant is consuming a healthful diet.
2. Outline three key factors that help determine when to introduce solid foods into an infant's diet.
3. Why should obesity in childhood be discouraged? What three factors are likely to contribute to this problem in a typical 6-year-old child?
4. Contrast the Dietary Guidelines issued for infants in this chapter with those for children over 2 and adults listed in Chapter 2. Which guidelines are similar? Do any contradict each other? If so, what would be the reason(s)?
5. Describe three pros and cons for snacking. What is the basic advice for healthful snacking from childhood through teen years?
6. What two nutrients are of particular interest in planning diets for teens? Why does each deserve to be singled out? What nutrient most deserves an "in moderation" warning?

REFERENCES

1. Albertson AM and others: Nutrient intake of 2- to 10-year-old American children: 10-year trends, *Journal of the American Dietetic Association* 92:1492, 1992.
2. Behrman RE and others: *Nelson textbook of pediatrics,* ed 13, Philadelphia, 1987, WB Saunders.
3. Birch LL: Children's preferences for high-fat foods, *Nutrition Reviews* 50:249, 1992.
4. Carroll P and others: Guidelines for counselling parents of young children with food sensitivities, *Journal of the American Dietetic Association* 92:602, 1992.
5. Colon AR, Dipalma JS: Colic, *American Family Physician* 40(6):122, 1989.
6. Forbes GB: Children and food: order amid chaos, *The New England Journal of Medicine* 324:262, 1991.
7. Hedges HH: The elimination diets as a diagnostic tool, *American Family Physician* 46(5):77S, 1992.
8. Hendricks KM, Badruddin SM: Weaning recommendations: the scientific basis, *Nutrition Reviews* 50:125, 1992.
9. Lloyd T and others: Calcium supplementation and bone mineral density in adolescent girls, *Journal of the American Medical Association* 270:841, 1993.
10. National Cholesterol Education Program: Highlights of the expert panel on blood cholesterol levels in children and adolescents, *American Family Physician* 45(5): 2127, 1992.
11. Oski FA: Iron deficiency in infancy and childhood, *New England Journal of Medicine* 329:190, 1993.
12. Phillips TJ, Dover JS: Recent advances in dermatology, *The New England Journal of Medicine* 326:167, 1992.
13. Pipes PL: *Nutrition in infancy and childhood,* St Louis, 1993, Mosby–Year Book.
14. Rees JM: Management of obesity in adolescence, *Medical Clinics of North America* 74:1275, 1990.
15. Sampson HA, Metcalfe DD: Food allergies, *Journal of the American Medical Association* 268:2840, 1992.
16. Satter EM: Childhood eating disorders, *Journal of The American Dietetic Association* 86:357, 1986.
17. Sigman-Grant M: Feeding preschoolers: balancing nutritional and developmental needs, *Nutrition Today,* p. 13, July/August 1992.
18. Snetselaar L, Lauer RM: Childhood, diet and the atherosclerotic process, *Nutrition Today,* p. 22, January/February 1992.
19. Stunkard AJ, Berkowitz RI: Treatment of obesity in children, *Journal of the American Medical Association* 264:2550, 1990.
20. Zeiger RS: Prevention of food allergy in infancy, *Annals of Allergy* 65:430, 1990.

RATE

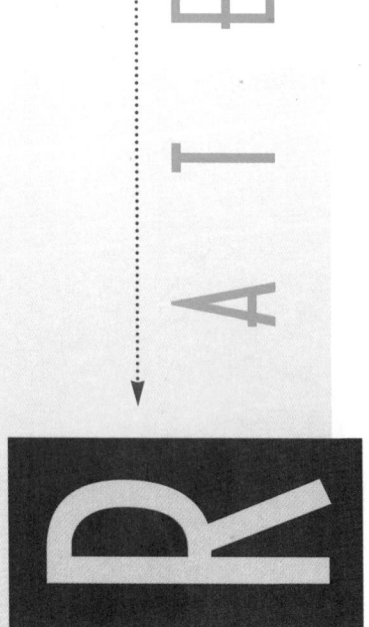

GETTING LITTLE BILLY TO EAT

Bill is 3 years old and his mother is worried about his eating habits. He absolutely refuses to eat vegetables, meat, and dinner in general. Some days he eats very little food. He wants to eat snacks most of time. His mother wants him to eat a formal lunch and dinner to make sure he gets all the nutrients he needs. Mealtime is a battle because Bill says that he isn't hungry, but his mother wants him to eat everything served on his plate. He drinks five or six glasses of whole milk per day because that is the one food he adores.

When his mother prepares dinner, she makes plenty of vegetables, boiling them until they are soft, hoping this will appeal to Bill. Bill's dad waits to eat his vegetables last, regularly telling the family that he eats them only because he has to. He also regularly complains about how dinner has been prepared. Bill saves his vegetables until last and usually gags when his mother orders him to eat them. Bill has been known to sit at the dinner table for an hour until the war of wills ends. Bill's mother serves casseroles and stews regularly because these are her best dishes. Bill likes to eat breakfast cereal, fruit, and cheese and will regularly request these foods for snacks. However, his mother tries to deny his requests so he will have an appetite for dinner. Bill's mother comes to you and asks you what she should do to get Bill to eat.

Analysis

1. List four mistakes Bill's parents are making that contribute to Bill's poor eating habits.

____

____

____

____

2. List four strategies they might try to promote good eating habits in Bill.

____

____

____

____

your plate

Nutrition ISSUE

FOOD ALLERGIES AND INTOLERANCES

Adverse reactions to foods—indicated by sneezing, coughing, nausea, vomiting, diarrhea, hives, and other rashes—are broadly classed as food allergies or food intolerances.[15] ***Allergies*** are reactions linked to immune system responses, such as the rapid increase in heart rate and shortness of breath that occur when susceptible people eat shrimp. The immune system senses what it considers "foreign proteins" and attempts to eliminate them. The symptoms experienced are the result of the battle.

On the other hand, symptoms of food intolerances—which include many of those listed previously—are not linked to an allergic mechanism. For example, symptoms of foodborne illness, such as *Salmonella* from infected egg products, are caused by toxins released by bacteria in food. These toxins directly affect intestinal cells. Let's examine each process, allergies and intolerances, separately so you can learn how to reduce your risk of becoming a victim.

Allergic reactions to foods are commonly reported and more frequently by females. The most common ages for food allergies are infancy and young adulthood. Allergic-related disease appears in about 30 to 40 million Americans. The following types of reactions are associated with food ingestion:

Classic—Itching, reddening skin, asthma, swelling, choking, and a runny nose
Gastrointestinal—Nausea, vomiting, diarrhea, intestinal gas, bloating, pain, constipation, and indigestion
General—Headache, skin reactions, tension and fatigue, tremors, and psychological problems

Allergic reaction symptoms vary with the location in the body, as noted previously. Timelines include from seconds to a few days. A generalized, all-systems reaction is called ***anaphylactic shock.*** This severe allergic response results in lowered blood pressure and respiratory and gastrointestinal tract distress. It can be fatal. A person with extreme sensitivity to a food may not be able to touch the food or even be in the same room where it is being cooked without responding to it.

About 90% of food allergies (also called *hypersensitivities*) are caused by milk, eggs, nuts (especially peanuts), corn, seafood, soy, and wheat. Other foods frequently identified with adverse reactions include alcoholic beverages, meat and meat products, vegetables, sugars, cereals, fish, fats and oils, fruits, chocolate, and cheese.[15] A family history of allergies greatly increases the risk.

Why Do Food Allergies Occur?

A food allergy is caused by an immune response to a food substance. ***Food sensitivity*** is a term often used today to describe milder reactions. Again, the word *allergy* specifies a disorder of the immune system. Allergens are usually large proteins with specific sizes and configurations.

Allergy
An immune response that occurs when immune bodies (antibodies) react with a foreign substance (antigen).

Anaphylactic Shock
A severe allergic reaction that results in greatly lowered blood pressure, as well as respiratory and gastrointestinal distress.

Food Sensitivity
A mild reaction to a substance in a food that might be noticed as slight twitching or redness of the skin.

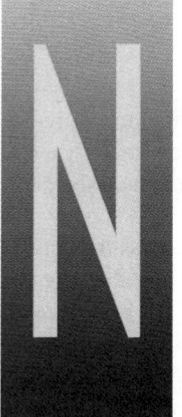

When an allergen enters an allergic-prone host for the first time, a specific immune reaction takes place, although it is not apparent. Subsequent exposures can then trigger various muscles to contract, increase permeability of blood vessels, and lead to nasal secretions, itching, and changes in dilation of the airways.

A big question concerning food allergies is how intact food proteins can cross the natural barriers of the GI tract to interact with the immune system. Considering the thoroughness of the digestive system, it seems that these particles would break down into amino acids that the body could then metabolize with no adverse effects. Evidence now shows, however, that minute amounts of large particles can gain access to the immune system through gaps between intestinal cells. These large particles can eventually be transported via the bloodstream to various body sites where they can cause a reaction.

In a nonallergic person, immune factors synthesized by intestinal cells act as a natural barrier against absorption and transportation of large molecules. This protection doesn't seem to function efficiently for people with food allergies. Because the immune systems and GI tracts of very young infants are not fully functioning yet, these organ systems are believed to contribute to the higher risk of allergic reactions in the very young.[15]

Testing for a Food Allergy

A bogus method used to test for food allergies is cytotoxic testing. In this test, blood cells from the allergic person are mixed with food proteins suspected of causing the problem. If cell damage is noted, sensitivity is suspected. This is not a reliable way to test for allergies. Don't be taken in by this form of health fraud.

The first step in determining the presence of a food allergy is to record in detail a history of symptoms, time from ingestion to onset of symptoms, most recent reaction, quantity of food needed to produce a reaction, and the food suspected of causing a reaction. A family history of allergic diseases can also help. The physician looks for signs of allergy, such as inflammation in the nasal cavity, skin diseases, and asthma. Skin testing can help pinpoint likely allergen suspects.

The next step usually is to eliminate from the diet all tested compounds that appear to cause allergic symptoms plus all other foods the person's history suggests may cause an allergy. If symptoms still persist, the person can restrict the diet even more severely or even use special formulas that are hypoallergenic. This type of elimination diet should eventually abolish all symptoms.[7]

After 2 to 4 weeks without symptoms, foods can be cautiously reintroduced, but not those thought to cause *anaphylactic shock.* Foods should be tried in small quantities at first—½ to 1 teaspoon (2.5 to 5 milliliters). The amount is increased until the dose approximates usual intake. In this way, allergenic substances can be identified if symptoms resume. In a clinical setting, this can be done using a double-blind approach where neither the patient nor the person scoring the results knows whether the diet contains the potentially offending food. This is especially needed when a psychological component might complicate the reaction or when symptoms are vague or ill-defined. Dried foods can be encapsulated and then given to the person.

Treatment of Food Allergies

Once potential allergens are identified, the best treatment is to avoid them, especially for people with zero tolerance. Careful reading of food labels is one excellent practice. Cromolyn sodium, a prescription medication given as an inhalant, can limit the extent of an immune reaction in the lungs.

A major challenge for the clinician treating a person with a food allergy is to make sure that what remains in the diet can still provide essential nutrients. Children especially, with their small food intake, permit less leeway in removing offending foods that may contain numerous nutrients. A registered dietitian can help guide the diet-planning process to ensure that what remains of the food choices still meets nutrient needs.[4]

If an allergic-prone woman is pregnant or breast-feeding, she should avoid offending foods—like eggs and peanuts—because antigens can cross the placenta during pregnancy. Antigens will also be secreted in her milk. She should work with her doctor to make sure an adequate diet is still consumed. In addition, when food allergies run in the family, women are advised to breast-feed their infants exclusively for 6 months. Human milk contains factors that may play a role in maturation of the small intestine. Formula-fed infants have a greater risk of developing allergies. Breast-feeding then should continue for as long as possible, preferably at least 1 year.[20]

The ***prognosis*** for food allergies that occur before 3 years of age is good. About 80% of children outgrow food allergies within 3 years. Food allergies diagnosed after age 3 years are often more long-lived, but not necessarily so.[15] In these cases about 33% of people outgrow their food allergies within 3 years. For others the symptoms are more long-lived. Occasional reintroduction of foods can be tried every 6 months or so to see whether the allergy symptoms have decreased, but not before 1 year of age. If no symptoms appear, tolerance to the food has developed.

Prognosis
A forecast of the course and end of a disease.

Food Intolerance
An adverse reaction to food that does not involve an allergic mechanism.

Food Intolerances

In addition to food allergies, ***food intolerances*** also cause adverse food reactions. Again, these do not involve the allergic mechanisms, and so it is important to treat them differently from actual food allergies. Food intolerance also differs from allergies in that more of the offending food is required to produce symptoms. Food intolerances can be caused by the following:

- Substances, such as in wine, tomatoes or pineapples, that can produce medicine-like activity, such as changes in blood pressure.
- Toxic contaminants, such as bacterial toxins; synthetic compounds, such as some food-coloring agents; antibiotics; and insect parts (see Chapter 17)
- Deficiencies in digestive enzymes, such as lactase
- Food poisoning caused by improper handling or cooking, as in *Clostridium botulinum* food-borne illness, or viral and bacterial infections, as in *Salmonella* food-borne illness.

Many of these conditions can lead to GI tract symptoms. In addition, anyone can expect to be sensitive to one or more of these causes of food intolerance.

Four other noteworthy food intolerances are induced by the presence of sulfites, monosodium glutamate (MSG), tartrazine, and tyramine in food. A sulfite reaction causes flushing, spasms of the airways, and a loss of blood pressure. Wine, dehydrated potatoes, dried fruits, gravy, soup mixes, and restaurant salad greens commonly contain sulfites. Evidence of reaction to MSG might be an increase in blood pressure, numbness, sweating, vomiting, headache, and facial pressure. MSG is commonly found in Chinese food and many processed foods, like soup. A reaction to tartrazine, a food color additive, includes spasm of the airways, itching, and reddening skin. Tyramine can cause high blood pressure in people taking monoamine-oxidase inhibitor medications (for mental depression). Tyramines are commonly found in "aged" foods, such as cheeses and red wines.

The basic treatment for food intolerances is to avoid specific offending components. However, this usually does not require total elimination, because people are generally not as sensitive to factors causing food intolerances as they would be to allergens. For instance, a slight amount of sulfites in a glass of wine may be tolerable, whereas a large dose from a chef's salad may cause a reaction. See Chapter 17 on food safety for more details about toxic reactions from foods.

How Many Children Are Sensitive to Food Additives?

In 1973, Dr. Benjamin Feingold suggested that food additives caused hyperactivity (now known as a part of the attention deficit hyperactivity disorder [ADHD]) in children. He theorized that because some children are allergic to aspirin-like compounds, and some food additives have aspirin-like structures, such children would also be allergic to certain food additives. Much research followed this proposal: generally, the research has not supported a strong or predictable association between the consumption of food additives and hyperactivity in children.

Today the incidence of ADHD is seen in approximately 2% to 4% of school-age children; boys are affected four to six times more than are girls. The initial identification of hyperactivity in children commonly occurs when they enter nursery or elementary school.

Teachers report that these students are uncontrollable, easily distracted, and unable to sit still; fail to finish assignments; act impulsively; bother other children; and, especially, intrude into other children's activities. Psychological testing can be used to further characterize the behaviors and reasons behind them.[2]

There are many pitfalls to both the diagnosis of ADHD and the study of links between diet and hyperactive behavior. By giving the child a special diet and observing behavior, parents are giving that child more attention. The extra attention alone can decrease disruptive behavior. In addition, an additive-free diet is likely to be more nutrient-rich, because it will contain more whole, less processed foods. So, it is difficult to know whether behavior changes in a hyperactive child on such a diet would result from eliminating additives or adding more nutrients.

The only definitive way to study this relationship is to use a double-blind protocol. A child would be given an additive-free food and then later a food full of additives. Neither the parents, the child, nor the researchers should know what is in the food. After the child has consumed the foods, the researchers score the child's behavior.

This procedure is much too cumbersome to be used in a school system or by a private pediatrician. Thus many suspected cases of food additive–linked hyperactivity are not tested in a definitive scientific manner. This is a real problem, because some diets used for hyperactive children eliminate more than just food additives. Some popular approaches eliminate dietary essentials, such as milk, fruit, and some grain products. The more limited the diet, the greater the risk of nutrient deficiencies and poor growth.

Chapter 5 noted that it is unlikely that use of sugar is the cause of hyperactivity or antisocial behavior in a child.

If an additive-free diet follows the Food Guide Pyramid and actually improves a child's attention span and behavior, there is no reason not to employ it. About 5% to 10% of cases may be helped by this treatment.[2] Eliminating food colors from the diet has no harmful effect as such.

A physician should agree that special diet restrictions are worth trying. Even then, diet changes must be handled carefully. In addition, a child should not be singled out as different from his or her peers and shouldn't end up feeling deprived as a result of dietary restrictions. The child should not see his or her own behavior as more directed by diet than by how he or she feels. Parents who look for excuses for a child's behavior may often find it easier to blame inappropriate behavior on something concrete, like food.

Will anything actually help the hyperactive child? Time is a very important therapy; hyperactivity tends to decrease as a child matures. When hyperactivity contributes to true ADHD, behavior therapies (especially to reinforce structure in one's life), frequent opportunities to dissipate excess energy, and stimulant medications (Ritalin, for example) can be used to treat the problem. The advice of a pediatrician skilled in the diagnosis and treatment of this disease should be sought.

chapter

15

NUTRITION DURING ADULTHOOD

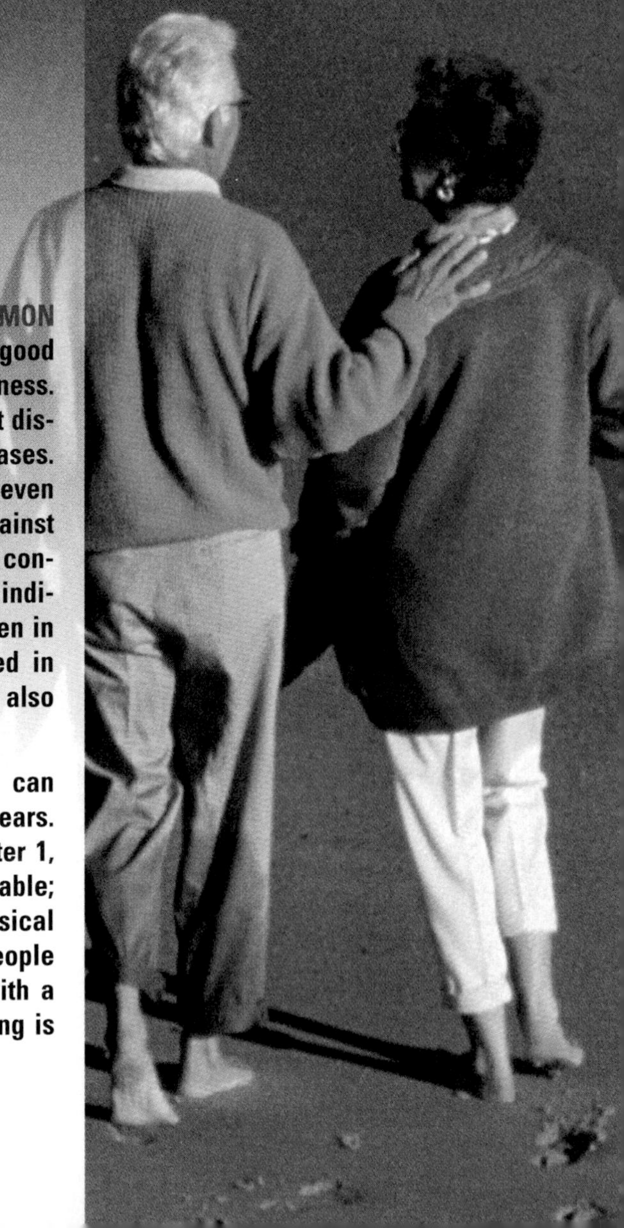

EATING IS ONE OF OUR GREAT PLEASURES. GUIDED BY COMMON sense and moderation, eating well is also a means to good health. Most of us want a long, productive life, free of illness. Yet, many people from early middle age onward suffer heart disease, strokes, diabetes, osteoporosis, or other chronic diseases. We can slow the development of, and in some cases even prevent, these diseases by pursuing a diet that works against them.[11] This action is most profitable if we begin early and continue throughout adulthood. We serve ourselves best—as individuals and as a nation—by striving to maintain vitality even in the later decades of life. This concept was first explored in Chapter 1. We will discuss it again in this chapter. We will also address the special nutrition needs of elderly persons.

Keep in mind that present day-to-day health practices can significantly influence health during a person's elderly years. Although genetics does play a role, as discussed in Chapter 1, many health problems that occur with age are not inevitable; they result from disease processes that influence physical health.[3] We have much to learn from healthy elderly people whose attention to health and physical activity—along with a little luck—keeps them active and vibrant. Successful aging is the goal. Age fast or slow—it is partly your choice.

ASSESS

TEST YOUR KNOWLEDGE

yourself

COULD YOU OR SOMEONE YOU KNOW HAVE A PROBLEM WITH ALCOHOL?

The Nutrition Issue in this chapter discusses ethanol, commonly known as alcohol. Problem drinking often has its seeds in the teen years. Significant health consequences of this typically arise in adulthood. Misuse of alcohol is one of our most preventable health problems. It is a prominent contributor to 5 of the 10 leading causes of death in the United States. The social consequences of alcohol dependency include divorce, unemployment, and poverty. The following questionnaire was developed by the National Council on Alcoholism. With this assessment you can examine whether you or someone you know might need help. Answer the following questions by placing an "X" in the appropriate blank.

	Yes	No
1. Do you occasionally drink heavily after disappointment, a quarrel, or when someone gives you a hard time?	______	______
2. When you have trouble or feel under pressure, do you drink more heavily than usual?	______	______
3. Have you ever noticed that you're able to handle liquor better than you did when you first started drinking?	______	______
4. Do you ever wake up the morning after you've been drinking and discover that you can't remember part of the evening before, even though your friends tell you that you didn't pass out?	______	______
5. When drinking with other people, do you try to have a few extra drinks when others won't know it?	______	______
6. Are there certain occasions when you feel uncomfortable if alcohol isn't available?	______	______
7. Have you recently noticed that when you begin drinking, you're in more of a hurry to get the first drink than you used to be?	______	______
8. Do you sometimes feel a little guilty about your drinking?	______	______
9. Are you secretly irritated when your family or friends discuss your drinking?	______	______
10. Have you recently noticed an increase in the frequency of memory blackouts?	______	______
11. Do you often find that you wish to continue drinking after your friends say they've had enough?	______	______

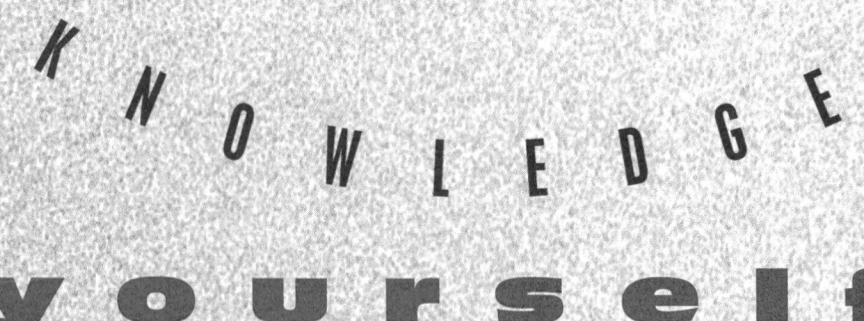

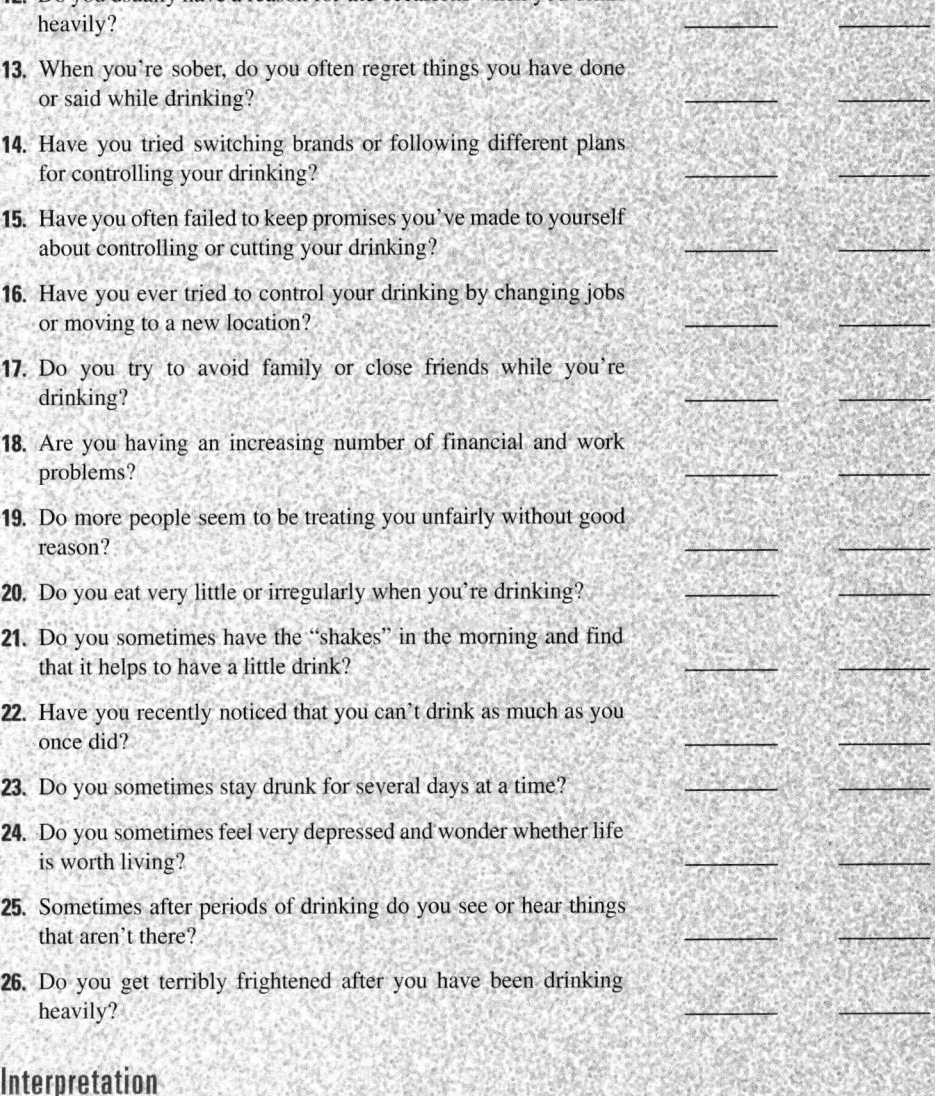

12. Do you usually have a reason for the occasions when you drink heavily? ______ ______

13. When you're sober, do you often regret things you have done or said while drinking? ______ ______

14. Have you tried switching brands or following different plans for controlling your drinking? ______ ______

15. Have you often failed to keep promises you've made to yourself about controlling or cutting your drinking? ______ ______

16. Have you ever tried to control your drinking by changing jobs or moving to a new location? ______ ______

17. Do you try to avoid family or close friends while you're drinking? ______ ______

18. Are you having an increasing number of financial and work problems? ______ ______

19. Do more people seem to be treating you unfairly without good reason? ______ ______

20. Do you eat very little or irregularly when you're drinking? ______ ______

21. Do you sometimes have the "shakes" in the morning and find that it helps to have a little drink? ______ ______

22. Have you recently noticed that you can't drink as much as you once did? ______ ______

23. Do you sometimes stay drunk for several days at a time? ______ ______

24. Do you sometimes feel very depressed and wonder whether life is worth living? ______ ______

25. Sometimes after periods of drinking do you see or hear things that aren't there? ______ ______

26. Do you get terribly frightened after you have been drinking heavily? ______ ______

Interpretation

These are all symptoms that may indicate alcoholism. "Yes" answers to several of the questions indicate the following stages of alcoholism:

Questions 1-8:	Potential drinking problem
Questions 9-21:	Drinking problem likely
Questions 22-26:	Definite drinking problem

It is vital that people assess themselves honestly. If you or someone you know demonstrates some or a number of these symptoms, it is important that help be pursued. If there is even a question in your mind, go talk to a professional about it. Alcohol abuse is one of many problems adults face.

YOUR ADULT YEARS

People who have healthful lifestyles and aim to prevent disease may or may not live longer. Heredity, accidents, and other events beyond our control influence longevity. However, health seekers often remain more active longer and spend less time immobilized. Many adults in America today have turned a healthful diet and moderate exercise regimen into lifetime pursuits of longevity. Coupled with avoiding tobacco products and limiting stress, these actions contribute to a healthful, long life.[3]

A DIET FOR THE ADULT YEARS

A diet that optimizes long-term nutritional health emphasizes low-fat dairy products, lean meats and plant proteins, a variety of fruits and vegetables, and whole-grain breads and cereals. The Food Guide Pyramid is a blueprint for this good diet.

To further refine food choices, recall also from Chapter 2 the Dietary Guidelines issued by the USDA/DHHS. The Surgeon General, the American Heart Association, the National Cancer Institute, and the National Academy of Sciences have added recommendations to the framework of the Dietary Guidelines. Following is a summary of the advice provided by the Dietary Guidelines, with additional comments from various health-related organizations.

A shortcut method for determining a healthful weight estimates 100 pounds for the first 60 inches for women and adds an extra 5 pounds for every inch thereafter. The corresponding values for males are 106 pounds for the first 60 inches and 6 additional pounds per inch thereafter.

1. **Eat a variety of foods.** Most groups specifically suggest variety and moderation in food choices. In addition, limit protein intake to no more than twice the RDA and do not take nutrient supplements in quantities greater than the RDA in any 1 day. Everyone should also meet the RDA for calcium, especially adolescent girls and women.
2. **Maintain healthful weight.** You can use the middle ranges of the Metropolitan Life Insurance Table as a standard or calculate your desirable weight using a Body Mass Index (BMI) of 19 to 25 for ages under 35, and 21 to 27 for ages over 35 (see Chapter 10). Emphasize balancing food intake with regular physical activity to avoid gradual weight gain that can lead to obesity.

   For those who are trying to lose weight, the recommended rate of weight loss is 1 to 2 pounds a week. To do this, increase physical activity and eat low-kcalorie, nutrient-rich foods: more fruits, vegetables, and grains; less fat and sugar; and fewer alcoholic beverages.
3. **Choose a diet low in fat, saturated fat, and cholesterol.** Limit fat intake to 30% of total kcalories and saturated fat to no more than one third of total fat intake (10% of total kcalories). A common dietary cholesterol limit is 300 milligrams per day. (The average American consumes 13% to 15% of total kcalories as saturated fat and about 400 to 500 milligrams of dietary cholesterol per day.) Choose lean meat, fish, poultry, and dry beans and peas as protein sources; use nonfat or low-fat milk and milk products; limit intake of fats and oils high in saturated fat; trim fat off meats; broil, bake, or boil instead of frying; and aim for moderate consumption of fat-containing foods, such as breaded or deep-fried items.
4. **Choose a diet with plenty of vegetables, fruits, and grain products.** Choose five or more servings of vegetables and fruits daily and six or more servings of a combination of breads, cereals, rice, and pasta daily. Aim for 20 to 30 grams of dietary fiber per day. These food choices should meet that goal. The current U.S. average for dietary fiber intake is closer to 15 grams per day. As mentioned in Chapter 1, dietary fiber is a term used to describe parts of plant foods that human digestive enzymes can't break down. There are several kinds of fiber, each with different chemical structures and biological effects (see Chapter 5 for details). Because foods differ in the kinds of fiber they contain, it's best to include a variety of fiber-rich foods.

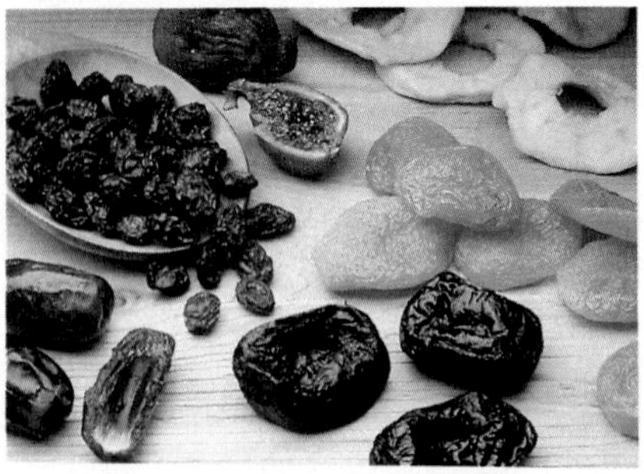

Eating dried fruit is an excellent way to increase your dietary fiber intake.

5. **Use sugars only in moderation.** Those people who are prone to dental caries (cavities), especially children, should limit the amount of sugary food they eat. Some authorities recommend that we eat no more than 10% to 15% of our total kcalories as sugars. This would amount to about 40 to 60 pounds per year, as opposed to our current per capita use of approximately 125 pounds per year. On a daily basis, this amounts to a limit of 10 to 15 teaspoons, less than a third of a cup, of sugar in a 2000-kcalorie diet.

6. **Use salt and sodium only in moderation.** Limit sodium intake to 3 grams per day. This is the amount of sodium contained in 6 grams of salt (40% of salt is sodium). The average person currently eats 4 to 7 grams of sodium per day. Limit the amount of salt in cooking and avoid adding it to food at the table. In addition, only very small amounts of salty, highly processed, salt-preserved, and salt-pickled foods should be eaten. A sodium restriction of 2.4 to 3 grams a day would require a great change in food habits for many of us. It would mean not eating processed (lunch) meats, salted snack foods, most canned and prepared soups, most types of cheese, and many tomato-based products.
7. **If you drink alcoholic beverages, do so in moderation.** Consume no more than two drinks daily—the equivalent of 8 ounces of wine, 24 ounces of beer, or 3 ounces of distilled spirits. Pregnant women should completely avoid alcohol. If you are concerned about excess kcalories and want a nutritious diet, keep in mind that alcoholic beverages are high in kcalories and low in or devoid of essential nutrients.

Beyond these overall recommendations, aim for moderate use of salt-cured, smoked, and ***nitrate***-cured foods, because they are suspected of increasing the risk of certain forms of cancer. Obtain adequate fluoride, particularly during the growing years, to strengthen tooth structure. Finally, children, adolescents, and women of childbearing age need to eat iron-rich foods, primarily to avoid developing iron-deficiency anemia.

Nitrate *A nitrogen-containing compound used to cure meats. Its use contributes a pink color to meats and confers some resistance to bacterial growth.*

This group of guidelines provide a good general focus for diet planning.[12] The practices recommended can accommodate many cultural dietary patterns. They are broad enough to allow you to include all the foods you enjoy in your eating plan—you may just have to eat some foods less frequently than others and/or in smaller portions, depending on your own health needs and preferences. Moderation, rather than elimination, is the overriding consideration.

Are Adults Following These Diet Recommendations?

In general, American adults—both young and old—are trying to follow many of the diet recommendations listed previously. Since the mid-1950s we have consumed less saturated fat as more people substitute skim and low-fat milk for cream and whole milk. However, we eat more cheese, which is usually a concentrated form of saturated fat. Since 1963 we eat less butter, eggs, and animal fat and more vegetable fats and oils and fish. We are also eating more fruits and vegetables. These changes generally follow the recommendations to reduce the intake of saturated fat and instead emphasize unsaturated fat. Today, animal breeders are raising much leaner cattle and hogs than in 1950. This helps us all. Our demand for chicken, a relatively lean source of animal protein, has also skyrocketed.

Other aspects of the average U.S. diet are more mixed. Nutritional surveys from the early 1980s (the most comprehensive to date) show that the major contributors of kcalories to the adult diet are as follows:

- White bread, rolls, and crackers
- Doughnuts, cakes, and cookies
- Alcoholic beverages
- Whole milk and beverages made with whole milk
- Hamburgers, cheeseburgers, and meatloaf

If the trend in diets were truly toward decreasing alcohol, sugar, and saturated fat and increasing fiber, these foods could hardly appear at the top of the list. Our suggestions for improvement would stress low-fat milk, whole-wheat bread and whole-grain cereals, lean meat and tuna, peanuts and kidney beans, and oranges and broccoli. What would your list look like?

Your task, as an adult, is to pinpoint the lifestyle practices most likely to cause you illness and chronic disease and to change those specifically. Whether these changes include switching to bran cereal, rice, pasta, fish, chicken, asparagus, and bok choy and walking 2 miles every other day is up to you. These practices all provide a means to promote and maintain nutritional and overall health.

FRANK & ERNEST® by Bob Thaves

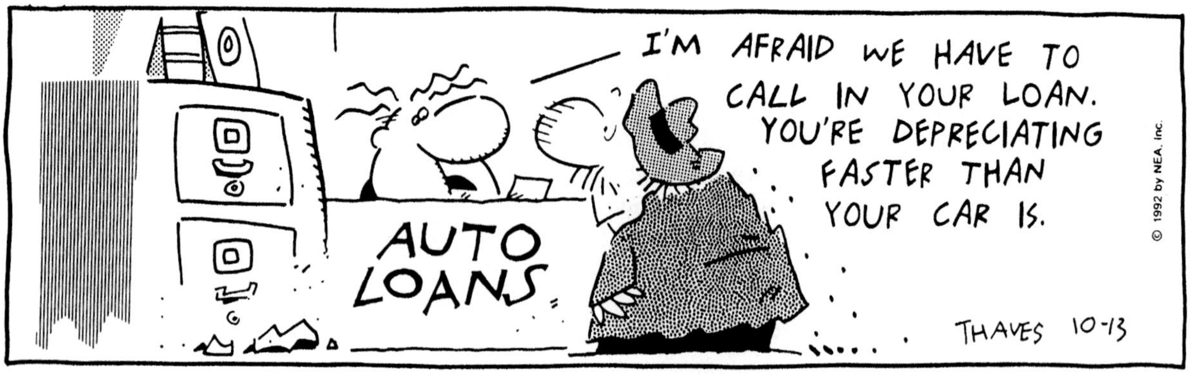

Reprinted by permission of NEA, Inc.

FIGURE 15-1
Frank and Ernest.

Keep in mind that an overall lifestyle that contains about an hour of physical activity each day, combined with a sensible dietary intake, reduces the risk of premature development of almost all the chronic diseases we adults face, including those that may develop in our elderly years.[20] The overriding consideration should be quality and length of life and the impact dietary changes might have on them. Now is the time to design and practice this plan (Figure 15-1). Learn more about the risk factors for chronic disease. Then review Chapter 16 for help in converting your plan into reality.

HEALTH OBJECTIVES FOR THE UNITED STATES FOR THE YEAR 2000

The Surgeon General's Report states that "for most of us, the more likely [health-related] problems are overeating too many kcalories for our activity levels and an imbalance in the nutrients consumed."

Health promotion and disease prevention became a public health strategy in the United States in the late 1970s. In 1979, a variety of health-related areas were highlighted as goals for national efforts in the document *Healthy People: The U.S. Surgeon General's Report on Health Promotion and Disease Prevention.*[21] Some goals in this document became the 1990 Health Objectives for the nation. Since this time, a new report, *Healthy People 2000,* issued in late 1990 by the U.S. Department of Health and Human Services' Public Health Service, has been released. This report consists of national health promotion and disease prevention objectives for the nation for the year 2000.

Healthy people 2000's nutrition-related challenges address the following[26]:

- Iron-deficiency anemia
- Poor growth in infants and children
- High fat intake
- Obesity
- High serum LDL-cholesterol levels
- High sodium intakes
- Low calcium intakes
- Low complex carbohydrate and dietary fiber intakes
- The need for more home-delivered meals for elderly persons
- A relative lack of breast-feeding, poor general nutrition knowledge, and the lack of nutrition education
- The need for more food labeling information
- The need for a comprehensive, nationwide, nutritional assessment and monitoring system in both health care and consumer settings.

The main objective of *Healthy People 2000* is to promote healthful lifestyles and reduce preventable death and disability in all Americans.

CONCEPT CHECK

The Dietary Guidelines form an effective framework for diet planning in adulthood. Additional recommendations for exercising regularly, not using tobacco products, and limiting stress can further maximize health potential. Surveys show that Americans are beginning to follow general health recommendations, but many goals still need more attention. Genetic background, medical conditions, and some lifestyle practices influence an individual's nutritional and health state. *Healthy People 2000* is a federal agenda aimed at disease prevention and health promotion for all Americans. Individual nutrition and health plans should be developed by all of us.

A FOCUS ON NUTRITION IN THE ELDERLY YEARS

How long do your family members generally live? Of those who died early in adulthood, can you pinpoint some causes? Do you plan to live longer than your parents did or will? How long will that be? Some basic statistics can help you predict this.

TABLE 15-1

Changes in the Causes of Death During This Century in the United States

Chronic diseases, rather than infectious diseases, are now the major "killers." AIDS is currently the eleventh leading cause of death.

Rank	Cause of Death	Percent Mortality*
1900		
1	Pneumonia and influenza	12
2	Tuberculosis	11
3	Diarrhea and enteritis	8
4	Heart disease	8
5	Cerebrovascular disease (stroke)	6
6	Nephritis	5
7	Accidents	4
8	Cancer	4
9	Diphtheria	2
10	Meningitis	2
1989		
1	Heart disease	34
2	Cancer	23
3	Cerebrovascular disease (stroke)	7
4	Accidents	4
5	Pulmonary (lung) disease	4
6	Pneumonia and influenza	4
7	Diabetes	2
8	Suicide	1
9	Liver disease and cirrhosis	1
10	Homicide and law enforcement	1

From National Center for Health Statistics: Monthly vital statistics report, *August 30, 1990.*
**Percent of all deaths in that year.*

Life Span The potential oldest age to which a person can survive.

Life Expectancy The average length of life for a given group of people born in a specific year, such as this year.

Life Span

Life span refers to the maximal number of years humans live. As far as we know, this hasn't changed in recorded time. The longest human life documented to date is 118 years. In contrast, the domestic dog has a life span of 20 years, and a rat, 5 years.

Life Expectancy

Life expectancy is the time an average person born in a specific year, such as 1994, can expect to live. In 1989, life expectancy in America was 71.8 years for men and 78.6 years for women. Worldwide, the highest average life expectancy is 82 years for women and 76 years for men in Japan. Researchers suggest that a diet based on rice, fish, vegetable protein sources, and some meat contributes to this record longevity.[22] Life expectancy hasn't always been this long; for primitive humans, it was about 30 to 35 years. It had increased to 49 years in Medieval England and remained so until the turn of this century. During the last 80 years, life expectancy for nearly all people has increased, mainly because of changes in the principal causes of death.

At the turn of this century, infectious diseases commonly caused death. Vaccines and antibiotics have tremendously lowered death from disease. The decline in infant and childhood deaths, coupled with better diets and health care, have allowed more people to age first into maturity and then into elderly years. Now the principal causes of death in Western societies are related to heart disease and cancer (Table 15-1).

Historically, the trend in America has been toward an ever-older population. During colonial times, half the population was over 16 years of age. By 1990, half were over 33. By 2050, half could be over 43, and approximately 20% of the entire U.S. population will be 65 years and older, twice as many as reach 65 years today (Figure 15-2). This age—65 years old—is arbitrarily listed as a dividing line for the beginning of the elderly years, because one can qualify for full Social Security benefits. But the timing of the elderly years for each of us varies with health and independence. Some people are quite healthy and independent at age 65, whereas others are disabled and greatly dependent on assistance for activities of daily living. Among the older population, the group constituting those aged 85+ years is the fastest growing segment. Between 1986 and 2050, the population aged 85+ years is expected to increase from about 1% to more than 5% of the total U.S. population. This is the first time in history our society will need to deal with such a large elderly population.[1]

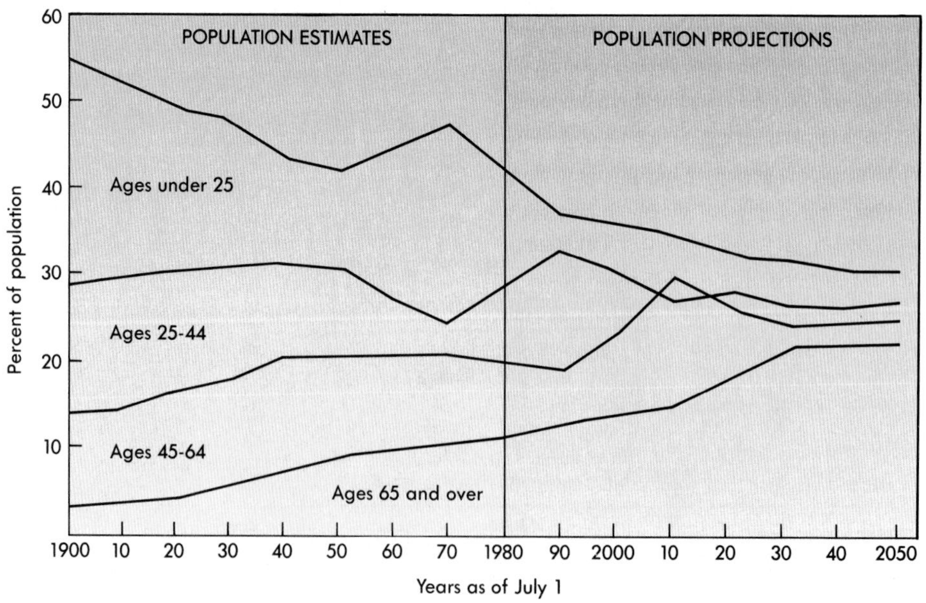

FIGURE 15-2
Trend in age distribution of U.S. population (including Armed Forces overseas), 1900-2050. The United States has never had a population with so many elderly people as it will soon have.

The "Graying" of America

The "graying" of America poses some problems. Today, while people older than age 65 account for 12% of the U.S. population, they account for more than 30% of all medications used, 40% of acute care hospital stays, and 50% of the federal health budget. Of elderly persons, 85% have nutrition-related problems, such as heart problems, diabetes, hypertension, osteoporosis, and obesity (Table 15-2).[3]

Postponing these chronic diseases for as long as possible will help control health care costs. The more independent, healthy years people live, the better life can be for them and the less they burden the health care system, which will increasingly have to scramble to accommodate a growing elderly population. Keep in mind that aging is not a disease, although the process of aging is still a mystery. It is difficult to design a model that predicts aging because so often disease speeds the process. But diseases that commonly accompany old age—osteoporosis and atherosclerosis, for example—are not an inevitable part of aging. Some people do die of old age, not as a direct result of disease.

What Actually Is Aging?

One view of aging describes it as processes of slow cell death beginning soon after fertilization. When we are young, aging is not apparent because the major metabolic activities are geared toward growth and maturation. We produce plenty of active cells to meet physiological needs. During late adolescence and adulthood, the body's major task is to maintain cells. But, inevitably, cells age and die. Eventually, as more cells die, the body cannot adjust to meet all physiological demands. Body functioning begins to decrease, but organs usually retain enough ***reserve capacity*** so that for a long time the body shows no outward disease. Although no symptoms appear, subclinical disease may develop, and if the disease is allowed to progress unchecked, organ function and then body function eventually deteriorate noticeably.[11]

Reserve Capacity *The extent to which an organ can preserve essentially normal function, despite decreasing cell number or activity.*

The aging process is clearly illustrated by changes for many people in the function of the enzyme lactase. For some people, lactase activity in the small intestine slows during childhood. Generally, however, clear symptoms of the deficiency—gas and bloating after milk consumption—do not appear until adulthood. Although lactase output decreases in these cases, perhaps from birth, enough enzyme is present to digest lactose until adulthood.

TABLE 15-2

Selected Disease Conditions Associated with Aging

	Rate of Occurrence Per 1000 Persons			
Chronic Condition	**Total**	**45-64 Years**	**65-74 Years**	**75+ Years**
Arthritis	131	280	460	508
Hypertension	124	265	408	395
Hearing impairments	91	149	261	381
Heart conditions	83	137	291	339
Visual impairments	35	46	72	136
Deformities or orthopedic impairments	121	175	191	198
Diabetes	26	55	98	92
Diverticula of intestines	8	15	36	45
Asthma	37	32	47	26

From the National Center for Health Statistics: Vital and health statistics, *May 24, 1988.*

NUTRITION insight

A PRESCRIPTION FOR LONGEVITY?

Some of us live longer and enjoy better health than others. Whole communities also show differences in longevity. In the United States, Seventh Day Adventist men live an average of 6 years longer than do other men. They have unusually low death rates from heart disease and cancer. When we examine their lifestyles, we find that most do not smoke or drink alcoholic beverages, and they eat less meat and more fruits, vegetables, and whole grains than do other men. These and other health habits are clearly identified as factors influencing how quickly we age (Figure 15-3).

FRANK & ERNEST® by Bob Thaves

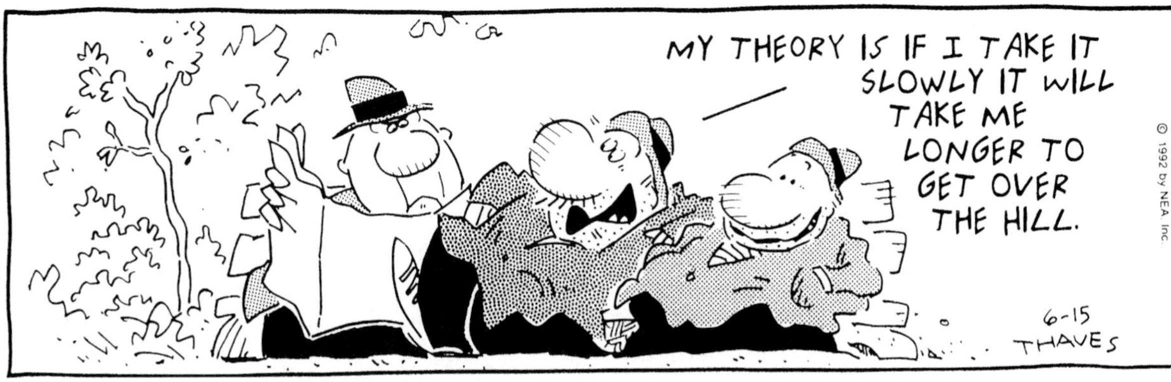

Reprinted by permission of NEA, Inc.

FIGURE 15-3
Frank and Ernest.

Studies show that people who followed seven simple health habits experienced a much lower death rate than those who did not. The long-lived group typically had the following habits: (1) they never smoked, (2) they moderated their alcohol consumption, (3) they ate breakfast regularly, (4) they didn't snack, (5) they slept 7 to 8 hours a night, (6) they exercised regularly, and (7) they maintained desirable body weights.

As we learned in the chapter on weight control, factors influencing weight—and hence longevity—appear to be related to nature as well as nurture. When researchers closely ex-

Cells age probably because of automatic cellular changes and environmental influences. Even in the most supportive of environments, cell structure and function inevitably change. Eventually, cells lose their ability to regenerate the internal parts they need, and they die. As more and more cells in an organ system die, organ function decreases. After age 14 months, human brain cells are continually lost, but we have enough reserve capacity to maintain mental function throughout life. ***Kidney nephrons*** are also continually lost. In some people, this loss leads to eventual kidney failure, but most of us maintain sufficient kidney function. Again, in aging, there is first a reduction in reserve capacity. Only after that is exhausted does actual organ function noticeably decrease.

Kidney Nephrons
Unit of kidney cells that filters wastes from the bloodstream and deposits them into the urine.

amine the genetic and lifestyle backgrounds of long-lived people, they surmise that vigorous physical activity, low-fat diets, and the prevention of excessive weight gain may be key factors of longevity.[12] Studies of families, and of twins in particular, also provide evidence for genetic control of human longevity. Identical twins tend to have very similar life spans and causes of death. Because identical twins have exactly the same genetic information, this argues strongly that longevity is determined at least partially by hereditary.

What Does Animal Research Tell Us About Longevity?

Animal studies on longevity are quite extensive. By limiting energy intake to about 60% of usual in rodents, life span can be increased by 35%.[15] The same treatment results in at least 50% lower incidence of cancer (see Chapter 8). Only energy should be limited; the rodent diet is supplemented with vitamins and minerals. Some studies have shown that food restriction can be started late in life and still extend the life span of rats. Scientists have found similar results using low-kcalorie diets in other species—including mice, hamsters, spiders, fish, and mollusks—and are optimistic that it may work in monkeys. A study of this possibility is currently under way. Many other hypotheses have been tested in animals, but none is as effective in extending life expectancy as is energy restriction.

There are many theories to explain how energy restriction increases life expectancy in rodents. It may be that a greatly reduced energy intake lowers the metabolic rate, which in turn reduces wear and tear on the body.[19] Or the mechanism may involve the immune system. Fewer kcalories may mean a delay in the natural aging of the immune system, thereby postponing the onset of diseases more commonly associated with old age.[4] Other theories focus on what happens to hormonal systems under conditions of severe energy restriction. Less insulin release, for example, could reduce cell turnover—a factor associated with aging. The ability of cells to repair damaged DNA could also be affected by energy intake. It is likely that several of these mechanisms come into play when animals are underfed. Other reasons for the longer life expectancy are also possible.

The extended life expectancies gained from reduced feeding may actually be equal to the natural life span of animals in the wild. Perhaps what we see in the laboratory is an acceleration of the aging process caused by ***ad libitum*** (and so overfeeding) that is typically allowed for laboratory animals. Might well-fed Western humans again look to long-lived rural people for the fountain of youth?

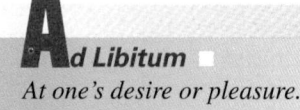

Ad Libitum *At one's desire or pleasure.*

Pass the Butter?

From animal studies, we can infer that many mammalian species—and maybe humans—might live longer by restricting energy intake. In every species studied so far, being thin has meant living longer. But, with humans the question is, are people willing to give up cheeseburgers and fries to have an unknown number of additional years of life? For most of us the deferred benefit of a longer, healthier life is overshadowed by the immediate pleasure of a hot fudge sundae. Clearly, we should consider striking a balance between immediate gratification and a pleasant long-term future. It is not just longevity, but quality of life that is lived, that is worth serious consideration.[11]

Theories on the Causes of Aging

Although the causes of aging remain a mystery, many hypotheses have been promoted to explain it[8,19]:

Errors crop up in copying the genetic blueprint (DNA)—Once enough errors in DNA copying accumulate, a cell can no longer synthesize the major proteins it needs to function, and therefore it dies.

Connective tissue stiffens—Collagen protein strands, found mostly in connective tissues, chemically bond to each other. The bonding decreases flexibility in key body components, altering organ function. Skin wrinkles and joints and arteries stiffen. The bonding may also restrict nutrients from entering cells.

Toxic products build up—Breakdown products of fats may act as intracellular sludge, hampering normal metabolic processes by clogging cells. Brown spots on the skin are a sign of this process.

Electron-seeking compounds damage cell parts—Electron-seeking compounds can break down cell membranes and proteins. One way to prevent some damage from these compounds is to consume adequate—not excessive—vitamins E and C, selenium, and beta-carotene. In contrast, it's not effective to consume cellular enzymes designed to break down the damaging compounds. The ingested enzymes are themselves broken down during digestion before they can act in the body. Despite that, some health food stores sell the enzyme superoxide dismutase, which is made by cells to destroy certain electron-seeking compounds.

Hormone function changes—The hormone dehydroepiandrosterone (DHEA), produced by adrenal glands (located near the kidneys), circulates at extremely high levels in young adults and falls sharply with age. This change has led to speculation that its decline may play a role in aging. Long-term effects of using products containing this hormone are unknown, but research is ongoing. The FDA has not approved use of DHEA, so marketing it is illegal in the United States. A fall in growth hormone levels is also being investigated as a potentially treatable hormonal effect of aging. Replacing growth hormone has wide-ranging, unpredictable effects, and it is very costly to obtain. The studies so far support the theory that growth hormone–related loss of lean body mass plays a role in aging.

The immune system loses some efficiency—The thymus gland (located in the upper chest) is a major component of the immune system. During adolescence the thymus gland reaches its maximal size, and by age 50 it is barely visible. The immune system itself runs a somewhat parallel course.[4] It is most efficient during childhood and young adulthood, but with advancing age, it is less able to recognize and counteract foreign substances—such as viruses—that enter the body. As we age, then, the immune system's ability to detect and destroy developing cancer cells decreases. Some cancer cells then can take advantage of the opportunity to multiply wildly.

Autoimmunity develops—***Autoimmune*** reactions occur when white blood cells and other immune bodies fail to distinguish between substances normally present in the body and invading foreign compounds. White blood cells and other immune bodies then begin to attack the body tissues in addition to foreign compounds. Many diseases, including some forms of diabetes and arthritis, involve this autoimmune response.

Death is programmed into the cell—Each human cell can divide only so many times, about 50. Once this number of divisions occurs, the cell automatically succumbs.

Glycosylation *of proteins*—Blood glucose, especially when chronically elevated—as occurs in poorly controlled diabetes—attaches to body proteins. This decreases protein function and can encourage immune system attack on such altered proteins. Eventually cell health declines.

Autoimmune *Immune reactions against normal body cells; self against self.*

Glycosylation *The process by which glucose attaches to other compounds, such as proteins.*

As the number of possible cell divisions increases, so does life span. The Galapagos tortoise, whose cells divide about 140 times, has a life span of perhaps 200 years.

CONCEPT CHECK

While life span has not changed, life expectancy has increased dramatically over the past century. For many societies this means an increasing proportion of the population is, and will be, over 65 years of age. Sidestepping continually rising health care costs and maximizing satisfaction with life require postponing chronic illness. Aging begins early in life and probably results from both automatic cellular changes and environmental influences. Some popular theories of aging suggest these possible causes: errors in DNA copying accumulate, connective tissue stiffens, fat by-products build up, electron-seeking compounds break down cell parts, hormonal and immune systems don't function well, and autoimmune responses and high blood glucose levels damage key body compounds.

Most likely, aging results from an interaction of these events and changes. Scientists point out that even very healthy people have a shortened life expectancy if they are exposed to sufficient environmental stresses such as radiation and certain chemical agents. Because cell aging and diseases like cancer are aggravated by environmental factors, it makes good sense to avoid such risks as excess sunlight and hazardous chemicals. Again, as we have stressed, we have some say in how fast we age.

THE EFFECTS OF AGING ON THE NUTRITIONAL HEALTH OF ELDERLY PERSONS

Elderly people vary more in health status among themselves than do persons in any other age-group. This means that chronological age is not so useful in predicting physical health status (physiological age) (Figure 15-4). As we said earlier, among people aged 65 and over, some are totally independent, healthy people, whereas others are frail and require almost total care. To predict the nutritional problems of an elderly person, it is necessary to know the extent of physiological change caused by aging (Figure 15-5) and whether the person shows early warning signs for long-term poor nutrition. As we examine how aging affects body systems and how these changes contribute to nutritional health, we will suggest ways to lessen the health risks in your life and parallel changes in diet to counteract problem conditions.

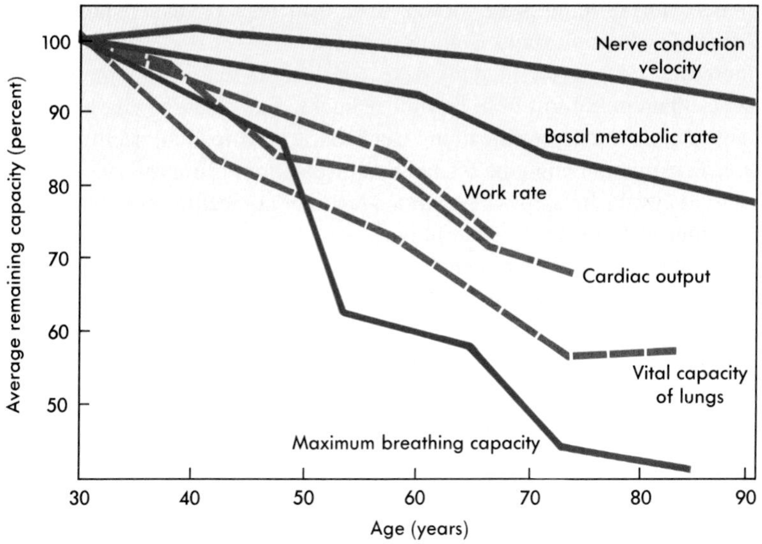

FIGURE 15-4
The decline in physiological function. Some physical and mental decline in aging is inevitable. But overall the decline is especially evident in sedentary people.

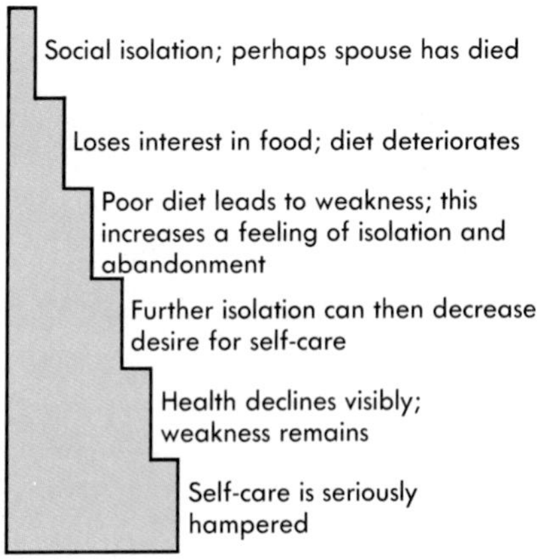

FIGURE 15-5
The decline of health in elderly persons. This decline needs to be prevented whenever possible.

The Senses of Taste and Smell

Sensitivity to taste and smell often decreases with age.[17] Stronger seasonings may be required to make foods taste good. Food companies are carving a niche in the marketplace by capitalizing on this change; by using a variety of flavor enhancers they make foods tastier for elderly persons. But for this group, a poor diet and possibly zinc deficiency can also contribute to a loss of taste.[25] Therefore a poor appetite should never be dismissed as a characteristic of old age. Many causes can be remedied.

Dental Health

About 50% of people over age 50 years in the United States have lost all their teeth.[6] Attention to dental hygiene and dental care throughout life greatly lessens this risk. Gum disease also is common and promotes tooth loss. Replacement dentures enable some to chew normally, but many elderly people—especially men—have denture problems. A pureed diet is not necessarily the remedy. Solving individual dietary needs requires identifying foods that need to be modified in consistency and can be eaten in a typical state. When people have problems chewing, nutrient-dense snacks like yogurt, bananas, and peanut butter can help. Sometimes just allowing extra time for chewing and swallowing encourages more eating.

Thirst

Elderly people often partially lose their sense of thirst and in turn don't drink enough fluids. They are then more likely to become dehydrated, a condition that leads to confusion. It is important for them to consume enough fluids, and if necessary, they should be monitored to ensure they do so. About 8 cups of fluid daily is a good goal. An approximate fluid recommendation is the same as for younger adults, 1 milliliter per kcalorie expended. This amount must be adjusted if diuretics are used or fluid is lost through other routes, such as through an ***ostomy*** (a surgically created opening in the body). Some important signs of dehydration—other than confusion—include dry lips, sunken eyes, increased body temperature, decreased blood pressure, constipation, decreased urine output, and nausea.

Ostomy
A surgically created short circuit in intestinal flow where the end point usually opens from the abdominal cavity rather than the anus, as is the case with a colostomy.

The Intestinal Tract

The main intestinal problem for elderly persons is constipation[3] (see Chapter 4 for a review of this problem). To keep the intestinal tract performing efficiently, elderly people generally need to consume more dietary fiber than they characteristically did in their youth. The goal is approximately 10 to 13 grams per 1000 kcalories in the diet, but generally no more than 35 grams on a daily basis. They should also drink more fluid to move along masses that could form from high fiber intake. Exercise likewise helps keep things moving smoothly. Because medications can induce constipation, a physician should be consulted if constipation might be related to a medication. If mineral oil is taken as a laxative, it should always be used with caution—and not at mealtimes—because it binds fat-soluble vitamins and limits their absorption.

As we noted earlier, lactase production frequently decreases with age. In Chapter 5 we list several options for people with lactose intolerance. The stomach slows its acid production as people age, usually limiting, in turn, the synthesis of intrinsic factor. These changes can contribute to poor absorption of vitamin B-12, and eventually, to pernicious anemia.[29]

Less stomach acid may also hamper iron absorption. Other conditions that affect the body's iron status occur with regular use of aspirin, which frequently causes blood loss in the stomach, and use of antacids, which may bind iron. Ulcers and hemorrhoids can also cause blood loss. Careful attention to iron status is needed in these cases.

Liver, Gallbladder, and Pancreas

With age, the liver functions less efficiently. When there is a history of significant alcohol consumption, fat buildup in the liver accounts for some decline. If cirrhosis develops, the liver functions even less efficiently (see the Nutrition Issue at the end of this chapter). When liver function deteriorates, it cannot efficiently detoxify many medications. The possibility for vitamin A toxicity in turn increases. Elderly people should be warned not to take excessive amounts of vitamin A, because toxic dosages can cause malaise, headache, bone pain, liver dysfunction, and a decrease in white blood cell count.[28]

The gallbladder also functions less efficiently as we age. Gallstones may dam up the bile to be secreted through the gallbladder, causing it to pool and back up into the liver instead. Gallstones can also interfere with fat digestion by allowing less bile into the small intestine. A low-fat diet or even surgery may be necessary.

Although the digestive function of the pancreas may decline with age, the pancreas has a large reserve capacity. A sign of a failing pancreas is high blood glucose, which occurs under several different conditions. Glucose may circulate in the bloodstream, instead of being taken up by cells, because the pancreas secretes less insulin or because cells resist insulin actions—especially adipose (fat) cells in obese people. Another cause can be insufficient chromium intake. Where appropriate, improved nutrient intake and weight loss can improve insulin action.

Kidney Function

Over time, the kidneys filter wastes more slowly as they lose nephrons (filters). As noted in Chapter 7, kidneys deteriorate more often in people who have regularly eaten excessive protein, and in some cases, excess energy (as inferred from studies on laboratory animals). The deterioration significantly decreases the kidneys' ability to excrete the products of protein breakdown. While an increased protein intake of 1 gram per kilogram of desirable body weight has been recommended for physically active elderly people,[30] that recommendation does not apply to people whose decreased kidney function causes urea—a main by-product of protein metabolism—to accumulate in the bloodstream.

Incontinence, the inability to control the muscle responsible for excretory functions, afflicts up to 20% of elderly persons living at home and 75% of those in nursing homes. The embarrassment of having to wear diapers causes many to avoid fluids (resulting in dehydration and constipation) and to become socially isolated.

Immune Function

With age, the immune system often operates less efficiently. Consuming adequate protein, the gamut of vitamins, and zinc helps maximize the health of the immune system.[25] Recurrent sicknesses and poor wound healing are warning signs of a diet deficient especially in protein and zinc. Eating too little food in general or too few animal proteins is usually the reason. Older people often eliminate meat from their diet because it's too hard to chew. Recall that animal proteins are an excellent source of zinc. On the other hand, overnutrition appears to be equally harmful to the immune system. For example, obesity and excessive fat, iron, and zinc can suppress the immune system.[4]

Lung Function

Lung efficiency declines somewhat with age[3] and is especially pronounced in elderly people who have smoked and continue to smoke tobacco products. Breathing becomes shallower and faster and more difficult as the number of lung air sacs decreases. Smoking often leads to emphysema and/or lung cancer. The decrease in lung efficiency contributes to a general downward spiral in body function; breathing difficulties limit physical activity and endurance and frequently discourage eating. These changes eventually cancel other efforts to maintain overall health.

Besides not smoking, exercise helps prevent lung problems. People need not lose their capacity to breathe deeply, as long as sufficient aerobic exercise is part of their regular routine. Otherwise, merely walking can demand the "exertion" of a marathon pace.[20] Coupled with poor muscle tone and decreased muscle mass, movement becomes continually more difficult. What is the answer? Stay physically active throughout life.

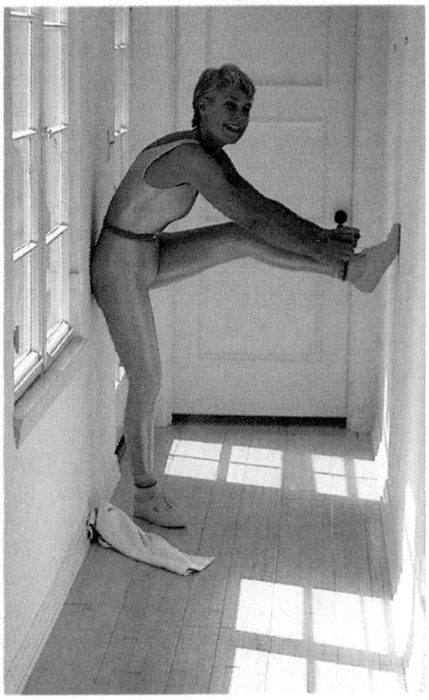

Age is no reason to stop exercising.

Hearing and Vision

Hearing and vision both decline as we age.[3] People differ as to when or whether these losses become disabling. Hearing impairment occurs mainly in members of industrial societies with urban traffic and aircraft noise and loud music. Degenerating eyesight, frequently caused by retinal degeneration, can affect a person's ability to physically get to a grocery store, locate the foods desired, read labels for nutritional content, and prepare the foods at home. Elderly people may also avoid social contacts because they can't hear. Such changes may make people afraid to socialize, be active, or take care of important routines of daily life, such as shopping. Recall from Chapter 8 the role for vitamin C in reducing cataracts in the eye. This provides another reason for adults to have a diet rich in fruits and vegetables.[27]

Decrease in Lean Tissue

Some muscle cells shrink and others are lost as muscles age; some muscles lose their ability to contract as they accumulate fat and collagen. Lifestyle greatly determines the rate of muscle mass deterioration. As you might predict, an active lifestyle tends to maintain muscle mass, whereas a very inactive one encourages its loss. Weight training has been shown to prevent muscle loss in elderly people.[7] Weight-training exercises can also be used to help elderly people regain some muscle strength. But in one study, when older adults stopped the weight-training program, any gains in muscle strength were quickly lost. This illustrates the importance of regular exercise throughout life.

Physical activity is also desirable for elderly people, because it allows them to eat more food, thereby increasing their chances of consuming adequate nutrients. Vitamin and mineral needs do not decrease to a great extent as we age, although food intake may. Another good practice is to decrease sugar and fat consumption to increase the diet's nutrient density. Elderly people may need to take a multivitamin and mineral supplement with a physician's guidance if they consume less than about 1500 kcalories daily (see Chapter 8).

Increase in Fat Stores

As lean tissue decreases with age, the body often takes on more fat. Some researchers feel that some extra fat stores in the elderly may be fine. Large population studies suggest that in otherwise healthy people, a little fat gain during the adult years does not pose

another BITE

In early adulthood and middle age, significant weight gain is a major problem. In the late elderly years, weight loss is more of a concern. Weight loss in elderly people often means increased risk of death. It may also indicate increased sickness and poor tolerance of medications. When assessing weight in elderly people, compare present weight with the previous year's weight.

TABLE 15-3

Suggested Desirable Weights for Adults

Height*	Weight in Pounds†	
	19 to 34 Years	35 Years and Over
5′0″	97-128‡	108-138
5′1″	101-132	111-143
5′2″	104-137	115-148
5′3″	107-141	119-152
5′4″	111-146	122-157
5′5″	114-150	126-162
5′6″	118-155	130-167
5′7″	121-160	134-172
5′8″	125-164	138-178
5′9″	129-169	142-183
5′10″	132-174	146-188
5′11″	136-179	151-194
6′0″	140-184	155-199
6′1″	144-189	159-205
6′2″	148-195	164-210
6′3″	152-200	168-216
6′4″	156-205	173-222
6′5″	160-211	177-228
6′6″	164-216	182-234

From USDA/DHHS: Dietary Guidelines for Americans, *1990.*

**Without shoes.*

†Without clothes.

‡The higher weights in the ranges generally apply to men, who tend to have more muscle and bone; the lower weights more often apply to women, who have less muscle and bone.

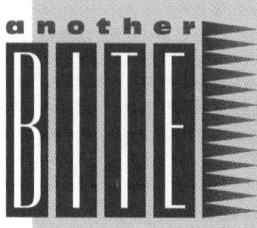

health risks. The booklet accompanying the 1990 Dietary Guidelines allows ranges for healthy body weights at given heights to begin climbing by 11 to 18 pounds in total once a person is over 35 years of age. The greater amounts are for taller people (Table 15-3). However, obesity is not desirable because it can raise blood pressure and blood glucose levels, as well as make it more difficult to walk and to care for oneself.

Cardiovascular Health

The heart often pumps blood less efficiently in elderly people, usually because of insufficient physical activity. Poor heart conditioning allows fatty and connective tissues to infiltrate the heart's muscular wall. This decline in ***cardiac output*** is not inevitable with aging and does not occur among elderly people who remain physically active.

Cardiac Output *The amount of blood pumped by the heart.*

Heart attack and stroke, the major causes of death in all adults, are caused primarily by atherosclerosis and high blood pressure. As one ages, atherosclerotic plaque accumulates in the arteries, reducing their elasticity, constricting blood flow, and consequently, elevating blood pressure.[2]

You already know the main way to limit the buildup of atherosclerotic plaque: keep your serum LDL-cholesterol level and total cholesterol/HDL-cholesterol ratio in the desirable range (see Chapter 6). New evidence is showing that even a diet very low in fat can cause some plaques to decrease in size.[24] Other studies use diet and medications or surgery to lower blood cholesterol levels, which, in turn, reduces the amount of plaque in the arteries supplying the heart. This suggests that a heart-healthy diet is more important during adult and elderly years than researchers previously thought.

High blood pressure, heavily implicated in both stroke and heart attack, can be lowered in most people by severe sodium restriction. A limit of 2 grams of sodium helps many people with hypertension, but that is a difficult diet to plan and follow. Alternatively, a mild sodium restriction (not to exceed 4 grams of sodium daily), while effective for salt-sensitive people, is not so helpful by itself for those who are not salt sensitive, but it aids the action of medications used to treat hypertension. (The Nutrition Issue in Chapter 9 reviews the effects of other nutrients on blood pressure.)

We can do much to prevent heart attack and stroke just by balanced eating, walking briskly or exercising regularly, controlling blood pressure, not smoking, and maintaining a desirable weight.[11]

Bone Health

In Chapter 9 we discussed the decline in bone density associated with aging. Recall that bone loss in women occurs especially after menopause. Bone loss in men is slow and steady from middle age throughout the elderly years. For women, increasing calcium intake to 1500 milligrams per day helps maintain density in some types of bones, such as the hip, but it does not predictably prevent bone loss from the spine. Other measures to prevent bone loss can be taken earlier and continued thereafter in life—maintaining adequate vitamin D nutriture, not smoking, drinking alcohol moderately or not at all (refer to Dietary Guidelines), and meeting the RDA for calcium. It should be noted that underweight women are at higher risk for developing osteoporosis. From laboratory animal studies, we infer that performing weight-bearing exercises also helps sustain bone. For adult women who are at higher risk or who may have osteoporosis, drug treatment should be considered—estrogen replacement therapy, active vitamin D hormone (calcitriol) therapy, or calcitonin therapy—administered with a physician's guidance.

If osteoporosis becomes very severe, it limits the ability of elderly people to exercise, shop, prepare food, and live normally.[6] They eat less and get fewer nutrients. There is additional concern that many elderly people may suffer from hidden osteomalacia, a condition that occurs primarily when there is not enough sun exposure and possibly poor vitamin D synthesis in the skin.[28] When they can't get regular sun exposure—during the winter or when they are homebound—elderly people need a source for 10 micrograms (400 IU) of vitamin D per day. Either fortified milk products or a vitamin supplement can provide this amount.

OTHER FACTORS THAT INFLUENCE NUTRIENT NEEDS IN ELDERLY PERSONS

Medications

Medications and old age often go together. Medications can improve health and quality of life, but some of them also profoundly affect nutrient needs at all ages, including the elderly years (Table 15-4). Forty-five percent of the elderly population regularly take multiple prescription drugs; many drugs affect appetite or absorption of nutrients.[6] Often, during later years people must take several medications for long periods. They should make sure to work with their physician and pharmacist to coordinate all medications taken. Pharmacists can advise when to take drugs—with or between meals—for greatest effectiveness.

Drug-related nutritional problems include (1) increased need for potassium when certain types of diuretics leach it out of the body and (2) changes in appetite caused by antidepressant agents or certain antibiotics. Blood loss from long-term use of aspirin or aspirin-like medications strains iron reserves and can lead to anemia. We recommend that people who must take one or more medications for more than just a few weeks should closely watch their diets, eating nutrient-dense foods and possibly taking nutrient supplements to counteract effects of certain medications.

Depression and Mental State

About 12% to 14% of elderly people experience significant depression. That—combined with isolation and loneliness as family and friends die, move away, or become less mobile—frequently contributes to apathetic eating and weight loss in older people. People living alone do not necessarily make poor food choices, but they often consume less energy in part from skipping meals, especially men. About one third of all elderly persons not in nursing homes live alone. Depression can be a downward spiral in which poor appetite produces weakness that leads to even poorer appetite. In elderly persons, the resulting poor nutritional state can produce further mental confusion and increased isolation and loneliness.[5]

TABLE 15-4

Some Potential Drug-Nutrient Interactions for Some Commonly Used Drugs

Drug	Use	Nutrient Affected	Potential Side Effect
Antacids (Maalox)	Reduce stomach acidity	Calcium, vitamin B-12, and iron	Decreased absorption due to altered gastrointestinal pH
Anticoagulants (Coumadin)	Prevent blood clots	Vitamin K	Poor utilization
Aspirin	Antiinflammatory; pain reduction	Iron	Anemia from blood loss
Cathartics (laxatives)	Induce bowel movement	Calcium and potassium	Poor absorption
Cholestyramine	Reduces blood cholesterol	Vitamins A, D, E, and K	Poor absorption
Cimetidine (Tagamet)	Treatment of ulcers	Vitamin B-12	Poor absorption
Colchicine	Treatment of gout	Vitamin B-12, carotenes, and magnesium	Decreased absorption due to damaged intestinal mucosa
Corticosteroids (prednisone)	Antiinflammatory	Zinc	Poor absorption
		Calcium	Poor utilization
Furosemide (Lasix)	Decreases hypertension; potassium-wasting diuretic	Potassium and sodium	Increased loss
Hydrochlorothiazide	Decreases hypertension; diuretic	Potassium and magnesium	Increased loss; decreased absorption
MAO inhibitors (Parnate)	Antidepressant	(Tyramine in aged foods)	Hypertension caused by poor tyramine metabolism
Tricyclic antidepressants (Elavil)	Antidepressant	—	Weight gain due to appetite stimulation

Nutrition has a role in preserving mental function in elderly persons. Specific nutritional deficiencies of thiamin, niacin, vitamins B-6 and B-12, and folate, as well as excessive alcohol use, cause well-recognized central nervous system disorders.[27] The subtle effects of eating minimal energy, leading to semistarvation, are often overlooked. In addition, as mentioned earlier, a poor fluid intake may lead to dehydration and, in turn, to confusion.

We know that mental illness can lead to a poor nutritional state, but the extent to which subtle nutritional deficiencies can lead to a poor mental state is not as clear cut. It is important to prevent overt nutrient deficiencies, especially those mentioned previously.

CONCEPT CHECK

Nutritional problems often accompany chronic diseases of elderly persons and intensify as organ function decreases over time. As we age, our senses of taste, smell, thirst, hearing, and sight lose some sensitivity; our abilities to digest and absorb lose efficiency; our organs—liver, gallbladder, pancreas, kidneys, lungs, and heart—work less effectively; and our immune system gradually loses capacity. In addition, muscle mass declines (largely because of inactivity), and bone mass gradually decreases. Diet changes and regular exercise can often help reduce the extent and impact of these typical results of aging.

DO THE RDAs INCREASE IN THE ELDERLY YEARS?

Currently, the RDAs for nutrients and energy include a category for both men and women who are 51 years of age and older. Because the lifestyle of an active 70-year-old person would differ considerably from that of a 90-year-old nursing home resident, this wide age range in the RDAs may be problematic. The recommendations for energy intake assume an active lifestyle, a characteristic the RDA committee supports. Note that nutrient recommendations have largely been projected from studies of young adults.

Only during the last few years has much research focused on this question. Because the RDAs apply only to healthy people, many elderly people—for example, those with ulcers or heavy aspirin users—are not covered by RDAs. Indeed it is particularly tricky to evolve RDAs valid for most older people, because many of them are ill and/or regularly take medications.

Recently, a noted research team suggested that the current RDAs for healthy elderly people are probably too high for vitamin A; too low in protein (for the active elders) and vitamins D, riboflavin, B-6, and B-12; and about right for the other nutrients.[28] In this case, the about right category may reflect either that studies suggest the RDA is adequate, or that we lack evidence to make a more definitive statement. Still, a well-planned diet that follows the Food Guide Pyramid can meet all nutrient needs of elderly people (Table 15-5).

There is a concern that the RDA for calcium should be increased to help slow the acceleration of bone loss suffered by elderly women. About 1500 milligrams per day is a common recommendation.

Elderly women need less iron because they no longer menstruate. However, chronic ulcers, hemorrhoids, and aspirin use may necessitate an increased iron intake.

Overall, nutrient needs for elderly persons resemble those for younger adults, but individual modifications are necessary to compensate for specific diseases.[4]

Planning a Diet for Elderly Persons

To supply energy needs for males aged 51 years and older, the current RDA suggestion is 2300 kcalories; for females, the recommendation is 1900 kcalories. (These values are

NUTRITION insight

ALZHEIMER'S DISEASE

Dementia General persistent loss or decrease in mental function.

Alzheimer's disease has become a dreaded possibility for many people approaching old age. Many of us have had first-hand experience as loved ones have been "lost" to this form of progressive ***dementia.*** Although it seems a disease of the times—with more and more people both in nursing homes and in families that devote more time to caring for these people—the disease has been around for quite a while.

In 1907 Dr. Alois Alzheimer documented several cases of what seemed to be early senility. Typical symptoms of the disease included personality changes, unreasonable fears, explosive outbursts, depression, and general forgetfulness. Today, the disease Dr. Alzheimer first described affects about 4 million people in the United States, including about 45% of all people over the age of 85 and 50% of all people in nursing homes.[10]

More reports on Alzheimer's disease surface every day. Is this a disease of modern society, or has it always been around but we didn't know how to diagnose it? Old age is often accompanied by a general decline in mental function. But what makes Alzheimer's disease different is that it can be diagnosed specifically by the presence of protein deposits and tangled masses of nerves in the areas of the brain that are linked to memory and thinking.[10] However, this type of diagnosis can be done only at autopsy, and so it is difficult to know precisely how many cases of dementia in old age are actually the Alzheimer's type. Clinical assessments can and should be made by an experienced physician. Because we know more about the typical course of the disease, clinical methods have become more reliable in differentiating between Alzheimer's disease and other causes of dementia.

Causes and Physical Effects

In general terms, Alzheimer's disease is best described as a progressive brain disorder marked by an inability to remember, reason, or understand what is going on. Age is the primary risk factor. Scientists propose causes, including altered cell development, altered brain proteins, and unidentified blood-borne agents. Genetic predisposition is closely linked to a minor form that occurs at about age 40, and scientists suspect this contributes to the major form as well.

In those with Alzheimer's disease, aluminum is highly concentrated in abnormal protein accumulations in the brain, but this high level of aluminum is more likely an effect rather than a cause of the disease. Evidence supporting this is that people mining aluminum develop cancer from aluminum toxicity but typically don't develop Alzheimer's disease.[16] Whether there are other, yet unknown, causes remains to be discovered.

Alzheimer's disease is progressive. Its course has been described as three stages, although these can vary in duration and intensity with individuals. Generally it (1) begins as confusion, depression, anxiety, and short-term memory loss, (2) develops into long-term memory loss and problems in communication and perception, and (3) may cause the individual to become bedridden and completely dependent. Wandering is a frequent reason that families put the person in a nursing home. Death in those with Alzheimer's disease is frequently attributable to bacterial infection or pneumonia associated with accidental food inhalation.

Treatment

Today, treatment of Alzheimer's disease is usually limited to the use of antidepressants and other drugs that target related symptoms of the disease. Therapies currently under investigation range from the use of aspirin to overlapping doses of potent, synthetically produced brain chemicals. A new medication under investigation is tacrine, a drug that may slow the brain's breakdown of acetylcholine, a major neurotransmitter used in sending nerve messages. Studies are encouraging, but side effects currently limit its usefulness.[9] In those with Alzheimer's disease, the decreased amount of neurotransmitter activity appears to relate strongly to the degree of memory impairment. But, to prevent a disease, we generally need to understand its causes. And unfortunately, we don't yet know as much as we need to about Alzheimer's disease.

Nutrition Considerations

The main nutrition goal for people with this disease is a healthful diet that maintains body weight. Forgetfulness may lead to irregular eating habits with associated weight loss. Because one characteristic of Alzheimer's disease is the death of cells that secrete acetylcholine, scientists once thought that a diet that provided choline and the related compound lecithin might correct this deficit. However, studies have found this to have no effect on Alzheimer's patients.

Abnormal food behaviors, such as gorging, are often seen early in the course of Alzheimer's disease. A craving for sweets may lead to a temporary weight gain that can be managed by offering lower-kcalorie snacks and meals. At the other extreme, there is often a partial or complete refusal to eat. Frequent, small meals and nutrient-dense snacks using favorite foods when possible may encourage more regular eating. People who are still leading reasonably independent lives may not be able to shop or to remember to eat meals. Congregate feeding programs and home-delivered meals may be helpful during the early stages of disease. Keep in mind that by the time the disease has been diagnosed, some people have already developed nutritional problems (see later section).

With the progression of the disease, there is more confusion and distractibility. At this stage, it is wise for others to oversee food planning and mealtimes. Measures should be taken to control distractions—such as television, radio, children, pets, and the telephone—that can disrupt a meal for someone with Alzheimer's disease. Others should monitor food temperatures, because victims may ignore discomfort and burn themselves. Tough, crunchy foods that may easily cause choking should be avoided. For those still capable of self-feeding, assistance devices should be used when appropriate: roller-rocker knives, bowls, plate guards, a damp washcloth under the plate to prevent skidding, cups with tops, flexible straws, and large bibs. These are available at medical supply houses. As people with Alzheimer's disease become less able to manage eating by themselves, it becomes more of a challenge to those trying to feed them. They may hold food in the mouth, forget how to eat or swallow, spit out food, and play with and then refuse food.

All of us need to pay attention to dietary recommendations to promote and maintain health. People with Alzheimer's disease may not be able to do this on their own. In later stages of this disease, people may not be tuned in to their own needs. The responsibility for providing good nutrition will ultimately fall to family, health care providers, and nursing home staff.[10]

The fastest-growing segment of the population is made up of people aged 85 and older. Thus, in the future, Alzheimer's disease could have devastating consequences for America's already strained health care system. The disease also takes an immense emotional toll on its victims and their family members[16] (Figure 15-6).

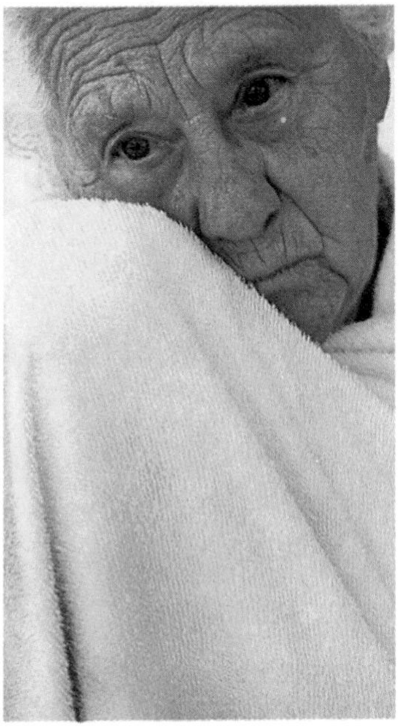

FIGURE 15-6
Alzheimer's disease. About 4 million American adults have Alzheimer's disease. This prevalence poses dire implications for public health in the future.

TABLE 15-5

Sample Diet of Nutrient-Dense Food Choices for Elderly Persons That Meets All RDAs for 1600 Kcalories

Breakfast
Crispy Wheat 'n Raisins, 1 cup
1% milk, 1 cup
Orange
Tea or coffee, if desired

Lunch
Turkey sandwich
- Whole-wheat bread, 2 slices
- Roasted turkey breast, 2 oz
- Mustard

Banana
Oatmeal raisin cookie, 1 cookie
1% milk, 1 cup

Dinner
Salad
- Romaine lettuce, 1 cup
- Tomatoes, ½ cup
- Italian dressing, 2 Tbsp
- Sunflower seeds, ¼ cup

Lean roast beef, 4 oz
Brown rice with meat broth, ½ cup
Carrot sticks, ¾ cup, steamed
Oatmeal raisin cookie, 1 cookie
Tea or coffee, if desired

NOTE: This diet follows the Food Guide Pyramid discussed in Chapter 2.

based on a 170-pound, 68-inch tall man and a 143-pound, 63-inch tall woman.) Studies show that elderly men eat closer to 1600 to 1900 kcalories, whereas women eat about 1250 to 1550 kcalories.

Diet plans for elderly persons should focus on nutrient density, especially of the following nutrients: vitamin D, along with sun exposure; vitamins E, thiamin, riboflavin, B-6, B-12, and C; and the minerals iron, calcium, and zinc. A sample diet that meets all these needs appears in Table 15-5. Ideally, some protein should come from lean meats to help meet vitamin B-6 and zinc needs, two nutrients of special concern. Because physical activity simultaneously increases appetite and uses energy, it allows the exerciser to eat more. Taking in more nutrients in general then simplifies the planning of an adequate diet.

Fluid needs are 1 milliliter per kcalorie expended or about 2 liters (8 cups) per day. A high-fiber diet can decrease constipation but increase fluid needs. Fiber intake should be slowly increased to about 35 grams a day, with each serving of fiber accompanied by a glass of water (or other fluid).

Singles of all ages face logistical problems with foods: purchasing, preparing, storing, and using foods with minimal waste are challenges. Economy packages of meats and vegetables are normally too large to be useful for a single person. Many singles live in small dwellings, some without kitchens and freezers. Gearing a diet to accommodate a limited budget and facilities and a single appetite requires special considerations.[4]

Following are some practical suggestions for diet planning for singles:

- If you own a freezer, cook large amounts, divide into portions, and freeze.
- Buy only what you can use; small containers may be expensive, but letting food spoil is also costly.
- Ask the grocer to break open a family-sized package of wrapped meat or fresh vegetables and separate it into smaller units.
- Buy only several pieces of a fruit—perhaps a ripe one, a medium-ripe one, and an unripe one—so that the fruit can be eaten over a period of several days.
- Keep a box of dry milk handy to add a nutritious punch to recipes for baked goods and whatever other foods for which this addition is acceptable.

another BITE

Regularly taking vitamin and mineral supplements can be expensive—an important consideration for people on fixed, and possibly inadequate, incomes. Too much of some supplements can lead to toxicity. Between about 35% and 70% of elderly people regularly take supplements, some at potentially toxic levels. If supplements are necessary, the elderly person should work closely with a physician or registered dietitian to determine which nutrients to include and the least amounts that are necessary.

Feeding sick, infirm, and/or mentally confused people is time-consuming and demanding work that requires special training.[14] Friends, relatives, and health personnel should look for poor nutrient intake in all elderly people, even those who live in nursing home settings. Research indicates that 43% of adults now aged 65 will spend some time in a nursing home. Family members have a unique opportunity to make sure nutrient needs of elderly people are met by looking for weight maintenance based on regular, healthful meal patterns. If problems arise in instituting a healthful diet, registered dietitians can offer professional and personalized advice.

From surveys it appears that the majority of elderly people like most vegetables, despite misconceptions that older people do not like broccoli (because it forms gas) or tomatoes (because they contain too much acid). By the time we reach adulthood, our eating habits reflect regional tastes, social class, ethnic group, and life experiences. There is no generic food list for elderly persons.

Overall, good nutrition benefits elderly persons in many ways. It delays the onset of some diseases; improves management of some existing diseases; hastens recovery from many illnesses; can increase mental, physical, and social well-being; and often decreases the need for and length of hospitalization.[6] Thus a good nutritional intake should be a

TABLE 15-6

Guidelines for Promoting Healthful Eating in Later Years

- Eat regularly; small frequent meals may be best.
- Find out which convenience foods and labor-saving devices can be of help.
- Try new foods, new seasonings, and new ways of preparing foods. Don't just use convenience foods and canned goods.
- Keep some easy-to-prepare foods on hand for times when tired.
- Add nonfat dry milk to recipes for baked goods and other appropriate foods to boost nutrition value.
- Have a treat occasionally, perhaps an expensive cut of meat or a favorite fresh fruit.
- Eat in a well-lit or sunny area; serve meals attractively; use foods with different flavors, colors, shapes, and textures.
- Arrange things so food preparation and clean-up are easier.
- Eat with friends or relatives or at a senior center when possible.
- Share cooking responsibilities with a neighbor.
- Use community resources for help in shopping and other daily care needs.
- Stay physically active.
- If possible, take a walk before eating to stimulate appetite.
- When necessary, chop, grind, or blend hard-to-chew foods. Softer, protein-rich foods can be substituted for meat when poor dental function limits normal food intake.
- If eating movements are limited, cut the food ahead of time, use utensils with deep sides or handles, and obtain more specialized utensils if needed.

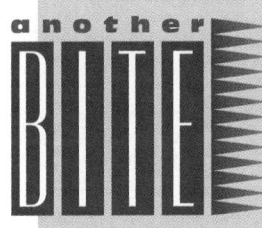

vital part of the health maintenance program for elderly people. A variety of strategies can promote healthful eating in the elderly years (Table 15-6). These should focus on presenting nutritious, tasty foods in a pleasant, friendly environment.

COMMUNITY NUTRITION SERVICES FOR ELDERLY PERSONS

Hospice *Hospital care that emphasizes comfort and dignity in death.*

Health care advice and services for elderly persons can come from clinics, private practitioners, hospitals, and health maintenance organizations. Home health care agencies, adult day-care programs, adult overnight-care programs, and ***hospice*** centers (for the terminally ill) can supply day-to-day care. Professionals in the above-mentioned organizations can help identify elders whose health needs require extra attention (Figure 15-7).

A Nutrition Self-Test For Older Adults

Here's a nutrition check for anyone over age 65. Circle the number of points for all statements that apply. Then check the total against the nutritional score.

1. The person has an ongoing illness or current condition has changed the kind or amount of food eaten. **(2 points)**
2. The person eats fewer than two full meals per day. **(3 points)**
3. The person eats few fruits, vegetables, or milk products. **(2 points)**
4. The person drinks three or more servings of beer, liquor, or wine almost every day. **(2 points)**
5. The person has tooth or mouth problems that make eating difficult. **(2 points)**
6. The person does not have enough money for food. **(4 points)**
7. The person eats alone most of the time. **(1 point)**
8. The person takes three or more different prescription or over-the-counter drugs each day. **(1 point)**
9. Without meaning to, the person has lost or gained 10 pounds in the last 6 months. **(2 points)**
10. The person cannot always shop, cook, or feed himself or herself. **(2 points)**

Nutritional Score:

0–2: Good. Recheck in 6 months.

3–5: Marginal. A local office on aging has information on nutrition programs for the elderly. The National Association of Area Agencies on Aging can assist in finding help; call (800)677-1116. Recheck in 6 months.

6 or more: High risk. A doctor should see this test and suggest how to improve nutritional health.

(Modified from the Nutrition Screening Initiative, 2626 Pennsylvania Avenue, NW, Suite 301, Washington, DC 20037.)

FIGURE 15-7
A nutrition checklist for elderly people.

Nutrition programs for those aged 60 and over offer congregate meal programs, which provide lunch at a central location, and home-delivered meals (often known as Meals-On-Wheels if sponsored by local private or public agencies) (Figure 15-8). Federal commodity distribution is available in some areas of the United States to low-income elderly people. Food stamps can also aid elderly persons who live below the poverty level. Food cooperatives and a variety of clubs and social organizations provide additional aid to them. The congregate meal programs and home-delivered meals are funded partially by the U.S. government under Title III of the Older Americans Act and through volunteer community efforts (Figure 15-9).

The U.S. government sets specific standards for home-delivered meals and for those served in congregate feeding centers. The meals are designed to provide one third of the RDA. The basic meal pattern is 3 ounces of meat or meat alternative, 2.5 cups of fruit or vegetable, 1 slice of bread or alternative, 1 teaspoon of butter or margarine, 1 cup of milk,

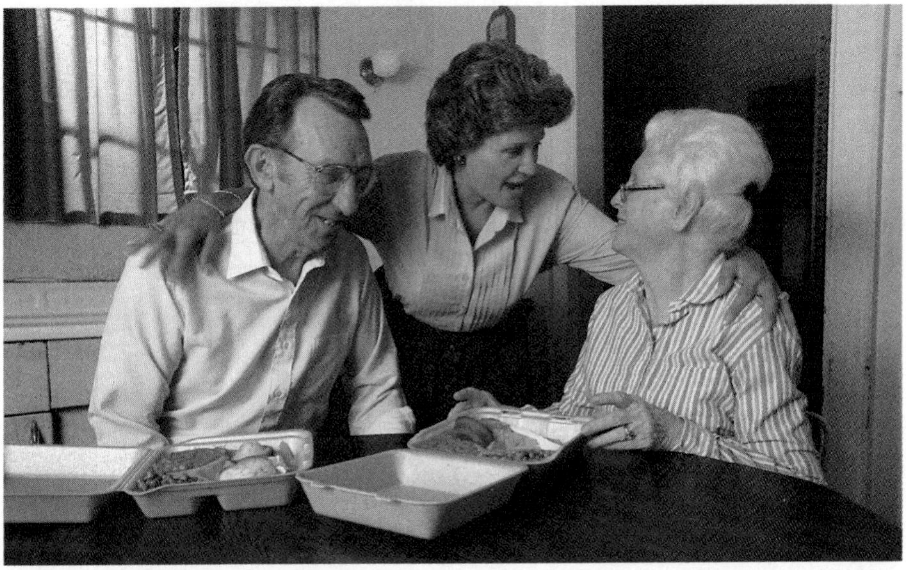

FIGURE 15-8
The home-delivered meals program represents a gift of nutrition and caring by a community to its elderly citizens.

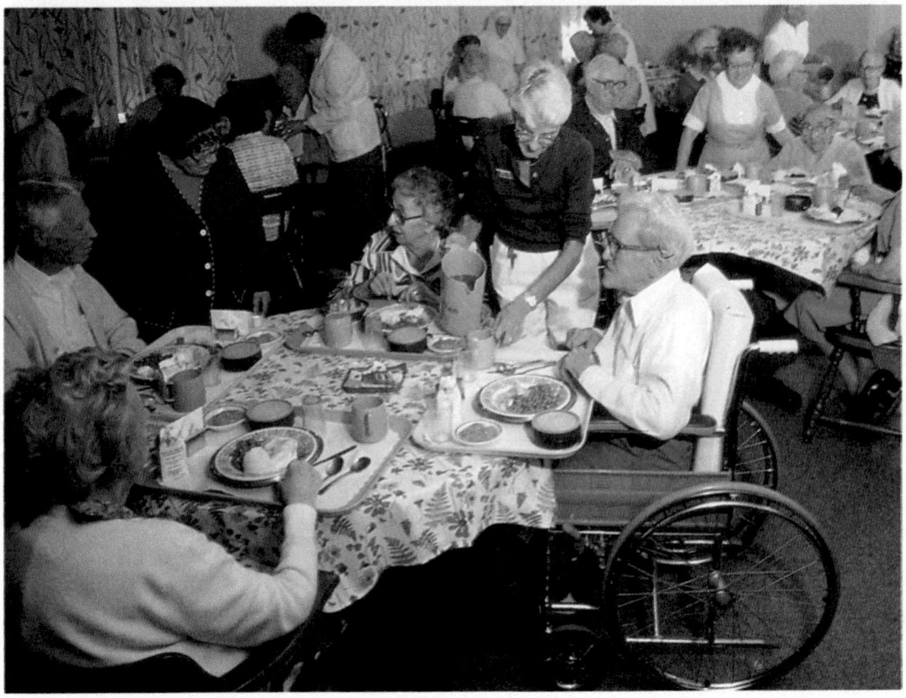

FIGURE 15-9
Congregate meals for elderly persons. Sites in many communities in the United States provide nutritious meals and an opportunity for socialization among elderly people.

and ½ cup of dessert. Foods rich in vitamins A and C are emphasized. The social aspect often improves an elderly person's appetite and general outlook.

Many eligible elderly people are missing meals and are poorly nourished, simply because they don't know of available programs. Irregular meal patterns and weight loss, often because of difficulties in preparing foods, are warning signs that undernutrition may be developing. An effort should be made to identify and inform these people of community services.

The ideal is to remain healthy and to live independently for as long as possible without becoming socially isolated. Personal living situations can greatly determine whether an elderly person is well-nourished.[5] For some, just getting to the store or having to carry groceries may be a major problem. Relatives and friends can be a real help. Special transportation arrangements may also be available through a local transit company or taxi service.

another BITE

Studies have found that congregate meal programs can positively influence the nutritional status of otherwise homebound people. Still, congregate meal programs provide at most one meal a day and usually not every day of the week. So if people come to depend on them exclusively, they eat too few meals. The problem with home-delivered meals is that the one or two meals delivered may never be eaten, and if not eaten on delivery and left at room temperature, they may become unsafe to eat later. Thus these programs help elderly persons, but even more help often is needed.

CONCEPT CHECK

Specific nutrient requirements for elderly persons are only now being extensively studied. Diet plans for elderly persons should be modified for decreased physical abilities, presence of drug-nutrient interactions, possible depression, and economic constraints. Particular attention should be paid to sun exposure and intake of the vitamins D, E, B-6, B-12, C, and thiamin, as well as the minerals iron, calcium, and zinc. A nutrient-dense diet helps to meet these needs. In the United States, many nutrition services—such as congregate and home-delivered meals—are available to help the elderly population obtain a healthful diet.

SUMMARY

- A goal for all of us should be to delay symptoms of and disabilities from chronic diseases for as many years as possible. Good nutritional habits, especially those that follow the Food Guide Pyramid and Dietary Guidelines, play a role in this process.
- A basic plan to promote health and prevent disease includes eating a proper diet, exercising regularly, abstaining from smoking, limiting alcohol intake, and limiting stress.
- The 1990 Dietary Guidelines for Americans recommend that individuals eat a variety of foods; maintain desirable weight; choose a diet low in fat, saturated fat, and cholesterol

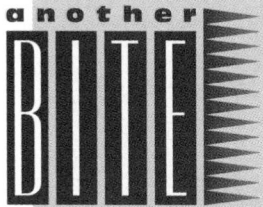

and rich in vegetables, fruits, and grains; use salt and sugar in moderation; and drink alcoholic beverages in moderation, if at all. Genetic background, medical conditions, and other lifestyle practices influence a person's optimal diet.

- While life span has not changed, life expectancy has increased dramatically over the past century. For many societies, this means that an increasing proportion of the population is over 65 years of age. As health care costs rise, the goal of delaying disease becomes even more important for all of us.
- Aging begins before birth. Cell aging probably results from automatic cellular changes and environmental influences, such as DNA damage. Add to this list damage caused by electron-seeking compounds, high blood glucose levels, hormonal changes, and alterations in the immune system as possible causes.
- Nutritional problems of elderly persons are related to the presence of chronic diseases and to the normal decreases in organ function that occur with time. These include loss of teeth, lessened sensitivity in the senses of taste and smell, changes in gastrointestinal tract function, and deterioration in heart and bone health. Although disease affects nutritional state, the reverse is also true. Immune function is adversely affected by undernutrition, setting the stage for infection.
- Alzheimer's disease is a progressive and irreversible brain disorder. Its causes are only beginning to be understood. It differs from other types of senile dementia in that the brain tissue accumulates abnormal protein plaques and tangled nerves (observable by autopsy). Nutritional health for people in advanced stages of disease is often complicated by special feeding problems.
- Specific nutrient needs for elderly persons are only now being studied extensively. Diet plans should be based on a nutrient-dense approach and individualized for existing health problems, decreased physical abilities, presence of drug-nutrient interactions, possible depression, and economic constraints. Specific nutrients—such as the vitamins D, E, B-6, C, B-12, riboflavin and thiamin, as well as the minerals iron, zinc, and calcium—often deserve special attention in diet planning.

Study Questions

1. How do nutrition needs of elderly persons differ from those of younger people? How are their needs similar? Be specific.
2. Define the term "reserve capacity" of organs and relate how this tends to hide the early effects of aging.
3. Describe two theories explaining the causes of aging and note evidence for each in your daily life experiences.
4. List four organ systems that can decline in function in the elderly years, along with a diet/lifestyle response to help cope with the decline.
5. What three resources in a community are widely available to aid elderly persons in maintaining nutritional health?

REFERENCES

1. Ahmed FE: Effect of nutrition on the health of the elderly, *Journal of the American Dietetic Association* 92:1102, 1992.
2. Biosca DG and others: The effect of nutritional prevention of cardiovascular diseases on longevity, *Nutrition Reviews* 50:407, 1992.
3. Carethers M: Health promotion in the elderly, *American Family Physician* 45:2253, 1992.
4. Chandra RK: Nutrition and immunity in the elderly, *Nutrition Reviews* 50:367, 1992.
5. Darnton-Hill I: Psychosocial aspects of nutrition and aging, *Nutrition Reviews* 50:476, 1992.
6. Dwyer JT and others: Assessing nutritional status in elderly patients, *American Family Physician* 47:613, 1993.
7. Evans WJ: Exercise, nutrition, and aging, *Journal of Nutrition* 122:796, 1992.
8. Ezzell C: A time to live, a time to die, *Science News* 142:344, 1992.
9. Farlow M and others: A controlled trial of tacrine in Alzheimer's disease, *Journal of the American Medical Association* 268:2523, 1992.
10. Flieger K: Alzheimer's mystery, *FDA Consumer,* p. 17, March 1992.
11. Fries JF: Strategies for reduction of morbidity, *American Journal of Clinical Nutrition* 55:1257S, 1992.
12. Gabel LL and others: Dietary prevention and treatment of disease, *American Family Physician* 46(5):41S, 1992.
13. Kendler KS and others: A population-based twin study of alcoholism in women, *Journal of the American Medical Association* 268:1877, 1992.
14. Kerstetter JE and others: Malnutrition in the institutionalized older adult, *Journal of the American Dietetic Association* 92:1109, 1992.
15. Kritchevsky D: Caloric restriction and experimental tumorigenesis, *Nutrition Today* p. 25, January/February 1993.
16. Larson EB and others: Cognitive impairment: dementia and Alzheimer's disease, *Annual Review of Public Health* 13:431, 1992.
17. Lewis R: When smell and taste go awry, *FDA Consumer,* p. 29, November 1991.
18. Lieber CS: Alcohol, liver, and nutrition, *Journal of the American College of Nutrition* 10:602, 1992.
19. Masoro EJ: Retardation of aging processes by food restriction: an experimental tool, *American Journal of Clinical Nutrition* 55:1250S, 1992.
20. McGinnis JM: The public health burden of a sedentary lifestyle, *Medicine and Science in Sports and Exercise* 24:S196, 1992.
21. McGinnis JM and others: Health progress in the United States, *Journal of the American Medical Association* 268:2545, 1992.
22. Matsuzaki T: Longevity, diet, and nutrition in Japan: epidemiological studies, *Nutrition Reviews* 50:355, 1992.
23. Morse RM, Flavin DK: The definition of alcoholism, *Journal of the American Medical Association* 268:1012, 1992.
24. Ornish D: Can lifestyle changes reverse coronary heart disease? *Lancet* 336:129, 1990.
25. Prasad AS: Zinc deficiency in elderly patients, *Nutrition* 9:218, 1993.
26. Rheinstein PH: Healthy people 2000 initiative, *American Family Physician* 46:1829, 1992.
27. Rosenberg IH, Miller JW: Nutritional factors in physical and cognitive functions of elderly people, *American Journal of Clinical Nutrition* 55:1237S, 1992.
28. Russell RM, Suter PM: Vitamin requirements of the elderly: an update, *American Journal of Clinical Nutrition* 58:4, 1993.
29. Russell RM: Changes in gastrointestinal function attributed to aging, *American Journal of Clinical Nutrition* 55:1203S, 1992.
30. Schlenker ED: *Nutrition in aging,* ed 2, St Louis, 1993, Mosby–Year Book.

HELPING THE ELDERLY EAT BETTER

During their lifetimes, most people usually eat meals with families or loved ones. As elderly people reach even older ages, many of them are faced with living and eating alone. In a study of the diets of 4400 older Americans, one man of every five living alone and over age 55 ate poorly. One of four women between the ages of 55 and 64 years followed a low-quality diet. These poor diets can contribute to deteriorating mental and physical health. Consider the following example of the living situation of an elderly person:

> Neal, a 70-year-old man, lives alone in a house in a local suburban area. He lost his wife 1 year ago. He doesn't have many friends; his wife was his primary confidante. His neighbors across the street and next door are friendly, and Neal used to help them with yard projects in his spare time. Neal's health has been good, but he has had trouble with his teeth recently. His diet has been poor, and in the last 3 months his physical and mental vigor has deteriorated. He has been slowly lapsing into a depression and so keeps the shades drawn and rarely leaves his house. Neal keeps very little food in the house, because his wife did most of the cooking and shopping and he just isn't that interested in food.

If you were one of Neal's relatives and learned of Neal's situation, what six things could you do or suggest to help improve his nutritional status and mental outlook? Look back into the chapter to get some ideas.

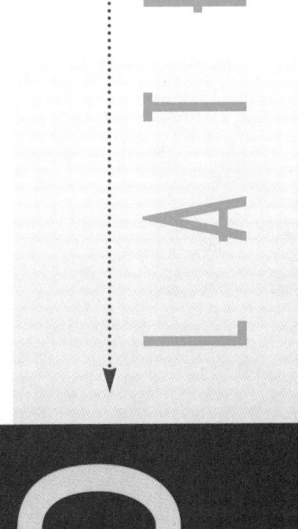

1. ______________________________

2. ______________________________

3. ______________________________

4. ______________________________

5. ______________________________

6. ______________________________

Nutrition ISSUE

ETHANOL—ITS METABOLISM AND POTENTIAL TO INFLUENCE HEALTH

Alcoholism is an important issue for all adults to examine carefully. From the teen years through early adulthood and on to the elderly years, alcohol's ability to tear away at nutritional and overall health is enormous (Figure 15-10). Alcohol, in excess, is by far the most common drug—wrecking families and friendships and filling jails. In 1990 the use of alcohol cost American society an estimated 136 billion dollars and more than 65,000 lives—22,000 of them on highways. Causes of alcoholism include genetic, psychosocial, and environmental factors.[23]

Alcohol Absorption and Action

After someone swallows an alcoholic beverage, the blood level of alcohol rises rapidly. Alcohol, also known as ethanol, is readily absorbed into the blood from all levels of the gastrointestinal tract. You've probably been warned, with good reason, not to drink on an empty stomach. Alcohol absorption depends partly on the rate of stomach emptying. Food, particularly fat, slows the stomach's emptying rate and stimulates secretions. These dilute the alcohol and slow its absorption into the bloodstream.

Some alcohol is metabolized in the cells lining the stomach, especially in men. Most of the remaining alcohol is metabolized in the liver.[18] About 10% of the ethanol in the body is directly eliminated by diffusion through the kidneys or lungs.

Alcohol affects the brain more than any other organ. Acting as a sedative, alcohol tends to relieve the drinker's anxiety, slur speech, reduce coordination in walking, impair judgment, and encourage uninhibited behavior. Because it lowers inhibitions, alcohol appears to act as a stimulant, but in fact it is a powerful depressant to the body. As William Shakespeare wrote: "It stirs up desire, but takes away the performance." Because it reduces secretion of the body's antidiuretic hormone, alcohol increases urination (see Chapter 9). It also causes the blood vessels to dilate, releasing body heat.

Metabolism

A social drinker who weighs 150 pounds and has normal liver function metabolizes about 7 to 14 grams (the equivalent of ½ to 1 12-ounce beer) of alcohol per hour (100 to 200 milligrams of alcohol per kilogram of body weight per hour). If a person drinks slightly less alcohol each hour than the amount that can be metabolized by the liver, the blood alcohol content remains low. In that case, a person can drink large amounts of alcohol over long periods without becoming noticeably intoxicated. When the rate of alcohol consumption exceeds the liver's metabolic capacity, the blood alcohol content rises and symptoms of intoxication appear (Table 15-7).

When a man and woman of similar size drink the same amount of alcohol, the woman retains more alcohol in her bloodstream; women cannot metabolize as much alcohol in their stomach cells. They have lower levels of the key alcohol-metabolizing enzyme, alcohol dehydrogenase. Women are also much quicker to develop alcohol-related ailments, such as cirrhosis of the liver, than are men with the same drinking history.[18]

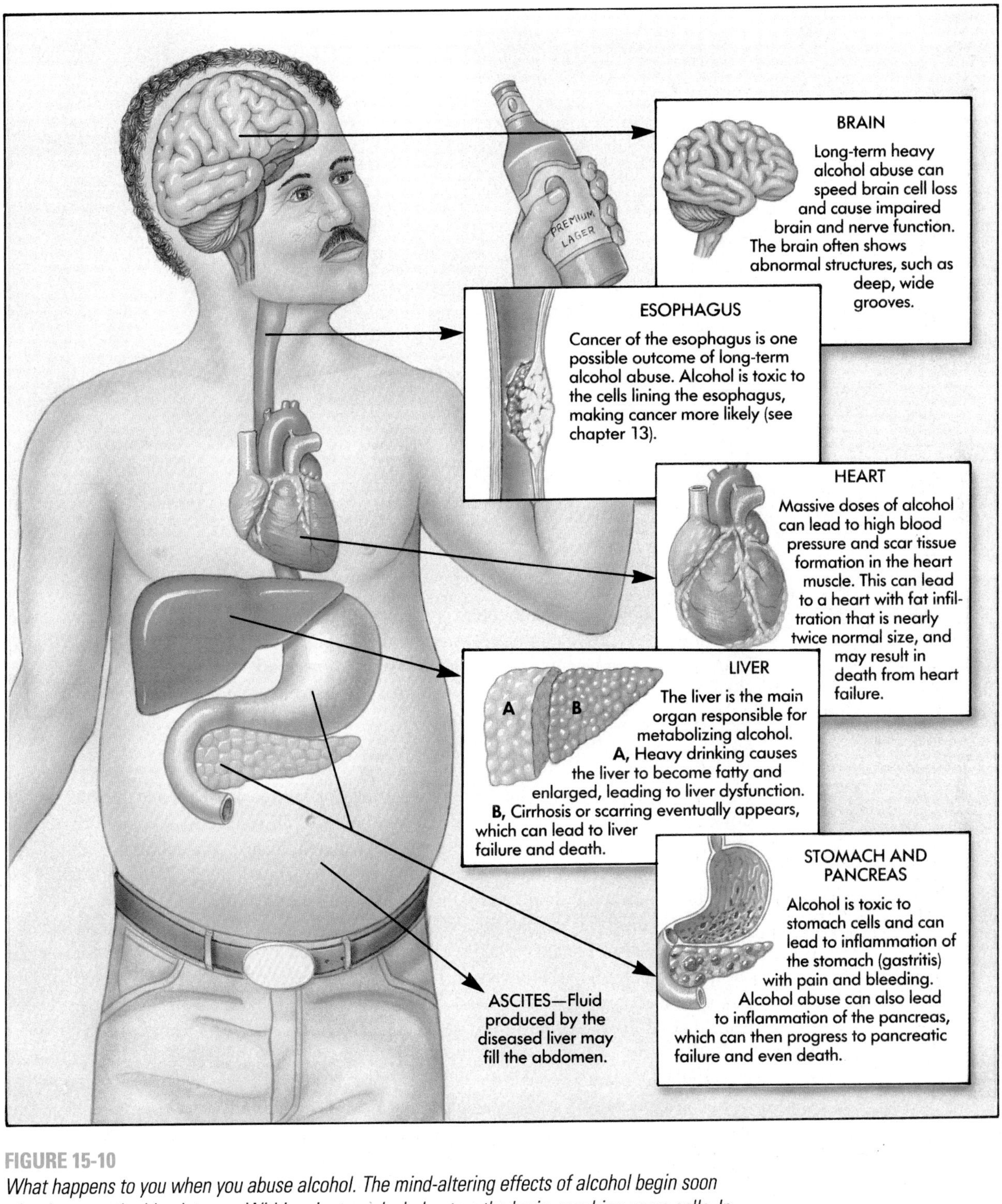
PREMIUM LAGER
BRAIN
Long-term heavy alcohol abuse can speed brain cell loss and cause impaired brain and nerve function. The brain often shows abnormal structures, such as deep, wide grooves.
ESOPHAGUS
Cancer of the esophagus is one possible outcome of long-term alcohol abuse. Alcohol is toxic to the cells lining the esophagus, making cancer more likely (see chapter 13).
HEART
Massive doses of alcohol can lead to high blood pressure and scar tissue formation in the heart muscle. This can lead to a heart with fat infiltration that is nearly twice normal size, and may result in death from heart failure.
LIVER
A
B
The liver is the main organ responsible for metabolizing alcohol.
A, Heavy drinking causes the liver to become fatty and enlarged, leading to liver dysfunction.
B, Cirrhosis or scarring eventually appears, which can lead to liver failure and death.
STOMACH AND PANCREAS
Alcohol is toxic to stomach cells and can lead to inflammation of the stomach (gastritis) with pain and bleeding. Alcohol abuse can also lead to inflammation of the pancreas, which can then progress to pancreatic failure and even death.
ASCITES—Fluid produced by the diseased liver may fill the abdomen.

FIGURE 15-10

What happens to you when you abuse alcohol. The mind-altering effects of alcohol begin soon after it enters the bloodstream. Within minutes, alcohol enters the brain, numbing nerve cells. In the heart, cardiac muscles strain to cope with alcohol's depressive action. If drinking continues, alcohol builds in the bloodstream, causing decrements in speech, vision, balance, and judgment. With extremely high levels of alcohol in the blood, respiratory failure becomes a possibility. In the long run, alcohol abuse increases the risk of certain forms of heart disease and cancer, and liver and pancreas failure.

TABLE 15-7

Blood Alcohol Levels and Symptoms

Level (mg/dl)	Sporadic Drinker	Chronic Drinker
50 (party level)	Congenial euphoria; decreased tension	No observable effect
75	Gregarious	Often no effect
100 (0.1%)	Uncoordinated; legally drunk (as in drunk driving) in most states; a level of 0.08% is legal drunkenness in some stricter locations	Minimal signs, such as slower reaction time
150	Unrestrained behavior; episodic dyscontrol; legally drunk at 0.15% in all states	Pleasurable euphoria or beginning of incoordination
200-250	Alertness lost; lethargic	Effort required to maintain emotional and motor control
300-350	Stupor to coma	Drowsy and slow
>500	Some will die	Coma

From Wyngaarden JB, Smith LH: Cecil textbook of medicine, *Philadelphia, 1988, WB Saunders.*

While the liver is metabolizing alcohol, it cannot rapidly metabolize medications, such as sedatives. Consequently, high amounts of alcohol mixed with some sedatives may cause a person to lapse into a coma and die.

When a person drinks a lot of alcohol, alcohol dehydrogenase in the liver cannot break it all down. For this and other reasons, another liver enzyme system begins to metabolize alcohol. The liver usually uses the same system to metabolize medications and other "foreign" compounds. Once the extra system is activated, alcohol tolerance increases because the rate of alcohol metabolism increases.[18]

Alcohol and Overall Health

About 32% of all Americans have three drinks or less each week, and 22% have two drinks or less a day. Only 11% have more than two drinks a day. Although the public health impact of alcohol abuse is still being calculated, misuse of alcohol, in and of itself, is one of the most preventable health problems in the United States. Drinking alcohol excessively contributes significantly to 5 of the 10 leading causes of death in the United States—certain forms of cancer, cirrhosis of the liver, motor vehicle and other accidents, suicides, and homicides. Tobacco reacts with alcohol in a way that reinforces its effects in causing esophageal and oral cancer. In addition, excessive alcohol drinking increases the risk of some types of heart disease, high blood pressure (especially in African-Americans), nerve diseases, nutritional deficiencies (discussed later), damage to a pregnant woman's fetus, and many other disorders. A major cause of lasting mental retardation that begins in infancy stems from fetal exposure to alcohol (see Chapter 13).

Social consequences of dependence on alcohol include divorce, unemployment, and poverty. An estimated 27 million American children are more likely to develop abnormally in psychosocial skills and relationships because their parents abuse alcohol.

For these reasons, alcohol should be used cautiously and in moderation, if at all. Drinking even small amounts of alcohol can lead to dependence on it. Approximately 10% of those who drink alcoholic beverages in the United States are alcoholics. As many as 18 million Americans are estimated to have alcohol problems. Of these, 41% (7.2 million) are alcohol abusers, drinkers who experienced at least one severe or moderately severe consequence of alcohol abuse—such as job loss, arrest, or illness—in the previous year.

The people who drink the most alcohol are those in the 20- to 40-year age-group. The practice often begins earlier. In a 1985 survey, 66% of the high school seniors interviewed reported that they had consumed alcohol in the past month and 5% described themselves as daily drinkers.

Studies indicate a genetic component in alcoholism.[13] On reaching adulthood, the biological children of alcoholic parents have a greater incidence of alcoholism than do the biological children of nonalcoholic parents.

Cirrhosis

Long-term alcohol use causes fatty liver, alcoholic hepatitis, and cirrhosis. Cirrhosis is a chronic and usually relentlessly progressive disease characterized by fatty infiltration of the liver. Eventually the fat chokes off the blood supply, depriving the liver cells of oxygen and nutrients. Liver cells then die and are replaced by connective (scar) tissue. This scarring process is what is called cirrhosis.[18] In America, most cases of cirrhosis are caused by alcohol consumption. Cirrhosis develops in 12% to 31% of cases of alcoholism. In addition to the amount and duration of alcohol consumption, genetic factors and individual differences determine the body's response to alcohol.

No specific amount of alcohol consumption guarantees cirrhosis of the liver. Rather, some people are very susceptible to its effects, and others are not. One observable pattern is that cirrhosis commonly results from a 15-year consumption of approximately 80 grams of alcohol per day (Table 15-8). This is equivalent to seven beers per day. Some evidence suggests that the dose may be effective in causing cirrhosis when it's as low as 40 grams a day for men and 20 grams a day for women. Early stages of alcoholic liver injury are reversible, whereas advanced stages usually are not. The only known prevention for alcoholic cirrhosis is to limit consumption of alcohol.

TABLE 15-8

Caloric, Carbohydrate, and Alcohol Content of Alcoholic Beverages

Beverage	Amount (ounces)	Alcohol (grams)	Carbohydrate (grams)	Energy (kcalories)
Beer				
Regular	12	13	14	150
Light	12	10	6	90
Extra light	12	8	3	70
Near	12	2	12	60
Distilled				
Gin, rum, vodka, whiskey	1.5	15	—	105
Brandy, cognac	1.0	11	—	75
Wine				
Red	4	12	1	85
Dry white	4	11	1	80
Sweet	4	12	5	105
Sherry	2	9	2	75
Port, muscatel	2	7	7	95
Vermouth, sweet	3	12	14	140
Vermouth, dry	3	13	4	105
Manhattan	3	21	2	165
Martini	3	19	1	140
Old-fashioned	3	21	1	180

From Guthrie HA: Introductory nutrition, *ed 7, St Louis, 1989, Mosby–Year Book.*

A poor nutritional status makes the liver more vulnerable to toxic substances by depleting supplies of antioxidants, such as vitamins E and C. A nutritious diet can help prevent some complications associated with alcoholism, but usually alcoholism wreaks serious destruction on the body with or without an adequate diet. Laboratory animal studies clearly show that even when consuming a nutritious diet, alcoholism can lead to cirrhosis of the liver.

Alcohol and Nutrition

Nutritional problems in a person with alcoholism result from deficiencies of a variety of nutrients[18]:

- *Vitamin A deficiency,* which may be caused by a poor diet, an inability of the liver to produce retinol-binding protein, or poor zinc status, which, in turn, reduces retinol-binding protein synthesis. In addition, the chemical-detoxifying systems in the liver induced by chronic alcohol consumption may hasten the degradation of vitamin A in the liver.
- *Thiamin deficiency,* which can be caused by decreased thiamin absorption or decreased liver synthesis of the active thiamin coenzyme. People with alcoholism often exhibit nervous system problems similar to those seen in someone with a thiamin deficiency.
- *Niacin deficiency* and resulting pellagra caused by a poor diet.
- *Vitamin B-6 deficiency,* probably stemming from a poor dietary intake of the vitamin and increased breakdown of the vitamin B-6 coenzyme.
- *Folate deficiency,* which can be caused by a poor diet and poor nutrient absorption. This, along with vitamin B-6 deficiency, are the two most common vitamin deficiencies of alcoholism.
- *Vitamin D deficiency,* usually caused by the liver's decreased capacity to convert vitamin D into the final usable form. Alcohol also may encourage bone cell dysfunction, which diminishes bone formation and reduces bone mineralization. This can lead to osteoporosis.
- *Vitamin C deficiency,* resulting primarily from a decrease in dietary intake or from altered liver metabolism, or both.
- *Vitamin K deficiency,* probably occurring because less of it is synthesized by intestinal bacteria, less is consumed, and less is absorbed.

General Recommendations for Drinking Alcohol

The Surgeon General's Office recommends that to reduce the risk of chronic disease, people should (1) drink alcohol only in moderation (no more than two drinks a day), if at all, (2) avoid drinking alcohol before or while driving, operating machinery, taking medications, or engaging in any other activity requiring judgment, and (3) avoid drinking alcohol while pregnant.

The National Academy of Science's report *Diet and Health* also does not recommend alcohol consumption. For those who do drink alcoholic beverages, the committee recommends limiting consumption to the equivalent of less than 1 ounce of pure alcohol in a single day. This is the equivalent of two cans of beer, two small glasses of wine, or two average cocktails. Again, pregnant women should avoid alcoholic beverages altogether.

This information is obviously not a plea for teetotalers to start drinking. It is important to note that people who drink casually and are not prone to abuse do not risk danger from moderate drinking. In fact, there are some benefits, such as a reduction in heart disease risk. The reasons for this are still unknown, but a reduction in blood clotting is one likely explanation. Unfortunately, however, when some of us open the door to alcohol, we walk through a door we wish we had never opened.

Do You Have a Problem with Alcohol?

Asking a person about the quantity and frequency of alcohol consumption is an important means of detecting abuse and dependence. The following questionnaire (CAGE) is popular for use in routine health care.

CAGE Questionnaire to Screen for Alcohol Abuse

C: Have you ever felt you ought to ***Cut*** down on drinking?
A: Have people ***A****nnoyed* you by criticizing your drinking?
G: Have you ever felt bad or ***G****uilty* about your drinking?
E: Have you ever had a drink first thing in the morning to steady your nerves or get rid of a hangover (***E****ye-opener*)?

Another key point to question is alcohol tolerance. Does it take more to make you inebriated than it did in the past? More than one positive response suggests an alcohol problem.

Treatment

Once a diagnosis of alcohol abuse or dependence is established, a physician should arrange appropriate treatment and counseling for the patient and family. The drinker must confront the immediate problem of how to stop the drinking. Total abstinence must be the primary goal. For people with alcoholism, there is no such thing as controlled drinking. A problem drinker cannot return safely to social drinking. The person should enter an Alcoholics Anonymous (AA) program or a reputable therapy program for people with alcoholism (one can check with a local mental health treatment center for programs available in the community). The spouse should join the treatment program as well. Success is usually proportionate to participation in AA, other social agencies and religious counseling. About 2 years of treatment should be expected.

Current research does not support the generally negative public opinion about the prognosis for alcoholism. In most industrial alcoholism treatment programs, where workers are socially stable and—because of the risk to jobs and pensions—well motivated, recovery rates run at the 70% to 80% level. This remarkably high cure rate is probably accounted for by early detection. Once a person moves from problem drinking to an advanced stage of alcoholism, success rates seldom exceed 40% to 50%. Early identification and intervention remain the most important steps in the treatment of alcoholism.

The medical deterrent drug disulfiram (Antabuse) can be of critical importance in helping the alcoholic to make the essential decision to stop drinking. An early step in alcohol metabolism is blocked by the action of this drug. As a result, a highly toxic alcohol by-product accumulates in the blood, producing prostrating nausea, vomiting, diffuse flushing, and a shocklike reaction when alcohol is consumed.

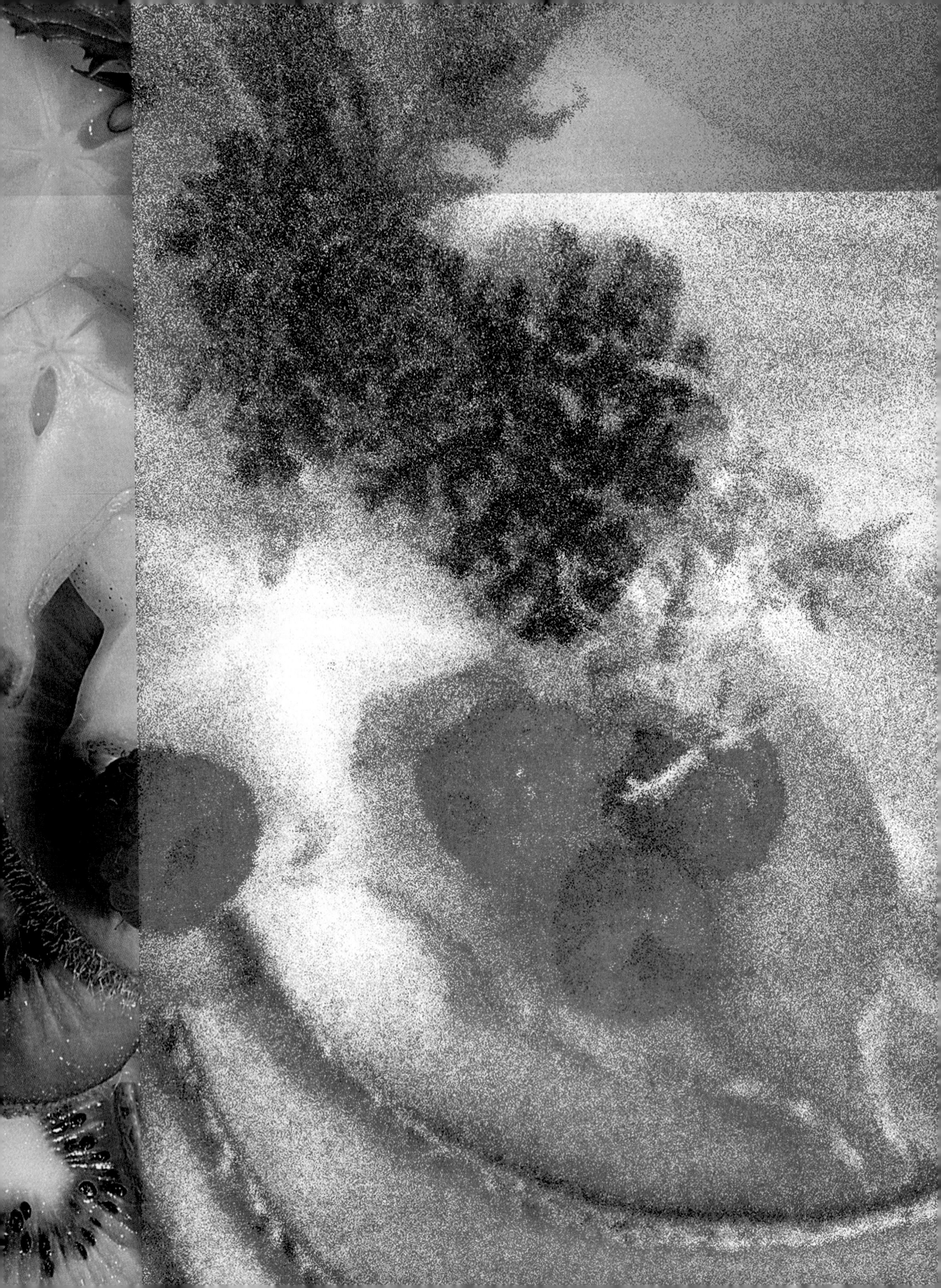

NUTRITION: BEYOND THE NUTRIENTS 5

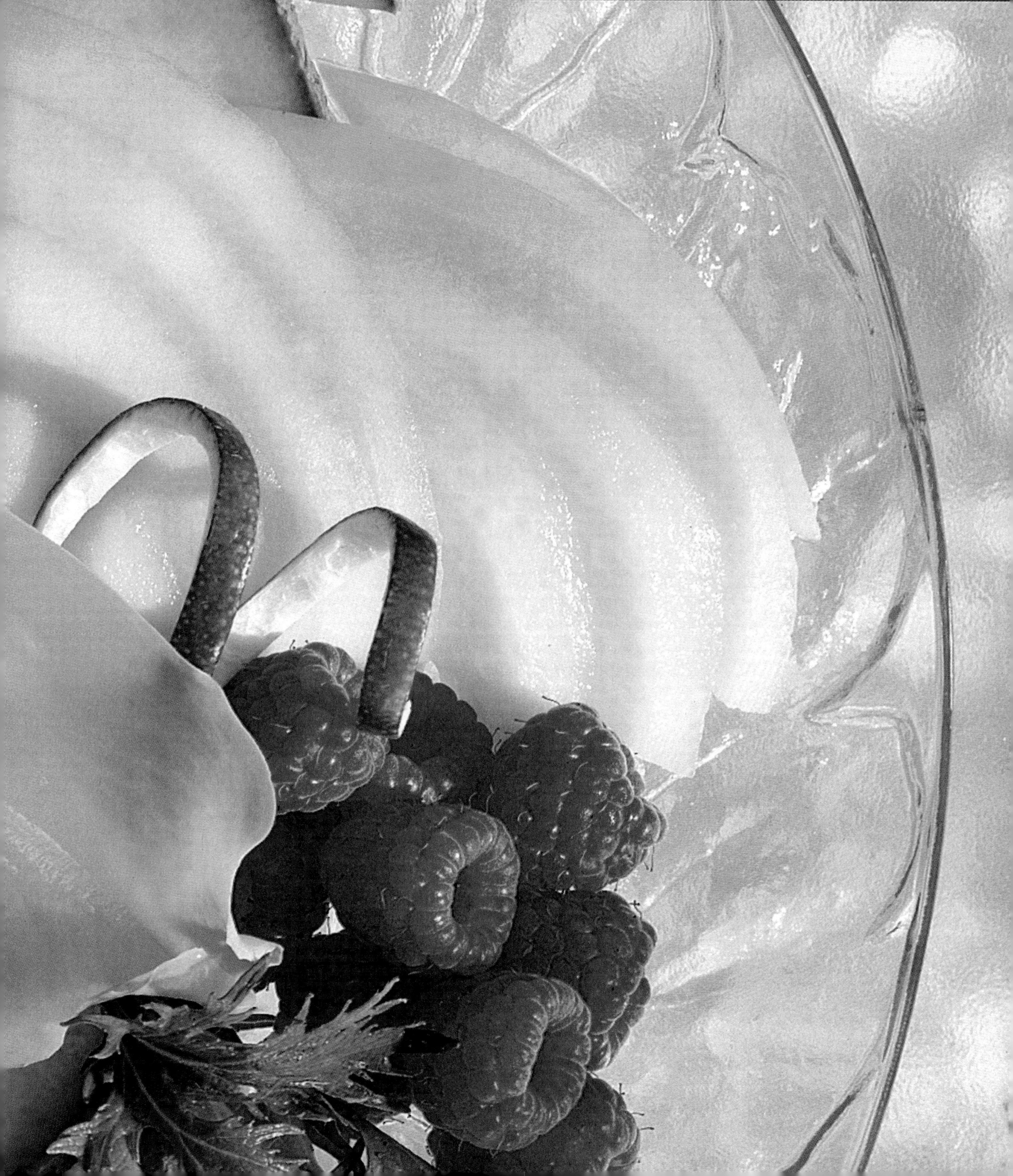

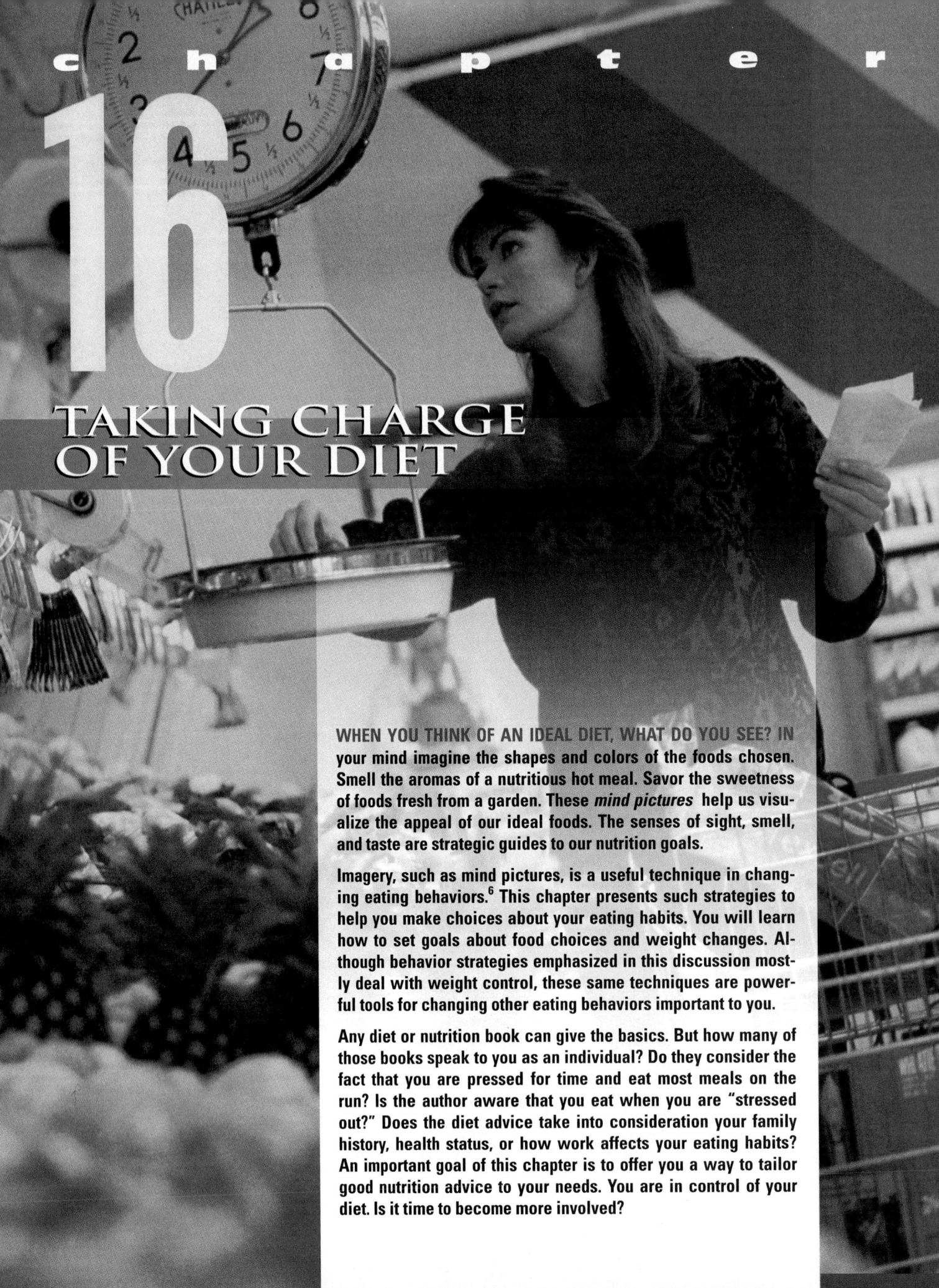

chapter 16

TAKING CHARGE OF YOUR DIET

WHEN YOU THINK OF AN IDEAL DIET, WHAT DO YOU SEE? IN your mind imagine the shapes and colors of the foods chosen. Smell the aromas of a nutritious hot meal. Savor the sweetness of foods fresh from a garden. These *mind pictures* help us visualize the appeal of our ideal foods. The senses of sight, smell, and taste are strategic guides to our nutrition goals.

Imagery, such as mind pictures, is a useful technique in changing eating behaviors.[6] This chapter presents such strategies to help you make choices about your eating habits. You will learn how to set goals about food choices and weight changes. Although behavior strategies emphasized in this discussion mostly deal with weight control, these same techniques are powerful tools for changing other eating behaviors important to you.

Any diet or nutrition book can give the basics. But how many of those books speak to you as an individual? Do they consider the fact that you are pressed for time and eat most meals on the run? Is the author aware that you eat when you are "stressed out?" Does the diet advice take into consideration your family history, health status, or how work affects your eating habits? An important goal of this chapter is to offer you a way to tailor good nutrition advice to your needs. You are in control of your diet. Is it time to become more involved?

DO YOUR EATING HABITS ENCOURAGE WEIGHT MAINTENANCE?

How often do you do the following (circle the appropriate number):

	Rarely	Sometimes	Often
1. Take 20 minutes or longer to eat a meal.	1	2	3
2. Eat foods that are baked, boiled, or broiled rather than fried.	1	2	3
3. Eat in one main place in your residence.	1	2	3
4. Drink six to eight glasses of water or other fluids daily.	1	2	3
5. Eat breakfast.	1	2	3
6. Store foods out of sight in your house or room.	1	2	3
7. Plan ahead of time the food you will eat.	1	2	3
8. Avoid skipping meals.	1	2	3
9. At a restaurant request salad dressing on the side or bring your own.	1	2	3
10. Eat until you are comfortably full rather than overeat.	1	2	3
11. Exercise regularly.	1	2	3
12. Choose low-fat foods.	1	2	3
13. Avoid the influence of friends and peers on your eating habits.	1	2	3
14. Leave food on your plate.	1	2	3
15. Do nothing else while eating (e.g., reading, watching television).	1	2	3

ADD TOGETHER THE NUMBERS YOU CIRCLED
AND ENTER THE TOTAL HERE ______________

Interpretation

Interpret your total score this way:

15-25 Dietary Doldrums:	Your eating habits need some attention.
26-35 Munching Mediocrity:	You are doing well for going to college, but it may not get you through to the "golden years."
36-45 Nutritional Stardom:	This score gets you into the nutrition hall of fame (however, don't reward yourself by overeating).

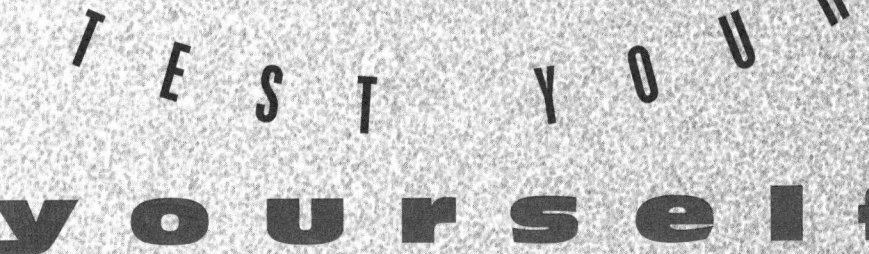

ASSESS

TEST YOUR KNOWLEDGE

yourself

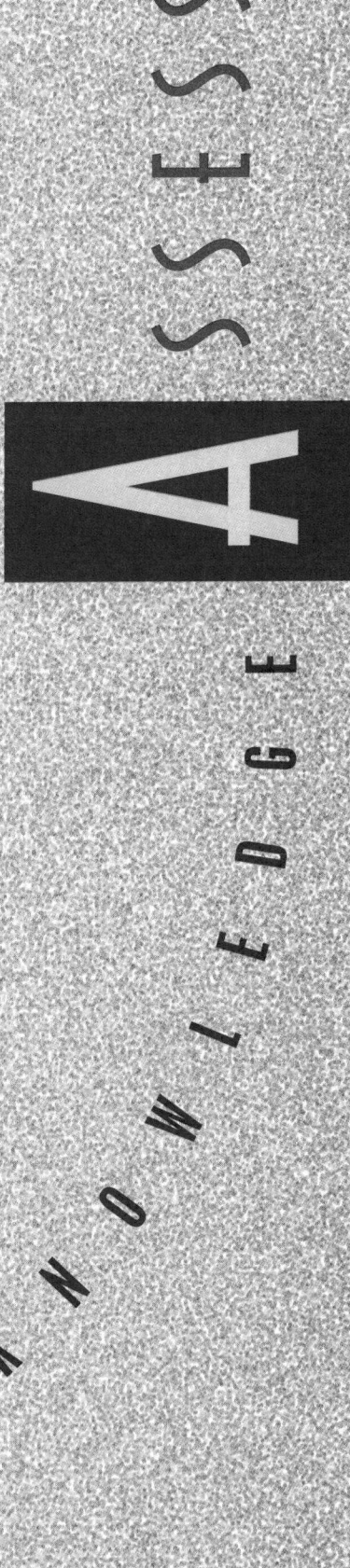

THE BEHAVIOR CHANGE PROCESS

Behavior patterns that have evolved throughout a lifetime do not change or disappear overnight. Planned behavior changes occur gradually and with some effort. First, a person must perceive that a problem exists.[6] For someone who is overweight, this might mean becoming more aware of health risks, recognizing a lack of physical stamina, or balking at the need to expand one's wardrobe.

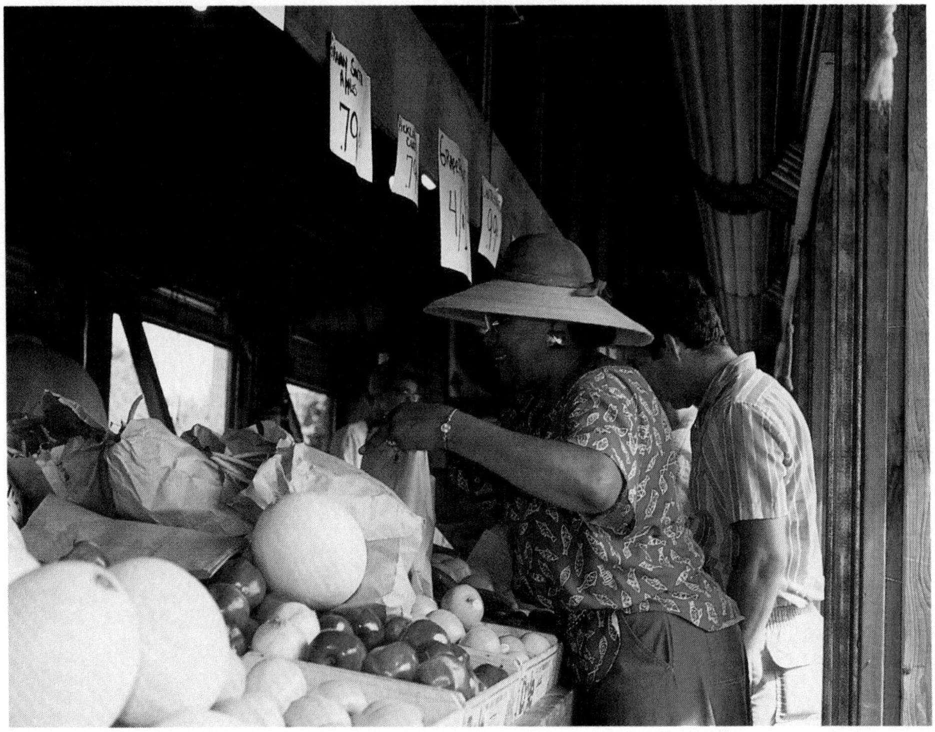

When considering a diet change, asking yourself if you eat enough fruits and vegetables is a good first step.

Receptive Framework for Learning *The process by which a person opens and responds to learning more about a problem—it usually involves seeking more information about an issue from books and people.*

After recognizing that a problem indeed exists, an interested person then develops a ***receptive framework for learning*** more about the problem. This might involve weighing the costs and benefits of changing behaviors; for example, balancing the time and effort required for exercising and sacrificing some favorite foods against the benefits of lowering weight, decreasing health risks, and feeling and looking better (Figure 16-1).

Having decided that the change is sufficiently beneficial, the person then must ask "Can I do it?" We know ourselves best. Is the change feasible? Can one's lifestyle accommodate the new goal? Can the person continue the new behaviors for years? Long-term commitment is a key part of any behavior change plan.[2] It may help a person to speak with others who have worked on similar health problems and to read about others' experiences. The changes then may seem less threatening and more possible. A health professional also can often provide the information and encouragement necessary to start the change process.

Starting on a New Path

Having decided to attempt a change, the person begins a trial run. Ideally, unwanted patterns are changed one step at a time, beginning with the easiest habit to discard. Changing too many habits too soon can be overwhelming, making it hard to adhere to a plan.[2] As we try new behaviors, we experience both difficulties and rewards: some hunger and discomfort versus compliments and greater self-esteem. Some experiences may be perceived as positive, but some will be perceived as negative—otherwise, the old practices would not have been cherished. Familiar foods now missing from the diet may leave a void.

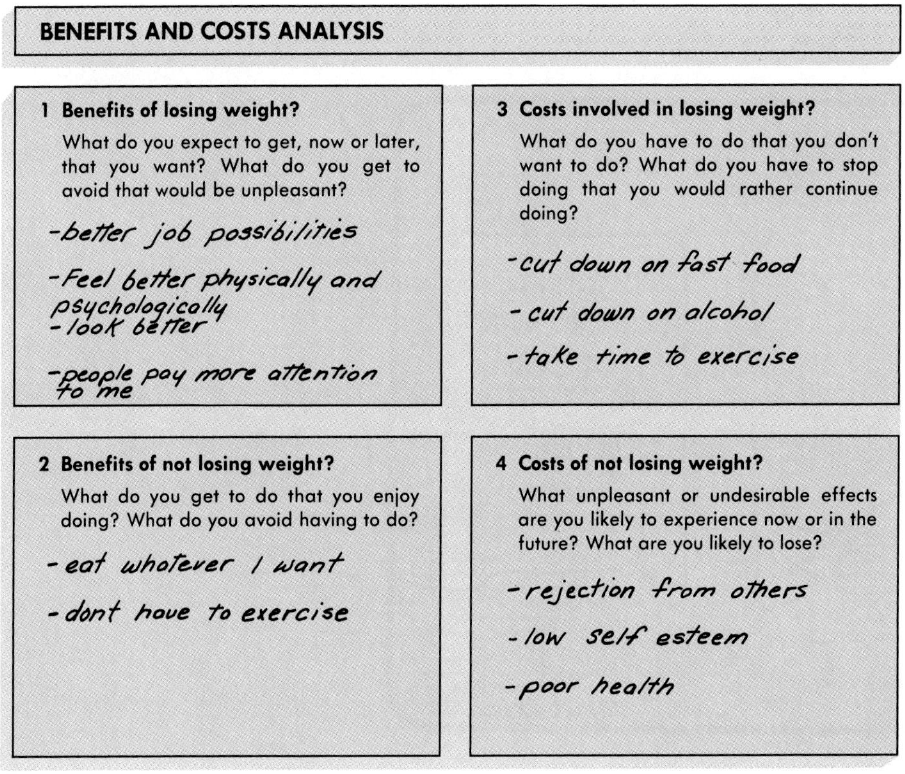

BENEFITS AND COSTS ANALYSIS

1 Benefits of losing weight?
What do you expect to get, now or later, that you want? What do you get to avoid that would be unpleasant?
-better job possibilities
-Feel better physically and psychologically
-look better
-people pay more attention to me

3 Costs involved in losing weight?
What do you have to do that you don't want to do? What do you have to stop doing that you would rather continue doing?
-cut down on fast food
-cut down on alcohol
-take time to exercise

2 Benefits of not losing weight?
What do you get to do that you enjoy doing? What do you avoid having to do?
-eat whatever I want
-dont have to exercise

4 Costs of not losing weight?
What unpleasant or undesirable effects are you likely to experience now or in the future? What are you likely to lose?
-rejection from others
-low self esteem
-poor health

FIGURE 16-1
Benefits and costs analysis applied to weight loss. This exercise helps put behavior change into the context of total lifestyle.

Are there parts of your health lifestyle that need improvement?

To deal with diet difficulties, positive ***reinforcement*** is critical (Figure 16-2).[2] This should be built into a diet plan. We deserve credit for attempting difficult tasks; we need rewards for hard work—perhaps a night at the movies, a new compact disc, an outing with friends, or a chance to sleep late. During this trial period, it is important to capitalize on success and learn how to derive psychological nourishment from conquering poor habits.

Finally, the person adopts and integrates the new behaviors into a total lifestyle. In the progression from becoming aware of a problem to adopting new behaviors, we can further take charge of our health. Now the possibilities for other improvements can be investigated, and the cycle repeated.

Reinforcement *A reaction by others in response to a person's behavior. Positive reinforcement entails encouragement; negative reinforcement entails criticism or penalty.*

CHARTING A PLAN FOR CHANGE

A good plan evolves over time. It is based on rational, deliberate decisions, coupled with trial and error experiences. Because a person can't know all possible strategies and tactics before beginning, a good plan incorporates all the information at hand.[6] Revisions will be necessary and should be expected.

If your goal is to control your weight, you should know that the typical restrictive diet not only fails to produce the desired results for most people but also can produce undesired results, such as fatigue and depression. As was discussed in Chapter 10, effective, long-range weight control programs encourage people to raise their activity levels and eat less fat, rather than to severely restrict their eating.[1] To discover the most effective options available, one can investigate some clinic programs and speak with registered dietitians.

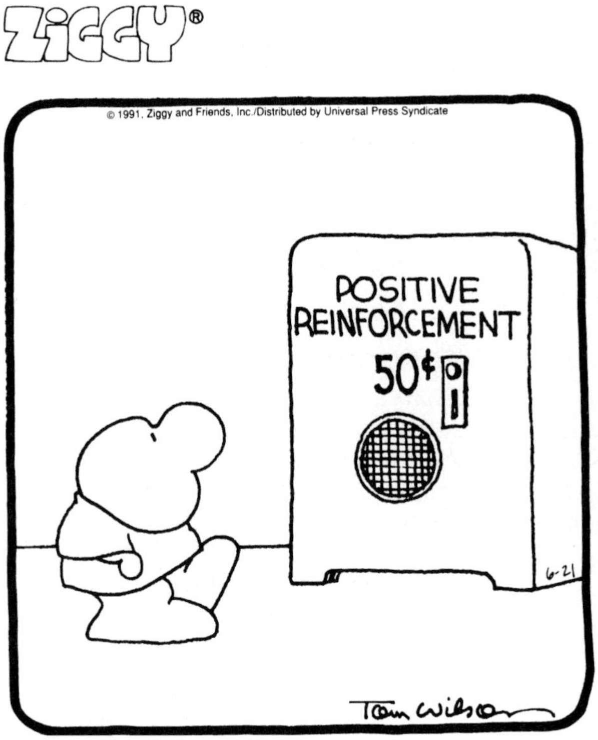

FIGURE 16-2
Ziggy.

BECOMING AWARE

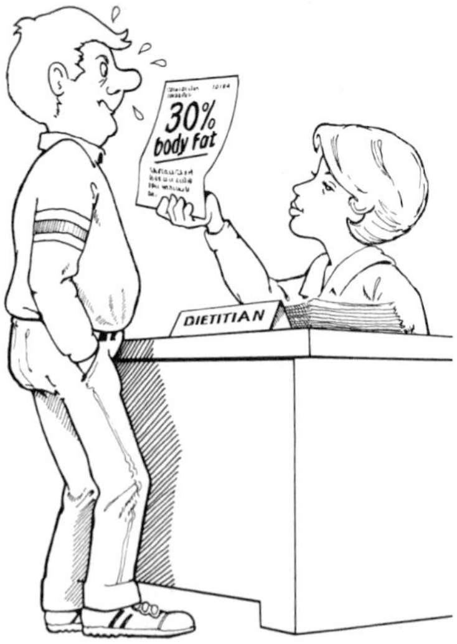

Alan is a 20-year-old male college student who has been steadily gaining weight since high school. At the YMCA a registered dietitian calculates that Alan stores about 50% more fat than is desirable. Alan is concerned about his long-term health and wants to correct his overfat problem before it leads to other health problems. Having seen his father change his diet and lose weight after a heart attack, Alan thinks that he too can make dietary changes with success.

Gathering Baseline Data

The next step in developing a personal plan for dietary change is to monitor eating behaviors, noting strengths and weaknesses.[4] Recording meals and snacks in a ***food diary*** may expose eating patterns previously unnoticed. Let's assume that you want to lower fat intake to help control your weight. You will have to adjust some habits, but which ones? In a diary, list any relevant behaviors, such as foods eaten, portion sizes, and amount of fat in the food eaten (Appendix C will help). Also, as you did in Chapter 1, record the intensity of hunger; the time and location of the meal or snack; any other activity performed, such as watching TV; whether others were present; and your reasons for choosing that particular food (Figure 16-3). A blank form for recording this information is included in Chapter 1 and Appendix C.

A review of the diary might reveal how both your outside environment and internal cues influence your nutrition and health habits. This is the time to look for patterns—identify both positive behaviors and ones that need changes. The patterns might suggest which food habits would be easy to change and which might be more difficult to alter. Consider classifying food choices as "ones you can't give up" versus "ones you can live without." See if certain eating habits are paired with other activities. For example, you may find that you often eat while visiting with friends, in response to an angry mood, or perhaps after 6 PM.[3] Subtle associations that influence eating habits can provide a good starting point for behavior changes.

Food Diary
A written record of sequential food intake for a period of time. Details associated with the food intake are often recorded as well.

another BITE

Let's assume information from your food diary, coupled with an evaluation of your current health status, reveals behaviors you need to change in order to establish better nutrition and health practices. You would like to take the next step, but are unsure of how to proceed. At this point a discussion with a physician or registered dietitian would be appropriate.

FIGURE 16-3
One day's food record. This activity can help one understand more about food habits.

Time	Minutes spent eating	M or S*	H†	Activity while eating	Place of eating	Food and quantity	Others present	Reason for choice
7:10 a.m.	15	M	2	standing, fixing lunch	kitchen	1 c orange juice 1 c corn flakes ¼ c 2% milk 2 t sugar black coffee	—	health habit health taste habit
10:00 a.m.	4	S	1	sitting, taking notes	classroom	12 oz diet cola	class	weight control
12:15 p.m.	40	M	2	sitting, talking	union	1 chicken sandwich 1 pear	friends	taste health
2:30 p.m.	10	S	1	sitting, studying	library	12 oz regular cola	friend	hunger
6:30 p.m.	35	M	3	sitting, talking	kitchen	1 pork chop 1 baked potato 2 T margarine lettuce 1 oz ranch dressing 1 c whole milk 1 piece cherry pie	boyfriend	convenience health taste health taste habit taste
9:10 p.m.	10	S	2	sitting, studying	living room	1 glass mineral water	—	weight control

*M or S: Meal or snack.
†H: Degree of hunger (0 = none; 3 = maximum).

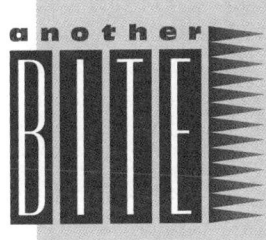

As we mentioned in Chapter 1, habit and sensory appeal—flavor, appearance, texture, and odor—usually determine both our intended and actual food choices. Of lesser importance in choosing foods to eat are health value, time constraints, social influence, energy value, and cost. After reevaluating your diary from Chapter 1, decide if this is true for you.

CONCEPT CHECK

In the process of changing behavior a person first becomes aware of a problem. Then the person studies the problem and develops a receptive frame of mind for making a change. He initiates a trial change. If he receives positive reinforcement, he may eventually incorporate the change into his lifestyle—he adopts it. Behavior change is most successful when tailored to specific personal needs. By carefully studying their own behaviors, people can more effectively change problem habits.

Setting Attainable Goals

If you're eating every dinner in quick-service restaurants and you want to change this habit, try fixing one dinner at home each week for a month. Consider this an experiment. Will it work for you?

What can we accomplish and how long will it take? Setting a realistic goal and allowing a reasonable amount of time to pursue it increase the likelihood of success.[9] For example, if one goal is to improve iron status, planning an iron-rich diet and taking iron supplements can show increased blood-iron levels within just a few months. Progress toward other types of goals, such as weight loss, might be apparent within a week and then progress from week to week. Seeing week-to-week progress can be the spark needed to continue moving ahead with a program.

If you aim to control a chronic disease, such as hypertension, diabetes or heart disease, health professionals can supply specific behavior goals. A clinical examination will confirm your degree of success. If the goal is broader, for example, to maintain or improve overall nutritional health, the path is not as well defined. Chapter 2 offers some suggestions.

Considering all these possible goals, it is best to change only a few specific behaviors at first—for example, lowering fat intake, using more whole-grain products, and not eat-

BASELINE

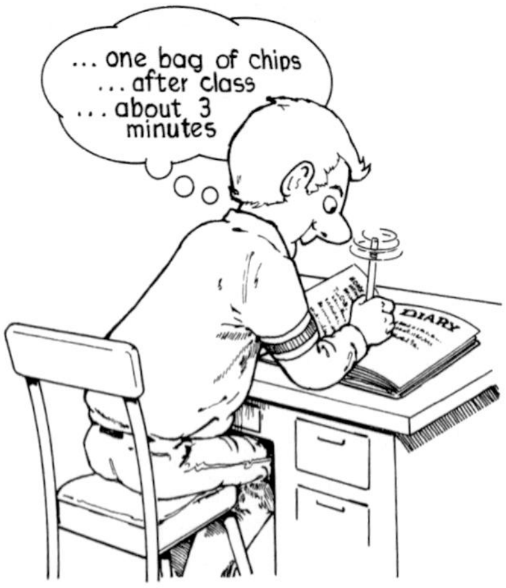

To better understand his eating habits, Alan keeps a food diary. In it he tracks what and how much he eats, how quickly he eats, the time, the environment, and his feelings at the time of eating. From this record he finds a previously unnoticed pattern—he starts snacking after his 2 PM class and does not stop until dinner. He is alarmed that he consumes so many kcalories almost unconsciously. In addition, Alan notes that his lunches usually are high in fat and his days lack much physical activity.

ing after 7 PM. By attempting small and perhaps easier dietary changes first, you reduce the scope of the problem and increase the likelihood of success.[7]

Measuring Commitment

The greater the personal commitment, the greater the chances of success. We need to examine the goals we set.[3] Are they worth pursuing? Are health benefits greater than the sacrifices to be made? Some people can ignore persistent ***arthritis*** in the knees, which is magnified by being overweight, because they derive great pleasure from eating. Others may love eating ice cream and chips and dips but finally realize that the price is too high. They realize that the benefit of keeping off unwanted pounds is greater than the momentary pleasure of immoderate snacking. They see that by changing eating habits, they feel better about themselves, move around more easily, feel less anxious in public, and most likely limit some future health problems.

Arthritis *Inflammation at a point where bones join together. The disease has many possible causes.*

People who are not strongly committed to changing a behavior often fail and become discouraged further. Usually, the more profound benefits from changing health and nutrition behaviors take time to achieve. This delayed success makes working toward long-term goals—improving fitness, lowering elevated blood pressure, and losing weight—difficult. As already noted, many long-term goals require a lifelong commitment. Only the person who contemplates the change can determine whether the value of good nutrition and good health is worth the price.[3]

Working Out the Details

Once a person establishes goals and discovers personal strengths and weaknesses in pursuing them, it is time to set the details of the plan. To do this, we need to know something about nutrition. The information contained in this book is a good place to start. Again, if you feel unable to work out a plan, seek professional help from a registered dietitian or physician.

One goal, as we have often suggested, is to reduce fat intake.[1] There are several means of doing this. You can eat less high-fat meat either by cutting your portion sizes or by eating these types of meat less frequently. You might eat high-fat meats only twice a week instead of every day. You can also search for new recipes and methods of preparation that yield leaner products and use less meat—broiling or stir frying for example—to reduce fat intake. Many more tactics for managing eating behavior exist (Table 16-1).[8] Once you control your consumption of high-fat meats, you can try other changes to help reach the overall goal.

PLANNING THE DETAILS

Alan addresses his overall weight problem in small steps. He plans to eat a better breakfast and lunch every day so he won't feel ravenous by midafternoon. He will keep low-kcalorie snack foods, such as oranges, handy in the apartment—instead of the usual bag of chips or cookies. He will start packing his lunch and limit visits to quick service restaurants to twice a week. In addition, at these restaurants he will make wiser selections from the menu, opting for such choices as the "create your own hamburger bar." He will use lots of tomato slices for juiciness and then choose low-fat milk. He will try to avoid eating his usual double-cheeseburger, fries, and milk shake. Finally, he plans to increase activity by both walking to class instead of driving and purchasing an exercise bike to ride each night while watching sports on television.

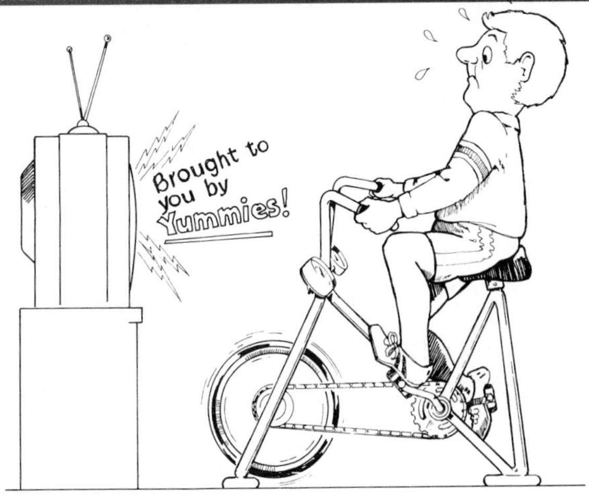

TABLE 16-1

Tactics for Managing Eating Behavior

Many things can trigger inappropriate eating behavior. But effective tactics can be used to gain control of eating. You may want to incorporate the tactics suggested below into a behavior change strategy.

Buying and Storing Food

Avoid market aisles of problem foods.
Don't pretend it's for the children or company.
Store problem food out of sight, or don't buy it.

Cooking, Preparing, and Serving Food

Broil, bake, or poach—don't fry.
Substitute low-fat and low-kcalorie ingredients for higher fat ones.
Don't sample while cooking.
Plan menus and measure portions.
Let others get their own snacks, desserts, and second helpings.

Eating Food

Drink plenty of water but little or no alcohol.
Eat more starches and avoid high-fat foods.
Eat three meals a day.
Replace impulse snacking with planned, healthful snacks.

Coping with *Problem Foods*

Make problem food temporarily off-limits, not forbidden forever.
Eat a little of a *problem food* when you aren't tempted to binge.

Eating Out in Restaurants

Choose a restaurant that offers healthful food choices.
Ask the waitress not to put bread and butter on the table before the meal.
Curb your appetite with an appetizer of broth-based soup.
Request no butter and no sauce on vegetables or entree.
Choose a broiled entree.
Request water with a meal.
Request salad dressing on the side or bring your own.
Don't look at the dessert list or dessert tray.

Coping with Others

Ask co-workers not to offer food.
Instead of eating to be polite, say, "No, thank you, I've had enough. It was delicious, and I'm full."

Coping with Emotions

Allow yourself an occasional treat; work it into your eating plan.
Avoid people and situations that upset you.
Go for a walk or use other exercise to unwind.
Lighten up; don't take it all so seriously.
Join a support group or seek counseling.

Managing Your Body

Exercise regularly.
Get adequate rest.

Modified from Nash JD: Maximize your body potential, *Palo Alto, Calif, 1986, Bull Publishing.*

Making It Official

Drawing up a ***behavior contract*** often adds incentive to follow through with a plan. The contract could list goal behaviors and objectives, milestones for measuring progress, and regular rewards for meeting the terms of the contract (Figure 16-4). After finishing a contract, the person should sign it in the presence of some friends (Figure 16-5).[3] This aids commitment.

We need to remember that positive reinforcement for following the contract contributes more to successful behavior change than negative reinforcement for not following it.[6] Initially, plans need to reward positive behaviors, and then they should focus on positive results. Positive behaviors, such as regular exercise, eventually lead to positive outcomes, such as weight loss. It may, however, take weeks to months to see the effects.

Behavior Contract *A written agreement that outlines intended behavior changes, plans for reinforcement, and witnesses to monitor progress.*

Name ______________________________

Goal

I agree to ______________________________
(specify behavior)
____

under the following circumstances ______________________________
(specify where, when, how much, etc.)
____

Substitute behavior and/or reinforcement schedule ______________________________
____

Environmental planning

In order to help me do this, I am going to (1) arrange my physical and social environment by ______________________________
____

and (2) control my internal environment (thoughts, images) by ______________________________
____

Reinforcements

Reinforcements provided by me daily or weekly (if contract is kept):
____
____

Reinforcements provided by others daily or weekly (if contract is kept):
____
____

Social support

Behavior change is more likely to take place when other people support you. During the quarter/semester please meet with the other person at least three times to discuss your progress.

The name of my "significant helper" is: ______________________________

This contract should include:

1. Baseline data (one week)
2. Well-defined goal
3. Simple method for charting progress (diary, counter, charts, etc.)
4. Reinforcements (immediate and long-term)
5. Evaluation method (summary of experiences, success, and/or new learnings about self).

FIGURE 16-4
A behavior contract. Completing a contract can help provide commitment for behavior change.

Name *Alan Young*

Goal

I agree to *ride my exercise bike*
(specify behavior)

under the following circumstances *for 30 minutes, 4 times per week*
(specify where, when, how much, etc.)
in the evening

Substitute behavior and/or reinforcement schedule *I will reinforce myself if I've achieved my goal after a month with a weekend off campus with my roommate.*

Environmental planning

In order to help me do this, I am going to (1) arrange my physical and social environment by *buying a new jogging suit at the local sporting goods store*

and (2) control my internal environment (thoughts, images) by *coordinating riding the bike with the first T.V. watching I do in the evening*

Reinforcements

Reinforcements provided by me daily or weekly (if contract is kept):
I will buy myself a new piece of clothing for off campus trip

Reinforcements provided by others daily or weekly (if contract is kept):
at the end of a month if I've completed my goal my parents will buy me a fitness club membership for winter.

Social support

Behavior change is more likely to take place when other people support you. During the quarter/semester please meet with the other person at least three times to discuss your progress.

The name of my "significant helper" is: *Mr. and Mrs. Young*

This contract should include:

1. Baseline data (one week)
2. Well-defined goal
3. Simple method for charting progress (diary, counter, charts, etc.)
4. Reinforcements (immediate and long-term)
5. Evaluation method (summary of experiences, success, and/or new learnings about self).

FIGURE 16-5
Alan's behavioral contract. What would your contract look like?

PSYCHING YOURSELF UP

While changing habits we are likely to get support from some friends, but others may prefer us the way we are. They may try to dissuade us from our plan. Even we may have moments when we want to abandon the plan. We all respond to others' opinions, especially about ourselves. We like approval, generally, and are influenced by others to behave in certain ways. No matter how committed we are to changing behaviors, we may need to mentally prepare ourselves to resist when others encourage behavior that defeats the desired goal.[6]

"Psyching yourself up" may enable you to pursue your goals in spite of others' expectations. Almost everyone benefits from some assertiveness training when it comes to changing behaviors. Here are a few suggestions:

Why might people try to block your success in changing your food habits?

- No one's feelings should be hurt if you say, "No, thank you," firmly and repeatedly, when others try to dissuade you from a plan. Rather, ask them—and yourself—why they want you to eat their way. Your needs are as important as someone else's.
- You don't have to eat a lot to accommodate anyone—your mother, business clients, or the chef. For example, going to a party with friends may make you feel like you have to eat a lot to participate, but you don't have to.[11] Also, ordering a lot just because someone else is paying for the meal is a trap.
- When entertaining, serve lighter, more healthful low-fat meals. Try some new recipes. This can be a useful step en route to changing your overall approach to cooking.
- Dealing with parties and social occasions built around food is difficult but possible. You can plan celebrations around a hike or a tennis court, rather than around chips, beer, and television. When you attend parties where food is everywhere, eat a low-fat salad (such as fruit salad) before you go, opt for pretzels or plain crackers,[12] converse far from the food table, and don't wear clothes that make it easy to overeat.
- Learn ways to handle "put-downs"—inadvertent or conscious. An effective response can be to communicate feelings honestly, without hostility. Tell criticizers that they have annoyed or offended you; that you are working to change your habits and would really like understanding and support from them.
- Fostering feelings of self-worth can empower you to change behavior. Ridding yourself of the habit of self-criticism requires strong self-restraint and retraining. Create and memorize lists of strengths, giving credit where it is deserved. Practice forgiving yourself. Instead of saying "I failed," practice saying "it didn't work out." Lower unrealistic expectations. Stop thinking negative thoughts about yourself; purposely switch to positive thoughts.
- If appropriate, persuade the cook to change the family or group diet. The best situation is when everyone wants to eat healthfully. The cook can influence healthful eating a great deal. It takes extra effort to find and develop new recipes and learn shortcuts and substitutions to cut fat and/or kcalories.[5] But the information can be found in cookbooks and newspaper recipes. Also, friends might have healthful recipes and food preparation tips.

DRAFTING A CONTRACT

To motivate himself, Alan drafts his plan into contract form. In the contract, he outlines his behavior changes and his choice of positive reinforcement for carrying out the plan: a weekend off campus with his roommates. He introduces his roommates to the plan, and one of them even wants to join him, knowing that he too will benefit from exercise and weight loss. Alan posts a chart on the refrigerator to record the amount of time spent on the exercise bike each night and his weekly body weight.

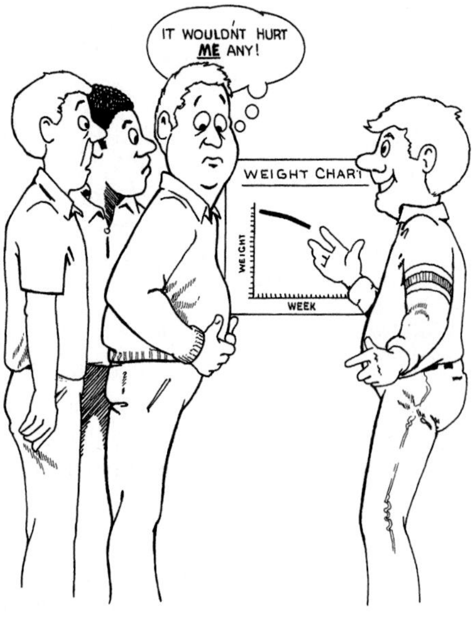

CONCEPT CHECK

To successfully change habits, a person should start by making small changes and providing rewards for sticking with the plan. At first, it is important to reward positive behaviors. Later, the focus switches to positive results, such as a loss of body weight or a lower blood cholesterol level. Before beginning a plan, one should determine the degree of commitment to it. Without commitment, the attempt to change habits will likely end up in failure.

PRACTICING THE PLAN

Once a person sets up a nutrition and health plan, the next step is to implement it. Start with a trial of at least 6 to 8 weeks. Thinking of a lifetime commitment can be overwhelming. Remember that we win the game one point at a time. Aim for a total duration of 6 months of new activities before giving up. It is difficult to overcome the habits of 5, 10, or 20 or more years.[3] More than once we may have to persuade ourselves of the value of continuing the behavior-change program. We may even backslide. That is not totally disastrous if we can learn to manage our thinking. Here are some suggestions to help keep a plan on track:

- Focus on reducing, but not necessarily extinguishing, undesirable behaviors—It is usually unrealistic to say "I will never eat a certain food again." Better to say "I will not eat that *problem* food as regularly as before."
- Monitor progress—Note progress in a diary and reward yourself according to your contract. Make sure to regularly prove to yourself that you are following the plan. While conquering some habits and seeing improvement, you may find yourself quite encouraged, even enthusiastic, about the plan of action. That can be the impetus to move ahead with the program.
- Control environments—In the early phases of behavior change, try to avoid problem situations, such as parties, coffee breaks, and favorite restaurants. Once new habits are firmly established, you can probably more successfully resist the temptations in these environments.
- Plan for failures—When faced with a situation or mood that may disrupt your plan, decide in advance what to do. If all else fails. . .
- Forgive and forget—Cultivate a long-term vision for a nutrition and health plan. Forgive occasional indiscretions. Focus on behaviors that have been established and performed day after day. Assume there will be setbacks, and work your way through them. An occasional lapse does not justify a relapse, and certainly not a collapse.[6]
- Recruit support from others—Have some family members, roommates, or friends witness your contract; educate them about the program and your needs. They can help prevent problem situations that encourage you to deviate from the plan (Figure 16-6).
- Watch for rationalization, the attempt to fool yourself—Distorting information and denying facts to support wishful thinking are ways we rationalize. Trying to justify backsliding by saying "I can't do it," when you have done it for 4 months already, is rationalizing. You won't fool even yourself.
- Be realistic—You cannot control every facet of your overall health. Genetic makeup and environment influence health, including body weight.[9] If you yearn for the body build of a sports hero or a movie star but have inherited other tendencies, reconsider. You may not achieve the shape you want, but can maintain a healthy body weight. Accept and like yourself for who you are.

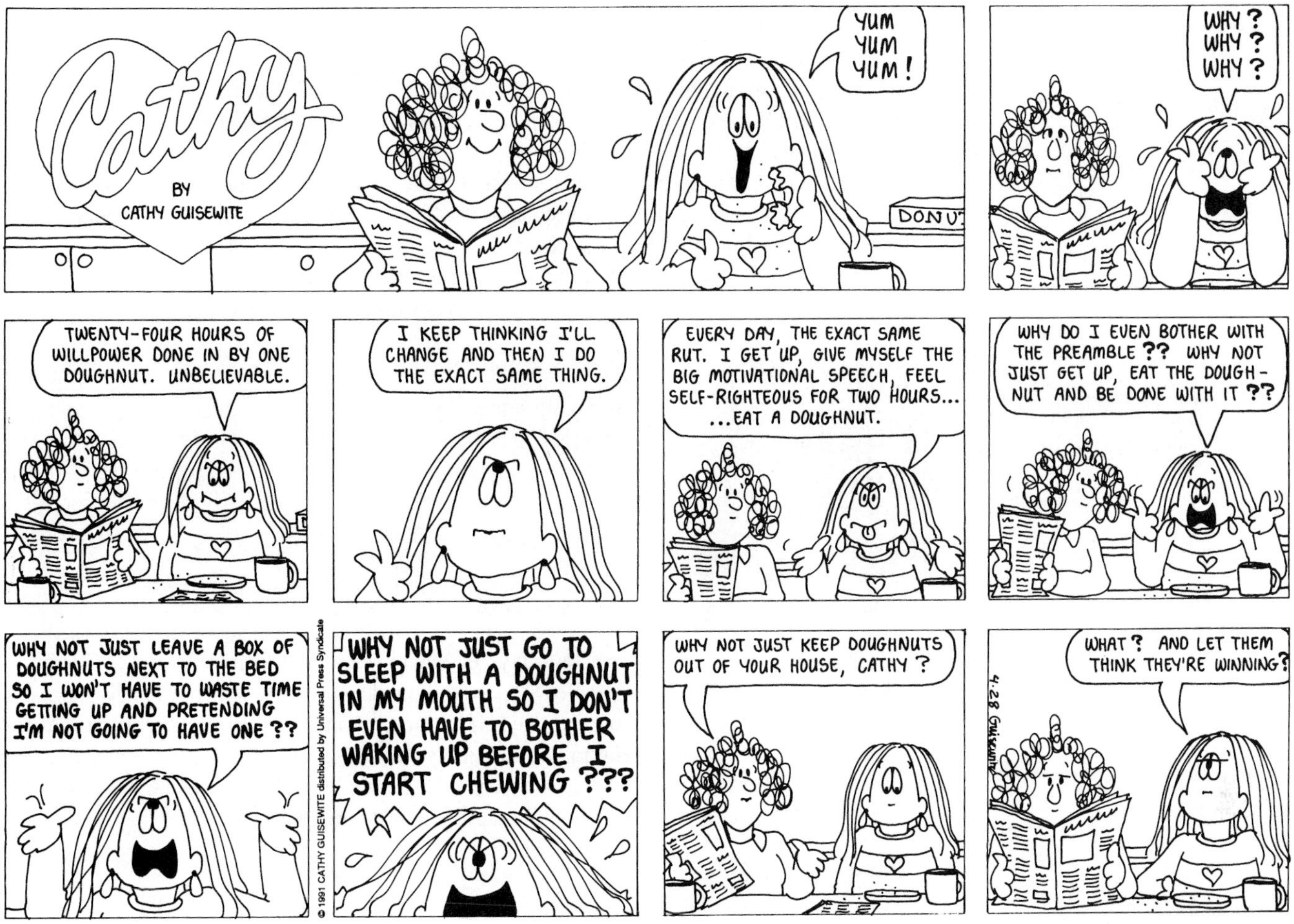

FIGURE 16-6
Cathy.

IMPLEMENTATION

As Alan pursues his new practices, unexpected obstacles arise. Friday night parties are a challenge, with their abundance of "munchies" and alcoholic beverages. Alan does not enjoy waking up earlier in the morning to pack his lunch, and he has to shop at the grocery store every few days for things he needs.

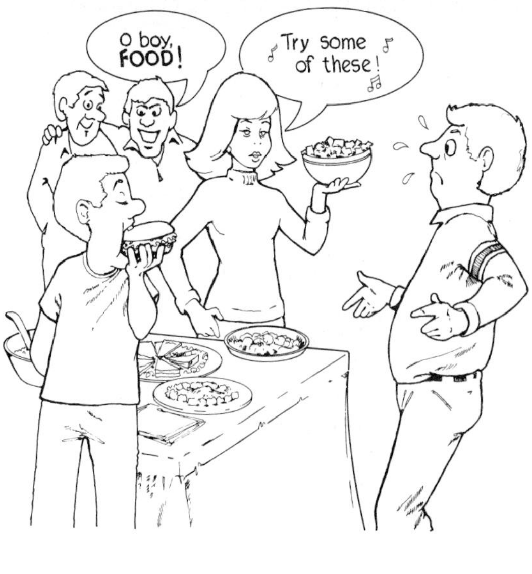

REEVALUATING A PLAN

After practicing a program for several months, a person needs to reevaluate it to clarify any issues. Does the plan of action actually lead to goals set? Are the goals in line with an overall nutrition and health plan? Reevaluation is especially in order if one's general lifestyle changes.

For example, as a person switches from a student lifestyle to that of a full-time worker, the level of physical activity may change drastically. A student may walk to classes and participate on intramural sports teams. But a job may require long hours at a desk. Though lifestyles change, the need for physical activity doesn't. Therefore the person may need to reevaluate plans for physical activity and adapt these to new situations.[2]

another BITE

Your friend with whom you often study makes a habit of eating potato chips during your study sessions. You frequently indulge yourself when offered the tempting snack. To stop this, think about buying an electric air-popper for a quick, almost-no-fat popcorn snack. This is a good alternative.[13]

Changing some habits for a few days or even a few months may be easy. Changing them forever is tough, unless we learn to enjoy the changes and identify the new habits as our own. But a lifetime change can pay off.[6] Many who trim fat from their waistlines report a higher energy level. Having extra energy, feeling good, and looking better provide further motivation to continue to follow the new habits. For many people these assets are much stronger incentives than the less tangible goal of preventing disease.

Preventing Relapse

Relapse often starts with a high-risk situation. Most people at first don't recognize the conditions that promote a relapse. One *slip* sometimes snowballs into a series of lapses that lead to complete reversion into old behaviors. The first lapse could be caused by stress, interpersonal conflicts, or inability to cope adequately with everyday events. These factors signal a high-risk situation. One or two slips are not fatal. Healthful behavior can

REEVALUATION

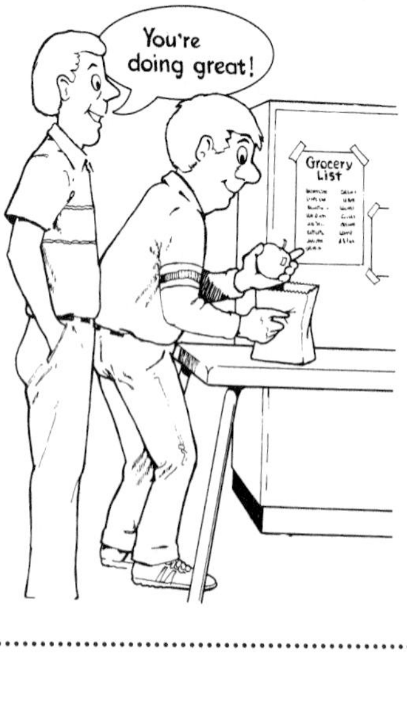
You're doing great!
Grocery List

Alan evaluates the obstacles he has encountered and brainstorms with his roommates to find ways to overcome them. He decides to cut back slightly on kcalories during the day on Fridays so at parties he can allow himself a limited number of snacks. He begins packing his lunch at night so he can grab it on the way to class and writes a complete grocery list that enables him to shop once each week.

Alan begins to notice how much more energy he has and so plans to continue the exercise program. He is even beginning to really enjoy it. He also realizes that he should move beyond his current food list so he doesn't get bored with his cooking and revert to relying on quick-service restaurants. After a month, he has not reached his desirable body weight, but friends are commenting on changes they see in him. This encouragement helps him to remain patient with his progress and focus on the ultimate goal, rather than the time needed to achieve it.

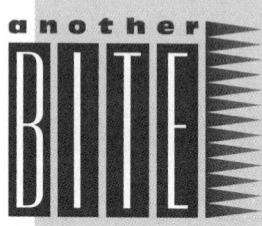

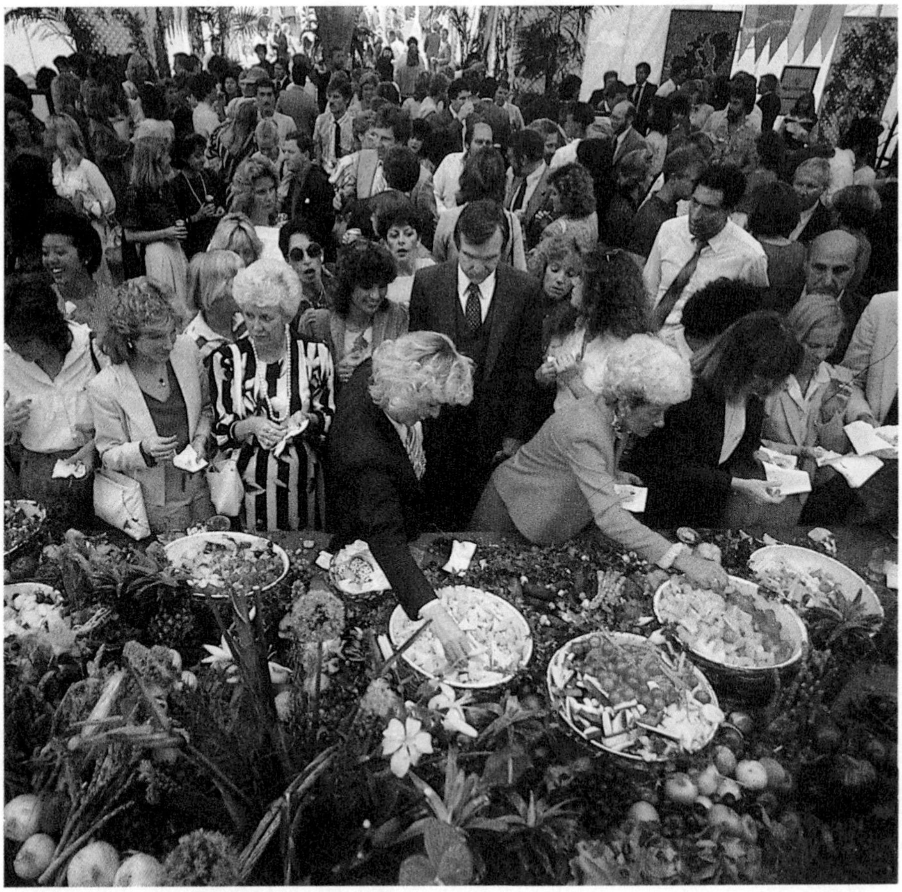

Behavior changes, such as choosing healthful food at a party, are one part of a successful weight-loss plan.

be recovered if the potential for relapse is planned in advance and even expected. Here are some suggestions[6]:

- Identify high-risk situations—As a backslide begins, determine the factors that contributed to the slide and analyze what provoked the high-risk situation. By focusing on the risks inherent in a situation, you can both plan to avoid them in the future and avoid the trap of dwelling on self-defeating guilt feelings.
- Mentally rehearse a response to a backsliding behavior—Imagine backsliding and seeing yourself taking positive action to recover. Rehearse responses to as many potential lapses as you can think of.
- Remember your goals—Keep in mind the reasons for making the commitment to change behaviors and the hard work it took to achieve them.

CONCEPT CHECK

To implement a behavior-change plan, a person can write a contract that identifies behaviors to practice, behavior rewards, and the time frame for accomplishing the plan. While trying to change behaviors, it is important to control the environment (to discourage deviation from the plan) and to get support from others. A plan for problems is needed—problems should not be an excuse for a relapse. The person needs to invoke a strategy that will allow one to move ahead despite a few failures along the way. Problems may require reconsidering the action plan—this is to be expected.

NUTRITION insight

BREAKING BEHAVIOR CHAINS

James Ferguson, M.D.

We are creatures of habit. All of our behaviors are linked, one to the next. Much like the chain that holds a boat to its anchor, our **behavior chains** can anchor us to relatively fixed conditions, like obesity. The behavior chain is a series of interconnected habitual behaviors.

The following is a good example of a behavior chain: Consider the businesswoman who comes home after a hard day at work. She puts down her briefcase, picks up the paper, turns on the television, and sits down. Soon she gets up and looks in the refrigerator, grabs a snack, again sits in front of the television, and, afterward, eats a meal. After dinner, she sits down to watch television, gets bored, walks into the kitchen, browses through the refrigerator, eats a piece of cheesecake, and wanders back to the television. Feeling guilty about the snack, she assuages her guilt with another piece of cheesecake. The initial event, such as stress or boredom, may seem innocuous, but the ending is typically the same—extra kcalories.

How many eating situations in your life can you describe in terms of behavior chains? A study of the series of linked events suggests a strategy for eliminating extra habitual eating or snacking. Break the chain! It's hard to just say no. The easy way to break the chain is to substitute an alternate activity. The earlier the chain is broken, the better and the easier it is to cut kcalories. Once the snack touches your taste buds, it's too late. When that cheesecake is only a gleam in your eye or, even better, a "pregleam," the awareness that you are headed for something to eat makes it easier to break the chain.

The way to cast off your chains is to identify them, pinpoint the weak links, break them, and substitute another behavior. Using alternate activities sounds easy, but it's hard to do on the spur of the moment. Figure 16-7 shows you how to use a diagram to identify the links in your behavior chains. It also gives you the opportunity to list substitute activities that can be used to break the links in the chain.

If your behavior chain is broken at any point, it will probably not continue. (The businesswoman's final behaviors—eating, feeling guilty, eating—probably won't occur.) The earlier in the chain you substitute a nonfood link, the easier it is to intervene.

Four types of behaviors can be substituted in an ongoing behavior chain:

1. Fun activities (grabbing your mate, taking a walk, reading a book)
2. Necessary activities (cleaning a room, balancing your checkbook)
3. Incompatible activities (taking a shower)
4. Urge-delaying activities (setting a kitchen timer for 20 minutes before allowing yourself to eat)

Using activities to interrupt behavior patterns that lead to inappropriate eating can be a powerful means of changing eating habits. This technique can also be useful when you are eating in response to environmental as well as to internal cues for eating, such as a television advertisement for food or a hunger pang that you feel at an odd time after a meal or before going to bed. If it's pushing you to eat, substitute!

Dr. Ferguson is a nationally prominent psychiatrist who specializes in weight control. He is the author of many books, including *Habits, Not Diets*.

ALTERNATE ACTIVITY SHEET:

SUBSTITUTE ACTIVITIES

Pleasant activities
1. Singing/washing hair
2. Playing piano/biking
3. Sewing/calling "shut-ins"

Necessary activities
1. Dusting
2. Vacuuming
3. Straightening house

Situations when used
1. Wanted ice cream—delayed with bath
2. Wanted wheat thins—cleaned up yard
3. Wanted snack—went for walk
4. Wanted cookies—did dishes first
5. Saw leftovers—went for bike ride
6. Tempted by cookies—set timer
7. Wanted snack—played piano

BEHAVIOR CHAIN

Identify the links in your eating response chain on the following diagram. Draw a line through the chain where it was interrupted. Add the link you substituted and the new chain of behaviors this substitution started.

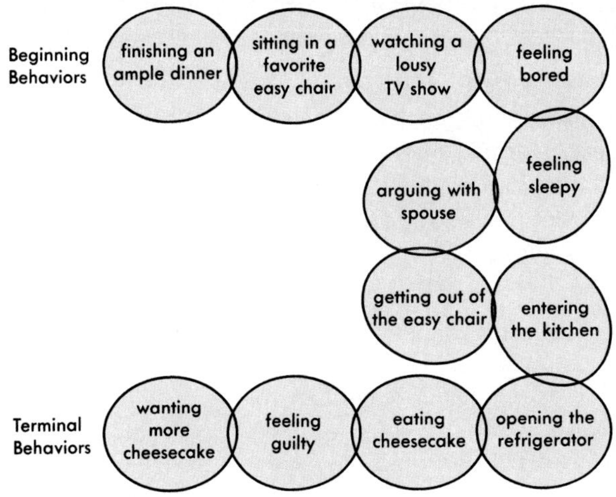

ALTERNATE ACTIVITY SHEET:

SUBSTITUTE ACTIVITIES

Pleasant activities
1. ______
2. ______
3. ______

Necessary activities
1. ______
2. ______
3. ______

Situations when used
1. ______
2. ______
3. ______
4. ______
5. ______
6. ______
7. ______

BEHAVIOR CHAIN

Identify the links in your eating response chain on the following diagram. Draw a line through the chain where it was interrupted. Add the link you substituted and the new chain of behaviors this substitution started.

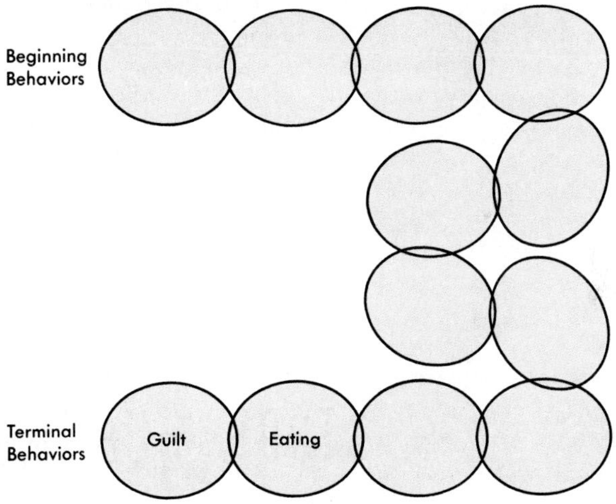

FIGURE 16-7

Identifying behavior chains. This is a good tool for understanding more about your habits and pinpointing ways to change unwanted habits.

SUMMARY

- Behavior change occurs in steps. First, a person becomes aware of a problem. Then the person openly receives new information about it, evolving a receptive framework for learning. That person then undertakes a trial period for the change, during which time positive reinforcement is critical. If an initial trial is successful, the person may permanently adopt new behaviors.
- Before charting a behavior-change plan, it is important to discover strengths and weaknesses regarding the intended behavior. A food diary kept for at least a week may show eating patterns and other behaviors that either contribute to or discourage new behaviors. The diary can reveal areas of one's outside environment that need to be altered to reduce temptation.
- When setting goals for a behavior plan, a key is to plan small steps that lead to the intended result and build in rewards to capitalize on achievements and maintain momentum.
- After you have set a plan of action, drawing up a contract that lists intended tasks, the incentive rewards, and the time frame for the behavior change is helpful. The contract should at first reward positive behaviors and later reward ultimate objectives.
- Before embarking on the behavior-change program, a person needs to evaluate personal commitment. A plan, no matter how skillfully developed, is not likely to succeed unless a person has a strong commitment to achieving the goals.
- When implementing a plan, the person needs to monitor progress and provide rewards. Controlling one's environment can reduce temptations to deviate from the plan. For example, deciding in advance to choose low-fat foods at a quick-service restaurant is helpful. The person should expect small failures and not consider them an excuse to abandon change. A forgive-and-forget attitude can prevent collapse of the whole strategy.
- It is necessary to plan for the possibility of relapse. Most people revert to old behaviors during periods of stress or interpersonal conflict. Identifying problem behavior chains and ways to substitute better links is recommended. Strategies to recover from relapse include identifying high-risk situations and mentally rehearsing a response.

STUDY QUESTIONS

1. Why does measuring commitment play a key part in any plan to change behavior?
2. What three parts should a behavior contract contain?
3. Describe one behavior strategy to use to avoid overeating at a party.
4. What is a behavior chain? How can this concept be used to aid behavior change?
5. Discuss two strategies for avoiding a relapse into old habits.

References

1. Atkinson RL: Treatment of obesity, *Nutrition Reviews* 50:338, 1992.
2. Brownell KD: *The LEARN program for weight control,* Philadelphia, 1989, KD Brownell.
3. Ferguson J: *Habits, not diets: the secret to lifetime weight control,* Palo Alto, Calif, 1988, Bull Publishing.
4. Ferguson KJ and others: Characteristics of successful dieters as measured by guided interview responses and restraint scale scores, *Journal of the American Dietetic Association* 92:1119, 1992.
5. Frankle RT, Yang M: *Obesity and weight control,* Rockville, Md, 1988, Aspen Publishers.
6. Insel PM, Roth WT: *Core concepts in health,* ed 6, Mountain View, Calif, 1994, Mayfield Publishing.
7. Kabatznick R: Towards a new psychology of dieting, *Nutrition Update* 2(3), Fall 1992.
8. Nash JD: *Maximize your body potential,* Palo Alto, Calif, 1986, Bull Publishing.
9. National Institutes of Health: Methods of voluntary weight loss and control, *Nutrition Today,* p. 27, July/August 1992.
10. Roberts C: Fast food fare, *New England Journal of Medicine,* 321:752, 1989.
11. Sweet CA: Rethinking eating out, *FDA Consumer,* p. 6, November 1989.
12. Warshaw HS: America eats out: nutrition in the chain and family restaurant industry, *Journal of the American Dietetic Association,* 93:17, 1993.
13. Weinstock CP: The grazing of America: a guide to healthy snacking, *FDA Consumer,* p. 8, March 1989.

RATE

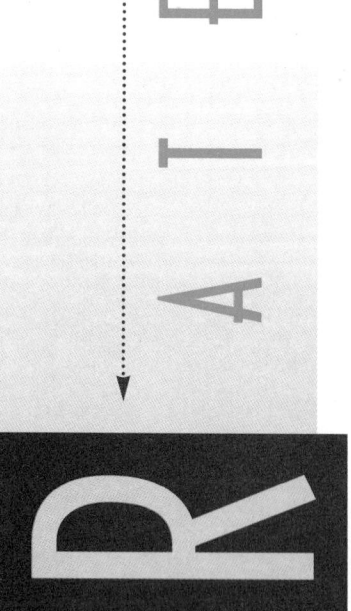

TAKING CHARGE OF FOOD PURCHASES

You may wonder what foods regularly end up on the grocery list of a nutrition professor and his family (which includes two elementary school children). Compare your latest list to Dr. Wardlaw's list. Note similarities and differences. Then customize the list below to your tastes. This is not the only list possible, but rather one that meets the nutrient needs and expectations of one family.

Vegetables

Potatoes
Carrots/celery
Fresh spinach
Green peppers
Broccoli/cauliflower
Lettuce: romaine
Asparagus
Mushrooms/zucchini
Tomatoes/green beans
Onions/garlic (lots)
Frozen: corn/peas
Other: ______

Dry goods

Flour: whole wheat/enriched white
Rice: white
Pasta
Sugar: white/brown
Cornmeal
Pancake mix
Yeast
Other: ______

Bread and crackers

Bread: whole wheat/buns/French
Crackers: whole wheat/saltine
Bagels/English muffins
Bran muffins
Tortillas: corn/flour
Other: ______

Fruit

Apples/bananas/pears
Oranges/grapes
Grapefruit/melon
Peaches/plums
Pineapple/cherries
Strawberries
Other: ______

Canned goods

Tomatoes
Tomato sauce
Tuna
Beans: kidney/pinto (refried)/baked
Soups: chicken noodle/minestrone
Other: ______

Breakfast cereal

Oatmeal/Oat Squares/Raisin Bran/Oatmeal Crisp/Wheaties
Other: ______

Dairy and spreads

1% milk
Nonfat yogurt
Cheese: cheddar/mozzarella/provolone
Mayonnaise
Tub margarine
Other: ______

Oil, condiments and spices

Oil: canola/corn/olive
Dry salad dressing mixes
Soy sauce/salsa/barbeque sauce
Vinegar/mustard/ketchup/steak sauce
Oregano/basil/curry
Peanut butter/jam
Pickle relish
Pancake syrup
Other: ______

Drinks

Frozen orange juice (calcium fortified)/juice boxes
Apple cider
Coffee: regular/decaf
Tea: regular/herbal
Sugar-free hot chocolate mix
Other: ______

Meat, seafood, and poultry

Chicken/ground round
Sliced meat: turkey/ham/salami/pepperoni
Low-fat hot dogs
Steak
Salmon/halibut/orange roughy
Low-fat bratwurst
Pork loin
Eggs
Other: ______

Desserts

Frozen yogurt
Cookies: chocolate chip/oatmeal/peanut butter
Other: ______

Snacks

Peanuts in the shell/raisins
Tortilla chips
Microwave popcorn
Low-fat granola bars
Diet soft drinks
Other: ______

your plate

Nutrition ISSUE

EATING ON THE RUN

Choosing healthful foods is not so difficult in many of today's quick-service restaurants. Some restaurants have evolved beyond hamburgers, French fries, and milk shakes to include a variety of vegetables, salad bars, and ethnic foods.[11] In addition, some restaurants are trying to cater to their more health-conscious clientele. If we buy more healthful foods, these restaurants will continue to meet this market demand.[13] Still, between 40% and 50% of the energy in most quick-service choices come from fat (Table 16-2). Thus many of these meal selections are high-kcalorie options when compared with the amount of other nutrients provided.

People who eat regularly at quick-service restaurants should choose meals carefully to meet their nutrient needs without exceeding their energy needs. Because these food outlets serve a need in our fast-paced society, they are probably a permanent part of the lifestyle of many Americans.[10] What follows is a list of suggestions for a good nutritional path among food choices in quick-service restaurants.

Breakfast

Before entering a local quick-service restaurant for breakfast, decide whether you can fix this meal at home. Can breakfast be prepared the night before so that it is ready for the next morning? The effort might be as simple as putting bread next to the toaster or cereal on the counter with a bowl. Breakfast can be a relaxing time, and many of us need time away from the fast pace of daily life. If you have abandoned breakfast at home, think again. Breakfast at home is usually faster than a visit to a quick-service restaurant.

If you still prefer breakfast out, we suggest a plain scrambled egg, or an English muffin with not more than 1 teaspoon of margarine. Add orange juice for a tasty breakfast. Substitute pancakes without the butter and minimal syrup instead of the egg and English muffin. Either way, you consume a lot less fat and kcalories than if you choose the typical meat, egg, and cheese-laden muffin or croissant. Be especially wary of croissants: they are loaded with fat. If you still want meat, consider Canadian bacon, a leaner breakfast meat.

Lunch and Dinner

A good choice for lunch or dinner is a sandwich made of whole-wheat bread and some lean meat or tuna. Pizza is a good idea once or twice a week. If ordered with vegetable toppings—mushrooms, green peppers, and onions—pizza provides a very nutritious lunch for a moderate amount of kcalories. The cheese used primarily is a low-fat variety. The next best choice is probably a hamburger, but not the king-size model. Consider buying the basic hamburger. Ideally, choose a restaurant that provides a plain hamburger on a bun and then allows you to create a masterpiece. At that point, emphasize lettuce, tomatoes, mustard, and a little ketchup. Be especially wary of mayonnaise, sauces, melted cheese, fried onions, or other sources of added fat. Chili is another alternative. It is lower in fat than a king-size hamburger, and the beans supply additional dietary fiber. Finally, soft burritos with beans or chicken are often low in fat. Cheese should be ordered on the side, if at all.

TABLE 16-2

Proceed with Caution. Many Food Choices in Quick-Service Restaurants Are High in Fat.*

Food (kcals)	% Fat
Arby's	
Deluxe roast beef sandwich (486)	42
French fries (211)	34
Ham 'n' cheese sandwich (353)	33
Broccoli and cheddar potato (541)	37
Chocolate milk shake (384)	26
Burger King	
Whopper with cheese (723)	60
Onion rings (274)	53
Apple pie (305)	35
Fish sandwich (488)	50
Chicken sandwich (688)	52
Scrambled egg platter (468)	58
KFC	
Drumstick (147)	55
Center breast (257)	49
Buttermilk biscuit (269)	47
Potato salad (141)	57
Cole slaw (103)	52
McDonald's	
Chicken McNuggets (323)	59
Egg McMuffin (340)	42
Chocolate chip cookies (342)	42
Taco Bell	
Beef burrito (466)	41
Taco (186)	39
Tostada (179)	40
Pizza Hut	
Cheese pizza (2 slices) (492)	33
Medium pan pizza—pepperoni (2 slices) (540)	37

**Hamburgers, French fries, milk shakes, etc. from quick-service outlets tend to have similar nutrient compositions. See Appendix A to evaluate your typical choices.*

Bite-size pieces should be made from chicken breast only, and not from processed chicken that can include ground chicken skin. Ask the restaurant manager from which parts of the chicken the entree is made. Let him or her know your nutrition and health interests. Broiled or baked chicken is the most healthful. If the chicken is fried, remove the coating. The same applies to fish: remove the coating. Actually, chicken and fish start out as low-fat protein sources, but by the time they are deep-fat fried, they resemble the protein:fat ratio of a typical hamburger sandwich. You do not save that many kcalories.

For side dishes, consider portion sizes. Order a small rather than a large portion of French fries. Order a baked potato, and to spice it up, put on plenty of chives but not more than a pat of margarine. Stay away from sour cream, cheese, and other toppings—you can save 300 kcalories.

At the salad bar, watch the addition of cheese, bacon bits, and dressing. Mayonnaise-based salads, such as macaroni and potato salad, are relatively high in kcalories. To minimize saturated fat intake, try the oil and vinegar and French dressings, rather than the creamy types such as bleu cheese dressing. Some people even find fresh-squeezed lemon juice is a satisfying alternative to dressing. Some restaurants do supply low-kcalorie dressings. Try these, or otherwise, add as little regular dressing as possible. You can always take your own with you too. Salad bars also offer fresh fruits and vegetables, which can contribute to a healthful meal.

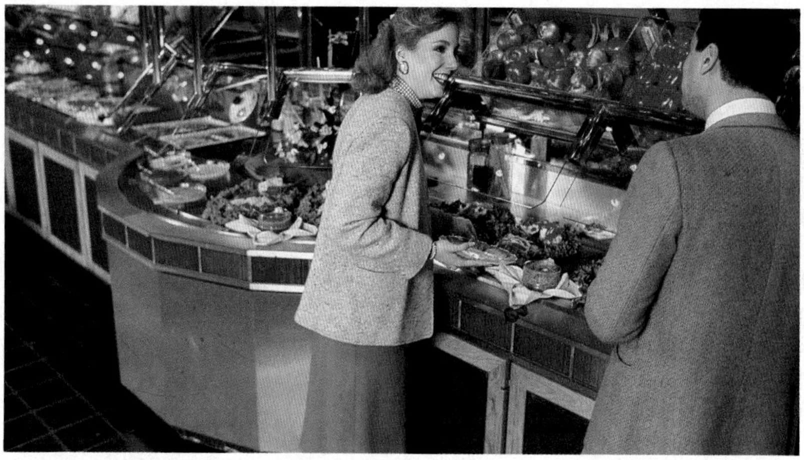

Salad bars contain both low-fat and high-fat choices—proceed with caution.

For beverages, consider low-fat (nonfat) milk, water, diet soft drinks, or ice tea. A typical milk shake contains about 350 to 400 kcalories. A cup of 2% milk has only 120 kcalories.

In all, focus on fat.[10] Its 9 kcalories per gram add up fast. But by all means, enjoy eating out. Look at the total diet, not at whether one food or another is going to ruin your health. We should think of eating as a pleasurable experience. There are some hurdles to clear, but once you learn the rules for eating on the run, you can find healthful, low-kcalorie meals even at quick-service restaurants.

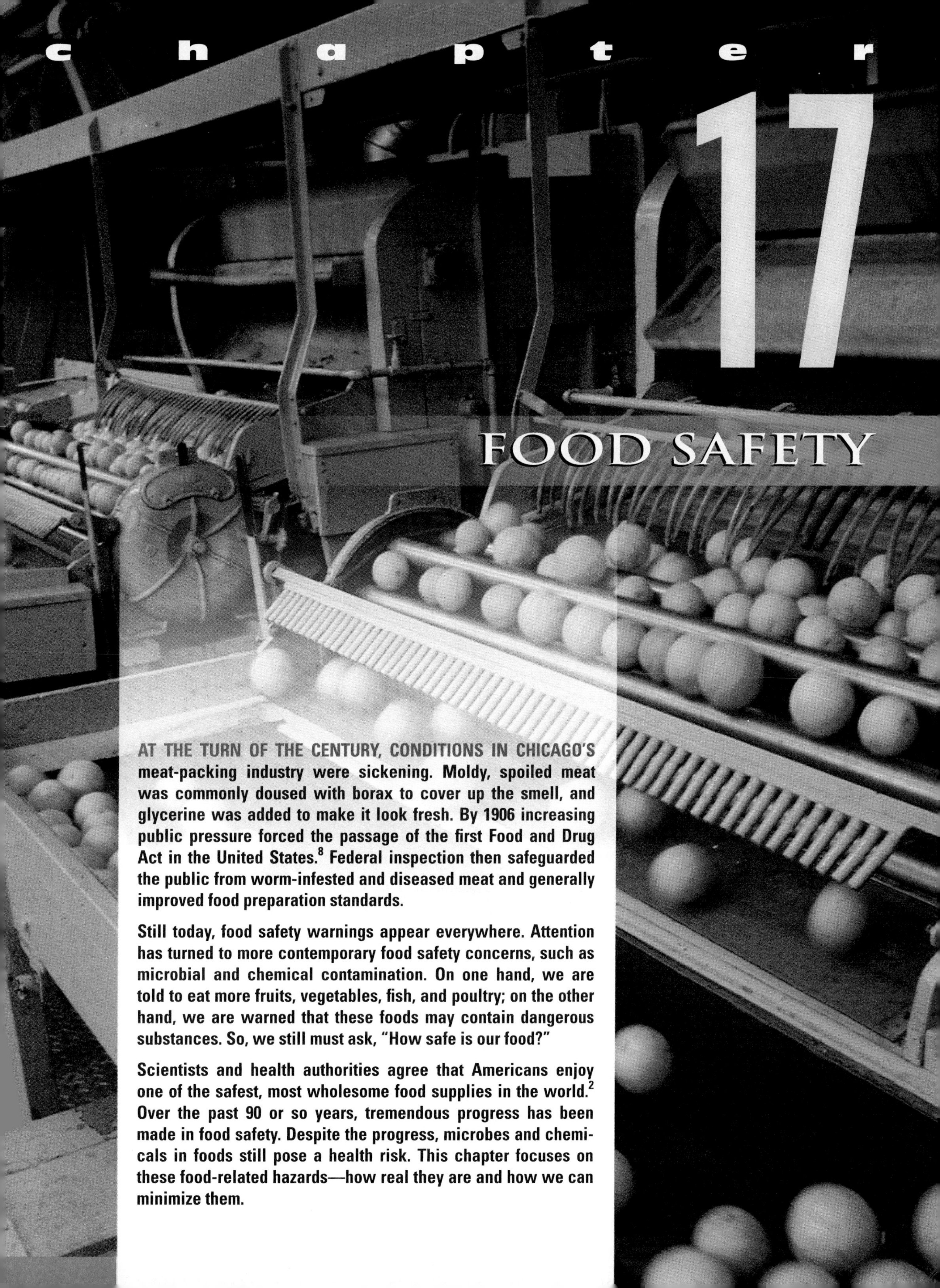

chapter 17

FOOD SAFETY

AT THE TURN OF THE CENTURY, CONDITIONS IN CHICAGO'S meat-packing industry were sickening. Moldy, spoiled meat was commonly doused with borax to cover up the smell, and glycerine was added to make it look fresh. By 1906 increasing public pressure forced the passage of the first Food and Drug Act in the United States.[8] Federal inspection then safeguarded the public from worm-infested and diseased meat and generally improved food preparation standards.

Still today, food safety warnings appear everywhere. Attention has turned to more contemporary food safety concerns, such as microbial and chemical contamination. On one hand, we are told to eat more fruits, vegetables, fish, and poultry; on the other hand, we are warned that these foods may contain dangerous substances. So, we still must ask, "How safe is our food?"

Scientists and health authorities agree that Americans enjoy one of the safest, most wholesome food supplies in the world.[2] Over the past 90 or so years, tremendous progress has been made in food safety. Despite the progress, microbes and chemicals in foods still pose a health risk. This chapter focuses on these food-related hazards—how real they are and how we can minimize them.

ASSESS YOURSELF

TEST YOUR KNOWLEDGE

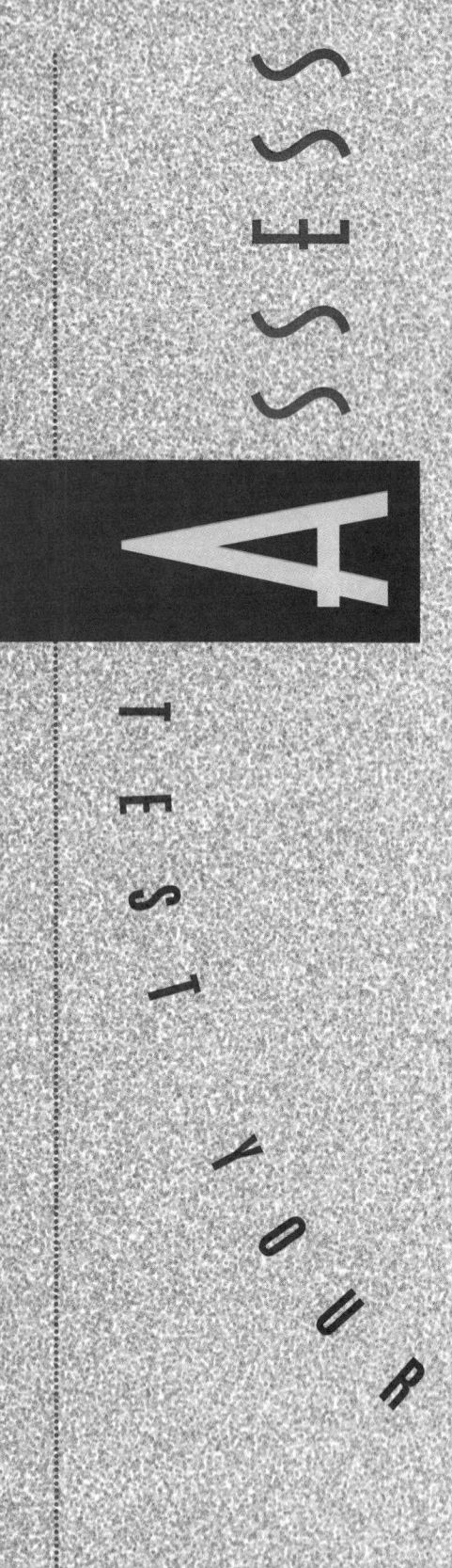

TEST YOUR FOOD SAFETY KNOWLEDGE

Take this quiz to see how aware you are about the safety of some basic foods. Place a check in the appropriate column to indicate whether you think the item is safe or risky to eat.

	Safe	Risky
1. Hot dogs that have been stored unopened in the refrigerator for over 7 days?		
2. A bruised piece of fruit?		
3. Frozen ham that was thawed on the counter?		
4. An opened jar of mayonnaise that has been in the refrigerator for 6 months?		
5. A foil-covered baked potato left out on the counter since the night before?		
6. Meat loaf that's pink in the middle after cooking?		
7. Raw ground beef that turns brown after 1 to 2 days of refrigeration?		
8. An uncooked potato with a greenish cast, eaten with the peel left on?		
9. Lettuce moistened by poultry drippings in a grocery bag?		
10. Steak that was thawed in the refrigerator and then refrozen with some ice crystals still present?		
11. Cooked shrimp that was never deveined?		
12. Mustard or ketchup with a black, crusty ring around the rim of the jar?		
13. Moldy or shriveled peanuts?		

Now that you've completed this assessment, check your answers below.

SAFE: 1, 2, 4, 7, 10, 11, 12.
RISKY: 3, 5, 6, 8, 9, 13.

Explanations of the safety or risk of these foods can be found in this chapter. It may have been hard for you to answer these questions. Many people don't know much about proper food preservation, handling, and cooking to avoid significant illness.

From *Tufts University Diet and Nutrition Letter* 3(11):7, 1986.

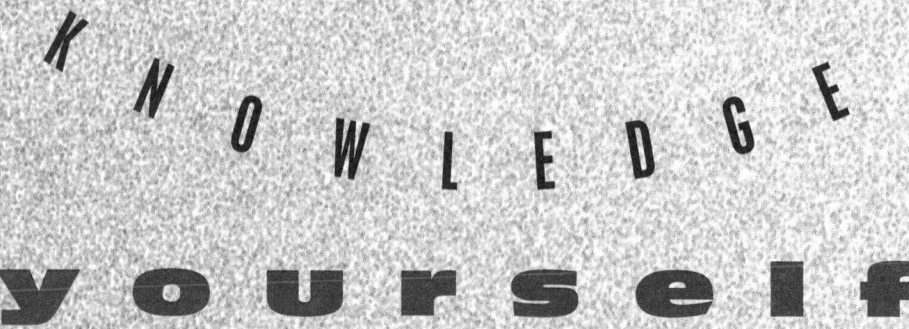

SETTING THE STAGE

During the early stages of urbanization in the United States, contaminated water and food—notably, milk—were responsible for many large outbreaks of typhoid fever, septic sore throat, scarlet fever, diphtheria, and other devastating human diseases. These spectacular experiences led to the development of processes for purifying water, treating sewage, and pasteurizing milk. Since that time, safe water and milk are universally available with only rare problems from either. The greatest health risk from food is contamination from ***bacteria*** and, to a lesser extent, from various forms of ***fungi*** and ***viruses.*** These microbes can all cause food-borne illness. But even though microbial contamination is the cause of most incidents of food-borne illness,[11] Americans seem more concerned about health risks from chemicals in foods. Of consumers surveyed in a recent Gallup poll, 75% said that pesticide contamination was a major concern to them. In the long run, there is some merit to this concern. But on a day-to-day basis, according to the Centers for Disease Control in Atlanta, Georgia, only 2% of all cases of food-borne illness in the United States is caused by food additives.

Microbial contamination of food is by far the more important issue for our day-to-day health. We will discuss it first. Then we will cover the use and safety of food additives.

Bacteria ■
A group of single-cell microorganisms, some of which produce poisonous substances called toxins that lead to ill health in humans. They contain only one chromosome and lack many organelles found in human cells. Bacteria produce enzymes that can digest substances around them. Some can live without oxygen and survive harsh conditions by means of spore formation.

Fungi ■
Simple parasitic life forms including molds, mildews, yeasts, and mushrooms. They live on dead or decaying organic matter. Fungi can grow as single cells, like yeast, or as multicellular colonies, as seen with molds.

Virus ■
The smallest known type of infectious agent, many of which cause disease in humans. They do not metabolize, grow, or move by themselves. They reproduce by the aid of a living cellular host. Viruses are essentially a piece of genetic material surrounded by a coat of protein.

FOOD-BORNE ILLNESS

About one third to one half of all cases of diarrhea in the United States, upward of 20 million each year, are induced by food-borne organisms.[11] It is estimated that diarrhea caused by these agents hits about 1 of every 10 to 35 Americans each year at a cost to the economy of $1 billion to $10 billion. For most of us, the typical result—a brief yet distressing episode of diarrhea, such as traveler's diarrhea—presents no real health risk. But for many, it can be more serious. Some people—especially children; elderly people; and those with alcoholism or with underlying health problems, such as cancer, a need to take an immunosuppressant agent, or acquired immunodeficiency syndrome (AIDS)—can suffer greatly from illnesses caused by food-borne microbes. Some bouts of this type of illness are lengthy and lead to food allergies, seizures, blood poisoning (from toxins or microbes in the bloodstream), or other illnesses. Annually about 9000 deaths occur from food-borne illness.

Because 30% of all such illness results from unsafe handling of food at home,[11] we each bear some responsibility for preventing food-borne illness. Usually you can't tell by taste, smell, or sight that a particular food contains harmful microbes. So you might not even be aware that food caused your distress. But, in fact, the last case of stomach or intestinal "flu" you had may have been caused by something you ate. The symptoms of both disorders are often the same: diarrhea, vomiting, fever, and weakness.

Why Is Food-Borne Illness So Common?

The risk of contracting food-borne illness is high, because—in addition to problems from consumers' mishandling food—the food industry tries to increase the shelf life of products. A longer shelf life at room temperature allows more time for bacteria in foods to multiply. Some bacteria grow even at refrigeration temperatures. Partially cooked—and some fully cooked—products pose a special risk, because refrigerated storage may only slow—not prevent—bacterial growth. FDA is especially concerned about this problem.[11]

The risk of illness from food-borne microbes increases as more centralized kitchens outside the home prepare our foods.[13] Supermarkets especially have become major food processors over the past decade and now offer a variety of prepared foods from specialty meat shops, salad bars, and bakeries. With so many two-income families, people are looking for convenient, easy-to-prepare nutritious foods. Supermarkets offer entrees that can be served immediately or reheated. The foods are usually prepared in central kitchens or processing plants and shipped to individual stores. If a food product is contaminated in the central kitchen or processing plant, patrons of stores over a wide area can suffer food-borne illness.

TABLE 17-1

Some Organisms That Cause Food-Borne Illness: Their Source, Symptoms, and Prevention

Organism	Source of Illness	Symptoms	Prevention Methods
Bacteria			
Staphylococcus aureus	Lives in nasal passages and in cuts on skin. Toxin is produced when food contaminated by bacteria is left for extended time at room temperature. Meats; poultry; egg products; tuna, potato, and macaroni salads; and cream-filled pastries are likely targets.	Onset: 2-6 hours after eating Diarrhea, vomiting, nausea, and abdominal cramps Mimics flu Lasts 24-48 hours Rarely fatal	• Handle foods in a sanitary manner. • Refrigerate foods promptly and properly. • Keep cuts on skin covered.
Salmonella	Found in raw meats, poultry, eggs, fish, milk, and products made with these items. Multiplies rapidly at room temperature. The bacteria themselves are toxic.	Onset: 5-72 hours after eating Nausea, fever, headache, abdominal cramps, diarrhea, and vomiting Can be fatal in infants, the elderly, and sick persons	• Handle foods in a sanitary manner. • Thoroughly cook foods. • Refrigerate foods promptly and properly. • Watch cross-contamination.
Clostridium perfringens	Widespread in environment. Generally found in meat and poultry dishes. Multiplies rapidly when foods are left for extended time at room temperature. The bacteria themselves are toxic.	Onset: 8-24 hours after eating (usually 12 hours) Abdominal pain and diarrhea Symptoms last a day or less, usually mild Can be more serious in older or already ill people	• Practice sanitary handling of foods, especially meat and meat dishes, gravies, and leftovers. • Thoroughly cook and reheat foods. • Refrigerate promptly and properly.
Clostridium botulinum	Widespread in the environment. However, bacteria produce toxin only in low-acid, anaerobic (oxygen-free) environments, such as in cans of green beans, mushrooms, spinach, olives, and beef. Honey may carry spores.	Onset: 12-36 hours after eating Double vision, inability to swallow, speech difficulty, and progressive paralysis of the respiratory system OBTAIN MEDICAL HELP IMMEDIATELY. BOTULISM CAN BE FATAL.	• Use proper methods for canning low-acid foods. • Avoid commercial cans of low-acid foods that have leaky seals or are bent, bulging, or broken. • Toxin can be destroyed after can or jar is opened by boiling contents hard for 20 minutes, but discard if suspect toxin is present because of off-odors.
Campylobacter jejuni	Found on poultry and beef and can contaminate meat and milk. Chief food sources are raw poultry and meat and unpasteurized milk.	Onset: 3-5 days after eating or longer Diarrhea, abdominal cramping, fever, and sometimes bloody stools Lasts 2-7 days.	• Thoroughly cook foods. • Handle foods in a sanitary manner. • Avoid unpasteurized milk.
Listeria monocytogenes	Found in soft cheeses and unpasteurized milk. Resists acid, heat, salt, and nitrate well.	Onset: 4-21 days Fever, headache, vomiting, and sometimes even more severe symptoms May be fatal Persons at increased risk: pregnant women, elderly persons, and those with immunosuppressive conditions	• Thoroughly cook foods. • Handle foods in a sanitary manner. • Avoid unpasteurized milk.
Yersinia enterocolitica	Common in nature; carried in food and water. They multiply rapidly at both room and refrigerator temperatures. Generally found in raw vegetables, meats, water, and unpasteurized milk.	Onset: 2-3 days after eating Fever, headache, nausea, diarrhea, and general malaise Mimics flu and appendicitis An important cause of intestinal distress in children	• Thoroughly cook foods. • Sanitize cutting instruments and cutting boards before preparing foods that are eaten raw. • Avoid unpasteurized milk and unchlorinated water.

TABLE 17-1 CONT'D

Some Organisms That Cause Food-Borne Illness: Their Source, Symptoms, and Prevention

Organism	Source of Illness	Symptoms	Prevention Methods
Bacteria			
Escherichia coli (some forms)	Found in raw ground beef, raw milk, and some types of soft cheeses.	Onset: 1-2 days after eating Diarrhea, abdominal cramps May cause kidney damage and death	• Avoid unpasteurized milk. • Thoroughly cook meat.
Viruses			
Hepatitis A virus	Chief food sources: shellfish harvested from contaminated areas and foods that are handled a lot during preparation and then eaten raw (such as vegetables).	Onset: 30 days Jaundice and fatigue May cause liver damage and death	• Handle foods in a sanitary manner. • Use treated drinking water. • Adequately cook foods.
Parasites			
Trichinella spiralis	Found in pork and wild game.	Onset: weeks-months Muscle weakness, fluid retention in face, fever, and flulike symptoms	• Thoroughly cook pork and wild game.
Anisakis	Found in raw fish.	Onset: 12 hours Stomach infection and severe stomach pain	• Thoroughly cook fish.
Tapeworms	Found in raw beef, pork, and fish.	Abdominal discomfort and diarrhea.	• Thoroughly cook all animal products.
Mycotoxins			
A group of toxic compounds produced by molds, such as aflatoxin	Produced in foods that are relatively high in moisture. Chief food sources: beans and grains that have been stored in a moist place.	May cause liver and/or kidney disease	• Check foods for visible mold and discard those that are contaminated. • Properly store susceptible foods.

A malfunction in a dairy plant in 1985 resulted in 16,284 confirmed cases of *Salmonella* bacteria infections and at least 2 deaths from contaminated milk. In 1987, lettuce shredded in a Texas plant and then placed in large plastic bags was the cause of the largest *Shigella* bacteria outbreak ever reported in the United States. At least 347 people were reported ill. The nutrients released when the lettuce was shredded, coupled with the moist environment provided by the plastic bags, allowed growth and reproduction of the organism. In 1993 at least 1 person died and 400 became ill in Washington State after eating at a specific chain of quick-service restaurants. The source of the problem was undercooked hamburger contaminated with the bacterium *Escherichia coli.* All the hamburger came from a central plant in California. All meat should be cooked thoroughly to limit risk from this and other causes of food-borne illness.

Still another cause of increased food-borne illness in America is greater consumption of ready-to-eat foods imported from foreign countries. In the past, food imports were mostly raw products processed here under strict sanitation standards. Now, however, we import more processed foods—such as cheese from France and seafood from Asia—some of which are contaminated.

Finally, more cases of food-borne disease are reported now because we are more aware of the role of various players in the process. Every decade the list of microorganisms suspected of causing food-borne illness expands (Table 17-1).[17] And we now know

Irradiation A process whereby radiation energy is applied to foods, creating compounds (ions) within the food that destroy cell membranes, break down DNA, link proteins together, limit enzyme activity, and alter a variety of other proteins and cell functions that can lead to food spoilage. This process does not make the food radioactive.

Food-borne Infection Food-borne illness that is caused directly by bacteria or other microbes in food.

food, besides serving as a good growth medium for some microorganisms, simply transmits many others as well.

Food Preservation—Past, Present, and Future

For centuries, salt, sugar, smoke, fermentation, and drying have been used to preserve food. Ancient Romans used sulfites to disinfect wine containers and preserve wine. In the age of exploration, European adventurers traveling to the New World preserved their meat by salting it. Most preserving methods work on the principle of decreasing free water—that is, the amount of water not bound to other components in the food. Salts and sugar decrease free water by binding to it. The process of drying drives off free water. Bacteria need abundant stores of water to grow; yeasts and molds can grow with less water, but some is still necessary.

Decreasing the water content of some rather high-moisture foods, however, causes them to lose essential characteristics. To preserve such foods—cucumber pickles, sauerkraut, milk (yogurt), and wine—fermentation has been a traditional alternative. Selected bacteria are used to ferment or pickle foods. The fermenting bacteria make acids and alcohol, which minimize the growth of other microbes. The acid produced is especially helpful in preventing the growth of the deadly bacterium *Clostridium botulinum.*

Today, we can add *pasteurization,* sterilization, refrigeration, freezing, ***irradiation,*** canning, and chemical preservatives to the list of food preservation techniques. A new method for food preservation—***aseptic processing***—simultaneously sterilizes the food and package separately before the food enters the package. Liquid foods, such as fruit juices, are especially easy to process in this manner. With aseptic packaging, boxes of sterile milk and juices can remain on supermarket shelves, free of microbial growth, for many years.

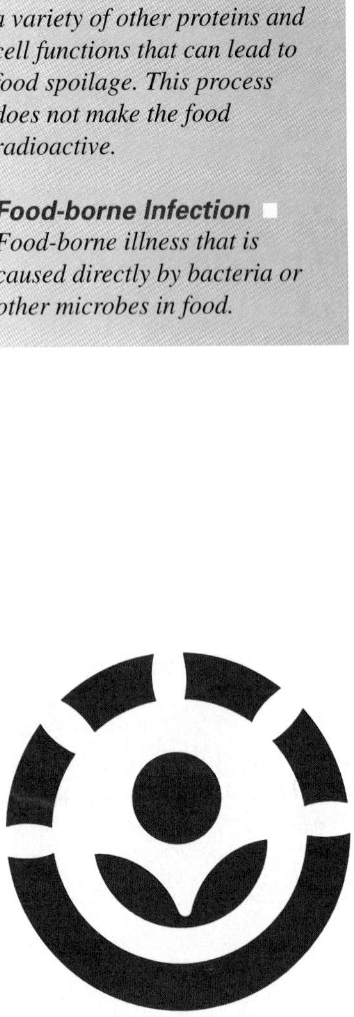

International label for noting prior irradiation of the food product.

Food irradiation is also a fairly recent development.[6] For over a decade FDA has permitted limited irradiation of wheat and wheat flour to control insect contamination. The gamma radiation used does not make the food radioactive. However, the energy is strong enough to break chemical bonds, destroy cell walls and cell membranes, break down DNA, and link proteins together. This allows irradiation to control growth of insects, microorganisms, and parasites in foods. This extends the shelf life and/or enhances the safety of spices, dry vegetable seasonings, pork products, fresh fruits and vegetables, and poultry.[15]

Irradiated food, except for dried seasonings, must be so labeled (see margin). Foods treated this way are safe in the opinion of FDA and many other health authorities.[15] Japan, France, Italy, and Mexico use food irradiation technology. To date, consumer acceptance of widespread use of food irradiation in the United States is still in question. Opponents of food irradiation point out that it is known to decrease the vitamin content of foods and to alter them chemically in ways that are both difficult to monitor and possibly harmful. Until recently no foods sold in the United States were irradiated except for a few spices. In January 1992 a food irradiation plant opened in Florida, and irradiated fruit was sold in Miami and several other cities. Sales were poor, and the future of the plant has become a political as well as scientific issue.[6]

Food-Borne Illness: When Undesirable Microbes Alter Foods

In 1871 an Italian scientist named Selmi proposed that food-borne illness was caused by ptomaines, breakdown residues of proteins produced during bacterial spoilage of food. Although people still refer to ptomaine poisoning, this idea has been rejected for a long time because ptomaines are not as poisonous as was once assumed. Today, we know that specific toxin-producing bacteria and other microbes cause food-borne illness. These organisms cause health problems either directly by invading the intestinal wall and producing an infection or indirectly by producing a toxin in the food that later harms us (called an intoxication).[11]

Salmonella organisms in contaminated food deliver a direct hit to the intestine, causing ***food-borne infections.*** The *Staphylococcus* bacterium produces a toxin, which in turn causes a ***food-borne intoxication.*** Many different types of bacteria cause food-borne illness, such as *Bacillus, Campylobacter, Clostridium, Escherichia, Listeria, Vibrio, Yersinia, Salmonella,* and *Staphylococcus.*[17,18] Because each teaspoon of soil contains about 2 billion bacteria, we are constantly at risk for food-borne illness. Luckily, only a small number of all bacteria actually pose a threat. Determining which microbe has caused an incident entails identifying the clinical features of the outbreak, the incubation period for symptoms, and the food source (see Table 17-1).

Food-borne Intoxication *Food-borne illness that is caused by toxins produced by bacteria or other microbes in food.*

General Rules for Preventing Food-Borne Illness

You can greatly reduce the risk of food-borne illness by following some very important rules[11]:

- Wash your hands thoroughly with hot, soapy water before handling food. Always wash your hands after handling raw meat, fish, poultry, or eggs, and after using the bathroom.
- When grocery shopping, select frozen foods and perishables, such as meat, poultry, or fish, last. Always put these products in separate plastic bags so that drippings don't contaminate other foods in the shopping cart. Then, don't let groceries sit in a warm car; this allows bacteria to grow. Refrigerate or freeze food promptly.
- Don't buy or use food from containers that leak, bulge, or are severely dented. Don't buy or use food from jars that are cracked or have loose or bulging lids. Don't taste or use food that has a foul odor or that spurts liquid when opened. The deadly *Clostridium botulinum* toxin is probably present.
- Wash thoroughly all counters, cutting boards, dishes, and other equipment in hot, soapy water and rinse. Do this both before preparing food and especially after foods come in contact with raw meat, fish, poultry, and eggs. This helps to rid *Salmonella* and other illness-causing microbes that may be present. Also, a sanitizing solution should be used to wipe off counters *at least* once a week. This can easily be made from household bleach diluted with water.
- Wash fresh fruit and vegetables carefully to remove dirt.
- If possible, cut foods to be eaten raw on a clean cutting board reserved for that purpose. If the same board must be used for both meat and other foods, cut the items to be eaten raw before cutting potentially contaminated items, such as meat.
- Cook animal foods thoroughly. Internal temperature for beef should reach 160° F or 71° C; for poultry, 180° F or 82° C; for fish and pork, 170° F or 77° C; and for eggs the yolk should at least be semisolid and the white hard. A good general precaution is to eat no raw animal products. This includes use of raw or undercooked eggs (cooked to less than 160° F or 71° C). Many people are poisoned each year by eating raw seafood (Figure 17-1). Undercooked pork can allow infection by the parasite that causes trichinosis. The U.S. Department of Agriculture (USDA) will answer questions on safe preparation and use of animal products by phone (1-800-535-4555).
- When possible, boil all canned foods when heating. Boiling for 10 minutes destroys the botulism toxin, if present.
- Once a food is cooked, cool it rapidly (to 40° F or 4° C) within 2 to 4 hours if it is not to be eaten immediately. Greater surface area allows quicker cooling, so separate foods into several pans. Don't recontaminate cooked food through contact with raw meat or juices that might be on your hands, cutting boards, or dirty utensils.
- Reheat leftovers to 165° F (74° C) and reheat gravy to a rolling boil to kill potential *Clostridium perfringens* bacteria present. Stopping at an acceptable eating temperature is not good enough.
- Keep hot foods hot and cold foods cold. Avoid time and temperature abuses. Store food below 40° F (4° C) or above 140° F (60° C) (Figure 17-2). Microbes that can cause illness thrive in more moderate temperatures (60° to 90° F or 16° to 32° C). Observe timelines for safe food storage (see Appendix M). This is important because some microbes can grow in the refrigerator. Do not leave cooked or refrigerated foods—such as meat and salads—at room temperature for more than 2 hours, because this allows microbes to grow and to cause food-borne illness.

By the end of 1993, all meats are slated to carry a label describing instructions for proper handling, cooking, and storage. Undercooked and mishandled meats lead to numerous cases of food-borne illness each year.

A seafood hot line is available through the American Seafood Institute. For free information on the purchase, preparation, and nutritional value of seafood products, call 1-800-328-3474 between 9 AM and 5 PM Eastern time on weekdays.

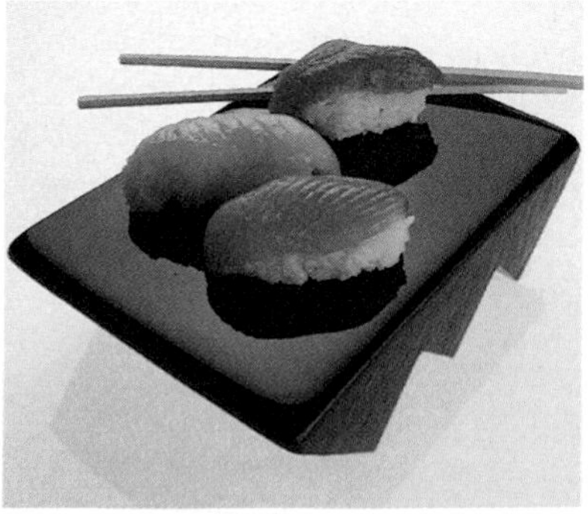

FIGURE 17-1
Sushi, like all raw animal food dishes, is a high-risk choice. Animal foods should be cooked thoroughly before eating.

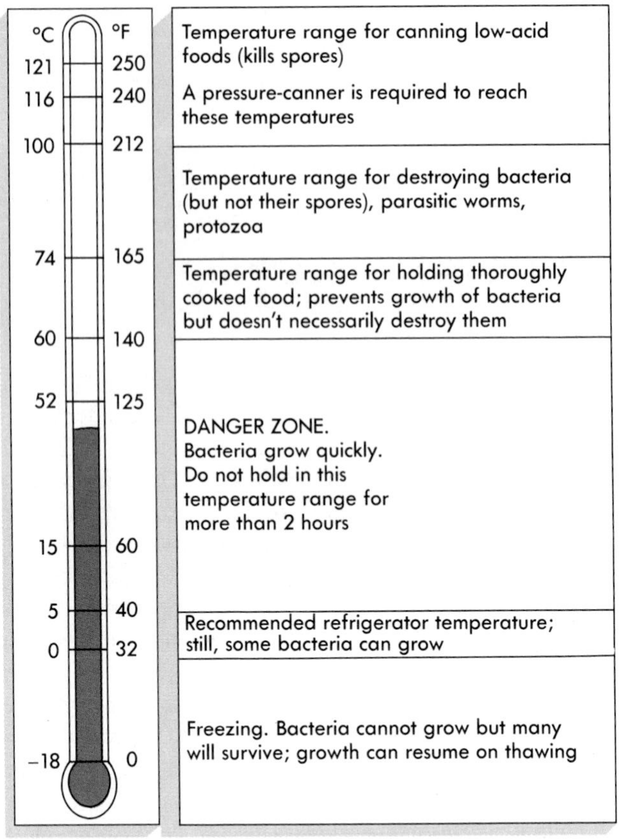

FIGURE 17-2

Effects of temperature on microbes that cause food-borne illness. (From Temperature Guide to Food Safety: Food and home notes, *Washington, DC, 1977, USDA.)*

USDA Food Safety "Musts"

- **Refrigerate perishable foods as quickly as possible after buying them.**
- **Wash raw vegetables thoroughly.**
- **Keep your kitchen or food preparation areas clean.**
- **Wash your hands before preparing food.**
- **Keep hot foods hot and cold foods cold after they are prepared.**

- Insulate perishable items if fresh-prepared food is taken on a picnic or other outing, or even if it is a long drive home from the store. Pack cold food in a cooler with plenty of ice. A cooler without ice can be used to keep hot food warmer.
- Avoid coughing and sneezing over foods, even when you are healthy. Cover cuts on hands. This helps stop *Staphylococcus aureus* from entering your food.
- Make sure the refrigerator stays below 40° F (4° C). Generally keep it as cold as possible without freezing the milk or lettuce.
- Cook stuffing separately from poultry; or wash the bird thoroughly, stuff it immediately before cooking, and then transfer the stuffing to a clean bowl immediately after cooking. Make sure the stuffing reaches a temperature of 165° F (74° C). *Salmonella* is the major concern with poultry.
- Consume only pasteurized milk and cheese. Using any raw milk poses a health risk.[12,23] This warning is especially important for pregnant women, because very toxic bacteria and viruses that thrive in unpasteurized milk—such as *Listeria*—can harm the fetus.
- Completely remove moldy portions of food by cutting deeply around the mold, or don't eat the food. When in doubt, throw the food out. Mold growth is prevented by properly storing foods at cold temperatures and using the foods within a reasonable time (see Appendix M).

Microbes that cause food-borne illness commonly enter food through cross-contamination (usually from improper food handling) and grow because they are maintained at temperatures favorable to them.[11] Many foods contain problem microbes. Most food-borne illness could be eliminated through sanitary food-handling procedures and appropriate storage.[17]

Watch for safe food-handling techniques when you eat out (Figure 17-3). Check that foods in a salad bar are iced, custard and pudding pies are chilled, hot foods served on a hot food bar are hot, and vending machines are checked regularly, especially those with sandwiches and milk. Foods stored and served in dormitories should be properly handled.

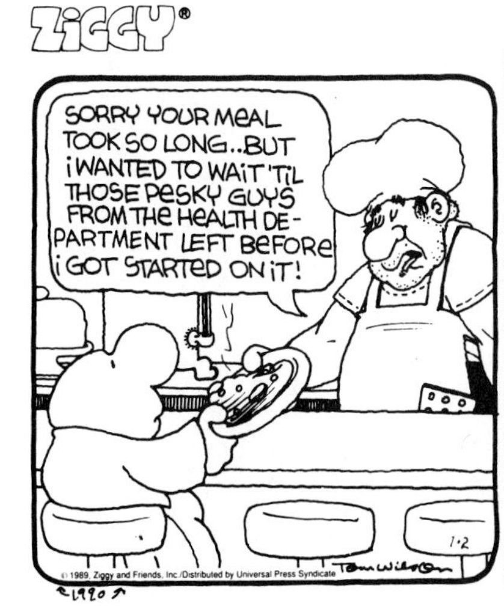

FIGURE 17-3
Ziggy.

another BITE

Several practices can reduce the risk of bacteria surviving during microwave cooking:

- Cover food with glass or ceramic when possible. The trapped steam helps decrease evaporation and heats the surface.
- Stir the product occasionally to avoid cold spots. Then allow microwaved food to stand, covered, after cooking is completed. The heat concentrated inside the food will radiate outward, helping to cook the exterior and equalize the temperature throughout.
- Thaw meats in the refrigerator. If thawed in the microwave, use the oven's defrost setting. Note that ice crystals in frozen foods are not heated well by the microwave oven and can create cold spots that later cook more slowly.

Treatment for Food-Borne Illness

If you suffer some food-borne illness, you can offset the effects of diarrhea by drinking a lot of fluids. Bed rest speeds recovery, and aspirin can ease the aches and pains. A fever of 102° F (39° C) or greater, blood in the stool, or dehydration from frequent vomiting or diarrhea (a sign of dehydration is dizziness when standing) deserves a physician's evaluation, especially if symptoms persist for more than 2 or 3 days. To prevent further contamination, wash your hands thoroughly and avoid handling food until the diarrhea disappears. In cases of suspected botulism, consult a physician immediately because an antitoxin may be available to speed recovery.

The USDA specifies three particular situations in which it is vital for consumers to report suspected food-borne illness to the local health department:

- If the food in question was eaten at a large gathering
- If the item came from a restaurant, delicatessen, sidewalk vendor, or a kitchen that serves large numbers of people
- If the suspected food was a commercial product, such as a canned good or a frozen, packaged item

CONCEPT CHECK

Bacteria and the toxins they produce cause most food-borne illness. Traditionally, several methods were commonly used to prevent the growth of microorganisms in food: sugar or salt was added to bind water or the foods were pickled, smoked, or dried before storage. Today, we have additional food processing methods, such as pasteurization, sterilization, canning, and irradiation. Also, food-handling practices—including cleanliness, storage of foods at proper temperatures, and thorough cooking of foods—help prevent contamination. All raw animal products and any cooked food must be treated with special care to reduce their potential to cause illness. Symptoms of food-borne illness resemble those associated with stomach or intestinal "flu": diarrhea, vomiting, abdominal bloating, and headache. Treatment in mild cases generally requires only bed rest and extra fluids. On the whole, we have a safe, sanitary food supply, and many of the public's food safety problems can be avoided if we use caution in food preparation.

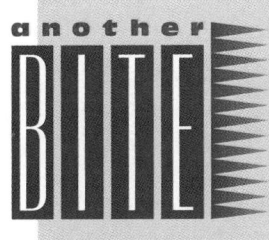

A CLOSER LOOK AT MICROBES THAT CAUSE FOOD-BORNE ILLNESS

We noted that finding the agent that led to food-borne illness requires some detective skills. Determining the agent depends on knowing the food source, the incubation time for and types of symptoms, and the duration of illness associated with an outbreak. Let's look at the characteristics of the major problem microbes individually.

Staphylococcus aureus (S. aureus)

The organism *Staphylococcus aureus (S. aureus)* causes 20% to 40% of food-borne illness cases each year. This microbe produces toxins in food, and so is classed as a food-borne intoxicant. Once ingested, the toxin causes nausea, vomiting, diarrhea, headaches, and abdominal cramps.[11] Symptoms usually develop within 2 to 6 hours of eating the contaminated food. The person rarely dies, but also develops no immunity against future attacks. Bed rest and fluids are generally the only treatment. Recovery takes place usually within 2 to 3 days.

S. aureus bacteria live mainly in the nasal passages and in skin sores. These microbes enter food when people sneeze and cough over food or handle food while they have open skin sores. Once present in significant numbers in a food, *S. aureus* can make enough toxin to cause human illness in about 4 hours if the food temperature stays near 100° F (38° C). The toxin is undetectable by flavor, odor, and appearance and can even withstand prolonged cooking.

Common foods associated with *S. aureus* intoxications are custard, ham, egg salad, cheese, seafood, cream-filled pastries, and milk. Whipped cream standing at room temperature for hours is a typical source. Keeping these and other foods above 140° F (60° C) or below 40° F (4° C) prevents both the bacterium's growth and further toxin production. To eliminate the spread of this microbe, it is important to work with clean hands, working surfaces, and utensils; direct coughs and sneezes away from food; and cover skin cuts on hands and arms when handling food.

Salmonella Food Poisoning

Many varieties of *Salmonella* bacteria cause food-borne illness. All 2000 types of *Salmonella* can be killed by normal cooking. Yet, they are responsible for almost 60% of cases of food-borne illness. These bacteria are commonly found in animal and human feces and enter food via infected water, contaminated cutting boards, contaminated meat products, cracked eggs, and actual bits of feces in food.[11] Ingesting the live bacteria causes the problem, and so is classed as a food-borne infection. The FDA calculates that

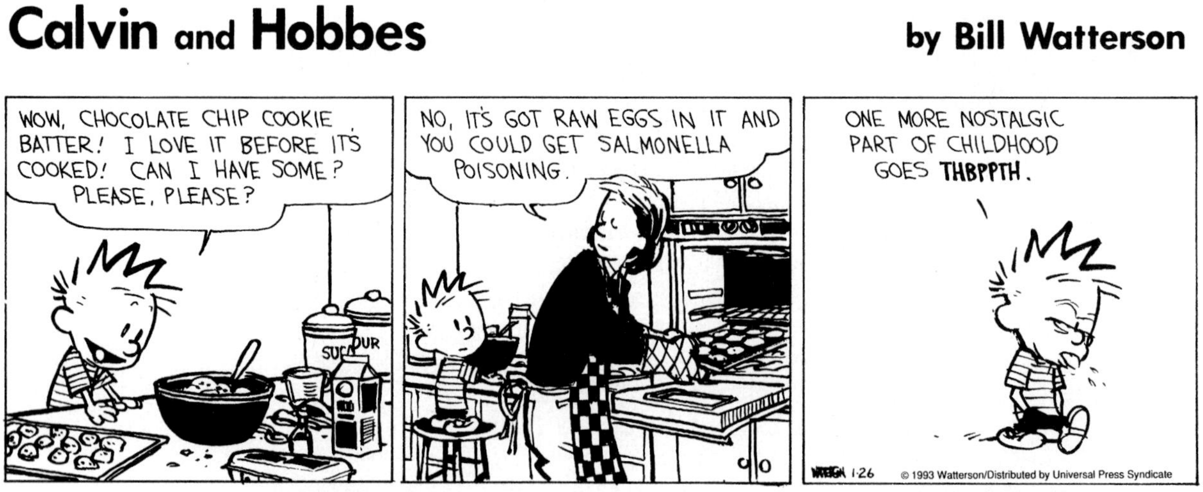

FIGURE 17-4
Calvin & Hobbes.

Salmonella-related illness costs more than $10 billion a year in medical care and lost work time in the United States.

Symptoms of *Salmonella* infections are the same as those of *S. aureus* food intoxications but can take longer to develop, from 5 to 72 hours. Again, bed rest and fluids are the only treatment, and recovery usually occurs within 2 to 3 days. Fatalities are rare. *Salmonella* attacks occur most frequently from consuming eggs, chicken, meat, meat products, custard made with infected eggs, raw milk, and inadequately refrigerated and reheated leftovers (Figure 17-4). Raw chicken is often contaminated, and undercooked food poses a special risk. Again, thorough cooking kills *Salmonella* bacteria.

To be safe, eggs should be boiled in water for 7 minutes, poached for 5 minutes (hard), or fried for 3 minutes on each side until the yolk is at least semisolid and the white is firm. Raw eggs should *not* be used in salads, sauces, eggnogs, or milk shakes. Hollandaise sauce, often warmed at low heat, is especially prey to *Salmonella,* as are eggs in uncooked homemade ice cream and mayonnaise. Recent research indicates that *Salmonella* can even be found in intact eggs, as well as cracked ones, especially if the egg has been left at room temperature for a few hours. This is a major concern for FDA and currently the focus of much research.[11]

Most outbreaks of *Salmonella* infections from foods can be traced to improper food handling. Picnics pose a special challenge, because food is frequently held for hours at a dangerous temperature (between 40° F and 140° F or 4° C and 60° C) (Figure 17-5). It takes only about 8 hours for *Salmonella* bacteria to multiply sufficiently to cause illness. Observing the temperature precautions for *S. aureus* organisms also prevents *Salmonella* bacteria growth.

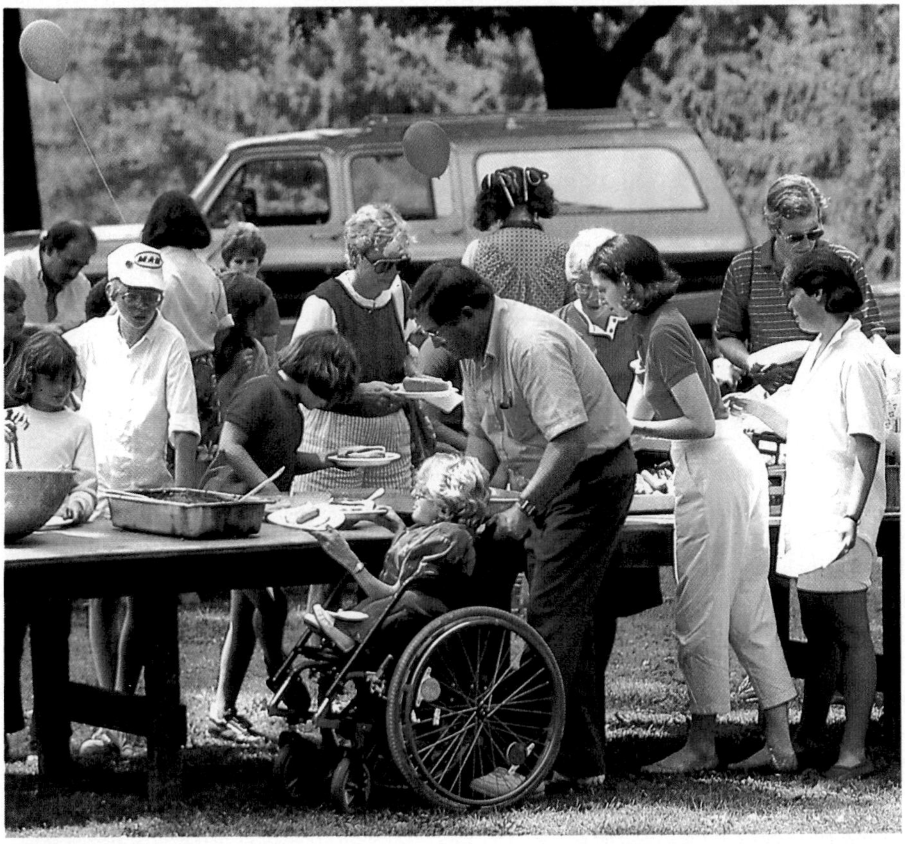

FIGURE 17-5

Picnics and other outdoor events demand special preventive measures. Many cases of food-borne illness happen at events like this family picnic. This is because foods may be out in the warm air for hours at a time.

Salmonella infections in foods are likely caused by cross-contamination of foods. To avoid outbreaks, keep hands and utensils clean when preparing foods and scrub a cutting board with a chlorinated cleanser after contact with raw meat or poultry. Store foods at temperatures either hot or cold enough to prevent bacterial growth. Do not allow susceptible foods to stand for more than 2 hours at room temperature. Marinate meat and seafood in the refrigerator. Finally, thaw foods in the refrigerator, in a microwave oven, or under a stream of cold water—not on the kitchen counter.

Clostridium perfringens (C. perfringens)

The bacterium *C. perfringens,* another major cause of food-borne infections, lives throughout the environment, especially in soil, the intestines of farm animals and humans, and sewage. It is called the "cafeteria germ," because most food-borne outbreaks by this organism are associated with the food service industry or with events where large quantities of food are prepared and served.[17] Symptoms of an infection resemble those of *Salmonella* food poisoning, but the victim usually doesn't vomit. Symptoms occur within 8 to 24 hours of consuming enough live bacteria. Again, bed rest and fluids are the only treatment, and recovery usually occurs within a day or so.

C. perfringens thrives in an oxygen-free environment. It forms heat-resistant spores that germinate and transform into bacteria at temperatures between 70° F and 120° F (21° C to 49° C). The bacteria then can quickly multiply to disease-causing levels. Foods stored in deep serving dishes are especially fertile media for growth of this bacteria, because the centers are isolated from air and stay warm.[11]

C. perfringens organisms are often found in cooked beef, turkey, gravy, dressing, stews, and casseroles. The best insurance against promoting their growth is to maintain proper holding temperatures and to divide large leftover portions into smaller ones. The more surface exposed to air, the less oxygen-deprived the centers will be. Be especially careful to cook meats completely and cool them rapidly in small containers. Thoroughly reheat leftover meat to 165° F (74° C) before serving. Always bring leftover gravy to a rolling boil. Refrigerate cold cuts and sliced meats at 40° F or 4° C, and serve them cold.

Clostridium botulinum (C. botulinum)

The *C. botulinum* bacterium can cause botulism, a food-borne illness that can be fatal. This microbe comes from soil and may exist as a bacterium or spore in all foods. As these bacteria multiply in food, they release a deadly toxin, and so lead to a food-borne intoxication.[11] The death rate for botulism receives much public attention; however, few cases are reported each year in the United States. At one time botulism was a serious problem of the canning industry, but now adequate heating and intact containers have virtually eliminated this danger from American manufactured canned foods.

Recently, researchers have noted botulism caused by spores (as opposed to bacteria) that enter the body. Infants between 2 and 6 months of age are at special risk, as are people with poor stomach acid production. Bacteria spores then germinate in the stomach and produce toxin. For this reason, honey—which can contain the *C. botulinum* spores—should not be given to infants under 1 year.

Symptoms of botulism appear within 12 to 36 hours of ingesting contaminated food. The toxin blocks nerve function, causing vomiting, abdominal pain, double vision, dizziness, and acute respiratory failure. If the person survives, recovery occurs within 10 days. Normally, bed rest is the only therapy. Sometimes, treatment for botulism requires intensive care, including mechanical ventilation; the early administration of antitoxin is recommended. Still, ultimate recovery may be slow.

C. botulinum grows only in the absence of air, and so it thrives primarily in canned food, especially improperly home-canned, low-acid foods, such as string beans, corn, mushrooms, beets, and asparagus. Recently, other foods with oxygen-deprived centers—such as potato salad, sauteed onions, stew, and chopped garlic—have caused botulism. The FDA now requires that chopped garlic in oil be acidified to protect against the hazard of *C. botulinum.* Cured meats also pose a risk for botulism; however, the nitrates and vitamin C used to preserve commercial products strongly inhibit bacterial growth.

Home-canned foods are the most common sources of botulism. While the canning process may kill all bacteria and the heat may drive out all oxygen, spores of *C. botulinum* can still survive if the heating is insufficient. When the can or jar cools, the spores germinate into bacteria that produce the toxin. Commercial canning factories are less likely to allow this to happen.

Always check all cans carefully. Look for rust on the seams, holes, and swollen sides or tops. Make sure the can sucks in air when opened and the liquid inside is clear and not milky and does not smell bad. If there are any signs of spoilage, return the can to the store or to the nearest public health department. Whatever you do, *do not taste the food. One string bean can contain enough toxin to kill you.*

• • • •

The bacteria discussed are the key offenders. However, the list of problem microbes—bacteria, fungi, molds, parasites, and viruses—as we noted earlier, is much longer.[7,17,18,23] Molds growing on foods can produce toxins that have a wide range of effects when consumed. Aflatoxins are produced by a mold that often grows on peanuts, corn, wheat, and oil seeds, such as cottonseed. Although aflatoxins cause cancer, FDA allows them at acceptable levels because they are considered unavoidable contaminants.

Parasites in foods pose additional problems. Most of us know to cook pork thoroughly. This kills a small parasitic worm, *Trichinella spiralis,* which can be live in raw or undercooked pork and cause the disease trichinosis[19] (Figure 17-6). Symptoms can take weeks or months to develop and include muscle weakness, fever, and fluid retention in the face. Equally harmful is the parasitic worm, *Anisakis,* found in its early growth stages in some raw fish. People who eat the popular Japanese dishes made of raw fish, sushi or sashimi, are particularly vulnerable to this type of food-borne illness. Symptoms usually occur within 12 hours of consumption and can include serious stomach pain if the young parasites penetrate the stomach lining. Thoroughly cooking fish or freezing it for at least 72 hours are reliable methods for eliminating the threat of *Anisakis* disease.

Viruses, such as hepatitis A, can also be transmitted in food. Symptoms include intestinal problems, weakness, fatigue, jaundice, and sometimes even development of serious liver disease requiring hospitalization. Because symptoms can take a month to show up, pinpointing the cause can be difficult. Unsanitary food handling in restaurants and raw seafood are the usual culprits.

THE FAR SIDE By GARY LARSON

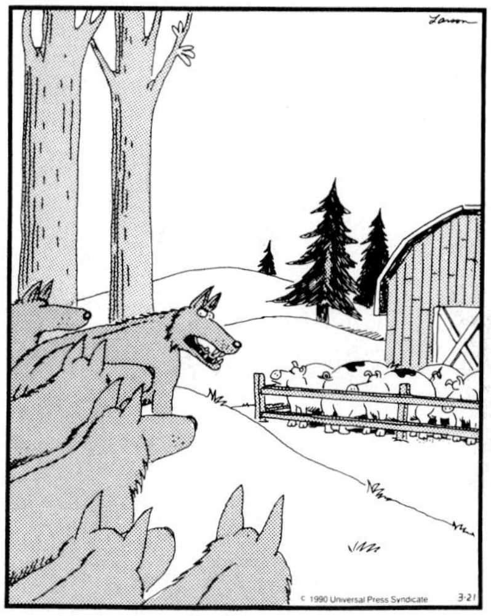

"I say we do it . . . and trichinosis be damned!"

FIGURE 17-6
The Far Side.

CONCEPT CHECK

To prevent food-borne intoxications from *Staphylococcus aureus* organisms, cover cuts on hands and avoid sneezing on foods. To avoid *Salmonella* food-borne infections, work with clean hands and utensils and separate raw meats, especially poultry products, from other foods. Thoroughly cook meat and poultry products to destroy any *Salmonella* present. To avoid infections from *Clostridium perfringens,* rapidly cool leftover foods and thoroughly reheat them. To avoid botulism from *Clostridium botulinum,* carefully examine canned foods and don't allow cooked foods to stand for more than 2 hours at room temperature. For other possible causes of food-borne illness, carefully handle raw animal products so that their juices do not contaminate other foods; thoroughly cook all foods, especially fish and other seafood; and consume only pasteurized dairy products.

FOOD ADDITIVES

By the time you see a food on the market shelf, it has usually had substances added to it to make it more palatable or to increase its nutrient content or shelf life. Manufacturers also add some substances to foods to make them easier to process.[8] Other substances may have found their way by accident into the foods you buy. All these extraneous substances are known as *additives,* and while some may be beneficial, others may be harmful. All added substances must be evaluated by FDA. Appendix N provides a comprehensive list of food additives and their purposes in foods.

Why Are Food Additives Used?

Limiting food spoilage accounts for the bulk of additive use. Food additives, such as potassium sorbate, are used to maintain the safety and acceptability of foods by retarding the growth of problem microbes implicated in food-borne illness.[20]

Additives are also used to combat some enzymes that lead to undesirable changes in color and flavor in foods but do not cause anything so serious as food-borne illness. This second type of food spoilage occurs when enzymes in a food react to oxygen—for example, when apple and peach slices darken or turn rust color as they are exposed to air. Antioxidants are a type of preservative that retards the action of oxygen-requiring enzymes on food surfaces. These preservatives are not necessarily novel chemicals. They include vitamins E and C and a variety of sulfites.[20]

another BITE

When buying products, especially perishables, check the product date for safety. Four types of dates are commonly used. The pack date is the day the product was manufactured. The pull or sell date indicates the last date the product should be sold. It allows some time for storing food at home before eating. Check the expiration date of foods stored at home, because that is the last date the food can safely be consumed. Last, baked goods may have a freshness date, indicating that the product may safely be eaten for a short time after the date but may not taste the same.

Intentional Food Additive
Additives knowingly (directly) incorporated into food products by manufacturers.

Incidental Food Additives
Contaminants that gain access to food products indirectly from environmental contamination of food ingredients or during the manufacturing process.

Generally Recognized As Safe (GRAS)
A group of food additives that in 1958 were considered safe, and therefore manufacturers were allowed to use them from then on when needed in food products. FDA bears responsibility for proving they are not safe.

Without the use of some food additives, it would be impossible to safely produce massive quantities of foods and distribute them nationwide or worldwide, as is now done. Despite consumer concerns about the safety of food additives, many have been extensively studied and proven safe when FDA guidelines for their use are followed.[20]

Intentional Versus Incidental Food Additives

Food additives are classified into two types: those that are ***intentionally*** (directly) added to foods and those that have ***incidentally*** (indirectly) entered foods as contaminants. Both types of agents are regulated by FDA. Currently, more than 2800 different substances are intentionally added to foods. As many as 10,000 other substances enter foods as contaminants. This includes substances that may reasonably be expected to enter food through surface contact with processing equipment or packaging materials.

The GRAS List

In 1958, all food additives used in the United States and considered safe at that time were put on a ***generally recognized as safe (GRAS)*** list.[8] Congress established the GRAS list because it felt manufacturers did not need to prove the safety of substances that were already generally regarded as safe by knowledgeable scientists. As is still the case, FDA was assigned responsibility for proving that a substance did not belong on the GRAS list. Since 1958, some substances on the list have been reviewed. A few, such as cyclamates, failed the review process and were removed from the list. Recently the additive red dye #3 was banned, because it is linked to cancer. Many chemicals on the GRAS list have not yet been rigorously tested, primarily because of expense. These chemicals have received a low priority for testing, mostly because they have long histories of use without evidence of harm and/or because their chemical structures do not suggest they are potential health hazards.

Are Synthetic Chemicals Always Bad?

Nothing about a natural product makes it inherently safer than a synthetic (man-made) product. Many synthetic products are simply laboratory copies of chemicals that also occur in nature (see the discussion in Chapter 18 on biotechnology for some examples).

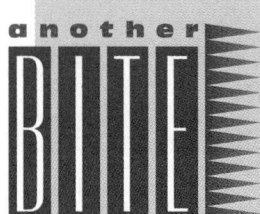

And although humans contribute some toxins to foods, such as synthetic pesticides and industrial chemicals, nature's poisons are often even more potent and prevalent. Some cancer researchers suggest that we ingest at least 10,000 times more (by weight) natural toxins produced by plants than we do man-made pesticide residues. This comparison doesn't make man-made chemicals any less toxic, but it does lend perspective.

Consider the familiar food additive baking powder, which is used to make the batter rise in cakes, pancakes, and other quick breads. When manufacturers list potassium acid tartrate, sodium aluminum phosphate, or monocalcium phosphate on cake mix labels, they are referring to baking powder by its chemical names. Baking soda could be listed by its proper name, sodium bicarbonate, just as ordinary table salt could be called sodium chloride. The question should not be whether a food additive—such as salt—is a chemical, but rather whether the chemical additive is safe to use.

Today, sugar, salt, corn syrup, and citric acid still constitute 98% of all additives by weight.

Vitamin E is often added to food to prevent rancidity of fats. This chemical is safe when used within certain limits. However, high doses have been associated with health problems (see Chapter 8). Thus even well-known chemicals we are comfortable using can be toxic in some circumstances and at some concentrations.

Testing Food Additives for Safety

Food additives are tested under FDA scrutiny for safety on at least two animal species, usually rats and mice. Scientists determine the highest dose of the additive that produces ***no observable effects*** in the animals. High doses are needed to reduce the cost and length of the tests. Still, these doses are proportionately much higher than humans are ever exposed to. The maximal dosage level is then divided by at least 100 to establish a margin of safety for human use.[8] The rationale for reducing the no observable effect level by a 100-fold margin is that we assume humans are at least 10 times more sensitive to food additives than laboratory animals and that any one person might be 10 times more sensitive than another. This very broad margin essentially ensures that the food additive in question will cause no deleterious health effects in humans. In fact, many synthetic chemicals are probably as harmless at these low doses as the natural compounds in apples or celery. Other terms used to express this margin of safety concept are *tolerance, allowable level,* and *acceptable level.*

No Observable Effect Level
This corresponds to the highest dose of an additive that produces no deleterious health effect in animals.

Delaney Clause
This clause to the 1958 Food Additives Amendment of the Pure Food and Drug Act in the United States prevents the intentional (direct) addition to foods of a compound introduced after that date that has been shown to cause cancer in animals or man.

One important exception applies to the schema for testing intentional food additives: if an additive is shown to cause cancer, even though caused by very high doses, no margin of safety is allowed. The food additive cannot be used, because it would violate the ***Delaney Clause*** in the 1958 Food Additive Amendments. This clause prohibits intentionally adding to foods a compound that was introduced after 1958 and causes cancer.[8] Evidence for cancer could come from either laboratory animal or human studies.

Recently, the value of animal cancer tests has been questioned. Research suggests that when rats are fed massive doses of chemicals, as they typically are in the tests, it may be the dose itself, rather than the chemical action, that causes cancer. The scientific community is currently debating which is the best method to test additives to evaluate cancer risk in humans.[8] The question boils down to how to test chemicals efficiently and how to apply data obtained from laboratory animals to humans. Nevertheless, we are left with our current approach until a better method is established.[19]

Incidental food additives are another matter altogether. The FDA cannot simply ban various industrial chemicals and mold toxins from foods, even though some of these contaminants can cause cancer. These products are not purposely added to foods—they are present whether we like it or not. The FDA sets an acceptable level for these substances. Basically, it establishes a cancer safety margin of 1 million, which means that a substance found in a food cannot contribute to more than one cancer case during the lifetimes of 1 million people.[8] If a higher risk exists, then the amount of the compound in a food must be reduced until the guideline is met. Currently some politicians and scientists want to see such a standard applied to all pesticides, which in effect would mean cancelling the Delaney Clause in the case of pesticides that have been linked to cancer risk. The Nutrition Issue on p. 564 covers this in more detail.

Note that the margin of safety for some vitamins and trace minerals is much lower than for additives. In a few cases, 5 to 10 times our needs for a nutrient can be toxic. So use of food additives is subjected to much stricter limits than are essential nutrients purchased in supplement form, such as copper and vitamin D.

NUTRITION insight

PROTECTING THE U.S. FOOD SUPPLY

A variety of federal, state, and local agencies in the United States monitor food safety. The history of the food laws they enforce is listed in Table 17-2. Some of the agencies involved are the following:

TABLE 17-2

Some Key U.S. Food Laws

1906: **Pure Food and Drug Act and Federal Meat Inspection Act**—This most importantly defined adulterated foods: those foods containing "any added poisons or other added deleterious ingredient which may render such article injurious to health."
1938: **Federal Food, Drug, and Cosmetic Act**—This provided for exemptions and safe tolerances for substances that, although not desirable in foods, were either necessary in production or unavoidable.
1958: **Food Additives Amendment (and the Color Additives Amendment of 1960)**—These made it necessary for manufacturers to demonstrate the safety of a new food additive before approval by FDA. The 1958 act also included the Delaney Clause: "No additive shall be deemed to be safe if it is found to produce cancer when ingested by man or animals, or if it is found after tests which are appropriate for the evaluation of the safety of the food additives to induce cancer in man or animals."
1990: **Nutrition Labeling and Education Act**—This law expanded the number of foods required to contain a nutrition label and formalized rules for label descriptors, such as "lite." It also set standards for health claims on foods, such as whether a food can lower the risk of heart disease.

From Expert Panel on Food Safety and Nutrition: Food Technology, *p. 73, January 1992.*

- *U.S. Department of Agriculture (USDA).* This agency enforces standards for wholesomeness and quality of grains, produce, meat, poultry, milk, and eggs produced in the United States. As part of this effort, more than 7000 inspectors visually examine the carcasses of more than 120 million animals a year in an effort to keep obviously diseased meat from going to market. Overall, activities include inspection of production plants and of grains, fruits, vegetables, meat, poultry, and dairy products.[10] USDA also routinely monitors animal foods for antibiotics.
- *Bureau of Alcohol, Tobacco, and Firearms.* This agency is responsible for enforcing laws first enacted in 1935 that cover the production, distribution, and labeling of most alcoholic beverages.
- *Environmental Protection Agency (EPA).* This agency regulates pesticides based on laws passed from 1947 through 1974. EPA must approve all pesticides before they are sold in the United States. It determines the safety of new pesticide products and sets allowable limits for pesticide residue in foods. This limit is not necessarily set at the maximal safe level of a pesticide in a food; EPA sets limits no higher than needed for a product's intended use. These levels are then enforced by FDA.[10] EPA also establishes water quality standards, including those for drinking water.
- *Food and Drug Administration (FDA).* This agency is responsible for ensuring the safety and wholesomeness of all foods sold in interstate commerce (except for meat and poultry, which are primarily under USDA jurisdiction). Follow their actions by

reading *FDA Consumer*. FDA also sets standards for specific foods and enforces federal regulations for labeling, food and color additives, food sanitation, and the safety of foods. The agency inspects food plants, imported food products, and mills that make feeds containing medications or nutritional supplements for animals destined for human consumption. Over 90,000 businesses are inspected each year; about half are food-related businesses.

FDA acts primarily when the public health is endangered or when proper medical care is being discouraged. It regulates products, not people. FDA cannot control what people say, just what is on the label and how a product is promoted. FDA gives low priority to simple economic deception by products.

To monitor foods for contaminants, FDA routinely samples items that are of dietary importance, such as produce. Foods suspected of containing illegal residues receive a more intensive evaluation.[9] An important part of FDA's safety sampling is a "market basket" study of foods that typify the American diet.[10] Four times a year, identical purchases of 234 foods—including processed foods—are analyzed for pesticide residues, radioactive elements, toxic metals, and other undesirable substances. Imported foods with illegal residues can be refused entry into the country by FDA.

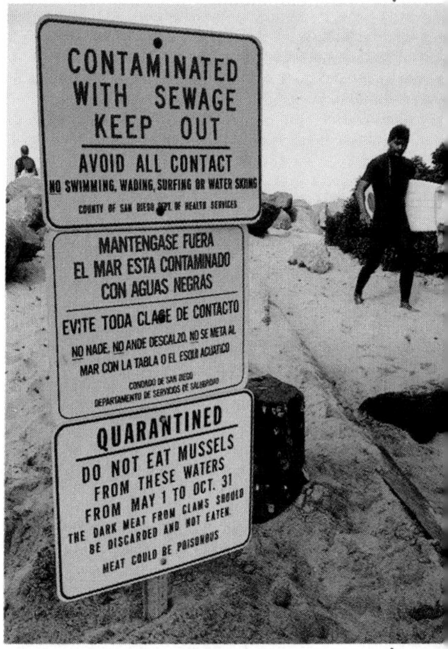

FIGURE 17-7
Purchase seafood from reputable suppliers. They must be able to guarantee that the food has been legally harvested.

another BITE

Traditionally, FDA does not regularly inspect food-processing plants. It relies instead on its "Good Manufacturers Procedures" plan that food processors and manufacturers are expected to follow. FDA inspectors may visit a specific food processing establishment only infrequently. The agency relies on consumer complaints to alert it to potential dangers—then it researches these in greater detail. There just isn't enough staff at FDA to carefully inspect all instances where federal regulations must be adhered to.

- *National Marine Fishery Service.* This agency is part of the Department of Commerce. It is responsible for seafood quality and other aspects of fisheries management. Its inspection program for fish products is voluntary, not mandatory. This is probably one reason that one fourth of all incidents of food-borne illness in the United States involve fish, according to the Centers for Disease Control in Atlanta (Figure 17-7). FDA does inspect seafood processing plants and spot-checks imported fish and seafood.
- *State and local government.* States inspect restaurants, retail food establishments, dairies, grain mills, and other food-related establishments within their borders. States have the primary responsibility for milk safety. FDA provides guidelines to state and local governments for regulating dairy products and restaurants.
- *Foreign governments.* Governments of at least 40 nations are now partners with the United States in ensuring food safety through agreements that cover 24 food products, including shellfish. International cooperation in food inspection and regulatory standards is expanding.

Again, the limited budgets of government enforcement agencies at all levels may limit the number and thoroughness of inspections. So individuals must assume some responsibility for these protective activities themselves. We must remain alert in cases of apparent abuse and contact the appropriate government agency.

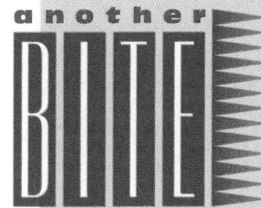

Obtaining Approval for a New Food Additive

Today, before a new substance can be added to foods, FDA must approve its use. Besides rigorously testing an additive to establish its safety margins, manufacturers must give the FDA information that (1) identifies the new additive, (2) gives its chemical composition, (3) states how it is manufactured, and (4) specifies laboratory methods used to measure its presence in the food supply at levels of intended use.

Manufacturers must also offer proof that the additive will accomplish its intended purpose in a food, that it is safe, and that the level present is no higher than needed. Additives cannot be used to hide defective food ingredients, such as rancid oils; deceive customers; or replace good manufacturing practices. A manufacturer must establish that the ingredient is necessary for producing a specific food product.

Common Food Additives

A list of food additive categories appears in Table 17-3, some of which serve the general function of preservatives: acidic or alkaline agents, antioxidants, antimicrobial agents, curing and pickling agents, and sequestrants. Let's look at some of the specific categories of additives to understand exactly why these are used and to learn more about the specific substances employed.[20]

Acidic or Alkaline Agents. Acids, such as calcium lactate, have many uses in foods. As flavor-enhancing agents, they impart a tart taste to soft drinks, sherbets, and cheese spreads, for example. As preservatives, they inhibit microbial growth. As antioxidants, they prevent discoloration and rancidity. They also adjust acid and base balance. Adding acids during food processing increases the margin of safety from botulism in naturally low-acid vegetables, such as beets.

Alkaline products, such as sodium hydroxide, can alter the texture and flavor of foods, including chocolate. In processing, alkaline products are sometimes used to produce a milder flavor by neutralizing the acids produced during fermentation.

Alternate Sweeteners. Currently, saccharin and acesulfame (Sunette) are the only nonnutritive sweeteners used in foods. Because aspartame (Nutrasweet) yields energy, it is considered a nutritive sweetener (see Chapter 5). Saccharin is carcinogenic to rats when administered over two generations. The cancers are found primarily in the bladder. However, population studies of humans have not found an increased risk of developing

TABLE 17-3

Food Additive Categories

Anticaking	Flour treating	Processing aids: clarifying, clouding, catalyst, flocculants, filter aids, crystallization inhibitors
Antimicrobial	Formulation aids: carriers, binders, fillers, plasticizers	Propellants
Antioxidants	Fumigants	Sequestrants
Colors and adjuncts	Humectants	Solvents and vehicles
Conditioners	Leavening	Stabilizers and thickeners
Curing and pickling	Lubricants and release agents	Surface active agents
Dough strengtheners	Nonnutritive sweeteners	Surface-finishing agents
Drying agents	Nutritive sweeteners	Synergists
Emulsifiers	Oxidizing and reducing	Texturizers
Enzymes	pH control	
Firming agents		
Flavor enhancers		
Flavoring agents		

From Hegarty V: Decisions in nutrition, St Louis, 1988, Mosby.
See Appendix N for examples of compounds that fall within these categories.

bladder cancer from exposure to saccharin. Congress has prevented FDA from banning saccharin due to the Delaney Clause, but a warning label must accompany any use.

Anticaking Agents. By absorbing moisture, such compounds as calcium silicate, ammonium citrate, magnesium stearate, and silicon dioxide keep table salt, baking powder, powdered sugar, and other powdered food products freeflowing. These chemicals prevent the caking and lumping that would make powdered or crystalline products hard to use.

Antimicrobial Agents. Sodium benzoate, sorbic acid, and calcium propionate are common preservatives. Sorbic acid is a potent inhibitor of molds and fungal growth. Calcium propionate, a natural part of some cheeses, inhibits mold growth.

Antioxidants. This type of food preservative helps delay food discoloration from oxygen exposure, such as occurs when potatoes are diced. It also helps keep fats from turning rancid. Two widely used antioxidants are BHA (butylated hydroxyanisole) and BHT (butylated hydroxytoluene). Vitamin E and related compounds also serve as antioxidants.

Sulfites also are widely used as antioxidants in foods. Sulfites are actually a group of sulfur-based chemicals—sulfur dioxide, gas, sodium and potassium bisulfite, and sodium and potassium meta bisulfite. After ingesting sulfites, people who are very sensitive to them may have difficulty breathing, wheeze, and vomit, as well as develop hives, diarrhea, abdominal pain, cramps, and dizziness. The FDA now limits the use of sulfites on raw fruits and vegetables—an action directed mainly at salad bars. Potatoes are not covered by that regulation. The FDA also requires manufacturers to declare the presence of sulfites on labels of packaged foods containing at least 10 parts per million of sulfites. Labels on wine bottles often list a sulfite warning.

Colors. Color additives do not improve nutritional qualities, but they can make foods more eye appealing. Food colorings cannot be used to deceive consumers—for example, by covering blemishes; to conceal inferiority; or to mislead people in any way. Although colorings are arguably unnecessary additives, manufacturers have satisfied FDA that color is "necessary" for the production of certain foods.

Controversy has surrounded the use of some food colors. Currently, the safety of using tartrazine (FD&C yellow No. 5) is disputed. It has caused allergic symptoms—such as hives, itching, and nasal discharge—in sensitive individuals, especially in people allergic to aspirin. Although few Americans are sensitive to tartrazine, FDA requires manufacturers to list FD&C yellow No. 5 on labels of food products containing it. Some red dyes have also raised alarms, and some have been banned.

Curing and Pickling Agents. Nitrates—and the related form, nitrites—are used as preservatives, especially to prevent growth of *Clostridium botulinum.* Sodium and potassium nitrates and nitrites are used to preserve meats, such as bacon, ham, salami, and hot dogs. Nitrates and nitrites have been used for centuries, in conjunction with salt, to preserve meat. An added effect of nitrates is their reaction with myoglobin pigments in meat to form a bright pink color. This gives the characteristic appearance to ham, hot dogs, and other cured meats.

Nitrate consumption from both cured foods and natural vegetables has been associated with the synthesis of nitrosamines in the stomach. Nitrosamines are potent cancer-causing agents, particularly for the stomach and esophagus. The actual risk appears to be low, however, except for people who secrete little stomach acid (some elderly people, for example). The FDA also feels that consumers take for granted a margin of microbial safety gained from nitrite use in cured meats. People often serve these meats cold or at least underheated. Consequently, government agencies have chosen not to ban nitrate or nitrite use in foods, but rather to change manufacturing practices to lower amounts of performed nitrosamines.

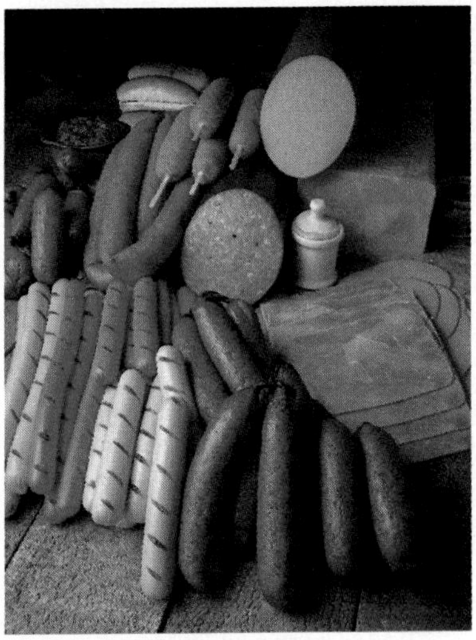
Cured meats rely on nitrates and/or nitrites for their pink color.

The addition of vitamin C to cured meats, such as bacon, is one way to reduce the amount of nitrosamines formed in foods. This is a common practice today. Other antioxidants, such as vitamin E, also inhibit synthesis of nitrosamines.

Most nitrites and nitrates in the U.S. food supply occur naturally in foods, primarily in vegetables and baked goods. About one third of nitrites and one seventh of nitrates in our food supply are added in manufacturing.

another BITE

If nitrates and nitrites form chemical substances that can cause cancer, why aren't they banned by the Delaney Clause? In the United States, USDA regulates the use of chemicals in meats. The laws that govern USDA functions are separate from the 1938 Federal Food, Drug, and Cosmetic Act. Because of this, the Delaney Clause, an amendment to the 1938 law, does not apply to USDA actions. Currently, USDA sees no clear threat to public safety from the regulated use of nitrates and nitrite in meats, and so no action has been taken.

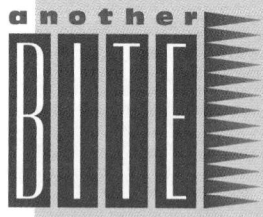

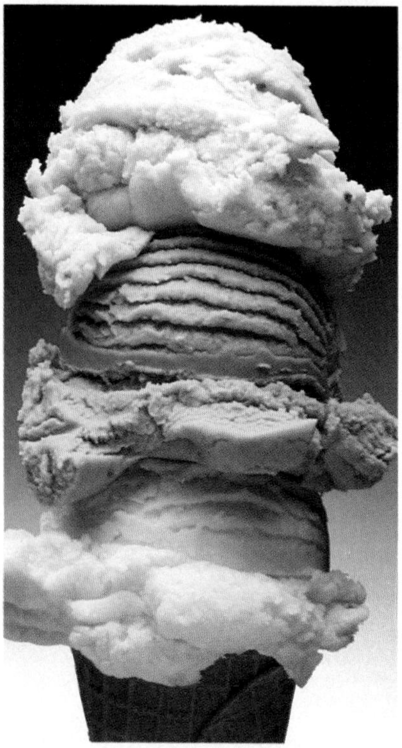

Ice cream often contains added emulsifiers and stabilizers.

Infants are more sensitive to MSG than adults, because infants have not yet developed a complete blood-brain barrier. This means they cannot fully exclude such substances as MSG from the brain.

Emulsifiers. These products, by distributing and suspending fat in water, improve the uniformity, smoothness, and body of foods, such as bakery goods, ice cream, and candies. In mayonnaise, for example, egg yolks act as emulsifiers in holding together the oil and the acids, such as vinegar or lemon juice. Lecithin, derived from soybeans, acts as an emulsifier in chocolate and margarine. Monoglycerides and diglycerides, found also as by-products of fat digestion, are used as emulsifiers in cake mixes.

Fat Replacements. Fat replacements—such as Paselli SA2, Dur-Low, Oatrim, and Sta-Slim 143—are being produced for commercial use. These carbohydrate-based products add to another major player—Simplesse—as we discussed in Chapter 6.

Flavors and Flavoring Agents. Naturally occurring and artificial agents can impart more flavor to foods. These agents include extracts from spices and herbs, as well as man-made agents. You probably have recognized flavors of some spices and of liquid derivatives of onion, garlic, cloves, and peppermint in foods. To meet the demand of industry, manufacturers have developed synthetic flavors that not only taste like natural flavors, but also have the advantage of stability. Often artificial flavors, such as butter or banana flavors, have the same chemical composition that makes up part of the natural flavor.

Flavor Enhancers. These substances—monosodium glutamate (MSG), for example—help bring out the natural flavors of foods. Some people are sensitive to MSG and experience flushing, chest pain, facial pressure, dizziness, sweating, rapid heart rate, nausea, vomiting, and high blood pressure after exposure. Because MSG is often used in Chinese food, reactions have been called *Chinese restaurant syndrome.* The onset of symptoms occurs about 10 to 20 minutes after ingestion and may last from 2 to 3 hours. People who find themselves sensitive to MSG should avoid it.

Humectants. These chemicals—such as glycerol, propylene glycol, and sorbitol—are added to foods to help retain proper moisture, fresh flavor, and texture. They are often used in candies, shredded coconut, and marshmallows.

Leavening Agents. Air and steam can be used to create a light texture in breads and cakes; however, carbon dioxide bubbles are much more reliable for this purpose. Common leavening agents that produce carbon dioxide gas include yeast, baking powder, and baking soda. Baking soda needs to react with acids to generate carbon dioxide. Baking powder can be used in either acid or alkaline conditions.

Maturing and Bleaching Agents. Such compounds as bromates, peroxides, and ammonium chloride hasten the natural aging and whitening processes of milled flour. This shortens the delay in using flour in baked products. Otherwise, freshly milled flour lacks the qualities necessary to make a stable, elastic dough and requires several months to be useful in baking.

Nutrient Supplements. Vitamin and mineral supplements are added to foods to improve their nutritional quality. Sometimes they replace nutrients lost in processing, as occurs when enriching flour. Vitamin A is added to margarine and to some forms of milk. Vitamin D is added to some dairy products. Potassium iodide is added to salt, and calcium to some flours. Breakfast cereals often contain a variety of added nutrients.

Stabilizers and Thickeners. These additives impart a smooth texture and uniform color and flavor to candies, ice creams and other frozen deserts, chocolate milk, and artificially sweetened beverages. Commonly used substances are pectins, vegetable gums (such as guar gum and carrageenan), gelatins, and agars. They work by absorbing water. Without stabilizers and thickeners, ice crystals form in ice cream and other frozen desserts, and particles of chocolate separate from chocolate milk. Stabilizers are also used to prevent evaporation and deterioration of flavorings used in cakes, puddings, and gelatin mixes.

Sequestrants. These compounds include EDTA and citric acid. They bind many free chemical ions, and by doing so, help preserve food quality by reducing the ability of ions to cause rancidity in products containing fat.

Sequestrants *Compounds that bind free metal ions; by so doing, they reduce the ability of ions to cause rancidity in foods containing fat.*

• • • •

In general, if you consume a variety of foods in moderation, the chances of food additives jeopardizing your health are minimal. Pay attention to your body. If you suspect an intolerance or sensitivity, consult your physician for further evaluation. Remember that, in the short run, you are more likely to suffer either from poor food-handling practices that allow bacteria to grow in food or from consuming raw animal foods than from eating additives. Excess energy, saturated fat, and other potential "problem" nutrients in our diets pose the greatest long-term risk.

another BITE

Look at the ingredients listed on a typical box of flavored gelatin dessert. Besides the expected sugar and gelatin, there is a long list of vitamins and minerals, adipic acid, disodium phosphate, fumaric acid, artificial color, and artificial flavor. You may wonder whether this is a smart food choice. If you are bewildered or concerned about all the additives generally creeping into your diet, you can easily avoid most of them by emphasizing unprocessed whole foods. However, no evidence shows that this will necessarily make you healthier. It amounts to a personal decision. Do you have faith that FDA and food manufacturers are adequately protecting your health and welfare, or do you want to take more personal control by minimizing your intake of compounds not naturally found in foods?

CONCEPT CHECK

Food additives are used to reduce spoilage caused by microbial growth, oxygen, some chemical ions, and other compounds. Additives are also used by food manufacturers to improve flavor and color, leaven, provide nutritional fortification, thicken, and emulsify food components. Additives are classified as intentional (direct)—those purposefully added to foods—and incidental (indirect)—those that end up in foods through environmental contamination or manufacturing practices. Additives in foods are limited to at most 1/100 of the highest amount that causes no observable effect when consumed by animals. The Delaney Clause further limits the intentional addition of cancer-causing compounds to foods regulated by FDA. Carcinogens that enter foods as contaminants have maximal levels set for them. These are monitored primarily by FDA.

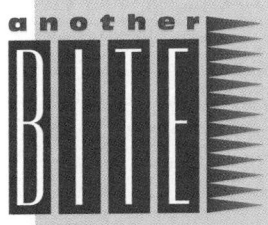

NUTRITION insight

ENVIRONMENTAL CONTAMINANTS IN FOOD

As we have alluded to, a variety of environmental contaminants may be found in foods. Aside from pesticide residue and products of fungal growth, other important contaminants deserve attention.

Lead

Ingesting this metal can cause anemia, kidney disease, and damage to the nervous system. Because it has a high atomic weight, it is a "heavy" metal. Many heavy metals are toxic at low doses. Lead toxicity is especially a problem for children because it curtails learning ability.[14] The U.S. Centers for Disease Control estimates that one in six U.S. children, up to 4 million, may suffer lowered intelligence and physiological problems as a result of blood-lead levels.[5] This is far greater than the number of children vecause it curtails childhood illnesses. It is important not to store food in a can with a lead solder joint after the can has been opened. Contact with air speeds degradation of the solder joint and the release of lead into the food product. This is especially important for acidic food products, such as tomatoes. If used for acidic products, such as soft drinks, cans today are often lead free.

Never store acidic products—such as fruit juice, sauerkraut, or pickled vegetables—in galvanized, tin, or other metal containers, except stainless steel. This includes opened tin cans. Acid can dissolve the metal, and lead will then leach into the food product. Lead can also leak out of solder joints in copper pipes, so let tap water run a minute or more before drinking it or cooking with it, especially first thing in the morning.

Lead can enter the food supply via leaded crystal and pottery glazes. Lead is no longer used in glazes on commercially produced dishes in the United States because of this hazard. However, there is no way to ensure the safety of homemade or imported pottery items. It is important not to use antiques or collectibles, including any leaded glass, for food or beverage storage because of the potential lead contamination.

Drinking water can be tested for lead for about $50 by laboratories certified by the Environmental Protection Agency (EPA). Avoid softening your drinking water, because soft water can leach lead from pipes. Use only cold water for drinking and cooking, and let it flow for a minute first if it has been off for an hour or more.

NATURALLY OCCURRING TOXINS IN FOODS

Foods contain a variety of naturally occurring toxic substances. Following are some of the more important examples[16]:

Mushrooms—some species are poisonous.

Safrole—found in sassafras, mace, and nutmeg; causes cancer.

Solanine—found in potato shoots and green spots on potato skins; inhibits nervous system action.

Aflatoxin—found on moldy grains and peanuts; causes cancer. The FDA rigorously inspects peanut butter to ensure that it's safe for consumption.

Avidin—found in raw egg whites; binds biotin, preventing its absorption. Cooking inactivates avidin.

Dioxin

This is an abbreviated name for a complex chemical defoliant. Dioxin is believed to cause cancer and other harmful effects in animals, even in small doses.[4] For Americans, major food sources of dioxin are bottom-feeding fish from the Great Lakes—an area with a great deal of industrial activity and chemical production. Dioxin is primarily a problem for people who frequently consume fish caught locally. People who eat commercial fish normally eat a variety, and even people who stick to one type of fish do not usually have a problem, because fish in interstate commerce generally come from different waters, only a few of which may contain dioxin.

Dioxin has also been detected in some paper products. Levels in milk cartons and coffee filters have currently been reduced to the point that they are so low they cannot be distinguished from "background" dioxin levels typically found in foods.

Mercury

The FDA first limited mercury, another heavy metal, in foods in 1969 after 120 people in Japan became ill from eating fish contaminated with high amounts. Birth defects in offspring of some of those people were also blamed on the mercury poisoning.[1] The fish most often contaminated was swordfish. Currently, swordfish shipments are automatically detained until they are shown to meet mercury standards. For freshwater fish in America, it is best to eat the younger, and hence smaller, fish. These have had less time to accumulate mercury than larger, older fish.

Urethane in Alcoholic Beverages

This chemical forms during fermentation of alcoholic beverages. If the fermented product is heated, as in the production of sherry and bourbon, urethane levels increase even more. Although urethane causes cancer in animals, it is unclear whether it causes cancer in humans. FDA research on urethane in food products is now a high priority. A prudent choice might be to limit consumption of products such as fruit brandies and sake, because these show consistently higher levels of urethane.

Polychlorinated Biphenyls (PCBs)

These chemicals were widely used for years in a variety of industrial products, but because they are linked to liver tumors and reproductive problems in animals, they are no longer produced. The FDA has banned their use in machinery associated with food and animal feed and has established limits for PCBs in susceptible foods and in paper used for food-packaging material.

The most significant food source of PCB residues is fish, primarily freshwater fish, such as coho and chinook salmon from the Great Lakes and bottom-feeding freshwater species from waters in other industrial areas. A key point in fish consumption is variety and moderation when local sources have the potential for contamination.

Goitrogens—found in raw rutabagas, turnips, brussels sprouts, broccoli, kale, and soybeans; inhibit thyroid hormone metabolism. Cooking destroys them.

Thiaminase—found in raw clams and mussels; it destroys the vitamin thiamin. Cooking inactivates thiaminase.

Glycyrrhizic acid—found in pure licorice extracts; causes hypertension.

Tetrodotoxin—found in puffer fish; causes respiratory paralysis.

Protease inhibitor—found in raw soybeans; inhibits digestive enzymes.

Saponins—found in alfalfa sprouts; destroy red blood cell membranes.

Tannins—found in tea; bind calcium and iron.

Oxalic acid—found in spinach; binds calcium.

Herbal teas—especially if they contain senna or comfrey, can cause diarrhea and liver damage. (See Chapter 3 for a list of other herbs that can threaten health.)

Nitrates—especially found in spinach, lettuce, and beets; can be converted into the carcinogen nitrosamine. (See Chapter 3 for a list of other herbs that can threaten health.)

Browning products—found in toasted grains; can cause genetic (DNA) changes.

People have coexisted for centuries with these naturally occurring toxins, learning to avoid some of them. Farmers know potatoes must be stored in the dark so that solanine won't be synthesized. Grain elevator operators check grain deliveries under ultraviolet light for the presence of aflatoxins. And we have naturally limited our consumption of other toxins and developed cooking and food preparation methods to limit their potency. Some are toxic only in doses higher than people ordinarily consume. For example, the amount of saponins in alfalfa sprouts eaten on a sandwich or salad daily will not harm you. Nevertheless, it is important to understand that some potentially harmful chemicals in foods occur naturally.

• • • •

Overall, the best practice with regard to minimizing exposure to environmental contaminants and naturally occurring toxins is to emphasize variety and moderation in selecting foods. A general program also includes (1) learning which foods pose risks, (2) thoroughly rinsing and scrubbing fruits and vegetables, (3) removing outer leaves of leafy vegetables, (4) eating smaller, rather than the larger, species of freshwater game fish (toxins accumulate more over the longer lifetime of the larger fish), (5) trimming fat and skin from meat, poultry, and fish, and (6) discarding any fat that is rendered from meat or fish during cooking. This practice helps, because many food contaminants dissolve in fat.[10]

SUMMARY

- Bacteria and other microbes in foods are the agents most likely to cause food-borne illness. To guard against this in the past, people used salt, sugar, smoke, fermentation, and drying to preserve foods. Today, we also recognize the importance of proper cooking and of keeping hot foods hot and cold foods cold. Pasteurization has also greatly improved the safety of dairy products.
- Cross-contamination commonly causes food-borne illness. It occurs when bacteria on raw animal products reach other foods that can support bacterial growth. Because of the risk of cross-contamination, no food should be kept at room temperature for more than 2 hours if it has come in contact with raw animal products and can support bacterial growth.
- Treatment for food-borne illness usually requires drinking a lot of fluids, avoiding food handling while diarrhea is present, thorough hand washing, and bed rest.
- The major causes of food-borne illness today are the bacteria *Salmonella, Staphylococcus aureus,* and *Clostridium perfringens.* To protect against these agents, cover cuts on the hands, do not sneeze on foods, avoid contact between raw meat or poultry products and other food products, and rapidly cool and then thoroughly reheat leftovers. Thorough cooking of foods and the use of pasteurized dairy products further protect against other problem microbes. Viruses, molds, and parasites also account for many cases of food-borne illness. Again, taking care to select, handle, and cook foods properly can prevent problems.

- Food additives are used primarily to extend shelf life by preventing microbial growth and destruction of food components by oxygen, certain chemical ions, and other substances. Food additives are classed as those intentionally added to foods and those that incidentally end up as contaminants in foods. An additive to a food is limited by FDA to at most 1/100 of the greatest amount that causes no observable effects in animals. In most cases, the Delaney Clause bans the use of any intentional food additive introduced after 1958 in the United States if it causes cancer.
- Antioxidants, such as vitamin E and sulfites, prevent oxygen and enzyme destruction of food products. Emulsifiers suspend fat in water, improving the uniformity, smoothness, and body of foods, such as ice cream. Common antimicrobial agents include sodium benzoate and sorbic acid, which prevent bacterial growth. Sequestrants bind free chemical ions, preventing them from causing fats to become rancid.
- A variety of environmental contaminants can be found in food. Because most of them dissolve in fat, trimming fat from meats and discarding fat that is rendered during cooking of meats, fish, and poultry are good steps to minimize exposure. In addition, it is helpful to wash fruits and vegetables thoroughly and to discard the outer leaves of leafy vegetables.
- Toxic substances occur naturally in a variety of foods, such as green potatoes, moldy grains, raw soybeans, and raw egg whites. Cooking foods limits their toxic effects. Over the centuries, people have purposely avoided some of these foods, such as moldy grains and the green parts of potatoes.

Study Questions

1. Identify three major classes of microorganisms that are responsible for food-borne illness and explain how each differs in one key aspect.
2. Which kinds of foods are most likely to be involved in food-borne illness? Why is this so?
3. Discuss five techniques that are important in preventing the spread of food-borne illness.
4. Define the term food additive and give examples of four intentional food additives. What is the specific function of each in foods? What is their relationship to the GRAS list?
5. Discuss the federal legislation that governs the use of food additives, including the Delaney clause?

References

1. Agency for Toxic Substances and Disease Registry: Mercury toxicity, *American Family Physician* 46:1731, 1992.
2. American Dietetic Association: Food and water safety, *Journal of the American Dietetic Association* 90:111, 1990.
3. Blair D: Uncertainties in pesticide risk estimation and consumer concern, *Nutrition Today,* p. 13, November/December 1989.
4. Blumenthal D: Deciding about dioxins, *FDA Consumer,* p. 10, February 1990.
5. Chao J, Kikano GE: Lead poisoning in children, *American Family Physician* 47:113, 1993.
6. Conley ST: What do consumers think about irradiated foods? *FSIS Food Safety Review,* p. 11, Fall 1992.
7. Czachor JS: Unusual aspects of bacterial water-borne illnesses, *American Family Physician* 46:797, 1992.
8. Expert Panel on Food Safety and Nutrition: Government regulation of food safety: interaction of scientific and societal forces, *Food Technology,* p. 73, January 1992.
9. Foulke JE: High-tech tools for food safety sleuths, *FDA Consumer,* p. 7, November 1992.
10. Foulke JE: FDA reports on pesticides in foods, *FDA Consumer,* p. 29, June 1993.
11. Hecht A: Preventing food-borne illness, *FDA Consumer,* p. 18, January/February 1991.
12. Hedberg CW and others: A multistate outbreak of *Salmonella javiana* and *Salmonella oranienburg* infections due to consumption of contaminated cheese, *Journal of the American Medical Association* 268:3203, 1992.
13. Hedberg CW and others: An international foodborne outbreak of *Shigellosis* associated with a commercial airline, *Journal of the American Medical Association* 268:3208, 1992.
14. Mahaffey KR: Exposure to lead in childhood, *The New England Journal of Medicine* 327:1308, 1992.
15. Mason J: Food irradiation: let's move ahead, *American Family Physician,* 47:1064, 1993.
16. Newberne PM: Naturally occurring foodborne toxicants. In Schills ME, Young VR, editors: *Modern nutrition in health and disease,* Philadelphia, 1988, Lea & Febiger.
17. Ryser ET, Marth EH: New food-borne pathogens of public health significance, *Journal of the American Dietetic Association* 89:948, 1989.
18. Schlech WF: Expanding the horizons of foodborne listeriosis, *Journal of the American Medical Association* 267:2081, 1992.
19. Segal M: Parasitic invaders, *FDA Consumer,* p. 7, July/August 1993.
20. Thayer AM: Food additives, *Chemical & Engineering News,* p. 26, June 15, 1992.
21. Thonney PR, Bisogni CA: Residues of agricultural chemicals on fruits and vegetables, *Nutrition Today,* p. 6, November/December, 1989.
22. Tritsch GL: Food irradiation, *Nutrition Reviews* 50:311, 1992.
23. Wood RC and others: *Campylobacter enteritis* outbreaks associated with drinking raw milk during youth activities, *Journal of the American Medical Association* 268:3228, 1992.

CAN YOU CHOOSE THE IMPROPER FOOD SAFETY PRACTICES?

In this chapter you learned the following facts:

- One third to one half of all diarrhea cases in America are induced by food-borne organisms.
- Diarrhea caused by food-borne illness hits about one of every ten to thirty-five Americans per year.

Carefully preparing foods to prevent food-borne illness can minimize its occurrence for most of us. Read the excerpt below and pick out the food safety violations that could contribute to food-borne illness.

John Noseguard, a local health department inspector, gives the following account of his visit to a local diner:

Workers at the Morningside Diner try hard to give good service and provide tasty, satisfying food. As I walked through the kitchen, I noticed that each food handler washed his/her hands thoroughly with hot, soapy water before handling the food, especially after handling raw meat, fish, poultry, or eggs. Before preparing raw foods they also thoroughly wash the cutting boards, dishes, and other equipment. As they use their cutting boards, after cutting food, they wipe them with a damp rag and use them again to cut more food.

When preparing fresh fruits and vegetables, they wash them but are careful to leave a little dirt on them for fear of washing important nutrients from the outside. The cooks generally cook meats to an internal temperature of 180° F (82° C). However, for pork, to preserve the flavor, it is cooked to an internal temperature of 140° F (60° C). Some cooked foods, which are to be served later, are cooled to 40° F (4° C) within 2 hours, and foods like beef stew are cooled in shallow pans.

To save the customer money, the management of the diner uses canned foods, even when the cans are dented. Often these can be purchased at lower prices. When leftovers are reheated, they are raised to an internal temperature of 150° F (66° C) and served. Food handlers take great care to remove moldy portions of food. The cooks prepare stuffing separately from the poultry. The temperature of their refrigerators was approximately 55° F (13° C).

1. Below, list the violations of food safety practices that could contribute to food-borne illness.

____

____

____

2. If you were writing a report describing ways the Morningside Diner could correct these practices, what would you say?

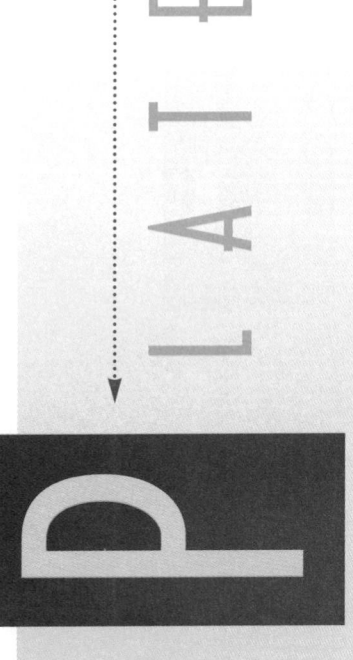

____

____

____

N u t r i t i o n ISSUE

PESTICIDES IN FOODS

Pesticides used in food production produce both good and unwanted effects. Most health authorities feel the benefits outweigh the risks. Pesticides help ensure an adequate food supply, make foods available at reasonable cost, and help ensure safety of the food supply. Alternatively, sentiment is growing nationwide that pesticides pose significant and avoidable health risks. Consumers have come to assume that man-made is dangerous and "organic" is safe. But such is not always the case. Some researchers believe this sentiment is grounded in fear and fueled by unbalanced reports. Other researchers say concern about pesticides is valid and overdue.[3]

The public is struggling to make sense of conflicting information. Most concern about pesticide residues in foods focuses on chronic rather than acute toxicity, because the amounts of residues, if present at all, are extremely small. These low concentrations found in foods are not known to produce adverse effects in the short term, although the high levels that occasionally result from accidents or misuse have done so. For humans, pesticides pose a danger mainly in their cumulative effects.[3] Hence, their threats to health are difficult to determine. However, growing evidence, including the problems of contamination of underground water supplies,[1] indicates that we would likely be better off as a nation if we could reduce our exposure to pesticides.

another BITE

Alar in apples illustrates the public's problem with conflicting information. Apple growers have routinely sprayed Alar on trees to control ripening. We now know that one component of Alar changes into a potential carcinogen when heated, as it is when apples are processed into juice. Manufacturers and apple growers have now moved quickly to eliminate the use of Alar. Still, as some school systems were taking apples off menus, the U.S. Environmental Protection Agency (EPA) stated that it is unlikely that a person would be harmed from eating apples containing Alar.

What Is a Pesticide?

Federal law defines a pesticide as any substance or mixture of substances intended to prevent, destroy, repel, or mitigate any pest.[21] Their built-in toxic properties lead to the possibility that other nontarget organisms, including humans, might also be harmed. The term *pesticide* tends to be used as a generic reference to many types of products, including insecticides, herbicides, fungicides, and rodenticides. A pesticide product may be chemical or bacterial, natural or man-made. For agriculture, EPA allows about 10,000 pesticide uses, involving some 300 active ingredients.[21] Pesticide use in general substantially contributes to the chemical load applied intentionally to the earth's surface. About 2.6 billion pounds of pesticides are used each year in the United States, 60% of which is applied to agricultural crops (Figure 17-8).[3]

Once a pesticide is applied, it can turn up in a number of unintended and unwanted places. It may be carried in the air and dust by wind currents, remain in soil attached to soil particles, be taken up by organisms in the soil, decompose to other compounds, be taken up by plant roots, or enter aquatic habitats. Each is a route to the food chain; some are more direct than others.

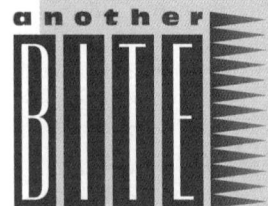

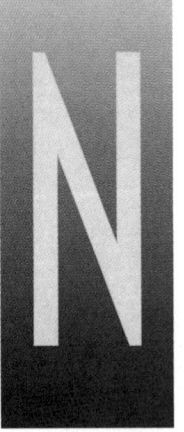

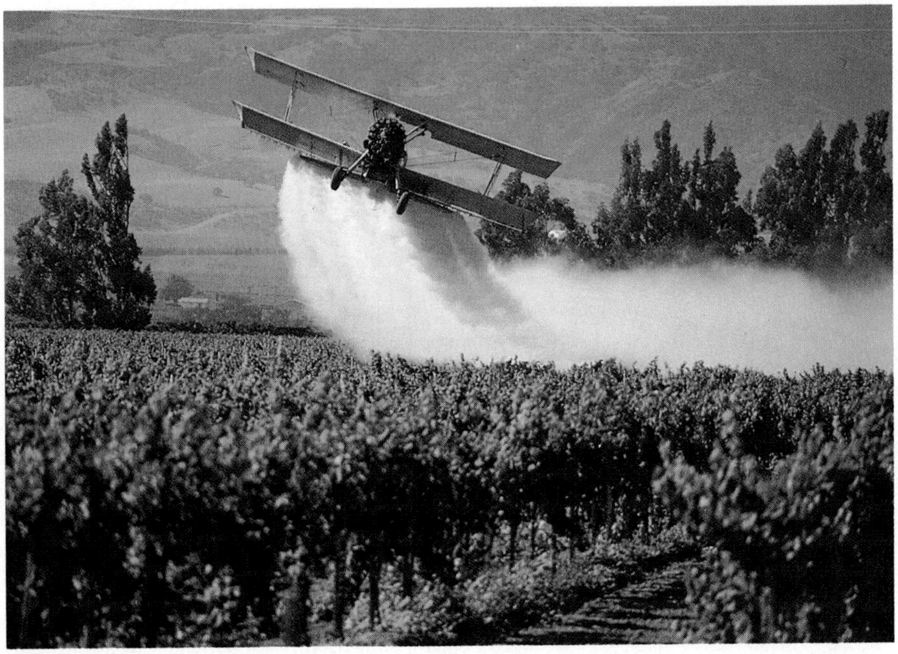

FIGURE 17-8
Pesticide use poses a risk versus benefit question. Each side raises points we need to consider.

Why Use Pesticides?

In the United States alone, pests destroy nearly $20 billion of food crops yearly, despite extensive pesticide use. The primary reason for using pesticides is economic—use of agricultural chemicals increases production and lowers the cost of food, at least in the short run. It decreases erosion by eliminating cultivation otherwise needed to get rid of weeds. Many farmers feel that they would have a tough time staying in business without pesticides. Quick and direct, pesticides help protect farmers from ruinous losses caused by a sudden pest outbreak. Unless pesticides are applied, farming must depend much more on crop rotation to limit damage from pests. Government subsidies in the United States that encourage planting the same crops year after year discourage crop rotation, and so stimulate pesticide use. (See the discussion on sustainable agriculture in Chapter 18. Crop rotation is a key feature of that farming technology.)

Still, pesticides also create new pests, because they destroy the spiders, wasps, and predatory beetles that naturally keep most plant-feeding insect populations in check. The brown plant hopper that has recently plagued Indonesian rice fields was not a serious problem before heavy insecticide use began in the early 1970s. In the United States, such major pests as spider mites and the cotton bollworm were merely nuisances until spraying decimated their predators.

About 40% of the pesticides are used by the homeowner and gardener. An important environmental problem is the improper disposal of the products by these users.

Consumer demands have also changed over the years. At one time we would not think twice about buying an apple with a worm hole; we simply took it home, cut out the wormy part, and ate the apple. Today, consumers find worm holes less acceptable, and so farmers rely more and more on pesticides to produce cosmetically attractive fruits and vegetables. On the practical side, pesticides can protect against rotting and decay of fresh fruits and vegetables. This is helpful, because our food distribution system does not usually permit consumer purchase within hours of harvest. Also, food grown without pesticides can contain naturally occurring organisms that produce carcinogens at levels far above current standards for pesticide residues. For example, fungicides help prevent the potent carcinogen aflatoxin (caused by growth of a fungus) from forming on some crops. So while some pesticides may improve the appearance of food products, others help keep some foods fresher and safer to eat.

Regulating Pesticides

Currently, a newly proposed pesticide is exhaustively tested, perhaps over 10 years or more, before it can be used. The EPA must decide both that the pesticide causes no unreasonable adverse effects to people and the environment and that benefits outweigh the risks of using it. However, there is concern about older chemicals registered before 1970, when less stringent testing conditions were permitted.[3] EPA is now asking chemical companies to retest the old compounds using more rigorous tests. But inadequate funding at EPA has hampered the review of older pesticides. The slow pace for this retesting has angered the critics of pesticide use. When weighing whether to approve or cancel a pesticide, EPA considers how much more it would cost the farmer to use an alternative pesticide or process and whether cancellation would decrease productivity. After determining the dollar cost to the farmer, EPA then looks at costs to processors and consumers as well.

If EPA suspects that any pesticide poses an imminent hazard to health, the agency can immediately stop its use.

Once a pesticide is approved for use, at least a 100-fold margin of safety is a standard requirement for contamination levels in food to minimize health effects other than cancer (such as kidney damage or birth defects).[8] These tolerances (limits) used for foods set the safety standard at 100 times less than the highest dose at which the pesticide causes no ill effects in animals—or lower. If the pesticide causes cancer, its use must not incur more than one cancer case in 1 million people. And, if the pesticide causes cancer and its level in finished foods is much greater than that allowed for use on crops, generally its use is banned by the Delaney Clause.[3] We noted earlier that there are proposals to stop the use of the Delaney Clause for pesticides and replace it with a simple standard such as a risk of "no more than one cancer case in one million people" as a guideline for use.

How Safe Are Pesticides?

A person's risk of poisoning from exposure to pesticides through food depends on how potent the chemical poison is, how concentrated it is in the food, how much and how frequently it's eaten, and the person's resistance or susceptibility to the substance. Pesticide use is clearly associated with impure water quality. Accumulating information also links pesticide use to increased cancer rates in farm communities. For U.S. rural counties, the incidence of lymph, genital, brain, and digestive tract cancers increases with higher-than-average herbicide use.[3] Respiratory cancer cases increase with greater insecticide use. In tests using laboratory animals, scientists have found that some of the chemicals present in pesticide residues cause birth defects, sterility, tumors, organ damage, and injury to the central nervous system. Some pesticides persist in the environment for years.

Still, some researchers argue that the cancer risk from pesticide residues is hundreds of times less than the risk of eating such common foods as peanut butter, brown mustard, and basil. Plants manufacture their own toxic substances to defend themselves against insects, birds, and grazing animals (including humans). When plants are stressed or damaged, they produce even more of these toxins. Because of this, many foods contain naturally occurring chemicals considered toxic, even carcinogenic. Other scientists argue that if natural carcinogens in large numbers are already in the food supply, then we should reduce the number of added carcinogens whenever possible. In other words, we should do what we can to decrease the problem.

The mere presence of a pesticide in food or water at any concentration frightens some people. But the levels of pesticide residues found in foods are almost always well below the tolerance levels that have been set to meet safety concerns. High and obviously hazardous concentrations are very rare and are usually the result of spills or improper uses. But the major challenge for scientists and regulators goes beyond detecting and measuring pesticide residues; it is rather a question of what, if any, biological significance they have.[21]

The Risks of Pesticides to Children

Any discussions of pesticides and associated health risks need to focus attention on children. They are not simply small adults in a biological sense. Hence, children face a higher risk from pesticides than adults for several reasons[3]:

1. Their exposure is greater; children eat more food in proportion to their body weight than do adults.
2. Children consume more foods that are potential sources of pesticide residues than do adults. They eat more fruit, for example.
3. Exposure at an early age carries a greater risk than does exposure later in life; residues accumulate to toxic levels over a longer period. Also, cancer has more time to develop.
4. Physiological susceptibility to the effects of carcinogens and neurotoxins in pesticides may be greater; the cells in children are dividing rapidly and the enzyme systems that detoxify chemicals are not fully developed.

Until recent years, EPA did not consider these factors in risk calculations. EPA now looks at age-level consumption data for approval of new pesticides. Although children are at greater risk from pesticides, the magnitude of that risk and how best to calculate it are open to debate. One general precaution is to keep children away from lawns, gardens, and flower beds that have been treated with pesticides and herbicides by the homeowner. Carefully washing fruits and vegetables and consuming a wide variety are other good recommendations.

Testing Levels of Pesticides in Foods

FDA tests thousands of raw products a year for pesticide residues and consistently finds 96% to 98% free of illegal residues. (A pesticide is considered illegal in this case if it is not approved for use on the crop in question or if the amount used exceeds the allowed levels.) Residues sometimes appear on the wrong crops or in excess amounts, because of contamination from nearby farms via wind or water. Still, actual crop residues are usually considerably lower than the legal limits, because worst-case scenarios of crop treatment and residue level are used to set the limits. When a problem is identified, FDA takes steps to make sure it's corrected and that the tainted food in question never reaches the consumer. However, of 600 pesticides available on international markets, many are not even detected by any of FDA's multiresidue tests.[3] This has raised concern by pesticide critics with regard to imported foods. Better tests that detect single residues are less frequently used because of cost.

Personal Action

We often take risks in our own lives, but we prefer to have a choice in the matter after weighing the pros and cons. For instance, we can choose not to immunize a child, but we do so with the understanding that the child might get sick. Or we can downhill ski or drive recklessly. These are personal risks that we choose to take. One can also choose to risk cancer from smoking or to avoid that risk. But in regard to pesticides in produce, someone else is deciding what is acceptable and what is not. Our only choice is whether to buy or avoid pesticide-containing foods. And in reality it is almost impossible to avoid pesticides entirely, because even organic produce often contains traces of pesticides, probably cross-contaminated from nearby farms.

Short-term studies of the effects of pesticides on laboratory animals cannot pinpoint long-term cancer risks precisely. But it should be clearly understood that the presence of minute traces of an environmental chemical in a food does not mean that any adverse effect will result from eating that food. FDA feels that the hazards are comparatively low and, in the short run, are less than the hazards of food-borne illness created in our own kitchens. We can't avoid the risks entirely, but we can limit pesticide exposure by following the advice previously given in this chapter.

In the future, we can encourage farmers to use fewer pesticides to protect our foods and water supplies and we will have to settle for produce that isn't perfect in appearance. Are you concerned enough about pesticides on food to change your shopping habits and take more political action?

c h a p t e r

18

UNDERNUTRITION THROUGHOUT THE WORLD

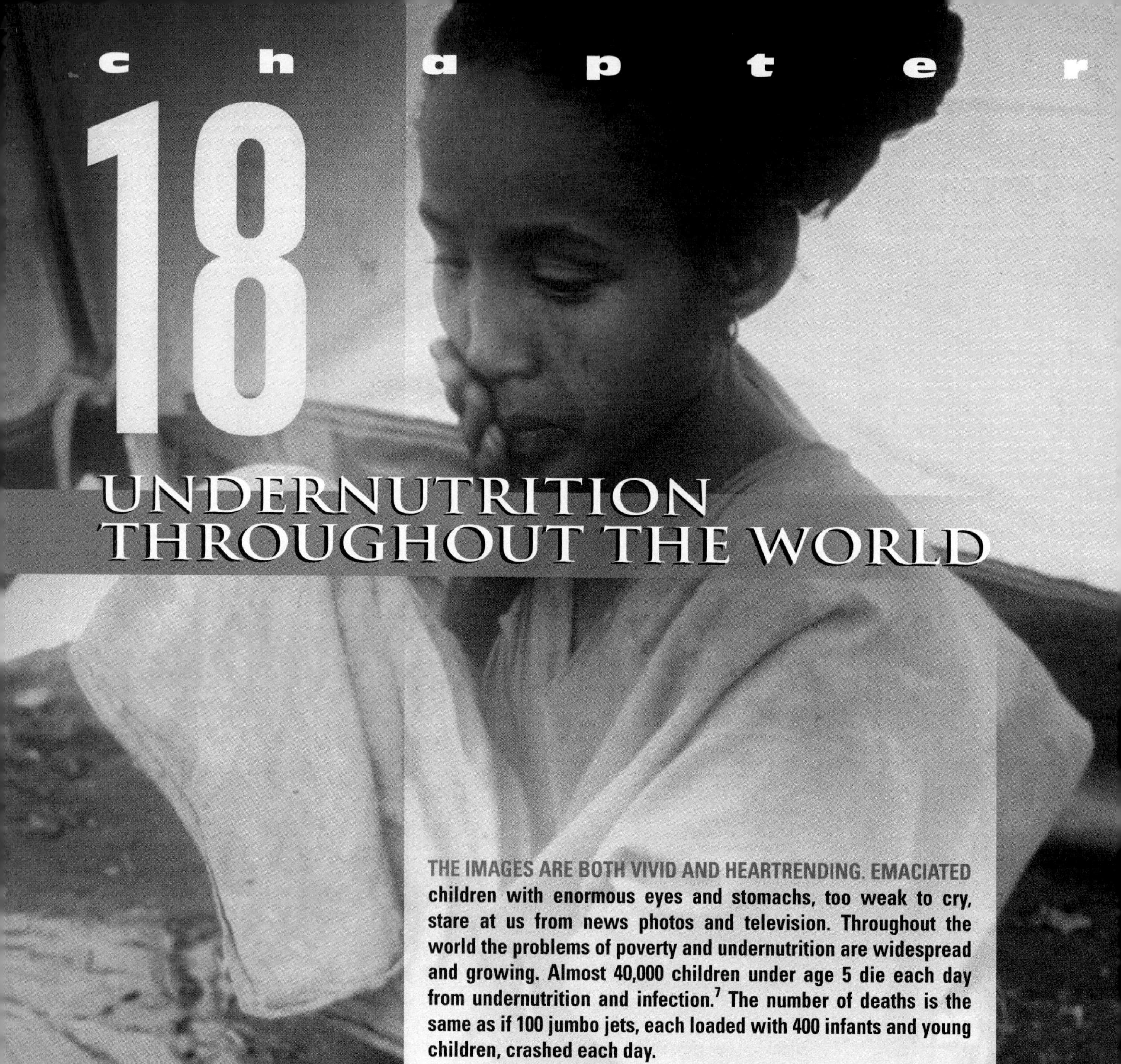

THE IMAGES ARE BOTH VIVID AND HEARTRENDING. EMACIATED children with enormous eyes and stomachs, too weak to cry, stare at us from news photos and television. Throughout the world the problems of poverty and undernutrition are widespread and growing. Almost 40,000 children under age 5 die each day from undernutrition and infection.[7] The number of deaths is the same as if 100 jumbo jets, each loaded with 400 infants and young children, crashed each day.

The majority (two thirds) of hungry people live in Asia.[7] Currently the largest increases in numbers of chronically hungry people occur each year in Africa, particularly in Chad, Sudan, Angola, Ethiopia, Mozambique, Somalia, Uganda, Zaire, and Zambia. At least 40% of the people in these countries are considered food insecure by the World Food Council. Theirs are just some of the eyes that haunt us.

In this chapter we examine the problem of undernutrition and the conditions that create it. We look at the causes, as well as some solutions. If we are to eradicate undernutrition, all of us will have to be responsible for supplying some answers to these problems, especially since Western societies have contributed to much of the economic and social destruction of the Third World.

ASSESS

TEST YOUR KNOWLEDGE yourself

BROADENING A NARROW VISION

Many people in the United States are unaware of the magnitude of undernutrition in the world, as well as in this country itself. Reading this chapter will open your eyes to the nutritional state of the world's peoples. You will discover what you can do to help correct the problem. But before you read this chapter, think about the following questions and provide the best answers you can.

1. Who is most likely to experience undernutrition in the United States?

2. What are the major causes of undernutrition in the United States?

3. What are the major causes of undernutrition in the developing countries of the world?

4. To what degree are you concerned about undernutrition in the United States and the world?

These questions are designed to spur you to think about the issues addressed in this chapter. As you read this chapter, these and other questions will be answered.

WORLD HUNGER CONTINUES TO PLAGUE US

In November 1974, the United Nations World Food Conference proclaimed the bold objective "that within a decade no child will go to bed hungry, that no family will fear for its next day's bread, and that no human being's future and capacities will be stunted by malnutrition." Not only does this promise remain unfulfilled, 17 years later hunger is a daily experience for one in eight people.[7]

The famines that occurred in Ethiopia in the 1980s called special attention to the problem of undernutrition in the developing world. The plight of millions of starving people consolidated widespread public support for immediate aid for the victims of famine. Still, hunger is not abated. It is still frequently in the news. Continuing civil wars in Africa, coupled with drought, have brought more than 30 million people to the brink of starvation. Relief aid has been arriving, but often too little, too late. The deadly combination of war and poor weather has also led to increasing hunger recently in Somalia, Sudan, Angola, Mozambique, Bangladesh, Afghanistan, the Philippines, and Cambodia.[7] As you might surmise, the problem of undernutrition in developing nations is ongoing and one that requires political and technological solutions.

UNDERNUTRITION AND POVERTY

Let's begin our look at these problems by first defining some key words:

Hunger is the physiological state that results when not enough food is eaten to meet energy needs. It also describes an uneasiness, discomfort, weakness, or pain caused by lack of food. If hunger is not attended to, the resulting medical and social costs from undernutrition are high—premature births and mental retardation, inadequate growth and development in childhood that contribute to poor school performance, decreased work output in adulthood, and chronic disease (Table 18-1).[5] Symptoms of chronic hunger are found not only in the developing world, but also in many people living at or below the poverty level in America.[2]

The primary cause of chronic hunger is poverty. Unemployment and underemployment, homelessness, drug addiction, functional illiteracy, single-parent families (often headed by a woman who has limited earning potential), wage discrimination, poor health,

TABLE 18-1

The Realities of Undernutrition

- Nearly one in five people worldwide is chronically undernourished—too hungry to lead a productive, active life.
- Today, 60,000 people will die of hunger—two thirds of them children.
- Approximately half of all children who die each year in developing countries do so from causes that could be prevented at low cost.
- At least 250,000 children are permanently blinded each year simply through lack of vitamin A.
- Women in poor countries average up to four times more births than women in the United States.
- Every day, the world produces about 3000 kcalories for each person, well above the average need of 2300 kcalories.
- Poor women in Third World countries face a 300-fold increased risk of death in pregnancy compared with women in the United States.
- In many developing countries, life expectancy of the population is one half to two thirds of that in the United States.
- Almost half of the world's people earn less than $200 a year—many use 80% to 90% of that income to obtain food. About $2000 to $3000 each year per person is needed for life expectancy to reach that seen the United States.
- Of the nearly 5.4 billion people on earth, more than 1.2 billion drink contaminated water.
- 1.8 billion people in the world are without proper sanitation facilities.
- Developing countries have two thirds of the 8 to 10 million AIDS cases worldwide.

inadequate governmental programs, and war/civil strife all contribute to this poverty. In developing nations the problems stemming from poverty, a lack of resources, and inadequate governmental programs are intensified.[7]

Malnutrition is a condition of impaired development or function caused by a long-term deficiency, excess, or imbalance in energy and/or nutrient intake. The occurrence of specific diseases of malnutrition depends mostly on the food/population ratio.[17] When food supplies are low and the population is large, undernutrition leading to nutritional deficiency diseases, such as goiter[20] and xerophthalmia (eye problems caused by a poor vitamin A intake), is common. However, when the food supply is ample or overabundant, poor food choices coupled with an excessive intake can lead to nutrition-related chronic diseases, such as certain forms of diabetes. Note, however, pockets of undernutrition among the poor may still be found in food-abundant areas, such as the United States.

Genetics contributes significantly to both forms of malnutrition. Not every child in Thailand who eats mainly rice develops ***protein-energy malnutrition (PEM)***; similarly, not every adult in New York City who consumes a high-fat, high-kcalorie diet suffers a heart attack.[17] Genetics influences the development of these diseases.

Undernutrition, referred to many times in this book, is the malnutrition that results from an inadequate intake, absorption, or use of the nutrients or energy needed for optimal growth, development, and body function. The earliest response to undernutrition is to reduce activity. This allows the individual to preserve energy for growth and other vital functions. With persistent undernutrition, the second response is a reduced rate of weight gain or poor weight maintenance. Later, in children, the rate of growth in height is reduced.[22]

Undernutrition is the most common form of malnutrition among the poor in both developing and developed countries. It is also the primary cause of specific nutrient deficiencies that in turn can result in muscle wasting, blindness (from xerophthalmia), scurvy, pellagra, beriberi, anemia, rickets, goiter, and a host of other effects[23] (Table 18-2). For example, more than 250,000 children develop blindness from xerophthalmia each year. This vitamin deficiency also raises the risk for other diseases, such as measles.[9] About half of all women in the Third World suffer from anemia caused by iron deficiency and malaria. Of the 5.4 billion people in the world, at least half a billion have some form of undernutrition.[7] Death and disease from infections, particularly those causing acute and prolonged diarrhea or acute lower respiratory disease, are dramatically increased when the infections are superimposed on a state of chronic undernutrition.[24]

Protein-energy malnutrition (PEM) is a form of undernutrition caused by an extremely deficient intake of energy and/or protein. The typically dramatic results of PEM—kwashiorkor and marasmus—were covered in Chapter 7. We will concentrate in this chapter on the more subtle effects of a chronic food insufficiency.

Malnutrition ■
Failing health that results from a long-standing dietary intake that either fails to meet or greatly exceeds nutritional needs.

Undernutrition ■
Failing health that results from a long-standing dietary intake that does not meet nutritional needs.

Protein-Energy Malnutrition (PEM) ■
This results when a person regularly consumes insufficient amounts of kcalories and protein. The deficiency eventually results in body wasting and an increased susceptibility to infections.

CONSEQUENCES OF UNDERNUTRITION—A CLOSER LOOK

Prolonged undernutrition is detrimental to health at any time throughout life, but consequences are more critical during some periods of growth and throughout the elderly years.

The Critical Periods

The human organism is particularly susceptible to the effects of undernutrition during periods of rapid growth, especially pregnancy, infancy, and childhood.

Pregnancy. The period of greatest health risk from undernutrition is during pregnancy. A pregnant woman needs extra nutrients to meet her own needs, as well as those of her developing fetus. If the mother's nutrient intake is inadequate during pregnancy, her own health can be seriously jeopardized. Stores of maternal nutrients may be depleted to provide for the baby. Maternal iron-deficiency anemia is one possible consequence. Pregnancy-induced hypertension (preeclampsia), a life-threatening condition involving rapid weight gain from fluid retention and a sharp increase in blood pressure, is also likely to be influenced by inadequate prenatal nutrition.

TABLE 18-2

Nutrient Deficiency Diseases Common Accompanying States of Undernutrition in the World

Disease and Key Nutrient Involved	Typical Result	Excellent Dietary Sources for the Nutrient
Xerophthalmia Vitamin A	Blindness, poor growth, increased infections	Liver, fortified milk, sweet potatoes, spinach, greens, carrots, cantaloupe, apricots
Rickets Vitamin D	Weakened bones, bow legs, fractures	Fortified milk, fish oils, sun exposure
Beriberi Thiamin	Nerve degeneration, poor muscle coordination, heart problems	Sunflower seeds, pork, whole and enriched grains, dried beans
Ariboflavinosis Riboflavin	Inflammation of face and oral cavity	Milk, mushrooms, spinach, liver, enriched grains
Pellagra Niacin	Diarrhea, skin inflammation, mental deterioration	Mushrooms, bran, tuna, chicken, beef, peanuts, whole and enriched grains
Scurvy Vitamin C	Poor wound healing, bleeding skin and gums	Citrus fruits, strawberries, broccoli
Iron-deficiency anemia Iron	Poor work output, poor growth, increased health risk in pregnancy	Meats, spinach, seafood, broccoli, peas, bran, whole-grain and enriched breads
Goiter Iodide	Enlarged thyroid gland, poor growth in infancy and childhood, possible mental retardation	Iodized salt, saltwater fish

Note that often two or more nutrition-deficiency diseases are found in an undernourished person in the Third World. This separate discussion of nutrients just makes it easier to see the important role of each nutrient.

In Africa, women give birth, on average, to more than six live babies. Coupled with chronic undernutrition, this high birthrate creates a 1 in 20 lifetime risk of dying from pregnancy-related causes for women. In contrast, American women face a risk of 1 death in about 6000 births from pregnancy-related causes. No other social indicator—literacy, life expectancy, and infant mortality included—shows a wider gap between the developing world and the industrialized world.[7]

Fetal and Infant Stages. The greatest risk from undernutrition during gestation is actually borne by the fetus. As it develops, a growing fetus requires a diet rich in protein, vitamins, and minerals. When these needs are not met, the infant is often born before 37 weeks of ***gestation***—about 40 weeks of gestation is ideal. Results of prematurity include poor lung function and a weakened immune response. These conditions lessen health and make death more likely. Long-term problems in growth and development can result if the infant does survive. At the extreme, low-birth-weight babies—2500 grams or less (about 5.5 pounds or less)—face 30 to 40 times the normal risk of dying before the age of 1 year, primarily because of their poor lung development. When low birth weight is accompanied by other physical abnormalities, medical intervention can cost $100,000 or more. When severe retardation occurs, the lifetime cost of care can be over $2 million.

Gestation *The time between conception and the birth of the infant.*

In the United States, low birth weight accounts for more than half of all infant deaths and for 75% of deaths of babies under 1 month of age. Worldwide, more than half of infant deaths stem from low birth weight.

Childhood. The rapid growth years of early childhood compose another period of high risk from undernutrition.[12] Because the human brain grows most rapidly from conception through early childhood, the brain and central nervous system are particularly vulnerable. After the preschool years, brain growth and development slow dramatically until maturity, when they stop. Nutritional deprivation, especially in early infancy, can lead to permanent brain impairment. Beyond early childhood, learning may be jeopardized by a deprived environment, but the basic size and structure of the brain are set.[11]

In general, poor children experience more nutritional deprivation and overall illness and are more severely affected by these effects than are other children. For example, iron-deficiency anemia, indicated by the presence of an abnormally low concentration of hemoglobin in the blood, is much more common among poor children than nonpoor children. This deficiency can lead to reduced stamina and learning problems. Undernutrition in childhood can also weaken resistance to infection, because immune function decreases when such nutrients as protein and zinc are very low in a diet.[6,21] Poorly nourished youngsters are then at risk for more frequent colds, ear infections, and other infectious diseases.

When adequate nutrients are restored to the diet of children, improvements in health can be obvious. For example, in recent years the height of several groups of growth-retarded children in the United States, including Hispanic children in Colorado, has been shown to increase after zinc supplementation. Note that nearly half of all black children in the United States live in poverty.

another BITE

Symptoms of undernutrition in children are not always obvious. Visitors to developing countries may not notice undernutrition in children—children who appear to be 3 or 4 years old actually may be 8 or 9 years old. Failure of children to grow is a common result of undernutrition and a warning sign that more extreme effects may follow. In a recent survey of 76 developing countries, stunting was seen in more than one third of children aged 2 to 5 years old.[2]

The Elderly. We need to consider one more group at risk for undernutrition—elderly and chronically ill persons. These people often require nutrient-dense foods, the amount depending on each person's state of health and level of activity. Because many have fixed incomes and significant medical costs, food can end up as a low-priority item. In addition, elderly and chronically ill people are often unable to take care of all their own needs, are sometimes isolated, and are more apt to be depressed—all important factors that can influence food intake.

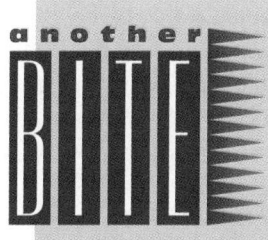

General Effects of Semistarvation

The results of undernutrition from semistarvation in the initial stages are often so mild that physical symptoms are absent, and blood tests typically do not detect the slight changes in metabolism. Even in the absence of clinical symptoms, however, undernourishment may affect reproductive capacity, resistance to or recovery from disease, activity and work output, and attitudes and behavior. Recall from Chapter 2 that as tissues continue to be depleted of nutrients, blood tests eventually detect biochemical changes, such as a drop in blood hemoglobin concentration. Physical symptoms, such as body weakness, become apparent with further depletion. Finally, the full-blown symptoms of the predominating deficiency become obvious enough to be recognized, such as edema associated with a protein deficiency.

In general, the occurrence of severe deficiency in a few people in a population represents the tip of the iceberg. This usually means that a much greater number have milder degrees of undernutrition. As we have noted, mild nutrient deficiencies, though perhaps not life threatening, can in certain critical combinations still cause very important practical difficulties in health, as well as in life in general. These should not, therefore, be dismissed as trivial, especially in the developing world.[5] It is becoming clear that combined deficiencies of certain vitamins, iron, and zinc, although less severe than those causing overt physical symptoms, can seriously reduce work performance. ***Marginal*** deficiencies of iodide, iron, and zinc are known to affect hundreds of millions of people worldwide.

Marginal *Noticeable, but not severe.*

Detailed experiments studying the effects of chronic undernutrition were performed by a group of scientists led by Dr. Ansel Keys in the 1940s. They maintained 32 previously healthy men on a diet averaging about 1600 kcalories daily for 6 months. During this time the men lost an average of 24% of their body weight. After about 3 months, the subjects complained of tiredness, muscle soreness, irritability, and hunger pains. They showed a loss of ambition, poor self-discipline, and poor concentration. They were often moody and depressed. Their ability to laugh heartily and sneeze was reduced, and they became intolerant to heat. Decreases in heart rate and muscle tone were also noted.

These cumulative stresses of undernutrition, then, eventually caused emotional instability and an overall apathetic frame of mind. Persistent hunger made it difficult for the subjects to pursue cultural interests, perform manual activities, and study. This in turn produced a frustrating discrepancy between their desire and ability to pursue activities. When they were permitted to eat normally again, even after 12 weeks of rehabilitation, the desire for more food and a feeling of tiredness continued for the subjects. By 20 weeks they had largely, but not fully, recovered—full recovery required about 33 weeks.

The effects of undernutrition in poor countries are likely even greater than that seen by Dr. Keys, because those subjects had adequate vitamin and mineral intakes. In addition, the populations in poorer countries must also contend with recurrent infections, poor sanitary conditions, extreme weather conditions, and regular exposure to very infectious diseases. Their greater nutrient requirements—especially iron—to combat rampant parasite and other infections compound the problem further. As mentioned before, both iron and zinc deficiency can lead to poor immune function and so increase the risk of disease caused by infections, such as diarrhea, pneumonia, and dysentery. This state of ill health in turn diminishes the ability of people, communities, and even whole countries to perform at peak levels of physical and mental capacity, robbing people and nations of human resources.[23]

As we mentioned earlier, a common consequence of undernutrition both in the United States and worldwide is an increased rate of infant mortality. The U.S. infant mortality rate is currently twenty-second worldwide. Contributing to infant mortality in the United States are teenage pregnancy and inadequate food intake. Young mothers frequently don't meet their nutrient needs, which in turn increases the risk of delivering a low-birth-weight infant. These babies have a much higher risk of catching life-threatening infections. And lack of food, whether for lack of money or poor food choices, compromises the health of many young children.

CONCEPT CHECK

Hunger is the uneasiness and pain that results when insufficient food is eaten to meet energy needs. Chronic hunger leads to undernutrition and, in turn, to growth failure for children and weakness in adults. Risk of infection increases and nutrient deficiency diseases also result. The primary cause of undernutrition is poverty. The critical periods when undernutrition most adversely influences health are pregnancy, infancy, childhood, and the elderly years. The effects in pregnancy and infancy are quite dramatic, as evidenced by mortality rates much higher than those of healthy populations.

UNDERNUTRITION IN THE UNITED STATES

About 36 million Americans live at or near the poverty level currently estimated at about $14,350 annually for a family of four, or earnings of $6,970 or less for an individual. More than two thirds of these people, or 9% of the total population of the United States, live in metropolitan areas. These poor include nearly a quarter of all children.[7] Overall, African-Americans have the highest poverty rate of any racial group—32%. The poverty rate for Caucasians is 11%; Hispanics, 28%; and Asians and Pacific Islanders, 12%.

About two thirds—24 million—of these Americans experience chronic hunger; 8 million are children—about 20% of all children. These citizens eat enough to prevent overt starvation, so undernutrition in the United States presents itself quite differently from that in the developing world. Kwashiorkor and marasmus, evident in the pictures of Ethiopian children in the mid-1980s and Somalian children in the 1990s, rarely occur. Undernutrition is instead reflected in the young child whose weight is several pounds below the low end of the normal range on a growth chart.[4] The untrained eye may not recognize the condition or may simply see the child as skinny. The trained professional will recognize that the child's size reflects growth failure.

Poor Americans often face difficult choices: whether to buy groceries for the family or pay this month's rent; whether to have dental work done or pay the current utility bill; or whether to replace clothes the children have outgrown or pay for transportation to apply for a job. Food is one of the few flexible items in a poor person's budget. Rents are fixed, utility costs aren't negotiable, the price of medical care and prescription drugs can't be bargained down, and bus drivers won't accept less than the going rate to transport riders. But a person can always eat less. The short-term consequences may be less dramatic than having the utilities shut off. The long-term cumulative effects, however, are disturbing.[16]

In sheer numbers, as well as the severity of health risks posed, undernutrition in the United States is a troubling problem. Its existence is all the more disturbing because the threat of undernutrition for most Americans was virtually eliminated in the 1970s.[4] The fact that major pockets of undernutrition were conquered and then reemerged and spread rapidly in the 1980s suggests that the roots of undernutrition are mainly political and socioeconomic, rather than technical. Resources are available for feeding all Americans.[2] In the developing world, far more factors complicate this problem, as we will discuss later.

another BITE

The presence of undernutrition in the United States raises a broad question for our society at large: Where can people in such situations turn when their own resources fail? The responsibility for helping those in need could lie with the federal, state, and local governments; religious groups; charitable organizations; and perhaps with the individuals themselves. All can be part of the solution.

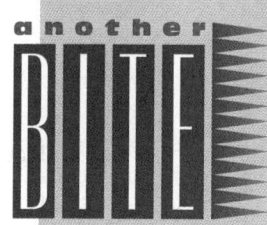

Undernutrition in the United States Is Not a New Problem

The problem of undernutrition in the United States actually began soon after the Pilgrims landed. Studies in the 1930s during the Depression documented both undernutrition and the existence of widespread pellagra (niacin deficiency) and rickets (vitamin D deficiency). In response, the government opened soup kitchens and began distributing food commodities.[14] Congress organized school lunch programs in 1946 after testimony by the United States Surgeon General that 70% of the men who had poor nutrition during the Depression era (10 to 12 years earlier) were being rejected for physical reasons by the draft.

In the 1950s, it was assumed that all Americans had enough to eat. Nevertheless, occasional reports of undernutrition surfaced, mostly among the chronic poor: migrant workers, Native Americans, Southern African-Americans, unemployed minorities, and some elderly people.

After observing extensive hunger and poverty during his presidential campaign, John F. Kennedy in the 1960s revitalized the food stamp program, a program begun two decades earlier, and expanded commodity distribution programs.[16] The program for low-income people, still in effect, allows recipients to use food stamps like cash to purchase food and seeds—but not tobacco, cleaning items, alcoholic beverages, or nonedible products—at stores authorized to accept them (Table 18-3).

The school breakfast program was passed in 1965 as politicians began to see firsthand the number of children coming to school hungry. Both school lunch and breakfast programs still enable low-income students to receive meals at reduced cost or no cost if certain income guidelines are met. In the same year Congress funded group noontime (called congregate) meals and home-delivered meals for all citizens over 60 years of age. Both are still active programs serving elderly persons.

Political and social awareness of hunger and undernutrition in the late 1960s was spurred on by the book *Hunger USA* and a resulting television documentary, *Hunger in America,* shown in May 1968. The film graphically demonstrated that hunger existed in all areas and ethnic groups in the United States.[14] The response was dramatic. Between 1969 and 1971, some already large federal food programs were expanded, and others were created. The Food Stamp program served only 2 million people in 1968, but by 1971 it was serving 11 million citizens. Today it serves more than 19 million people. The School Lunch program, which served only 2 million poor children before 1970, was serving 8 million children by 1971. In 1990 about 12 million children had the cost of their lunch fully or partly subsidized by the program. The School Breakfast program, which was still only a pilot program for children living in poverty areas, became nationally available by 1975.

In the early 1970s the Special Supplemental Feeding Program for Women, Infants, and Children (WIC) was authorized. This program provides food vouchers and nutrition education to low-income pregnant and lactating women and their young children. WIC has been repeatedly shown to be cost effective, especially in reducing the numbers of premature, low-birth-weight babies.[14] WIC is also credited for the widespread drop in iron-deficiency anemia among children in the last decade. The current federal budget shortfalls have over the last few years threatened both the scope and the existence of this program. This raises a yearly struggle for support of the program. "Of all the dumb ways of saving money, not feeding pregnant women and kids is the dumbest," said the late Dr. Jean Mayer, one of the world's leading pioneers in nutrition.[14]

Undernutrition in United States—A Reevaluation

In 1977, a team of physicians resurveyed areas of undernutrition studied 10 years earlier. They found that the degree of poverty in regions like Appalachia and the slums of big cities had not changed. If anything, poverty was often worse than in 1967. Yet undernutrition had essentially disappeared as a social phenomenon.[4] As a population, Americans had more food resources available to them. The large federal food programs—Food Stamps, the School Lunch and School Breakfast programs, and WIC—contributed to this

TABLE 18-3

Some Federally Subsidized Programs That Supply Food for Americans

Program	Eligibility	Description
Food Stamps	Low income	Coupons are given to purchase food at grocery stores, the amount based on size of household and income.
Emergency Food System	Low income	Food stamps issued on 24-hour notice for 1 month while eligibility for further use of the program can be investigated.
Commodity Supplemental Food Program	Certain low-income populations, such as pregnant women and young children	USDA surplus foods are distributed by county agencies.
Special Supplemental Feeding Program for Women, Infants, and Children (WIC)	Low-income pregnant/lactating women, infants, and children less than 5 years old at nutritional risk	Coupons are given to purchase milk, cheese, fruit juice, cereal, infant formula, and other specific food items at grocery stores
School Lunch	Low income	Free or reduced-price lunch distributed by the school; meal follows USDA pattern based on the Food Guide Pyramid; cost for the child depends on family income. In schools without a lunch program, special milk programs may be available.
School Breakfast	Low income	Free or reduced-price breakfast distributed by the school; meal follows USDA pattern; cost for the child depends on family income.
Child Care Food Program	Child enrolled in organized child care program; income guidelines are the same as School Lunch Program	Reimbursement given for meals supplied to children at the site; meals must follow USDA guidelines based on the Food Guide Pyramid.
Congregate Meals for the Elderly	Age 60 or over (no income guidelines)	Free noon meal is furnished at a site; meal follows specific pattern based on ⅓ of the RDA.
Home-delivered Meals	Age 60 or over, homebound	Noon meal is delivered at no cost or for a fee, depending on income, at least 5 days a week. Sometimes other meals for later consumption are delivered at the same time; private organizations that sponsor these problems often refer to them as "Meals on Wheels."

difference. Politicians had responded to the demands of the American people by directing federal resources toward a massive human problem, and the effort succeeded. Certainly some Americans still fell through the cracks, but a food "safety net" was catching many whose needs had not been met before.

The 1980s

The first official recognition that widespread hunger had reappeared in the United States came from a conference of mayors in 1982. While the news media had been reporting the appearance of soup kitchens and bread lines in the nation's cities since the beginning of the decade, the mayors identified growing hunger as a national problem.[4]

Why was there a sudden increase in hungry people in the United States? First, unemployment in the United States rose from 6.2% in early 1980 to 10.8% in 1983. Although the rate has since fallen to about 6% to 7%, more Americans are unemployed today than were unemployed in 1980, partly because of population expansion. Second, in every year but one since 1976, the scope of the Food Stamp program has been narrowed and eligibility tightened, so that participants lost $7 to $10 billion worth of foods in the period from 1982 to 1985. In 1981, the School Lunch program was reduced by one third. In addition, during that time, funding levels for the senior citizen meals programs lagged far behind the increases in food and operating costs, as well as behind the increasing numbers in this age-group.[14]

In a 1985 report, *Hunger in America: The Growing Epidemic,* a group of physicians associated the reappearance of widespread hunger in the United States with government policies and budget cutbacks.[4] Other contemporary reports pointed out that for the majority of food programs, at least half the clients were families with children—those most at risk from undernutrition.

another BITE

Although cuts in the Food Stamp and school meal programs were made in the early 1980s, attempts to cut WIC were not successful. A bipartisan coalition in Congress protected WIC against proposed funding reductions. This coalition maintained and even increased WIC participation in the mid-1980s in the face of annual efforts to cut funds. This points to the political nature of the problems we discuss in the United States. Who went hungry depended very heavily on political decisions.

Congress Acts Again

During 1986 and 1987, Congressional leaders became more concerned over undernutrition and associated adverse health outcomes. They added back $400 million to the Food Stamp and school meals programs and increased funding for WIC.[14] These changes, however, while signaling a growing awareness of undernutrition, still fall far short of the amount needed to end the problem. For instance, the need for WIC services still greatly outstrips resources allocated to the program. This forces children out of the program, because pregnant women and infants are given the highest priority.

The 1990s

The number of hungry people increased in the United States in the early 1990s. The U.S. Conference of Mayors reported that 1990 emergency food requests were up 22% and shelter requests up 24% over 1989. The Salvation Army said requests for aid increased by 20% in 1990. There are currently more than 180 food banks, 23,000 food pantries, and 3300 soup kitchens trying to cope with this problem. Just over two of every three people requesting emergency food assistance in the survey cities were members of families—children and their parents. Across the nation the problem of hunger among some citizens remains.[16]

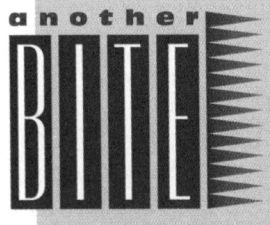

Poverty Is Also at the Heart of the Current Problem

The root cause of hunger and undernutrition in the United States continues to be poverty. In 1992 there were more than 36 million Americans living at or below the poverty threshold. Many families have suffered economic hardship due to massive layoffs in U.S. industries in the late 1980s and early 1990s. And the limited budget that results affects a person's food purchases. In response, many women who were caregivers have returned to work to help support family income. But of the 13 million jobs created between 1980 and 1985, most were in the service sector, such as in quick-service restaurants. If both parents have such full-time, low-paying jobs, the family may still operate at or below the poverty level, currently $14,350 for a family of four. Note that parents in most poor families do work—nearly two in three poor families include at least one worker. In sum, not only have impoverished people in the United States had to exist with less federal assistance, they have also netted a dwindling amount of family income.

HOMELESSNESS IN THE UNITED STATES

The economics of poverty and undernutrition has recently changed in one more very important way. Homelessness is much more evident now than in 1980. Estimates of the number of homeless vary widely, ranging from 350,000 to 3 million.[7] Homelessness exists partly because the cost of housing has substantially increased and partly because federal support for subsidized housing was cut dramatically during the 1980s. In 1969 the average American spent about 33% of his or her income on housing. In 1989, half of all poor renter households paid at least 70% of their income in rent and utilities.[14] Many families below the poverty line pay 80%. But the government considers housing costs, which include rent and utilities, to be affordable if they consume no more than 30% of a family's income. When so much is spent for shelter, almost every other expense is pushed aside, including enough food for children. The larger the family, the less money left to feed each child. Other important causes of homelessness include release of mentally ill persons from mental institutions in the 1980s, unemployment, substance abuse, and personal crises.

The availability of cooking facilities affects nutrient intake of the poor. In the absence of cooking facilities, people may buy expensive foods that require no preparation. These typically are processed snack foods, which provide energy but often limited nutrients.

The stereotypical image of a homeless person is someone out of step with society who might refuse to work. However, each year, as more and more typical Americans find themselves on the streets, we are having to rethink this stereotype.[7] Of the 10,562 people who used structures funded by the Community Shelter Board in Columbus, Ohio, over a 9-month period in 1989, 47% had at least a high school diploma, 22% were employed, 17% had recently been employed, and 18% were children; the total included 513 families. In an affluent California community (Contra Costa County), investigators found that 48% of emergency food recipients were members of families with children; only 2% were transients; and 45% of adult emergency food recipients were employed in low-paying jobs or had recently lost a job. Many emergency food recipients were disabled (16% of survey respondents), raising dependent children alone (27%), or children themselves (33%).

FOOD AND SHELTER FOR ALL AMERICANS

The reasons for both homelessness and undernutrition in America are many. Blaming the victims obscures the real issues. These problems increased dramatically in the 1980s, linked to political and economic factors. Opponents of federal nutrition programs raise the issue of cost, often citing the federal deficit as a reason for limiting spending and stating that much money is wasted by bureaucrats and drug-addicted recipients. In our opinion, these factors do not outweigh the even greater need to meet the nutritional and housing needs of American citizens. Consider that when money was needed for the Gulf War, it was there, and when it was needed for the savings and loan bailout, it was there. If we decided to do something about homelessness and poverty, the money would be there too. The approximately $1.2 trillion budget of the United States allows for many choices.

Undernutrition especially is a condition that need not exist. Nutrition programs and community intervention, if used fully and effectively, could go a long way toward meeting the food needs of those at highest risk.[14] More employment opportunities could then help solidify the improvements. The near elimination of large-scale undernutrition in the United States in the 1970s demonstrates that this national problem can be solved. Until the economy can accept all of us, a federal food safety net is important.

Private emergency food network systems are also important but are not sufficient to meet all food needs in the United States. Private donations often taper off during economic hardship in a given geographical area. In addition, much of what is donated is limited in nutritional value. Of necessity, processed and canned grocery items predominate, rather than protein-rich foods or perishable items, such as fresh produce and milk. During recent years, an extensive network of private agencies to feed the hungry has emerged.[7] There are numerous food banks around the United States in the Second Harvest system. These food banks distribute corporate surplus to thousands of soup kitchens and food pantries operating out of church basements and social service agencies. Yet despite this extraordinary effort, a huge gap remains between food aid and human need. There is no escaping the fact that federal assistance is the most effective way to help poor Americans get adequate nutrition. When federal assistance is a priority, undernutrition can be beaten.

As part of this discussion, we should consider the responsibility of both the the poor themselves and the well off. All citizens have a responsibility to contribute answers to our economic and social problems if we are to remain a moral and just society. The government must often step in with its programs when individual members of society fail to shoulder responsibility for themselves and others around them. Is the government to blame when a father walks out on his wife and children, leaving them without adequate resources to buy food and clothing, or when an unwed 16-year-old woman is pregnant with her second child? Out-of-wedlock births range from 17% to 67% for different racial groups in the United States. As well, 28% of children live in single-parent homes. The long-term solution to these problems is partly governmental in nature and partly social; all citizens should develop a sense of ethical responsibility. Political leaders, inlcuding Hillary Rodham Clinton and the Reverend Jesse Jackson see this second thrust as a key goal for American society as a whole. We all have a role and a stake in ending this national scourge.

It is not fair to solely blame the victims of poverty. Unemployment and expensive housing are formidable foes. Even while they desire a better life, and most do, people do not strive indefinitely against circumstances sure to defeat them.[7] Many of the poor are ill equipped for the battle—elderly, sick, and handicapped persons; single female heads of households; and young children. But it is also not fair for the government to shoulder all the blame. In terms of undernutrition in America, is there so much blame that it goes around and touches almost all of us? Until the economy can accept all of us, it is important for all of society to take the initiative and reach out to others in need.[2]

CONCEPT CHECK

Hunger and undernutrition in the United States were recognized by political leaders in the 1960s. In response, federally subsidized food programs—such as food stamps, school lunch, and congregate meals for elderly persons—were started or received substantially increased funding. This federal response greatly reduced undernutrition in the United States. The number of at-risk people increased in the 1980s because funding for these programs was reduced and an economic recession took place. Since 1985 some funding has been restored, but elimination of undernutrition remains a challenge for the United States—government and citizens alike.

UNDERNUTRITION IN THE THIRD WORLD

Undernutrition in the Third World is also tied to poverty, so any true solution must address this problem. However, the countries that are considered to be Third World nations—that neither are industrialized nor have a planned economy as the former Soviet Union supported—have a multitude of problems so complex and interrelated that they cannot be treated separately. Programs that have proven immensely helpful in the United States would be only a starting point in the Third World. Solutions have to consider major obstacles, such as the following:[23]

- Extreme imbalances in the food/population ratio in different regions of a country
- The rapid depletion of natural resources
- Cultural attitudes toward certain foods
- Poor ***infrastructure,*** especially poor housing, sanitation and storage facilities, education, communications, and transportation systems
- War and political/civil unrest
- Mounting external debt

Infrastructure *The basic framework of a system of organization. For a society, this includes roads, bridges, telephones, and other basic technologies.*

Let's examine each problem individually. In this context, Figure 18-1 depicts key factors relating to a person's food intake.

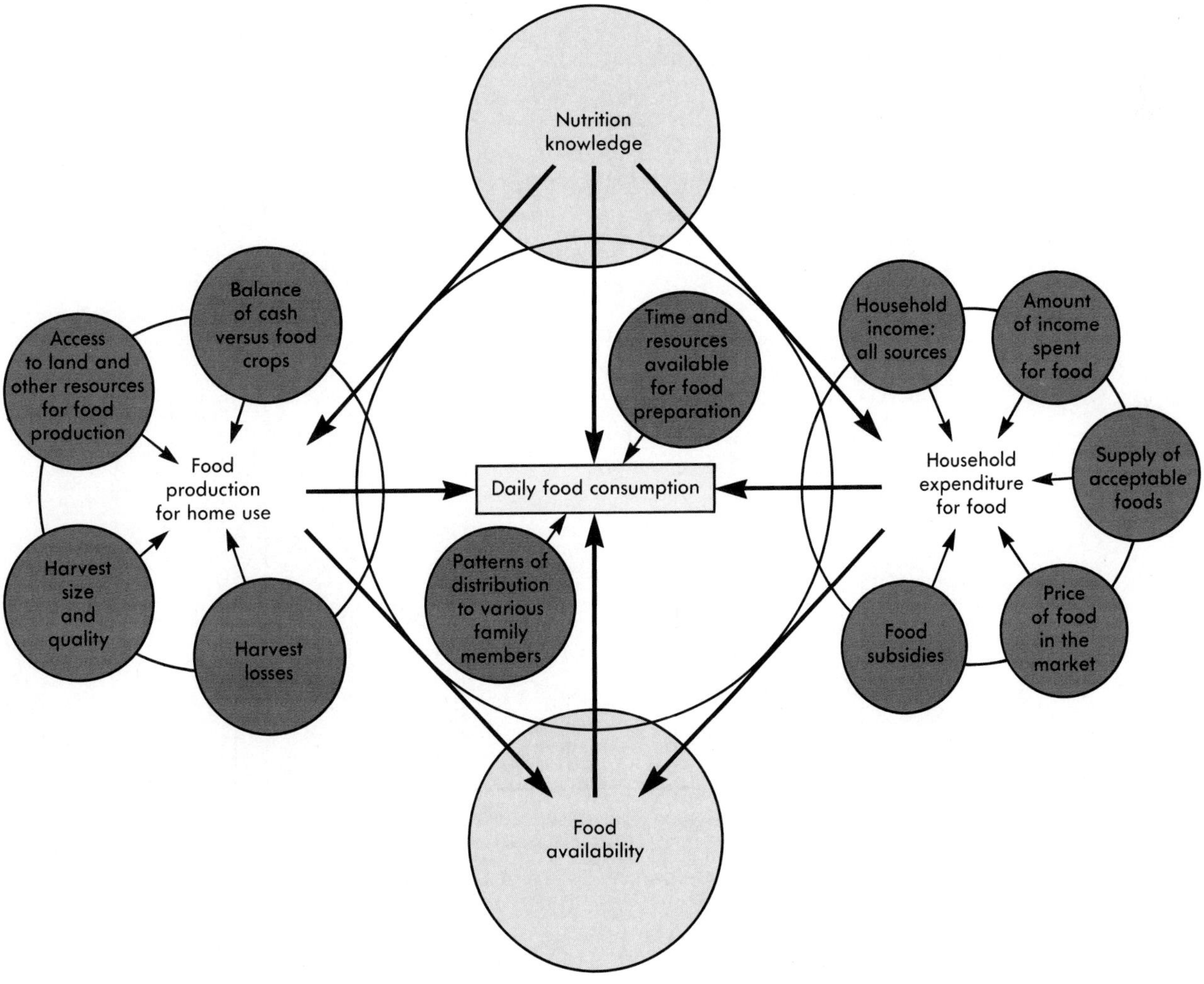

FIGURE 18-1
The many factors affecting household food consumption.

THE FOOD/POPULATION RATIO

Geometric Ratio
A group of numbers where the division of each number by the one to the left of it yields the same answer.

Arithmetic Ratio
A group of numbers where the difference between each number is the same.

Whether the earth can yield enough food for all people has been a long-standing question. As early as 1798, the English clergyman and political economist, Thomas Malthus, proposed a rather pessimistic view of the prospects for humans. He said that given the passion between the genders (which he felt was something to be counseled against), the population would always increase in a ***geometric ratio***—2, 4, 8, 16, 32, and so on. Meanwhile, at best, the food supply would increase only ***arithmetically***—2, 4, 6, 8, 10, and so on. This prediction means that while the food/population ratio might begin at 2/2, eventually population will grow to 32 while food supplies will only increase to feed 10.[17]

Malthus felt that in the likely absence of sexual restraint, the growing population would be subject to recurring checks imposed by widespread starvation, war, or natural catastrophe brought on by disease. His proposals became the object of intense controversy in England and elsewhere, often meeting vigorous opposition. Eminent scientists in Britain pointed out that scientific advances in agriculture would greatly increase food production. In fact, that has been true. Nevertheless, the population explosion is just that.[7] Malthus was correct in his prediction of geometric growth in the world population. So far this growth has not slowed significantly through either natural checks or recent human interventions, such as birth control (Figure 18-2).

Birth control programs have been effective in developed countries but have been relatively ineffective in developing countries that could really profit from them. Whereas women in the United States average 1.9 live births each, women in Rwanda (in eastern Africa) average 8.5 live births each (Figure 18-3).

At this time, there are about 5.4 billion persons in the world. About three quarters live

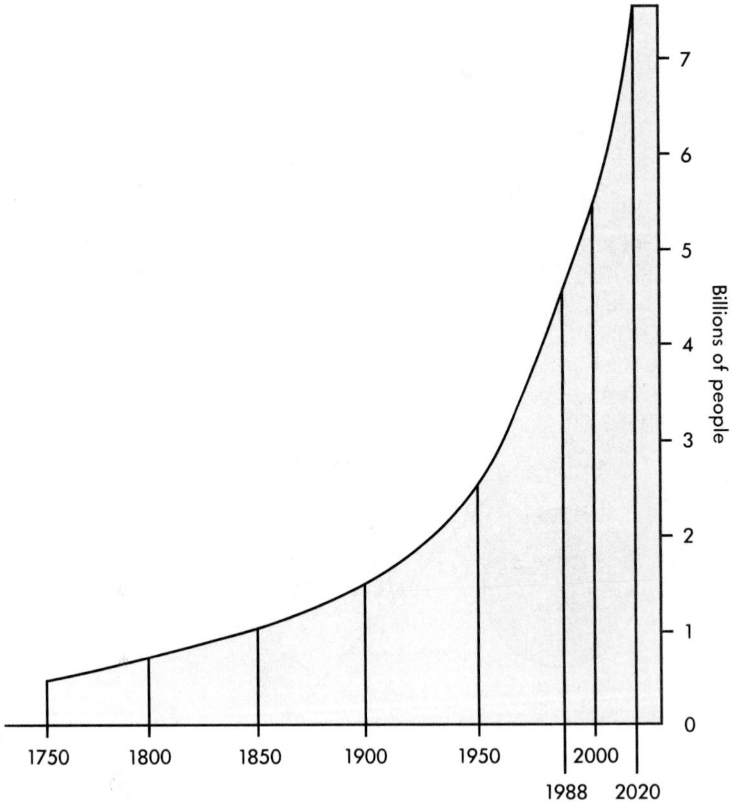

FIGURE 18-2
World population trends since 1750. (From Ehrlich PR, Ehrlich AH: National Geographic, *p. 913, December 1988.)*

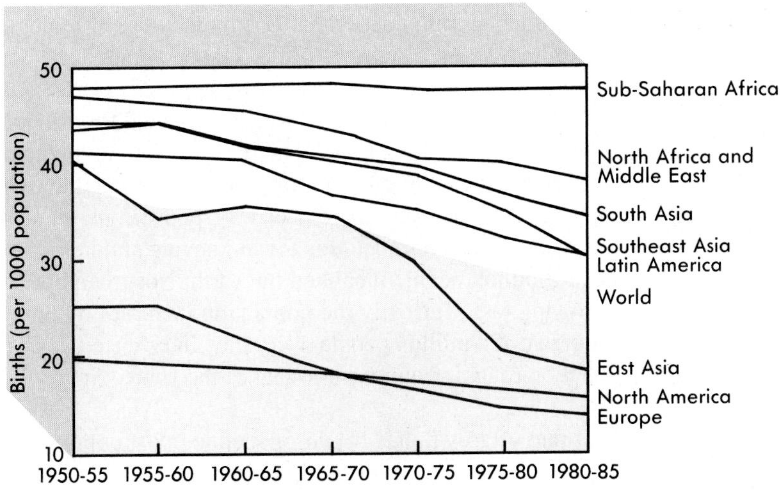

FIGURE 18-3

Birthrates in regions throughout the world. Rates have declined since the end of World War II. The only exception to this trend is in sub-Saharan Africa. As a result, Africa may account for nearly one fourth of the world's population by the late twenty-first century.

in developing Third World countries. Many experts believe that the global supply of food would provide adequate nutrition for all 5.4 billion of us, about 3000 kcalories each per day. But food supplies are not distributed equally among consumers.[7] Gross disparities exist between developed and developing countries, among the rich and poor within countries, and even within families. In some instances, women and children get less to eat than do men, and sometimes girl children get less than do boy children.

As well, food supply and population trends within the developing world itself clearly differ. Latin America and Asia both have had declining population growth rates since 1970, and their share of the world population will have risen only marginally between 1950 and 2025. On the other hand, the population in Africa will have more than doubled to 19% of the world population over the same 75-year period. The population will likely rise from 650 million in 1992 to 900 million by the year 2000.

Economists estimate that world food production will continue to increase more rapidly than the world population in the near future, allowing the food/population ratio to increase through the year 2000. In the short run then, the primary problem appears not to be food production, but distribution and use, especially in poverty-stricken areas of the developing nations.[7]

Eventually, though, it is likely that food production will begin to lag behind population growth. And we are currently drifting in that direction, especially when one examines worldwide grain reserves. Most good farmland in the world is already in use, and because of poor farming practices or competing land-use demands, the number of farmable acres worldwide decreases annually. For many reasons, sustainable world food output—that which does *not* deplete the earth's resources—is now running well behind food consumption. This suggests that food production in less-developed countries will barely keep up with population growth and will soon lag behind. That in turn will reduce the reserves needed to both combat and help stave off undernutrition, particularly widespread starvation, in poor countries.

A Renewed Focus on Population Control

While efforts on the supply side of the food/population ratio are essential, some—but not all—scientists in this area of research feel there is no substitute for reducing the demand side. They argue that the survival of our civilization depends on limiting reproduction.

For millions of years, maximizing reproduction has been a measure of biological success. Because disease and difficult living conditions often claimed young lives, producing many offspring by couples was one strategy for carrying on the family. These conditions still hold in Third World countries and constitute as well a key method for providing support in old age. More children also means more helpers to farm, hunt, and prepare food. Traditionally, poorer people bear more children—contrary to what you might predict.

Now, in an evolutionary blink of the eye—mere decades—poor people in developing nations are being asked to change their entire attitude toward having children. It is a difficult undertaking. In 1888, 1.5 billion people inhabited the earth. Now the population exceeds 5.4 billion and is growing fast. Currently the population increases by three people every second, or about a quarter of a million people every day. In essence the world must accommodate a new population roughly equivalent to that of the United States and Canada every 3 years!

Even though the overall rate of growth has begun to decline, most population experts believe population size will still pass 8 billion during the next 50 years. The poorest countries are increasing the most, further straining their ability to cope. And, if population growth continues as predicted, governments will be forced to confront problems that they could more easily finesse in less crowded times. A 1988 United Nations World Food Council report concluded that earlier progress in fighting undernutrition and poverty has either come to a halt or is being reversed in many parts of the world. This is particularly evident in Africa.[7] The pressure of more people to feed will intensify the problems.

Attempts to Stem the Human Tide

Attempts to implement family-planning programs in Third World nations have met only partial success. Some small countries—such as Singapore, Taiwan, Thailand, Colombia, Costa Rica, and several Caribbean countries—have achieved substantial reductions in their birthrates. Larger countries, including India and Mexico, are struggling.

China has explicitly recognized that it is already overpopulated—22% of the world's population is living on 7% of the world's arable land. It has the world's most stringent family-planning program; the government allows only one child per urban couple—two at most in rural areas. The birth rate is now 1.8 children in a woman's lifetime. Penalties for having extra children include restricted housing and employment opportunities. China's program, though successful by world standards, has encountered opposition. A new policy that allows families to earn private income, while very successful in increasing food production, has unexpectedly created an incentive to have more children to help earn the income. The overall result has been a recent surge in the birthrate, which has been countered by new efforts to impose restraints.

In the final analysis, successful birth control programs have to recognize that only when people have enough to eat and are financially secure will they feel safe having fewer children. By providing the poor with a livelihood that allows access to food, shelter, health care, and enough money to support themselves in old age, experts believe more couples will then *choose* to have fewer children. Increasing per capita income and education level are currently held out as the most likely long-term solutions to excessive population growth.[7]

another BITE

Promoting breast-feeding is important to family health. It helps naturally space births farther apart. Solely breast-feeding an infant lessens ovulation in women, and so fertilization, for an average of about 6 months (though it cannot be relied on totally as a form of birth control). When childbirths are more widely spaced, the health of mother and infant is aided, and fewer total births occur. In addition, in Third World Countries, breast-feeding cuts infant mortality by providing some of the mother's immune factors for the infant, while also lessening the risk from water-borne diseases.

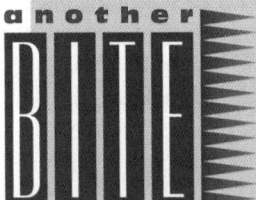

In 1960 families in South Korea averaged six children each. Economic policies, coupled with a strong family-planning program, transformed South Korea from a struggling country to an economic success. Today, Korean families average slightly fewer than two children each, and the population will soon stabilize. However, nations do not have to wait to become industrialized before launching population control programs. Indonesia, South Korea, and Thailand made great economic strides and at the same time controlled population growth. Still, to date, population stabilization—as in Western countries—has mainly been accompanied by relative wealth and security.

In addition to economics, another unavoidable roadblock to family-planning programs lies with ancient cultural, religious, and traditional beliefs. In sub-Saharan Africa, being childless not only carries an aura of evil for the woman, but also marks the end of a line of descent. The Yoruba believe, for example, that a childless woman has made a pact with evil spirits before her own birth to kill her children and, devoid of descendants, will return to join these evil spirits in some other-worldly sphere. These women are almost as afraid of being rendered functionally infertile by the death of all their children as they are of bearing none. Thus female sterilization and even contraception are widely feared. Even women with four or five children fear, not unreasonably, that all the children may suddenly die.

In India, a rigid class structure that leaves those in the lower classes destitute encourages these families to have more children for many of the economic reasons discussed previously. Also, Moslem religious practices typically promote a large, abundant family as a sign of prosperity and health.

Malthus' gloomy mathematical prediction may soon become fact. If we cannot find ways of humanely controlling population growth, nature may solve the problem by killing off large portions of humanity in the ways Malthus predicted. Only the future will tell.

CONCEPT CHECK

Currently, world food production is sufficient to meet the energy needs of the world's population. Undernutrition exists despite adequate food resources, because of poverty, politics, and unequal distribution. In addition, projected population growth may soon overwhelm food production. Limiting population growth, especially in Third World countries where birth rates are high, is a challenging priority encouraged by some scientists.

THE DECLINING STATE OF AGRICULTURAL RESOURCES

Population control has become more critical lately as we quickly deplete, and in some cases exhaust, the earth's resources. The productive capacity of agriculture is approaching its limits worldwide. As we mentioned, food production—especially in parts of the Third World—is being undermined by environmentally unsustainable farming methods.[7]

The term ***green revolution*** describes a phenomenon starting in the 1960s where a dramatic rise in crop yields in some countries—such as the Philippines, India, and Mexico—was made possible because of increased use of fertilizers and the development of superior crops through careful plant breeding. Many green revolution technologies have now achieved most of their potential. One example is that rice yield has not increased significantly since the release of superior varieties in 1966. Wheat is another example. India more than tripled its wheat harvest between 1965 and 1983, a period when high-yielding crop strains were introduced. Since then its grain output has not increased. Future gains in productivity may be much harder to accomplish because of the need to farm less productive soils. Until the introduction of yet another superior wheat or rice strain, developing countries will not benefit greatly from recent, more modest breakthroughs in biotechnology

Green Revolution *A time during the 1960s when there was much emphasis on improving strains and cultivation practices of cereal grains, such as rice, wheat, and corn.*

NUTRITION insight

PROTECTING THE ENVIRONMENT WITH LOW-INPUT SUSTAINABLE AGRICULTURE

Low-Input Sustainable Agriculture (LISA) *A form of farming that attempts to limit use of purchased inputs, such as manufactured fertilizers and pesticides. Use of manure and crop rotation are typical substitute inputs.*

Herbicide *A compound that reduces the growth and reproduction of plants.*

The recent consumer uprisings over pesticides in food and water, incidents of farmer and farm worker poisonings, and the rising cost of crop production have led to a broad base of public support for changing agricultural production systems. Concern particularly targets those systems that deliver detrimental environmental and public health side effects. Note that today a Midwestern corn farmer spends at least $46 per acre for fertilizer and $17 per acre for pesticides each year. Can these costs be reduced?

Low-input sustainable agriculture (LISA) seeks to reduce use of purchased inputs (chemicals, machinery, and so on), while maintaining or increasing yields and farm profits. The overall objective is to reduce costs, environmental and health hazards, and natural resource degradation. Sustainable agriculture offers a system of farm production that relies chiefly on working with nature, rather than trying to conquer it. The biological and stewardship techniques employed have already demonstrated adequate agricultural returns, without locking farmers into an expensive and environmentally damaging array of new farm inputs. Pesticides, fertilizers, water, and soil erosion are all receiving special attention. The LISA concept is gaining support in both the United States and Third World countries, because water and soil conservation are needs that exist worldwide.

Reduction in Pesticide Use

LISA is especially effective in offering solutions to the problems of pesticides in the environment and in food. In the United States there is a growing market for meat and other agricultural products that are free of pesticide residues, as well as added growth hormones and antibiotics. Farmers can grow crops profitably on a commercial scale using technologies that substantially reduce the need for pesticides. Rather than resorting to ***herbicide*** exclusively to knock out weeds, farmers can combine timely cultivation with variations in planting dates and seeding rates to produce thicker canopies at the right time to shade out weeds. LISA is also reintroducing crop rotation—a traditional farming practice that provides effective pest control with sufficient economic returns. In many instances, commercial pesticides are still the best, most cost-effective, or only means for growing a successful crop. But LISA techniques can substantially reduce use of chemical pesticides.

Exporting agrichemicals made in the United States to Third World countries is a time bomb in the area of worker safety. Pesticide use in Third World countries differs totally from pesticide use in America. Virtually all chemical use in those countries is by hand application, and controls are virtually nonexistent. Many extremely hazardous toxic materials, such as methyl parathion, are virtually impossible to apply safely by hand under tropical conditions. Sooner or later, political—if not moral—pressure will force industry to respond to this very real problem.

Reducing Fertilizer Use

Today, the conventional emphasis on maximal yields relies on heavy additions of fertilizers. The LISA farm community is seeking soil nutrient management practices that focus instead on long-term soil health rather than short-term yields. This in turn allows for maximal economic return, use of the soil's internal capacity for regeneration, and minimal damage to ground and surface water. Crop rotation is an important tool in this effort.

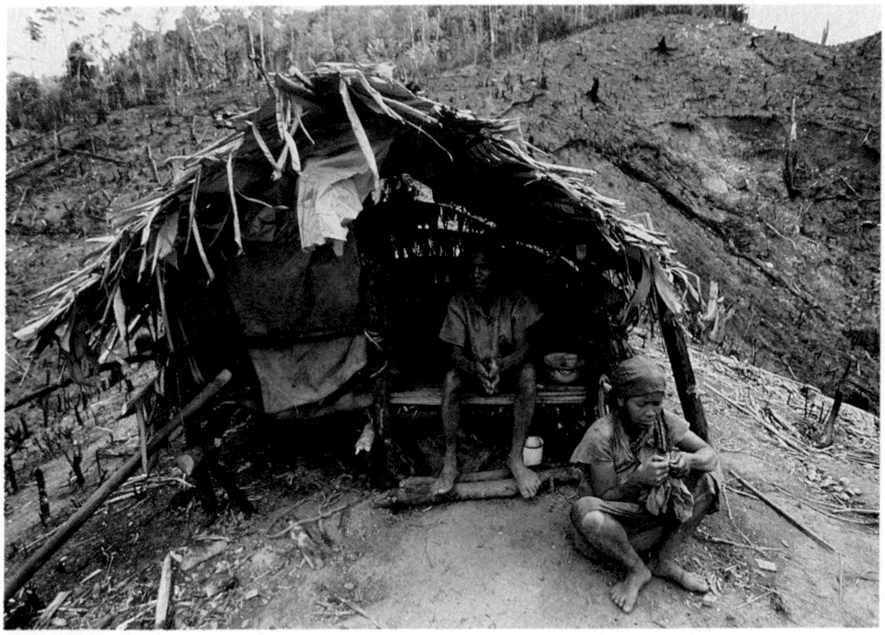

FIGURE 18-4
The need for LISA exists worldwide. Losing ground in their effort to grow rice, farmers in Madagascar survey erosion on hills cleared of rain forest. Farming further depletes the soil, and in turn new land must be cleared. Slash-and-burn farming destroys 50 acres of rain forest an hour worldwide.

Lessening Water and Soil Erosion

Although not widely recognized at this time, recent world food output has increased unsustainable methods, such as plowing highly erodible land and depleting water tables through over-irrigation. In Africa, a land area twice the size of New Jersey is turned into unproductive desert each year because of soil erosion (Figure 18-4). The erosion is caused by over-grazing livestock, destructive farming techniques, and destroying mature rain forests. Soil erosion is also a problem in the United States. LISA can help slow this erosion.

Many of Africa's ***cash crops*** damage the land, draining the soil of vital nutrients. Then, when the land has been used up, farmers move on to other areas, leaving behind desolated land ripe for soil erosion. In the short run, farmers can over-plow and over-pump with impressive results, but in doing so they use up the natural resources on which long-term productivity depends.

Nearly all available irrigation water worldwide is currently used, and groundwater supplies are becoming depleted at rapid rates in many regions. China, which has more than 20% of the world's irrigated land, is plagued with a growing scarcity of fresh water. Third World countries often over-concentrate poultry, swine, and milk production around metropolitan areas, in turn polluting and over-drawing ground water.

Cash Crop
Crop grown by countries with specific intent to export in order to gain the ability to purchase goods from other countries, rather than to feed the country's citizens. Examples are coffee, tea, cocoa, and bananas.

A World View

The Food and Agriculture Organization (FAO) of the United Nations works on this principle: "The fight to ensure that all people have enough nutritious food to eat is worthy of our greatest efforts, but it must be fought with the full recognition that it cannot be won unless agricultural, fisheries, and forestry production returns to the earth as much—or more—than it takes." These words suggest we need to take immediate steps to protect an already fragile environment from further deterioration if the world is to feed a population of 6 billion by the year 2000. LISA is one alternative for the future.

(see the Nutrition Issue at the end of this chapter). Actually, the green revolution was never intended to solve the world's food problems, according to Dr. Norman Borlaug, its chief architect. It was just a stopgap measure until world leaders could get population growth under control.

Ecosystem *A community in nature that includes plants and animals and the environment associated with them.*

Areas of the world that remain uncultivated or ungrazed are mostly of poor quality: rocky, steep, infertile, too dry, too wet, or inaccessible. Much of this land is invaluable for providing crucial ***ecosystem*** benefits. This is particularly true for humid tropical areas, such as the Amazon basin rain forests, which significantly influence the earth's climate, notably through oxygen production. Some nations, such as Brazil, can still expand onto land that will sustain cultivation, but such countries are in the distinct minority. And even then, this expansion in Brazil comes at the expense of further rain forest devastation. The overwhelming experience over the last few decades has been overextension of agriculture onto erodible land, followed by predictable degradation, erosion, and abandonment. Currently farmland equivalent to the size of Ireland is lost to erosion every year.

The prospects of obtaining substantially more food from the oceans are also poor. Since 1989 the world fish catch per person has been declining. Clearly, we can exploit the earth's resources only so far—world population likely cannot continue to expand as it does today without potentially invoking serious famine and death.

ATTITUDES TOWARD FOODS

Culture affects food use just as it does family size. In India, for example, the Hindu reverence for cattle has multiplied some already significant nutrition problems. These sacred cows consume food rather than provide it; the wandering cows also considerably damage vegetation that could otherwise feed humans. Although the cows provide milk, there is no effort to improve milk production through selective breeding practices.

In the United States, many people shun potential foods such as horse meat, insects, textured soy protein, and algae.

In certain areas of India, a child may not be fed milk curds because of a superstitious belief that these inhibit growth, or bananas because they supposedly cause convulsions. These are obstacles, but not roadblocks, to good nutrition. Given enough food resources, a healthful diet that allows for individual food taboos and prejudices is possible.

THE EFFECTS OF POOR INFRASTRUCTURE ON HEALTH: SHELTER AND SANITATION IN THE THIRD WORLD

When people die from undernutrition in Third World countries, other influences almost always contribute, such as inadequate shelter and sanitation. Poor sanitation raises the risk for infection, as does undernutrition. Together these represent a lethal combination (Figure 18-5). More than one billion people today occupy inadequate and deteriorating shelter with poor conditions. The future looks even worse. By the year 2000, Mexico City will house more than 26 million people, with Sao Paulo, Calcutta, and Bombay not far behind. Many of the 15 million child deaths each year in developing countries (half of them in children under 5 years old) could be prevented if standards of environmental hygiene were improved.

In Brazil, migrants displaced by multinational land developers have flooded from the North and Northeast into Rio de Janeiro and São Paulo, attracted by the prospect of jobs. There they have built shanty towns next to apartment towers and affluent suburbs, but the jobs do not materialize and the desperate poverty begets more poverty.

Urban populations of some developing countries are currently growing at an annual rate of 5% to 7%. This urban explosion is the result of both high birthrates and continuing migration of people to the cities from the countryside.[7] People come to the cities to find employment and resources the countryside can no longer provide. It is estimated that by the year 2000 about half the world's population will live in cities and towns. Such a skewed population distribution will result in further impoverishment.

In Third World countries, the poor make up most of the urban population, and their needs for housing and community services often outstrip available governmental resources. Most of these urban poor live in over-crowded, self-made shelters that are only partially served by public utilities and lack a safe and adequate water supply. The shanty towns and ghettos of the Third World provide surroundings that are often worse than the rural areas the people left behind (Figure 18-6). And because the people now need cash to purchase food, they find themselves with diets that are even more meager than the home-

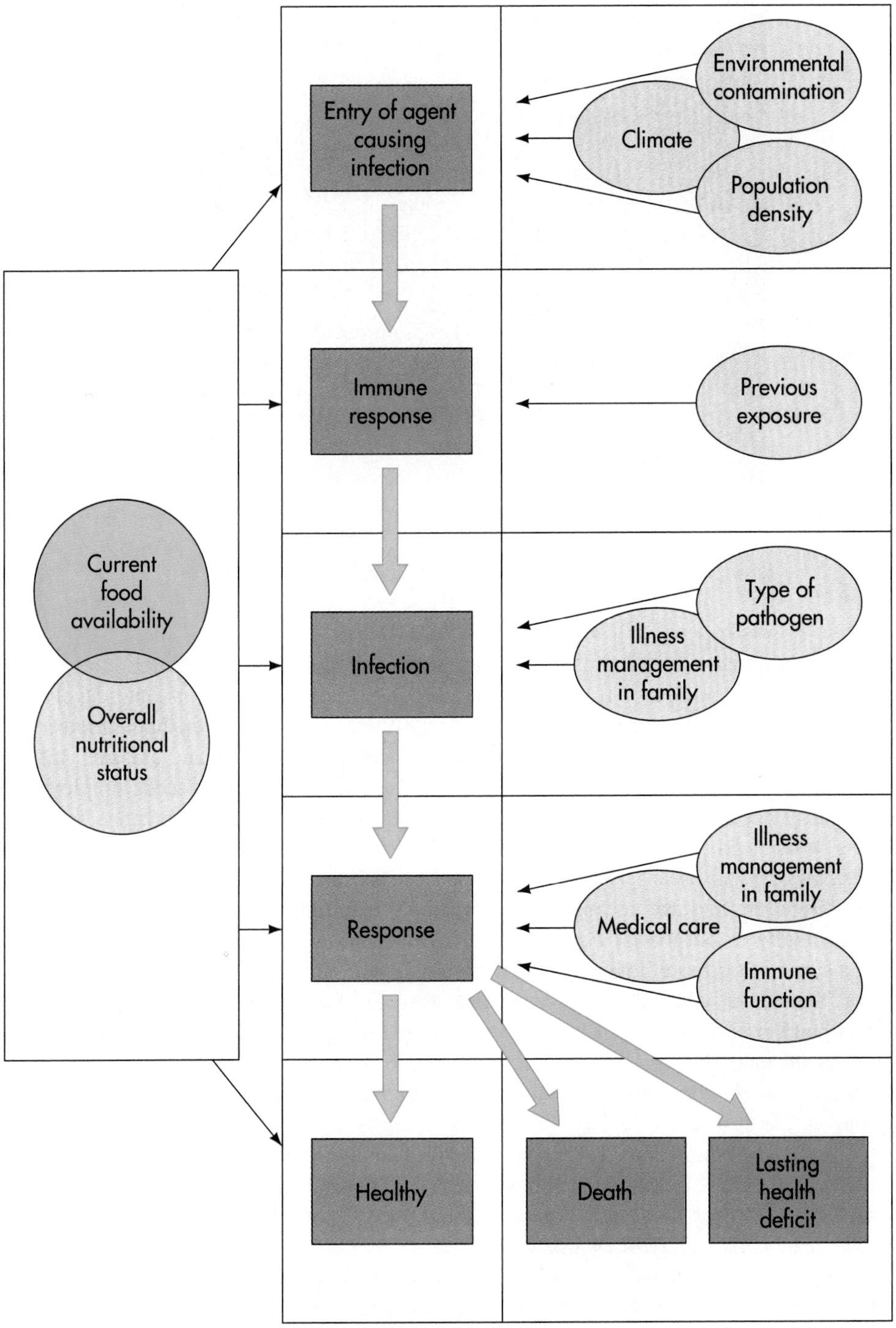

FIGURE 18-5
Nutritional status and overall food supply combine with a variety of environmental factors to influence the risk of infection and ultimate outcome.

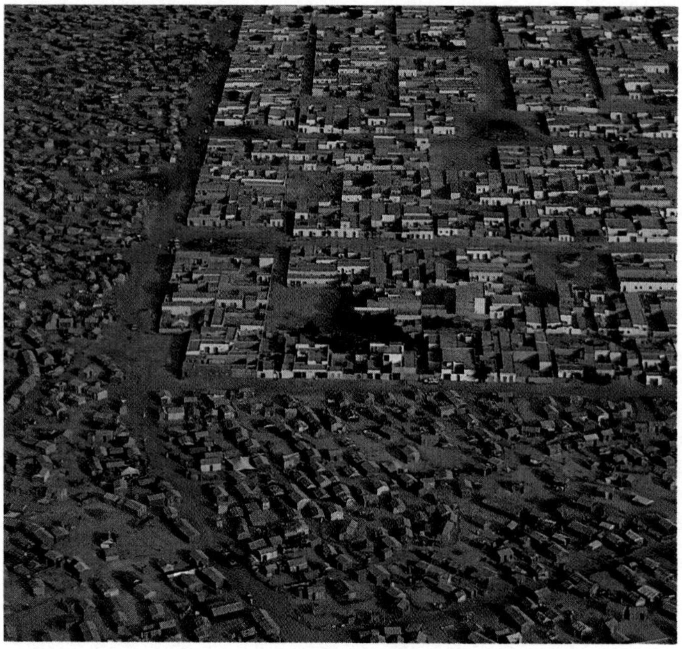

FIGURE 18-6
Urban centers in Africa can bear little resemblance to Western experiences.

grown rural fare.[12] To make matters worse, makeshift shelters often lack facilities to protect food from spoilage or from the ravages of insects and rodents. In some developing countries, food losses can amount to as much as 30% to 40% of the perishable foods.

A move from rural to urban life takes its greatest toll on infants and children. Infants are often weaned early from the breast, partly because the mother seeks employment and partly because she may be trying to emulate the image of sophisticated, formula-using women promoted in advertisements. Unfortunately, infant formulas are relatively expensive, and so poor parents may use too little to meet the baby's needs, or they may over-dilute the mixture. Because the water supply may not be safe, the prepared formula is also likely to be grossly contaminated with bacteria. In many nations, bottle-fed infants contract far more illnesses and are as much as 25 times more likely to die in childhood than those who are exclusively breast-fed for the first 6 months of life. On the other hand, breastmilk is generally much more hygienic, readily available, and nutritionally sound and again provides infants with some immune factors. In spite of the grim statistics, major corporations continue to heavily market infant formulas in these regions.

Overall, the single most effective health advantage that can be gained for people, wherever they live, is a safe and convenient water supply. The World Health Organization (WHO) estimates that 1.2 billion people, about one fifth of all people, have an unsafe and inadequate water supply in 1990.

Poor sanitation, another example of inadequate infrastructure in the Third World, creates a further critical public health problem. It is common to see human feces, rotting garbage, and associated insect and rodent infestations in Third World cities. Human urine and feces are potent sources of disease organisms, and so are two of the most dangerous substances people encounter in routine daily living. In some developing countries, diarrheal diseases account for as many as one third of all deaths in children under 5 years of age. WHO estimates that even with progress in housing, 1.8 billion people in the world were still without proper sanitation in 1990.

To this already unbalanced equation, add the threat of sickness from acquired immuno-deficiency syndrome (AIDS), a disease with no cure. Developing countries currently have two thirds of the world's 13 million human immunodeficiency virus (HIV) infections, and numbers are increasing rapidly. The economic and social impact as more people contract AIDS will be enormous.[3] In an already undernourished population, the long-term effects may rival those of a prolonged war.

CONCEPT CHECK

Poor housing conditions, impure water, and inadequate sanitation worldwide increase the risk for infection and disease. Infection then combines with undernutrition to further compromise health status. A healthful diet, clean drinking water, and sanitary handling of human waste all contribute to health—these should be the rights of every human being.

WAR AND POLITICAL/CIVIL UNREST

The president of Mali recently stated, "Only by translating our sense of common destiny into action will we be able to resolve the paradox of currently spending $1000 billion each year in the production of lethal weapons, while only a fraction of that sum would make our planet a land of prosperity for millions of people who today suffer from illness, hunger, thirst and ignorance."

Worldwide military spending has doubled over the past 20 years to more than $2 million per minute. The amount spent on weapons every minute could feed 2000 undernourished children for a year. The Third World's share of the global arms budget increased from 9% to 16% from 1977 to 1987, draining resources that could be used to combat poverty and hunger. Although Africa has been ravaged by economic decay and famines for years, military spending in Africa more than doubled in the 1970s and held firm in the early 1980s. Presently, less than one half of 1% of the total world yearly production of goods and services is devoted to economic development assistance, while approximately 6% goes to military expenditures.

In the worst cases, civil disruptions and war contribute in large measure to massive undernutrition.[18] War-related famine affects at least 20 million people in southern and northeastern Africa. In southern Sudan, 3 to 4 million men, women, and children were starving in 1991 because civil war prevented them from planting their fields and restocking their herds. Even when food might be available, political divisions may well impede distribution to the point that undernutrition will plague many people for years into the future. In addition, aid programs aimed at the poor, especially during emergencies, have been undermined by poor administration, corruption, and political influence. In the 1970s the problem of undernutrition was perceived as a technical one—how to produce enough food for the growing world population. Today, the problem is largely a political one—how to achieve cooperation among and within nations such that gains in food production and infrastructure are not wiped out by war. Today in Africa, war is destroying what the last 30 years of aid helped to build. Somalia and Angola are prime examples.

EXTERNAL DEBT

At a recent meeting of the United Nations, many developing countries asserted that they were on the verge of economic collapse and felt that a major contributing factor was the $1.3 trillion external debt they collectively owed. Latin American debt represents 45% of the region's gross regional output of goods and services. Nearly 40% of total export earnings are spent in paying off this debt. One option is for Latin American nations to form a comprehensive plan aimed at renegotiating the external debt on more realistic terms. The

NUTRITION insight

THE HUMAN IMPACT OF AIDS WORLDWIDE

The Black Plague, which left its grim mark on human civilization, took the lives of approximately 25 million people in the fourteenth century. By the year 2000, an estimated 30 to 120 million people around the world will be infected with the human immunodeficiency virus (HIV), and possibly 25 million people will have acquired immunodeficiency syndrome (AIDS). A disease currently with no cure, the majority of people infected with HIV—the twentieth century plague—face certain death from it.

The devastating impact of AIDS on human civilization has been very rapid when measured on Earth's scale of time, and the true costs to societies—other than the cost of human lives—have yet to be borne.[3] Though AIDS has not replaced heart disease and stroke as the primary cause of death in America, the very nature of the disease is likely to wreak significant human devastation here and worldwide, partly because its primary route of transmission is a basic human behavior—sexual activity.

The Route of Infection

Can eating a balanced diet prevent HIV or stave off AIDS? The answer is no. Again, there is no known cure for HIV and AIDS. Prevention is based on safe sexual practices and avoidance of contact with infected blood products and body fluids. Eating a balanced diet helps lessen the impact of infections but does not cure the disease or prevent ultimate death from it. And a poor nutritional status only contributes to quicker onset of such symptoms as wasting and ultimately leads to a quicker demise.

The vectors, or vehicles of transmission, for HIV are blood and body fluids, including sexual secretions. Most cases have been transmitted through homosexual and heterosexual contact and intravenous drug use, when a needle infected with the virus is shared. After initial contact with HIV, a person may notice no symptoms for as long as 5 to 10 years, and so may be an unsuspecting carrier. When the immune system can no longer fight off related opportunistic infections, such as tuberculosis and pneumonia, the condition of AIDS is well on its way.

Who Is Affected?

The belief that AIDS is a novel disease affecting a limited population of homosexual males on the east and west coasts in the United States is dangerously inaccurate. Though homosexual people currently account for more than half the cases in America, the number of AIDS cases in heterosexual people—especially women and the children that HIV-infected women bear—is rapidly increasing. This is evidenced by recent studies showing that about 20% of people in some South Florida towns have HIV infections, with heterosexual contact being the main method of contracting the virus.

AIDS needs no passport. Heterosexually transmitted HIV flows freely in Thai sex parlors, along the truck routes of India, around Dominican Republic sugar cane plantations, and in the copper mines of Zambia.[3] It is likely that ¼ of all adults in Zambia are infected with HIV. Heterosexual contact accounts for the majority of cases. A recent study warns us that 57 countries risk major HIV outbreaks. Reported HIV cases are increasing in both China and Russia, and the rate of infection is expected to surge in these countries by the year 2000.

current debt of the United States limits its ability to correct this problem (and to help its own poor as well).

Many African nations carry large debt burdens. Recent drops in prices for raw commodities, higher prices for imported oil, and embezzlement of funds by high political officials are at the root of this problem. Still countries need to import—and pay for—machinery, concrete, trucks, and consumer goods. To make up the difference between export income and import expenses, countries have been forced to borrow billions of dollars

What Are the Costs of AIDS?

Though human life can't be tagged with a price, the cost of AIDS research and medical care for AIDS patients, the loss of labor force to industry, and the economic hardship experienced by families of victims can be quantified. By 2000 the AIDS plague could siphon off an estimated $81 to $107 billion from the American economy and may drain $356 to $514 billion from the global economy. This is money that could be spent on goods and services to help maintain stable economies around the world.

The impact of AIDS will hit poor countries worst, because their economies are already small and their living standards low. Brazil, for example, would need to spend $600 million to adequately help its AIDS victims today. Such an economic burden would certainly mean rising budget deficits and expanding levels of debt, especially for a country that is still struggling with a foreign debt load of more than $100 billion. Such situations may well be the plight of other developing nations.

Hidden Costs

Behind the mind-reeling statistics of AIDS are the costs to businesses, families, and society in general that aren't so obvious.[3] In India and Thailand, for example, a significant number of the adult male populations will be forfeited to AIDS. Worker productivity will plummet because AIDS victims produce less and demand more, especially as they wither and waste away in the latter stages of the disease. Business productivity drops even further when relatives take time away from work or school to care for family members afflicted with AIDS. And AIDS demands a considerable amount of family income. Hard-pressed families that have to devote much of their income to doctors and medicines have little left for living expenses. Other family members must strain to keep up with daily duties because they must care for orphans left behind in the disease's wake. The number of youngsters orphaned by AIDS could more than double in the next 3 years to 3.7 million worldwide.

Individual and Government Response—Has It Been Adequate?

Governments worldwide have come under fire for their slow response in fighting AIDS. At present, neither governments nor the medical profession in developing countries has taken the lead to stem the AIDS tide. In India, for example, Bombay's first AIDS clinic was opened in January 1993 by a private interest group. And governments of developing nations frequently can't afford to supply AIDS counseling or treatment. Even worse, they continue to act as if their countries remain immune to the scourge. Such a weak response on the part of government leaders and resigned attitudes of citizens will undoubtedly lead to a greater degree of poverty and illness worldwide. We all must act in concert to stop the spread of HIV.[3]

from international banks. While the African debts are much smaller in absolute terms than the debts of Brazil, Argentina, and Mexico, for example, the actual burden is greater when national incomes and export earnings are considered. Nearly half the money African nations earn from exports goes to paying off the continent's multi-billion dollar debt. As a result, African nations have had to impose austerity programs. The effects of wage cuts and the increased prices for food and consumer goods can push many of these poor nations over the edge into widespread undernutrition.

SOLUTIONS TO UNDERNUTRITION IN THE THIRD WORLD

As you have probably guessed, eliminating undernutrition in the Third World will be complicated. In the 1980s it was a common practice for the more abundant nations of the world to supply famished areas with direct food aid. Though highly publicized and praised at the time, direct food aid is not a long-term solution.[19] While reducing the number of deaths from famine, it can also reduce incentives for local production by driving down local prices. In addition, the affected countries may have little or no means of transporting the food to those who need it most. Furthermore, the donated foods may meet with little cultural acceptance.

In the short run, there is no choice—aid must be given because people are starving. Still, improving the infrastructure for poor people, especially rural people, needs to be the long-term focus. This is because the most significant factor affecting undernutrition of people in impoverished areas of the world is their reliance on outside sources for basic needs. Their dependence makes them constantly vulnerable.

One American federal program that has helped improve the infrastructure of developing nations is the Peace Corps, which provides such services as assisting education, distributing food and medical supplies, and building structures for local use. The aim of the Peace Corps is to provide infrastructure and education to help create independent, self-sustaining economies around the world.

Recall that in the last 20 years, world food supplies have grown faster than the population. Thus the increase in undernutrition during this period is caused by an increase in the number of people cut off from their fair share of this supply. Millions of farmers are losing access to resources they need to be self-reliant. And the number of households with insufficient means to support themselves is growing. In response, careful small-scale, regional development is needed. There is a growing realization that the rural landless will flock to the overcrowded cities unless economic opportunities can be created for them.[7]

Small-scale rural enterprises and off-farm activities would ensure that poor people in rural areas who have no access to land or other assets can acquire entitlement to food. Such enterprises can be run by the people who stand to benefit, either as individuals or as members of small groups, using very limited capital. A prerequisite would be access to credit, appropriate technologies, a market, and the ability to transport the product to that market. Households that presently have land could be helped in different ways so that they would be able to feed themselves.

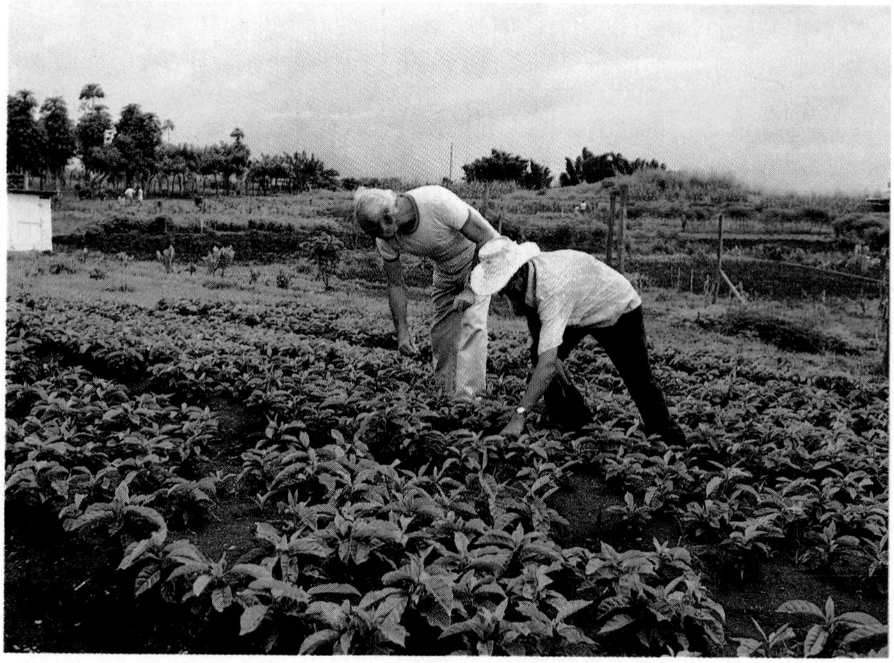

Poor people in less developed countries benefit from access to the land to help maintain food security.

For the most part, the problem is one of helping people produce much of their own needs and directing them to resources and employment opportunities. Experience has shown that credit—along with training, food storage facilities, and marketing—allows rural people to participate in development to their benefit and the benefit of their families and communities. Suitable technologies for processing, preserving, marketing, and distributing nutritious local staples need to be encouraged so small farmers—men and women—can flourish.

Land ownership brings many advantages, particularly available food. But if food resources instead become concentrated in the hands of a few, as often happens in unequal land ownership, these won't be equally distributed unless efficient transportation systems are in place. Inequitable distribution then proves a very difficult problem to resolve.

Raising the economic status of impoverished people by employing them turns out to be as important as is expanding the food supply. If an increase in food supply is achieved without an accompanying rise in employment, then there may be no long-term change in the number of undernourished people. It is possible to see food prices fall with increased mechanization, use of fertilizers, and other modern technologies. But these very same advances can also displace people from jobs. When this happens, the food that is produced will still be out of reach for those who need it most.

A shipment of high-technology tractors, for example, might put local laborers out of work. Rice might be planted more efficiently using farm machinery, but using human power eventually leaves more humans with the resources to buy food. Success in reducing undernutrition in the Third World must occur by employing more poor people more productively on available land or by providing other jobs. From a Third World point of view, it is of little consequence that these jobs are technologically primitive by Western standards. As we mentioned before, an effort to increase both per capita income and education is needed. Employment must be part of that effort.

SOME CONCLUDING THOUGHTS

It is also prudent to assume that the developing world will have to rely largely on its own resources to finance development, especially in light of the current budget deficit in the United States. For decades, countries in Africa could count on the cold war as an economic resource. The United States and the former Soviet Union opposed each other through African proxies, pouring money to prop up pro-Western or pro-Communist governments. Now the big powers' priorities have turned inward. It is even more essential then to make full use of human resources available in the developing world itself. The right choice for production ends up depending on the relative need to employ people and the number of people available to do the work.

Over-emphasizing cash crops, such as coffee, tea, rubber, and cocoa—as some developing countries have done, especially Latin American ones—is not likely to solve the nutritional problems of poor people. Cash crops are usually grown at the expense of food crops, on the assumption that money earned from the cash crops will be used to purchase enough food for the families of the workers. However, this is not always the case.[12] Food can be bought, but it may not be enough and it would be more expensive. In such a situation, poorer families are at greater risk than others, because the money earned from cash crops is often not enough to meet other basic family needs, let alone their food needs. As with poor families in the United States, buying quality foods often takes second priority, resulting in nutritional deprivation.

Also detrimental are the economics of drug crops, such as cocaine, marijuana, or opium poppy seeds. Frequently viewing drugs as valuable cash crops, workers often believe that the large sums of money netted from these crops—which are often more easily grown than food crops—can meet family needs and increase the standard of living. An unfortunate reality is that many workers see little or no cash earnings and so become victims of their trade. Cash from drug crops often lines the pockets of criminals and corrupt government officials and results in little incentive to initiate subsistence-level food crops that could provide employment and nourishment for many.

The battle against world undernutrition then is twofold: to supply nutrients to the undernourished and to reduce the number of people in danger of undernutrition. The second part of this battle is a very real one. Many delegates to a recent Food and Agriculture Organization of the United Nations (FAO) conference stressed the need for strategies that could supply food to vulnerable households, subsidize basic commodities purchased by the poor, and raise the levels of education, employment, and income-generating capacity of the poor.

Today, one third of the earth's population does not receive enough food to maintain an active working life, though enough grain is still produced to supply 3000 kcalories daily for every man, woman, and child on the planet. More than half of it is grown in the Third World. The economic loss from undernutrition is staggering, and the amount of human pain and suffering is incalculable. With all the international relief efforts, government assistance, and private organizations combined, we are still operating in the Dark Ages in our battle against undernutrition (Figure 18-7).

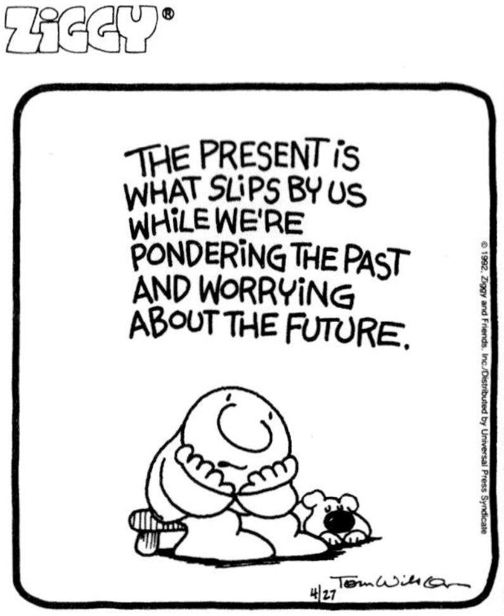
ZIGGY®
THE PRESENT IS WHAT SLIPS BY US WHILE WE'RE PONDERING THE PAST AND WORRYING ABOUT THE FUTURE.

FIGURE 18-7
Ziggy.

PREVENTING FAMINE

Policies to prevent famine must focus on increasing the productivity of rural people and reducing war and civil strife.[10] Then as agricultural surpluses grow, producers can sell some, rather than consume all, of their harvest. Livestock numbers will grow, absorbing surplus grain and providing animal protein. As rural wealth grows, food becomes a smaller portion of the household budget. If disaster strikes, food stocks will be adequate, livestock can be slaughtered, and price swings will be more tolerable. The conditions of scarcity that characterize famine then cease to arise. In the end, it is positive government action that must strengthen the rural economies, thus ending the kind of desperate poverty that links natural or man-made disasters to famine and ultimately to widespread death. Little such preparedness planning exists in Africa today. Famine-prone African countries are very fully dependent on international sources of supply for food, medicine, transport, and famine management. However, these usually arrive on the scene after the famine has already peaked. Local remedies, such as food reserves, can be put into action much sooner. Perhaps if we rid ourselves of negative government actions worldwide, the task could become easier.

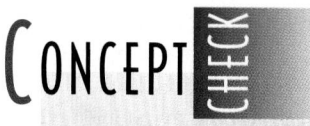

CONCEPT CHECK

War, civil strife, and external debt contribute to the difficulty of ending undernutrition in many Third World countries. Overall, the solution seems to lie in providing sufficient employment so that people can purchase the food their family needs and/or providing access to land and other food production resources. Programs must be sensitive to regional conditions to ensure that new technologies introduced don't intensify existing problems for the poorest people. Simple approaches are appropriate if people using them are left with the resources needed to feed their families.

SUMMARY

- Poverty is a common thread wherever people suffer from undernutrition. Malnutrition can occur when the food supply is either scarce or abundant. The resulting deficiency conditions or degenerative diseases are influenced by genetic makeup.
- Undernutrition is the most common form of malnutrition in developing countries. It results from inadequate intake, absorption, or use of nutrients or food energy. Many deficiency conditions then appear and infectious diseases thrive, because the immune system cannot function properly.
- The greatest risk of undernutrition occurs during critical periods of growth and development: gestation, infancy, and childhood. Low birth weight is a leading cause of infant deaths worldwide. Many developmental problems are caused by nutritional deprivation during critical periods of brain growth.
- Undernutrition diminishes both physical and mental capabilities. In poor countries, this is worsened by recurrent infections, poor sanitary conditions, extreme weather, inadequate shelter, and exposure to diseases.
- In the United States, famine has been nonexistent since the 1930s, but undernutrition is present. Soup kitchens, food stamps, school lunch and breakfast programs, and the Supplemental Feeding Program for Women, Infants, and Children (WIC) have focused on improving the nutritional health of poor and at-risk people. These programs have proven effective in reducing undernutrition when adequately funded.
- Multiple factors contribute to the problem of undernutrition in Third World countries. In densely populated countries, food resources may be inadequate and the means for distributing food may be poor. Farming methods often encourage erosion, which deprives the soil of valuable nutrients, thus defeating future efforts to grow food. Poor water availability hampers food production. Naturally occurring devastation from droughts, excessive rainfall, fire, crop infestation, and human causes—such as urbanization, civil unrest, war, debt, and poor sanitation—all contribute to the major problem of undernutrition.
- Any proposed solutions to the problem of world undernutrition must consider the interaction of multiple factors, many of which are thoroughly embedded in cultural traditions. Family planning efforts, for example, may not succeed until life expectancy can be raised. Through education, efforts should be made to improve farming methods, encourage breast-feeding, and improve sanitation and hygiene. Direct food aid is only a short-term solution. In what may appear to be a step backward, a focus on subsistence-level farming, away from the specialization of cash crops, is needed to increase the economic status of poor people. This and small scale industrial development are ways to gain meaningful employment and purchasing power for vast numbers of the rural poor.

STUDY QUESTIONS

1. Describe in a short paragraph evidence of undernutrition that you have seen in the society around you while you were growing up. What are/were the roots of these problems?
2. Why is solving the problem of undernutrition a key factor in development of the ulti-

mate potential of Third World countries? What basic nutrients are keys to the health of these people?

3. Choose one problem that contributes to the complex picture of famine. In one page, describe the problem and discuss possible solutions.
4. What do you believe contributes to undernutrition in wealthy nations, such as the United States? What are some solutions to these problems?
5. A person you recently met asks you where to find food and shelter. Where would you first direct this person in your community for help? If you are unsure, try to find out.

REFERENCES

1. ADA Reports: Position of The American Dietetic Association: Biotechnology and the future of food, *Journal of The American Dietetic Association* 93:189, 1993.
2. Anonymous: The Medford Declaration to End Hunger in the United States, *Nutrition Reviews* 50:240, 1992.
3. Berkley SF: AIDS in the global village, *Journal of the American Medical Association* 268:3368, 1992.
4. Brown JL, Allen D: Hunger in America, *Annual Review of Public Health* 9:503, 1988.
5. Buzina R and others: Workshop on functional significance of mild-to-moderate malnutrition, *American Journal of Clinical Nutrition* 50:172, 1989.
6. Chandra RK: Protein-energy malnutrition and immunological responses, *Journal of Nutrition* 122:597, 1992.
7. Cohen MJ, Hoehn RA: *Hunger 1993,* Washington, DC, 1992, Bread of the World Institute.
8. Etherton TD and others: Recombinant bovine and porcine somatotropin: safety and benefits of these biotechnologies, *Journal of The American Dietetic Association* 93:177, 1993.
9. Fawzi WW and others: Vitamin A supplementation and child mortality, *Journal of The American Medical Association* 269:898, 1993.
10. Field JO: Famine: a perspective for the nutrition community, *Nutrition Reviews* 49:144, 1991.
11. Grantham-McGregor SM: Assessments of the effects of nutrition on mental development and behavior in Jamaican studies, *American Journal of Clinical Nutrition* 57:303S, 1993.
12. Lewis S: Food security, environment, poverty, and the world's children, *Journal of Nutrition Education* 24:3S, 1992.
13. Maryanski J: Genetically engineered foods: fears & facts, *FDA Consumer,* p. 11, January/February 1993.
14. Mayer J: Nutritional problems in the United States: then and now two decades later, *Nutrition Today,* p. 15, January/February 1990.
15. Miller HI: Foods of the future: the new biotechnology and FDA regulation, *Journal of The American Medical Association* 269:910, 1993.
16. Nestle M, Guttmacher S: Hunger in the United States: policy implications, *Nutrition Reviews* 50:242, 1992.
17. Olson RE: World food production and problems in human nutrition, *Nutrition Today,* p. 18, January/February 1989.
18. Schaller JG, Nightengale EO: Children and childhoods: hidden casualties of war and civil unrest, *Journal of The American Medical Association* 268:642, 1992.
19. Singer HW: The African food crisis and the role of food aid, *Food Policy,* p. 196, August 1989.
20. Tebeb HN: Goiter problems in Ethiopia, *American Journal of Clinical Nutrition* 57:315S, 1993.
21. Udomkesmalee E and others: Effect of vitamin A and zinc supplementation on the nutriture of children in Northeast Thailand, *American Journal of Clinical Nutrition* 56:50, 1992.
22. Walker SP and others: Morbidity and the growth of stunted and nonstunted children, and the effect of supplementation, *American Journal of Clinical Nutrition* 56:504, 1992.
23. World Declaration on Nutrition, *Nutrition Reviews* 51:41, 1993.
24. Yip R, Sharp TW: Acute malnutrition and high childhood mortality related to diarrhea, *Journal of the American Dietetic Association* 270:587, 1993.

FIGHTING WORLD UNDERNUTRITION ON A PERSONAL LEVEL

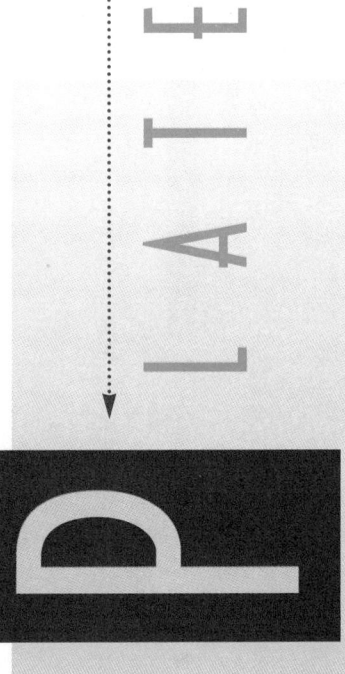

The following are suggested activities for doing something about world and domestic undernutrition. We encourage you to try to make a difference, even if it represents just one small step. Like any change in behavior, don't try to do too many things at once. Try one or two of them, representing your personal stand against this gigantic problem.

1. Fast for 1 or 2 days. Keep a diary of how you feel physically and emotionally through the day. At the end of the fasting period record what you learned about being without food. NOTE: *If you have a medical problem that demands regular consumption of food, like diabetes, or you are pregnant, do not choose this activity.*
2. Fast one meal per day for a month (e.g., lunch). Save an amount of money equivalent to the amount you would spend eating this meal out (e.g., $4.00). Donate the money to a voluntary agency that does anti-hunger work, such as those listed below:

   Bread for the World
   802 Rhode Island Ave., NE
   Washington, DC 20018

   Oxfam America
   115 Broadway
   Boston, MA 02116

   Seeds
   222 East Lake Dr.
   Decatur, GA 30030

   Food Research and Action Center
   1875 Connecticut Ave., NW #540
   Washington, DC 20009

   Save the Children Federation
   P.O. Box 970
   Westport, CT 06881

   The Hunger Project
   2015 Steiner St.
   San Francisco, CA 94115

   Institute for Food and
   Development Policy
   1885 Mission St.
   San Francisco, CA 94103

   Interreligious Taskforce
   on U.S. Food Policy
   110 Maryland Ave., NE
   Washington, DC 20002

   Catholic Relief Services
   209 W Fayette St.
   Baltimore, MD 21201

   CARE
   660 First Ave.
   New York, NY 10016

   Second Harvest
   116 Michigan Ave.
   Suite #4
   Chicago, IL 60603

3. Write a letter to a senator or member of congress asking what he or she is doing about ending domestic and world undernutrition.
4. Volunteer at a local soup kitchen or homeless shelter for a time-limited period (1 month).
5. Call your local social service agency and ask what services are available locally to deal with hunger and undernutrition in the community. Then ask about how to donate money or volunteer your services.
6. Sponsor a child in a foreign country with monthly financial aid for food and clothing. To do this you can write to the following organization:

   World Vision International
   Box O
   Pasadena, CA 91109

7. Contribute to World Food Day activities each October 16th.
8. Organize students on your campus. At Miami University in Oxford, Ohio, two students saw the successful culmination of a year-long effort to provide food for the homeless in the suburban Cincinnati area by distributing excess food from the university's dining halls. Let us know about your efforts!

Nutrition ISSUE

BIOTECHNOLOGY AS AN ANSWER TO FOOD SHORTAGES?

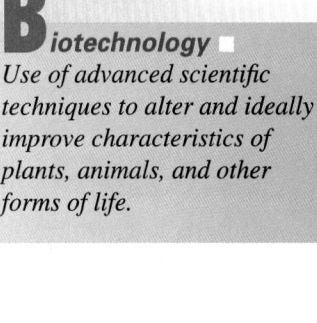

Biotechnology Use of advanced scientific techniques to alter and ideally improve characteristics of plants, animals, and other forms of life.

The human ability to manipulate nature has enabled us to improve the production and yield of many important foods. Traditional ***biotechnology*** is almost as old as agriculture. The first farmer to selectively improve his stock by breeding the best bull with the best cows was implementing biotechnology in a simple sense. The first baker who used yeast to make bread rise likewise used biotechnology to produce an improved product.

By the 1930s, biotechnology made it possible to selectively breed better plant hybrids; as a result, corn production in the United States quickly doubled. Through similar methods, agricultural wheat was crossed with wild grasses to acquire more desirable properties, such as greater yield, increased resistance to mildew and bacterial diseases, and tolerance to salt or adverse climatic conditions (Figure 18-8).

Another type of biotechnology uses hormones rather than breeding. In the last decade, Canadian salmon have been treated with a hormone that allows them to mature three times faster than normal—without changing the fish in any other way. Overall, then, biotechnology is the use of living things—plants, animals, bacteria—to manufacture products.[15]

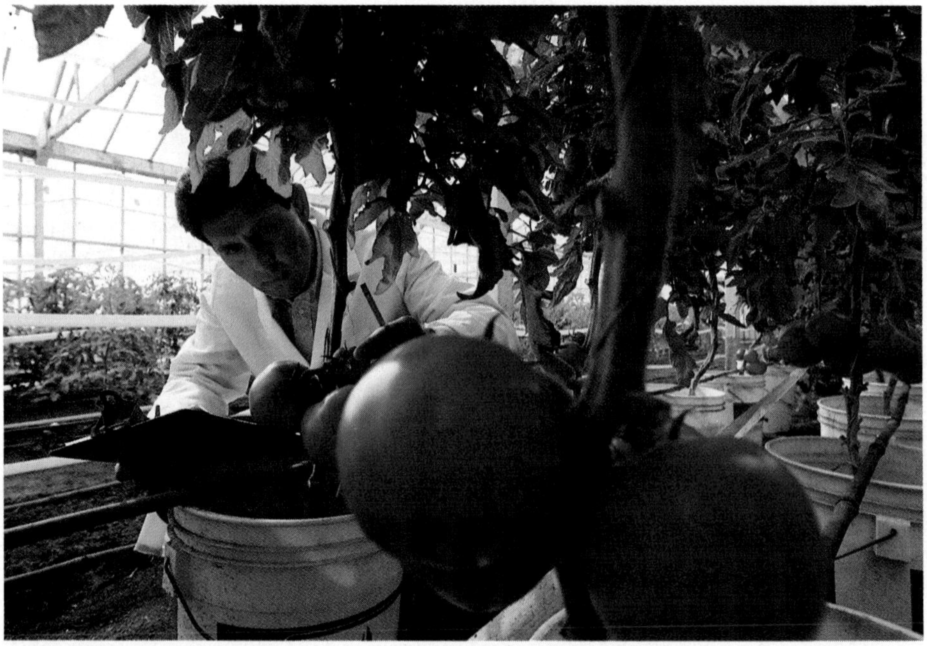

FIGURE 18-8
Much traditional biotechnology has gone into the tomato we enjoy today.

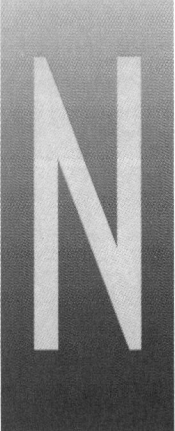

The New Biotechnology

The *new biotechnology* that is part of agriculture today includes a number of methods that directly modify products. It differs from traditional methods because it directly changes some of the genetic material (DNA) of organisms to improve characteristics. No longer is cross-breeding plants or animals the only tool. The new process, called ***genetic engineering,*** was developed mostly in the 1970s. It now covers a wide range of cell and subcell techniques for synthesizing and then placing genetic material in organisms.[15] This allows access to a wider gene pool, and it permits faster and more accurate production of new and more useful microbial, plant, and animal species. Traditional breeding has been hit or miss. But biotechnology is precise—scientists select the traits they want and genetically engineer or introduce the gene that produces the desired trait into animals. However, it is important to note that genetic engineering does not replace conventional breeding practices; both work together.[15]

Genetic Engineering *Alteration of genetic material in plants or animals with the intent of improving growth, disease resistance, or other characteristics.*

Currently, genetic engineering at the farm level has led to new types of seeds, availability of new growth hormones, and application of microbial inoculants to stop pests and frost damage. Biotechnology is also used to develop drought-tolerant crops, as well as for methods to better detect *Listeria* and other microbes that cause food-borne illness. Plants are being engineered to grow without chemical pesticides, and new forms of potatoes can last without preservatives. There is even interest in putting certain animal genes into plants to improve various plant characteristics. To our eyes and palates, these first benefits of the new biotechnology will seem only subtly different because cautious use is the current order of the day. But the ultimate benefits could be substantial.[1]

Questions surround the use of the new biotechnology. Take, for instance, research on a new tomato that is genetically engineered to allow it to stay firm longer. Is it still a tomato? It looks the same, feels the same, tastes the same, and even has the identical nutritional value as that of the original product. The only change researchers have made is to counteract the action of a single gene in the DNA that makes tomatoes rot rapidly. The reversal of just one gene out of 10,000 is the only change needed to make the *biotech* tomato significantly different from the standard garden variety.

Still, ultimately the question remains—how many and which properties can be changed in a plant, animal, or bacterium before it becomes something else? A tomato altered in only one specific way still seems to be a tomato, but does it remain one if it is improved in 10 or 20 ways? When traditional methods crossed a tangerine with a grapefruit, the new genetic structure was clearly something else, now commonly known as a tangelo.

Is the New Biotechnology Safe?

New biotechnology continues to develop under protest. Although genetically modified organisms offer the possibility of reducing environmentally detrimental activities, such as the use of chemical pesticides, critics point out past mistakes of releasing foreign agents, such as insects and plants, into areas with no natural predators. While the risks may appear to be momentarily negligible, they may be cumulative, and so, dangerous in the long run. Still, FDA will carefully scrutinize all products developed using this technology.[13]

Public opinion has long been turning against processes perceived as harmful to the environment, such as producing unnatural products. Because food reserves are high in the United States, Canada, and Europe, increasing food production has been questioned. The prime example of skepticism concerning unnatural products is Western Europe's ban of the growth hormone previously used in beef production there. They felt the increase in meat supply was not worth the perceived risks posed by the product. In the United States, FDA has recently approved the first genetically engineered food product for humans, an enzyme called renin, traditionally used in making cheese. Will a protest arise over its use?

Other potentially beneficial applications of the new biotechnology are currently being studied by both scientists and concerned consumer groups.[8] Bovine somatotropin (BST), a hormone produced by cattle, has been known since the 1930s to increase milk production when injected into dairy cattle. Today an identical BST produced through genetic engineering can be used to greatly increase milk yield. Because it is a protein, any BST in the milk produced would be digested and, therefore, inactivated when eaten. People even produce their own form of somatotropin, but it is structured considerably differently from that in BST. Because cows produce BST naturally, it has always been present in their milk. Treating the animals with the proposed higher levels of BST won't increase the level of hormone occurring naturally in the milk nor will it alter the milk's nutrient composition.

While FDA is still evaluating the animal and environmental safety of BST, the agency has determined that milk from treated animals is safe for humans. One question is whether the increased milk production will stress the health of the cows themselves, leading farmers to use more antibiotics, which can show up in milk. The public already appears to oppose it, and the European Economic Community has banned its use. Again, with milk surpluses in the United States and Europe, there is little to help garner public support. Furthermore, dairy farmers in Wisconsin—as well as other dairy-producing regions—are generally opposed to the introduction of the hormone, because they fear negative consumer reaction will lower milk consumption. The industry is also concerned that a sharp increase in milk output would adversely affect prices and, in turn, harm thousands of small dairy farms facing an already precarious economic situation.

Will the New Biotechnology Help Reduce Third World Undernutrition?

Whether genetically engineered applications will help reduce Third World undernutrition remains to be seen. Unless price cuts parallel the increased production, landowners and suppliers of biotechnology will capture the benefits of biotechnology, and so its rewards will most likely remain unshared. This principle needs to be emphasized; the person who couldn't afford a tangelo yesterday probably won't be able to afford one tomorrow. The same can be said for improved tomatoes. And as with most innovations, the more successful farmers, often those with larger farms, will adopt the new biotechnology first. Because of this, the present trend to fewer, larger farms will continue in the Third World—a trend that is counterproductive in addressing the most pressing undernutrition issues there. Furthermore, biotechnology does not promise dramatic gains in grain production, the primary food resource in the world.

For the Third World, the focus needs to be on providing people with resources to produce and/or purchase their own food rather than on simply growing more food. Biotechnology is merely a useful tool against, not a panacea for, the complex scourge of world undernutrition.

APPENDIXES

APPENDIX A

FOOD COMPOSITION TABLES

WT, weight; **KCAL,** kcalories; **PROT,** protein; **CARB,** carbohydrate; **FIBR,** fiber; **FAT,** fat; **SATF,** saturated fat; **MONO,** monosaturated fat; **POLY,** polyunsaturated fat; **CHOL,** cholesterol; **SOD,** sodium; **POT,** potassium;

Food Name	Portion	WT (Gm)	KCAL	PROT (Gm)	CARB (Gm)	FIBR (Gm)	FAT (Gm)	SATF (Gm)	MONO (Gm)	POLY (Gm)
Baby Foods										
BABY FOOD-CEREAL-OATMEAL-MILK	OUNCE	28.4	33	1	4	0.7	1	0.4	0.8	0.9
BABY FOOD-CEREAL-RICE-MILK	OUNCE	28.4	33	1	5	0.3	1	t	t	t
BABY FOOD-DESSERT-BANANAS & TAPIOCA	OUNCE	28.4	16	t	4	0.7	0	0	0	0
BABY FOOD-DESSERT-CUSTARD CHOCOLATE-USDA	OUNCE	28.4	24	1	5	0.1	1	0.3	0.2	t
BABY FOOD-DESSERT-CUSTARD-VANILLA	OUNCE	28.4	24	t	5	0.1	1	0.3	0.2	t
BABY FOOD-DESSERT-MANGO/TAPIOCA	OUNCE	28.4	23	t	6	0	t	0	0	0
BABY FOOD-DESSERT-ORANGE PUDDING	OUNCE	28.4	23	t	5	0.1	t	0.2	0.1	t
BABY FOOD-DESSERT-PAPAYA/APPLE/TAPIOCA	OUNCE	28.4	20	t	5	0.1	0	0	0	0
BABY FOOD-DESSERT-PLUMS & TAPIOCA	OUNCE	28.4	20	0	6	0.3	0	0	0	0
BABY FOOD-DESSERT-PRUNES & TAPIOCA	OUNCE	28.4	20	t	5	0.7	0	0	0	0
BABY FOOD-EGG YOLKS	SERVING	28.4	58	3	t	0	5	1.5	1.8	0.5
BABY FOOD-FRUIT JUICE-APPLE	FL OZ	31	14	0	4	0.3	0	0	0	0
BABY FOOD-FRUIT JUICE-APPLE BLUEBERRY	OUNCE	28.4	17	t	5	0.1	t	0	0	0
BABY FOOD-FRUIT JUICE-APPLE PEACH-USDA	FL OZ	31	13	0	3	0.3	0	0	0	0
BABY FOOD-FRUIT JUICE-APPLE PRUNE-USDA	FL OZ	31	23	t	6	0.5	0	0	0	0
BABY FOOD-FRUIT JUICE-MIXED FRUIT-USDA	FL OZ	31	14	0	4	0.3	0	0	0	0
BABY FOOD-FRUIT JUICE-ORANGE	FL OZ	31	14	t	3	0.3	t	0	0	0
BABY FOOD-FRUIT-APPLESAUCE	OUNCE	28.4	12	t	3	0.7	0	0	0	0
BABY FOOD-FRUIT-PEACHES	OUNCE	28.4	20	t	5	0.7	0	0	0	0
BABY FOOD-FRUIT-PEARS	OUNCE	28.4	12	t	3	0.3	0	0	0	0
BABY FOOD-FRUIT-PEARS & PINEAPPLE	OUNCE	28.4	12	t	3	0.3	0	0	0	0
BABY FOOD-MEAT-BEEF	OUNCE	28.4	30	4	0	0	2	0.7	0.6	0.1
BABY FOOD-MEAT-BEEF & EGG NOODLES-STR	OUNCE	28.4	15	1	2	0.1	1	0.2	0.2	t
BABY FOOD-MEAT-BEEF STEW	OUNCE	28.4	14	1	2	0.3	t	0.2	0.1	t
BABY FOOD-MEAT-CHICKEN STEW-STR	OUNCE	28.4	22	2	2	0.2	1	0.3	0.5	0.2
BABY FOOD-MEAT-LAMB	OUNCE	28.4	29	4	0	0	1	0.7	0.5	0.1
BABY FOOD-MEAT-LIVER	OUNCE	28.4	29	4	t	0	1	0.4	0.2	t
BABY FOOD-MEAT-PORK	OUNCE	28.4	35	4	0	0	2	0.7	1	0.2
BABY FOOD-MEAT-VEAL	OUNCE	28.4	29	4	0	0	1	0.7	0.6	0.1
BABY FOOD-VEGETABLES-BEANS-GREEN	OUNCE	28.4	7	t	2	0.4	0	0	0	0
BABY FOOD-VEGETABLES-BEANS-GREEN/BU-STR	OUNCE	28.4	9	t	2	0.7	t	t	0	t
BABY FOOD-VEGETABLES-CARROTS-STR-USDA	OUNCE	28.4	8	t	2	0.7	0	0	0	0
BABY FOOD-VEGETABLES-GARDEN	OUNCE	28.4	11	1	2	0.7	t	0	0	0
BABY FOOD-VEGETABLES-PEAS	OUNCE	28.4	11	1	2	0.7	t	0	0	0
BABY FOOD-VEGETABLES-SQUASH	OUNCE	28.4	7	t	2	0.7	t	0	0	0
BABY FOOD-VEGETABLES-SWEET POTATOES	OUNCE	28.4	16	t	4	0.7	0	0	0	0
Beverages										
ALE-MILD-AMERICAN	CUP	230	98	1	8	0	0	0	0	0
BEER-BUDWEISER	FL OZ	30	13	t	1	0.2	0	0	0	0
BEER-LIGHT	FL OZ	29.5	8	t	t	0	0	0	0	0
BEER-MICHELOB	FL OZ	30	13	t	1	0.1	0	0	0	0
BEER-NATURAL LIGHT	FL OZ	30	8	t	1	0	0	0	0	0
BEER-REGULAR	FL OZ	29.7	12	t	1	0.1	0	0	0	0
BRANDY-CALIFORNIA	ITEM	30	73	*	*	0	0	0	0	0
BRANDY-COGNAC-PONY	ITEM	30	73	0	0	0	0	0	0	0
CARNATION INSTANT BREAKFAST-CHOCOLATE	ITEM	36	130	7	23	*	1	*	*	*
CARNATION INSTANT BREAKFAST-EGGNOG	ITEM	34	130	7	23	*	0	0	0	0
CARNATION INSTANT BREAKFAST-VANILLA	ITEM	35	130	7	24	*	0	0	0	0
CHAMPAGNE-DOMESTIC-GLASSFUL	ITEM	120	84	t	3	0	0	0	0	0
CHOCOLATE BEVERAGE POWDER-DRY MILK ADDED	OUNCE	28.4	100	5	20	0.5	1	0.5	0.3	0
CHOCOLATE BEVERAGE POWDER-NO DRY MILK	OUNCE	28.4	99	1	26	12	1	0.5	0.3	t
CIDER-FERMENTED	FL OZ	30	12	t	t	0	0	0	0	0

t = Trace of nutrient present ** = Not available*

MAG, magnesium; **IRON,** iron; **ZINC,** zinc; **VITA,** vitamin A; **VITC,** vitamin C; **THIA,** thiamin; **RIBO,** riboflavin; **NIAC,** niacin; **VB6,** vitamin B-6; **FOL,** folate; **VB12,** vitamin B-12; **CALC,** calcium; **PHOS,** phosphorus; **SEL,** selenium; **VE-a,** alpha tocopherol equivalents.

CHOL (mg)	SOD (mg)	POT (mg)	MAG (mg)	IRON (mg)	ZINC (mg)	VITA (RE)	VITC (mg)	THIA (mg)	RIBO (mg)	NIAC (mg)	VB6 (mg)	FOL (μg)	VB12 (μg)	CALC (mg)	PHOS (mg)	SEL (μg)	VE-a (mg)
0	13	58	10	3.4	0.3	6	t	0.14	0.16	1.7	0.02	3	0.09	62	45	1	0.2
0	13	54	13	3.5	0.2	6	t	0.13	0.14	1.5	0.03	2	0.09	68	50	1	0.2
0	3	25	3	0.1	t	1	5	t	0.01	0.1	0.03	2	0	1	2	0	0.2
0	7	24	3	0.1	0.1	1	t	t	0.03	t	t	1	t	17	14	0	0.1
0	8	19	2	0.1	0.1	2	t	t	0.02	t	0.01	2	t	16	13	0	0.1
0	1	17	1	t	t	19	35	0.01	0.01	0.1	0.03	1	0	1	2	0	0.2
0	6	24	2	t	t	3	3	0.01	0.02	t	0.01	2	0	9	8	0	0.1
0	1	22	1	0.1	t	2	32	t	0.01	t	0.01	1	0	2	2	0	0.2
0	2	24	1	0.1	t	3	t	t	0.01	0.1	0.01	t	0	2	2	0	0.2
0	1	50	3	0.1	t	13	t	0.01	0.02	0.1	0.02	t	0	4	4	0	0.2
223	11	22	2	0.8	0.5	107	t	0.02	0.08	t	0.05	26	0.44	22	81	5	0.5
0	1	28	1	0.2	t	1	18	t	0.01	t	0.01	0	0	1	2	0	0.2
0	0	20	1	0.1	t	1	8	0.01	0.01	t	0.01	1	0	1	2	0	0.2
0	t	30	1	0.2	t	2	18	t	t	0.1	0.01	t	0	1	1	0	0.2
0	2	46	2	0.3	t	1	21	t	t	0.1	0.01	0	0	3	5	0	0.2
0	1	31	2	0.1	t	1	20	0.01	t	t	0.01	2	0	2	2	0	0.2
0	0	57	3	0.1	t	2	19	0.01	0.01	0.1	0.02	8	0	4	3	0	0.2
0	1	20	1	0.1	t	0	11	t	0.01	t	0.01	1	0	1	2	0	0.2
0	2	46	2	0.1	t	5	9	t	0.01	0.2	t	1	0	2	3	0	0.2
0	1	37	2	0.1	t	1	7	t	0.01	0.1	t	1	0	2	3	0	0.2
0	1	33	2	0.1	t	1	8	0.01	0.01	0.1	0.01	1	0	3	2	0	0.2
4	23	62	5	0.4	0.7	16	1	t	0.04	0.8	0.04	2	0.4	2	24	3	0.1
2	8	13	2	0.1	0.1	31	t	0.01	0.01	0.2	0.01	1	0.03	3	8	3	0.1
4	98	40	3	0.2	0.2	95	1	t	0.02	0.4	0.02	2	0.15	3	12	3	0.1
8	114	26	3	0.2	0.1	50	1	0.01	0.02	0.3	0.01	t	0.04	10	14	3	0.1
0	18	58	4	0.4	0.8	7	t	0.01	0.06	0.8	0.04	1	0.62	2	27	4	0.1
52	21	64	4	1.5	0.8	3247	6	0.01	0.51	2.4	0.1	96	0.61	1	58	7	0.1
14	12	63	3	0.3	0.6	3	1	0.04	0.06	0.6	0.06	1	0.28	1	27	4	0.1
11	18	61	4	0.4	0.6	4	1	0.01	0.05	1	0.04	2	0.37	2	28	3	0.1
0	1	45	7	0.2	0.1	13	2	0.01	0.02	0.1	0.01	10	0	11	6	0	0.2
0	1	45	7	0.4	0.1	13	2	0.01	0.03	0.1	0.01	8	0	18	6	170	0.2
0	11	56	3	0.1	t	325	2	0.01	0.01	0.1	0.02	4	0	6	6	0	0.2
0	10	48	6	0.2	0.1	172	2	0.02	0.02	0.2	0.03	11	0	8	8	0	0.2
0	1	32	4	0.3	0.1	16	2	0.02	0.02	0.3	0.02	7	0	6	12	0	0.2
0	1	51	3	0.1	t	57	2	t	0.02	0.1	0.02	4	0	7	4	0	0.2
0	6	75	4	0.1	0.1	183	3	0.01	0.01	0.1	0.03	3	0	4	7	0	0.2
0	16	*	*	0.2	*	0	0	0	0.07	0.5	*	*	*	30	41	1	*
0	2	7	2	t	0	0	0	t	0.01	0.1	0.02	2	0.01	1	4	0	0
0	1	5	1	t	t	0	0	t	0.01	0.1	0.01	1	t	1	4	0	0
0	2	7	2	t	0	0	0	t	0.01	0.1	0.02	2	0.01	1	4	0	0
0	2	5	1	t	t	0	0	t	0.01	0.1	0.01	1	0	1	4	0	0
0	1	7	2	t	t	0	0	t	0.01	0.1	0.02	2	0.01	1	4	*	0
0	*	*	*	*	*	*	*	*	*	*	*	*	*	*	*	*	*
0	t	1	0	t	t	0	0	t	t	t	0	0	0	0	1	*	0
*	136	422	80	4.5	3	525	27	0.3	0.07	5	0.4	0	0.6	100	150	*	5
0	196	266	80	4.5	3	525	27	0.3	0.07	5	0.4	0	0.6	100	150	*	5
0	145	382	80	4.5	3	525	27	0.3	0.07	5	0.4	0	0.6	100	150	*	5
0	*	*	*	*	*	*	*	*	*	*	*	*	*	*	*	*	*
2	147	227	23	0.5	0.3	3	1	0.04	0.21	0.2	t	12	0.68	167	155	*	0.1
0	60	168	28	0.9	0.4	1	t	0.01	0.04	0.1	t	2	0	11	36	*	0.1
0	0	36	1	0.1	t	0	t	0.01	0.01	t	0.01	t	0	2	2	*	t

WT, weight; **KCAL,** kcalories; **PROT,** protein; **CARB,** carbohydrate; **FIBR,** fiber; **FAT,** fat; **SATF,** saturated fat; **MONO,** monosaturated fat; **POLY,** polyunsaturated fat; **CHOR,** cholesterol; **SOD,** sodium; **POT,** potassium;

Food Name	Portion	WT (Gm)	KCAL	PROT (Gm)	CARB (Gm)	FIBR (Gm)	FAT (Gm)	SATF (Gm)	MONO (Gm)	POLY (Gm)
COCKTAIL-DAIQUIRI	ITEM	100	186	t	7	0	t	t	t	t
COCKTAIL-EGGNOG	ITEM	123	335	4	18	0	16	1.8	1.3	0.3
COCKTAIL-GIN RICKEY	ITEM	120	150	0	1	0	0	0	0	0
COCKTAIL-HIGHBALL	FL OZ	29	26	0	0	0	0	0	0	0
COCKTAIL-MANHATTAN	FL OZ	28.5	64	t	1	0	0	0	0	0
COCKTAIL-MARTINI	FL OZ	28.2	63	0	t	0	0	0	0	0
COCKTAIL-MINT JULEP	ITEM	300	212	0	3	0	0	0	0	0
COCKTAIL-OLD FASHIONED	ITEM	100	180	0	4	0	0	0	0	0
COCKTAIL-PINA COLADA-HOME RECIPE	FL OZ	31.4	58	t	9	0.1	1	0.3	0.1	0.1
COCKTAIL-PLANTERS PUNCH	ITEM	100	175	t	8	0	0	0	0	0
COCKTAIL-RUM SOUR	ITEM	100	165	0	0	0	0	0	0	0
COCKTAIL-TOM COLLINS	FL OZ	29.6	16	0	t	0	0	0	0	0
COFFEE SUBSTITUTE-PREPARED	FL OZ	30.3	2	t	t	0	0	0	0	0
COFFEE-BREWED	FL OZ	29.6	1	t	t	0	0	t	0	t
COFFEE-INSTANT-PREPARED	CUP	239	5	t	1	0	0	t	0	t
CORDIALS/LIQUEUR-54 PROOF	FL OZ	34	97	t	12	0	0	0	0	0
FRUIT PUNCH DRINK-CANNED	FL OZ	31	15	0	4	0	0	t	t	t
FRUIT PUNCH-POWDERED-PREPARED WITH WATER	CUP	262	97	0	25	*	t	t	t	t
GATORADE-THIRST QUENCHING DRINK	FL OZ	30.1	8	0	2	0	0	0	0	0
HOT COCOA-PREPARED WITH MILK-HOME RECIPE	CUP	250	218	9	26	3	9	5.6	2.7	0.3
LIQUEURS-ANISETTE	ITEM	20	74	0	7	0	0	0	0	0
LIQUEURS-APRICOT BRANDY	ITEM	20	64	t	6	0	0	0	0	0
LIQUEURS-BENEDICTINE	ITEM	20	69	*	7	0	0	0	0	0
LIQUEURS-CREME DE MENTHE	FL OZ	33.6	125	0	14	0	t	t	t	0.1
LIQUEURS-CURACAO	ITEM	20	54	*	6	0	0	0	0	0
OVALTINE-CHOCOLATE FLAVOR-PREPARED/MILK	CUP	265	227	10	29	0.2	9	5.5	2.6	0.4
OVALTINE-MALT FLAVOR-PREPARED WITH MILK	CUP	265	228	10	29	0.1	8	5.4	2.5	0.4
POSTUM-INSTANT GRAIN BEVERAGE-DRY MIX	OUNCE	28.4	103	2	24	0	t	0	0	0
SANKA-DECAFFEINATED COFFEE-PREPARED	FL OZ	29.8	t	0	t	0	0	0	0	0
SODA-CLUB-CARBONATED	FL OZ	29.6	0	0	0	0	0	0	0	0
SODA-COLA TYPE-CARBONATED	FL OZ	30.8	13	0	3	0	0	t	0	0
SODA-CREAM FLAVORED-CARBONATED	FL OZ	30.9	16	0	4	0	0	0	0	0
SODA-DIET COLA-NUTRASWEET-CARBONATED	FL OZ	29.6	t	t	t	0	0	0	0	0
SODA-DR. PEPPER TYPE COLA-CARBONATED	FL OZ	30.8	13	0	3	0	t	t	0	0
SODA-GINGER ALE-CARBONATED	FL OZ	30.5	10	0	3	0	0	0	0	0
SODA-GRAPE-CARBONATED	FL OZ	31	13	0	3	0	0	0	0	0
SODA-ROOT BEER-CARBONATED	FL OZ	30.8	13	0	3	0	0	0	0	0
SODA-TAB-LOW CALORIE COLA-CARBONATED	CUP	236	0	0	0	0	0	0	0	0
SODA-TONIC WATER/QUININE-CARBONATED	FL OZ	30.5	10	0	3	0	0	0	0	0
TANG-INSTANT BREAKFAST DRINK-ORANGE-DRY	OUNCE	28.4	104	0	26	*	0	0	0	0
TEA-BREWED	FL OZ	29.6	t	0	t	0	0	t	0	t
TEA-HERBAL-BREWED	FL OZ	29.6	t	0	t	0	0	t	0	t
TEA-INSTANT-PREPARED-SWEETENED	CUP	259	88	t	22	0	0	t	t	t
TEA-INSTANT-PREPARED-UNSWEETENED	CUP	237	2	0	t	0	0	0	0	0
WATER-MINERAL-PERRIER	CUP	237	0	0	0	0	0	0	0	0
WATER-MUNICIPAL TAP	CUP	237	0	0	0	0	0	0	0	0
WHISKEY/GIN/RUM/VODKA-100 PROOF	FL OZ	27.8	82	0	0	0	0	0	0	0
WHISKEY/GIN/RUM/VODKA-80 PROOF	FL OZ	27.8	64	0	0	0	0	0	0	0
WHISKEY/GIN/RUM/VODKA-86 PROOF	FL OZ	27.8	70	0	t	0	0	0	0	0
WHISKEY/GIN/RUM/VODKA-90 PROOF	FL OZ	27.7	73	0	0	0	0	0	0	0
WHISKEY/GIN/RUM/VODKA-94 PROOF	FL OZ	27.8	77	0	0	0	0	0	0	0
WINE COOLER-WHITE WINE AND 7UP	SERVING	102	55	t	6	0	0	0	0	0
WINE-CALIFORNIA/RED-GLASSFUL	ITEM	102	85	t	3	0	0	0	0	0
WINE-DESSERT	FL OZ	30	46	t	4	0	0	0	0	0
WINE-MADEIRA-GLASSFUL	ITEM	100	105	t	1	0	0	0	0	0
WINE-MUSCATEL/PORT-GLASSFUL	ITEM	100	158	t	14	0	0	0	0	0
WINE-RED-TABLE	FL OZ	29.5	21	t	1	0	0	0	0	0
WINE-ROSE-TABLE	FL OZ	29.5	21	t	t	0	0	0	0	0
WINE-SAUTERNE-GLASSFUL	ITEM	100	84	t	4	0	0	0	0	0
WINE-SHERRY-DRY-GLASSFUL	ITEM	60	84	t	5	0	0	0	0	0
WINE-VERMOUTH-DRY-GLASSFUL	ITEM	100	105	0	1	0	0	0	0	0
WINE-VERMOUTH-SWEET-GLASSFUL	ITEM	100	167	0	12	0	0	0	0	0
WINE-WHITE-TABLE	FL OZ	29.5	20	t	t	0	0	0	0	0

t = Trace of nutrient present ** = Not available*

MAG, magnesium; **IRON,** iron; **ZINC,** zinc; **VITA,** vitamin A; **VITC,** vitamin C; **THIA,** thiamin; **RIBO,** riboflavin; **NIAC,** niacin; **VB6,** vitamin B-6; **FOL,** folate; **VB12,** vitamin B-12; **CALC,** calcium; **PHOS,** phosphorus; **SEL,** selenium; **VE-a,** alpha tocopherol equivalents.

CHOL (mg)	SOD (mg)	POT (mg)	MAG (mg)	IRON (mg)	ZINC (mg)	VITA (RE)	VITC (mg)	THIA (mg)	RIBO (mg)	NIAC (mg)	VB6 (mg)	FOL (μg)	VB12 (μg)	CALC (mg)	PHOS (mg)	SEL (μg)	VE-a (mg)
0	5	21	2	0.2	0.1	1	2	0.01	t	t	0.01	2	0	3	6	*	t
94	75	178	16	0.7	0.6	25	0	0.04	0.11	0	0.07	15	0.57	44	74	*	0.2
0	19	12	1	0	0.1	t	4	0.01	0	0	t	1	0	2	1	*	t
0	4	1	t	t	t	0	0	t	0	t	0	0	0	1	1	*	*
0	1	7	1	t	t	0	0	t	t	t	0	t	0	1	2	*	0
0	1	5	1	t	t	0	0	0	t	t	t	t	0	1	1	*	0
0	0	6	t	0.1	0.1	0	0	0.02	0.01	t	t	0	0	t	10	*	0
0	1	2	0	t	t	0	0	0.01	t	t	t	0	0	0	4	*	0
0	2	22	3	0.1	t	t	1	0.01	t	t	0.01	3	0	3	2	*	t
0	*	*	*	0.1	*	0	8	0.1	0	0	*	*	*	4	3	*	*
0	1	2	0	t	t	0	0	0.01	t	t	t	0	0	0	4	*	0
0	5	2	t	t	t	0	1	t	0	t	t	t	0	1	t	*	t
0	1	7	1	t	t	0	0	t	0	0.1	t	t	0	1	2	*	0
0	1	16	1	t	t	0	0	0	0	0.1	0	t	0	1	t	0	0
0	7	86	10	0.1	0.1	0	0	0	t	0.7	0	0	0	7	7	0	0
0	1	1	0	t	t	0	0	t	t	t	0	0	0	0	0	*	0
0	7	8	1	0.1	t	1	9	0.01	0.01	t	0	t	0	2	t	0	0
0	37	3	3	0.1	0.1	t	31	0	0.01	t	0	t	0	42	52	*	*
0	12	3	t	t	t	0	0	t	0	0	0	0	0	0	3	*	0
33	123	480	56	0.8	1.2	96	2	0.1	0.44	0.4	0.11	12	0.87	298	270	*	0.3
0	*	*	*	*	*	*	*	*	*	*	*	*	*	*	*	*	*
0	2	11	1	t	t	t	3	0.01	t	t	t	1	0	1	1	*	t
0	*	*	*	*	*	*	*	*	*	*	*	*	*	*	*	*	*
0	2	0	0	t	t	0	0	0	0	t	0	0	0	0	0	*	*
0	*	*	*	*	*	*	*	*	*	*	*	*	*	*	*	*	*
34	228	600	52	4.8	1.1	700	29	0.63	0.97	12.7	0.77	29	0.87	392	302	*	0.4
37	201	576	47	4.5	1.1	770	30	0.67	1.16	11.9	0.75	29	0.87	371	308	*	0.3
0	28	896	*	1.9	*	0	0	0.17	0.08	6.8	*	*	*	77	189	*	*
0	0	10	1	t	t	0	0	0	0	t	0	0	0	1	1	*	0
0	6	0	0	t	t	0	0	0	0	0	0	0	0	1	0	*	0
0	1	t	t	t	t	0	0	0	0	0	0	0	0	1	4	*	0
0	4	t	t	t	t	0	0	0	0	0	0	0	0	2	0	*	0
0	2	0	t	t	t	0	0	t	0.01	0	0	0	0	1	3	*	*
0	3	t	0	t	t	0	0	0	0	0	0	0	0	1	3	*	0
0	2	t	t	0.1	t	0	0	0	0	0	0	0	0	1	0	*	0
0	5	t	t	t	t	0	0	0	0	0	0	0	0	1	0	*	0
0	4	t	t	t	t	0	0	0	0	0	0	0	0	2	0	*	0
0	30	*	*	*	*	*	*	*	*	*	*	*	*	*	30	*	*
0	1	0	0	t	t	0	0	0	0	0	0	0	0	t	0	*	0
0	13	81	*	t	*	535	107	0	0	0	*	*	*	71	76	*	*
0	1	11	1	t	t	0	0	0	t	0	0	2	0	0	t	0	*
0	t	3	t	t	t	0	0	t	t	0	0	t	0	1	0	*	0
0	8	49	5	0.1	0.1	0	0	0	0.05	0.1	0.01	10	0	5	3	0	0
0	7	47	5	t	0.1	0	0	0	0.01	0.1	0.01	1	0	5	2	0	0
0	3	0	1	0	0	0	0	0	0	0	0	0	0	32	0	*	0
0	7	1	2	t	0.1	0	0	0	0	0	0	0	0	5	0	*	0
0	0	0	0	t	t	0	0	t	t	t	0	0	0	0	1	*	0
0	0	1	0	t	t	0	0	t	0	0	0	0	0	0	1	0	0
0	t	1	0	t	t	0	0	t	0	t	0	0	0	0	1	0	0
0	1	0	0	0	0	0	0	0	0	0	0	0	0	0	0	0	0
0	0	0	0	t	t	0	0	t	t	t	0	0	0	0	1	*	0
0	7	41	5	0.2	0.1	t	2	t	t	t	0.01	t	0	6	7	*	t
0	10	116	11	1	0.1	0	0	0.01	0.03	0.1	0.04	1	0.01	8	13	*	0
0	3	28	3	0.1	t	0	0	0.01	0.01	0.1	0	t	0	2	3	*	0
0	5	92	9	0.2	0.1	0	0	0.02	0.02	0.2	0	t	0	8	9	*	0
0	4	75	4	1.6	0.1	0	0	0.01	0.01	0.2	0.05	2	0	8	9	*	0
0	19	41	4	0.1	t	0	0	t	0.01	t	0.01	1	0	2	4	*	0
0	1	29	3	0.1	t	0	0	t	0.01	t	0.01	t	t	2	4	*	0
0	2	89	10	0.4	0.1	0	0	t	0.02	0.1	0.02	1	0.01	8	14	*	0
0	2	45	6	0.2	t	0	0	0.01	0.01	0.1	0.01	1	0.01	5	8	3	0
0	4	75	10	0.4	0.1	0	0	0.01	0.01	0.2	0.02	1	0.01	8	14	5	0
0	9	92	9	0.2	0.1	0	0	0.02	0.02	0.2	0	t	0	8	9	*	0
0	1	24	3	0.1	t	0	0	t	t	t	t	t	0	3	4	*	0

WT, weight; **KCAL,** kcalories; **PROT,** protein; **CARB,** carbohydrate; **FIBR,** fiber; **FAT,** fat; **SATF,** saturated fat; **MONO,** monosaturated fat; **POLY,** polyunsaturated fat; **CHOR,** cholesterol; **SOD,** sodium; **POT,** potassium;

Food Name	Portion	WT (Gm)	KCAL	PROT (Gm)	CARB (Gm)	FIBR (Gm)	FAT (Gm)	SATF (Gm)	MONO (Gm)	POLY (Gm)
Breads										
BAGEL-EGG-3 INCH DIAMETER	ITEM	55	163	6	31	1.2	1	*	*	*
BAGEL-WATER-3 INCH DIAMETER	ITEM	55	163	6	31	1.2	1	0.2	0.4	0.6
BISCUITS-BAKING POWDER-FROM HOME RECIPE	ITEM	28.4	105	2	13	0.4	5	1.2	2	1.2
BISCUITS-BAKING POWDER-PREPARED FROM MIX	ITEM	28.4	104	2	13	0.5	5	3.3	1.3	0.2
BREAD STICKS-VIENNA TYPE	ITEM	35	106	3	20	1	1	*	*	*
BREAD-CRACKED WHEAT-ENRICHED	SLICE	25	66	2	13	1.3	1	0.1	0.2	0.2
BREAD-FRENCH-ENRICHED	SLICE	35	98	3	18	0.8	1	0.2	0.4	0.4
BREAD-ITALIAN-ENRICHED	SLICE	30	85	3	17	0.8	0	0	0	0
BREAD-MELBA TOAST-PLAIN	SLICE	4.67	16	1	3	0.3	0	0	0	0
BREAD-MELBA TOAST-WHEAT	SLICE	4.67	16	1	3	0.3	0	0	0	0
BREAD-MIXED GRAIN-UNTOASTED	SLICE	25	64	2	12	1.6	1	*	*	*
BREAD-PITA	ITEM	38	105	4	21	0.6	1	0.1	t	0.1
BREAD-PUMPERNICKEL	SLICE	32	82	3	15	1.9	1	*	*	*
BREAD-RAISIN-ENRICHED	SLICE	25	70	2	13	0.6	1	0.2	0.3	0.2
BREAD-RYE-AMERICAN-LIGHT	SLICE	25	66	2	12	1.6	1	*	*	*
BREAD-VIENNA-ENRICHED	SLICE	25	70	2	13	0.8	1	0.2	0.3	0.3
BREAD-WHEAT-FIRM	SLICE	21	59	2	11	2.4	1	0.1	0.2	0.3
BREAD-WHEAT-TOASTED	SLICE	22	68	2	12	2.5	2	0.2	0.3	0.8
BREAD-WHITE-FIRM	SLICE	23	61	2	11	0.4	1	0.2	0.3	0.3
BREAD-WHITE-FIRM-ENRICHED-TOASTED	SLICE	20	65	2	12	0.5	1	0.2	0.3	0.3
BREAD-WHITE-SOFT-ENRICHED-CRUMBS	CUP	45	120	4	22	1.2	2	0.3	0.5	0.5
BREAD-WHOLE WHEAT-FIRM	SLICE	25	61	2	11	2.8	1	0.1	0.2	0.3
BREAD-WHOLE WHEAT	SLICE	25	67	2	12	2.8	2	0.2	0.3	0.8
BREADCRUMBS-DRY-GRATED-ENRICHED	CUP	100	390	13	73	3.7	5	1	1.6	1.4
CORNBREAD-HOME RECIPE	SLICE	45	108	2	16	1.2	4	1.5	1.9	1.1
CRACKERS-ANIMAL	ITEM	1.9	9	t	1	t	t	0.1	0.1	t
CRACKERS-CHEDDAR SNACKS	ITEM	1.6	7	t	1	0.1	t	*	*	*
CRACKERS-CHEESE	ITEM	1	5	t	1	t	t	0.1	0.1	t
CRACKERS-CHEESE SNACKS	ITEM	1.13	6	t	1	t	t	0.1	0.1	t
CRACKERS-GRAHAM-PLAIN	ITEM	7	28	1	5	0.2	1	0.1	0.3	0.2
CRACKERS-GRAHAM-SUGAR-HONEY	ITEM	7	30	1	5	0.1	1	0.1	0.4	0.1
CRACKERS-OYSTER	ITEM	0.45	2	t	t	t	t	0	0	0
CRACKERS-RITZ	ITEM	3.33	18	t	2	0.1	1	*	*	*
CRACKERS-RY KRISP-NATURAL	ITEM	2.1	8	t	2	0.3	t	0	0	0
CRACKERS-RYE WAFERS	ITEM	6.5	23	1	5	1.1	0	0	0	0
CRACKERS-SALTINES	ITEM	2.75	13	t	2	0.1	t	0.1	0.1	0.1
CRACKERS-SESAME AND WHEAT-RALSTON	ITEM	1.9	9	t	1	0.2	t	*	*	*
CRACKERS-SNACKERS-RALSTON	ITEM	3.5	18	t	2	0.1	1	*	*	*
CRACKERS-TRISCUITS	ITEM	4.5	21	t	3	0.2	1	0.2	0.2	0.2
CRACKERS-WHEAT THINS	ITEM	1.8	9	t	1	0.1	t	*	*	*
FRENCH TOAST-FROM HOME RECIPE	SLICE	65	153	6	17	2	7	0.5	0.9	0.5
MUFFIN-BLUEBERRY-FROM HOME RECIPE	ITEM	40	110	3	17	0.9	4	1.1	1.4	0.7
MUFFIN-BRAN-FROM HOME RECIPE	ITEM	40	112	3	17	2.5	5	1.2	1.4	0.8
MUFFIN-CORN-FROM HOME RECIPE	ITEM	40	125	3	19	1	4	1.2	1.6	0.9
MUFFIN-ENGLISH-PLAIN-TOASTED	ITEM	53	154	5	30	1.5	1	0.3	0.4	0.4
MUFFIN-ENGLISH-PLAIN	ITEM	56	133	4	26	1.3	1	1.9	2.6	1.5
MUFFIN-PLAIN-FROM HOME RECIPE	ITEM	40	120	3	17	0.9	4	1	1.7	1
MUFFIN-SOY	ITEM	40	119	4	17	0.8	4	*	*	*
PANCAKES-BUCKWHEAT-FROM MIX	ITEM	27	55	2	6	0.6	2	0.8	0.9	0.4
PANCAKES-PLAIN-FROM HOME RECIPE	ITEM	27	60	2	9	0.5	2	0.5	0.8	0.5
PANCAKES-PLAIN-FROM MIX	ITEM	27	59	2	8	0.4	2	0.7	0.7	0.3
ROLL-BROWN & SERVE-ENRICHED	ITEM	26	85	2	14	1	2	0.4	0.7	0.5
ROLL-CINNAMON	ITEM	26	100	2	14	0.7	4	0.6	1.2	0.5
ROLL-CROISSANT-SARA LEE	ITEM	26	109	2	11	0.6	6	3.3	1.6	0.3
ROLL-HAMBURGER/HOTDOG-COMMERCIAL	ITEM	40	114	3	20	1	2	0.5	0.8	0.6
ROLL-HARD-COMMERCIAL-ENRICHED	ITEM	50	155	5	30	1.5	2	0.4	0.6	0.5
ROLL-SUBMARINE/HOAGIE-ENRICHED	ITEM	135	390	12	75	3.8	4	0.9	1.4	1.4
ROLL-WHOLE WHEAT-HOMEMADE	ITEM	35	90	4	18	1.8	1	0.4	0.6	1.4
WAFFLES-ENRICHED-FROM HOME RECIPE	ITEM	75	245	7	26	1.1	13	2.3	2.8	1.4
WAFFLES-FROZEN	ITEM	37	103	2	16	0.9	4	*	*	*
WAFFLES-OAT BRAN-NO CHOLESTEROL-EGGO	ITEM	39	110	3	16	2	4	0.7	1.1	2.1

t= Trace of nutrient present **= Not available*

MAG, magnesium; **IRON,** iron; **ZINC,** zinc; **VITA,** vitamin A; **VITC,** vitamin C; **THIA,** thiamin; **RIBO,** riboflavin; **NIAC,** niacin; **VB6,** vitamin B-6; **FOL,** folate; **VB12,** vitamin B-12; **CALC,** calcium; **PHOS,** phosphorus; **SEL,** selenium; **VE-a,** alpha tocopherol equivalents.

CHOL (mg)	SOD (mg)	POT (mg)	MAG (mg)	IRON (mg)	ZINC (mg)	VITA (RE)	VITC (mg)	THIA (mg)	RIBO (mg)	NIAC (mg)	VB6 (mg)	FOL (μg)	VB12 (μg)	CALC (mg)	PHOS (mg)	SEL (μg)	VE-a (mg)
8	198	41	11	1.5	0.3	24	0	0.21	0.16	1.9	0.02	13	0.05	23	37	*	*
0	198	41	11	1.5	0.3	0	0	0.21	0.16	1.9	0.02	13	0	23	37	18	*
0	175	33	6	0.4	*	0	0	0.08	0.08	0.7	*	*	*	34	49	5	1
1	221	33	3	0.6	0.1	37	0	0.1	0.07	1.8	0.01	2	0.04	34	99	5	1
0	548	33	*	0.3	*	0	0	0.02	0.03	0.3	*	*	*	16	31	*	*
0	108	33	9	0.7	*	0	0	0.1	0.1	0.8	0.02	*	0	16	32	11	t
0	193	30	7	1.1	0.2	0	0	0.16	0.12	1.4	0.02	13	0	39	28	10	t
0	152	22	*	0.7	*	0	0	0.12	0.07	1	0.02	11	0	5	23	8	t
0	30	11	2	0.1	0.1	0	0	0.01	0.01	0.1	t	1	0	5	10	*	t
0	30	11	3	0.1	0.1	0	0	0.01	0.01	0.1	0.01	1	0	5	10	*	t
0	103	55	12	0.8	0.3	0	0	0.1	0.1	1	0.03	16	0	26	53	11	t
0	215	45	8	0.9	0.3	0	0	0.17	0.08	1.4	0.04	22	0	31	38	*	t
0	173	139	22	0.9	0.4	0	0	0.11	0.17	1.1	0.05	*	0	23	70	14	0
0	94	60	6	0.8	0.2	0	0	0.08	0.16	1	0.01	9	0	26	23	*	*
0	174	51	6	0.7	0.3	0	0	0.1	0.08	0.8	0.02	10	0	20	36	9	*
0	138	22	5	0.8	0.2	0	0	0.12	0.09	1	0.01	9	0	28	20	7	t
0	153	42	23	0.8	0.4	0	0	0.07	0.05	0.9	0.05	13	0	17	63	11	t
0	91	87	24	0.7	0.6	t	0	0.06	0.04	0.8	0.05	13	0.03	20	64	11	t
0	118	26	5	0.7	0.1	0	0	0.11	0.07	0.9	0.01	8	0	29	25	6	t
0	117	28	5	0.6	0.1	0	0	0.07	0.06	0.8	0.01	8	0	22	23	6	t
0	231	50	9	1.3	0.3	0	0	0.21	0.14	1.7	0.02	16	0	57	49	13	0.1
0	159	44	23	0.9	0.4	0	0	0.09	0.05	1	0.05	14	0	18	65	11	t
0	89	85	23	0.7	0.6	11	0	0.07	0.04	0.8	0.05	12	0.03	20	63	11	t
0	736	152	32	3.6	*	0	0	0.35	0.35	4.8	*	*	*	122	141	20	*
0	126	42	8	0.7	0.2	7	0	0.08	0.08	0.7	0.03	5	0.08	49	44	5	0.6
0	8	2	t	0.1	t	0	0	0.01	0.01	0.1	0	t	t	t	1	0	t
*	14	2	t	0.1	t	t	0	0.01	0.01	0.1	t	t	0.01	1	2	1	t
t	12	2	t	t	t	t	0	t	t	0.1	t	t	0.01	1	2	0	t
t	10	2	t	0.1	t	t	0	0.01	0.01	t	t	t	0.04	1	1	1	t
0	33	28	4	0.3	0.1	0	0	0.01	0.04	0.3	0.01	1	0	3	11	1	t
0	33	12	2	0.2	0.1	0	0	0.02	0.02	0.2	0.01	1	0	3	8	1	t
0	5	1	t	t	t	0	0	t	t	t	0	t	0	t	t	0	t
0	32	3	*	0.1	*	*	*	0.01	0.01	0.1	*	*	*	5	8	*	t
0	19	10	3	0.1	0.1	*	*	0.01	0.01	t	0.01	1	*	1	7	1	t
0	57	39	*	0.3	*	0	0	0.02	0.02	0.1	*	*	*	4	25	1	t
1	37	3	1	0.1	t	0	0	0.13	0.01	0.1	t	t	0	1	3	4	t
0	17	4	1	0.1	t	0	0	0.01	0.01	0.1	t	t	0.01	1	3	1	t
0	24	4	t	0.1	t	t	0	0.01	0.02	0.2	t	t	t	1	3	1	t
0	24	6	3	0.2	0.1	0	0	0.02	0.01	0.2	0.01	1	0.04	1	9	1	t
0	*	*	*	*	*	*	*	*	*	*	*	*	*	*	*	0	t
t	257	86	12	1.3	0.6	22	0	0.12	0.16	1	0.04	18	0.29	72	85	*	0.4
21	252	46	10	0.6	*	18	0	0.09	0.1	0.7	*	*	*	34	53	*	*
21	168	99	35	1.3	1.1	40	2	0.1	0.11	1.3	0.11	17	0.09	54	111	*	*
21	192	54	18	0.7	*	25	0	0.1	0.1	0.7	*	*	*	42	68	*	*
0	414	364	12	1.8	0.5	0	0	0.24	0.21	2.4	0.03	21	0	105	73	15	0.1
0	358	314	11	1.6	0.4	0	0	0.26	0.18	2.1	0.02	18	0	91	63	15	0.9
21	176	50	11	0.6	*	8	0	0.09	0.12	0.9	*	*	*	42	60	*	*
0	*	*	52	0.9	*	40	0	0.08	0.1	0.5	*	*	*	35	56	*	*
20	160	66	5	0.4	0.2	12	0	0.04	0.05	0.2	0.06	3	0.36	59	91	2	*
20	160	33	5	0.4	0.2	6	0	0.06	0.07	0.5	0.06	3	0.36	27	38	2	*
20	160	43	5	0.3	0.2	8	0	0.04	0.06	0.3	0.06	3	0.36	36	71	3	*
0	144	25	5	0.8	0.2	0	0	0.1	0.06	0.9	0.02	10	*	20	23	8	0.2
0	96	36	5	0.5	0.1	4	t	0.07	0.07	0.4	0.02	6	t	8	22	5	0.3
29	140	40	7	1	0.2	8	0	0.28	0.1	1.2	0.02	9	0.05	12	32	*	0.1
0	241	37	8	1.2	0.2	0	0	0.2	0.13	1.6	0.01	15	*	54	33	12	t
0	312	49	12	1.2	0.3	0	0	0.2	0.12	1.7	0.02	30	0	24	46	15	t
0	761	122	*	3	*	0	0	0.54	0.32	4.5	0.05	*	*	58	115	41	0.1
0	197	102	40	0.8	0.6	0	0	0.12	0.05	1.1	0.08	16	0.05	34	98	16	t
45	445	129	17	1.5	0.7	28	0	0.18	0.24	1.5	0.05	14	0.37	154	135	11	*
0	256	78	8	1.8	0.3	95	0	0.17	0.2	1.9	0.1	1	*	30	141	*	*
0	220	194	39	1.8	0.7	100	0	0.15	0.17	0.8	0.2	16	0.6	20	135	*	0.6

WT, weight; **KCAL,** kcalories; **PROT,** protein; **CARB,** carbohydrate; **FIBR,** fiber; **FAT,** fat; **SATF,** saturated fat; **MONO,** monosaturated fat; **POLY,** polyunsaturated fat; **CHOR,** cholesterol; **SOD,** sodium; **POT,** potassium;

Food Name	Portion	WT (Gm)	KCAL	PROT (Gm)	CARB (Gm)	FIBR (Gm)	FAT (Gm)	SATF (Gm)	MONO (Gm)	POLY (Gm)
Breakfast Cereals										
CEREAL-100% BRAN	CUP	66	178	8	48	19.5	3	0.6	0.6	1.9
CEREAL-100% NATURAL-PLAIN	CUP	104	489	12	65	3.8	22	15.1	4.3	2
CEREAL-40% BRAN FLAKES-KELLOGGS	CUP	39	127	5	31	5.5	1	0	0	0
CEREAL-40% BRAN FLAKES-POST	CUP	47	152	5	37	6.5	1	0	0	0
CEREAL-ALL BRAN	CUP	85.2	212	12	63	25.5	2	0.2	0.2	0.8
CEREAL-ALPHA BITS	CUP	28.4	111	2	25	0.3	1	0.1	0.2	0.3
CEREAL-APPLE JACKS	CUP	28.4	110	2	26	0.2	t	0	0	0
CEREAL-BRAN BUDS	CUP	85.2	220	12	65	23.6	2	0.3	0.3	1.1
CEREAL-BRAN CHEX	CUP	49	156	5	39	7.9	1	0.2	0.2	0.7
CEREAL-BRAN FLAKES-RALSTON	CUP	49	159	6	39	6	1	0	0	0
CEREAL-C.W. POST-PLAIN	CUP	97	432	9	69	2.2	15	11.3	1.7	1.4
CEREAL-C.W. POST-WITH RAISINS	CUP	103	446	9	74	2	15	11	1.7	1.4
CEREAL-CAP'N CRUNCH	CUP	37	156	2	30	0.4	3	2.2	0.4	0.5
CEREAL-CAP'N CRUNCH-CRUNCHBERRIES	CUP	35	146	2	29	0.4	3	1.9	0.4	0.5
CEREAL-CHEERIOS	CUP	22.7	89	3	16	0.9	1	0.3	0.5	0.6
CEREAL-COCOA KRISPIES	CUP	36	139	2	32	0.2	1	0	0	0
CEREAL-COCOA PEBBLES	CUP	32.5	133	2	28	0.2	2	1	0.6	0.1
CEREAL-CORN BRAN	CUP	36	125	2	30	6.8	1	*	*	*
CEREAL-CORN CHEX	CUP	28.4	111	2	25	0.5	t	0	0	0
CEREAL-CORN FLAKES-KELLOGGS	CUP	22.7	88	2	20	0.5	t	0	0	0
CEREAL-CORN FLAKES-LOW SODIUM	CUP	25	100	2	22	0.3	t	0	0	0
CEREAL-CORN FLAKES-RALSTON	CUP	25	98	2	22	0.5	t	0	0	0
CEREAL-CORN GRITS-REGULAR-ENRICHED-HOT	CUP	242	145	3	32	0.6	t	0.1	0.1	0.2
CEREAL-CORN GRITS-REGULAR-UNENRICHED-HOT	CUP	242	145	3	32	0.6	t	0.1	0.1	0.2
CEREAL-CORN-SHREDDED-ADDED SUGAR	CUP	25	95	2	22	1.5	0	0	0	0
CEREAL-CRACKLIN BRAN	CUP	60	229	6	41	9.1	9	5.6	0.8	1.5
CEREAL-CRACKLIN OAT BRAN-KELLOGGS	SERVING	28.4	110	3	20	2	4	1	3	0
CEREAL-CREAM OF RICE-COOKED	CUP	244	127	2	28	0.4	t	0	0	0
CEREAL-CREAM OF WHEAT-INSTANT	CUP	241	153	4	32	2.2	1	0	0	0
CEREAL-CREAM OF WHEAT-PACKET SIZE	ITEM	150	132	3	29	2	t	0	0	0
CEREAL-CREAM OF WHEAT-REGULAR-HOT	CUP	251	133	4	28	1.9	1	0	0	0
CEREAL-CRISP RICE-LOW SODIUM	CUP	26	105	1	24	0.4	t	0	0	0
CEREAL-CRISPY RICE	CUP	28.4	112	2	25	1	t	0	0	0
CEREAL-CRISPY WHEATS AND RAISINS	CUP	43	150	3	35	2	1	0	0	0
CEREAL-FARINA-COOKED-ENRICHED-HOT	CUP	233	117	3	25	3.3	t	t	t	0.1
CEREAL-FORTIFIED OAT FLAKES	CUP	48	177	9	35	1.2	1	0	0	0
CEREAL-FROOT LOOPS-GENERAL MILLS	CUP	28.4	111	2	25	0.3	1	0	0	0
CEREAL-FROSTED FLAKES-KELLOGGS	CUP	35	133	2	32	0.8	t	0	0	0
CEREAL-FROSTED FLAKES-RALSTON	CUP	38	149	2	34	0.8	1	0	0	0
CEREAL-FROSTED MINI WHEATS-KELLOGGS	ITEM	7.1	26	1	6	0.5	t	0	0	0
CEREAL-FROSTED RICE KRISPIES-KELLOGGS	CUP	28.4	109	1	26	0.1	t	0	0	0
CEREAL-GRANOLA-HOMEMADE	CUP	122	594	15	67	12.8	33	5.8	9.4	17.2
CEREAL-GRANOLA-NATURE VALLEY	CUP	113	503	12	76	4.2	20	13	2.9	2.8
CEREAL-GRAPE NUTS FLAKES-POST	CUP	32.5	116	3	27	2.1	t	0	0	0
CEREAL-GRAPE NUTS-POST	CUP	114	407	13	94	5.5	t	0	0	0
CEREAL-HEARTLAND NATURAL-PLAIN	CUP	115	499	12	79	5.4	18	9.5	3.5	3.7
CEREAL-HONEY BRAN	CUP	35	119	3	29	3.9	1	0	0	0
CEREAL-HONEY NUT CHEERIOS-GENERAL MILLS	CUP	33	125	4	27	1.3	1	0.1	0.3	0.3
CEREAL-HONEYCOMB-POST	CUP	22	86	1	20	0.3	t	t	0.1	0.2
CEREAL-KING VITAMAN	CUP	21	85	1	18	0.3	1	0.7	0.2	0.2
CEREAL-KIX	CUP	18.9	74	2	16	0.3	t	0.1	0.1	0.2
CEREAL-LIFE-PLAIN/CINNAMON	CUP	44	162	8	32	1.4	1	0	0	0
CEREAL-LUCKY CHARMS	CUP	32	125	3	26	0.6	1	0.2	0.4	0.5
CEREAL-MALT O MEAL-COOKED	CUP	240	122	4	26	0.6	t	0	0	0
CEREAL-MAYPO-COOKED-HOT	CUP	240	170	6	32	1.2	2	*	*	*
CEREAL-NUTRI GRAIN-BARLEY	CUP	41	153	5	34	2.4	t	0	0	0
CEREAL-NUTRI GRAIN-CORN	CUP	42	160	3	36	2.6	1	0.1	0.2	0.5
CEREAL-NUTRI GRAIN-RYE	CUP	40	144	4	34	2.6	t	0	0	0
CEREAL-NUTRI GRAIN-WHEAT	CUP	44	158	4	37	2.8	1	0	0	0
CEREAL-OAT BRAN-COOKED	CUP	219	88	7	25	1.8	2	0.4	0.6	0.7
CEREAL-OAT BRAN-KELLOGGS	SERVING	28.4	100	4	22	1.5	1	*	*	*
CEREAL-OAT BRAN-QUAKER	CUP	85	270	18	51	12.3	6	0.8	1.7	2.1

t = Trace of nutrient present   ** = Not available*

MAG, magnesium; **IRON,** iron; **ZINC,** zinc; **VITA,** vitamin A; **VITC,** vitamin C; **THIA,** thiamin; **RIBO,** riboflavin; **NIAC,** niacin; **VB6,** vitamin B-6; **FOL,** folate; **VB12,** vitamin B-12; **CALC,** calcium; **PHOS,** phosphorus; **SEL,** selenium; **VE-a,** alpha tocopherol equivalents.

CHOL (mg)	SOD (mg)	POT (mg)	MAG (mg)	IRON (mg)	ZINC (mg)	VITA (RE)	VITC (mg)	THIA (mg)	RIBO (mg)	NIAC (mg)	VB6 (mg)	FOL (μg)	VB12 (μg)	CALC (mg)	PHOS (mg)	SEL (μg)	VE-a (mg)
0	457	824	312	8.1	5.7	0	63	1.6	1.8	20.9	2.1	47	6.3	46	801	20	1.5
0	45	514	125	3.1	2.4	6	0	0.31	0.56	2.4	0.19	31	0.13	181	383	*	0.7
0	363	248	71	11.2	5.1	516	0	0.5	0.6	6.9	0.7	138	2.1	19	192	4	0.2
0	431	251	102	7.5	2.5	622	0	0.6	0.7	8.3	0.8	166	2.5	21	296	5	0.2
0	961	1051	318	13.5	11.2	1125	45	1.11	1.28	15	1.53	301	0	69	794	25	1.3
0	219	110	17	1.8	1.5	375	0	0.4	0.4	5	0.5	100	1.5	8	51	10	t
0	125	23	6	4.5	3.7	375	15	0.4	0.4	5	0.5	100	0	3	30	18	0.1
0	523	1425	271	13.5	11.2	1125	45	1.11	1.28	15	1.53	301	0	57	740	25	0.9
0	455	394	126	7.8	2.1	11	26	0.6	0.26	8.6	0.9	173	2.6	29	327	10	0.6
0	456	191	118	7.8	2	649	26	0.6	0.7	8.6	0.9	173	2.6	27	273	*	1
0	167	198	67	15.4	1.6	1284	0	1.3	1.5	17.1	1.7	342	5.1	47	224	*	0.7
0	160	260	74	16.4	1.6	1364	0	1.3	1.5	18.1	1.9	364	5.5	51	232	*	0.7
0	278	48	15	9.8	4	5	0	0.66	0.71	8.6	1	238	2.34	6	47	*	0.2
0	243	49	14	9	3.6	5	0	0.59	0.67	8.1	0.93	128	2.51	11	47	*	0.2
0	246	81	31	3.6	0.6	300	12	0.3	0.34	4	0.41	5	1.2	39	107	10	0.2
0	275	53	12	2.3	1.9	477	19	0.5	0.5	6.3	0.6	127	0.02	6	47	*	t
0	155	54	13	2.1	1.7	430	0	0.42	0.49	5.7	0.59	115	1.72	6	25	*	t
0	310	70	18	12.2	4	8	0	0.37	0.7	10.9	0.86	232	1.39	41	52	2	*
0	271	23	4	1.8	0.1	14	15	0.4	0.07	5	0.5	100	1.5	3	11	2	0.1
0	281	21	3	1.4	0.1	300	12	0.3	0.34	4	0.41	80	0	1	14	1	t
0	3	18	3	0.6	0.1	10	0	t	0.05	0.1	0.02	2	0	11	12	1	t
0	239	22	3	0.6	0.1	10	13	0.1	0	1.1	0.02	2	0	2	10	1	0.1
0	0	53	10	1.6	0.2	*	*	0.24	0.15	2	0.06	2	0	0	29	24	t
0	0	53	10	1.6	0.2	*	*	0.24	0.15	2	0.06	2	0	0	29	24	t
0	247	*	4	0.6	0.1	0	13	0.33	0.05	4.4	0.45	88	1.33	1	10	2	0.1
0	487	355	116	3.8	3.2	794	32	0.8	0.9	10.6	1.1	212	0	40	241	10	0.7
0	140	160	60	1.8	1.5	180	15	0.38	0.43	5	0.5	100	1.5	20	150	*	1.2
0	2	49	7	0.5	0.4	0	0	0	0	1	0.07	7	0	7	42	*	*
0	6	48	14	12	0.4	0	0	0.2	0.1	1.8	0.03	11	0	59	43	*	t
0	241	55	9	8.1	0.2	1250	0	0.4	0.2	5	0.5	100	0	40	20	*	0.7
0	2	43	10	10.3	0.3	0	0	0.25	0	1.5	0.04	10	0	50	42	*	t
0	3	20	10	0.8	0.4	0	0	0	0.05	0.4	0.04	3	0	17	27	4	t
0	208	27	12	0.7	0.5	0	1	0.11	0.03	2	0.04	3	0.08	5	31	4	t
0	204	174	35	6.8	0.5	569	0	0.6	0.6	7.6	0.8	15	2.3	71	117	6	11.4
0	0	30	5	1.2	0.2	*	*	0.19	0.12	1.3	0.02	5	0	5	28	*	2
0	429	343	58	13.7	1.5	636	0	0.6	0.7	8.4	0.9	169	2.5	68	176	10	0.3
0	145	26	7	4.5	3.7	375	15	0.4	0.4	5	0.5	100	0	3	24	18	0.1
0	284	22	3	2.2	0.1	463	19	0.5	0.5	6.2	0.6	124	0	1	26	*	*
0	247	24	3	1	0.8	503	20	0.5	0.6	6.7	0.7	3	2	4	9	*	*
0	2	24	56	0.4	0.4	94	4	0.09	0.11	1.3	0.13	25	0	2	19	*	t
0	240	21	5	1.8	0.3	375	15	0.4	0.4	5	0.5	100	0	1	27	4	t
0	12	612	141	4.8	4.5	10	1	0.73	0.31	2.1	0.43	99	0	76	494	3	5.7
0	232	389	116	3.8	2.2	8	0	0.39	0.19	0.8	0.09	85	0	71	354	37	3.4
0	250	113	36	5.2	0.7	430	0	0.42	0.49	5.7	0.59	115	1.72	13	97	10	0.1
0	792	381	76	5	2.5	1500	0	1.48	1.71	20.1	2.05	402	6.04	43	286	34	0.3
0	294	385	147		3	7	1	0.36	0.16	1.6	0.19	64	0	75	416	*	0.8
0	202	151	46	5.6	0.9	463	19	0.5	0.5	6.2	0.6	23	1.9	16	132	*	0.8
0	299	115	39	5.2	0.9	437	17	0.4	0.5	5.8	0.6	22	1.7	23	122	*	0.2
0	166	70	8	1.4	1.2	291	0	0.3	0.3	3.9	0.4	78	1.2	4	22	*	0.1
0	161	26	7	12.7	0.2	717	33	0.92	1.06	12.9	1.18	286	4.13	2	27	*	6.7
0	226	30	8	5.4	0.2	250	10	0.25	0.28	3.3	0.34	67	1	24	26	*	t
0	229	197	14	11.6	1.5	3	1	0.95	1	11.6	0.08	37	0	154	238	*	0.3
0	227	66	27	5.1	0.6	424	17	0.4	0.5	5.6	0.6	6	1.7	36	88	*	0.2
0	2	31	5	9.5	0.2	0	0	0.4	0.3	5.9	0.02	6	0	5	23	*	0.3
0	9	211	51	8.4	1.5	702	28	0.7	0.8	9.4	0.9	9	2.8	125	248	*	*
0	277	108	32	1.5	5.4	543	22	0.5	0.6	7.2	0.7	145	2.2	11	126	27	10.8
0	276	98	27	0.9	5.5	556	22	0.5	0.6	7.4	0.8	148	2.2	1	120	3	t
0	272	72	31	1.1	5.3	530	21	0.5	0.6	7	0.7	141	2.1	8	104	*	t
0	299	120	34	1.2	5.8	583	23	0.6	0.7	7.7	0.8	155	2.3	12	164	7	t
0	2	201	88	1.9	1.2	0	0	0.35	0.07	0.3	0.06	13	0	22	261	*	0.4
0	270	115	40	4.5	3.8	180	*	0.38	0.43	5	0.5	*	1.5	*	150	*	*
0	15	540	180	5.4	3.6	1028	0	0.9	0.31	15	1.49	48	5.18	60	600	*	2

WT, weight; **KCAL**, kcalories; **PROT**, protein; **CARB**, carbohydrate; **FIBR**, fiber; **FAT**, fat; **SATF**, saturated fat; **MONO**, monosaturated fat; **POLY**, polyunsaturated fat; **CHOR**, cholesterol; **SOD**, sodium; **POT**, potassium;

Food Name	Portion	WT (Gm)	KCAL	PROT (Gm)	CARB (Gm)	FIBR (Gm)	FAT (Gm)	SATF (Gm)	MONO (Gm)	POLY (Gm)
CEREAL-OAT BRAN-RAISIN/SPICE-HOT	OUNCE	28.4	100	3	19	3.8	1	*	*	*
CEREAL-OATMEAL-COOKED	CUP	234	145	6	25	2.1	2	0.4	0.8	0.9
CEREAL-OATMEAL-RAW	CUP	81	311	13	54	4.6	5	0.9	1.8	2.1
CEREAL-OATS-APPLE/CINNAMON-QUAKER-PACKET	ITEM	149	135	4	26	1.4	2	0.3	0.6	0.7
CEREAL-OATS-BRAN/RAISIN-QUAKER-PACKET	ITEM	195	158	5	30	1.8	2	0.3	0.7	0.8
CEREAL-OATS-CINNAMON/SPICE-QUAKER-PACKET	ITEM	161	177	5	35	1.5	2	0.3	0.7	0.8
CEREAL-OATS-MAPLE/SUGAR-QUAKER-PACKET	ITEM	155	163	5	32	1.4	2	0.3	0.7	0.8
CEREAL-OATS-PLAIN-QUAKER-INSTANT-PACKET	ITEM	177	104	4	18	1.6	2	0.3	0.6	0.7
CEREAL-OATS-PUFFED-ADDED SUGAR	CUP	25	100	3	19	2.7	1	0.2	0.1	0.5
CEREAL-PRODUCT 19-KELLOGGS	CUP	33	126	3	27	0.4	t	0	0	0
CEREAL-RAISIN BRAN-KELLOGGS	CUP	49.2	154	5	37	5.3	1	0.1	0.1	0.5
CEREAL-RAISIN BRAN-POST	CUP	56.8	174	5	43	6	1	0.2	0.2	0.5
CEREAL-RAISIN BRAN-RALSTON	CUP	56	178	4	47	7.1	t	0	0	0
CEREAL-RALSTON-COOKED-HOT	CUP	253	134	6	28	4.2	1	0	0	0
CEREAL-RICE CHEX	CUP	25.2	100	1	23	0.2	t	0	0	0
CEREAL-RICE KRISPIES-KELLOGGS	CUP	28.4	112	2	25	0.1	t	0	0	0
CEREAL-RICE-PUFFED-ADDED SUGAR	CUP	28.4	115	1	26	0.2	0	0	0	0
CEREAL-RICE-PUFFED-PLAIN	CUP	14	56	1	13	0.1	t	0	0	0
CEREAL-ROMAN MEAL-COOKED	CUP	241	147	7	33	2.3	1	*	*	*
CEREAL-SPECIAL K-KELLOGGS	CUP	21.3	83	4	16	0.2	t	0	0	0
CEREAL-SUGAR CORN POPS-KELLOGGS	CUP	28.4	108	1	26	0.2	t	0	0	0
CEREAL-SUGAR SMACKS-KELLOGGS	CUP	37.9	141	3	33	0.5	1	0	0	0
CEREAL-SUPER SUGAR CRISP-POST	CUP	33	123	2	30	0.5	t	0	0	0
CEREAL-TASTEEOS	CUP	24	94	3	19	0.8	1	0	0	0
CEREAL-TEAM	CUP	42	164	3	36	0.4	1	0	0	0
CEREAL-TOASTIES-POST	CUP	22.7	88	2	20	0.4	t	0	0	0
CEREAL-TOTAL-GENERAL MILLS	CUP	33	116	3	26	2.4	1	0.1	0.1	0.3
CEREAL-TRIX-GENERAL MILLS	CUP	28.4	109	2	25	0.3	t	0	0	0
CEREAL-WHEAT CHEX	CUP	46	169	5	38	3.4	1	0.5	0.1	0.3
CEREAL-WHEAT FLAKES-ADDED SUGAR	CUP	30	105	3	24	2.7	0	0	0	0
CEREAL-WHEAT GERM-BROWN SUGAR AND HONEY	CUP	113	426	25	69	5.7	9	1.6	1.3	5.5
CEREAL-WHEAT GERM-TOASTED	CUP	113	432	33	56	14.6	12	2.1	1.7	7.5
CEREAL-WHEAT-PUFFED-ADDED SUGAR	SERVING	38	138	6	30	2.1	t	*	0.1	0.1
CEREAL-WHEAT-PUFFED-PLAIN	CUP	12	44	2	10	0.4	t	0	0	0
CEREAL-WHEAT-ROLLED-COOKED-HOT	CUP	240	180	5	41	2.9	1	0.2	0.1	0.5
CEREAL-WHEAT-SHREDDED-BISCUIT	ITEM	23.6	83	3	19	2.2	t	0	0	0
CEREAL-WHEAT-WHOLE MEAL-COOKED-HOT	CUP	245	110	4	23	1.6	1	0.2	0.1	0.5
CEREAL-WHEATENA-COOKED	CUP	243	136	5	29	2.6	1	*	*	*
CEREAL-WHEATIES	CUP	29	101	3	23	2	1	0.1	0.1	0.2
CEREAL-WHOLE WHEAT NATURAL	CUP	242	150	5	33	2.7	1	0.2	0.2	0.4
OATS-ROLLED OR OATMEAL-DRY	CUP	81	311	13	54	3.8	5	0.9	1.6	1.9
Combination Foods										
BEEF POTPIE-HOME RECIPE-1/3 OF 9" PIE	SLICE	210	515	21	39	3.9	30	7.9	12.9	7.4
BEEF STEW-WITH VEGETABLES	CUP	245	220	16	15	3.2	11	4.9	4.5	0.5
BEEF-RAVIOLIOS-CANNED WITH MEAT SAUCE	OUNCE	28.4	28	1	4	0.2	1	0.1	0.2	0.3
BURRITO-BEANS AND CHEESE	ITEM	93	189	8	28	8.3	6	3.4	1.2	0.9
CHEESE SOUFFLE-HOME RECIPE	CUP	95	207	9	6	0.1	16	6.6	5.8	2.5
CHICKEN A LA KING-COOKED-HOME RECIPE	CUP	245	470	27	12	1.2	34	12.9	13.4	6.2
CHICKEN AND NOODLES-COOKED-HOME RECIPE	CUP	240	365	22	26	1.3	18	5.9	7.1	3.5
CHICKEN CHOW MEIN-CANNED	CUP	250	95	7	18	0.9	0	0	0	0
CHICKEN CHOW MEIN-HOME RECIPE	CUP	250	255	31	10	0.5	10	2.4	3.4	3.1
CHICKEN POTPIE-BAKED-HOME RECIPE	SLICE	232	545	23	42	4.2	31	11	13.5	5.5
CHILI CON CARNE-WITH BEANS-CANNED	CUP	255	340	19	31	5	16	7.5	7.2	1
CHILI WITH BEANS-CANNED	CUP	255	286	15	30	6.9	14	6	6	0.9
CHIMICHANGA-BEEF	ITEM	174	425	20	43	4.3	20	8.5	8.1	1.1
CHOP SUEY-WITH BEEF AND PORK-HOME RECIPE	CUP	250	300	26	13	*	17	8.5	6.2	0.7
CORN DOG-PLAIN	ITEM	175	460	17	56	2.8	19	5.2	9.1	3.5
ENCHILADA-CHEESE	ITEM	163	320	10	29	3.2	19	10.6	6.3	0.8
ENCHIRITO-CHEESE/BEEF/BEAN	ITEM	193	344	18	34	3.4	16	8	6.5	0.3
HAMBURGER-BACON AND CHEESE-GENERIC	ITEM	150	464	25	29	1.8	27	*	*	*
HOT DOG-PLAIN WITH BUN-GENERIC	ITEM	98	242	10	18	0.9	15	5.1	6.9	1.7
MACARONI & CHEESE-BAKED-HOME RECIPE	CUP	200	430	17	40	*	22	11.9	7.3	1

t = Trace of nutrient present ** = Not available*

MAG, magnesium; **IRON,** iron; **ZINC,** zinc; **VITA,** vitamin A; **VITC,** vitamin C; **THIA,** thiamin; **RIBO,** riboflavin; **NIAC,** niacin; **VB6,** vitamin B-6; **FOL,** folate; **VB12,** vitamin B-12; **CALC,** calcium; **PHOS,** phosphorus; **SEL,** selenium; **VE-a,** alpha tocopherol equivalents.

CHOL (mg)	SOD (mg)	POT (mg)	MAG (mg)	IRON (mg)	ZINC (mg)	VITA (RE)	VITC (mg)	THIA (mg)	RIBO (mg)	NIAC (mg)	VB6 (mg)	FOL (µg)	VB12 (µg)	CALC (mg)	PHOS (mg)	SEL (µg)	VE-a (mg)
0	10	100	43	0.7	0.8	0	t	0.06	0.05	1.2	0.08	24	0	16	148	*	0
0	1	132	56	1.6	1.2	7	*	0.26	0.05	0.3	0.05	9	0	20	178	20	3.5
0	3	284	120	3.4	2.5	10	0	0.59	0.11	0.6	0.1	26	0	42	384	22	0.2
0	222	107	34	6.1	0.7	435	0	0.48	0.28	5.1	0.7	137	0	158	117	13	0.9
0	247	236	57	7.6	1.4	479	0	0.56	0.63	8.1	0.76	155	0	173	206	17	1.2
0	280	104	51	6.7	1	475	0	0.56	0.34	5.7	0.77	153	0	172	146	14	1
0	280	102	42	6.4	0.9	451	0	0.53	0.32	5.4	0.74	145	0	162	143	13	0.9
0	286	100	43	6.3	0.9	455	0	0.53	0.29	5.5	0.74	150	0	163	133	15	1.1
0	294	*	28	4	0.7	275	13	0.33	0.38	4.4	0.45	6	1.33	44	102	6	0.2
0	378	51	12	21	0.5	1748	70	1.7	2	23.3	2.3	466	7	4	47	*	34.9
0	359	256	64	6	5	500	0	0.49	0.59	6.7	0.69	133	2.02	17	183	5	1.1
0	370	350	97	9	3	750	0	0.74	0.85	10	1.02	201	3.01	27	238	6	1.3
0	486	287	84	6.7	1.7	556	2	0.6	0.6	7.4	0.7	148	2.2	27	247	6	*
0	4	153	59	1.6	1.4	0	0	0.2	0.18	2.1	0.11	18	0.11	14	148	*	2
0	211	29	6	1.6	0.3	2	13	0.33	0.01	4.4	0.45	89	1.34	4	25	4	t
0	340	30	10	1.8	0.5	375	15	0.4	0.4	5	0.5	100	0	4	34	4	t
0	21	43	8	0	1.5	300	15	0	0	0	0.5	99	1.48	3	14	2	0.2
0	t	16	4	0.1	0.1	0	0	0.02	0.01	0.4	0.01	3	0	1	14	1	0.1
0	3	302	109	2.1	1.8	0	0	0.24	0.12	3.1	0.11	24	0	30	215	*	*
0	199	37	12	3.4	2.8	280	11	0.28	0.32	3.8	0.38	75	0.01	6	41	13	0.1
0	103	17	2	1.8	1.5	375	15	0.4	0.4	5	0.5	100	0	1	28	*	t
0	100	56	18	2.4	0.4	500	20	0.49	0.57	6.7	0.68	134	0	4	41	*	*
0	29	123	20	2.1	1.7	437	0	0.4	0.5	5.8	0.6	116	1.7	7	60	26	0.1
0	183	71	26	3.8	0.7	318	13	0.31	0.36	4.2	0.43	9	1.27	11	96	10	0.2
0	259	71	19	2.6	0.6	556	22	0.5	0.6	7.4	0.8	7	2.2	6	65	7	0.1
0	238	26	3	0.6	0.1	300	0	0.3	0.34	4	0.41	80	1.2	1	10	*	0.1
0	409	123	37	21	0.8	1748	70	1.7	2	23.3	2.3	466	7	56	137	*	34.9
0	181	27	6	4.5	0.1	371	15	0.37	0.43	5	0.51	3	1.51	6	19	*	0.1
0	308	174	58	7.3	1.2	0	24	0.6	0.17	8.1	0.8	162	2.4	18	182	*	0.2
0	368	81	33	4.8	0.7	330	16	0.4	0.45	5.3	0.54	9	1.59	12	83	3	0.1
0	3	803	272	7.7	14.1	0	0	1.41	0.7	4.7	0.83	298	0	38	971	*	20.5
0	5	1070	362	10.3	18.8	50	7	1.89	0.93	6.3	1.11	398	0	51	1295	*	15.9
0	2	132	55	1.8	0.9	0	0	0.08	0.09	4.1	0.07	12	0	11	135	*	*
0	t	42	17	0.6	0.3	0	0	0.02	0.03	1.3	0.02	4	0	3	43	*	0.1
0	535	202	53	1.7	1.2	0	0	0.17	0.07	2.2	*	26	*	19	182	*	2.5
0	t	77	40	0.7	0.6	0	0	0.07	0.06	1.1	0.06	12	0	10	86	*	0.1
0	535	118	54	1.2	1.2	0	0	0.15	0.05	1.5	*	27	*	17	127	*	2.6
0	5	187	49	1.4	1.7	0	0	0.02	0.05	1.3	0.05	17	0	10	146	58	*
0	363	108	32	4.6	0.7	384	15	0.4	0.4	5.1	0.5	9	1.5	44	100	3	0.1
0	1	171	54	1.5	1.2	0	0	0.17	0.12	2.2	0.18	27	0	17	167	58	2.6
0	3	284	120	3.4	2.5	20	0	0.59	0.11	0.6	0.1	26	0	42	384	43	1.2
44	596	334	*	3.8	*	344	6	0.3	0.3	5.5	*	*	*	29	149	*	1.2
72	1006	613	*	2.9	*	480	17	0.15	0.17	4.7	*	*	t	29	184	*	0.5
*	131	46	*	0.3	*	50	t	0.03	0.02	0.4	*	*	*	5	*	*	t
14	583	248	40	1.1	0.8	118	1	0.11	0.36	1.8	0.13	41	0.45	107	90	*	0.9
137	346	115	14	1	1	152	0	0.05	0.23	0.2	0.06	14	0.35	191	185	*	1.4
186	759	404	*	2.5	*	226	12	0.1	0.42	5.4	*	*	*	127	358	*	0.9
96	600	149	*	2.2	*	80	0	0.05	0.17	4.3	*	*	*	26	247	*	0.2
98	722	418	*	1.3	*	30	13	0.05	0.1	1	*	*	*	45	85	*	0
98	717	473	*	2.5	*	56	10	0.08	0.23	4.3	*	*	*	58	293	*	0
72	593	343	*	3	*	618	5	0.34	0.31	5.5	*	*	*	70	232	32	0.9
38	1354	594	*	4.3	*	30	*	0.08	0.18	3.3	0.26	*	*	82	321	*	*
43	1330	932	115	8.8	5.1	86	4	0.12	0.27	0.9	0.34	58	0.03	119	393	*	1.4
9	910	587	62	4.6	5	15	5	0.48	0.64	5.8	0.27	31	1.52	63	123	*	4.5
64	1052	425	*	4.8	*	120	33	0.28	0.38	5	*	*	*	60	248	*	0
79	972	262	17	6.2	1.3	36	0	0.29	0.71	4.2	0.1	60	0.44	101	166	*	1.3
44	784	240	50	1.3	2.5	186	1	0.09	0.42	1.9	0.39	34	0.74	324	133	*	1.7
49	1251	560	71	2.4	2.8	134	5	0.18	0.69	3	0.21	254	1.63	217	224	*	*
68	660	339	35	3.7	5.3	75	2	0.15	0.27	4.9	0.24	26	1.8	116	302	23	0.1
44	671	143	13	2.3	2	0	t	0.24	0.27	3.7	0.05	30	0.51	24	97	*	*
68	1086	240	36	1.6	1.8	258	1	0.15	0.31	1.5	0.15	17	0.46	362	322	*	1

WT, weight; **KCAL,** kcalories; **PROT,** protein; **CARB,** carbohydrate; **FIBR,** fiber; **FAT,** fat; **SATF,** saturated fat;
MONO, monosaturated fat; **POLY,** polyunsaturated fat; **CHOR,** cholesterol; **SOD,** sodium; **POT,** potassium;

Food Name	Portion	WT (Gm)	KCAL	PROT (Gm)	CARB (Gm)	FIBR (Gm)	FAT (Gm)	SATF (Gm)	MONO (Gm)	POLY (Gm)
MACARONI & CHEESE-ENRICHED-CANNED	CUP	240	230	9	26	1.4	10	4.2	3.1	1.4
MACARONI & CHEESE-ENRICHED-HOME RECIPE	CUP	200	430	17	40	1.2	22	8.9	8.8	2.9
MEAT LOAF-WITH CELERY AND ONIONS	SERVING	87.6	213	16	5	0.1	14	5.3	5.9	0.6
MIXED FRUIT-CANNED-HEAVY SYRUP PACK	CUP	255	184	1	48	2.9	t	t	t	0.1
MIXED FRUIT-FROZEN-SWEETENED	CUP	250	245	4	61	3	t	0.1	0.1	0.2
NACHOS-CHEESE	SERVING	113	345	9	36	2.2	19	7.8	8	2.2
PEAS & CARROTS-CANNED-DIETARY-LOW SODIUM	CUP	255	96	6	22	7.1	1	0.1	0.1	0.3
PEAS AND CARROTS-CANNED	CUP	255	97	6	22	8.6	1	0.1	0.1	0.3
PEAS AND CARROTS-FROZEN-BOILED	CUP	160	77	5	16	7.1	1	0.1	0.1	0.3
PEAS AND ONIONS-CANNED	CUP	120	61	4	10	4.3	t	0.1	t	0.2
PEAS AND ONIONS-FROZEN-BOILED	CUP	180	81	5	16	4.7	t	0.1	t	0.2
PIZZA-CHEESE-BAKED	SLICE	63	140	8	21	1.6	3	1.5	1	0.5
PIZZA-CHEESE/MEAT/VEGETABLE	SLICE	79	184	13	21	1.8	5	1.5	2.5	0.9
PIZZA-PEPPERONI-BAKED	SLICE	71	181	10	20	1.5	7	2.2	3.1	1.2
PORK AND BEANS WITH FRANKFURTERS-CANNED	CUP	257	365	17	40	12.8	17	6.1	7.3	2.2
PORK AND BEANS WITH SWEET SAUCE-CANNED	CUP	253	281	13	53	14	4	1.4	1.6	0.5
PORK AND BEANS WITH TOMATO SAUCE-CANNED	CUP	253	248	13	49	13.8	3	1	1.1	0.3
RICE-FRIED (NASI GORENG)	OUNCE	28.3	55	1	7	t	2	0.3	0.5	1.1
SALAD-CARROT RAISIN-HOME RECIPE	CUP	268	306	4	56	16.7	12	6.8	12.8	23.4
SALAD-CHEF-WITH HAM AND CHEESE	SERVING	200	196	13	7	2.4	13	7	4.1	0.7
SALAD-CHICKEN	CUP	205	502	26	17	2.2	36	4.3	7.2	10.1
SALAD-COLESLAW	TBSP	8	6	t	1	0.3	t	t	0.1	0.1
SALAD-CRAB	SERVING	100	145	12	5	0.3	9	1	1.7	3.5
SALAD-FRUIT-CANNED-JUICE PACK	CUP	249	125	1	33	1.6	t	t	t	t
SALAD-FRUIT-CANNED-WATER PACK	CUP	245	74	1	19	4.5	t	t	t	0.1
SALAD-GREEN SALAD-TOSSED	SERVING	207	32	3	7	2.1	t	t	t	0.1
SALAD-MACARONI	SERVING	28.4	51	1	5	0.3	3	0.2	0.4	0.7
SALAD-MANDARIN ORANGE GELATIN	SERVING	28.4	23	t	6	0.6	0	0	0	0
SALAD-POTATO	CUP	250	358	7	28	5.3	21	3.6	6.2	9.3
SALAD-TACO	SERVING	198	279	13	24	2.8	15	6.8	5.2	1.8
SALAD-THREE BEAN-ALEX	SERVING	28.4	33	1	7	2.1	t	*	*	*
SALAD-THREE BEAN-CANNED-DEL MONTE	OUNCE	28.4	22	1	5	1.5	t	0	0	0
SALAD-WALDORF GELATIN	SERVING	28.4	27	2	5	0.3	t	0	0	0
SANDWICH-BLT-WITH MAYONNAISE	ITEM	148	282	7	29	2.9	16	6.8	5.5	4.9
SANDWICH-CHICKEN/SALAD/MAYONNAISE	OUNCE	28.3	81	6	3	0.4	5	0.6	1	1.4
SANDWICH-CLUB	ITEM	315	590	36	42	4.2	21	14.5	11.6	10.5
SANDWICH-HAM AND CHEESE	ITEM	146	353	21	33	3.3	16	6.4	6.7	1.4
SANDWICH-ROAST BEEF-PLAIN	ITEM	139	346	22	34	3.4	14	3.6	6.8	1.7
SANDWICH-ROAST BEEF-WITH CHEESE	ITEM	176	402	32	27	2.7	18	9	3.7	3.5
SANDWICH-STEAK	ITEM	204	459	30	52	5.2	14	3.8	5.4	3.4
SANDWICH-SUBMARINE-ROAST BEEF	ITEM	216	411	29	44	4.4	13	7.1	1.8	2.6
SANDWICH-SUBMARINE-WITH COLDCUTS	ITEM	228	456	22	51	5.1	19	6.8	8.2	2.3
SANDWICH-TUNA/SALAD/MAYONNAISE	OUNCE	28.3	64	5	5	0.3	3	0.4	0.7	1.1
SPAGHETTI IN SAUCE/CHEESE-FRANCO	OUNCE	28.4	11	1	5	*	t	*	*	*
SPAGHETTI/TOMATO/CHEESE-CANNED	CUP	250	190	6	39	2.5	2	0.5	0.3	0.4
SPAGHETTI/TOMATO/CHEESE-FROM HOME RECIPE	CUP	250	260	9	37	2.5	9	2	5.4	0.7
SPAGHETTI/TOMATO/MEAT-CANNED	CUP	250	260	12	29	2.8	10	2.2	3.3	3.9
SPAGHETTI/TOMATO/MEAT-FROM HOME RECIPE	CUP	248	330	19	39	2.7	12	3.3	6.3	0.9
SPINACH SOUFFLE	CUP	136	219	11	3	0.8	18	7.2	6.8	3.1
TACO	ITEM	171	370	21	27	2.7	21	11.4	6.6	1
TUNA-SALAD-CELERY/MAYONNAISE/PICKLE/EGG	CUP	205	350	30	7	1	22	4.3	6.3	6.7
VEGETABLES-MIXED-CANNED-DRAINED	CUP	163	77	4	15	8.1	t	0.1	t	0.2
VEGETABLES-MIXED-FROZEN-BOILED	CUP	182	107	5	24	6.9	t	0.1	t	0.1
Dairy Products										
CHEESE FOOD-AMERICAN-PASTEURIZED PROCESS	OUNCE	28.4	93	6	2	0	7	4.4	2	0.2
CHEESE SPREAD-AMERICAN-PROCESSED	OUNCE	28.4	82	5	2	0	6	3.8	1.8	0.2
CHEESE-AMERICAN-PASTEURIZED PROCESS	OUNCE	28.4	106	6	t	0	9	5.6	2.5	0.3
CHEESE-BLUE	OUNCE	28.4	100	6	1	0	8	5.3	2.2	0.2
CHEESE-BLUE-CRUMBLED-UNPACKED	CUP	135	477	29	3	0	39	25.2	10.5	1.1
CHEESE-BRICK	OUNCE	28.4	105	7	1	0	8	5.3	2.4	0.2
CHEESE-BRIE	OUNCE	28.4	95	6	t	0	8	4.9	2.3	0.2
CHEESE-CAMEMBERT-WEDGE	ITEM	38	114	8	t	0	9	5.8	2.7	0.3
CHEESE-CARAWAY	OUNCE	28.4	107	7	1	0	8	5.3	2.4	0.2

t= Trace of nutrient present   **= Not available*

MAG, magnesium; **IRON,** iron; **ZINC,** zinc; **VITA,** vitamin A; **VITC,** vitamin C; **THIA,** thiamin; **RIBO,** riboflavin; **NIAC,** niacin; **VB6,** vitamin B-6; **FOL,** folate; **VB12,** vitamin B-12; **CALC,** calcium; **PHOS,** phosphorus; **SEL,** selenium; **VE-a,** alpha tocopherol equivalents.

CHOL (mg)	SOD (mg)	POT (mg)	MAG (mg)	IRON (mg)	ZINC (mg)	VITA (RE)	VITC (mg)	THIA (mg)	RIBO (mg)	NIAC (mg)	VB6 (mg)	FOL (μg)	VB12 (μg)	CALC (mg)	PHOS (mg)	SEL (μg)	VE-a (mg)
42	729	139	*	1	*	52	0	0.12	0.24	1	*	*	*	199	182	*	0.4
42	1086	240	52	1.8	*	172	0	0.2	0.4	1.8	*	*	*	362	322	28	0.3
107	103	182	14	1.9	3.1	12	1	0.05	0.15	3.2	0.16	11	1.52	23	112	1	0.1
0	10	214	13	0.9	0.2	49	176	0.04	0.1	1.5	0.09	8	0	3	26	1	0.7
0	8	327	14	0.7	0.1	81	188	0.04	0.09	1	0.06	19	0	18	30	1	*
18	816	172	55	1.3	1.8	92	1	0.19	0.37	1.5	0.2	10	0.82	272	276	*	3
0	10	256	37	1.9	1.5	1471	17	0.19	0.14	1.5	0.22	47	0	58	116	3	0.1
0	663	255	36	1.9	1.5	1471	17	0.19	0.14	1.5	0.22	47	0	59	117	*	0.1
0	109	253	26	1.5	0.7	1242	13	0.36	0.1	1.9	0.14	42	0	37	78	*	0.2
0	530	115	19	1	0.7	19	4	0.12	0.08	1.5	0.23	32	0	20	61	*	t
0	67	211	23	1.6	0.5	63	12	0.27	0.12	1.9	0.16	36	0	25	61	*	0.2
9	336	110	16	0.6	0.8	74	1	0.18	0.16	2.5	0.04	59	0.33	116	113	*	*
21	382	178	18	1.5	1.1	101	2	0.21	0.17	2	0.09	27	0.36	101	131	*	0.8
14	267	153	8	0.9	0.5	54	2	0.14	0.23	3.1	0.05	53	0.19	65	75	*	*
15	1105	604	72	4.5	4.8	39	6	0.15	0.14	2.3	0.12	77	0	123	267	*	0.6
18	850	673	86	4.2	3.8	28	8	0.12	0.15	0.9	0.22	95	0	154	266	*	0.6
17	1113	759	88	8.3	14.8	62	8	0.13	0.12	1.3	0.18	57	0	141	297	*	0.6
7	126	41	4	2.2	0.1	70	0	0.01	0.01	0.5	0.02	3	0.02	6	15	*	0.4
33	377	928	42	3	0.5	1100	12	0.16	0.16	1	0.68	28	0.14	96	130	*	16
46	567	415	28	1.2	1.7	740	24	0.34	0.24	2.2	0.21	46	0.47	227	251	19	0.7
67	1395	521	40	3.7	2	30	2	0.47	0.42	7.7	0.34	39	0.2	128	207	*	5.6
1	2	15	1	t	t	7	3	0.01	0.01	t	0.01	2	0	4	3	*	0.4
69	487	260	26	0.6	2.8	9	2	0.06	0.06	1.3	0.12	35	4.74	38	129	*	1.4
0	13	288	21	0.6	0.4	149	8	0.03	0.04	0.9	0.07	6	0	28	36	1	*
0	7	191	12	0.7	0.2	108	5	0.04	0.05	0.9	0.08	6	0	17	22	1	*
0	53	356	22	1.3	0.4	235	48	0.06	0.1	1.2	0.16	77	0	26	80	1	0.5
1	148	21	3	0.3	0.1	4	1	0.03	0.02	0.2	0.02	2	0.01	5	12	*	0.2
0	14	9	*	*	*	*	*	*	*	*	*	*	*	*	*	*	*
171	1323	635	39	1.6	0.8	82	25	0.19	0.15	2.2	0.35	17	0.39	48	130	*	5.9
44	763	416	52	2.3	2.7	78	4	0.1	0.35	2.5	0.21	40	0.64	192	143	*	2.3
*	107	63	*	*	*	*	*	*	*	*	*	*	*	*	*	*	*
0	101	38	6	0.3	0.1	8	1	0.01	0.01	0.1	0.01	10	0.01	10	16	*	0.3
0	16	14	5	0.1	0.1	5	1	0.01	0.01	t	0.02	2	0.01	5	10	*	0.3
44	1222	274	27	1.5	1.8	174	13	0.16	0.14	1.6	0.23	26	0.55	53	89	*	1.9
9	75	27	6	0.3	0.3	11	t	0.02	0.04	0.8	0.05	5	0.03	7	26	*	0.8
93	2601	583	58	4.3	3.9	350	27	0.38	0.41	10.2	0.5	55	1.17	103	394	*	4.1
58	772	290	16	3.3	1.4	77	3	0.31	0.49	2.7	0.2	71	0.54	130	152	*	1.1
52	792	316	31	4.2	3.4	21	2	0.38	0.31	5.9	0.27	40	1.22	54	239	*	0.2
77	1634	345	40	5.1	5.4	46	0	0.38	0.46	5.9	0.34	41	2.05	183	401	*	0.4
73	798	525	49	5.2	4.5	44	6	0.4	0.37	7.3	0.37	89	1.57	91	297	*	0.4
73	845	330	67	2.8	4.4	50	6	0.42	0.42	6	0.32	45	1.82	41	193	*	5.2
35	1650	394	68	2.5	2.6	79	12	1	0.8	5.5	0.13	54	1.09	189	287	*	5.4
3	93	31	5	1.4	0.1	11	t	0.02	0.04	0.9	0.03	6	0.21	10	34	*	0.7
*	114	*	*	0.2	*	11	0	0.03	0.02	0.3	*	*	*	3	*	*	*
4	955	303	28	2.8	*	186	10	0.35	0.28	4.5	*	*	*	40	88	25	*
4	955	408	*	2.3	*	216	13	0.25	0.18	2.3	*	*	*	80	135	*	*
39	1220	245	28	3.3	*	200	5	0.15	0.18	2.3	*	*	*	53	113	*	*
75	1009	665	*	3.7	*	1590	22	0.25	0.3	4	*	*	*	124	236	22	*
184	763	201	38	1.3	1.3	675	3	0.09	0.31	0.5	0.12	62	1.36	230	231	*	1.8
57	802	473	71	2.4	3.9	147	2	0.15	0.45	3.2	0.24	23	1.04	221	203	*	1.7
68	434	*	*	2.7	*	118	2	0.08	0.23	10.3	*	*	*	41	291	*	0
0	243	474	26	1.7	0.7	1899	8	0.08	0.08	0.9	0.13	39	0	44	69	1	1
0	64	308	40	1.5	0.9	778	6	0.13	0.22	1.6	0.14	35	0	46	93	1	*
18	337	79	9	0.2	0.9	78	0	0.01	0.13	t	0.04	2	0.32	163	130	6	0.2
16	381	69	8	0.1	0.7	67	0	0.01	0.12	t	0.03	2	0.11	159	202	6	0.2
27	406	46	6	0.1	0.9	103	0	0.01	0.1	t	0.02	2	0.2	174	211	3	0.2
21	396	73	7	0.1	0.8	61	0	0.01	0.11	0.3	0.05	10	0.35	150	110	6	0.2
102	1884	346	31	0.4	3.6	292	0	0.04	0.52	1.4	0.22	49	1.64	712	523	27	0.9
27	159	38	7	0.1	0.7	92	0	t	0.1	t	0.02	6	0.36	191	128	3	0.2
28	178	43	6	0.1	0.7	57	0	0.02	0.15	0.1	0.07	18	0.47	52	53	*	0.2
27	320	71	8	0.1	0.9	105	0	0.01	0.19	0.2	0.09	24	0.49	147	132	8	0.2
26	196	26	6	0.2	0.8	90	0	0.01	0.13	0.1	0.02	5	0.08	191	139	*	0.2

WT, weight; **KCAL,** kcalories; **PROT,** protein; **CARB,** carbohydrate; **FIBR,** fiber; **FAT,** fat; **SATF,** saturated fat; **MONO,** monosaturated fat; **POLY,** polyunsaturated fat; **CHOR,** cholesterol; **SOD,** sodium; **POT,** potassium;

Food Name	Portion	WT (Gm)	KCAL	PROT (Gm)	CARB (Gm)	FIBR (Gm)	FAT (Gm)	SATF (Gm)	MONO (Gm)	POLY (Gm)
CHEESE-CHEDDAR-CUT PIECES	OUNCE	28.4	114	7	t	0	9	6	2.7	0.3
CHEESE-CHEDDAR-INCH CUBES	ITEM	17.2	69	5	t	0	6	3.6	1.6	0.2
CHEESE-CHEDDAR-LOWFAT-LOW SODIUM-PAULY	OUNCE	28.4	83	9	1	0	5	1.3	0.6	0.1
CHEESE-CHEDDAR-SHREDDED	CUP	113	455	28	1	0	38	23.8	10.6	1.1
CHEESE-CHESHIRE	OUNCE	28.4	110	7	1	0	9	5.5	2.5	0.2
CHEESE-COLBY	OUNCE	28.4	112	7	1	0	9	5.7	2.6	0.3
CHEESE-COTTAGE-1% LOWFAT-UNPACKED	CUP	226	164	28	6	0	2	1.5	0.7	0.1
CHEESE-COTTAGE-2% LOWFAT-UNPACKED	CUP	226	203	31	8	0	4	2.8	1.2	0.1
CHEESE-COTTAGE-4% FAT-LARGE CURD-UNPACK	CUP	225	232	28	6	0	10	6.4	2.9	0.3
CHEESE-COTTAGE-4% FAT-SMALL CURD-UNPACK	CUP	210	217	26	6	0	9	6	2.7	0.3
CHEESE-COTTAGE-DRY CURD-UNCREAMED	CUP	145	123	25	3	0	1	0.4	0.2	t
CHEESE-COTTAGE-WITH FRUIT-UNPACKED	CUP	226	279	22	30	0	8	4.9	2.2	0.2
CHEESE-CREAM	OUNCE	28.4	100	2	1	0	10	6.3	2.8	0.4
CHEESE-EDAM	OUNCE	28.4	101	7	t	0	8	5	2.3	0.2
CHEESE-FETA	OUNCE	28.4	75	4	1	0	6	4.2	1.3	0.2
CHEESE-FONTINA	OUNCE	28.4	110	7	t	0	9	5.4	2.5	0.5
CHEESE-GARLIC-LOWFAT-LOW SODIUM-PAULY	OUNCE	28.4	80	8	0	0	6	3	*	2.5
CHEESE-GJETOST	OUNCE	28.4	132	3	12	0	8	5.4	2.2	0.3
CHEESE-GOUDA	OUNCE	28.4	101	7	1	0	8	5	2.2	0.2
CHEESE-GRUYERE	OUNCE	28.4	117	8	t	0	9	5.4	2.9	0.5
CHEESE-LIMBURGER	OUNCE	28.4	93	6	t	0	8	4.8	2.4	0.1
CHEESE-MONTEREY JACK	OUNCE	28.4	106	7	t	0	9	5.4	2.5	0.3
CHEESE-MONTEREY JACK-LOWFAT-LOW SODIUM	OUNCE	28.4	80	8	0	0	6	3	*	2.5
CHEESE-MOZZARELLA-MADE FROM SKIM MILK	OUNCE	28.4	72	7	1	0	5	2.9	1.3	0.1
CHEESE-MOZZARELLA-MADE FROM WHOLE MILK	OUNCE	28.4	80	6	1	0	6	3.7	1.9	0.2
CHEESE-MUENSTER	OUNCE	28.4	104	7	t	0	9	5.4	2.5	0.2
CHEESE-NEUFCHATEL	OUNCE	28.4	74	3	1	0	7	4.2	1.9	0.2
CHEESE-PARMESAN-GRATED	CUP	100	456	42	4	0	30	19.1	8.7	0.7
CHEESE-PIMENTO-PROCESSED	OUNCE	28.4	106	6	t	0	9	5.6	2.5	0.3
CHEESE-PORT DU SALUT	OUNCE	28.4	100	7	t	0	8	4.7	2.7	0.2
CHEESE-PROVOLONE	OUNCE	28.4	100	7	1	0	8	4.8	2.1	0.2
CHEESE-RICOTTA-MADE WITH PART SKIM MILK	CUP	246	340	28	13	0	20	12.1	5.7	0.6
CHEESE-RICOTTA-MADE WITH WHOLE MILK	CUP	246	428	28	7	0	32	20.4	8.9	1
CHEESE-ROMANO	OUNCE	28.4	110	9	1	0	8	4.9	2.2	0.2
CHEESE-ROQUEFORT	OUNCE	28.4	105	6	1	0	9	5.5	2.4	0.4
CHEESE-SWISS	OUNCE	28.4	107	8	1	0	8	5	2.1	0.3
CHEESE-SWISS-LOWFAT-LOW SODIUM-PAULY	OUNCE	28.4	97	9	1	0	7	5.1	2.1	0.3
CHEESE-SWISS-PASTEURIZED PROCESS	OUNCE	28.4	95	7	1	0	7	4.6	2	0.2
CHEESE-TILSIT	OUNCE	28.4	96	7	1	0	7	4.8	2	0.2
CREAM-COFFEE-TABLE-LIGHT-FLUID	CUP	240	469	6	9	0	46	28.9	13.4	1.7
CREAM-HALF & HALF-MILK AND CREAM-FLUID	CUP	242	315	7	10	0	28	17.3	8	1
CREAM-IMITATION-LIQUID-NON DAIRY-FROZEN	CUP	245	333	2	28	0	24	4.8	18.5	0.1
CREAM-IMITATION-NON DAIRY-POWDERED	CUP	94	514	5	52	0	33	30.6	0.9	t
CREAM-MOCHA MIX-NON DAIRY	TBSP	15	20	1	1	t	2	0.8	0.8	0.8
CREAM-SOUR-CULTURED	CUP	230	493	7	10	0	48	30	13.9	1.8
CREAM-SOUR-HALF & HALF	TBSP	15	20	t	1	0	2	1.1	0.5	0.1
CREAM-SOUR-IMITATION	OUNCE	28.4	59	1	2	0	6	5	0.2	t
CREAM-SOUR-IMITATION-NONFAT DRY MILK	CUP	235	415	8	11	0	39	31.2	5	1.2
CREAM-WHIPPED-IMITATION-NON DAIRY-FROZEN	CUP	75	239	1	17	0	19	16.3	1.2	0.4
CREAM-WHIPPED-IMITATION-NON DAIRY-POWDER	CUP	80	151	3	13	0	10	8.6	0.7	0.2
CREAM-WHIPPED-IMITATION-PRESSURIZED	CUP	60	154	2	7	0	13	8.3	3.9	0.5
CREAM-WHIPPED-IMITATION-PRESSURIZED	CUP	70	184	1	11	0	16	13.2	1.4	0.2
CREAM-WHIPPING-HEAVY-UNWHIPPED-FLUID	CUP	238	821	5	7	0	88	54.8	25.4	3.3
CREAM-WHIPPING-LIGHT-UNWHIPPED-FLUID	CUP	239	699	5	7	0	74	46.2	21.7	2.1
MILK-1% FAT-LOWFAT-FLUID	CUP	244	102	8	12	0	3	1.6	0.8	0.1
MILK-1% FAT-NONFAT MILK SOLIDS ADDED	CUP	245	104	9	12	0	2	1.5	0.7	0.1
MILK-1% FAT-PROTEIN FORTIFIED	CUP	246	119	10	14	0	3	1.8	0.8	0.1
MILK-2% FAT-FLUID-PROTEIN FORTIFIED	CUP	246	137	10	14	0	5	3	1.4	0.2
MILK-2% FAT-LOWFAT-FLUID	CUP	244	121	8	12	0	5	2.9	1.4	0.2
MILK-2% FAT-NONFAT MILK SOLIDS ADDED	CUP	245	125	9	12	0	5	2.9	1.4	0.2
MILK-BUTTERMILK-CULTURED-FLUID	CUP	245	99	8	12	0	2	1.3	0.6	0.1
MILK-BUTTERMILK-DRIED-SWEET CREAM	CUP	120	464	41	59	0	7	4.3	2	0.3
MILK-CHOCOLATE-1% FAT-FLUID	CUP	250	158	8	26	0.2	3	1.5	0.8	0.1
MILK-CHOCOLATE-2% FAT-FLUID	CUP	250	179	8	26	0.2	5	3.1	1.5	0.2

t = Trace of nutrient present   ** = Not available*

MAG, magnesium; **IRON,** iron; **ZINC,** zinc; **VITA,** vitamin A; **VITC,** vitamin C; **THIA,** thiamin; **RIBO,** riboflavin; **NIAC,** niacin; **VB6,** vitamin B-6; **FOL,** folate; **VB12,** vitamin B-12; **CALC,** calcium; **PHOS,** phosphorus; **SEL,** selenium; **VE-a,** alpha tocopherol equivalents.

CHOL (mg)	SOD (mg)	POT (mg)	MAG (mg)	IRON (mg)	ZINC (mg)	VITA (RE)	VITC (mg)	THIA (mg)	RIBO (mg)	NIAC (mg)	VB6 (mg)	FOL (μg)	VB12 (μg)	CALC (mg)	PHOS (mg)	SEL (μg)	VE-a (mg)
30	176	28	8	0.2	0.9	90	0	0.01	0.11	t	0.02	5	0.23	204	145	5	0.2
18	107	17	5	0.1	0.5	55	0	0.01	0.07	t	0.01	3	0.14	124	88	3	0.1
14	68	32	8	0.2	0.9	18	0	0.01	0.01	t	0.02	5	0.24	200	137	*	0.1
119	701	111	31	0.8	3.5	359	0	0.03	0.42	0.1	0.08	21	0.94	815	579	18	0.7
29	198	27	6	0.1	0.8	84	0	0.01	0.08	t	0.02	5	0.23	182	131	*	0.2
27	171	36	7	0.2	0.9	88	0	t	0.11	t	0.02	5	0.23	194	129	16	0.2
10	918	193	12	0.3	0.9	25	0	0.05	0.37	0.3	0.15	28	1.43	138	302	52	1.5
19	918	217	14	0.4	1	47	0	0.05	0.42	0.3	0.17	30	1.61	155	340	52	1.5
34	911	189	11	0.3	0.8	110	0	0.05	0.37	0.3	0.15	27	1.4	135	297	52	1.4
31	850	177	11	0.3	0.8	103	0	0.04	0.34	0.3	0.14	26	1.31	126	277	48	1.3
10	19	47	6	0.3	0.7	13	0	0.04	0.21	0.2	0.12	21	1.2	46	151	34	0.9
25	915	151	9	0.3	0.7	84	0	0.04	0.29	0.2	0.12	22	1.12	108	236	4	*
31	85	34	2	0.3	0.2	122	0	0.01	0.06	t	0.01	4	0.12	23	30	1	0.2
25	274	53	8	0.1	1.1	78	0	0.01	0.11	t	0.02	5	0.44	207	152	1	0.2
25	316	18	5	0.2	0.8	36	0	0.04	0.24	0.3	0.12	9	0.48	140	96	*	0.2
33	227	18	4	0.1	1	100	0	0.01	0.06	t	0.02	2	0.48	156	98	*	0.2
20	95	*	*	*	*	*	*	*	*	*	*	*	*	*	*	*	*
27	170	399	20	0.1	0.3	78	0	0.09	0.39	0.2	0.08	1	0.69	113	126	*	0.2
32	232	34	8	0.1	1.1	55	0	0.01	0.1	t	0.02	6	0.44	198	155	0	0.2
31	95	23	10	t	1.1	104	0	0.02	0.08	t	0.02	3	0.45	287	172	1	0.2
26	227	36	6	t	0.6	109	0	0.02	0.14	t	0.02	16	0.3	141	111	*	0.2
25	152	23	8	0.2	0.9	81	0	t	0.11	t	0.02	5	0.23	212	126	13	0.2
20	95	*	*	*	*	*	*	*	*	*	*	*	*	*	*	*	*
16	132	24	7	0.1	0.8	50	0	0.01	0.09	t	0.02	2	0.23	183	131	3	0.2
22	106	19	5	0.1	0.6	68	0	t	0.07	t	0.02	2	0.19	147	105	3	0.2
27	178	38	8	0.1	0.8	96	0	t	0.09	t	0.02	3	0.42	203	133	*	0.2
22	113	32	2	0.1	0.2	96	0	t	0.06	t	0.01	3	0.08	21	39	*	0.2
79	1862	107	51	1	3.2	211	0	0.05	0.39	0.3	0.11	8	1.4	1376	807	24	0.6
27	405	46	6	0.1	0.8	108	1	0.01	0.1	t	0.02	2	0.2	174	211	6	0.2
35	151	39	7	0.1	0.7	114	0	t	0.07	t	0.02	5	0.43	184	102	*	0.2
20	248	39	8	0.2	0.9	69	0	0.01	0.09	t	0.02	3	0.42	214	141	*	0.2
76	307	308	36	1.1	3.3	319	0	0.05	0.46	0.2	0.05	32	0.72	669	449	*	1.6
124	207	257	28	0.9	2.9	362	0	0.03	0.48	0.3	0.11	30	0.83	509	389	*	1.6
29	340	25	12	0.2	0.7	49	0	0.01	0.11	t	0.02	2	0.32	302	215	*	0.2
26	513	26	8	0.2	0.6	89	0	0.01	0.17	0.2	0.04	14	0.18	188	111	*	0.2
26	74	31	10	0.1	1.1	72	0	0.01	0.1	t	0.02	2	0.48	272	171	2	0.2
19	32	32	10	t	1.1	72	0	0.01	0.11	t	0.02	2	0.48	273	172	*	0.2
24	388	61	8	0.2	1	69	0	t	0.08	t	0.01	2	0.35	219	216	2	0.2
29	213	18	4	0.1	1	89	0	0.02	0.1	0.1	0.02	6	0.6	198	142	*	0.2
159	95	292	21	0.1	0.7	519	2	0.08	0.36	0.1	0.08	6	0.53	231	192	1	2
89	98	314	25	0.2	1.2	315	2	0.09	0.36	0.2	0.09	6	0.8	254	230	1	2
0	194	466	0	0.1	t	66	0	0	0	0	0	0	0	22	157	*	*
0	170	763	4	1.1	0.5	57	0	0	0.16	0	0	0	0	21	397	*	*
0	5	20	*	*	*	*	*	*	*	*	*	*	*	*	*	*	*
102	123	331	26	0.1	0.6	546	2	0.08	0.34	0.2	0.04	25	0.69	268	195	*	*
6	6	19	2	t	0.1	20	t	0.01	0.02	t	t	2	0.05	16	14	*	t
0	29	46	2	0.1	0.3	0	0	0	0	0	0	0	0	1	13	*	0
0	240	380	*	0.1	*	6	2	0.09	0.38	0.2	*	*	*	266	205	*	*
0	19	14	1	0.1	t	194	0	0	0	0	0	0	0	5	6	*	*
8	53	121	8	t	0.2	87	1	0.02	0.09	t	0.02	3	0.21	72	69	*	*
46	78	88	6	t	0.2	165	0	0.02	0.04	t	0.03	2	0.18	61	54	*	*
0	43	13	1	t	t	99	0	0	0	0	0	0	0	4	13	*	*
326	89	179	17	0.1	0.6	1051	1	0.05	0.26	0.1	0.06	9	0.43	154	149	*	2
265	82	231	17	0.1	0.6	809	1	0.06	0.3	0.1	0.07	9	0.47	166	146	*	2
10	123	381	34	0.1	1	150	2	0.1	0.41	0.2	0.11	12	0.9	300	235	3	0.1
10	128	397	35	0.1	1	150	2	0.1	0.42	0.2	0.11	13	0.94	313	245	3	0.1
10	143	444	39	0.2	1.1	150	3	0.11	0.47	0.2	0.12	15	1.05	349	273	3	0.1
19	145	447	40	0.2	1.1	150	3	0.11	0.48	0.2	0.13	15	1.05	352	276	6	0.1
18	122	377	33	0.1	1	150	2	0.1	0.4	0.2	0.11	12	0.89	297	232	7	0.1
18	128	397	35	0.1	1	150	2	0.1	0.42	0.2	0.11	13	0.94	313	245	7	0.1
9	257	371	27	0.1	1	24	2	0.08	0.38	0.1	0.08	12	0.54	285	219	3	1
83	621	1910	131	0.4	4.8	79	7	0.47	1.9	1.1	0.41	57	4.59	1421	1119	*	0
7	152	426	33	0.6	1	150	2	0.1	0.42	0.3	0.1	12	0.86	287	256	3	0.2
17	150	422	33	0.6	1	150	2	0.09	0.41	0.3	0.1	12	0.85	284	254	3	0.2

WT, weight; **KCAL,** kcalories; **PROT,** protein; **CARB,** carbohydrate; **FIBR,** fiber; **FAT,** fat; **SATF,** saturated fat; **MONO,** monosaturated fat; **POLY,** polyunsaturated fat; **CHOR,** cholesterol; **SOD,** sodium; **POT,** potassium;

Food Name	Portion	WT (Gm)	KCAL	PROT (Gm)	CARB (Gm)	FIBR (Gm)	FAT (Gm)	SATF (Gm)	MONO (Gm)	POLY (Gm)
MILK-CHOCOLATE-WHOLE-FLUID	CUP	250	208	8	26	0.2	8	5.3	2.5	0.3
MILK-CONDENSED-SWEETENED-CANNED	CUP	306	982	24	166	0	27	16.8	7.4	1
MILK-EGGNOG-COMMERCIAL	CUP	254	342	10	34	0	19	11.3	5.7	0.9
MILK-EVAPORATED-SKIM-CANNED	CUP	255	199	19	29	0	1	0.3	0.2	t
MILK-EVAPORATED-WHOLE-CANNED	CUP	252	338	17	25	0	19	11.6	5.9	0.6
MILK-GOAT-WHOLE-FLUID	CUP	244	168	9	11	0	10	6.5	2.7	0.4
MILK-HUMAN-WHOLE-MATURE	CUP	246	171	3	17	0	11	4.9	4.1	1.2
MILK-IMITATION	CUP	244	150	4	15	0	8	1.9	4.9	1.2
MILK-INDIAN BUFFALO-WHOLE	CUP	244	236	9	13	0	17	11.2	4.4	0.4
MILK-MALTED-CHOCOLATE FLAVOR-PREPARED	CUP	265	229	9	30	0.1	9	5.5	2.6	0.4
MILK-MALTED-NATURAL FLAVOR-PREPARED	CUP	265	237	10	27	0.2	10	6	2.8	0.6
MILK-NONFAT/SKIM-FLUID	CUP	245	86	8	12	0	t	0.3	0.1	t
MILK-NONFAT/SKIM-INSTANTIZED-DRIED	CUP	68	244	24	36	0	t	0.3	0.1	t
MILK-NONFAT/SKIM-INSTANTIZED-ENVELOPE	ITEM	91	326	32	48	0	1	0.4	0.2	t
MILK-NONFAT/SKIM-MILK SOLIDS ADDED	CUP	245	90	9	12	0	1	0.4	0.2	t
MILK-NONFAT/SKIM-PROTEIN FORTIFIED	CUP	246	100	10	14	0	1	0.4	0.2	t
MILK-SHEEP-WHOLE-FLUID	CUP	245	264	15	13	0	17	11.3	4.2	0.8
MILK-SOY-FLUID	CUP	240	79	7	4	3.1	5	0.5	0.8	2
MILK-WHOLE-DRY	CUP	128	635	34	49	0	34	21.4	10.1	0.9
MILK-WHOLE-LOW SODIUM	CUP	244	149	8	11	0	8	5.3	2.4	0.3
MILK-WHOLE-REGULAR-3.3% FAT-FLUID	CUP	244	150	8	11	0	8	5.1	2.4	0.3
MILKSHAKE-CHOCOLATE-THICK	ITEM	300	356	9	64	0.8	8	5	2.3	0.3
MILKSHAKE-VANILLA-THICK	ITEM	313	350	12	56	0.2	9	5.9	2.7	0.4
WHEY-ACID-DRY	TBSP	2.9	10	t	2	0	t	t	t	t
WHEY-ACID-FLUID	CUP	246	59	2	13	0	t	0.1	0.1	t
WHEY-SWEET-DRY	TBSP	7.5	26	1	6	0	t	0.1	t	t
WHEY-SWEET-FLUID	CUP	246	66	2	13	0	1	0.6	0.2	t
YOGURT-FRUIT FLAVORS-LOWFAT-ADDED SOLIDS	CUP	227	231	10	43	0.8	2	1.6	0.7	0.1
YOGURT-ORIGINAL COFFEE-LOWFAT-DANNON	SERVING	227	200	10	34	0	3	1.8	0.8	0.1
YOGURT-PLAIN-LOWFAT-MILK SOLIDS ADDED	CUP	227	144	12	16	0	4	2.3	1	0.1
YOGURT-PLAIN-NONFAT-MILK SOLIDS ADDED	CUP	227	127	13	17	0	t	0.3	0.1	t
YOGURT-PLAIN-WHOLE MILK-NO SOLIDS	CUP	227	139	8	11	0	7	4.8	2	0.2
Desserts										
BROWNIES WITH NUTS-HOME RECIPE	ITEM	20	95	1	10	0.5	6	1.5	3	1.2
BROWNIES-COMMERCIALLY PREPARED	ITEM	60	243	3	39	1.3	10	3.1	3.8	2.6
CAKE-ANGEL FOOD-PREPARED FROM MIX	SLICE	53	142	4	32	t	t	*	*	*
CAKE-CHEESECAKE-COMMERCIAL	SLICE	85	257	5	24	1.8	16	6.7	6	2.9
CAKE-COFFEE-PREPARED FROM MIX	SLICE	72	230	5	38	2.4	7	2	2.7	1.5
CAKE-DEVILS FOOD WITH ICING-FROM MIX	SLICE	69	235	3	40	1.5	8	3.1	2.8	1.1
CAKE-GINGERBREAD-PREPARED FROM MIX	SLICE	63	175	2	32	1.8	4	1.1	1.8	1.1
CAKE-PINEAPPLE UPSIDE DOWN-HOME RECIPE	SLICE	70	221	2	35	1.2	9	1.9	3.9	2.1
CAKE-POUND-HOME RECIPE	SLICE	33	160	2	16	0.1	10	5.9	3	0.6
CAKE-SHEET-NO ICING-HOME RECIPE	SLICE	86	315	4	48	1	12	3.3	4.9	2.6
CAKE-SPONGE-HOME RECIPE	SLICE	66	188	5	36	0	3	1.1	1.3	0.5
CAKE-STRAWBERRY SHORTCAKE	SERVING	175	344	5	61	2.1	9	*	*	*
CAKE-STREUSEL TYPE-WITH ICING-FROM MIX	SLICE	50	172	2	25	0.9	8	*	*	*
CAKE-WHITE/CHOCOLATE ICING-HOME RECIPE	SLICE	71	271	3	42	0.8	11	3	2.9	1.3
CAKE-YELLOW/CHOCOLATE ICING-HOME RECIPE	SLICE	69	268	3	40	0.6	11	3	3	1.4
COOKIE-CHOCOLATE CHIP-BAKED FROM MIX	ITEM	10.5	50	1	7	0.3	2	0.7	0.9	0.6
COOKIE-CHOCOLATE CHIP-FROM HOME RECIPE	ITEM	10	46	1	6	0.3	3	0.6	1.2	0.8
COOKIE-FIG BAR-COMMERCIAL	ITEM	14	53	1	11	0.6	1	0.2	0.3	0.2
COOKIE-GINGERSNAP-FROM HOME RECIPE	ITEM	7	34	t	5	0.3	2	*	*	*
COOKIE-MACAROON	ITEM	19	90	1	13	0.4	5	*	*	*
COOKIE-OATMEAL/RAISIN-PREPARED FROM MIX	ITEM	13	62	1	9	0.4	3	0.5	0.8	0.5
COOKIE-PEANUT BUTTER-FROM MIX	ITEM	10	50	1	6	0.2	3	0.6	1.2	0.7
COOKIE-SANDWICH-CHOCOLATE/VANILLA	ITEM	10	50	1	7	0.2	2	0.6	1	0.6
COOKIE-SUGAR-FROM MIX	ITEM	20	99	1	13	0.3	5	*	*	*
COOKIE-VANILLA WAFER	ITEM	4	19	t	3	t	1	0.1	0.2	0.1
CUPCAKE WITH CHOCOLATE ICING	ITEM	36	130	2	21	0.4	5	2	1.7	0.7
CUPCAKE-NO ICING	ITEM	25	90	1	14	0.3	3	0.8	1.2	0.7
CUSTARD-BAKED	CUP	265	305	14	29	1	15	6.8	5.4	0.7
DANISH PASTRY-CHEESE	ITEM	91	353	6	29	0.6	25	5.1	15.6	2.4
DANISH PASTRY-FRUIT	ITEM	94	335	5	45	1.8	16	3.3	10.1	1.6

t = Trace of nutrient present   ** = Not available*

MAG, magnesium; **IRON,** iron; **ZINC,** zinc; **VITA,** vitamin A; **VITC,** vitamin C; **THIA,** thiamin; **RIBO,** riboflavin; **NIAC,** niacin; **VB6,** vitamin B-6; **FOL,** folate; **VB12,** vitamin B-12; **CALC,** calcium; **PHOS,** phosphorus; **SEL,** selenium; **VE-a,** alpha tocopherol equivalents.

CHOL (mg)	SOD (mg)	POT (mg)	MAG (mg)	IRON (mg)	ZINC (mg)	VITA (RE)	VITC (mg)	THIA (mg)	RIBO (mg)	NIAC (mg)	VB6 (mg)	FOL (μg)	VB12 (μg)	CALC (mg)	PHOS (mg)	SEL (μg)	VE-a (mg)
30	149	417	33	0.6	1	91	2	0.09	0.41	0.3	0.1	12	0.84	280	251	3	0.2
104	389	1136	78	0.6	2.9	302	8	0.28	1.27	0.6	0.16	34	1.36	868	775	3	0
149	138	420	47	0.5	1.2	268	4	0.09	0.48	0.3	0.13	2	1.14	330	278	3	*
10	293	847	69	0.7	2.3	300	3	0.12	0.79	0.4	0.14	23	0.61	740	497	3	0
73	267	764	61	0.5	1.9	184	5	0.12	0.8	0.5	0.13	20	0.41	658	509	3	0
28	122	499	34	0.1	0.7	135	3	0.12	0.34	0.7	0.11	1	0.16	326	270	*	0
34	42	126	8	0.1	0.4	178	12	0.03	0.09	0.4	0.03	13	0.11	79	34	4	2.2
0	191	279	16	1	2.9	0	0	0.03	0.22	0	0	0	0	79	181	*	2.6
46	127	434	76	0.3	0.5	130	5	0.13	0.33	0.2	0.06	14	0.89	412	286	*	*
34	172	499	47	0.5	1.1	80	3	0.13	0.44	0.6	0.14	16	0.91	304	265	3	0.2
37	223	529	52	0.3	1.1	94	3	0.2	0.59	1.3	0.19	22	1.03	354	303	3	*
4	126	406	28	0.1	1	150	2	0.09	0.34	0.2	0.1	13	0.93	302	247	7	0.1
12	373	1160	80	0.2	3	484	4	0.28	1.19	0.6	0.24	34	2.72	837	670	*	*
17	499	1552	107	0.3	4	648	5	0.38	1.59	0.8	0.31	45	3.63	1120	896	22	*
5	130	418	36	0.1	1	150	2	0.1	0.43	0.2	0.11	13	0.95	316	255	3	0.1
5	144	446	40	0.2	1.1	150	3	0.11	0.48	0.2	0.12	15	1.05	352	275	3	0.1
66	108	334	45	0.2	1.3	108	10	0.16	0.87	1	0.15	17	1.74	474	387	*	0
0	29	338	46	1.4	0.6	7	0	0.39	0.17	0.4	0.1	4	0	10	118	*	t
124	475	1702	108	0.6	4.3	354	11	0.36	1.54	0.8	0.39	47	4.16	1168	993	*	0.2
33	6	617	12	0.1	0.9	95	2	0.05	0.26	0.1	0.08	12	0.88	246	209	3	0.1
33	120	370	33	0.1	0.9	92	2	0.09	0.4	0.2	0.1	12	0.87	291	228	3	0.1
32	333	672	48	0.9	1.4	78	0	0.14	0.67	0.4	0.08	15	0.95	396	378	5	*
37	299	572	37	0.3	1.2	107	0	0.09	0.61	0.5	0.13	21	1.63	457	361	5	*
t	28	66	6	t	0.2	1	t	0.02	0.06	t	0.02	1	0.07	59	39	*	t
1	118	352	24	0.2	1.1	5	t	0.1	0.34	0.2	0.1	5	0.44	253	191	*	*
t	80	155	13	0.1	0.2	1	t	0.04	0.17	0.1	0.04	1	0.18	59	70	*	t
5	132	396	20	0.2	0.3	12	t	0.09	0.39	0.2	0.08	2	0.68	115	112	*	*
10	133	442	33	0.2	1.7	31	2	0.08	0.4	0.2	0.09	21	1.06	345	271	11	*
11	140	498	37	0.2	1.9	30	2	0.1	0.46	0.2	0.1	24	1.2	389	306	*	0.1
14	159	531	40	0.2	2	45	2	0.1	0.49	0.3	0.11	25	1.28	415	326	11	*
4	174	579	43	0.2	2.2	5	2	0.11	0.53	0.3	0.12	28	1.39	452	355	11	*
29	105	351	26	0.1	1.3	84	1	0.07	0.32	0.2	0.07	17	0.84	274	215	11	*
0	50	38	3	0.4	*	7	0	0.04	0.03	0.2	*	*	*	8	30	1	0.5
9	153	83	16	1.3	0.6	3	3	0.07	0.13	0.6	0.03	4	0.15	25	87	3	*
0	142	52	6	0.5	0.1	0	0	0.06	0.12	0.6	0.01	5	0.02	50	63	3	1.4
57	189	83	9	0.4	0.4	43	4	0.03	0.11	0.4	0.05	15	0.42	48	75	*	1.5
*	310	78	*	1.2	*	24	0	0.14	0.15	1.3	*	*	*	44	125	5	1.9
33	180	90	*	1	*	20	0	0.07	0.1	0.6	*	4	*	41	72	4	1.9
1	90	173	14	0.9	0.3	0	0	0.09	0.11	0.8	0.05	5	0.07	57	63	4	*
20	167	119	12	1.1	0.4	54	4	0.11	0.08	0.7	0.04	8	0.06	50	44	*	0.6
68	58	20	*	0.5	*	16	0	0.05	0.06	0.4	*	2	*	6	24	2	0.9
1	382	68	12	0.9	0.3	30	0	0.13	0.15	1.1	0.02	6	0.09	55	88	6	2.3
162	164	59	7	1.1	0.8	25	0	0.09	0.13	0.7	0.04	15	0.33	25	65	4	1.8
*	*	*	*	2	*	86	89	0.17	0.21	1.3	*	*	*	73	84	*	*
*	214	55	7	0.7	0.2	6	0	0.06	0.06	0.5	0.02	5	0.1	27	99	*	0.4
3	200	77	14	0.7	0.3	4	0	0.07	0.11	0.7	0.02	4	0.06	70	127	5	1.9
36	191	73	13	0.8	0.3	10	0	0.08	0.1	0.7	0.02	6	0.12	57	61	4	1.9
6	38	14	3	0.2	0.1	6	0	0.01	0.02	0.2	t	1	*	3	7	1	0.3
5	21	21	4	0.2	t	1	0	0.02	0.02	0.1	t	1	0.01	3	8	1	0.3
0	45	41	4	0.3	0.1	3	0	0.02	0.02	0.2	0.02	1	0	10	8	1	0.4
0	20	14	1	0.2	t	1	0	0.01	0.01	0.1	t	1	0.01	3	4	1	0.2
0	6	88	*	0.2	*	0	0	0.01	0.03	0.1	*	*	*	5	16	1	0.5
0	37	23	4	0.3	0.1	2	0	0.02	0.02	0.2	0.01	2	*	4	14	1	0.3
3	57	19	4	0.2	0.8	3	0	0.02	0.02	0.4	0.01	2	0.01	12	24	*	0.3
0	63	4	5	0.2	0.1	0	0	0.02	0.03	0.2	t	t	0	3	24	1	0.3
*	109	14	2	0.4	0.1	3	0	0.04	0.02	0.5	0.01	2	*	21	38	1	0.5
3	10	3	1	0.1	*	1	0	0.01	0.01	0.1	*	*	*	2	3	0	0.1
15	120	42	*	0.4	*	12	0	0.05	0.06	0.4	*	*	*	47	71	3	0.1
0	113	21	*	0.3	*	8	0	0.05	0.05	0.4	*	*	*	40	59	2	0.7
278	209	387	*	1.1	*	87	1	0.11	0.5	0.3	*	*	*	297	310	3	*
20	320	116	16	1.9	0.6	43	3	0.27	0.21	2.6	0.06	15	0.23	70	80	*	3.2
19	333	110	14	1.4	0.5	24	2	0.29	0.21	1.8	0.06	15	0.23	22	69	*	2.3

WT, weight; **KCAL,** kcalories; **PROT,** protein; **CARB,** carbohydrate; **FIBR,** fiber; **FAT,** fat; **SATF,** saturated fat; **MONO,** monosaturated fat; **POLY,** polyunsaturated fat; **CHOR,** cholesterol; **SOD,** sodium; **POT,** potassium;

Food Name	Portion	WT (Gm)	KCAL	PROT (Gm)	CARB (Gm)	FIBR (Gm)	FAT (Gm)	SATF (Gm)	MONO (Gm)	POLY (Gm)
DANISH PASTRY-PLAIN	ITEM	65	250	4	29	0.6	14	4.7	6.1	3.2
DOUGHNUTS-CAKE-PLAIN	ITEM	25	104	1	12	0.3	6	1.2	1.2	2
DOUGHNUTS-YEAST-GLAZED	ITEM	50	205	3	22	1.1	11	3	5.8	3.3
ECLAIR-CUSTARD WITH CHOCOLATE ICING	ITEM	100	239	6	23	0.5	14	*	*	*
FROZEN YOGURT-FRUIT VARIETIES	CUP	226	216	7	42	*	2	*	*	*
FRUIT BAR-OAT BRAN-NUTS-HEALTH VALLEY	ITEM	43	150	4	28	2.9	4	*	*	*
GRANOLA BAR	ITEM	24	109	2	16	1	4	*	*	*
ICE CREAM SUNDAE-CARAMEL	ITEM	165	323	8	53	*	10	4.8	3.2	1.1
ICE CREAM SUNDAE-HOT FUDGE	ITEM	165	297	6	50	1.2	9	5.3	2.4	0.8
ICE CREAM SUNDAE-STRAWBERRY	ITEM	165	289	7	48	0.7	8	4	2.9	1.1
ICE CREAM-FRENCH VANILLA-SOFT SERVE	CUP	173	377	7	38	0	23	13.5	5.9	0.7
ICE CREAM-VANILLA-HARDENED-10% FAT	CUP	133	269	5	32	0	14	8.9	3.6	0.3
ICE CREAM-VANILLA-RICH-HARDENED-16% FAT	CUP	148	349	4	32	0	24	14.7	6.8	0.9
ICE MILK-VANILLA-HARDENED-4.3% FAT	CUP	131	184	5	29	0	6	3.5	1.4	0.1
ICE MILK-VANILLA-SOFT SERVE-2.6% FAT	CUP	175	223	8	38	0	5	2.9	1.2	0.1
PIE-APPLE-FROM HOME RECIPE	SLICE	135	323	3	49	2.2	14	3.9	6.4	3.6
PIE-BANANA CREAM-FROM HOME RECIPE	SLICE	130	285	6	40	1.4	12	3.8	4.7	2.3
PIE-BLUEBERRY-FROM HOME RECIPE	SLICE	135	325	3	47	1.7	15	3.5	6.2	3.6
PIE-BOSTON CREAM-HOME RECIPE	SLICE	69	210	3	34	1	6	1.9	2.5	1.3
PIE-CHERRY-FROM HOME RECIPE	SLICE	135	350	4	52	1.1	15	4	6.4	3.6
PIE-CUSTARD-FROM HOME RECIPE	SLICE	130	285	8	30	2.1	14	4.8	5.5	2.5
PIE-LEMON MERINGUE-FROM HOME RECIPE	SLICE	120	300	4	47	1.4	11	3.7	4.8	2.3
PIE-MINCE-FROM HOME RECIPE	SLICE	135	365	3	56	2	16	4	6.6	3.6
PIE-PEACH-FROM HOME RECIPE	SLICE	135	345	3	52	1.8	14	3.5	6.2	3.6
PIE-PECAN-FROM HOME RECIPE	SLICE	118	495	6	61	4.1	27	4	14.4	6.3
PIE-PUMPKIN-FROM HOME RECIPE	SLICE	130	275	5	32	3.5	15	5.4	5.4	2.4
PUDDING-BANANA CREAM-INSTANT MIX-JELLO	OUNCE	28.4	106	0	27	0	0	0	0	0
PUDDING-BUTTERSCOTCH-INSTANT MIX-JELLO	OUNCE	28.4	105	0	27	0	0	0	0	0
PUDDING-CHOCOLATE-COOKED-FROM MIX & MILK	CUP	260	320	9	59	0	8	4.3	2.6	2
PUDDING-CHOCOLATE-INSTANT-FROM MIX	CUP	260	325	8	63	0	7	3.6	2.2	0.3
PUDDING-CHOCOLATE-SUGAR FREE-2% MILK	SERVING	133	100	5	14	0.3	3	*	*	*
PUDDING-LEMON-INSTANT MIX-JELLO	OUNCE	28.4	105	t	27	0.3	t	0	0	0
PUDDING-RICE WITH RAISINS	CUP	265	387	10	71	1.4	8	*	*	*
PUDDING-TAPIOCA CREAM-HOME RECIPE-STARCH	CUP	165	220	8	28	0.6	8	4.1	2.5	0.5
PUDDING-VANILLA (BLANCMANGE)-HOME RECIPE	CUP	255	285	9	41	0	10	6.2	2.5	0.2
PUDDING-VANILLA-SUGAR FREE-WITH 2% MILK	SERVING	133	90	4	12	0.2	2	*	*	*
SHERBET-ORANGE-2% FAT	CUP	193	270	2	59	0	4	2.4	1	0.1
TURNOVER-APPLE	OUNCE	28.4	85	1	11	0.2	5	1.3	2.3	1.4
TURNOVER-CHERRY	OUNCE	28.4	84	1	11	0.2	5	1.1	1.9	1.1
TWINKIE-HOSTESS	ITEM	42	143	1	26	*	4	*	*	*
Eggs										
EGG SUBSTITUTE-FROZEN	CUP	240	384	27	8	0	27	4.6	5.8	15
EGG SUBSTITUTE-LIQUID	CUP	251	211	30	2	0	8	1.7	2.3	4
EGG SUBSTITUTE-POWDER	SERVING	28.4	126	16	6	0	4	1.1	1.5	0.5
EGG-DUCK-WHOLE-FRESH-RAW	ITEM	70	130	9	1	0	10	2.6	4.6	0.9
EGG-FRIED IN BUTTER-WHOLE-LARGE-CHICKEN	ITEM	46	92	6	1	0	7	1.9	2.8	1.3
EGG-HARD COOKED-NO SHELL-LARGE-CHICKEN	ITEM	50	77	6	1	0	5	1.6	2	0.7
EGG-POACHED-WHOLE-LARGE-CHICKEN	ITEM	50	74	6	1	0	5	1.5	1.9	0.7
EGG-RAW-WHITE-LARGE-CHICKEN	ITEM	33.4	17	4	t	0	0	0	0	0
EGG-RAW-WHOLE-LARGE-CHICKEN	ITEM	50	75	6	1	0	5	1.6	1.9	0.7
EGG-RAW-YOLK-LARGE-CHICKEN	ITEM	16.6	59	3	t	0	5	1.6	2	0.7
EGG-SCRAMBLED-WITH MILK & BUTTER-CHICKEN	ITEM	61	101	7	1	0	7	2.2	2.9	1.3
OMELET-TWO EGG-HAM AND CHEESE	ITEM	120	266	19	2	0	20	7.3	7.5	2.9
Fast Foods										
ARBY'S-BEEF AND CHEESE SANDWCH	ITEM	176	402	32	27	1.1	18	9	3.7	3.5
ARBY'S-CHICKEN BREAST SANDWICH	ITEM	184	493	23	48	1.6	25	5.1	9.6	10.3
ARBY'S-CLUB SANDWICH	ITEM	252	560	30	43	2.3	30	11.6	9.3	8.4
ARBY'S-HAM AND CHEESE SANDWICH	ITEM	146	353	21	33	1	16	6.4	6.7	1.4
ARBY'S-ROAST BEEF SANDWICH	ITEM	139	346	22	34	1	14	3.6	6.8	1.7
ARBY'S-SUPER ROAST BEEF SANDWICH	ITEM	234	501	25	50	1.6	22	8.5	8.2	5.4
ARBY'S-TURKEY DELUXE	ITEM	236	510	28	46	*	24	*	*	*

t = Trace of nutrient present ** = Not available*

MAG, magnesium; **IRON,** iron; **ZINC,** zinc; **VITA,** vitamin A; **VITC,** vitamin C; **THIA,** thiamin; **RIBO,** riboflavin; **NIAC,** niacin; **VB6,** vitamin B-6; **FOL,** folate; **VB12,** vitamin B-12; **CALC,** calcium; **PHOS,** phosphorus; **SEL,** selenium; **VE-a,** alpha tocopherol equivalents.

CHOL (mg)	SOD (mg)	POT (mg)	MAG (mg)	IRON (mg)	ZINC (mg)	VITA (RE)	VITC (mg)	THIA (mg)	RIBO (mg)	NIAC (mg)	VB6 (mg)	FOL (μg)	VB12 (μg)	CALC (mg)	PHOS (mg)	SEL (μg)	VE-a (mg)
0	249	61	10	1.2	0.5	11	0	0.16	0.15	1.5	*	*	*	69	66	*	*
10	139	27	6	0.4	0.1	2	0	0.06	0.05	0.4	0.01	2	*	11	55	2	0.2
13	117	34	10	0.6	*	5	0	0.1	0.1	0.8	*	11	*	16	33	4	0.4
*	82	122	*	0.7	*	68	0	0.04	0.16	0.1	*	*	*	80	112	*	*
*	*	*	24	0	*	0	0	0.01	0.26	0	*	*	*	200	200	*	*
0	5	230	40	1.4	0.8	0	10	0.19	0.06	0.7	0.06	19	0	25	134	*	3
*	67	78	*	0.8	*	*	*	0.07	0.03	*	*	*	0	14	67	*	*
26	208	338	30	0.2	0.9	56	4	0.07	0.31	1	0.05	13	0.64	201	231	*	1
22	190	413	35	0.6	1	46	2	0.07	0.31	1.1	0.13	10	0.68	216	238	*	0.7
23	99	292	26	0.3	0.7	48	2	0.07	0.3	1	0.08	20	0.69	173	167	*	0.8
153	153	338	25	0.4	2	199	1	0.08	0.45	0.2	0.1	9	1	236	199	2	0.1
59	116	257	18	0.1	1.4	133	1	0.05	0.33	0.1	0.06	3	0.63	176	134	2	0.1
88	108	221	16	0.1	1.2	207	1	0.04	0.28	0.1	0.05	2	0.54	151	115	3	0.1
18	105	265	19	0.2	0.6	52	1	0.08	0.35	0.1	0.09	3	0.88	176	129	2	0.1
13	163	412	29	0.3	0.9	44	1	0.12	0.54	0.2	0.13	5	1.37	274	202	3	1
0	207	115	11	1.2	0.2	5	2	0.15	0.11	1.2	0.04	7	0	12	31	15	2.2
40	252	264	*	1	*	66	1	0.11	0.22	1	*	*	*	86	107	15	*
0	361	88	9	1.4	*	8	4	0.15	0.11	1.4	*	*	0	15	31	15	2.2
0	128	61	*	0.7	*	28	0	0.09	0.11	0.8	*	*	*	46	70	5	*
0	410	142	9	0.9	*	118	0	0.16	0.12	1.4	*	*	0	19	34	15	2.2
*	373	178	*	1.2	*	60	0	0.11	0.27	0.8	*	*	*	125	147	15	2.1
0	223	53	7	0.9	0.3	33	4	0.1	0.12	0.7	0.03	11	0.19	16	48	13	1.9
0	604	240	24	1.9	*	0	1	0.14	0.12	1.4	*	*	*	38	51	15	2.2
0	361	21	9	1.2	*	198	4	0.15	0.14	2	*	*	0	14	39	15	2.2
0	260	145	*	3.7	*	40	0	0.26	0.14	1	*	*	*	55	122	12	*
0	278	208	17	1	*	320	0	0.11	0.18	1	*	*	*	66	90	15	2.1
0	190	1	*	t	*	0	0	0	0	0	*	*	*	1	111	*	*
0	244	1	*	t	*	0	0	0	0	0	*	*	*	1	102	*	*
32	335	354	*	0.8	*	68	2	0.05	0.39	0.3	*	*	*	265	247	*	*
28	322	335	*	1.3	*	68	2	0.08	0.39	0.3	*	*	*	374	237	*	*
*	310	*	*	0.7	*	40	*	0.06	0.26	*	*	*	*	150	300	*	*
0	190	1	*	t	*	0	0	0	0	0	*	*	*	1	111	*	*
*	188	469	*	1.1	*	35	0	0.08	0.37	0.5	*	*	*	260	249	*	*
80	257	223	*	0.7	*	60	2	0.07	0.3	0.2	*	*	*	173	180	*	*
36	165	352	*	0	*	82	2	0.08	0.41	0.3	*	*	*	298	232	*	*
*	380	*	*	*	*	40	*	0.03	0.17	*	*	*	*	150	200	*	*
14	88	198	15	0.3	1.3	39	4	0.03	0.09	0.1	0.03	14	0.16	103	74	*	*
1	109	14	3	0.3	0.1	2	t	0.03	0.02	0.3	0.01	1	0.03	4	11	*	0.5
4	124	20	3	0.2	0.1	12	t	0.02	0.02	0.2	0.01	1	0	4	14	*	0.5
21	189	*	*	0.5	*	8	0	0.06	0.06	0.5	*	*	*	19	*	*	*
5	479	512	36	4.8	2.4	324	1	0.29	0.93	0.3	0.32	39	0.81	175	172	*	1.3
3	444	828	22	5.3	3.3	542	0	0.28	0.75	0.3	0.01	37	0.75	133	304	*	1.4
162	227	211	18	0.9	0.5	105	t	0.06	0.5	0.2	0.04	35	1	92	136	*	0.2
619	102	156	12	2.7	1	279	0	0.11	0.28	0.1	0.18	56	3.78	45	154	*	0.6
211	162	61	5	0.7	0.5	114	0	0.03	0.24	t	0.07	18	0.42	25	89	12	*
213	62	63	5	0.6	0.5	84	0	0.03	0.26	t	0.06	22	0.56	25	86	12	0.4
212	140	60	5	0.7	0.6	95	0	0.03	0.22	t	0.06	18	0.4	25	89	12	0.4
0	55	48	4	t	0	0	0	t	0.15	t	t	1	0.07	2	4	5	0
213	63	60	5	0.7	0.6	95	0	0.03	0.25	t	0.07	23	0.5	25	89	22	0.4
213	7	16	1	0.6	0.5	323	0	0.03	0.11	t	0.07	24	0.52	23	81	7	0.3
215	171	84	7	0.7	0.6	119	t	0.03	0.27	t	0.07	18	0.47	44	104	*	1.3
445	598	182	17	1.7	1.8	273	4	0.18	0.57	0.8	0.19	38	1.08	153	286	33	0.1
77	1634	345	40	5.1	5.4	58	0	0.38	0.46	5.9	0.34	41	2.05	183	401	*	0.4
91	1019	330	46	3.5	1.7	15	0	0.45	0.39	14.8	0.65	32	0.34	111	290	*	2.6
100	1610	466	46	3.6	3.1	127	28	0.68	0.43	7	0.4	44	0.94	200	433	*	3.3
58	772	290	16	3.3	1.4	96	3	0.31	0.49	2.7	0.2	71	0.54	130	152	*	1.1
52	792	316	31	4.2	3.4	63	2	0.38	0.31	5.9	0.27	40	1.22	54	239	*	0.2
40	798	503	58	6.4	10.7	0	0	0.53	0.6	9.4	0.48	41	4.29	115	402	*	0.4
70	1220	*	*	2.7	*	*	*	0.45	0.34	8	*	*	*	80	*	*	*

WT, weight; **KCAL,** kcalories; **PROT,** protein; **CARB,** carbohydrate; **FIBR,** fiber; **FAT,** fat; **SATF,** saturated fat;
MONO, monosaturated fat; **POLY,** polyunsaturated fat; **CHOR,** cholesterol; **SOD,** sodium; **POT,** potassium;

Food Name	Portion	WT (Gm)	KCAL	PROT (Gm)	CARB (Gm)	FIBR (Gm)	FAT (Gm)	SATF (Gm)	MONO (Gm)	POLY (Gm)
ARBYS-SOUP-BOSTON CLAM CHOWDER	SERVING	227	207	10	18	1.4	11	4	5	2
ARBYS-SOUP-CREAM OF BROCCOLI	SERVING	227	180	9	19	1.8	8	5	2	1
ARBYS-SOUP-FRENCH ONION	SERVING	227	67	2	7	0.9	3	1	2	1
ARBYS-SOUP-LUMBERJACK MIXED VEGETABLE	SERVING	227	89	2	13	1.3	4	2	1	1
ARBYS-SOUP-OLD FASHIONED CHICKEN NOODLE	SERVING	227	99	6	15	0.7	2	1	1	1
ARBYS-SOUP-PILGRIM CLAM CHOWDER	SERVING	227	193	10	18	1.9	11	4	5	2
ARBYS-SOUP-ROAST BEEF AND VEGETABLE	SERVING	227	96	5	14	0.5	3	1	1	1
ARBYS-SOUP-SPLIT PEA AND HAM	SERVING	227	200	8	21	3.9	10	5	1	1
ARBYS-SOUP-TOMATO FLORENTINE	SERVING	227	84	3	15	0.5	2	1	1	1
ARBYS-SOUP-WISCONSIN CHEESE	SERVING	227	287	9	19	1.8	19	8	8	3
ARTHUR TREACHER-CHICKEN SANDWICH	ITEM	156	413	16	44	*	19	*	*	6.7
BEEF BURGER-FAST FOOD	OUNCE	28.3	72	5	7	t	3	*	*	*
BUN-HAMBURGER/HOTDOG-FAST FOOD	OUNCE	28.3	98	3	16	0	2	*	*	*
BURGER KING-BACON DOUBLE CHEESE-DELUXE	SERVING	195	592	33	28	1.1	39	16	14	6
BURGER KING-BARBECUE BACON DOUBLE CHEESE	ITEM	174	536	32	31	0.8	31	14	13	2
BURGER KING-BK BROILER	ITEM	168	379	24	31	1.8	18	3	8	3.8
BURGER KING-BK BROILER SAUCE	SERVING	14	90	0	0	0	10	1	2	5
BURGER KING-CHICKEN TENDERS	PIECE	90	39	3	2	0.3	2	0.5	0.8	0.5
BURGER KING-CROISSANT-EGG AND CHEESE	ITEM	127	369	13	24	2.1	25	14.1	7.5	1.4
BURGER KING-CROISSANT-EGG/CHEESE/HAM	ITEM	152	475	19	24	*	34	17.5	11.4	2.4
BURGER KING-DOUBLE CHEESEBURGER	ITEM	172	483	30	29	1.4	27	13	11	2
BURGER KING-FISH TENDERS	SERVING	99	267	12	18	1.1	16	3	7	4
BURGER KING-MUSHROOM SWISS DOUBLE CHEESE	ITEM	176	473	31	27	*	27	12	11	2
BURGER KING-RANCH DIP SAUCE	SERVING	28	171	0	2	*	18	3	4	10
BURGER KING-SWEET & SOUR SAUCE	SERVING	28	45	0	11	t	0	0	0	0
BURGER KING-TARTAR DIP SAUCE	SERVING	28	174	0	3	t	18	3	4	11
BURGER KING-TATER TENDERS	SERVING	71	213	2	25	*	12	3	6	3
BURGER KING-WHOPPER HAMBURGER	ITEM	261	630	26	50	2.5	36	16.5	13.8	2.2
CHEESE BURGER-FAST FOOD	OUNCE	28.3	78	6	7	0.1	3	1.7	1.7	0.2
CHICKEN-BREAST AND WING-BREADED-FRIED	SERVING	163	494	36	20	0.3	30	7.8	12.2	6.8
CHICKEN-BREAST-FAST FOOD	OUNCE	28.3	73	8	3	0	4	0.6	0.9	0.5
CHICKEN-DRUMSTICK & THIGH-BREADED-FRIED	SERVING	148	430	30	16	0.2	27	7.1	10.9	6.3
CHICKEN-DRUMSTICK-FAST FOOD	OUNCE	28.3	59	7	4	0	2	0.9	1.2	0.7
CHICKEN-FRIED-FAST FOOD-VARIOUS PORTIONS	OUNCE	28.3	82	5	6	0	5	1.1	1.7	1
CHICKEN-MEAT-SHAPED-FRIED-FAST FOOD	OUNCE	28.3	82	5	5	0	5	*	*	*
CHICKEN-SHOULDER-FAST FOOD	OUNCE	28.3	92	5	3	0	6	*	*	*
CHICKEN-THIGH-FAST FOOD	OUNCE	28.3	104	7	3	0	7	1.2	1.7	1
CHICKEN-WING-FAST FOOD	OUNCE	28.3	92	8	3	0	5	*	*	*
CHURCHS CHICKEN-WHITE MEAT	ITEM	100	327	21	10	*	23	*	*	*
COLESLAW-FAST FOOD	OUNCE	28.3	24	1	3	0	1	0.2	0.4	0.8
DAIRY QUEEN-BANANA SPLIT	ITEM	383	540	10	91	*	15	*	*	*
DAIRY QUEEN-DIP ICE CREAM CONE-REGULAR	ITEM	156	300	7	40	*	13	*	*	*
DAIRY QUEEN-FLOAT	ITEM	397	330	6	59	*	8	*	*	*
DAIRY QUEEN-ICE CREAM CONE-REGULAR	ITEM	142	226	5	33	*	8	4.9	2.5	0.5
DAIRY QUEEN-ICE CREAM SUNDAE-REGULAR	ITEM	177	319	6	53	2.2	10	5.6	2.6	0.9
DAIRY QUEEN-MALT-REGULAR	ITEM	418	600	15	89	*	20	*	*	*
DOUBLE CHEESE BURGER-FAST FOOD	OUNCE	28.3	66	4	7	0.1	3	2.2	1.9	0.2
FAST FOOD-PIZZA WITH CHEESE	OUNCE	28.4	63	3	9	0.6	1	0.7	0.4	0.2
FAST FOOD-PIZZA WITH PEPPERONI	OUNCE	28.4	72	4	8	0.6	3	0.9	1.3	0.5
FISH CAKE-FRIED-WITH BUN-FAST FOOD	OUNCE	28.3	85	3	8	0	5	0.4	0.8	0.5
FRANKFURTER-CONEY DOG-FAST FOOD	OUNCE	28.3	69	3	7	0	3	3.1	4	0.8
FRANKFURTER-HOT DOG-FAST FOOD	OUNCE	28.3	78	3	7	0	4	3.1	4	0.8
HAMBURGER-DOUBLE PATTY-EVERYTHING ON IT	OUNCE	28.4	68	4	5	0.3	3	1.3	1.3	0.4
HARDEE-BACON AND EGG BISCUIT	SERVING	124	410	15	35	0.6	24	5	14	5
HARDEE-BACON EGG AND CHEESE BISCUIT	SERVING	137	460	17	35	0.7	28	8	15	5
HARDEE-BIG COUNTRY BREAKFAST-COUNTRY HAM	SERVING	254	670	29	52	*	38	9	21	8
HARDEE-BIG COUNTRY BREAKFAST-SAUSAGE	SERVING	274	850	33	51	*	57	16	31	11
HARDEE-BIG COUNTRY BREAKFAST-WITH BACON	SERVING	217	660	24	51	0	40	10	22	8
HARDEE-BIG COUNTRY BREAKFAST-WITH HAM	SERVING	251	620	28	51	*	33	7	19	8
HARDEE-BIG ROAST BEEF SANDWICH	SERVING	134	300	18	32	0.9	11	5	5	2
HARDEE-BIG TWIN HAMBURGER	SERVING	173	450	23	34	1.7	25	11	9	5
HARDEE-BISCUIT N GRAVY	SERVING	221	440	9	45	*	24	6	14	5
HARDEE-CHICKEN N PASTA SALAD	SERVING	414	230	27	23	*	3	1	1	1

t = Trace of nutrient present   ** = Not available*

MAG, magnesium; **IRON,** iron; **ZINC,** zinc; **VITA,** vitamin A; **VITC,** vitamin C; **THIA,** thiamin; **RIBO,** riboflavin; **NIAC,** niacin; **VB6,** vitamin B-6; **FOL,** folate; **VB12,** vitamin B-12; **CALC,** calcium; **PHOS,** phosphorus; **SEL,** selenium; **VE-a,** alpha tocopherol equivalents.

CHOL (mg)	SOD (mg)	POT (mg)	MAG (mg)	IRON (mg)	ZINC (mg)	VITA (RE)	VITC (mg)	THIA (mg)	RIBO (mg)	NIAC (mg)	VB6 (mg)	FOL (μg)	VB12 (μg)	CALC (mg)	PHOS (mg)	SEL (μg)	VE-a (mg)
28	1157	319	20	1.4	0.7	100	4	0.06	0.22	0.9	0.12	9	9.38	170	143	*	0.1
3	1113	455	55	0.8	0.7	50	9	0.11	0.42	0.8	0.18	46	0.59	237	193	*	1.4
0	1248	106	2	0.6	0.6	10	2	0.03	0.02	0.6	0.05	14	0	25	11	*	0.3
4	1075	268	6	1.9	2.7	250	9	0.06	0.1	1.9	0.15	14	0.3	41	91	*	0.4
25	929	78	5	0.7	0.4	200	1	0.05	0.06	1.3	0.03	2	0.14	16	34	*	0.1
28	1157	379	19	2	1.1	350	4	0.06	0.16	1.3	0.15	9	9.67	134	126	*	0.2
10	996	211	5	1	1.4	300	5	0.03	0.05	1	0.07	10	0.3	16	39	*	0.3
30	1029	272	36	2	3	300	1	0.11	0.09	2.4	0.2	4	0.23	32	168	*	0.1
2	910	221	10	1.6	0.2	100	12	0.09	0.09	1.3	0.12	15	0.1	45	58	*	2.3
31	1129	441	7	1.3	1.1	90	2	0.03	0.24	0.7	0.05	7	0	252	241	*	0.4
*	708	279	27	1.7	*	37	19	0.17	0.24	8.1	*	*	*	59	147	*	*
*	55	46	*	0.3	*	8	t	0.02	0.04	0.8	*	*	*	3	25	*	*
*	22	31	*	0.2	*	0	t	0.07	0.02	0.4	*	*	*	9	13	*	*
111	804	463	38	4	6.4	71	8	0.3	0.39	8.1	0.37	31	3.24	156	373	*	1.5
105	795	429	36	4	6.5	49	4	0.29	0.39	8.3	0.35	27	3.34	158	379	*	0.6
53	764	324	29	3.2	3.2	44	6	0.27	0.26	5.2	0.24	38	1.52	74	153	*	2.6
7	95	*	*	*	*	*	*	*	*	*	*	*	*	*	*	*	*
8	90	249	22	1	0.7	25	0	0.14	0.12	6.2	0.32	9	0.3	9	234	*	0.3
216	551	174	22	2.2	1.8	300	t	0.19	0.38	1.5	0.1	36	0.78	244	349	*	0.7
213	1080	272	26	2.1	2.2	135	11	0.52	0.3	3.2	0.23	36	1.01	144	336	*	*
100	851	344	31	3	4	100	6	0.22	0.31	4.9	0.24	31	1.81	189	305	*	1.8
28	870	176	33	1.7	0.6	20	t	0.23	0.17	2.3	0.06	23	1.05	60	191	*	1.3
95	746	*	*	4.1	*	*	*	*	*	*	*	*	*	*	*	*	*
0	208	*	*	*	*	*	*	*	*	*	*	*	*	*	*	*	*
0	52	9	2	0.1	t	0	0	t	t	0.1	t	t	0	1	3	*	0
16	302	14	1	0.3	0.1	26	t	t	0.01	t	0.08	2	0.06	7	8	*	3.9
3	318	*	*	*	*	*	*	*	*	*	*	*	*	*	*	*	*
104	990	520	50	6	5.3	192	13	0.02	0.03	5.2	0.31	31	2.81	104	312	*	3.9
12	198	68	6	0.6	0.7	9	t	0.02	0.05	0.6	0.04	7	0.31	25	33	*	0.1
149	975	566	38	1.5	1.6	58	0	0.14	0.3	12	0.57	9	0.67	60	307	*	1
24	142	85	8	0.2	0.3	9	1	0.02	0.05	2	0.16	1	0.09	4	52	*	0.1
165	756	446	37	1.6	3.2	67	0	0.14	0.43	7.2	0.33	10	0.83	36	240	*	1.3
26	133	74	6	0.3	0.8	7	t	0.02	0.06	1.4	0.1	2	0.09	4	41	*	0.1
25	153	71	7	0.3	0.6	7	t	0.02	0.05	1.6	0.12	2	0.09	4	39	*	0.2
*	141	40	*	0.3	*	6	t	0.01	0.01	0.8	*	*	*	4	34	*	*
*	150	74	*	0.1	*	4	t	0.02	0.04	1.9	*	*	*	4	32	*	*
26	139	68	6	0.1	0.7	6	t	0.02	0.07	1.4	0.09	2	0.08	4	37	*	0.1
*	198	54	*	0.2	*	7	1	0.02	0.04	1.5	*	*	*	5	31	*	*
*	498	186	*	1	*	48	1	0.1	0.18	7.2	*	*	*	94	*	*	*
1	77	45	4	0.5	t	8	t	0.01	t	t	0.02	9	0.01	10	9	*	0.4
30	*	*	*	1.8	*	225	18	0.6	0.6	0.8	*	*	0.9	350	250	*	*
20	*	*	*	0.4	*	90	0	0.09	0.34	0	*	*	0.6	200	150	*	*
20	*	*	*	0	*	30	0	0.12	0.17	0	*	*	0.6	200	200	*	*
38	126	233	21	0.2	0.8	87	2	0.07	0.36	0.4	0.09	7	0.28	212	192	*	*
23	204	443	37	0.7	1.1	75	3	0.07	0.34	1.2	0.14	11	0.73	232	255	*	1.6
50	*	*	*	3.6	*	225	4	0.12	0.6	0.8	*	*	1.8	500	400	*	*
17	50	85	6	0.6	0.9	8	t	0.02	0.04	0.8	0.05	5	0.42	3	31	*	0.1
4	151	49	7	0.3	0.4	33	1	0.08	0.07	1.1	0.02	26	0.15	52	51	*	0.3
6	107	61	3	0.4	0.2	22	1	0.05	0.09	1.2	0.02	21	0.07	26	30	*	*
20	167	52	8	0.5	0.7	6	t	0.02	0.04	1.4	0.03	12	0.85	14	34	*	0.3
15	242	49	3	1	0.6	7	1	0.07	0.07	1.1	0.03	1	0.33	12	30	*	0.1
15	219	48	3	0.6	0.6	5	t	0.01	0.01	0.6	0.03	1	0.33	6	33	*	0.1
15	99	71	6	0.7	0.7	1	t	0.05	0.05	1	0.07	6	0.51	13	39	*	0.1
155	990	180	25	2.2	1.4	116	3	0.33	0.45	3	0.14	14	0.47	253	358	*	1.2
165	1220	200	27	2.4	1.5	129	3	0.37	0.49	3.3	0.15	15	0.52	279	396	*	1.3
345	2870	710	*	*	*	*	*	*	*	*	*	*	*	*	*	*	*
340	1980	670	*	*	*	*	*	*	*	*	*	*	*	*	*	*	*
305	1540	530	23	2.5	2.5	333	0	0.31	0.8	1.8	0.34	53	1.5	78	347	*	4.7
325	1780	620	*	*	*	*	*	*	*	*	*	*	*	*	*	*	*
45	880	320	33	3.7	6.1	0	0	0.3	0.34	5.4	0.28	24	2.45	66	230	*	0.2
55	580	280	35	4	4.6	17	3	0.28	0.31	6.7	0.27	34	2.27	80	197	*	0.9
15	1250	210	*	*	*	*	*	*	*	*	*	*	*	*	*	*	*
55	380	620	*	9	*	*	*	*	*	*	*	*	*	*	*	*	*

WT, weight; **KCAL**, kcalories; **PROT**, protein; **CARB**, carbohydrate; **FIBR**, fiber; **FAT**, fat; **SATF**, saturated fat; **MONO**, monosaturated fat; **POLY**, polyunsaturated fat; **CHOR**, cholesterol; **SOD**, sodium; **POT**, potassium;

Food Name	Portion	WT (Gm)	KCAL	PROT (Gm)	CARB (Gm)	FIBR (Gm)	FAT (Gm)	SATF (Gm)	MONO (Gm)	POLY (Gm)
HARDEE-CRISPY CURLS	SERVING	85	300	4	36	*	16	3	8	5
HARDEE-GRILLED CHICKEN SANDWICH	SERVING	192	310	24	34	2.2	9	1	3	5
HARDEE-HAM & EGG BISCUIT	SERVING	138	370	15	35	1.1	19	4	12	4
HARDEE-HAM EGG & CHEESE BISCUIT	SERVING	151	420	18	35	0.8	23	6	13	4
HARDEE-MUSHROOM N SWISS HAMBURGER	SERVING	186	490	30	33	*	27	13	12	2
HARDEE-REGULAR ROAST BEEF SANDWICH	SERVING	114	260	15	31	0.8	9	4	4	2
HARDEE-THE LEAN ONE SANDWICH	ITEM	220	420	27	37	*	18	8	8	2
HARDEE-THREE PANCAKES	SERVING	137	280	8	56	1.4	2	1	1	1
JACK IN THE BOX-BREAKFAST JACK SANDWICH	ITEM	121	301	18	28	*	13	*	*	*
JACK IN THE BOX-JUMBO JACK CHEESEBURGER	ITEM	272	628	32	45	*	35	15	12.6	2
JACK IN THE BOX-JUMBO JACK HAMBURGER	ITEM	246	551	28	45	*	29	11.4	12.6	2.4
JACK IN THE BOX-MOBY JACK SANDWICH	ITEM	141	455	17	38	*	26	*	*	*
JACK IN THE BOX-ONION RINGS-BAG	ITEM	83	275	4	31	1.3	16	7	6.7	0.7
KFC-CHICKEN HOT WINGS	PIECE	119	63	4	3	0.1	4	0.8	10.3	0.7
KFC-CHICKEN SANDWICH	SERVING	166	482	21	39	1.4	27	6	3.9	9
KFC-CRISPY CHICKEN-BREAST	PIECE	135	342	33	12	0.1	20	5	4.7	2
KFC-CRISPY CHICKEN-DRUMSTICK	PIECE	69	204	14	6	t	14	3	3.7	2
KFC-CRISPY CHICKEN-THIGH	PIECE	119	406	20	14	0.1	30	8	7	4
KFC-CRISPY CHICKEN-WING	PIECE	65	254	12	9	0.1	19	4	5.7	3
LONG JOHN SILVER-BATTERED SHRIMP-9 PIECE	PIECE	357	95	3	10	1.8	5	1.1	3.2	0.6
LONG JOHN SILVER-BREADED SHRIMP	PIECE	420	51	1	6	2.1	2	0.5	1.6	0.3
LONG JOHN SILVER-CATFISH FILLET	SERVING	373	860	28	90	0.1	42	10	26	6
LONG JOHN SILVER-CHICKEN PLANK-4 PIECE	SERVING	415	940	39	94	*	44	10	29	5
LONG JOHN SILVER-CHICKEN-LIGHT HERB	SERVING	498	630	35	85	0	17	3	5	7
LONG JOHN SILVER-CLAM CHOWDER WITH COD	SERVING	198	140	11	10	1.7	6	2	3	2
LONG JOHN SILVER-CLAM DINNER	SERVING	363	980	21	122	0	45	10	30	6
LONG JOHN SILVER-COLE SLAW	SERVING	98	140	1	20	2.3	6	1	2	4
LONG JOHN SILVER-FISH & CHICKEN ENTREE	SERVING	398	870	35	91	*	40	9	26	5
LONG JOHN SILVER-FISH & MORE ENTREE	SERVING	381	800	31	88	1.7	37	8	23	5
LONG JOHN SILVER-FISH AND FRYES-3 PIECE	SERVING	358	810	42	77	*	38	9	27	2
LONG JOHN SILVER-FISH SANDWICH PLATTER	SERVING	379	870	26	108	4.1	38	8	22	7
LONG JOHN SILVER-FRIES	SERVING	85	220	3	30	2.9	10	3	7	1
LONG JOHN SILVER-GARDEN SALAD	SERVING	246	170	9	13	2.1	9	0.8	1	0.8
LONG JOHN SILVER-GUMBO-COD & SHRIMP BOBS	SERVING	198	120	9	4	3	8	2	3	3
LONG JOHN SILVER-HOMESTYLE FISH SANDWICH	SERVING	196	510	22	58	2.1	22	5	13	3
LONG JOHN SILVER-HOMESTYLE FISH-3 PIECE	SERVING	456	960	43	97	2	44	10	29	5
LONG JOHN SILVER-HOMESTYLE FISH-6 PIECE	SERVING	513	1260	49	124	2.3	64	14	43	6
LONG JOHN SILVER-HUSHPUPPIES	PIECE	24	70	2	10	*	2	1	1	1
LONG JOHN SILVER-LIGHT FISH-LEMON	SERVING	291	320	24	49	2.4	4	1	1	1
LONG JOHN SILVER-LIGHT FISH-PAPRIKA	SERVING	284	300	24	45	1.3	2	1	1	1
LONG JOHN SILVER-MIXED VEGETABLES	SERVING	113	60	2	9	5.9	2	1	1	1
LONG JOHN SILVER-OCEAN CHEF SALAD	SERVING	321	250	24	19	*	9	2	2	2
LONG JOHN SILVER-RICE PILAF	SERVING	142	210	5	43	0.8	2	1	1	1
LONG JOHN SILVER-SEAFOOD PLATTER	SERVING	400	970	30	109	5.3	46	10	30	6
LONG JOHN SILVER-SEAFOOD SALAD	SERVING	337	270	16	36	1.3	7	1	2	3
LONG JOHN SILVER-SEAFOOD SALAD-SCOOP	SERVING	142	210	14	26	0.6	5	1	2	3
LONG JOHN SILVER-SHRIMP & FISH DINNER	SERVING	348	770	25	85	7.3	37	8	23	5
LONG JOHN SILVER-SHRIMP FISH & CHICKEN	SERVING	380	840	31	89	*	40	9	26	5
LONG JOHN SILVER-SHRIMP SCAMPI	SERVING	529	610	25	87	0	18	3	6	7
MCDONALDS-APPLE BRAN MUFFIN	SERVING	85	190	5	46	4.5	0	0	0	0
MCDONALDS-APPLE DANISH	SLICE	115	390	6	51	1.6	18	3.5	10.8	2
MCDONALDS-APPLE PIE	SERVING	83	260	2	30	1.1	15	4.8	9.1	0.9
MCDONALDS-BACON AND EGG BISCUIT	SERVING	156	440	18	33	0.8	26	8.2	16.1	2
MCDONALDS-BACON BITS	SERVING	3	16	1	t	0	1	0	1.2	0
MCDONALDS-BARBEQUE (BARBECUE) SAUCE	SERVING	32	50	t	12	1.9	1	0.1	0.2	0.2
MCDONALDS-BIG MAC HAMBURGER	ITEM	215	560	25	43	*	32	10.1	20.1	1.5
MCDONALDS-BISCUIT WITH SPREAD	SERVING	75	260	5	32	1	13	3.4	8.6	0.6
MCDONALDS-CHEESEBURGER	ITEM	116	310	15	31	*	14	5.2	7.7	0.9
MCDONALDS-CHEF SALAD	SERVING	283	230	21	8	*	13	5.9	6.5	0.9
MCDONALDS-CHICKEN MCNUGGETS-6 PIECE	SERVING	113	290	19	17	*	16	4.1	10.4	1.8
MCDONALDS-CHOCOLATE MILKSHAKE-LOWFAT	SERVING	293	320	12	66	*	2	0.8	0.9	0.1
MCDONALDS-CHUNKY CHICKEN SALAD	SERVING	250	140	23	5	1	3	0.9	2	0.5
MCDONALDS-CINNAMON AND RAISIN DANISH	ITEM	110	440	6	58	*	21	4.2	13	1.6
MCDONALDS-COOKIE-CHOCOLATY	SERVING	56	330	4	42	1.1	16	5	10.2	0.4

t= Trace of nutrient present **= Not available*

MAG, magnesium; **IRON,** iron; **ZINC,** zinc; **VITA,** vitamin A; **VITC,** vitamin C; **THIA,** thiamin; **RIBO,** riboflavin; **NIAC,** niacin; **VB6,** vitamin B-6; **FOL,** folate; **VB12,** vitamin B-12; **CALC,** calcium; **PHOS,** phosphorus; **SEL,** selenium; **VE-a,** alpha tocopherol equivalents.

CHOL (mg)	SOD (mg)	POT (mg)	MAG (mg)	IRON (mg)	ZINC (mg)	VITA (RE)	VITC (mg)	THIA (mg)	RIBO (mg)	NIAC (mg)	VB6 (mg)	FOL (μg)	VB12 (μg)	CALC (mg)	PHOS (mg)	SEL (μg)	VE-a (mg)
0	840	370	*	*	*	*	*	*	*	*	*	*	*	*	*	*	*
60	890	410	44	3	2.7	413	t	0.43	0.59	4.2	0.1	31	0.47	542	611	*	3.4
160	1050	210	26	2.8	1.6	127	9	0.56	0.54	3.9	0.21	39	0.73	95	234	*	1.9
170	1270	230	30	2.7	1.7	142	4	0.4	0.54	3.7	0.17	17	0.57	308	436	*	1.5
70	940	370	*	*	*	*	*	*	*	*	*	*	*	*	*	*	*
35	730	260	28	3.1	5.2	0	0	0.26	0.29	4.6	0.24	20	2.09	56	196	*	0.2
85	760	510	*	*	*	*	*	*	*	*	*	*	*	*	*	*	*
15	890	240	25	1.9	0.9	63	1	0.22	0.39	1.4	0.1	14	0.42	341	411	*	1.6
182	1037	190	24	2.5	1.8	133	3	0.41	0.47	5.1	0.14	*	1.1	177	310	*	*
110	1666	499	49	4.6	4.8	220	5	0.52	0.38	11.3	0.31	*	3.05	273	411	*	*
80	1134	492	44	4.5	4.2	74	4	0.47	0.34	11.6	0.3	*	2.68	134	261	*	*
56	837	246	30	1.7	1.1	72	1	0.3	0.21	4.5	0.12	*	1.1	167	263	*	*
14	430	129	15	0.9	0.4	2	1	0.09	0.1	0.9	0.06	11	0.12	73	86	*	0.6
25	113	218	22	1.5	2.1	63	t	0.05	0.15	7.7	0.49	4	0.33	18	175	*	0.9
47	1060	297	41	3.1	1.5	14	0	0.4	0.35	13.4	0.59	29	0.31	100	261	*	2.3
114	790	347	40	1.6	1.5	20	0	0.11	0.17	18.4	0.77	5	0.46	21	312	*	0.6
71	324	157	16	0.9	2	17	0	0.06	0.16	4.1	0.24	6	0.22	8	120	*	0.5
129	688	280	29	1.8	3	35	0	0.11	0.29	8.2	0.4	10	0.36	16	221	*	0.6
67	422	115	12	0.8	1.1	25	0	0.04	0.09	4.3	0.27	2	0.18	10	97	*	0.6
14	163	94	132	10.3	4.2	242	5	0.3	0.5	9.9	0.36	34	3.4	214	764	*	14.1
6	85	41	156	12.1	5	285	6	0.35	0.58	11.6	0.43	39	3.99	252	899	*	16.6
65	990	1180	121	4.6	3.4	317	11	0.2	0.49	9.7	0.87	67	9.41	200	1017	*	5.7
70	1660	1320	*	*	*	*	*	*	*	*	*	*	*	*	*	*	*
85	2170	790	95	4.8	3.6	120	0	0.32	0.65	26.3	1.05	10	0.75	214	782	*	1.3
20	590	380	17	1.7	0.9	74	4	0.05	0.14	1.2	0.13	8	8.44	117	110	*	0.2
15	1200	870	41	56.7	6.2	365	47	0.34	0.91	7.2	0.26	54	201	209	572	*	4.5
15	260	190	13	0.5	0.1	225	30	0.04	0.03	0.3	0.13	37	0.03	36	23	*	4.4
70	1520	1290	*	*	*	*	*	*	*	*	*	*	*	*	*	*	*
70	1390	1260	131	3.3	2.1	71	5	0.39	0.5	12.3	0.72	46	5.17	133	769	*	7.7
85	1630	1340	*	*	*	*	*	*	*	*	*	*	*	*	*	*	*
55	1110	1050	94	6.4	2.3	65	2	0.87	0.65	11.1	0.42	89	2.29	238	488	*	5.7
5	60	390	29	0.6	0.3	0	9	0.15	0.02	2.8	0.2	25	0	16	79	*	0.2
5	380	20	40	1.7	1.1	239	26	0.14	0.15	11.4	0.56	66	0.27	42	217	*	0.9
25	740	310	41	2.3	0.8	300	21	0.12	0.08	2	0.17	47	0.24	100	105	*	1.7
45	780	470	48	18	1.2	33	1	0.45	0.34	5.7	0.22	46	1.19	123	252	*	2.9
100	1890	1540	157	3.9	2.6	85	6	0.47	0.59	14.7	0.87	56	6.19	159	920	*	9.3
130	1590	1660	177	4.4	2.9	96	7	0.53	0.67	16.6	0.98	62	6.97	179	1035	*	10.4
5	25	65	*	*	*	*	*	*	*	*	*	*	*	*	*	*	*
75	900	470	56	2.3	1.4	80	10	0.29	0.15	3.4	0.34	46	0.58	40	238	*	3.1
70	650	460	98	2.4	1.6	53	4	0.29	0.37	9.2	0.54	35	3.86	99	573	*	5.8
0	330	120	24	0.9	0.5	75	4	0.08	0.13	0.9	0.08	21	t	29	56	*	0.8
80	1340	160	*	*	*	*	*	*	*	*	*	*	*	*	*	*	*
0	570	140	17	1.8	0.6	60	1	0.15	0.02	1.5	0.08	5	0.01	17	45	*	0.8
70	1540	1100	114	4.1	2.2	59	13	0.42	0.37	8.2	0.88	37	1.68	109	484	*	4.3
90	670	100	86	3.2	5.2	129	20	0.13	0.16	3.7	0.27	47	2.89	148	444	*	7.4
90	570	100	36	1.4	2.2	250	8	0.05	0.07	1.6	0.11	20	1.22	63	187	*	3.1
80	1250	1030	82	3.5	1.6	28	17	0.37	0.21	6.6	0.64	35	1.06	54	422	*	4.4
80	1450	1170	*	*	*	*	*	*	*	*	*	*	*	*	*	*	*
220	2120	560	203	13.6	6.2	364	11	0.13	0.2	13.6	0.55	10	5.57	299	1156	*	12.9
0	230	202	55	0.6	1.2	1	1	0.02	0.08	0.4	0.37	77	0.78	31	178	*	0.4
26	370	69	8	1.4	0.2	35	16	0.28	0.2	2.2	0.03	3	0	14	31	*	3.8
0	240	50	6	0.7	0.2	0	11	0.06	0.02	0.3	0.02	2	0	11	22	*	2.7
253	1230	237	31	2.6	1.7	160	0	0.36	0.33	2.5	0.17	18	0.59	185	451	*	1.5
0	95	4	3	0	0.1	0	0	0	0	0	t	4	0.04	0	7	*	0.2
0	340	56	6	0.3	0.1	30	2	0.01	0.01	0.2	0.02	1	0	13	6	*	1.8
103	950	237	38	4	4.7	106	2	0.48	0.41	6.8	0.27	21	1.8	256	314	*	*
1	730	100	14	1.3	0.7	0	0	0.23	0.11	1.7	0.03	6	0.1	75	168	*	1.8
53	750	223	21	2.3	2.1	118	2	0.29	0.21	3.9	0.12	18	0.94	199	177	*	0.5
128	490	*	*	1.5	*	411	14	0.31	0.29	3.6	*	*	*	256	*	*	*
65	520	*	*	1	*	0	0	0.11	0.12	9	*	*	*	13	*	*	*
10	240	*	*	0.8	*	92	0	0.13	0.5	0.4	*	*	*	332	*	*	*
78	230	436	37	1	2.9	366	20	0.22	0.17	8.5	0.6	27	0.63	34	257	*	10.8
35	430	*	*	1.8	*	33	3	0.32	0.24	2.8	*	*	*	35	*	*	*
4	280	72	20	2.2	0.5	0	0	0.18	0.21	2.5	0.03	5	0.07	24	71	*	1.4

WT, weight; **KCAL,** kcalories; **PROT,** protein; **CARB,** carbohydrate; **FIBR,** fiber; **FAT,** fat; **SATF,** saturated fat; **MONO,** monosaturated fat; **POLY,** polyunsaturated fat; **CHOR,** cholesterol; **SOD,** sodium; **POT,** potassium;

Food Name	Portion	WT (Gm)	KCAL	PROT (Gm)	CARB (Gm)	FIBR (Gm)	FAT (Gm)	SATF (Gm)	MONO (Gm)	POLY (Gm)
MCDONALDS-COOKIE-MCDONALDLAND	SERVING	56	290	4	47	0.6	9	1.9	6.8	0.5
MCDONALDS-CROUTONS	SERVING	11	50	1	7	0.5	2	0.5	1.3	0.1
MCDONALDS-EGG MCMUFFIN	ITEM	138	290	18	28	1.4	11	3.8	6.1	1.3
MCDONALDS-ENGLISH MUFFIN	SERVING	59	170	5	27	1.6	5	2.4	1.7	0.5
MCDONALDS-FILET O FISH	ITEM	142	440	14	38	1.1	26	5.2	10.2	10.8
MCDONALDS-FRENCH FRIES-LARGE	SERVING	122	400	6	46	4.2	22	9.1	11.6	0.9
MCDONALDS-FRENCH FRIES-MEDIUM	SERVING	97	320	4	36	3.4	17	7.2	9.2	0.7
MCDONALDS-FRENCH FRIES-REGULAR ORDER	SERVING	68	220	3	26	*	12	5.1	6.5	0.5
MCDONALDS-GARDEN SALAD	SERVING	213	110	7	6	1.8	7	2.9	3.2	0.5
MCDONALDS-HAMBURGER	ITEM	102	260	12	31	*	10	3.6	5.1	0.8
MCDONALDS-HASHBROWN POTATO	SERVING	55	130	1	15	1.1	7	3.2	3.7	0.4
MCDONALDS-HONEY SAUCE	SERVING	14	45	0	12	*	0	0	0	0
MCDONALDS-HOT CAKES WITH SYRUP	SERVING	176	410	8	74	*	9	3.7	3.1	2.5
MCDONALDS-HOT CARAMEL SUNDAE	SERVING	174	270	7	59	1	3	1.5	1.2	0.1
MCDONALDS-HOT FUDGE SUNDAE	SERVING	169	240	7	51	1.3	3	2.4	0.8	0.1
MCDONALDS-HOT MUSTARD SAUCE	SERVING	30	70	1	8	0.3	4	0.5	1.2	1.9
MCDONALDS-ICED CHEESE DANISH	SERVING	110	390	7	42	*	22	6	12.1	1.8
MCDONALDS-McCHICKEN SANDWICH	SERVING	190	490	19	40	1.6	29	5.4	11.5	11.6
MCDONALDS-McDLT HAMBURGER	ITEM	234	580	26	36	*	37	11.5	16.7	8.5
MCDONALDS-MCLEAN DELUXE HAMBURGER	SERVING	206	320	22	35	2.4	10	4	5	1
MCDONALDS-MILKSHAKE-CHOCOLATE-LOWFAT	SERVING	293	320	12	66	*	2	1	1	0
MCDONALDS-MILKSHAKE-STRAWBERRY-LOWFAT	SERVING	293	320	11	67	*	1	1	1	0
MCDONALDS-MILKSHAKE-VANILLA-LOWFAT	SERVING	293	290	11	60	0	1	1	1	0
MCDONALDS-PORK SAUSAGE	SERVING	48	180	8	0	0	16	5.9	8.5	1.9
MCDONALDS-QUARTER POUND CHEESEBURGER	ITEM	194	520	29	35	*	29	11.2	16.5	1.5
MCDONALDS-QUARTER POUNDER HAMBURGER	ITEM	166	410	23	34	*	21	8.1	11.4	1.2
MCDONALDS-RASPBERRY DANISH	ITEM	117	410	6	62	*	16	3.1	10.2	1.1
MCDONALDS-SALAD DRESSING-PEPPERCORN	OUNCE	28.4	160	0	2	0	18	2	4	10
MCDONALDS-SALAD DRESSING-RED FRENCH	OUNCE	28.4	80	0	10	0	4	0	2	2
MCDONALDS-SAUSAGE AND EGG BISCUIT	ITEM	180	520	20	33	*	35	11.2	20	2.5
MCDONALDS-SAUSAGE BISCUIT	ITEM	123	440	13	32	1.4	29	9.3	17.2	2.5
MCDONALDS-SAUSAGE MCMUFFIN	ITEM	117	370	17	27	1.1	22	7.8	11.7	2.4
MCDONALDS-SAUSAGE MCMUFFIN WITH EGG	ITEM	167	440	23	28	1.6	27	9.5	14.2	3.2
MCDONALDS-SCRAMBLED EGGS	SERVING	98	140	12	1	0	10	3.3	5	1.4
MCDONALDS-SIDE SALAD	SERVING	115	60	4	3	1.2	3	1.5	1.6	0.3
MCDONALDS-STRAWBERRY MILKSHAKE-LOWFAT	SERVING	293	320	11	67	*	1	0.6	0.6	0.1
MCDONALDS-STRAWBERRY SUNDAE	SERVING	171	210	6	49	0.7	1	0.6	0.4	t
MCDONALDS-SWEET AND SOUR SAUCE	SERVING	32	60	t	14	t	t	t	0.1	0.1
MCDONALDS-VANILLA MILKSHAKE-LOWFAT	SERVING	293	290	11	60	*	1	0.6	0.7	0.1
MCDONALDS-VANILLA-FROZEN YOGURT	SERVING	80	100	4	22	*	1	0.4	0.3	0.1
PIZZA-BEEF/CHICKEN/ONION	OUNCE	28.3	73	6	7	t	2	*	*	*
PIZZA-BEEF/ONION	OUNCE	28.3	73	4	8	0.1	3	*	*	*
PIZZA-CHICKEN CURRY/PEAS	OUNCE	28.3	82	4	9	0.2	3	*	*	*
PIZZA-CHICKEN/MUSHROOM/TOMATO	OUNCE	28.3	61	5	7	0.1	1	*	*	*
PIZZA-CHICKEN/PINEAPPLE	OUNCE	28.3	81	4	6	0.1	4	*	*	*
PIZZA-COMBINATION SUPREME	OUNCE	28.3	51	4	7	0.2	1	1.3	1.5	0.4
PIZZA-CURRY BEEF/PEAS	OUNCE	28.3	71	5	7	0.2	3	0.9	1.6	1
PIZZA-ONION/TOMATO/GREEN PEPPER/MUSHROOM	OUNCE	28.3	45	3	7	0.2	1	*	*	*
PIZZA-PEPPERONI/BEEF/SALAMI/MUSHROOM/ETC	OUNCE	28.3	83	5	5	0.1	5	*	*	*
PIZZA-SHRIMP/CUCUMBER	OUNCE	28.3	69	4	7	0.1	3	*	*	*
PIZZA-SHRIMP/SQUID/MUSHROOM	OUNCE	28.3	70	5	7	0.1	2	*	*	*
POTATOES-FRENCH FRIED-FAST FOOD	OUNCE	28.3	91	1	10	0	5	1.8	1.9	0.8
POTATOES-MASHED-FAST FOOD	OUNCE	28.3	26	1	5	0	t	0.3	0.5	0.3
RAX-GRILLED CHICKEN SANDWICH	ITEM	190	440	24	36	1.6	19	2.9	4.5	5.4
SALAD-FAST FOOD	OUNCE	28.3	34	t	3	0	2	*	*	*
SPAGHETTI-VEGETABLES/SAUCE/CHEESE	OUNCE	28.3	28	4	3	0.3	t	*	*	*
SUBWAY SANDWICH-HAM AND CHEESE-ON WHEAT	ITEM	194	673	39	86	6	22	7	8	4
SUBWAY-BMT SANDWICH-ON HONEY WHEAT ROLL	ITEM	220	1011	45	88	6	57	20	25	7
SUBWAY-BMT SANDWICH-ON ITALIAN ROLL	ITEM	213	982	44	83	5	55	20	24	7
SUBWAY-CLUB SANDWICH-ON HONEY WHEAT	ITEM	220	722	47	89	6	23	7	9	4
SUBWAY-CLUB SANDWICH-ON ITALIAN ROLL	ITEM	213	693	46	83	5	22	7	8	4
SUBWAY-COLD CUT COMBO SANDWICH-ITALIAN	ITEM	184	853	46	83	5	40	12	15	10
SUBWAY-COLD CUT COMBO SANDWICH-ON WHEAT	ITEM	191	883	48	88	6	41	12	15	10

t = Trace of nutrient present ** = Not available*

MAG, magnesium; **IRON,** iron; **ZINC,** zinc; **VITA,** vitamin A; **VITC,** vitamin C; **THIA,** thiamin; **RIBO,** riboflavin; **NIAC,** niacin; **VB6,** vitamin B-6; **FOL,** folate; **VB12,** vitamin B-12; **CALC,** calcium; **PHOS,** phosphorus; **SEL,** selenium; **VE-a,** alpha tocopherol equivalents.

CHOL (mg)	SOD (mg)	POT (mg)	MAG (mg)	IRON (mg)	ZINC (mg)	VITA (RE)	VITC (mg)	THIA (mg)	RIBO (mg)	NIAC (mg)	VB6 (mg)	FOL (μg)	VB12 (μg)	CALC (mg)	PHOS (mg)	SEL (μg)	VE-a (mg)
0	300	38	13	2.1	0.3	0	0	0.25	0.18	2.5	0.03	4	0.07	9	91	*	1.4
0	140	20	5	0.4	0.1	0	t	0.05	0.03	0.4	0.01	3	0	6	15	*	0.1
226	740	213	33	2.8	1.8	150	1	0.47	0.33	3.7	0.16	44	0.8	256	319	*	1.8
9	270	74	12	1.6	0.4	37	0	0.33	0.14	2.5	0.1	51	t	151	60	*	0.1
50	1030	150	27	1.8	0.9	44	t	0.3	0.15	2.7	0.1	20	0.82	165	229	*	*
16	200	866	40	0.9	0.6	0	15	0.24	0	3.3	0.32	40	0.15	18	162	*	0.3
12	150	692	32	0.7	0.5	0	12	0.19	0	2.6	0.25	32	0.12	14	129	*	0.2
9	110	484	22	0.5	0.4	0	8	0.14	0	1.8	0.18	22	0.08	10	90	*	*
83	160	450	35	1.3	1	391	14	0.1	0.16	0.6	0.49	57	0.23	149	188	*	0.8
37	500	215	23	2.3	2.1	46	2	0.28	0.16	3.8	0.12	17	0.84	122	110	*	0.4
9	330	238	9	0.3	0.2	0	2	0.06	0.02	0.9	0.07	4	0	6	39	*	0.1
0	0	*	*	0.1	*	0	t	0	0.01	t	*	*	*	*	*	*	*
21	640	187	25	2.1	0.6	52	5	0.32	0.33	2.8	0.12	9	0.19	114	501	*	*
13	180	414	51	0.1	1.1	87	0	0.08	0.35	0.3	0.38	19	0.66	222	198	*	1.2
6	170	274	32	0.5	1.3	64	0	0.08	0.35	0.3	0.07	7	0.6	235	178	*	1.1
5	250	26	5	0.2	0.1	2	t	0.01	0.01	0.2	0.01	1	0	15	7	*	1.2
47	420	*	*	1.4	*	38	1	0.29	0.23	2.1	*	*	*	33	*	*	*
43	780	340	47	2.6	1.7	31	2	0.96	0.21	8.9	0.67	33	0.35	143	299	*	2.7
109	990	*	*	3.9	*	226	7	0.39	0.36	6.9	*	*	*	225	*	*	*
60	670	290	35	3.8	3.2	67	10	0.35	0.31	5.8	0.26	48	1.48	93	170	*	2.7
10	240	*	*	*	*	*	*	*	*	*	*	*	*	332	*	*	*
10	170	*	*	*	*	*	*	*	*	*	*	*	*	327	*	*	*
10	170	643	48	0.2	2.4	38	2	0.12	0.59	0.3	0.13	31	1.54	327	394	*	0.1
48	350	*	*	0.7	*	0	0	0.27	0.1	2.3	*	*	*	8	*	*	*
118	1150	341	41	3.7	5.7	211	3	0.37	0.39	6.7	0.23	23	2.15	295	382	*	*
86	660	322	37	3.7	5.1	67	3	0.36	0.29	6.7	0.27	23	1.88	142	249	*	*
26	310	*	*	1.5	*	35	3	0.33	0.21	2.1	*	*	*	14	*	*	*
14	170	22	0	0.1	t	6	0	t	0.01	t	t	1	0.04	3	4	*	2.4
0	220	22	0	0.1	t	6	0	t	0.01	t	t	1	0.04	3	4	*	2.4
275	1250	319	25	3.2	2.2	88	t	0.53	0.35	4	0.2	40	1.37	116	490	*	*
49	1080	196	20	2	1.5	0	0	0.49	0.21	4	0.11	9	0.5	83	443	*	3.1
64	830	179	20	2.3	1.7	72	1	0.6	0.29	4.8	0.13	48	0.5	235	273	*	1.6
263	980	255	29	3.3	2.4	150	0	0.64	0.42	4.8	0.19	68	0.72	263	390	*	2.3
399	290	102	10	2.1	1.1	156	1	0.07	0.26	0.1	0.08	27	1.68	57	136	*	2.9
41	85	219	12	0.7	0.3	217	7	0.05	0.08	0.3	0.06	40	0	76	26	*	0.4
10	170	*	*	0.1	*	92	0	0.13	0.48	0.3	*	*	*	327	*	*	*
5	95	263	19	0.2	1.2	64	1	0.07	0.29	0.3	0.07	9	0.54	190	127	*	0.6
0	190	10	2	0.2	t	65	1	0	0.01	0.1	t	t	0	11	3	*	0
10	170	*	*	0.1	*	92	0	0.13	0.48	0.3	*	*	*	327	*	*	*
3	80	*	*	0.2	*	38	0	0.04	0.18	0.4	*	*	*	112	*	*	*
*	267	49	*	0.7	*	23	1	0.03	0.02	1.3	*	*	*	73	53	*	*
*	132	50	*	0.2	*	23	t	0.01	0.02	0.9	*	*	*	21	36	*	*
*	146	45	*	0.2	*	30	t	0.02	0.03	1.7	*	*	*	19	37	*	*
*	167	44	*	0.2	*	23	t	0.01	0.01	0.8	*	*	*	24	37	*	*
*	267	37	*	0.4	*	25	1	0.03	0.03	2.1	*	*	*	86	114	*	*
6	165	45	6	0.2	0.3	10	1	0.02	0.02	1.8	0.04	7	0.08	27	39	*	0.3
8	130	47	7	0.2	0.7	29	1	0.02	0.02	3.6	0.06	2	0.37	24	38	*	0.7
*	136	43	*	0.2	*	9	t	0.01	0.02	1.6	*	*	*	25	33	*	*
*	367	61	*	0.2	*	22	t	0.02	t	3.1	*	*	*	76	59	*	*
*	143	46	*	0.2	*	12	t	0.01	0.01	2.3	*	*	*	25	48	*	*
*	160	33	*	0.2	*	13	t	0.01	0.01	0.9	*	*	*	22	38	*	*
3	17	130	10	0.6	0.1	6	t	0.02	0.01	0.4	0.07	8	0	2	20	*	0.1
1	82	48	5	0.8	0.1	15	t	0.02	0.01	0.2	0.06	2	0.02	3	14	*	0.2
88	1050	340	47	3.6	1.7	16	0	0.46	0.4	15.3	0.67	33	0.35	114	299	*	2.7
*	128	40	*	0.7	*	4	1	0.02	0.01	t	*	*	*	5	14	*	*
*	84	52	*	0.3	*	4	t	0.01	0.01	0.2	*	*	*	4	10	*	*
73	2508	918	*	*	*	*	*	*	*	*	*	*	*	*	*	*	*
133	3199	1002	*	*	*	*	*	*	*	*	*	*	*	*	*	*	*
133	3139	917	66	4.3	6.1	67	5	0.27	0.34	5.1	0.48	63	2.33	64	308	*	5.1
84	2777	1055	40	3.2	1.4	83	15	0.49	0.35	9.3	0.46	43	0.44	96	247	*	4.2
84	2717	971	66	3.1	2.5	74	20	0.48	0.33	12.5	0.58	47	0.95	58	384	*	1.3
166	2218	876	28	2.9	2.7	87	17	0.36	0.33	3.8	0.2	39	1.23	227	315	*	0.9
166	2278	1010	29	3	2.8	90	18	0.37	0.35	3.9	0.21	41	1.28	235	327	*	0.9

WT, weight; **KCAL,** kcalories; **PROT,** protein; **CARB,** carbohydrate; **FIBR,** fiber; **FAT,** fat; **SATF,** saturated fat; **MONO,** monosaturated fat; **POLY,** polyunsaturated fat; **CHOR,** cholesterol; **SOD,** sodium; **POT,** potassium;

Food Name	Portion	WT (Gm)	KCAL	PROT (Gm)	CARB (Gm)	FIBR (Gm)	FAT (Gm)	SATF (Gm)	MONO (Gm)	POLY (Gm)
SUBWAY-HAM & CHEESE SANDWICH-ON ITALIAN	ITEM	184	643	38	81	5	18	7	8	4
SUBWAY-MEATBALL SANDWICH-ON ITALIAN ROLL	ITEM	215	918	42	96	3	44	17	17	4
SUBWAY-MEATBALL-ON HONEY WHEAT ROLL	ITEM	224	947	44	101	*	45	17	18	4
SUBWAY-ROAST BEEF SANDWICH-ITALIAN ROLL	ITEM	184	689	42	84	5	23	8	9	4
SUBWAY-ROAST BEEF SANDWICH-ON WHEAT ROLL	ITEM	189	717	41	89	6	24	8	9	4
SUBWAY-SALAD DRESSING-BUTTERMILK RANCH	SERVING	56.7	348	1	2	0	37	5	7	24
SUBWAY-SALAD DRESSING-LITE ITALIAN	SERVING	56.7	23	1	4	0	1	4	6.4	15.9
SUBWAY-SEAFOOD/CRAB SANDWICH-ON ITALIAN	ITEM	210	986	29	94	*	57	11	15	28
SUBWAY-SEAFOOD/CRAB SANDWICH-ON WHEAT	ITEM	219	1015	31	100	2.5	58	11	16	28
SUBWAY-SPICY ITALIAN SANDWICH-ON ITALIAN	ITEM	213	1043	42	83	5	63	23	28	7
SUBWAY-STEAK & CHEESE SANDWICH-ITALIAN	ITEM	213	765	43	83	6	32	12	12	4
SUBWAY-TURKEY BREAST SANDWICH-WHEAT ROLL	ITEM	192	674	42	88	7	20	6	7	7
TACO BELL-BEAN BURRITO	ITEM	168	332	17	43	6.4	12	5.6	4.2	0.6
TACO BELL-BEEF BURRITO	ITEM	110	262	13	29	1.3	10	5.2	3.7	0.4
TACO BELL-BEEFY TOSTADA	ITEM	225	334	16	30	5.2	17	11.5	3.5	0.5
TACO BELL-BURRITO SUPREME	ITEM	225	457	21	43	5	22	7.7	7.4	1.7
TACO BELL-DOUBLE BEEF BURRITO SUPREME	ITEM	255	457	24	42	5.7	22	10.1	15.4	2.1
TACO BELL-ENCHIRITO	ITEM	213	382	20	31	*	20	9.3	*	1.5
TACO BELL-MEXICAN PIZZA	SERVING	223	575	21	40	5.8	37	11.4	8.2	9.7
TACO BELL-NACHOS	SERVING	106	346	7	38	1.4	19	5.7	10	1.6
TACO BELL-NACHOS BELLGRANDE	SERVING	287	649	22	61	*	35	12.3	*	2.6
TACO BELL-PINTOS & CHEESE	SERVING	128	190	9	19	4.9	9	3.6	4.9	0.8
TACO BELL-SOFT TACO	ITEM	92.1	228	12	18	2.6	12	5.4	3.7	1.2
TACO BELL-TACO BELLGRANDE	ITEM	163	355	18	18	4.5	23	10.9	6.6	1.3
TACO BELL-TACO LIGHT	ITEM	170	410	19	18	*	29	11.6	*	5.4
TACO BELL-TACO SALAD WITH SALSA/NO SHELL	SERVING	530	520	31	30	7	31	14.4	19.2	1.7
TACO BELL-TACO SALAD WITH SALSA/SHELL	SERVING	595	941	36	63	7.9	61	18.7	21.6	12.1
TACO BELL-TACO SALAD-NO SALSA-NO SHELL	SERVING	530	502	30	26	7	31	14.4	19.2	1.7
TACO BELL-TACO-REGULAR	ITEM	171	370	21	27	1.2	21	11.4	6.6	1
TACO BELL-TOSTADA-REGULAR	ITEM	144	223	10	27	4	10	5.4	3.1	0.7
WENDYS-BACON AND CHEESE POTATO	SERVING	347	450	15	57	9.9	18	37.1	38.2	14.1
WENDYS-BIG CLASSIC-QUARTER POUND BURGER	SERVING	277	570	27	46	2.3	33	15.9	14.8	4.3
WENDYS-BROCCOLI AND CHEESE POTATO	SERVING	377	400	9	59	*	16	*	*	*
WENDYS-CHEESE POTATO	SERVING	348	470	13	57	3.6	21	12.1	9.3	4
WENDYS-CHEESE SAUCE	SERVING	56	40	1	5	0.2	2	1.9	1.1	0.3
WENDYS-CHEESE TORTELLINI/SPAGHETTI SAUCE	SERVING	112	120	4	24	1	1	2.8	2.2	0.9
WENDYS-CHICKEN CLUB SANDWICH	SERVING	231	500	30	42	2.3	24	5.5	8.5	8
WENDYS-CHICKEN SALAD	SERVING	56	120	7	4	0.2	8	3	2.8	3
WENDYS-CHILI	SERVING	255	220	21	23	6	7	3	5.7	1.1
WENDYS-DOUBLE HAMBURGER	ITEM	226	540	34	40	2.3	27	10.5	10.3	2.8
WENDYS-FRENCH FRIES-REGULAR SIZE	SERVING	134	440	5	53	4.6	23	8.5	9.1	3.6
WENDYS-KIDS MEAL HAMBURGER	SERVING	104	260	14	30	1.3	9	3.5	4.8	0.8
WENDYS-REFRIED BEANS	SERVING	56	70	4	10	3	3	1	2.2	1
WENDYS-SEAFOOD SALAD	SERVING	56	110	4	7	0.2	7	1	4.5	4
WENDYS-SINGLE CHEESEBURGER/EVERYTHING	SERVING	252	490	29	35	2.7	27	10.8	11.2	4.6
WENDYS-SINGLE HAMBURGER	ITEM	218	511	26	40	2.8	27	10.4	11.4	2.2
WENDYS-SINGLE HAMBURGER/EVERYTHING	SERVING	234	420	25	35	2.7	21	6.7	9.4	4.4
WENDYS-SPANISH RICE	SERVING	56	70	2	13	0.7	1	0.1	0.3	1
WENDYS-TACO SALAD WITH TACO CHIPS	SERVING	791	660	40	46	10.5	37	28.8	28.7	15.4
WENDYS-TRIPLE HAMBURGER	ITEM	259	693	50	29	*	42	15.9	18.2	2.7
WENDYS-TUNA SALAD	SERVING	56	100	8	4	0.3	6	1	0.8	3

Fats & Oils

Food Name	Portion	WT (Gm)	KCAL	PROT (Gm)	CARB (Gm)	FIBR (Gm)	FAT (Gm)	SATF (Gm)	MONO (Gm)	POLY (Gm)
BUTTER-REGULAR-PAT	ITEM	5	36	t	t	0	4	2.5	1.2	0.2
BUTTER-REGULAR-STICK	ITEM	113	813	1	t	0	92	57.3	26.6	3.4
BUTTER-REGULAR-TABLESPOON	TBSP	14	100	t	t	0	11	7.1	3.3	0.4
BUTTER-UNSALTED-PAT	ITEM	5	36	t	t	0.1	4	2.5	1.2	0.2
FAT-ANIMAL-CHICKEN-FOR COOKING	TBSP	12.8	115	0	0	0	13	3.8	5.7	2.7
FAT-ANIMAL-LARD (PORK)	CUP	205	1849	0	0	0	205	80.4	92.5	23
MARGARINE-DIET/LOW CALORIE-MAZOLA	TBSP	14	50	0	0	0	6	1	2.1	2.6
MARGARINE-IMITATION-40% FAT	TSP	4.8	17	0	0	0	2	0.4	0.8	0.7
MARGARINE-IMITATION-SPREAD-60% FAT	TSP	4.8	26	0	0	0	3	0.6	1.5	0.7
MARGARINE-NO STICK-SPRAY-MAZOLA	SERVING	0.72	6	0	0	0	1	0.1	0.2	0.4

t = Trace of nutrient present   ** = Not available*

MAG, magnesium; **IRON,** iron; **ZINC,** zinc; **VITA,** vitamin A; **VITC,** vitamin C; **THIA,** thiamin; **RIBO,** riboflavin; **NIAC,** niacin; **VB6,** vitamin B-6; **FOL,** folate; **VB12,** vitamin B-12; **CALC,** calcium; **PHOS,** phosphorus; **SEL,** selenium; **VE-a,** alpha tocopherol equivalents.

CHOL (mg)	SOD (mg)	POT (mg)	MAG (mg)	IRON (mg)	ZINC (mg)	VITA (RE)	VITC (mg)	THIA (mg)	RIBO (mg)	NIAC (mg)	VB6 (mg)	FOL (μg)	VB12 (μg)	CALC (mg)	PHOS (mg)	SEL (μg)	VE-a (mg)
73	1710	834	50	2.2	2.8	174	17	0.53	0.39	3.6	0.34	45	0.76	304	527	*	3.8
88	2022	1210	47	5	6.2	72	19	0.33	0.39	9.4	0.4	35	3.21	78	263	*	1
88	2082	1498	*	*	*	*	*	*	*	*	*	*	*	*	*	*	*
83	2288	910	57	3.7	5.3	58	5	0.23	0.29	4.4	0.42	54	2.01	55	266	*	4.4
75	2348	994	59	3.8	5.4	59	5	0.24	0.3	4.5	0.43	56	2.07	56	273	*	4.5
6	492	17	1	0.1	0.1	48	0	0.01	0.01	t	0.01	4	0.12	8	15	*	2.3
0	952	13	t	0.1	0.1	14	0	0.01	0.01	t	0.01	3	0.09	6	3	*	4.9
56	2027	641	62	4.4	5.3	107	5	0.51	0.38	7	0.26	91	6.54	230	336	*	2.5
56	1967	557	*	*	*	*	*	*	*	*	*	*	*	*	*	*	*
137	2282	880	*	*	*	*	*	*	*	*	*	*	*	*	*	*	*
82	1556	909	43	4.2	6.8	119	6	0.33	0.46	5.1	0.38	36	2.54	231	456	*	0.8
67	2520	605	*	*	*	*	*	*	*	*	*	*	*	*	*	*	*
79	1030	405	t	3.8	3	240	3	0.28	0.6	3.9	0.21	73	1	144	143	*	1.9
33	746	370	41	3.1	2.4	42	1	0.12	0.46	3.2	0.16	20	0.99	42	88	*	0.9
75	870	490	68	2.5	3.2	383	4	0.09	0.5	2.9	0.26	t	1.13	190	173	*	2
126	367	350	52	3.8	5.9	216	8	0.45	0.92	6.2	0.27	43	1.53	146	245	*	2.1
57	1053	431	87	4	5.9	286	9	0.43	2.19	3.7	0.35	132	2.18	145	548	*	2.3
54	1243	*	*	2.8	*	290	28	0.26	0.42	2.3	*	*	*	269	*	*	*
52	1031	408	63	3.7	2.3	295	31	0.32	0.33	3	0.27	113	0.2	257	360	*	2.5
9	399	159	43	0.9	2.6	169	2	0.01	0.16	0.7	0.12	16	0.62	191	439	*	2.8
36	997	674	*	3.5	*	341	58	0.1	0.34	2.2	*	*	*	297	*	*	*
16	642	399	50	1.4	1.1	132	51	0.05	0.15	0.4	0.19	98	0.08	156	175	*	1.4
32	516	178	31	2.3	1.4	64	1	0.39	0.22	2.7	0.16	40	0.31	116	132	*	0.9
56	472	334	54	1.9	2.4	254	5	0.11	0.29	2	0.28	71	0.55	182	234	*	1.6
56	594	316	*	2.4	*	199	5	0.2	0.33	2.5	*	*	*	155	*	*	*
80	1431	1151	111	5.1	9.1	908	76	0.26	0.64	3.2	0.78	99	4.29	367	567	*	6
80	1662	1212	125	7.1	10.3	888	77	0.51	0.75	4.8	0.88	111	4.82	398	637	*	6.8
80	1056	988	111	4.5	9.1	572	74	0.25	0.5	3.2	0.78	99	4.29	331	567	*	6
57	802	473	71	2.4	3.9	257	2	0.15	0.45	3.2	0.24	23	1.04	221	203	*	0.8
30	543	403	59	1.9	1.9	187	1	0.1	0.33	1.3	0.17	75	0.68	211	116	*	1.4
10	1125	1580	167	15.3	7	266	77	1.04	0.81	14.5	1.94	75	2.26	713	1015	*	4.9
85	1075	590	49	4.8	6.4	162	9	0.35	0.5	8	0.38	51	2.92	304	491	*	2.9
0	470	1555	*	*	*	*	*	*	*	*	*	*	*	*	*	*	*
0	580	1435	72	2.3	2.4	288	34	0.22	0.43	3.5	0.57	31	0.3	417	398	*	2.3
0	300	70	10	0.1	0.2	24	t	0.03	0.11	0.1	0.03	3	0.22	114	88	*	0.1
5	280	110	14	1.3	0.6	110	4	0.12	0.18	1.2	0.09	12	0.17	75	92	*	0.9
75	950	515	42	14.4	1.5	87	16	0.51	0.37	16	0.48	45	0.46	101	259	*	4.4
0	215	60	8	0.5	0.7	22	1	0.02	0.08	1.8	0.13	6	0.14	13	58	*	2.4
45	750	495	53	6.3	4.1	146	19	0.16	0.26	4.8	0.23	41	1.46	55	228	*	1.8
122	791	569	49	6	5.7	31	1	0.36	0.39	7.6	0.54	27	4.07	102	314	*	1.1
25	265	855	46	1	0.5	0	14	0.24	0.04	4.4	0.32	39	0	26	125	*	0.3
35	545	205	22	2.5	2.2	7	1	0.23	0.2	3.8	0.14	25	1	63	110	*	0.5
0	215	210	25	1.2	0.5	0	2	0.08	0.04	0.2	0.09	71	0	25	72	*	0.5
0	455	40	14	0.5	0.9	21	3	0.02	0.03	0.6	0.05	8	0.48	25	74	*	1.2
90	1155	495	44	4.3	4.3	136	11	0.4	0.42	6.5	0.3	55	1.8	234	348	*	3.2
86	825	479	43	4.9	4.9	93	3	0.42	0.38	7.3	0.33	36	2.38	96	233	*	1.1
70	865	495	40	4.3	3.7	76	11	0.4	0.35	6.6	0.29	54	1.68	105	193	*	3
0	440	130	9	0.7	0.2	24	9	0.05	0.02	0.6	0.06	4	0	15	17	*	0.3
35	1110	1330	166	9.2	13.6	1478	67	0.4	0.93	15.2	1.16	147	6.41	532	847	*	9
142	713	785	55	8.3	10.8	47	1	0.31	0.56	11	0.62	31	4.92	65	393	*	*
0	290	90	10	0.6	0.2	15	1	0.02	0.04	3.8	0.05	4	0.68	9	62	*	0.5
11	41	1	t	t	t	8	0	0	t	t	0	t	0.01	1	1	0	0.1
248	937	29	2	0.2	0.1	855	0	0.01	0.04	t	t	3	0.14	27	26	3	1.8
31	116	4	t	t	t	105	0	t	0.01	t	0	t	0.02	3	3	0	0.2
11	1	1	t	t	t	38	0	0	t	t	0	t	0.01	1	1	*	0.1
11	0	0	0	0	0	0	0	0	0	0	0	0	0	0	0	*	2.7
195	t	t	t	0	0.2	0	0	0	0	0	0	0	0	t	0	86	2.5
0	130	1	t	0	t	130	0	0	0	0	0	0	0	0	t	0	0.1
0	46	1	t	0	0	48	t	0	t	t	0	t	t	1	1	*	0.4
0	48	1	t	0	0	48	t	0	t	t	0	t	t	1	1	*	0.4
0	0	*	*	0	*	0	0	0	0	0	*	*	*	0	0	*	*

WT, weight; **KCAL,** kcalories; **PROT,** protein; **CARB,** carbohydrate; **FIBR,** fiber; **FAT,** fat; **SATF,** saturated fat; **MONO,** monosaturated fat; **POLY,** polyunsaturated fat; **CHOR,** cholesterol; **SOD,** sodium; **POT,** potassium;

Food Name	Portion	WT (Gm)	KCAL	PROT (Gm)	CARB (Gm)	FIBR (Gm)	FAT (Gm)	SATF (Gm)	MONO (Gm)	POLY (Gm)
MARGARINE-REGULAR-HARD-UNSALTED	TSP	4.7	34	0	0	0	4	0.7	1.7	1.2
MARGARINE-REGULAR-SOFT-UNSALTED	TSP	4.7	34	0	0	0	4	0.6	1.8	1.2
MARGARINE-SOYBEAN-SOFT-TUB-UNSALTED	TSP	4.7	34	0	0	0	4	0.6	1.7	1.3
MARGARINE-WHIPPED	TBSP	9	70	0	0	0	8	1.4	2.5	3.1
MAYONNAISE-IMITATION-MILK CREAM	TBSP	15	15	t	2	0	1	0.4	0.3	0.1
MAYONNAISE-LIGHT-LOW CALORIE-KRAFT	TBSP	14	40	0	1	0	4	0.5	0.6	1.4
MAYONNAISE-SOYBEAN-COMMERCIAL	TBSP	14	99	t	t	0	11	1.6	3.1	5.7
OIL-VEGETABLE-CORN	CUP	218	1927	0	0	0	218	27.7	52.7	128
OIL-VEGETABLE-OLIVE	CUP	216	1909	0	0	0	216	30.7	159	18.2
OIL-VEGETABLE-PEANUT	CUP	216	1909	0	0	0	216	36.4	99.9	69.2
OIL-VEGETABLE-SAFFLOWER	CUP	218	1927	0	0	0	218	20.5	26.3	162
OIL-VEGETABLE-SESAME	TBSP	13.6	120	0	0	0	14	1.9	5.4	5.7
OIL-VEGETABLE-SOYBEAN	CUP	218	1927	0	0	0	218	31.8	93.8	82
SALAD DRESSING-BLUE CHEESE	TBSP	15.3	77	1	1	0.1	8	1.5	1.9	4.3
SALAD DRESSING-BLUE CHEESE-LOW CALORIE	TBSP	16	10	0	1	0	1	0.5	0.3	0
SALAD DRESSING-CAESAR	TBSP	15	70	0	1	t	7	*	*	*
SALAD DRESSING-FRENCH	TBSP	15.6	67	t	3	0.1	6	1.5	1.2	3.4
SALAD DRESSING-FRENCH-LOW CALORIE	TBSP	16.3	22	0	4	0.1	1	0.1	0.2	0.5
SALAD DRESSING-ITALIAN	TBSP	14.7	69	0	2	0.1	7	1	1.7	4.1
SALAD DRESSING-ITALIAN-LOW CALORIE	TBSP	15	16	0	1	0.1	2	0.2	0.3	0.9
SALAD DRESSING-MAYONNAISE TYPE	TBSP	14.7	57	0	4	0	5	0.7	1.3	2.6
SALAD DRESSING-MAYONNAISE-LOW CALORIE	TBSP	16	20	0	2	0	2	0.4	0.4	1
SALAD DRESSING-MIRACLE WHIP LIGHT	TBSP	14	45	0	2	0	4	*	*	*
SALAD DRESSING-OIL/VINEGAR-HOME RECIPE	TBSP	15.6	70	0	t	0	8	1.4	2.3	3.8
SALAD DRESSING-RANCH STYLE	TBSP	15	54	t	1	0	6	0.7	1.4	2.7
SALAD DRESSING-RUSSIAN	TBSP	15.3	76	t	2	0	8	1.1	1.8	4.5
SALAD DRESSING-RUSSIAN-LOW CALORIE	TBSP	16.3	23	t	5	0.2	1	0.1	0.2	0.4
SALAD DRESSING-THOUSAND ISLAND	TBSP	15.6	59	0	2	0.6	6	0.9	1.3	3.1
SALAD DRESSING-THOUSAND-LOW CALORIE	TBSP	15.3	24	t	3	0.3	2	0.2	0.4	1
SANDWICH SPREAD-COMMERCIAL	TBSP	15.3	60	t	3	t	5	0.8	1.1	3.1
SHORTENING-VEGETABLE-SOYBEAN/COTTONSEED	CUP	205	1812	0	0	0	205	51.2	89	52.2
VEGETABLE SPRAY-PAM-BUTTER FLAVORED	SERVING	0.9	7	0	0	0	1	0.1	0.2	0.5
VEGETABLE SPRAY-PAM-UNFLAVORED	SERVING	0.9	7	0	0	0	1	0.1	0.2	0.5

Fish

Food Name	Portion	WT (Gm)	KCAL	PROT (Gm)	CARB (Gm)	FIBR (Gm)	FAT (Gm)	SATF (Gm)	MONO (Gm)	POLY (Gm)
FISH STICKS-BREADED-FROZEN-COOKED	OUNCE	28.4	77	4	7	0.7	3	0.9	1.4	0.9
FISH-ANCHOVY-FILLET-CANNED	ITEM	4	8	1	0	0	t	0.1	0.2	0.1
FISH-BLUEFISH-BAKED WITH BUTTER	ITEM	155	246	41	0	0	8	1.8	1.8	3.9
FISH-CARP-COOKED-DRY HEAT	SERVING	85	138	19	0	0	6	1.2	2.5	1.6
FISH-CATFISH-BREADED-FRIED	SERVING	85	195	15	7	0.8	11	2.8	4.8	2.8
FISH-CLAMS-BREADED-FRIED	SERVING	85	172	12	9	0.3	9	2.3	3.9	2.4
FISH-CLAMS-CANNED-SOLIDS AND LIQUIDS	OUNCE	28.4	13	2	1	0	t	0.1	0	0
FISH-CLAMS-COOKED-MOIST HEAT	SERVING	85	126	22	4	0	2	0.2	0.1	0.5
FISH-CLAMS-RAW-MEAT ONLY	SERVING	85	63	11	2	0	1	0.1	0.1	0.2
FISH-COD-ATLANTIC-COOKED-DRY HEAT	PIECE	180	189	41	0	0	2	0.3	0.2	0.5
FISH-CRAB CAKE	ITEM	60	93	12	t	t	5	0.9	1.7	1.4
FISH-CRAB MEAT-KING-CANNED-UNPACKED	CUP	135	135	24	1	0	3	0.6	0.6	2
FISH-CRAB-ALASKA KING-RAW	SERVING	85	71	16	0	0	1	0.1	0.1	0.1
FISH-CRAB-BLUE-CANNED	CUP	135	134	28	0	0	2	0.3	0.3	0.6
FISH-CRAB-BLUE-COOKED-MOIST HEAT	CUP	135	138	27	0	0	2	0.3	0.4	0.9
FISH-CRAB-DEVILED	CUP	240	451	27	32	2.3	23	4.8	9.6	7.1
FISH-CRAB-IMITATION-SURIMI	SERVING	85	87	10	9	0	1	0.2	0.2	0.6
FISH-CRAB-IMPERIAL	CUP	220	323	32	9	0	17	4.2	6.7	4.8
FISH-CRAB-STEAMED-PIECES	CUP	155	150	30	0	0	2	0.2	0.3	0.8
FISH-CRAYFISH-COOKED-MOIST HEAT	SERVING	85	97	20	0	0	1	0.2	0.3	0.3
FISH-CROAKER-BREADED-FRIED	SERVING	85	188	16	6	0.3	11	3	4.5	2.5
FISH-EEL-COOKED-DRY HEAT	SERVING	85	201	20	0	0	13	2.6	7.8	1
FISH-FLATFISH-COOKED-DRY HEAT	SERVING	85	100	21	0	0	1	0.3	0.3	0.4
FISH-GEFILTEFISH-COMMERCIAL-WITH BROTH	PIECE	42	35	4	3	t	1	0.2	0.3	0.1
FISH-GROUPER-COOKED-DRY HEAT	SERVING	85	100	21	0	0	1	0.3	0.2	0.3
FISH-HADDOCK-BREADED-FRIED	PIECE	85	140	17	5	0.3	5	1.4	2.2	1.2
FISH-HADDOCK-BROILED	SERVING	85	95	21	0	0	1	0.1	0.1	0.3
FISH-HALIBUT-ALL TYPES-BROILED IN BUTTER	PIECE	125	214	32	0	0	9	*	*	*
FISH-HALIBUT-COOKED-BROILED	SERVING	85	119	23	0	0	2	0.4	0.8	0.8

t= Trace of nutrient present **= Not available*

MAG, magnesium; **IRON,** iron; **ZINC,** zinc; **VITA,** vitamin A; **VITC,** vitamin C; **THIA,** thiamin; **RIBO,** riboflavin; **NIAC,** niacin; **VB6,** vitamin B-6; **FOL,** folate; **VB12,** vitamin B-12; **CALC,** calcium; **PHOS,** phosphorus; **SEL,** selenium; **VE-a,** alpha tocopherol equivalents.

CHOL (mg)	SOD (mg)	POT (mg)	MAG (mg)	IRON (mg)	ZINC (mg)	VITA (RE)	VITC (mg)	THIA (mg)	RIBO (mg)	NIAC (mg)	VB6 (mg)	FOL (μg)	VB12 (μg)	CALC (mg)	PHOS (mg)	SEL (μg)	VE-a (mg)
0	t	1	t	0	0	47	t	0	t	t	0	t	t	1	1	0	0.6
0	1	2	t	0	0	47	t	0	t	t	0	t	t	1	1	0	0.5
0	1	2	t	0	0	47	t	0	t	t	0	t	t	1	1	0	0.1
0	97	2	t	0	0	310	0	0	0	0	t	t	0.01	2	2	0	1.1
6	76	15	1	0.1	t	t	t	t	0.02	t	t	t	0.04	11	9	*	0.1
5	15	1	0	0	t	1	0	0	t	0	0	t	0.01	0	0	*	2.9
8	78	5	t	0.1	t	12	0	0	0	0	0.08	1	0.04	2	4	*	2.9
0	0	0	0	0	0	0	0	0	0	0	0	0	0	0	0	*	31.1
0	t	0	t	0.8	0.1	0	0	0	0	0	0	0	0	t	3	*	25.7
0	t	t	t	0.1	t	0	0	0	0	0	0	0	0	t	0	*	25.1
0	0	0	0	0	0	0	0	0	0	0	0	0	0	0	0	*	74.2
0	0	0	0	0	0	0	0	0	0	0	0	0	0	0	0	*	0.2
0	0	0	0	0	0	0	0	0	0	0	0	0	0	0	0	*	17.7
9	167	6	0	0	0	10	t	0	0.02	0	0.01	1	0.04	12	11	*	0.9
4	177	5	*	0	*	9	0	0	0.01	0	*	*	*	10	8	*	8
*	*	*	*	*	*	*	*	*	*	*	*	*	*	*	*	*	7
2	214	12	0	0.1	t	3	0	t	t	0	t	1	0.02	2	2	*	0.8
1	128	13	0	0.1	t	0	0	0	0	0	0	0	0	2	2	*	0.2
0	116	2	t	0	t	4	0	0	0	0	t	1	0.02	1	1	*	0.7
1	118	2	0	0	t	0	0	0	0	0	0	0	0	0	1	*	0
4	104	1	t	0	t	10	0	0	0	0	t	1	0.03	2	4	*	0.6
2	44	1	*	0	*	12	*	0	0	0	*	*	*	3	4	*	5
5	95	*	*	*	*	*	*	*	*	*	*	*	*	*	*	*	4
0	t	1	0	0	0	0	0	0	0	0	0	0	0	2	1	*	0.6
4	97	1	t	t	t	13	0	t	t	t	t	1	0.03	2	4	*	0.6
0	133	24	t	0.1	0.1	32	1	0.01	0.01	0.1	0.01	2	0.05	3	6	*	0.9
1	141	26	t	0.1	t	3	1	t	t	0	t	1	0.02	3	6	*	0.1
5	109	18	t	0.1	t	15	0	0	0	0	t	1	0.03	2	3	*	0.6
2	153	17	t	0.1	t	15	0	0	0	0	t	1	0.03	2	3	*	0.2
12	153	5	0	0	0	0	0	0	0	0	0	0	0	0	0	*	0.6
0	0	0	0	0	0	0	0	0	0	0	0	0	0	0	0	*	27.9
0	0	0	*	0	*	0	0	*	*	*	*	*	*	0	0	*	*
0	0	0	*	0	*	0	0	*	*	*	*	*	*	0	0	*	*

CHOL (mg)	SOD (mg)	POT (mg)	MAG (mg)	IRON (mg)	ZINC (mg)	VITA (RE)	VITC (mg)	THIA (mg)	RIBO (mg)	NIAC (mg)	VB6 (mg)	FOL (μg)	VB12 (μg)	CALC (mg)	PHOS (mg)	SEL (μg)	VE-a (mg)
32	165	74	7	0.2	0.2	9	0	0.04	0.05	0.6	0.02	5	0.51	6	51	3	*
3	147	22	3	0.2	0.1	1	0	t	0.02	0.8	0.01	1	0.04	9	10	2	t
108	161	*	43	1.1	*	24	*	0.17	0.16	2.9	*	*	1.64	45	445	47	*
72	54	363	32	1.4	1.6	8	1	0.12	0.06	1.8	0.19	15	1.25	44	451	26	1.8
69	238	289	23	1.2	0.7	7	0	0.06	0.11	1.9	0.16	14	1.62	37	184	*	1.8
52	309	277	12	11.8	1.2	77	9	0.09	0.21	1.8	0.05	16	34.2	54	160	*	1.7
18	15	40	*	1.2	0.3	*	*	t	0.03	0.3	*	*	5.4	16	39	46	0.6
57	95	534	16	23.8	2.3	145	19	0.13	0.36	2.9	0.09	16	84.1	78	287	*	1.7
29	48	267	8	11.9	1.2	77	11	0.07	0.18	1.5	0.05	14	42	39	144	16	0.2
99	141	440	76	0.9	1	25	2	0.16	0.14	4.5	0.51	15	1.89	25	248	81	0.1
90	198	195	20	0.7	2.5	49	2	0.05	0.05	1.7	0.1	25	3.56	63	128	13	1.2
135	675	149	29	1.1	5.8	*	*	0.11	0.11	2.6	*	*	13.5	61	246	30	1.7
36	711	173	42	0.5	5.1	6	6	0.04	0.04	0.9	0.13	37	7.65	39	186	19	*
120	450	505	53	1.1	5.4	3	4	0.11	0.11	1.9	0.2	57	0.62	136	351	30	1.4
135	376	437	45	1.2	5.7	3	4	0.14	0.07	4.5	0.24	69	9.86	140	278	30	1.4
223	2081	398	64	2.9	5.5	330	14	0.19	0.26	3.6	0.31	88	8.69	113	329	53	5.3
17	715	77	37	0.3	0.3	17	0	0.03	0.02	0.2	0.03	1	1.36	11	240	19	0.1
275	1602	288	57	2	6.4	211	11	0.13	0.26	2.4	0.31	83	10.6	132	365	48	3.5
82	1662	406	53	1.2	11.8	14	12	0.08	0.09	2.1	0.28	79	17.8	92	434	34	1.5
151	58	298	26	2.7	1.4	19	3	0.15	0.07	2.5	0.15	3	2.94	26	281	*	1.3
71	296	289	35	0.7	0.4	19	0	0.08	0.11	3.7	0.22	15	1.79	27	184	*	2.3
137	55	297	22	0.5	1.8	966	2	0.16	0.04	3.8	0.07	15	2.45	22	235	43	4.5
58	89	292	49	0.3	0.5	9	0	0.07	0.1	1.9	0.2	8	2.13	15	246	*	*
13	220	38	4	1	0.3	11	t	0.03	0.03	0.4	0.03	1	0.35	10	31	*	0
40	45	403	32	1	0.4	43	0	0.07	0.01	0.3	0.3	9	0.59	18	121	*	*
42	150	296	*	1	*	*	2	0.03	0.06	2.7	*	*	1.1	34	210	41	0.5
63	74	339	43	1.2	0.4	16	0	0.03	0.04	3.9	0.29	11	1.18	36	205	25	0.5
75	168	656	*	1	*	255	*	0.06	0.09	10.4	*	*	*	20	310	41	0.5
35	59	490	91	0.9	0.5	46	0	0.06	0.08	6.1	0.34	12	1.16	51	242	51	*

WT, weight; **KCAL,** kcalories; **PROT,** protein; **CARB,** carbohydrate; **FIBR,** fiber; **FAT,** fat; **SATF,** saturated fat; **MONO,** monosaturated fat; **POLY,** polyunsaturated fat; **CHOR,** cholesterol; **SOD,** sodium; **POT,** potassium;

Food Name	Portion	WT (Gm)	KCAL	PROT (Gm)	CARB (Gm)	FIBR (Gm)	FAT (Gm)	SATF (Gm)	MONO (Gm)	POLY (Gm)
FISH-HERRING-ATLANTIC-BROILED	SERVING	85	173	20	0	0	10	2.2	4.1	2.3
FISH-HERRING-ATLANTIC-RAW	SERVING	85	134	15	0	0	8	1.7	3.2	1.8
FISH-HERRING-CANNED-SOLIDS AND LIQUIDS	SERVING	100	208	20	0	0	14	*	*	2
FISH-HERRING-PICKLED-BISMARCK TYPE	ITEM	50	131	7	5	0	9	1.2	6	0.8
FISH-LOBSTER NEWBURG	CUP	250	485	46	13	0	27	30.1	14.9	2.3
FISH-LOBSTER THERMIDOR	SERVING	157	405	29	15	0	27	18.9	9.4	1.5
FISH-LOBSTER-COOKED-MOIST HEAT	OUNCE	28.4	28	6	t	0	t	t	t	t
FISH-LOBSTER-NORTHERN-RAW	OUNCE	28.4	26	5	t	0	t	0.1	0.1	t
FISH-MACKEREL-ATLANTIC-CANNED	CUP	190	296	44	0	0	12	3.4	5.2	0.2
FISH-MACKEREL-ATLANTIC-RAW	OUNCE	28.4	58	5	0	0	4	0.9	1.2	1.4
FISH-MACKEREL-COOKED-DRY HEAT	SERVING	85	223	20	0	0	15	3.6	6	3.7
FISH-MULLET-COOKED-DRY HEAT	SERVING	85	128	21	0	0	4	1.2	1.2	0.8
FISH-MUSSELS-BLUE-RAW	CUP	150	129	18	6	0	3	0.6	0.8	0.9
FISH-OCEAN PERCH-BREADED-FRIED	PIECE	85	195	16	6	0.1	11	2.7	4.4	2.3
FISH-OCEAN PERCH-COOKED-DRY HEAT	SERVING	85	103	20	0	0	2	0.3	0.7	0.5
FISH-OYSTER-EASTERN-CANNED	CUP	248	171	18	10	0	6	1.6	0.6	1.8
FISH-OYSTER-EASTERN-COOKED-MOIST HEAT	SERVING	85	117	12	7	0	4	1.1	0.4	1.3
FISH-OYSTERS-BREADED-FRIED	SERVING	85	167	7	10	0.1	11	2.7	4	2.8
FISH-OYSTERS-EASTERN-RAW-MEAT ONLY	CUP	248	171	18	10	0	6	1.6	0.6	1.8
FISH-OYSTERS-PACIFIC-RAW	SERVING	85	69	8	4	0	2	0.4	0.3	0.8
FISH-PERCH-COOKED-DRY HEAT	SERVING	85	100	21	0	0	1	0.2	0.2	0.4
FISH-PIKE-COOKED-DRY HEAT	SERVING	85	96	21	0	0	1	0.1	0.2	0.2
FISH-POLLOCK-ATLANTIC-RAW	SERVING	85	78	17	0	0	1	0.1	0.1	0.4
FISH-POLLOCK-COOKED-DRY HEAT	SERVING	85	96	20	0	0	1	0.2	0.1	0.4
FISH-POMPANO-COOKED-DRY HEAT	SERVING	85	179	20	0	0	10	3.8	2.8	1.2
FISH-RED SNAPPER-COOKED-DRY HEAT	SERVING	85	109	22	0	0	1	0.3	0.3	0.5
FISH-RED SNAPPER-RAW	SERVING	85	85	17	0	0	1	0.2	0.2	0.4
FISH-ROCKFISH-COOKED-DRY HEAT	SERVING	100	121	24	0	0	2	0.5	0.4	0.6
FISH-SALMON PATTY	SERVING	100	239	16	16	1	12	3.5	5.3	3.6
FISH-SALMON-BROILED OR BAKED-WITH BUTTER	SERVING	100	182	27	0	0	7	1.4	2.7	2.7
FISH-SALMON-COOKED-MOIST HEAT	SERVING	85	157	23	0	0	6	1.2	2.2	1.9
FISH-SALMON-PINK-CANNED-SOLIDS & LIQUIDS	SERVING	85	118	17	0	0	5	1.3	1.5	1.7
FISH-SALMON-SMOKED	SERVING	100	117	18	0	0	4	0.9	2	1
FISH-SARDINES-ATLANTIC-CANNED IN OIL	ITEM	12	25	3	0	0	1	0.2	0.5	0.6
FISH-SARDINES-CANNED IN TOMATO SAUCE	ITEM	38	68	6	0	0.1	5	1.2	1.4	1.6
FISH-SCALLOPS-BAY AND SEA-STEAMED	OUNCE	28.4	32	7	1	0	t	*	*	*
FISH-SCALLOPS-FROZEN-BREADED-FRIED	ITEM	15	32	3	2	0.1	2	0.4	0.7	0.4
FISH-SCALLOPS-RAW	SERVING	85	75	14	2	0	1	0.1	t	0.2
FISH-SEA BASS-COOKED-DRY HEAT	SERVING	85	105	20	0	0	2	0.6	0.5	0.8
FISH-SHAD-BAKED-BUTTER/MARGARINE & BACON	SERVING	100	201	23	0	0	11	2.5	2.2	5.9
FISH-SHRIMP-CANNED MEAT	CUP	128	154	30	1	0	3	0.5	0.4	1
FISH-SHRIMP-COOKED-MOIST HEAT	SERVING	85	84	18	0	0	1	0.2	0.2	0.4
FISH-SHRIMP-FRENCH FRIED	SERVING	85	206	18	10	0.5	10	1.8	3.2	3.8
FISH-SMELT-ATLANTIC-CANNED	ITEM	20	40	4	0	0	3	*	*	*
FISH-SMELT-COOKED-DRY HEAT	SERVING	85	105	19	0	0	3	0.5	0.7	1
FISH-SOLE/FLOUNDER-BAKED	SERVING	127	148	31	0	0	2	0.5	0.4	0.5
FISH-SQUID-COOKED-FRIED	SERVING	85	149	15	7	0.3	6	1.6	2.3	1.8
FISH-SQUID-RAW	SERVING	85	78	13	3	0	1	0.3	0.1	0.4
FISH-STURGEON-STEAMED	SERVING	100	135	21	0	0	5	1.2	2.5	0.9
FISH-SURIMI	SERVING	85	84	13	6	0	1	0.2	0.1	0.4
FISH-SWORDFISH-BROILED-BUTTER/MARGARINE	SERVING	100	174	28	0	0	6	2	3.4	2.2
FISH-SWORDFISH-COOKED-DRY HEAT	SERVING	85	132	22	0	0	4	1.2	1.7	1
FISH-TILEFISH-COOKED-DRY HEAT	SERVING	85	125	21	0	0	4	0.7	1.1	1.1
FISH-TROUT-BROOK-COOKED	SERVING	100	196	24	t	0	11	1.5	2.8	2.6
FISH-TROUT-RAINBOW-COOKED-DRY HEAT	SERVING	85	128	22	0	0	4	0.7	1.1	1.3
FISH-TUNA-BLUEFIN-COOKED-DRY HEAT	SERVING	85	156	25	0	0	5	1.4	1.8	1.6
FISH-TUNA-CANNED IN OIL-DRAINED SOLIDS	SERVING	85	168	25	0	0	7	1.3	2.5	2.5
FISH-TUNA-DIETETIC-LOW SODIUM-DRAINED	OUNCE	28.4	36	8	t	0	1	0.1	0.2	0.2
FISH-TUNA-LIGHT-CANNED IN WATER-DRAINED	SERVING	85	111	25	0	0	t	0.1	0.1	0.1
FISH-TUNA-WHITE-ALBACORE-CANNED IN WATER	SERVING	85	116	23	0	0	2	0.6	0.6	0.8
FISH-TUNA-YELLOWFIN-RAW	SERVING	85	92	20	0	0	1	0.2	0.1	0.2
FISH-WHITE PERCH-FRIED FILET	ITEM	65	108	13	0	0	5	*	*	*
FISH-WHITEFISH-LAKE-BAKED-STUFFED	SERVING	100	215	15	6	0.6	14	*	*	*
FISH-WHITING-COOKED-DRY HEAT	SERVING	85	98	20	0	0	1	0.3	0.3	0.5

t= Trace of nutrient present **= Not available*

MAG, magnesium; **IRON,** iron; **ZINC,** zinc; **VITA,** vitamin A; **VITC,** vitamin C; **THIA,** thiamin; **RIBO,** riboflavin; **NIAC,** niacin; **VB6,** vitamin B-6; **FOL,** folate; **VB12,** vitamin B-12; **CALC,** calcium; **PHOS,** phosphorus; **SEL,** selenium; **VE-a,** alpha tocopherol equivalents.

CHOL (mg)	SOD (mg)	POT (mg)	MAG (mg)	IRON (mg)	ZINC (mg)	VITA (RE)	VITC (mg)	THIA (mg)	RIBO (mg)	NIAC (mg)	VB6 (mg)	FOL (μg)	VB12 (μg)	CALC (mg)	PHOS (mg)	SEL (μg)	VE-a (mg)
66	98	356	35	1.2	1.1	26	1	0.1	0.25	3.5	0.3	10	11.2	63	258	52	0.9
51	76	278	27	0.9	0.8	24	1	0.08	0.2	2.7	0.26	9	11.6	49	201	85	0.9
98	*	*	*	1.8	*	*	*	0.18	*	*	*	*	*	147	297	58	*
7	435	35	4	0.6	0.3	129	0	0.02	0.07	1.7	0.09	1	2.14	39	45	50	0.5
376	573	428	56	2.3	4.2	530	1	0.18	0.28	1.6	0.17	32	4.11	218	480	188	2.6
236	360	388	35	1.9	2.6	295	0	0.15	0.51	4.8	0.11	20	2.58	290	451	118	1.7
20	108	100	10	0.1	0.8	7	0	t	0.02	0.3	0.02	3	0.88	17	53	23	0.3
27	84	78	8	0.1	0.9	6	0	t	0.01	0.4	0.02	3	0.26	14	41	21	*
150	720	369	70	3.9	1.9	248	2	0.08	0.4	11.7	0.4	10	13.2	458	572	89	3.2
20	26	89	22	0.5	0.2	14	t	0.05	0.09	2.6	0.11	t	2.47	3	62	*	0.4
64	71	341	83	1.3	0.8	46	t	0.14	0.35	5.8	0.39	1	16.2	13	236	30	1.9
54	60	389	28	1.2	0.7	36	1	0.09	0.09	5.4	0.42	8	0.21	26	207	*	2.1
42	429	479	51	5.9	2.4	72	12	0.24	0.32	2.4	0.08	63	18	39	296	84	1.1
32	128	242	*	1.1	*	*	*	0.1	0.1	1.6	*	*	0.85	28	192	20	1.1
46	82	298	33	1	0.5	12	1	0.11	0.11	2.1	0.23	9	0.98	117	235	30	1.6
136	278	568	134	16.6	226	223	12	0.37	0.41	3.1	0.24	22	47.5	112	344	149	2.6
93	190	389	93	11.4	155	145	7	0.25	0.28	2.1	0.08	15	32.5	76	236	51	*
69	355	208	49	5.9	74.1	77	3	0.13	0.17	1.4	0.05	12	13.3	53	135	*	1.9
136	277	568	135	16.6	226	222	12	0.34	0.41	3.3	0.12	25	47.5	111	344	141	2
43	90	143	19	4.3	14.1	69	7	0.06	0.2	1.7	0.04	9	13.6	7	138	56	0.7
98	67	292	32	1	1.2	9	1	0.07	0.1	1.6	0.12	5	1.87	87	218	30	1.6
43	42	281	34	0.6	0.7	20	3	0.06	0.07	2.4	0.12	15	1.96	62	239	32	1.4
60	73	303	57	0.4	0.4	9	0	0.04	0.16	2.8	0.24	3	2.71	51	188	*	*
82	99	329	62	0.2	0.5	20	0	0.06	0.07	1.4	0.06	3	3.57	5	410	*	*
54	65	541	27	0.6	0.6	31	0	0.58	0.13	3.2	0.2	15	1.02	36	290	*	0.9
40	48	444	31	0.2	0.4	30	1	0.05	t	0.3	0.39	5	2.98	34	171	*	*
31	54	355	27	0.2	0.3	26	1	0.04	t	0.2	0.34	4	2.55	27	169	*	*
44	77	520	34	0.5	0.5	66	1	0.04	0.08	3.9	0.27	10	1.2	12	228	39	*
64	96	89	34	1.2	0.8	20	4	0.12	0.22	4	0.07	13	3	78	104	*	2.1
47	116	443	32	1.2	0.7	48	2	0.16	0.06	9.8	0.22	5	2.71	18	418	48	1.4
42	50	454	32	0.8	0.4	15	1	0.16	0.17	7.1	0.39	4	3.06	39	248	26	1.2
47	471	277	29	0.7	0.8	14	0	0.02	0.16	5.6	0.26	13	5.85	181	279	45	1.2
23	784	175	18	0.9	0.3	26	0	0.02	0.1	4.7	0.28	2	3.26	11	164	61	1.4
17	61	48	5	0.4	0.2	8	0	0.01	0.03	0.6	0.02	1	1.07	46	59	6	*
23	157	130	13	0.9	0.5	27	t	0.02	0.09	1.6	0.05	9	3.42	91	139	*	0.2
15	75	135	*	0.9	*	*	*	*	*	*	*	*	*	33	96	15	*
9	70	50	9	0.1	0.2	3	t	0.01	0.02	0.2	0.02	3	0.2	6	35	12	0.1
28	137	274	48	0.2	0.8	13	3	0.01	0.06	1	0.13	14	1.3	20	186	65	*
45	74	279	45	0.3	0.4	54	0	0.11	0.13	1.6	0.39	5	0.26	11	211	*	1
69	79	377	*	0.6	*	9	*	0.13	0.26	8.6	*	*	*	24	313	*	2
222	216	269	53	3.5	1.6	23	3	0.04	0.05	3.5	0.14	2	1.44	75	299	41	3.6
166	190	155	29	2.6	1.3	56	2	0.03	0.03	2.2	0.11	3	1.26	33	116	54	3.2
150	292	191	34	1.1	1.2	48	1	0.11	0.12	2.6	0.08	7	1.59	57	185	27	0.8
*	*	*	*	0.3	*	*	*	*	*	*	*	*	*	72	74	10	0.1
77	66	316	32	1	1.8	15	0	0.63	0.12	1.5	0.15	4	3.37	66	251	105	1.7
86	133	436	74	0.4	0.8	14	4	0.1	0.15	2.8	0.31	11	3.19	23	368	160	1.5
221	260	237	33	0.9	1.5	9	4	0.05	0.39	2.2	0.05	5	1.04	33	213	*	1.9
198	37	209	28	0.6	1.3	9	4	0.02	0.35	1.9	0.05	4	1.1	27	188	*	1
75	108	364	35	2	0.5	243	0	0.08	0.09	9.8	0.22	17	2.6	40	263	49	0.6
26	122	95	37	0.2	0.3	17	0	0.02	0.02	0.2	0.03	1	1.36	8	240	*	*
4	478	354	33	1.3	1.4	616	3	0.04	0.05	10.9	0.36	3	1.9	7	275	47	1.2
43	98	314	29	0.9	1.3	35	1	0.04	0.1	10	0.32	2	1.72	5	287	*	1
54	50	435	28	0.3	0.5	18	0	0.12	0.16	3	0.26	15	2.13	22	201	*	*
69	79	602	35	1.1	1.3	96	1	0.12	0.06	2.5	0.44	17	3.25	218	272	*	0.8
62	29	539	33	2.1	1.2	19	3	0.07	0.19	5.9	0.39	15	2.98	73	273	*	0.7
42	43	275	54	1.1	0.7	643	0	0.24	0.26	9	0.45	2	9.25	9	277	85	0.9
15	301	176	26	1.2	0.8	20	0	0.03	0.1	10.5	0.09	5	1.87	11	264	61	1.4
10	11	74	9	0.3	0.1	7	*	0.01	0.01	3.5	0.11	0	0.4	1	63	33	1
15	303	267	25	2.7	0.4	20	0	0.03	0.1	10.5	0.32	4	1.87	10	158	61	*
35	333	241	29	0.5	0.4	20	0	t	0.04	4.9	0.37	4	1.87	3	227	61	*
38	32	377	43	0.6	0.4	15	1	0.37	0.04	8.3	0.77	2	0.44	14	162	85	0.4
*	*	*	*	0.7	*	0	0	0.04	0.05	2.7	*	*	*	9	113	16	0.8
*	195	291	*	0.5	*	601	0	0.11	0.11	2.3	*	*	*	*	246	*	*
71	113	369	23	0.4	0.5	29	0	0.06	0.05	1.4	0.15	13	2.21	53	242	*	*

WT, weight; **KCAL,** kcalories; **PROT,** protein; **CARB,** carbohydrate; **FIBR,** fiber; **FAT,** fat; **SATF,** saturated fat;
MONO, monosaturated fat; **POLY,** polyunsaturated fat; **CHOR,** cholesterol; **SOD,** sodium; **POT,** potassium;

Frozen Dinners

Food Name	Portion	WT (Gm)	KCAL	PROT (Gm)	CARB (Gm)	FIBR (Gm)	FAT (Gm)	SATF (Gm)	MONO (Gm)	POLY (Gm)
BEEF AND GREEN PEPPERS-STOUFFER DINNER	ITEM	220	225	10	18	*	11	*	*	*
BEEF AND SPINACH PASTA SHELLS-STOUFFER	ITEM	255	290	19	28	*	11	*	*	*
BEEF BURGUNDY-FROZEN DINNER-EFFICIENC	ITEM	142	144	17	6	*	5	*	*	*
BEEF CUBES IN WINE SAUCE-HORMEL ENTREE	OUNCE	28.4	52	4	1	*	4	1.9	1.6	0.1
BEEF DINNER-SWANSON FROZEN DINNER	ITEM	326	320	25	34	3.3	9	9.6	12.7	4.1
BEEF SHORT RIBS IN BARBECUE SAUCE-HORMEL	OUNCE	28.4	54	5	1	0.8	3	1.7	1.4	0.2
BEEF SIRLOIN TIPS-LE MENU FROZEN DINNER	ITEM	326	400	29	27	*	19	*	*	*
BEEF STEW-HORMEL ENTREE	OUNCE	28.4	29	2	2	*	1	0.5	0.5	t
BEEF STROGANOFF-FROZEN DINNER-EFFICIENC	ITEM	170	192	20	8	*	8	*	*	*
BEEF TERIYAKI-LIGHT AND ELEGANT	ITEM	227	240	18	37	*	3	*	*	*
CHICKEN AND BROCCOLI-LIGHT AND ELEGANT	ITEM	270	290	19	30	*	11	*	*	*
CHICKEN AND DUMPLINGS WITH GRAVY-HORMEL	OUNCE	28.4	31	3	2	0.3	1	0.4	0.6	0.2
CHICKEN BURGUNDY-CLASSIC LITE DINNER	ITEM	319	240	23	24	*	5	*	*	*
CHICKEN CACCIATORE-STOUFFER DINNER	ITEM	319	310	25	29	2.9	11	8.4	12.2	9.7
CHICKEN CHOW MEIN-LEAN CUISINE DINNER	ITEM	319	250	14	36	*	5	*	*	*
CHICKEN CREPES/MUSHROOM SAUCE-STOUFFER	ITEM	234	390	30	19	2.3	22	7.3	3.8	0.9
CHICKEN DINNER-SWANSON FROZEN DINNER	ITEM	326	660	26	64	6.2	33	7.4	10.5	6.9
CHICKEN DIVAN-STOUFFER FROZEN DINNER	ITEM	241	335	21	14	1	22	9.2	8.2	3.3
CHICKEN FLORENTINE-LE MENU FROZEN DINNER	ITEM	354	510	28	35	6.7	28	8	11.4	7.5
CHICKEN KIEV-LE MENU FROZEN DINNER	ITEM	234	500	21	35	4.4	30	5.3	7.6	5
CHICKEN PARMIGIANA-LE MENU FROZEN DINNER	ITEM	333	390	26	28	*	19	*	*	*
CHICKEN PASTA SHELLS-STOUFFER DINNER	ITEM	255	400	26	24	3	22	2.5	3.2	2
CHICKEN-GLAZED-WITH RICE-LEAN CUISINE	ITEM	241	270	26	23	*	8	*	*	*
CHICKEN-SWEET AND SOUR-BUDGET GOURMET	SERVING	284	350	18	53	1.7	7	1.3	1.7	3.3
CORN SOUFFLE-STOUFFER FROZEN SIDE DISH	ITEM	113	155	4	19	*	7	*	*	*
EGG ROLL-BEEF AND SHRIMP-FROZEN-LA CHOY	ITEM	12	27	1	4	0.1	1	0.1	0.2	0.1
FETTUCINI ALFREDO-STOUFFER FROZEN DINNER	ITEM	142	270	8	19	*	18	*	*	*
FETTUCINI-CHICKEN-BUDGET GOURMET	SERVING	284	400	23	29	*	21	*	*	*
FILET OF FISH DIVAN-LEAN CUISINE DINNER	ITEM	351	270	31	16	*	10	*	*	*
FILET OF FISH FLORENTINE-LEAN CUISINE	ITEM	255	240	26	13	*	9	*	*	*
FISH AND CHIPS-VAN DE KAMPS DINNER	ITEM	224	500	16	45	4.7	30	6.2	7	6.9
FLOUNDER FILET-LE MENU FROZEN DINNER	ITEM	298	350	22	27	*	17	*	*	*
GLAZED CHICKEN-LIGHT AND ELEGANT	ITEM	227	230	24	25	*	4	*	*	*
HAM-BANQUET FROZEN DINNER	ITEM	284	369	17	48	2.6	12	2	3.4	3.1
LASAGNA-SAUSAGE-BUDGET GOURMET	SERVING	284	284	20	38	3.8	20	9	5.8	0.9
LINGUINI WITH CLAM SAUCE-STOUFFER DINNER	ITEM	298	285	17	36	*	8	*	*	*
MACARONI AND CHEESE-LIGHT AND ELEGANT	ITEM	255	300	15	37	*	9	*	*	*
MANICOTTI-CHEESE/MEAT-BUDGET GOURMET	SERVING	284	450	20	33	2.4	26	11.1	6	1.3
MEATBALLS AND NOODLES-STOUFFER DINNER	ITEM	312	475	25	33	*	27	*	*	*
MEATLOAF-BANQUET FROZEN DINNER	ITEM	312	412	21	29	5.4	24	7.5	9.1	2.9
MEXICAN DINNER-SWANSON FROZEN DINNER	ITEM	454	590	20	64	6.7	29	9.5	13	8.5
NOODLES ROMANOFF-STOUFFER FROZEN DINNER	ITEM	113	170	6	16	*	9	*	*	*
OCEAN FISH WITH LEMON SAUCE-EFFICIENC	SERVING	113	262	14	3	0.9	21	1.6	0.9	1.5
ORIENTAL BEEF-LEAN CUISINE FROZEN DINNER	ITEM	245	250	18	28	*	7	*	*	*
PEPPER STEAK WITH RICE-BUDGET GOURMET	SERVING	284	300	15	39	1.4	9	5.8	8.2	11.8
PORK LOIN AND GRAVY-HORMEL ENTREE	OUNCE	28.4	40	5	1	*	2	0.9	0.7	0.3
QUICHE LORRAINE-FROZEN DINNER-MRS SMITHS	ITEM	269	720	34	54	0.8	41	*	*	*
SALISBURY STEAK-LEAN CUISINE	ITEM	269	280	25	11	*	15	*	*	*
SCALLOPED POTATOES AND HAM-HORMEL ENTREE	OUNCE	28.4	28	2	3	0.6	1	0.6	0.4	0.1
SCALLOPS/VEGETABLES/RICE-LEAN CUISINE	ITEM	312	220	17	32	*	3	*	*	*
SEAFOOD GUMBO-HORMEL ENTREE	OUNCE	28.4	10	1	1	*	t	t	t	t
SHRIMP CREOLE-LIGHT AND ELEGANT	ITEM	283	200	11	31	2.2	2	2.9	5.6	5.1
SIRLOIN TIP/VEGETABLES-BUDGET GOURMET	SERVING	284	310	16	21	2.6	18	1.9	2	0.4
SOLE-LIGHT-VAN DE KAMP'S FROZEN DINNER	ITEM	142	293	16	17	1.9	18	0.4	0.3	0.5
SPAGHETTI-BEEF AND MUSHROOM-LEAN CUISINE	ITEM	326	280	15	38	*	7	*	*	*
SPAGHETTI-LIGHT AND ELEGANT	ITEM	290	290	16	40	*	8	*	*	*
SWEDISH MEATBALLS IN SAUCE-HORMEL ENTREE	SERVING	28.4	44	3	2	0.1	3	1.7	1.1	0.2
SWISS STEAK IN GRAVY-HORMEL ENTREE	OUNCE	28.4	34	4	1	0.4	2	0.7	1	0.2
TUNA NOODLE CASSEROLE-STOUFFER DINNER	ITEM	163	200	10	18	0.5	9	*	*	*
TURKEY & GRAVY-FROZEN	CUP	240	160	14	11	2.7	6	2	2.3	1.1
TURKEY BREAST-LE MENU FROZEN DINNER	ITEM	319	470	27	36	*	24	*	*	*
TURKEY PIE-STOUFFER FROZEN DINNER	ITEM	284	460	20	35	*	26	*	*	*

t = Trace of nutrient present ** = Not available*

MAG, magnesium; **IRON,** iron; **ZINC,** zinc; **VITA,** vitamin A; **VITC,** vitamin C; **THIA,** thiamin; **RIBO,** riboflavin; **NIAC,** niacin; **VB6,** vitamin B-6; **FOL,** folate; **VB12,** vitamin B-12; **CALC,** calcium; **PHOS,** phosphorus; **SEL,** selenium; **VE-a,** alpha tocopherol equivalents.

CHOL (mg)	SOD (mg)	POT (mg)	MAG (mg)	IRON (mg)	ZINC (mg)	VITA (RE)	VITC (mg)	THIA (mg)	RIBO (mg)	NIAC (mg)	VB6 (mg)	FOL (μg)	VB12 (μg)	CALC (mg)	PHOS (mg)	SEL (μg)	VE-a (mg)
*	960	420	*	2.3	*	136	0	0.08	0.16	3.9	*	*	*	0	*	*	*
*	1315	485	*	*	*	*	*	*	*	*	*	*	*	*	*	*	*
411	147	*	0.6	*	449	0	0.04	0.24	4.1	*	*	*	5	*	*	*	*
15	106	71	4	0.5	1.3	*	t	0.77	0.05	0.5	0.02	4	0.41	3	23	*	*
84	1085	616	42	4	4.7	1140	6	0.14	0.27	4.9	0.52	24	2.1	36	283	*	2
15	176	92	5	0.7	1.7	11	t	0.01	0.07	0.7	0.03	11	0.52	3	28	*	0.8
*	1100	*	*	*	*	*	*	*	*	*	*	*	*	*	*	*	*
7	106	51	3	0.2	0.5	*	t	0.01	0.02	0.3	0.01	6	0.15	4	15	*	t
*	785	316	*	2.9	*	68	2	0.05	0.32	2.9	*	*	*	23	*	*	*
*	625	215	*	5.6	*	24	2	0.4	0.1	2.5	*	*	*	30	152	*	*
*	805	180	*	1.6	*	75	1	0.11	0.21	1.8	*	*	*	204	240	*	*
9	116	45	3	0.2	0.2	65	t	0.01	0.03	0.6	0.04	11	0.06	5	29	*	0
*	*	*	*	*	*	*	*	*	*	*	*	*	*	*	*	*	*
166	1135	300	73	3.9	4.1	176	33	0.24	0.42	18.2	0.95	22	0.57	75	398	*	2.9
25	1030	270	*	*	*	*	*	*	*	*	*	*	*	*	*	*	*
76	1040	420	50	2.6	1.1	910	33	0.15	0.19	8	0.46	28	0.19	54	192	*	0.9
111	1610	602	60	2.7	2.6	323	12	0.33	0.39	10.3	0.45	30	0.36	112	295	*	2.8
86	830	415	52	1.7	2	221	20	0.13	0.44	4.6	0.29	41	0.74	269	295	*	0.9
121	985	653	66	2.9	2.9	351	13	0.36	0.42	11.2	0.49	33	0.39	122	320	*	3.1
80	745	432	43	1.9	1.9	232	9	0.24	0.28	7.4	0.33	22	0.26	80	212	*	2
*	900	*	*	*	*	*	*	*	*	*	*	*	*	*	*	*	*
165	1060	350	47	3.7	2.2	177	28	0.3	0.43	7.5	0.35	28	0.39	59	226	*	1.3
55	810	380	*	*	*	*	*	*	*	*	*	*	*	*	*	*	*
40	640	429	45	0.7	1.4	80	2	0.12	0.34	3	0.38	13	0.17	60	163	*	1.3
*	510	190	*	0.4	*	94	0	0.08	0.16	0.8	*	34	*	48	*	*	*
2	81	15	1	0.1	0.1	12	2	0.01	0.01	0.1	0.01	1	0.02	2	5	*	0.1
*	1195	240	*	*	*	*	*	*	*	*	*	*	*	*	*	*	*
100	740	*	*	1.8	*	350	2	0.15	0.43	6	*	*	*	200	*	*	*
85	780	850	*	*	*	*	*	*	*	*	*	*	*	*	*	*	*
100	700	540	*	*	*	*	*	*	*	*	*	*	*	*	*	*	*
33	551	785	53	2.2	1	18	11	0.24	0.14	4.3	0.41	23	0.68	35	271	*	2.8
*	1125	*	*	*	*	*	*	*	*	*	*	*	*	*	*	*	*
*	655	300	*	4.8	*	31	*	0.21	0.07	7.7	*	*	*	18	348	*	*
36	1590	125	38	2.5	2.5	1311	57	0.57	0.23	3.4	0.48	21	0.45	151	278	*	4.4
80	950	591	54	2.7	3.7	183	18	0.45	0.43	4	0.28	23	0.91	400	348	*	1.1
*	1010	115	*	*	*	*	*	*	*	*	*	*	*	*	*	*	*
*	1015	210	*	2	*	60	t	0.34	0.43	1.5	*	*	*	238	334	*	*
50	920	484	45	2.7	2.3	280	10	0.45	0.51	4	0.23	31	0.72	450	376	*	2
*	1620	395	*	*	*	*	*	*	*	*	*	*	*	*	*	*	*
79	1991	468	64	4.3	3.4	427	8	0.16	0.22	4.2	0.36	48	1.21	84	243	*	1.7
44	1865	603	75	5.1	3.6	93	7	0.35	0.3	3.8	0.3	135	0.83	198	340	*	4
*	675	95	*	0.8	*	61	*	0.08	0.16	0.8	*	*	*	88	*	*	*
16	370	224	22	0.7	0.5	0	0	0.17	0.18	2.8	0.13	18	0.22	15	93	*	1.2
35	1150	270	*	*	*	*	*	*	*	*	*	*	*	*	*	*	*
25	800	729	49	0.7	6	60	2	0.15	0.17	3	0.59	22	3.9	40	350	*	4
9	133	82	5	0.2	0.4	*	t	2.61	0.04	0.9	0.06	10	0.07	2	32	*	*
95	1965	610	*	2.7	*	67	0	0.33	1.01	6	*	*	*	97	*	*	*
95	800	650	*	*	*	*	*	*	*	*	*	*	*	*	*	*	*
4	146	68	4	0.1	0.2	8	1	0.05	0.03	0.4	0.02	6	0.06	8	23	*	0.4
20	1200	360	*	*	*	*	*	*	*	*	*	*	*	*	*	*	*
6	146	82	5	0.2	0.1	*	t	0.01	0.02	0.2	0.03	6	0.09z	8	16	*	*
293	1045	200	88	2.5	2.4	889	1	0.22	0.03	3.3	0.32	14	1.91Z	54	225	*	6.5
40	570	504	35	0.4	4.4	150	2	0.15	0.17	4	0.44	16	1.87	60	195	*	0.4
45	412	453	39	0.9	0.6	10	21	0.13	0.13	3.3	0.25	36	1.35	39	200	*	0.7
20	1450	580	*	*	*	*	*	*	*	*	*	*	*	*	*	*	*
*	700	273	*	6	*	157	10	0.25	0.15	3.4	*	*	*	100	252	*	*
8	165	87	6	0.5	0.4	11	t	1.07	0.06	0.5	0.03	9	0.18	15	39	*	0.1
8	110	86	5	0.5	0.6	76	t	0.02	0.05	0.9	0.04	27	0.32	5	15	*	0.1
*	670	210	*	1.2	*	54	*	0.17	0.23	3.5	*	*	*	98	*	*	*
43	1328	146	20	2.2	1.7	20	0	0.06	0.31	4.3	0.23	10	0.58	33	194	*	2
*	1165	*	*	*	*	*	*	*	*	*	*	*	*	*	*	*	*
*	1735	270	*	*	*	*	*	*	*	*	*	*	*	*	*	*	*

WT, weight; **KCAL,** kcalories; **PROT,** protein; **CARB,** carbohydrate; **FIBR,** fiber; **FAT,** fat; **SATF,** saturated fat; **MONO,** monosaturated fat; **POLY,** polyunsaturated fat; **CHOR,** cholesterol; **SOD,** sodium; **POT,** potassium;

Food Name	Portion	WT (Gm)	KCAL	PROT (Gm)	CARB (Gm)	FIBR (Gm)	FAT (Gm)	SATF (Gm)	MONO (Gm)	POLY (Gm)
TURKEY TETRAZZINI-STOUFFER FROZEN DINNER	ITEM	170	240	12	17	*	14	*	*	*
TURKEY-SLICED-LIGHT AND ELEGANT	ITEM	227	230	20	25	*	5	*	*	*
VEAL PARMIGIANA-EFFICIENC ENTREE	ITEM	213	296	24	17	1.6	14	9	7.6	4.8
VEAL STEAK-CLASSIC LITE FROZEN DINNER	ITEM	312	280	25	27	5.8	8	5.9	6.9	3.6
VEGETABLE LASAGNA-LE MENU FROZEN DINNER	ITEM	312	400	15	30	5.1	24	9.4	6.7	4.2
Fruits										
APPLES-RAW-PEELED	ITEM	128	73	t	19	2.4	t	0.1	t	0.1
APPLES-RAW-PEELED-BOILED	CUP	171	91	t	23	4.1	1	0.1	t	0.2
APPLES-RAW-SLICED-WITH SKIN	CUP	110	65	t	17	2.4	t	0.1	t	0.1
APPLESAUCE-CANNED-SWEETENED	CUP	255	194	t	51	3.1	t	0.1	t	0.1
APPLESAUCE-CANNED-UNSWEETENED	CUP	244	105	t	28	3.7	t	t	t	t
APRICOT-RAW-WITHOUT PIT	ITEM	35.3	17	t	4	0.7	t	t	0.1	t
APRICOTS-CANNED-JUICE PACK	CUP	248	119	2	31	2.8	t	t	t	t
APRICOTS-DRIED-SULFURED-COOKED-NO SUGAR	CUP	250	213	3	55	19.5	t	t	0.2	0.1
APRICOTS-DRIED-SULFURED-UNCOOKED	CUP	130	309	5	80	10.1	1	t	0.3	0.1
AVOCADO-RAW-CALIFORNIA	ITEM	173	306	4	12	6.1	30	4.5	19.4	3.5
BANANAS-RAW-PEELED	ITEM	114	105	1	27	1.8	1	0.2	t	0.1
BLACKBERRIES-FROZEN-UNSWEETENED	CUP	151	97	2	24	7.6	1	t	0.1	0.4
BLACKBERRIES-RAW	CUP	144	75	1	18	8.9	1	0.1	0.2	0.3
BLUEBERRIES-CANNED-HEAVY SYRUP PACK	CUP	256	225	2	57	2.8	1	0.1	0.1	0.3
BLUEBERRIES-FROZEN-UNSWEETENED	CUP	155	79	1	19	4.9	1	t	0.1	0.6
BLUEBERRIES-RAW	CUP	145	81	1	21	3.3	1	0.1	0.2	0.3
BOYSENBERRIES-FROZEN-UNSWEETENED	CUP	132	66	1	16	5.2	t	t	t	0.2
CHERRIES-SWEET-RAW	ITEM	6.8	5	t	1	0.1	t	t	t	t
CRANAPPLE JUICE-CANNED	CUP	253	170	t	43	0	0	0	0	0
CRANBERRY JUICE COCKTAIL-BOTTLED	CUP	253	144	0	36	0	t	0	0	0
CRANBERRY SAUCE-CANNED-SWEETENED	CUP	277	418	1	108	3.2	t	0.1	0.1	0.2
DATES-DOMESTIC-NATURAL AND DRY-WHOLE	ITEM	8.3	23	t	6	0.7	t	0	0	0
FIGS-DRIED-UNCOOKED	CUP	199	507	6	130	18.5	2	0.5	0.5	1.1
FRUIT COCKTAIL-CANNED-JUICE PACK	CUP	248	114	1	29	1.5	t	t	t	t
FRUIT ROLL UP-CHERRY	ITEM	14.4	50	0	12	*	1	*	*	*
GRAPE DRINK-CANNED	CUP	253	154	1	38	0	t	0.1	t	0.1
GRAPEFRUIT-CANNED-JUICE PACK	CUP	249	92	2	23	1.6	t	t	t	0.1
GRAPEFRUIT-PINK & RED-RAW	ITEM	246	74	1	19	3.2	t	t	t	0.1
GRAPEFRUIT-WHITE-RAW	ITEM	236	78	2	20	2.5	t	t	t	0.1
GRAPES-RAW-SLIP SKIN (AMERICAN) TYPE	CUP	92	58	1	16	1.5	t	0.1	t	0.1
JUICE APPLE-CANNED OR BOTTLED	CUP	248	116	t	29	0.5	t	t	t	0.1
JUICE-APPLE-FROZEN-DILUTED	CUP	239	112	t	28	0.6	t	t	t	0.1
JUICE-GRAPE-CANNED & BOTTLED	CUP	253	154	1	38	0	t	0.1	t	0.1
JUICE-GRAPE-FROZEN CONCENTRATE	ITEM	216	387	1	96	0.6	1	0.2	t	0.2
JUICE-GRAPEFRUIT-CANNED-SWEETENED	CUP	250	115	1	28	0	t	t	t	0.1
JUICE-GRAPEFRUIT-CANNED-UNSWEETENED	CUP	247	94	1	22	0.4	t	t	t	0.1
JUICE-GRAPEFRUIT-FROZEN CONCENTRATE	ITEM	207	302	4	72	0	1	0.1	0.1	0.2
JUICE-LEMON-CANNED & BOTTLED	CUP	244	51	1	16	0.7	1	0.1	t	0.2
JUICE-LEMON-FROZEN-SINGLE STRENGTH	CUP	244	54	1	16	0.7	1	0.1	t	0.2
JUICE-LEMON-RAW	CUP	244	61	1	21	0.7	0	0	0	0
JUICE-ORANGE GRAPEFRUIT-CANNED	CUP	247	106	1	25	0.5	t	t	t	t
JUICE-ORANGE GRAPEFRUIT-FROZEN-DILUTED	CUP	248	110	1	26	0	0	0	0	0
JUICE-ORANGE-CANNED	CUP	249	104	1	25	0.3	t	t	0.1	0.1
JUICE-ORANGE-CANNED-FROZEN CONCENTRATE	ITEM	213	339	5	81	1.7	t	0.1	0.1	0.1
JUICE-PINEAPPLE-CANNED	CUP	250	140	1	35	0.3	t	t	t	0.1
JUICE-PINEAPPLE-FROZEN-DILUTED	CUP	250	130	1	32	0.3	t	t	t	t
JUICE-PRUNE-CANNED & BOTTLED	CUP	256	182	2	45	2.6	t	t	0.1	t
LEMONADE-CANNED-FROZEN CONCENTRATE	ITEM	219	425	0	112	5.6	0	0	0	0
LEMONADE-FROZEN CONCENTRATE-DILUTED	CUP	248	105	0	28	0.6	0	0	0	0
LEMONS-RAW-UNPEELED	ITEM	108	22	1	12	1	t	t	t	0.1
MELONS-CANTALOUPE-RAW-CUBED PIECES	CUP	160	56	1	13	1.3	t	0	0	0
MELONS-CASABA-RAW	CUP	170	44	2	11	2	t	0	0	0
MELONS-HONEYDEW-RAW-CUBED PIECES	CUP	170	60	1	16	1.5	t	0	0	0
NECTARINES-RAW	ITEM	136	67	1	16	2.2	1	0.1	0.2	0.3
ORANGES-RAW-ALL COMMON VARIETIES-WHOLE	ITEM	131	62	1	15	3.1	t	t	t	t
PAPAYA NECTAR-CANNED	CUP	250	143	t	36	1.2	t	0.1	0.1	0.1
PAPAYAS-RAW	CUP	140	55	1	14	1.3	t	0.1	0.1	t

t= Trace of nutrient present **= Not available*

MAG, magnesium; **IRON,** iron; **ZINC,** zinc; **VITA,** vitamin A; **VITC,** vitamin C; **THIA,** thiamin; **RIBO,** riboflavin; **NIAC,** niacin; **VB6,** vitamin B-6; **FOL,** folate; **VB12,** vitamin B-12; **CALC,** calcium; **PHOS,** phosphorus; **SEL,** selenium; **VE-a,** alpha tocopherol equivalents.

CHOL (mg)	SOD (mg)	POT (mg)	MAG (mg)	IRON (mg)	ZINC (mg)	VITA (RE)	VITC (mg)	THIA (mg)	RIBO (mg)	NIAC (mg)	VB6 (mg)	FOL (μg)	VB12 (μg)	CALC (mg)	PHOS (mg)	SEL (μg)	VE-a (mg)
*	620	200	*	0.6	*	41	*	0.12	0.24	2.4	*	*	*	72	*	*	*
*	1020	280	*	1	*	171	1	0.12	0.14	4.6	*	*	*	18	121	*	*
162	973	466	49	2.3	3.6	123	6	0.3	0.38	6.8	0.43	25	1.21	97	401	*	2.6
60	1738	932	81	3.6	4.2	241	33	0.36	0.43	6.5	0.53	62	0.85	171	299	*	2.7
39	1135	519	82	3.2	1.5	723	62	0.23	0.47	3.3	0.34	78	0.2	296	274	*	2.5
0	0	144	4	0.1	0.1	6	5	0.02	0.01	0.1	0.06	1	0	5	9	1	0.3
0	2	150	5	0.3	0.1	8	t	0.03	0.02	0.2	0.08	1	0	9	13	1	0.1
0	0	126	5	0.2	t	6	6	0.02	0.02	0.1	0.05	3	0	8	8	1	0.6
0	8	156	7	0.9	0.1	3	4	0.03	0.07	0.5	0.07	2	0	9	17	1	0.2
0	5	183	7	0.3	0.1	7	3	0.03	0.06	0.5	0.06	1	0	7	17	1	0.2
0	t	104	3	0.2	0.1	92	4	0.01	0.01	0.2	0.02	3	0	5	7	0	0.3
0	9	409	24	0.7	0.3	420	12	0.05	0.05	0.9	0.13	4	0	30	50	1	2.2
0	9	1222	42	4.2	0.7	591	4	0.02	0.08	2.4	0.29	0	0	40	104	*	*
0	13	1791	61	6.1	1	941	3	0.01	0.2	3.9	0.2	13	0	59	152	*	*
0	21	1097	70	2	0.7	106	14	0.19	0.21	3.3	0.48	113	0	19	73	*	3.7
0	1	451	33	0.4	0.2	9	10	0.05	0.11	0.6	0.66	22	0	7	22	1	0.3
0	2	211	33	1.2	0.4	17	5	0.04	0.07	1.8	0.09	51	0	44	45	1	1.1
0	0	282	29	0.8	0.4	24	30	0.04	0.06	0.6	0.08	49	0	46	30	1	0.9
0	9	102	9	0.8	0.2	16	3	0.09	0.14	0.3	0.09	4	0	14	26	2	1.7
0	2	84	8	0.3	0.1	13	4	0.05	0.06	0.8	0.09	10	0	12	17	1	1.6
0	9	129	7	0.2	0.2	15	19	0.07	0.07	0.5	0.05	9	0	9	15	1	*
0	2	183	21	1.1	0.3	9	4	0.07	0.05	1	0.07	84	0	36	36	1	0.6
0	0	15	1	t	t	1	t	t	t	t	t	t	0	1	1	0	t
0	5	68	5	0.2	0.1	0	81	0.01	0.05	0.2	0.05	1	0	18	8	1	*
0	10	46	5	0.4	0.2	0	90	0.02	0.02	0.1	0.05	1	0	8	5	1	*
0	80	72	8	0.6	0.1	6	11	0.04	0.06	0.3	0.04	*	0	11	17	1	*
0	t	54	3	0.1	t	t	0	0.01	0.01	0.2	0.02	1	0	3	3	*	*
0	22	1417	117	4.4	1	26	2	0.14	0.18	1.4	0.45	15	0	287	135	*	0
0	10	236	17	0.5	0.2	76	7	0.03	0.04	1	0.13	6	0	20	35	1	0.5
0	5	45	*	*	*	*	*	*	*	*	*	*	0	*	*	*	*
0	8	334	25	0.6	0.1	2	t	0.07	0.09	0.7	0.16	7	0	23	28	*	*
0	19	420	26	0.5	0.2	0	84	0.07	0.05	0.6	0.05	22	0	37	30	1	0.6
0	0	312	20	0.3	0.2	64	91	0.1	0.05	0.5	0.1	23	0	36	22	1	0.6
0	0	350	21	0.1	0.2	2	79	0.09	0.05	0.6	0.1	24	0	28	18	1	0.6
0	2	176	5	0.3	t	9	4	0.09	0.05	0.3	0.1	4	0	13	9	1	0.6
0	7	296	8	0.9	0.1	t	2	0.05	0.04	0.2	0.07	t	0	16	18	2	t
0	17	301	12	0.6	0.1	*	1	0.01	0.04	0.1	0.08	1	0	14	17	2	t
0	8	334	25	0.6	0.1	2	t	0.07	0.09	0.7	0.16	7	0	23	28	1	*
0	15	160	32	0.8	0.3	6	179	0.11	0.2	0.9	0.32	10	0	28	32	2	*
0	5	405	25	0.9	0.2	0	67	0.1	0.06	0.8	0.05	26	0	20	28	1	0.1
0	2	378	25	0.5	0.2	2	72	0.1	0.05	0.6	0.05	26	0	17	27	1	0.1
0	6	1002	78	1	0.4	7	248	0.3	0.16	1.6	0.32	26	0	56	101	1	0.1
0	51	249	20	0.3	0.1	4	61	0.1	0.02	0.5	0.11	25	0	27	22	1	*
0	2	217	20	0.3	0.1	3	77	0.14	0.03	0.3	0.15	23	0	20	20	1	*
0	2	303	15	0.1	0.1	5	112	0.07	0.02	0.2	0.12	32	0	17	15	1	*
0	7	390	25	1.1	0.2	29	72	0.14	0.07	0.8	0.06	35	0	20	35	1	0.1
0	2	439	24	0.2	0.2	27	102	0.15	0.02	0.7	0.06	*	0	20	32	1	0.1
0	6	436	27	1.1	0.2	44	86	0.15	0.07	0.8	0.22	136	0	21	36	1	0.1
0	7	1435	73	0.7	0.4	59	294	0.6	0.14	1.5	0.33	331	0	67	122	1	*
0	3	335	33	0.7	0.3	1	27	0.14	0.06	0.6	0.24	58	0	43	20	2	*
0	3	340	23	0.8	0.3	3	30	0.18	0.05	0.5	0.19	27	0	28	20	2	0.1
0	10	707	36	3	0.5	1	11	0.04	0.18	2	0.56	1	0	31	64	1	*
0	4	153	*	0.4	*	4	66	0.05	0.06	0.7	*	*	0	9	13	1	*
0	0	40	*	0.1	*	1	17	0.01	0.02	0.2	*	12	0	2	3	1	*
0	3	157	13	0.8	0.1	3	83	0.05	0.04	0.2	0.12	11	0	66	16	1	0.3
0	14	494	18	0.3	0.3	516	68	0.06	0.03	0.9	0.18	27	0	18	27	1	0.2
0	20	357	14	0.7	0.3	5	27	0.1	0.03	0.7	0.2	29	0	9	12	1	0.2
0	17	461	12	0.1	*	7	42	0.13	0.03	1	0.1	*	0	10	17	1	0.2
0	0	288	11	0.2	0.1	100	7	0.02	0.06	1.4	0.03	5	0	7	22	1	1.2
0	0	237	13	0.1	0.1	27	70	0.11	0.05	0.4	0.08	40	0	52	18	2	0.3
0	13	78	8	0.9	0.4	28	8	0.02	0.01	0.4	0.02	5	0	25	0	1	1.9
0	4	359	14	0.1	0.1	282	87	0.04	0.05	0.5	0.03	53	0	34	7	1	*

WT, weight; **KCAL,** kcalories; **PROT,** protein; **CARB,** carbohydrate; **FIBR,** fiber; **FAT,** fat; **SATF,** saturated fat; **MONO,** monosaturated fat; **POLY,** polyunsaturated fat; **CHOR,** cholesterol; **SOD,** sodium; **POT,** potassium;

Food Name	Portion	WT (Gm)	KCAL	PROT (Gm)	CARB (Gm)	FIBR (Gm)	FAT (Gm)	SATF (Gm)	MONO (Gm)	POLY (Gm)	
PEACHES-CANNED-HEAVY SYRUP PACK	CUP	256	189	1	51	1.1	t	t	0.1	0.1	
PEACHES-RAW-SLICED	CUP	170	73	1	19	2.7	t	t	0.1	0.1	
PEACHES-RAW-WHOLE	ITEM	87	37	1	10	1.4	t	t	t	t	
PEAR NECTAR-CANNED	CUP	250	150	t	39	1.6	t	t	t	t	
PEARS-CANNED-HEAVY SYRUP PACK	CUP	255	189	1	49	2.4	t	t	0.1	0.1	
PEARS-RAW-BARTLETT WITH SKIN	ITEM	166	98	1	25	4.3	1	t	0.1	0.2	
PINEAPPLE GRAPEFRUIT DRINK	CUP	253	129	1	32	0	t	t	t	0.1	
PINEAPPLE ORANGE DRINK	CUP	253	134	1	32	0	0	0	0	0	
PINEAPPLE-BITS-CANNED IN SYRUP	CUP	252	131	1	34	1.9	t	t	t	0.1	
PINEAPPLE-FROZEN-SWEETENED	CUP	245	208	1	54	5.4	t	t	t	0.1	
PINEAPPLE-RAW-DICED	CUP	155	76	1	19	1.9	1	0.1	0.1	0.2	
PLUMS-PURPLE-CANNED-HEAVY SYRUP PACK	CUP	258	230	1	60	1.1	t	t	0.2	0.1	
PLUMS-RAW-JAPANESE & HYBRID	ITEM	66	36	1	9	1.4	t	t	0.3	0.1	
PLUMS-RAW-PRUNE TYPE	ITEM	28.4	20	0	6	0.6	0	0	0	0	
POMEGRANATES-RAW	ITEM	154	105	1	26	1.1	t	0.1	t	0.1	
PRUNES-CANNED-HEAVY SYRUP PACK	CUP	234	246	2	65	8.6	t	t	0.3	0.1	
PRUNES-DRIED-COOKED-WITH SUGAR	CUP	238	295	3	78	7.6	1	t	0.3	0.1	
PRUNES-DRIED-COOKED-WITHOUT SUGAR	CUP	212	227	2	60	7.5	t	t	0.3	0.1	
PRUNES-DRIED-UNCOOKED	CUP	161	385	4	101	11	1	0.1	0.5	0.2	
RAISINS-SEEDLESS	CUP	145	435	5	115	7.7	1	0.2	t	0.2	
RAISINS-SEEDLESS-PACKET	ITEM	14	42	t	11	0.7	t	t	t	t	
RASPBERRIES-CANNED-HEAVY SYRUP PACK	CUP	256	234	2	60	6.5	t	t	t	0.2	
RASPBERRIES-FROZEN-SWEETENED	CUP	250	258	2	65	11	t	t	t	0.2	
RASPBERRIES-RAW	CUP	123	60	1	14	5.5	1	t	0.1	0.4	
RHUBARB-COOKED FROM RAW-ADDED SUGAR	CUP	270	380	1	97	5.4	0	0	0	0	
STRAWBERRIES-CANNED-HEAVY SYRUP PACK	CUP	254	234	1	60	3.1	1	t	0.1	0.3	
STRAWBERRIES-FROZEN-SWEETENED-SLICED	CUP	255	245	1	66	19.8	t	t	t	0.2	
STRAWBERRIES-FROZEN-SWEETENED-WHOLE	CUP	255	199	1	54	5.6	t	t	t	0.2	
STRAWBERRIES-FROZEN-UNSWEETENED	CUP	149	52	1	14	3.9	t	t	t	0.1	
STRAWBERRIES-RAW-WHOLE	CUP	149	45	1	11	3.9	1	t	0.1	0.3	
TANGERINES-CANNED-LIGHT SYRUP PACK	CUP	252	154	1	41	1.4	t	t	t	0.1	
TANGERINES-RAW-PEELED	ITEM	84	37	1	9	1.7	t	t	t	t	
WATERMELON-RAW	CUP	160	51	1	12	0.6	1	*	*	*	

Grains

Food Name	Portion	WT (Gm)	KCAL	PROT (Gm)	CARB (Gm)	FIBR (Gm)	FAT (Gm)	SATF (Gm)	MONO (Gm)	POLY (Gm)	
BISQUICK MIX-DRY	CUP	112	480	8	76	3	16	*	*	*	
CORN CHIPS	OUNCE	28.4	155	2	17	1.7	9	1.5	3.4	4.3	
CORN GRITS-DRY	CUP	156	579	14	124	18.6	2	0.3	0.5	0.8	
CORNMEAL-DEGERMED-ENRICHED-COOKED	CUP	240	878	20	186	1.9	4	0.5	1	1.7	
CROUTONS-HERB SEASONED	CUP	30	100	4	20	1.4	0	0	0	0	
FLOUR-WHEAT-ENRICHED-SIFTED	CUP	115	419	12	88	3.1	1	0.2	0.1	0.5	
FLOUR-WHEAT-WHITE-FOR BREAD	CUP	137	495	16	99	4.5	2	0.3	0.2	1	
MACARONI-COOKED-FIRM STAGE-HOT	CUP	130	183	6	37	2.1	1	0.1	0.1	0.4	
NOODLES-EGG-COOKED	CUP	160	213	8	40	3	2	0.5	0.7	0.7	
NOODLES-EGG-SPINACH-COOKED	CUP	160	211	8	39	0.4	3	0.6	0.8	0.6	
NOODLES-RAMEN-ORIENTAL	CUP	227	207	6	31	2	9	0.4	0.4	0.4	
OAT BRAN-RAW	CUP	94	231	16	62	12.5	7	1.3	2.2	2.6	
OATS-WHOLE GRAIN-UNCOOKED	CUP	156	607	26	104	20.8	11	1.9	3.4	4	
PASTA-FRESH-PLAIN-COOKED	OUNCE	28.4	38	1	7	0.3	t	t	t	0.1	
POPCORN-POPPED-OIL & SALT	CUP	9		40	1	5	0.4	2	1.5	0.2	0.2
POPCORN-POPPED-PLAIN	CUP	6		25	1	5	0.4	0	0	0	0
POPCORN-POPPED-SUGAR COATED	CUP	35	135	2	30	1.4	1	0.5	0.2	0.4	
PRETZEL-DUTCH-TWISTED	ITEM	16	60	2	12	*	1	*	*	*	
PRETZEL-THIN-STICK	ITEM	0.3	1	t	t	*	t	0	0	0	
PRETZEL-THIN-TWISTED	ITEM	6		24	1	5	*	t	*	*	*
RICE CAKE-LOW SODIUM	ITEM	9.31	35	1	8	0.2	t	1.2	0.1	t	
RICE CAKE-REGULAR	ITEM	9.31	35	1	8	0.2	t	1.2	0.1	t	
RICE-BROWN-LONG GRAIN-COOKED	CUP	195	216	5	45	3.3	2	0.4	0.6	0.6	
RICE-BROWN-LONG GRAIN-RAW	CUP	185	685	15	143	10.7	5	1.1	2	1.9	
RICE-WHITE-INSTANT-HOT	CUP	165	162	3	35	1.3	t	0.1	0.1	0.1	
RICE-WHITE-LONG GRAIN-COOKED	CUP	205	264	6	57	2.1	1	0.2	0.2	0.2	
RICE-WHITE-LONG GRAIN-RAW	CUP	185	675	13	148	1.9	1	0.3	0.4	0.3	
RICE-WILD-COOKED	CUP	164	166	7	35	2.6	1	0.1	0.1	0.4	
RYE-WHOLE-DRY	CUP	169	566	25	118	8.9	4	0.5	0.5	0.9	

t = Trace of nutrient present   ** = Not available*

MAG, magnesium; **IRON,** iron; **ZINC,** zinc; **VITA,** vitamin A; **VITC,** vitamin C; **THIA,** thiamin; **RIBO,** riboflavin; **NIAC,** niacin; **VB6,** vitamin B-6; **FOL,** folate; **VB12,** vitamin B-12; **CALC,** calcium; **PHOS,** phosphorus; **SEL,** selenium; **VE-a,** alpha tocopherol equivalents.

CHOL (mg)	SOD (mg)	POT (mg)	MAG (mg)	IRON (mg)	ZINC (mg)	VITA (RE)	VITC (mg)	THIA (mg)	RIBO (mg)	NIAC (mg)	VB6 (mg)	FOL (μg)	VB12 (μg)	CALC (mg)	PHOS (mg)	SEL (μg)	VE-a (mg)
0	15	235	13	0.7	0.1	85	7	0.03	0.06	1.6	0.05	8	0	8	28	1	*
0	0	335	12	0.2	0.2	91	11	0.03	0.07	1.7	0.03	6	0	9	20	1	0.2
0	0	171	6	0.1	0.1	47	6	0.02	0.04	0.9	0.02	3	0	4	10	1	0.1
0	10	33	8	0.7	0.2	t	3	0.01	0.03	0.3	0.04	3	0	13	8	1	t
0	13	166	10	0.6	0.2	0	3	0.03	0.06	0.6	0.04	3	0	13	18	1	0.3
0	0	208	10	0.4	0.2	3	7	0.03	0.07	0.2	0.03	12	0	18	18	1	0.8
0	56	139	15	0.8	0.1	0	68	0.05	0.05	0.6	2.02	25	0	15	10	2	0.2
0	8	121	15	0.7	0.2	134	63	0.08	0.05	0.5	0.12	28	0	13	10	2	0
0	3	266	40	1	0.3	4	19	0.23	0.06	0.7	0.19	12	0	36	17	3	0.3
0	5	245	25	1	0.3	7	20	0.25	0.07	0.7	0.18	26	0	22	10	2	0.2
0	2	175	22	0.6	0.1	4	24	0.14	0.06	0.7	0.14	16	0	11	11	1	0.2
0	50	234	13	2.2	0.2	67	1	0.04	0.1	0.8	0.07	7	0	24	33	1	*
0	0	114	5	0.1	0.1	21	6	0.03	0.06	0.3	0.05	1	0	3	7	0	0.5
0	0	48	2	0.1	t	8	1	0.01	0.01	0.1	0.02	1	0	3	5	0	0.2
0	5	399	5	0.5	0.2	0	9	0.05	0.05	0.5	0.16	9	0	5	12	1	0.8
0	7	529	35	1	0.4	187	7	0.08	0.29	2	0.48	t	0	40	61	1	*
0	4	741	45	2.5	0.5	68	6	0.05	0.22	1.6	0.48	t	0	51	78	1	*
0	4	708	43	2.4	0.5	65	6	0.05	0.21	1.5	0.46	t	0	48	75	1	*
0	6	1200	73	4	0.9	320	5	0.13	0.26	3.2	0.43	6	0	82	127	1	*
0	17	1089	48	3	0.4	1	5	0.23	0.13	1.2	0.36	5	0	71	141	1	1
0	2	105	5	0.3	t	t	t	0.02	0.01	0.1	0.04	t	0	7	14	0	0.1
0	9	241	31	1.1	0.4	9	22	0.05	0.08	1.1	0.11	27	0	27	23	1	1.2
0	3	285	33	1.6	0.5	15	41	0.05	0.11	0.6	0.09	65	0	38	43	1	0.8
0	0	187	22	0.7	0.6	16	31	0.04	0.11	1.1	0.07	32	0	27	15	1	0.4
0	5	548	32	1.6	0.2	22	16	0.05	0.14	0.8	0.05	14	0	211	41	1	0.5
0	9	218	22	1.2	0.2	7	80	0.05	0.09	0.1	0.12	01	0	33	29	1	0.4
0	8	249	18	1.5	0.1	6	106	0.04	0.13	1	0.08	38	0	28	32	1	0.5
0	3	250	15	1.2	0.1	7	101	0.04	0.2	0.7	0.07	10	0	28	31	1	0.5
0	3	221	16	1.1	0.2	7	61	0.03	0.06	0.7	0.04	25	0	24	19	1	0.3
0	1	247	15	0.6	0.2	4	85	0.03	0.1	0.3	0.09	26	0	21	28	1	0.2
0	15	197	20	0.9	0.6	212	50	0.13	0.11	1.1	0.11	12	0	18	25	1	*
0	1	132	10	0.1	0.2	77	26	0.09	0.02	0.1	0.06	17	0	12	8	1	*
0	3	186	18	0.3	0.1	59	15	0.13	0.03	0.3	0.23	4	0	13	14	1	*
*	1400	*	*	*	*	*	*	*	*	*	*	*	*	*	*	*	0.3
0	164	43	22	0.4	0.4	11	1	0.05	0.03	0.6	0.05	2	0	37	55	2	1.9
0	1	213	42	6.1	0.6	0	0	1	0.59	7.7	0.23	7	0	3	114	*	0.2
0	7	389	96	9.9	1.7	98	0	1.72	0.98	12.1	0.62	115	0	12	202	6	0.4
0	372	39	11	1.5	0.3	0	0	0.13	0.2	1.7	0	0	0	29	42	*	0.3
0	2	123	25	5.3	0.8	0	0	0.9	0.57	6.8	0.05	30	0	17	124	5	t
0	2	136	34	6	1.2	0	0	1.11	0.7	10.4	0.05	40	0	21	133	*	*
0	1	41	23	1.8	0.7	0	0	0.27	0.13	2.2	0.05	1	0	1	71	32	t
53	11	45	30	2.5	1	10	0	0.3	0.13	2.4	0.06	11	0.14	19	110	*	*
52	20	59	38	1.7	1	17	0	0.39	0.2	2.4	0.18	34	0.22	30	91	*	12.7
36	829	69	17	1.8	0.6	221	t	0.16	0.1	1.4	0.07	8	0.01	18	70	*	0.2
0	4	532	221	5.1	2.9	0	0	1.1	0.21	0.9	0.16	49	0	55	690	*	1.6
0	3	669	276	7.4	6.2	0	0	1.19	0.22	1.5	0.19	87	0	84	816	*	1.7
10	2	7	5	0.3	0.2	2	0	0.06	0.04	0.3	0.01	2	0.04	2	18	*	0.1
0	174	*	16	0.2	0.4	*	0	*	0.01	0.2	*	*	*	1	19	2	*
0	0	*	*	0.2	0.5	*	0	*	0.01	0.1	0.01	*	0	1	17	1	*
0	0	*	*	0.5	*	*	0	*	0.02	0.4	*	*	*	2	47	7	*
0	258	21	4	0.2	0.2	0	0	0.05	0.04	0.7	t	3	0	4	21	*	t
0	5	t	t	t	t	0	0	t	t	t	0	t	0	t	t	*	0
0	97	6	1	0.1	0.1	0	0	0.02	0.02	0.3	t	1	0	2	5	*	t
0	t	26	3	0.2	0.1	0	t	t	t	0.1	0.01	1	0	7	10	*	t
0	11	27	3	0.2	0.1	0	t	t	t	0.1	0.01	1	0	7	10	*	t
0	9	83	83	0.8	1.2	0	0	0.19	0.05	3	0.28	8	0	20	161	76	1.3
0	13	413	265	2.7	3.7	0	0	0.74	0.17	9.4	0.94	36	0	43	616	*	1.3
0	5	7	8	1	0.4	0	0	0.12	0.08	1.5	0.02	6	0	13	23	33	0.2
0	4	80	26	2.3	0.9	0	0	0.33	0.03	3	0.19	7	0	23	95	41	0.2
0	9	213	46	8	2	0	0	1.07	0.09	7.8	0.3	16	0	52	213	37	0.2
0	6	166	53	1	2.2	0	0	0.09	0.14	2.1	0.22	43	0	5	134	*	0.3
0	10	4462	204	4.5	6.3	0	0	0.53	0.42	7.2	0.5	101	0	56	632	*	2.2

WT, weight; **KCAL,** kcalories; **PROT,** protein; **CARB,** carbohydrate; **FIBR,** fiber; **FAT,** fat; **SATF,** saturated fat;
MONO, monosaturated fat; **POLY,** polyunsaturated fat; **CHOR,** cholesterol; **SOD,** sodium; **POT,** potassium;

Food Name	Portion	WT (Gm)	KCAL	PROT (Gm)	CARB (Gm)	FIBR (Gm)	FAT (Gm)	SATF (Gm)	MONO (Gm)	POLY (Gm)
SHAKE 'N BAKE-PACKAGE-GENERAL FOODS	OUNCE	28.4	116	2	18	*	4	*	*	*
SORGHUM-WHOLE-DRY	CUP	192	651	22	143	28.6	6	0.9	1.9	2.6
SPAGHETTI-COOKED-TENDER STAGE-HOT	CUP	140	155	5	32	2.2	1	*	*	*
STUFFING MIX-DRY FORM	CUP	30	111	4	22	*	1	*	*	*
STUFFING MIX-PREPARED	CUP	140	501	9	50	*	31	*	*	*
TACO SHELLS	ITEM	11	50	1	7	0.9	2	0.3	1.2	0.5
TORTILLA CHIPS-DORITOS	OUNCE	28.4	139	2	19	1.9	7	1.4	3.2	1.8
Meats										
BACON BITS	TBSP	6	27	2	2	0.6	2	0.2	0.4	0.8
BACON-PORK-BROILED/PAN-FRIED/ROASTED	SLICE	6.3	36	2	t	0	3	1.1	1.5	0.4
BARBECUE LOAF-PORK AND BEEF	SLICE	23	40	4	1	*	2	0.7	1	0.2
BEEF CUTS-LEAN AND FAT-SIMMERED/ROASTED	SLICE	85	297	21	0	0	23	9.5	10.2	0.9
BEEF CUTS-LEAN ONLY-SIMMERED/ROASTED	SLICE	85	347	19	0	0	30	12.3	13.7	1
BEEF-DRIED-CURED-CHIPPED	SERVING	71	117	21	1	0	3	1.1	1.1	0.1
BEEF-HEART-COOKED-SIMMERED	SLICE	85	149	25	t	0	5	1.4	1.1	1.2
BEEF-LIVER-FRIED IN MARGARINE	SLICE	85	184	23	7	0	7	2.4	1.5	1.5
BEEF-POT ROAST-CHUCK-ARM CUT-COOKED	SLICE	100	231	33	0	0	10	3.8	4.4	0.4
BEEF-POT ROAST-CHUCK-BLADE CUT-COOKED	SLICE	100	270	31	0	0	15	6.2	6.8	0.5
BEEF-RIB STEAK-COOKED	ITEM	100	221	28	0	0	11	4.8	4.9	0.3
BEEF-STEAK-CHICKEN FRIED	ITEM	100	389	18	12	0	30	6.6	7.4	1.1
BEEF-TENDERLOIN STEAK-BROILED	ITEM	100	204	28	0	0	9	3.6	3.6	0.4
BEERWURST-BEER SALAMI-BEEF	SLICE	6	20	1	t	0	2	0.8	0.8	0.1
BEERWURST-BEER SALAMI-PORK	SLICE	6	14	1	t	0	1	0.4	0.5	0.1
BOCKWURST-RAW-PORK-LINK	ITEM	65	200	9	t	0	18	6.6	8.5	1.9
BOLOGNA-CURED PORK-4 BY 1/8 INCH SLICE	SLICE	23	57	4	t	0	5	1.6	2.3	0.5
BRATWURST-PORK-COOKED-LINK	ITEM	85	256	12	2	0	22	7.9	10.4	2.3
BRAUNSCHWEIGER-LIVER SAUSAGE-CURED PORK	SLICE	18	65	2	1	0	6	2	2.7	0.7
BRISKET-LEAN-COOKED	SLICE	100	241	29	0	0	13	4.6	5.8	0.4
CANADIAN BACON-PORK-GRILLED	SLICE	23.3	43	6	t	0	2	0.7	0.9	0.2
CHEESEFURTER-PORK AND BEEF	ITEM	43	141	6	1	0	13	4.5	5.9	1.3
CHITTERLINGS-PORK-SIMMERED	OUNCE	28.4	86	3	0	0	8	2.9	2.8	2.1
CHORIZO-PORK AND BEEF-LINK	ITEM	60	273	15	1	0	23	8.6	11	2.1
CORNED BEEF HASH-CANNED	CUP	220	400	19	24	*	25	11.9	10.9	0.5
CORNED BEEF LOAF-JELLIED	SLICE	28.4	44	7	0	0	2	0.7	0.8	0.1
CORNED BEEF-CANNED	SERVING	85	213	23	1	0	13	5.3	5.1	0.5
FRANKFURTER (HOT DOG)-NO BUN-BEEF & PORK	ITEM	57	183	6	1	0	17	6.1	7.8	1.6
FROG LEGS-FRIED-FLOUR COATED	ITEM	24	70	4	2	0.2	5	0.7	1.2	0.7
HAM AND CHEESE LOAF/ROLL	SLICE	28.4	74	5	t	0.5	6	2.1	2.6	0.6
HAM AND CHEESE SPREAD	TBSP	15	37	2	t	*	3	1.3	1.1	0.2
HAM SALAD SPREAD	TBSP	15	32	1	2	0	2	0.8	1.1	0.4
HAM-BOILED-REGULAR-11% FAT-LUNCHEON MEAT	SLICE	28.4	52	5	1	0	3	1	1.4	0.3
HAM-CANNED-CHOPPED-LUNCHEON MEAT	SLICE	21	50	3	t	0	4	1.3	1.9	0.4
HAM-CANNED-EXTRA LEAN-4% FAT	CUP	140	190	30	1	0	7	2.2	3.5	0.6
HAM-CANNED-PORK-ROASTED-13% FAT	CUP	140	316	29	1	0	21	7.1	9.9	2.5
HAM-DEVILED-CANNED-LUNCHEON MEAT	TBSP	13	45	2	0	0	4	1.5	1.8	0.4
HAM-EXTRA LEAN-5% FAT-ROASTED	CUP	140	203	29	2	0	8	2.5	3.7	0.8
HAM-LEAN ONLY-ROASTED	CUP	140	220	35	0	0	8	2.6	3.5	0.9
HAM-MINCED-PORK	SLICE	21	55	3	t	0	4	1.5	2	0.5
HAM-ROASTED-REGULAR-11% FAT-BONELESS	CUP	140	249	32	0	0	13	4.4	6.2	2
HAMBURGER PATTY-BROILED-EXTRA LEAN BEEF	ITEM	85	218	22	0	0	14	5.5	6.1	0.5
HAMBURGER PATTY-BROILED-MEDIUM-LEAN BEEF	ITEM	85	231	21	0	0	16	6.2	6.9	0.6
HAMBURGER-GROUND-REGULAR-BAKED	SERVING	85	244	20	0	0	18	7	7.8	0.7
HAMBURGER-GROUND-REGULAR-FRIED	SERVING	85	260	20	0	0	19	7.5	8.4	0.7
HEADCHEESE-PORK	SLICE	28.4	60	5	t	0	4	1.4	2.3	0.5
ITALIAN SAUSAGE-PORK-LINK	ITEM	67	216	13	1	0	17	6.1	8	2.2
KIELBASA-PORK AND BEEF	SLICE	26	81	3	1	0	7	2.6	3.4	0.8
KNOCKWURST-PORK AND BEEF-LINK	ITEM	68	209	8	1	0	19	6.9	8.7	2
LAMB CHOP-RIB-BROILED-LEAN AND FAT	SERVING	85	307	19	0	0	25	10.8	10.3	2
LAMB CHOP-RIB-BROILED-LEAN ONLY	SERVING	57	134	16	0	0	7	2.7	3	0.7
LAMB-LEG-ROASTED-LEAN AND FAT	SLICE	85	219	22	0	0	14	5.9	5.9	1
LAMB-LEG-ROASTED-LEAN ONLY	SLICE	71	136	20	0	0	6	2	2.4	0.4
LAMB-SHOULDER-ROASTED-LEAN AND FAT	SLICE	85	235	19	0	0	17	7.2	6.9	1.4
LAMB-SHOULDER-ROASTED-LEAN ONLY	SLICE	64	131	16	0	0	7	2.6	2.8	0.6

t= Trace of nutrient present **= Not available*

MAG, magnesium; **IRON,** iron; **ZINC,** zinc; **VITA,** vitamin A; **VITC,** vitamin C; **THIA,** thiamin; **RIBO,** riboflavin; **NIAC,** niacin; **VB6,** vitamin B-6; **FOL,** folate; **VB12,** vitamin B-12; **CALC,** calcium; **PHOS,** phosphorus; **SEL,** selenium; **VE-a,** alpha tocopherol equivalents.

CHOL (mg)	SOD (mg)	POT (mg)	MAG (mg)	IRON (mg)	ZINC (mg)	VITA (RE)	VITC (mg)	THIA (mg)	RIBO (mg)	NIAC (mg)	VB6 (mg)	FOL (μg)	VB12 (μg)	CALC (mg)	PHOS (mg)	SEL (μg)	VE-a (mg)
*	984	57	*	0.7	*	62	t	0.16	0.18	2.2	*	*	*	14	44	*	*
0	12	672	*	8.5	*	0	0	0.46	0.27	5.6	*	*	0	54	551	*	*
0	1	85	24	1.3	0.7	0	0	0.2	0.11	1.5	0.09	17	0	11	70	85	0.1
*	399	52	*	1	*	0	0	0.07	0.08	1	*	*	*	37	57	*	*
*	1254	126	*	2.2	*	91	0	0.13	0.17	2.1	*	*	*	92	136	*	*
0	20	27	11	0.3	0.1	5	0	0.03	0.02	0.2	0.04	3	0	16	25	*	0.5
0	180	51	21	0.5	0.2	5	0	0.03	0.03	t	0.1	4	0	30	59	*	1.2
0	165	9	6	0.3	0.1	0	t	0.03	0.02	0.1	0.01	8	0.07	8	18	*	0.4
5	101	31	2	0.1	0.2	0	2	0.04	0.02	0.5	0.02	t	0.11	1	21	1	t
9	307	76	4	0.3	0.6	2	4	0.08	0.06	0.5	0.06	2	0.39	13	30	3	*
78	50	244	18	2.2	4.7	0	0	0.07	0.18	2.9	0.26	6	2.03	8	164	25	0.1
78	55	186	14	1.9	4.5	0	0	0.05	0.15	2.4	0.2	5	1.91	8	147	25	0.1
65	2464	315	23	3.2	3.7	*	0	0.05	0.23	2.7	*	*	1.31	4	124	38	*
164	54	198	21	6.4	2.7	0	1	0.12	1.31	3.5	0.18	2	12.2	5	213	48	0.5
410	90	309	20	5.3	4.6	9216	19	0.18	3.52	12.3	1.22	187	95	9	392	48	0.5
101	66	289	24	3.8	8.7	0	0	0.08	0.29	3.7	0.33	11	3.4	9	268	6	0.1
106	71	263	23	3.7	10.3	0	0	0.08	0.28	2.7	0.29	6	2.47	13	235	6	0.1
80	69	394	27	2.6	7	0	0	0.11	0.22	4.8	0.4	8	3.32	13	208	6	0.1
97	815	126	30	2.3	4.9	8	0	0.11	0.14	2.7	0.5	11	3.27	11	110	*	0.1
84	63	419	30	3.6	5.6	0	0	0.13	0.3	3.9	0.38	8	0.44	7	238	*	0.2
4	62	10	1	0.1	0.1	0	1	t	0.01	0.2	0.01	t	0.12	1	6	2	t
4	74	15	1	t	0.1	0	2	0.03	0.01	0.2	0.02	t	0.05	t	6	2	t
38	718	176	12	0.4	1	4	0	0.27	0.11	2.7	0.15	4	0.53	10	95	10	*
14	272	65	3	0.2	0.5	0	8	0.12	0.04	0.9	0.06	1	0.21	3	32	4	t
51	473	180	12	1.1	2	0	1	0.43	0.16	2.7	0.18	2	0.81	38	126	25	*
28	206	36	2	1.7	0.5	759	2	0.05	0.28	1.5	0.06	8	3.62	2	30	2	0.1
93	72	287	23	2.8	6.9	0	0	0.07	0.22	3.8	0.3	8	2.55	6	239	5	0.1
14	360	91	5	0.2	0.4	0	5	0.19	0.05	1.6	0.11	1	0.18	3	69	3	0.1
29	465	89	5	0.5	1	16	8	0.11	0.07	1.3	0.05	1	0.74	25	76	10	0.1
41	11	2	3	1.1	1.4	0	0	0	0.02	t	t	1	0.29	8	13	*	0.1
53	741	239	11	1	2.1	0	0	0.38	0.18	3.1	0.32	1	1.2	5	90	10	0.1
50	1188	440	*	4.4	*	*	*	0.02	0.2	4.6	*	*	*	29	147	*	0.1
13	270	29	3	0.6	1.2	0	2	0	0.03	0.5	0.03	2	0.36	3	21	7	0.1
73	855	116	12	1.8	3	0	t	0.02	0.2	2.9	0.11	3	1.38	17	94	21	0.1
29	639	95	6	0.7	1.1	0	15	0.11	0.07	1.5	0.08	2	0.74	6	49	5	0.1
32	119	65	6	0.3	0.3	0	1	0.03	0.06	0.3	0.03	6	0.11	5	39	*	0.5
16	381	84	5	0.3	0.6	7	7	0.17	0.05	1	0.07	1	0.23	17	72	*	t
9	179	24	3	0.1	0.3	14	1	0.05	0.03	0.3	0.02	t	0.11	33	74	*	0
6	137	23	2	0.1	0.2	0	1	0.07	0.02	0.3	0.02	t	0.11	1	18	*	0
16	373	94	5	0.3	0.6	0	8	0.24	0.07	1.5	0.1	1	0.24	2	70	13	0
10	287	60	3	0.2	0.4	0	0	0.11	0.04	0.7	0.07	1	0.15	1	29	10	0
42	1589	487	29	1.3	3.1	0	39	1.45	0.35	6.9	0.63	7	0.99	8	293	66	0.4
87	1317	500	24	1.9	3.5	0	20	1.15	0.36	7.4	0.42	7	1.48	11	340	66	0.4
10	160	*	2	0.3	0.2	0	*	0.02	0.01	0.2	0.04	*	0.09	1	12	2	0
74	1684	402	20	2.1	4	0	29	1.06	0.28	5.6	0.56	5	0.91	11	275	66	0.4
77	1858	442	31	1.3	3.6	0	t	0.95	0.36	7	0.66	6	0.98	10	318	66	0.4
15	261	65	3	0.2	0.4	0	6	0.15	0.04	0.9	0.06	t	0.2	2	33	10	*
83	2100	573	30	1.9	3.5	0	32	1.02	0.46	8.6	0.43	4	0.98	12	393	66	0.4
71	60	266	18	2	4.6	6	0	0.05	0.23	4.2	0.23	8	1.84	6	137	20	0.3
74	65	256	18	1.8	4.6	9	0	0.04	0.18	4.4	0.22	8	2	9	134	20	0.3
74	51	188	13	2.1	4.2	0	0	0.03	0.14	4	0.2	7	1.99	8	117	*	0.3
75	71	255	17	2.1	4.3	0	0	0.03	0.17	5	0.2	8	2.3	10	145	*	0.3
23	357	9	3	0.3	0.4	*	6	0.01	0.05	0.3	0.05	1	0.3	5	17	5	*
52	618	204	12	1	1.6	0	1	0.42	0.16	2.8	0.22	3	0.87	16	114	22	0.1
17	280	71	4	0.4	0.5	0	5	0.06	0.06	0.7	0.05	1	0.42	11	39	4	t
39	687	136	8	0.6	1.1	0	18	0.23	0.1	1.9	0.11	1	0.8	7	67	10	0
84	64	230	20	1.6	3.4	0	0	0.08	0.19	6	0.09	12	2.16	16	151	14	0.1
52	49	178	17	1.3	3	0	0	0.06	0.14	3.7	0.09	12	1.5	9	121	10	0.1
79	56	266	20	1.7	3.7	*	*	0.09	0.23	5.6	0.13	17	2.2	9	162	14	t
63	48	240	19	1.5	3.5	*	*	0.08	0.21	4.5	0.12	16	1.87	6	146	12	t
78	56	214	19	1.7	4.4	*	*	0.08	0.2	5.2	0.11	18	2.24	17	156	14	0.1
56	44	170	16	1.4	3.9	*	*	0.06	0.17	3.7	0.1	16	1.73	12	128	11	0.1

WT, weight; **KCAL,** kcalories; **PROT,** protein; **CARB,** carbohydrate; **FIBR,** fiber; **FAT,** fat; **SATF,** saturated fat; **MONO,** monosaturated fat; **POLY,** polyunsaturated fat; **CHOR,** cholesterol; **SOD,** sodium; **POT,** potassium;

Food Name	Portion	WT (Gm)	KCAL	PROT (Gm)	CARB (Gm)	FIBR (Gm)	FAT (Gm)	SATF (Gm)	MONO (Gm)	POLY (Gm)
LIVER CHEESE-PORK	SLICE	38	116	6	1	0	10	3.4	4.7	1.3
LIVERWURST-LIVER SAUSAGE-PORK	SLICE	18	59	3	t	0	5	1.9	2.4	0.5
MORTADELLA-PORK AND BEEF	SLICE	15	47	2	t	0	4	1.4	1.7	0.5
OLIVE LOAF-PORK	SLICE	28.4	67	3	3	0	5	1.7	2.2	0.6
PEPPERONI-PORK AND BEEF	SLICE	5.5	27	1	t	0	2	0.9	1.2	0.2
PIMENTO/PICKLE LOAF-PORK	SLICE	28.4	74	3	2	*	6	2.2	2.7	0.7
POLISH SAUSAGE-PORK	ITEM	227	740	32	4	0	65	23.4	30.6	7
PORK CHOP-LOIN-BROILED-LEAN AND FAT	ITEM	82	284	19	0	0	22	8.1	10.2	2.5
PORK CHOP-LOIN-BROILED-LEAN ONLY	ITEM	66	169	18	0	0	10	3.5	4.5	1.2
PORK-CENTER LOIN-ROASTED-LEAN AND FAT	ITEM	88	268	22	0	0	19	6.9	8.8	2.2
PORK-CENTER LOIN-ROASTED-LEAN ONLY	SLICE	72	173	21	0	0	9	3.3	4.2	1.1
PORK-FEET-PICKLED	OUNCE	28.4	58	4	t	0	5	1.6	2.2	0.5
PORK-FEET-SIMMERED	OUNCE	28.4	55	5	0	0	4	1.2	1.7	0.4
PORK-KIDNEYS-BRAISED	CUP	140	211	36	0	0	7	2.1	2.2	0.5
PORK-LIVER-BRAISED	OUNCE	28.4	47	7	1	0	1	0.4	0.2	0.3
PORK-SHOULDER-ROASTED-LEAN ONLY	CUP	140	342	36	0	0	21	7.2	9.4	2.6
PORK-SPARERIBS-BRAISED	OUNCE	28.4	113	8	0	0	9	3.3	4	1
PORK-TENDERLOIN-ROASTED-LEAN ONLY	OUNCE	28.4	47	8	0	0	1	0.5	0.6	0.2
PORK-TONGUE-BRAISED	SERVING	85	230	21	0	0	16	5.5	7.5	1.6
POTTED MEAT-CANNED-BEEF/CHICKEN/TURKEY	TBSP	13	30	2	0	0	2	0.8	0.9	0.1
RABBIT-STEWED-BONELESS-SKINLESS	SERVING	85	175	26	0	0	7	2.1	1.9	1.4
ROAST BEEF-BOTTOM ROUND-COOKED-LEAN ONLY	SLICE	78	173	25	0	0	8	2.7	3.4	0.3
ROAST BEEF-BOTTOM ROUND-LEAN AND FAT	SLICE	85	222	25	0	0	13	4.8	5.7	0.5
ROAST BEEF-RIB-BROILED-LEAN AND FAT	SLICE	85	308	18	0	0	26	10.8	11.4	0.9
ROAST BEEF-RIB-BROILED-LEAN ONLY	SLICE	51	122	14	0	0	7	3	3.1	0.2
SALAMI-COOKED-BEEF-4 BY 1/8 INCH SLICE	SLICE	23	60	3	1	0	5	2.1	2.2	0.2
SALAMI-DRY OR HARD-PORK-SLICE	SLICE	10	41	2	t	0	3	1.2	1.6	0.4
SAUSAGE-LINK-COOKED-PORK	ITEM	13	48	3	t	0	4	1.4	1.8	0.5
SAUSAGE-PATTY-COOKED-FRESH PORK	ITEM	27	100	5	t	0	8	2.9	3.8	1
SAUSAGE-VIENNA-CANNED-BEEF AND PORK	ITEM	16	45	2	t	0	4	1.5	2	0.3
STEAK-SIRLOIN-BROILED-LEAN AND FAT	ITEM	85	238	23	0	0	15	6.4	6.9	0.6
STEAK-SIRLOIN-BROILED-LEAN ONLY	ITEM	56	116	17	0	0	5	2	2.2	0.2
STEAK-TOP ROUND-BROILED-LEAN AND FAT	SLICE	85	179	26	0	0	7	2.8	3.1	0.3
STEAK-TOP ROUND-BROILED-LEAN ONLY	SLICE	68	130	22	0	0	4	1.5	1.7	0.2
SWEETBREADS-CALF-BRAISED	SERVING	85	143	28	0	0	3	*	*	*
THURINGER/CERVELAT-PORK	SLICE	23	77	4	t	0	7	2.8	3	0.3
VEAL-LEG-TOP ROUND-PAN FRIED	SERVING	85	179	27	0	0	7	2.7	2.8	0.5
VEAL-RIB-SEPARABLE LEAN ONLY-BRAISED	SERVING	85	185	29	0	0	7	2.2	2.2	0.6
VEAL-SHOULDER-ARM-LEAN ONLY-ROASTED	SERVING	85	139	22	0	0	5	2	1.8	0.4
VENISON-DRIED-SALTED	SERVING	100	142	31	0	0	1	*	*	0.1
VENISON-ROASTED	SLICE	100	146	30	0	0	2	2.1	1.1	1.9
Miscellaneous										
BAKING POWDER-LOW SODIUM	TSP	4.3	7	t	2	*	0	0	0	0
BAKING POWDER-NO CALCIUM SULFATE	TSP	3	4	t	1	*	0	0	0	0
BAKING POWDER-STRAIGHT PHOSPHATE	TSP	3.8	5	t	1	*	0	0	0	0
BAKING POWDER-WITH CALCIUM SULFATE	TSP	2.9	3	t	1	*	0	0	0	0
BAKING SODA	TSP	3	0	0	0	0	0	0	0	0
CHEWING GUM-CANDY COATED	ITEM	1.7	5	0	2	0	t	0	0	0
CHEWING GUM-WRIGLEYS	ITEM	3	10	0	2	0	0	0	0	0
GELATIN DESSERT-PREPARED	CUP	240	140	4	34	0	0	0	0	0
GELATIN-D ZERTA-LOW CALORIE-PREPARED	CUP	240	16	4	0	0	0	0	0	0
GELATIN-DRY-ENVELOPE	ITEM	7	25	6	0	0	0	0	0	0
GELATIN-JELLO-SUGAR FREE-PREPARED	CUP	240	16	2	0	0	0	0	0	0
OLIVES-GREEN-PICKLED-CANNED	ITEM	4	4	t	t	0.1	1	0.1	0.4	t
OLIVES-MISSION-RIPE-CANNED	ITEM	3	5	t	t	0.1	1	0.1	0.4	t
PICKLE RELISH-HAMBURGER-HEINZ	OUNCE	28.4	30	0	7	*	0	0	0	0
PICKLE RELISH-HOT DOG-HEINZ	OUNCE	28.4	35	0	8	*	0	0	0	0
PICKLE RELISH-SWEET-CHOPPED	TBSP	15	20	0	5	0.3	0	0	0	0
PICKLE-DILL-CUCUMBER-MEDIUM SIZED	ITEM	65	5	0	1	0.8	0	0	0	0
PICKLE-FRESH PACK-CUCUMBER-SLICED	ITEM	7.5	5	0	2	0.1	0	0	0	0
PICKLE-SWEET/GHERKIN-SMALL-WHOLE	ITEM	15	20	0	5	0.2	0	0	0	0
POPSICLE	ITEM	95	70	0	18	0	0	0	0	0

t = Trace of nutrient present   ** = Not available*

MAG, magnesium; **IRON,** iron; **ZINC,** zinc; **VITA,** vitamin A; **VITC,** vitamin C; **THIA,** thiamin; **RIBO,** riboflavin; **NIAC,** niacin; **VB6,** vitamin B-6; **FOL,** folate; **VB12,** vitamin B-12; **CALC,** calcium; **PHOS,** phosphorus; **SEL,** selenium; **VE-a,** alpha tocopherol equivalents.

CHOL (mg)	SOD (mg)	POT (mg)	MAG (mg)	IRON (mg)	ZINC (mg)	VITA (RE)	VITC (mg)	THIA (mg)	RIBO (mg)	NIAC (mg)	VB6 (mg)	FOL (μg)	VB12 (μg)	CALC (mg)	PHOS (mg)	SEL (μg)	VE-a (mg)
66	466	86	5	4.1	1.4	1996	1	0.08	0.85	4.5	0.18	40	9.33	3	79	6	0.1
28	215	36	2	1.2	0.5	760	2	0.05	0.19	1.5	0.03	5	2.42	5	41	3	0.1
8	187	25	2	0.2	0.3	0	4	0.02	0.02	0.4	0.02	t	0.22	3	15	2	t
11	421	84	5	0.2	0.4	6	3	0.08	0.07	0.5	0.07	1	0.36	31	36	4	0.1
4	112	19	1	0.1	0.1	0	0	0.02	0.01	0.3	0.01	t	0.14	1	7	1	t
11	394	97	5	0.3	0.4	2	4	0.08	0.07	0.6	0.05	1	0.34	27	40	4	*
159	1989	538	32	3.3	4.4	0	2	1.14	0.34	7.8	0.43	5	2.22	27	309	66	0.4
77	54	287	20	0.7	2	2	t	0.69	0.29	4.3	0.31	4	0.81	5	193	14	0.1
63	49	276	19	0.6	1.9	2	t	0.64	0.28	3.9	0.3	4	0.71	5	184	11	0.1
80	56	284	17	0.9	1.8	2	t	0.73	0.21	4.4	0.35	1	0.53	5	173	28	0.1
66	50	261	15	0.8	1.6	2	t	0.65	0.19	3.9	0.32	1	0.43	4	158	23	0.1
26	262	67	1	0.2	0.4	0	0	t	0.01	0.1	0.11	1	0.18	9	10	*	0.1
28	9	42	1	0.1	0.3	0	0	t	0.02	0.1	0.03	t	0.05	13	14	*	0.1
673	111	200	25	7.4	5.8	109	15	0.55	2.22	8.1	0.65	57	10.9	18	337	294	0.6
101	14	43	4	5.1	1.9	1531	7	0.07	0.62	2.4	0.16	46	5.3	3	68	20	0.1
136	106	493	28	2.1	5.9	3	t	0.82	0.51	6	0.56	7	1.23	11	323	43	0.2
34	26	91	7	0.5	1.3	1	0	0.12	0.11	1.6	0.1	1	0.31	13	74	5	t
26	19	153	7	0.4	0.9	1	t	0.27	0.11	1.3	0.12	2	0.16	3	82	9	0.1
124	93	201	17	4.2	3.9	0	1	0.27	0.43	4.5	0.2	3	2.03	16	148	*	0.3
15	156	*	*	*	*	*	*	0	0.03	0.2	*	*	*	*	*	2	0
73	32	255	17	2	2	0	0	0.05	0.15	6.1	0.29	8	5.53	17	192	*	1.6
75	40	240	20	2.7	4.3	0	0	0.06	0.2	3.2	0.28	9	1.93	4	212	19	0.1
81	43	248	20	2.8	4.4	0	0	0.06	0.21	3.3	0.29	9	2.04	5	217	20	0.1
73	52	257	17	1.8	4.3	0	0	0.07	0.15	2.7	0.25	5	2.37	10	140	20	0.1
41	38	192	13	1.3	3.5	0	0	0.04	0.11	2.1	0.15	4	1.49	5	109	12	0.1
15	270	52	3	0.5	0.5	0	4	0.02	0.04	0.7	0.05	t	1.11	2	26	4	t
8	226	38	2	0.1	0.4	0	0	0.09	0.03	0.6	0.06	t	0.28	1	23	2	t
11	168	47	2	0.2	0.3	0	0	0.1	0.03	0.6	0.04	t	0.22	4	24	4	t
22	349	97	5	0.3	0.7	0	0	0.2	0.07	1.2	0.09	1	0.47	9	50	3	t
8	152	16	1	0.1	0.3	0	0	0.01	0.02	0.3	0.02	1	0.16	2	8	8	0
77	54	306	24	2.6	4.9	15	0	0.1	0.22	3.3	0.34	8	2.26	9	185	29	0.1
50	37	226	18	1.9	3.7	3	0	0.07	0.17	2.4	0.25	6	1.6	6	137	19	0.1
72	51	365	26	2.4	4.6	0	0	0.1	0.22	5	0.46	10	2.08	5	203	29	0.1
57	42	301	21	2	3.8	0	0	0.08	0.18	4.1	0.38	8	1.69	4	167	23	0.1
*	*	*	*	*	*	*	*	0.05	0.14	2.5	*	*	*	*	*	*	*
17	286	62	3	0.6	0.6	0	5	0.04	0.08	1	0.06	t	1.27	3	26	3	t
89	64	362	26	0.8	2.8	0	t	0.06	0.3	1	0.41	13	1.23	5	237	10	t
123	84	270	22	1.2	5.1	0	0	0.05	0.26	6.7	0.29	14	1.3	20	186	10	t
93	77	302	23	1	3.7	0	0	0.06	0.28	7	0.25	15	1.33	23	192	*	0.3
*	*	*	*	1.9	*	*	*	0.09	0.34	10	*	*	*	60	298	*	*
82	70	336	29	3.5	4.5	0	0	0.37	0.28	7.4	0.26	7	6.22	20	264	*	t
0	t	471	*	0	*	0	0	0	0	0	*	*	*	207	314	*	*
0	329	5	*	0	*	0	0	0	0	0	*	*	*	58	87	*	*
0	312	6	*	0	*	0	0	0	0	0	*	*	*	239	359	*	*
0	290	4	*	0	*	0	0	0	0	0	*	*	*	183	45	*	*
0	821	*	*	*	*	0	0	0	0	0	0	0	0	*	*	*	0
0	t	0	0	0	0	0	0	0	0	0	0	0	0	t	0	*	0
0	0	0	0	0	0	0	0	0	0	0	0	0	0	3	0	*	0
0	0	0	0	0	0	0	0	0	0	0	0	0	0	5	46	16	0
0	20	3	2	t	0.1	0	0	0	0	0	t	0	0	6	0	*	0
0	8	180	0	0.4	0	0	4	0	0	0	0	0	0	0	0	2	0
0	120	*	*	*	*	*	*	*	*	*	*	*	*	*	*	*	*
0	81	2	1	0.1	t	1	0	0	0	t	0	t	0	2	1	0	0.1
0	19	1	1	t	t	1	0	0	0	t	0	t	0	3	t	0	0.1
0	325	*	*	0.2	*	*	*	*	*	*	*	*	*	6	4	0	*
0	200	*	*	0.2	*	*	*	*	*	*	*	*	*	6	4	0	*
0	124	30	1	0.1	t	2	1	0	t	0	t	1	0	3	2	0	t
0	928	130	8	0.7	0.2	7	4	0	0.01	0	0.01	1	0	17	14	0	0.1
0	50	15	t	0.2	t	1	1	0	0	0	t	t	0	3	2	0	t
0	128	30	t	0.2	t	1	1	0	0	0	t	t	0	2	2	0	t
0	0	4	0	0	0	0	0	0	0	0	0	0	0	0	0	*	0

WT, weight; **KCAL,** kcalories; **PROT,** protein; **CARB,** carbohydrate; **FIBR,** fiber; **FAT,** fat; **SATF,** saturated fat; **MONO,** monosaturated fat; **POLY,** polyunsaturated fat; **CHOR,** cholesterol; **SOD,** sodium; **POT,** potassium;

Food Name	Portion	WT (Gm)	KCAL	PROT (Gm)	CARB (Gm)	FIBR (Gm)	FAT (Gm)	SATF (Gm)	MONO (Gm)	POLY (Gm)
VANILLA-PURE	TSP	4.7	14	0	1	0	0	0	0	0
VINEGAR-CIDER	TBSP	15	0	0	1	0	0	0	0	0
VINEGAR-DISTILLED	CUP	240	29	0	12	0	0	0	0	0
YEAST-BAKER'S-DRY-ACTIVE-PACKAGE	SERVING	7	20	3	3	2.2	0	0	0	0
YEAST-BREWER'S-DRY	TBSP	8	25	3	3	2.5	0	0	0	0
Nuts & Seeds										
ALMOND BUTTER-PLAIN	TBSP	16	101	2	3	1.8	9	0.9	6.1	2
NUT-FILBERT/HAZEL-DRIED-CHOPPED	CUP	115	727	15	18	9.8	72	5.3	56.5	6.9
NUT-WALNUT-PERSIAN/ENGLISH	CUP	120	770	17	22	5.8	74	6.7	17	47
NUTS-ALMONDS-UNBLANCHED-SHELLED-CHOPPED	CUP	130	766	26	27	12.1	68	6.4	44.1	14.2
NUTS-ALMONDS-UNBLANCHED-SHELLED-SLIVERED	CUP	115	677	23	24	10.7	60	5.7	39	12.6
NUTS-BEECHNUTS-DRIED	OUNCE	28.4	164	2	10	2.6	14	1.6	6.2	5.7
NUTS-BRAZIL-DRIED-SHELLED	CUP	140	918	20	18	10.8	93	22.6	32.2	33.8
NUTS-BUTTERNUTS-DRIED	OUNCE	28.4	174	7	3	2.4	16	0.4	3	12.1
NUTS-CASHEWS-DRY ROASTED	CUP	137	786	21	45	10	64	12.5	37.4	10.7
NUTS-CASHEWS-OIL ROASTED	CUP	130	749	21	37	7.8	63	12.4	36.9	10.6
NUTS-HICKORY-DRIED	OUNCE	28.4	187	4	5	2.4	18	2	9.3	6.2
NUTS-MACADAMIA-DRIED	CUP	134	941	11	18	12.4	99	14.8	77.9	1.7
NUTS-MACADAMIA-OIL ROASTED	CUP	134	962	10	17	9.3	103	15.4	80.9	1.8
NUTS-MIXED-DRY ROASTED	CUP	137	814	24	35	11.6	71	9.5	43	14.8
NUTS-MIXED-OIL ROASTED	CUP	142	876	24	30	12.8	80	12.4	45	18.9
NUTS-PEANUTS-OIL ROASTED	CUP	144	837	38	27	12.8	71	9.9	35.2	22.4
NUTS-PEANUTS-OIL ROASTED-SALTED	CUP	144	837	38	27	12.8	71	9.9	35.2	22.4
NUTS-PEANUTS-SPANISH-DRIED	CUP	146	828	38	24	11.7	72	10	35.7	22.7
NUTS-PECANS-DRIED-HALVES	CUP	108	720	8	20	7	73	5.9	45.5	18.1
NUTS-PECANS-OIL ROASTED	CUP	110	754	8	18	8.5	78	6.3	48.8	19.4
NUTS-PISTACHIO-DRIED	CUP	128	739	26	32	13.8	62	7.8	41.8	9.4
NUTS-PISTACHIO-DRY ROASTED	CUP	128	776	19	35	13.8	68	8.6	45.6	10.2
NUTS-SOYBEAN KERNELS-ROASTED	CUP	108	489	40	33	9.2	26	3.4	6	13.8
NUTS-WALNUT-BLACK-DRIED-CHOPPED	CUP	125	759	30	15	8.1	71	4.5	15.9	46.9
NUTS-WALNUTS-FINELY GROUND	CUP	80	486	20	10	5.2	45	2.9	10.2	29.9
PEANUT BUTTER-CHUNK STYLE	TBSP	16.1	95	4	3	1.1	8	1.5	3.8	2.3
PEANUT BUTTER-LOW SODIUM-PETER PAN	TBSP	16	95	5	3	1.7	9	1.4	4	2.5
PEANUT BUTTER-OLD FASHIONED	TBSP	16	95	4	3	1.1	8	1.5	3.8	2.7
PEANUT BUTTER-SMOOTH TYPE	TBSP	16	94	4	3	1	8	1.5	3.8	2.3
SEEDS-BREADFRUIT-ROASTED	OUNCE	28.4	59	2	11	8	1	0.2	0.1	0.4
SEEDS-PUMPKIN/SQUASH-DRIED	CUP	138	747	34	25	14.8	63	12	19.7	28.8
SEEDS-PUMPKIN/SQUASH-ROASTED	CUP	64	285	12	34	29.4	12	2.4	3.9	5.7
SEEDS-SESAME-DRIED-WHOLE	CUP	144	825	26	34	21.6	72	10	27	31.4
SEEDS-SESAME-ROASTED-WHOLE	OUNCE	28.4	161	5	7	5.3	14	1.9	5.2	6
SEEDS-SUNFLOWER-DRIED	CUP	144	821	33	27	9.8	71	7.5	13.6	47.1
SEEDS-SUNFLOWER-OIL ROASTED	CUP	135	830	29	20	9.2	78	8.1	14.8	51.2
Poultry										
CHICK-BREAST-NO SKIN-ROASTED	ITEM	172	284	53	0	0	6	1.7	2.1	1.3
CHICK-THIGH-NO SKIN-ROASTED	ITEM	52	109	14	0	0	6	1.6	2.2	1.3
CHICKEN FRANKFURTER	ITEM	45	116	6	3	0	9	2.5	3.8	1.8
CHICKEN ROLL-LIGHT	SLICE	28.4	45	6	1	0	2	0.6	0.8	0.5
CHICKEN SPREAD-CANNED	TBSP	13	25	2	1	0	2	1.7	0.8	0.1
CHICKEN-BACK-FRIED-FLOUR COATED	ITEM	144	477	40	9	0.2	30	8.1	11.8	6.9
CHICKEN-BACK-STEWED	ITEM	122	316	27	0	0	22	6.1	8.7	4.9
CHICKEN-BREAST-NO SKIN-FRIED	ITEM	172	322	58	1	0	8	2.2	3	1.8
CHICKEN-BREAST-ROASTED	ITEM	196	386	58	0	0	15	4.3	5.9	3.3
CHICKEN-BREAST-STEWED	ITEM	220	404	60	0	0	16	4.6	6.4	3.5
CHICKEN-BREAST-WITH SKIN-FRIED IN BATTER	ITEM	280	728	70	25	*	37	9.9	15.3	8.6
CHICKEN-BREAST-WITH SKIN-FRIED IN FLOUR	ITEM	196	436	62	3	0.1	17	4.8	6.9	3.8
CHICKEN-CANNED-BONELESS-WITH BROTH	ITEM	142	234	31	0	0	11	3.1	4.5	2.5
CHICKEN-CAPON-ROASTED	ITEM	1274	2914	369	0	0	148	41.6	60.5	32.1
CHICKEN-DRUMSTICK-WITH SKIN-FRIED/FLOUR	ITEM	49	120	13	1	0	7	1.8	2.7	1.6
CHICKEN-GIBLETS-FRIED-FLOUR COATED	CUP	145	402	47	6	*	20	5.5	6.4	4.9
CHICKEN-GIBLETS-SIMMERED	CUP	145	228	38	1	0	7	2.2	1.7	1.6
CHICKEN-GIZZARD-SIMMERED	CUP	145	222	39	2	0	5	1.5	1.4	1.5

t= Trace of nutrient present **= Not available*

MAG, magnesium; **IRON,** iron; **ZINC,** zinc; **VITA,** vitamin A; **VITC,** vitamin C; **THIA,** thiamin; **RIBO,** riboflavin; **NIAC,** niacin; **VB6,** vitamin B-6; **FOL,** folate; **VB12,** vitamin B-12; **CALC,** calcium; **PHOS,** phosphorus; **SEL,** selenium; **VE-a,** alpha tocopherol equivalents.

CHOL (mg)	SOD (mg)	POT (mg)	MAG (mg)	IRON (mg)	ZINC (mg)	VITA (RE)	VITC (mg)	THIA (mg)	RIBO (mg)	NIAC (mg)	VB6 (mg)	FOL (μg)	VB12 (μg)	CALC (mg)	PHOS (mg)	SEL (μg)	VE-a (mg)
0	0	0	*	0	*	0	0	0	0	0	*	*	0	0	*	*	*
0	t	15	3	0.1	t	0	0	0	0	0	0	0	0	1	1	13	0
0	2	36	0	1.4	0	0	0	0	0	0	0	0	0	14	22	74	0
0	1	140	4	1.1	*	0	0	0.16	0.38	2.6	0.14	286	0	3	90	0	t
0	9	152	18	1.4	0.6	0	0	1.25	0.34	3	0.2	313	0	17	140	0	t
0	2	121	48	0.6	0.5	0	t	0.02	0.1	0.5	0.01	10	0	43	84	*	1.5
0	3	512	328	3.8	2.8	8	1	0.58	0.13	1.3	0.7	83	0	216	359	2	27.3
0	12	602	203	2.9	3.3	15	4	0.46	0.18	1.3	0.67	79	0	113	380	23	3.1
0	14	952	385	4.8	3.8	0	1	0.27	1.01	4.4	0.15	76	0	346	676	5	31.1
0	13	842	340	4.2	3.4	0	1	0.24	0.9	3.9	0.13	68	0	306	598	5	27.6
0	11	289	0	0.7	0.1	0	4	0.09	0.11	0.2	0.19	32	0	t	0	2	*
0	3	840	315	4.8	6.4	0	1	1.4	0.17	2.3	0.35	6	0	246	840	2260	9
0	0	119	67	1.1	0.9	3	1	0.11	0.04	0.3	0.16	19	0	15	127	2	*
0	22	774	356	8.2	7.7	0	0	0.27	0.27	1.9	0.35	95	0	62	671	7	0.8
0	22	689	332	5.3	6.2	0	0	0.55	0.23	2.3	0.33	88	0	53	554	88	0.2
0	t	124	49	0.6	1.2	4	1	0.25	0.04	0.3	0.06	11	0	17	95	2	1.5
0	7	493	155	3.2	2.3	0	0	0.47	0.15	2.9	0.26	21	0	94	182	7	4.7
0	9	441	157	2.4	1.5	1	0	0.29	0.15	2.7	0.27	21	0	60	268	7	4.7
0	16	817	308	5.1	5.2	2	1	0.27	0.27	6.4	0.41	69	0	96	596	7	8.2
0	16	825	333	4.6	7.2	3	1	0.71	0.32	7.2	0.34	118	0	153	659	7	8.5
0	8	982	266	2.6	9.6	0	0	0.36	0.16	20.6	0.37	181	0	127	744	55	10
0	624	982	266	2.6	9.6	0	0	0.36	0.16	20.6	0.37	181	0	127	744	55	10
0	26	1029	245	6.7	4.8	0	0	0.93	0.2	17.6	0.51	350	0	134	549	7	12.2
0	1	423	138	2.3	5.9	14	2	0.92	0.14	1	0.2	42	0	39	314	3	3.4
0	1	395	142	2.3	6.1	*	2	0.34	0.11	1	0.21	43	0	37	324	6	1.4
0	7	1399	203	8.7	1.7	30	9	1.05	0.22	1.4	0.32	74	0	173	644	7	6.7
0	8	1242	166	4.1	1.7	31	9	0.54	0.32	1.8	0.33	76	0	90	609	7	6.7
0	4	1588	187	4.8	3.9	22	2	0.11	0.16	1.9	0.32	244	0	149	392	*	*
0	2	655	252	3.8	4.3	37	4	0.27	0.14	0.9	0.69	82	0	72	580	24	1.1
0	1	419	161	2.5	2.7	24	3	0.18	0.09	0.6	0.44	52	0	46	371	15	0.7
0	78	121	26	0.3	0.4	0	0	0.02	0.02	2.2	0.07	15	0	7	51	1	1
0	5	110	28	0.3	0.5	0	0	0.02	0.02	2.2	0.06	13	0	5	60	2	1.1
0	75	110	30	0.3	0.5	0	0	0.01	0.01	2.3	0.06	13	0	5	60	2	1
0	77	115	25	0.3	0.4	*	0	0.02	0.02	2.1	0.06	13	0	5	52	2	1.1
0	8	307	18	0.3	0.3	8	2	0.12	0.07	2.1	0.12	17	0	24	50	4	*
0	24	1114	738	20.7	10.3	53	3	0.29	0.44	2.4	0.12	79	0	59	1620	*	1.4
0	12	588	168	2.1	6.6	4	t	0.02	0.03	0.2	0.02	6	0	35	59	*	0.6
0	16	674	505	21	11.2	1	0	1.14	0.36	6.5	1.14	139	0	1404	906	*	3.3
0	3	135	101	4.2	2	t	0	0.23	0.07	1.3	0.23	28	0	281	181	*	0.6
0	4	992	509	9.8	7.3	7	2	3.29	0.36	6.5	1.81	327	0	168	1015	111	71.7
0	4	652	171	9.1	7	7	2	0.43	0.38	5.6	1.07	316	0	76	1538	104	66.8
146	126	440	50	1.8	1.7	11	0	0.12	0.2	23.6	1.02	6	0.58	26	392	46	0.6
49	46	124	12	0.7	1.3	10	0	0.04	0.12	3.4	0.18	4	0.16	6	95	21	0.2
45	617	38	5	0.9	0.5	17	0	0.03	0.05	1.4	0.14	2	0.11	43	48	10	0.1
14	166	65	5	0.3	0.2	7	0	0.02	0.04	1.5	0.06	1	0.04	12	45	*	0.1
7	50	14	2	0.3	0.2	3	0	t	0.02	0.4	0.02	t	0.02	16	12	*	t
128	130	325	33	2.3	3.6	53	0	0.15	0.34	10.5	0.44	12	0.4	35	239	25	0.5
96	78	178	20	1.5	2.4	113	0	0.05	0.18	5.3	0.18	6	0.22	22	146	25	0.4
156	136	474	54	2	1.9	12	0	0.14	0.22	25.4	1.1	8	0.62	28	424	31	0.6
166	138	480	54	2.1	2	55	0	0.13	0.23	24.9	1.08	6	0.64	28	420	53	0.7
166	136	390	48	2	2.1	54	0	0.09	0.25	17.2	0.64	6	0.46	28	344	53	0.8
238	770	564	68	3.5	2.7	57	0	0.32	0.41	29.5	1.2	16	0.82	56	516	30	1
176	150	506	58	2.3	2.1	29	0	0.16	0.26	26.9	1.14	8	0.68	32	456	21	0.7
78	714	196	17	2.3	2	100	3	0.02	0.18	9	0.5	6	0.42	20	350	20	0.4
1098	626	3252	308	18.9	22.1	260	0	0.89	2.17	114	5.5	70	4.14	182	3140	227	4.5
44	44	112	11	0.7	1.4	12	0	0.04	0.11	3	0.17	4	0.16	6	86	5	0.2
647	164	478	37	15	9.1	5195	13	0.14	2.21	15.9	0.88	550	19.3	26	414	25	2
570	85	229	30	9.3	6.6	3234	12	0.13	1.38	6	0.49	545	14.7	18	331	25	2
281	97	259	29	6	6.4	82	2	0.04	0.35	5.8	0.17	77	2.81	14	225	25	*

WT, weight; **KCAL,** kcalories; **PROT,** protein; **CARB,** carbohydrate; **FIBR,** fiber; **FAT,** fat; **SATF,** saturated fat; **MONO,** monosaturated fat; **POLY,** polyunsaturated fat; **CHOR,** cholesterol; **SOD,** sodium; **POT,** potassium;

Food Name	Portion	WT (Gm)	KCAL	PROT (Gm)	CARB (Gm)	FIBR (Gm)	FAT (Gm)	SATF (Gm)	MONO (Gm)	POLY (Gm)
CHICKEN-HEART-SIMMERED	CUP	145	268	38	t	0	12	3.3	2.9	3.3
CHICKEN-LEG-NO SKIN-ROASTED	ITEM	95	182	26	0	0	8	2.2	2.9	1.9
CHICKEN-LEG-NO SKIN-STEWED	ITEM	101	187	27	0	0	8	2.2	3	1.9
CHICKEN-LEG-ROASTED	ITEM	114	265	30	0	0	15	4.2	6	3.4
CHICKEN-LIVER PATE-CANNED	TBSP	13	26	2	1	0	2	0.5	0.7	0.3
CHICKEN-LIVER-SIMMERED	CUP	140	219	34	1	0	8	2.6	1.9	1.3
CHICKEN-THIGH-FRIED-FLOUR COATED	ITEM	62	162	17	2	t	9	2.5	3.6	2.1
CHICKEN-THIN SLICED-SMOKED-LAND O FROST	SERVING	28.4	60	5	1	0	4	1	1.4	0.8
CHICKEN-WING-FRIED-FLOUR COATED	ITEM	32	103	8	1	0	7	1.9	2.8	1.6
CHICKEN-WING-ROASTED	ITEM	34	99	9	0	0	7	1.9	2.6	1.4
CHICKEN-WING-STEWED	ITEM	40	100	9	0	0	7	1.9	2.6	1.4
DUCK-FLESH & SKIN-ROASTED	ITEM	764	2574	145	0	0	217	73.9	98.6	27.9
DUCK-NO SKIN-ROASTED	ITEM	442	890	104	0	0	50	18.4	16.4	6.3
GOOSE-FLESH & SKIN-ROASTED	ITEM	1548	4721	389	0	0	339	106	159	39
GOOSE-LIVER PATE-SMOKED-CANNED	TBSP	13	60	1	1	0	6	*	*	*
GOOSE-NO SKIN-ROASTED	ITEM	1182	2813	342	0	0	150	53.9	51.3	18.3
TURKEY HAM-CURED THIGH MEAT	SLICE	28.4	37	5	t	0	1	0.5	0.3	0.4
TURKEY LOAF-BREAST	SERVING	28.4	31	6	0	0	t	0.1	0.1	0.1
TURKEY PASTRAMI	SLICE	28.4	40	5	t	0	2	1	0.6	0.5
TURKEY ROLL-LIGHT	OUNCE	28.4	42	5	t	0	2	0.6	0.7	0.5
TURKEY ROLL-LIGHT AND DARK	OUNCE	28.4	42	5	1	0	2	0.6	0.7	0.5
TURKEY-BREAST-NO SKIN-ROASTED	ITEM	612	826	184	0	0	5	1.4	0.8	1.2
TURKEY-DARK MEAT-NO SKIN-ROASTED	CUP	140	262	40	0	0	10	3.4	2.3	3
TURKEY-GIBLETS-SIMMERED	CUP	145	242	39	3	0	7	2.2	1.7	1.7
TURKEY-GIZZARD-SIMMERED	CUP	145	236	43	1	0	6	1.6	1.1	1.6
TURKEY-LIGHT MEAT-NO SKIN-ROASTED	CUP	140	219	42	0	0	5	1.4	0.8	1.2
TURKEY-LIGHT/DARK MEAT-NO SKIN-ROASTED	CUP	140	238	41	0	0	7	2.3	1.5	2
TURKEY-LIVER-SIMMERED	CUP	140	237	34	5	0	8	2.6	2.1	1.5
TURKEY-THIN SLICED-SMOKED-LAND O FROST	SERVING	28.4	50	5	1	0	3	0.8	0.9	0.7
Sauces & Dips										
CATSUP-TOMATO-HEINZ LITE	TBSP	15	8	t	2	*	0	0	0	0
CATSUP-TOMATO-LOW SODIUM-HEINZ	TBSP	15	8	t	2	*	0	0	0	0
DIP-BACON AND HORSERADISH-KRAFT	TBSP	15	30	1	2	*	3	*	*	*
DIP-BUTTERMILK-KRAFT	TBSP	15	40	1	1	*	4	*	*	*
DIP-CLAM-KRAFT	TBSP	15	30	1	2	*	2	*	*	*
DIP-FRENCH ONION-KRAFT	TBSP	15	30	1	2	*	2	*	*	*
DIP-GARLIC-KRAFT	TBSP	15	30	1	2	*	2	*	*	*
DIP-GREEN ONION-KRAFT	TBSP	15	25	1	2	*	2	*	*	*
DIP-GUACAMOLE-KRAFT	TBSP	15	25	1	2	*	2	*	*	*
DIP-JALAPENO BEAN-FRITOS	OUNCE	28.4	33	2	3	1.9	1	0.2	0.4	0.9
DIP-JALAPENO PEPPER-KRAFT	TBSP	15	25	1	2	*	2	*	*	*
GRAVY-BEEF-CANNED	CUP	233	123	9	11	0.1	5	2.7	2.2	0.2
GRAVY-BROWN-FROM DRY-PREPARED WITH WATER	CUP	258	75	2	13	t	2	0.8	0.7	0.1
GRAVY-CHICKEN-CANNED	CUP	238	188	5	13	2.1	14	3.4	6.1	3.4
GRAVY-MUSHROOM-CANNED	CUP	238	119	3	13	1	6	1	2.8	2.4
GRAVY-PORK-FROM DRY-PREPARED WITH WATER	CUP	258	77	2	13	*	2	0.7	0.9	0.2
GRAVY-TURKEY-CANNED	CUP	238	121	6	12	*	5	1.5	2.1	1.2
HORSERADISH-PREPARED	TBSP	15	6	t	1	0.3	0	0	0	0
MUSTARD-BROWN-PREPARED	CUP	250	228	15	13	2.1	16	7.7	14	30.8
MUSTARD-LOW SODIUM-FEATHERWEIGHT	TSP	5	4	t	t	*	t	*	*	*
MUSTARD-YELLOW-PREPARED	TSP	5	5	t	t	0.1	t	0	0	0
SAUCE-BARBECUE-READY TO SERVE	CUP	250	188	5	32	2.3	5	0.7	1.9	1.7
SAUCE-BEARNAISE-FROM DRY MIX-MILK/BUTTER	CUP	255	701	8	18	0.1	68	41.8	19.9	3
SAUCE-CHEESE-FROM DRY MIX-MILK/BUTTER	CUP	279	307	16	23	0.1	17	9.3	5.3	1.6
SAUCE-CHILI-BOTTLED	TBSP	15	16	t	4	*	0	0	0	0
SAUCE-CHILI-LOW SODIUM	TBSP	14.2	8	0	2	*	0	0	0	0
SAUCE-CURRY-FROM DRY MIX-MADE WITH MILK	CUP	272	269	11	26	0.9	15	6	5.1	2.8
SAUCE-HOLLANDAISE-DRY MIX-MADE WITH MILK	CUP	255	703	8	18	0.1	68	41.9	20	2.9
SAUCE-MARINARA-CANNED	CUP	250	170	4	26	*	8	1.2	4.3	2.3
SAUCE-MUSHROOM-DRY MIX-MADE WITH MILK	CUP	267	227	11	24	0.5	10	5.4	3.3	1.1
SAUCE-PICANTE-CANNED	FL OZ	16	9	t	2	*	1	0	0	0
SAUCE-SALSA WITH GREEN CHILIES-CANNED	FL OZ	16	10	t	2	*	1	0	0	0
SAUCE-SOUR CREAM-FROM MIX-WITH MILK	CUP	314	509	19	45	*	30	16.1	9.9	2.8

t= Trace of nutrient present   **= Not available*

MAG, magnesium; **IRON,** iron; **ZINC,** zinc; **VITA,** vitamin A; **VITC,** vitamin C; **THIA,** thiamin; **RIBO,** riboflavin; **NIAC,** niacin; **VB6,** vitamin B-6; **FOL,** folate; **VB12,** vitamin B-12; **CALC,** calcium; **PHOS,** phosphorus; **SEL,** selenium; **VE-a,** alpha tocopherol equivalents.

CHOL (mg)	SOD (mg)	POT (mg)	MAG (mg)	IRON (mg)	ZINC (mg)	VITA (RE)	VITC (mg)	THIA (mg)	RIBO (mg)	NIAC (mg)	VB6 (mg)	FOL (μg)	VB12 (μg)	CALC (mg)	PHOS (mg)	SEL (μg)	VE-a (mg)
350	70	192	29	13.1	10.6	12	3	0.1	1.07	4.1	0.47	116	10.6	27	289	71	1.7
89	87	230	23	1.2	2.7	18	0	0.07	0.22	6	0.35	8	0.31	12	174	13	0.3
90	78	192	21	1.4	2.8	18	0	0.06	0.22	4.9	0.22	8	0.23	11	151	13	0.4
105	99	256	26	1.5	3	46	0	0.08	0.24	7.1	0.37	8	0.35	14	199	16	0.4
51	50	12	2	1.2	0.3	28	1	0.01	0.18	1	0.03	42	1.05	1	23	*	t
883	71	196	29	11.9	6.1	6886	22	0.21	2.45	6.2	0.82	1077	27.1	20	437	99	3.4
60	55	147	15	0.9	1.6	18	0	0.06	0.15	4.3	0.21	5	0.19	8	116	11	0.2
21	182	49	5	0.4	0.5	0	0	0	0.03	1.6	0.07	2	0.06	0	39	*	0.1
26	25	57	6	0.4	0.6	12	0	0.02	0.04	2.1	0.13	1	0.09	5	48	6	0.1
29	28	62	7	0.4	0.6	16	0	0.01	0.04	2.3	0.14	1	0.1	5	51	6	0.1
28	27	56	6	0.5	0.7	16	0	0.02	0.04	1.9	0.09	1	0.07	5	48	6	0.1
640	454	1560	124	20.6	14.2	483	0	1.33	2.06	36.9	1.4	50	2.26	86	1190	*	5.3
396	286	1114	88	11.9	11.5	103	0	1.15	2.08	22.5	1.1	44	1.76	52	898	*	3.1
1416	1084	5092	341	43.8	40.6	325	0	1.19	5	64.5	5.73	31	6.35	201	4180	*	26.8
20	91	18	2	0.7	0.1	130	t	0.01	0.04	0.3	0.01	8	1.22	9	26	*	0
1138	898	4586	296	33.9	499	142	0	1.09	4.61	48.2	5.5	142	5.56	165	3652	*	21
16	283	92	5	0.8	0.8	0	0	0.02	0.07	1	0.07	2	0.07	3	54	*	0.2
12	406	79	6	0.1	0.3	0	0	0.01	0.03	2.4	0.1	1	0.57	2	65	*	0.1
15	297	74	4	0.5	0.6	0	0	0.02	0.07	1	0.08	1	0.07	3	57	*	0.1
12	139	71	5	0.4	0.4	0	0	0.03	0.06	2	0.09	1	0.07	11	52	*	0.1
16	166	77	5	0.4	0.6	0	0	0.03	0.08	1.4	0.08	1	0.07	9	48	*	0.1
510	318	1784	178	9.4	10.6	0	0	0.26	0.8	45.9	3.42	38	2.36	76	1370	49	0.6
119	110	406	34	3.3	6.3	0	0	0.09	0.35	5.1	0.5	13	0.52	45	286	35	0.9
606	86	290	25	9.7	5.3	2629	3	0.07	1.31	6.5	0.47	501	34.8	19	296	*	0.2
336	79	306	27	7.9	6	81	2	0.05	0.47	4.5	0.17	75	2.76	22	186	*	3.4
97	89	426	39	1.9	2.9	0	0	0.09	0.18	9.6	0.75	8	0.52	27	307	*	0.1
107	99	418	37	2.5	4.3	0	0	0.09	0.26	7.6	0.64	10	0.52	35	298	35	0.9
876	89	272	21	10.9	4.3	5288	3	0.07	1.99	8.3	0.73	932	66.5	15	381	*	4
23	283	80	7	0.4	0.8	0	0	0	0.03	1.2	0.12	2	0.1	40	58	*	0.1
0	110	54	*	0.1	*	21	2	0.01	0.01	0.2	*	*	*	7	8	0	*
0	90	54	*	0.1	*	21	2	0.01	0.01	0.2	*	*	*	7	8	0	*
0	100	*	*	*	*	*	*	*	*	*	*	*	*	*	*	*	*
3	135	*	*	*	*	*	*	*	*	*	*	*	*	*	*	*	*
5	115	*	*	*	*	*	*	*	*	*	*	*	*	*	*	*	*
0	120	*	*	*	*	*	*	*	*	*	*	*	*	*	*	*	*
0	80	*	*	*	*	*	*	*	*	*	*	*	*	*	*	*	*
0	85	*	*	*	*	*	*	*	*	*	*	*	*	*	*	*	*
0	108	*	*	*	*	*	*	*	*	*	*	*	*	*	*	*	*
1	163	77	9	0.4	0.1	4	0	0.02	0.03	1.1	0.03	20	0	7	23	6	0.3
0	80	*	*	*	*	*	*	*	*	*	*	*	*	*	*	*	*
7	1305	189	5	1.6	2.3	0	0	0.08	0.08	1.5	0.02	5	0.23	14	70	*	*
3	1076	57	10	0.2	0.3	0	0	0.04	0.09	0.8	0	0	0	66	44	*	*
5	1373	260	5	1.1	1.9	264	0	0.04	0.1	1.1	0.02	5	0.24	48	69	*	1.7
0	1357	252	5	1.6	1.7	0	0	0.08	0.15	1.6	0.05	29	0	17	36	*	t
3	1235	57	10	0.3	0.3	0	2	0.05	0.06	0.8	0.03	3	0.16	31	44	*	*
5	1373	259	5	1.7	1.9	0	0	0.05	0.19	3.1	0.02	5	0	10	69	*	*
0	165	44	3	0.1	0.1	0	3	t	t	t	0.01	t	0	9	5	*	t
0	3268	325	46	4.5	0.8	0	2	0.07	0.02	0.4	0.09	11	0	310	335	*	4.4
0	1	7	*	0.1	*	*	*	*	*	*	*	*	*	4	4	3	0.1
0	65	7	2	0.1	*	*	*	*	*	*	*	*	*	4	4	0	0.1
0	2032	435	45	2.3	0.5	218	18	0.08	0.05	2.3	0.19	10	0	48	50	*	3.3
189	1265	298	26	0.3	0.8	757	2	0.08	0.26	0.3	0.08	10	0.51	230	186	*	*
53	1566	554	47	0.3	1	117	2	0.15	0.56	0.3	0.14	13	1.12	570	437	*	*
0	201	56	*	0.1	*	21	2	0.01	0.01	0.2	*	*	*	3	8	0	*
0	10	*	*	*	*	*	*	*	*	*	*	*	*	*	*	*	*
35	1276	495	46	1.1	1.1	41	3	0.11	0.54	0.5	0.11	16	1.09	484	280	*	*
189	1134	309	26	0.2	0.8	696	2	0.08	0.33	0.2	0.08	10	0.51	240	194	*	*
0	1573	1060	60	2	0.7	240	32	0.11	0.15	4	0.62	34	0	45	88	*	*
34	1535	494	37	0.5	1.3	94	2	0.19	0.8	4.8	0.19	40	0.8	302	166	*	0.7
0	218	77	*	0.3	*	23	9	0.02	0.01	0.2	*	*	*	4	8	*	*
0	111	87	*	0.3	*	39	9	0.02	0.01	0.3	*	*	*	4	9	*	*
91	1007	733	44	0.6	1.4	144	3	0.13	0.7	0.6	0.13	16	0.94	546	*	*	*

WT, weight; **KCAL,** kcalories; **PROT,** protein; **CARB,** carbohydrate; **FIBR,** fiber; **FAT,** fat; **SATF,** saturated fat; **MONO,** monosaturated fat; **POLY,** polyunsaturated fat; **CHOR,** cholesterol; **SOD,** sodium; **POT,** potassium;

Food Name	Portion	WT (Gm)	KCAL	PROT (Gm)	CARB (Gm)	FIBR (Gm)	FAT (Gm)	SATF (Gm)	MONO (Gm)	POLY (Gm)
SAUCE-SOY	TBSP	18	10	1	2	0	t	t	t	t
SAUCE-SOY-TAMARI	TBSP	18	11	2	1	0	t	t	t	t
SAUCE-SPAGHETTI-TOMATO BASED-CANNED	CUP	249	271	5	40	*	12	1.7	6.1	3.3
SAUCE-STEAK-HEINZ 57	TBSP	15	15	t	3	*	t	0	0	0
SAUCE-STROGANOFF-FROM MIX-PREPARED	CUP	296	272	12	34	1.2	11	6.8	3	0.4
SAUCE-SWEET/SOUR-FROM MIX-PREPARED	CUP	313	294	1	73	1.9	t	t	t	t
SAUCE-TABASCO	TSP	5	0	t	t	0	0	0	0	0
SAUCE-TACO-CANNED	FL OZ	16	11	t	2	*	1	*	*	*
SAUCE-TARTAR-REGULAR	TBSP	14	75	0	1	*	8	1.5	1.8	4.1
SAUCE-TERIYAKI-BOTTLED-READY TO SERVE	TBSP	18	15	1	3	t	0	0	0	0
SAUCE-TERIYAKI-FROM MIX-PREPARED-WATER	CUP	283	130	4	28	0.1	1	0.1	0.2	0.5
SAUCE-TOMATO-CANNED-LOW SODIUM-S&W	CUP	226	90	4	18	3.4	0	0	0	0
SAUCE-TOMATO-CANNED-SALT ADDED	CUP	245	74	3	18	3.7	t	0.1	0.1	0.2
SAUCE-TOMATO-SPANISH-CANNED	CUP	244	81	4	18	3.7	1	0.1	0.1	0.3
SAUCE-TOMATO-WITH HERBS/CHEESE-CANNED	CUP	244	144	5	25	3.7	5	1.5	0.9	2
SAUCE-TOMATO-WITH MUSHROOMS-CANNED	CUP	245	86	4	21	3.7	t	t	t	0.1
SAUCE-TOMATO-WITH ONIONS-CANNED	CUP	245	103	4	24	3.7	t	0.1	0.1	0.2
SAUCE-WHITE-DEHYDRATED-PREPARED-MILK	CUP	264	240	10	21	0.1	14	6.4	4.7	1.7
SAUCE-WHITE-MEDIUM-WITH ENRICHED FLOUR	CUP	250	405	10	22	0.4	31	19.3	7.8	0.8
SAUCE-WORCESTERSHIRE	TBSP	15	12	t	3	0	0	0	0	0
TOMATO CATSUP	TBSP	15	15	0	4	0.2	0	0	0	0
Soups										
SOUP-BEAN WITH BACON-CANNED-WITH WATER	CUP	253	173	8	23	3.2	6	1.5	2.2	1.8
SOUP-BEEF BROTH-CANNED-READY TO EAT	CUP	240	17	3	t	0	1	0.3	0.2	t
SOUP-BEEF BROTH-DEHYDRATED-CUBED	ITEM	3.6	6	1	1	0	t	0.1	0.1	t
SOUP-BEEF NOODLE-CANNED-PREPARED-WATER	CUP	244	84	5	9	1.5	3	1.2	1.2	0.5
SOUP-BEEF-CHUNKY-CANNED-READY TO SERVE	CUP	240	170	12	20	*	5	2.6	2.1	0.2
SOUP-BLACK BEAN-CANNED-PREPARED-WATER	CUP	247	116	6	20	*	2	0.4	0.5	0.5
SOUP-CHEESE-CANNED-PREPARED WITH MILK	CUP	251	230	9	16	2	15	9.1	4.1	0.4
SOUP-CHICKEN AND DUMPLINGS-CANNED-MILK	CUP	241	96	6	6	0.7	6	1.3	2.5	1.3
SOUP-CHICKEN BROTH-CANNED-PREPARED-WATER	CUP	244	39	5	1	0	1	0.4	0.6	0.3
SOUP-CHICKEN NOODLE-CANNED-WITH WATER	CUP	241	75	4	9	1.5	2	0.7	1.1	0.6
SOUP-CHICKEN NOODLE-LOW SODIUM	CUP	240	91	5	10	1.4	2	0.7	1.1	0.6
SOUP-CHICKEN NOODLE-PREPARED FROM DRY	CUP	252	53	3	7	0.2	1	0.3	0.5	0.4
SOUP-CHICKEN-CHUNKY-CANNED-READY TO EAT	CUP	251	178	13	17	0.8	7	2	3	1.4
SOUP-CHICKEN-CHUNKY-LOW SODIUM	CUP	251	173	13	15	*	5	*	*	*
SOUP-CHICKEN/RICE-CANNED-READY TO SERVE	CUP	240	127	12	13	1.4	3	1	1.4	0.7
SOUP-CHILI-BEEF-CANNED-PREPARED-WATER	CUP	250	170	7	22	*	7	3.4	2.8	0.3
SOUP-CLAM CHOWDER-MANHATTAN STYLE-WATER	CUP	244	78	2	12	2.1	2	0.4	0.4	1.3
SOUP-CLAM CHOWDER-NEW ENGLAND-WITH MILK	CUP	248	163	9	17	1.5	7	3	2.3	1.1
SOUP-CLAM CHOWDER-NEW ENGLAND-WITH WATER	CUP	244	95	5	12	1.5	3	0.4	1.2	1.1
SOUP-CONSOMME-CANNED-PREPARED WITH WATER	CUP	241	29	5	2	*	0	0	0	*
SOUP-CORN-CANNED-LOW SODIUM-CAMPBELLS	SERVING	305	191	3	31	*	5	*	*	*
SOUP-CRAB-CANNED-READY TO SERVE	CUP	244	76	5	10	*	2	0.4	0.7	0.4
SOUP-CREAM OF ASPARAGUS-CANNED-WITH MILK	CUP	248	161	6	16	0.8	8	3.3	2.1	2.2
SOUP-CREAM OF CELERY-CANNED-WITH MILK	CUP	248	164	6	15	0.8	10	3.9	2.5	2.7
SOUP-CREAM OF CHICKEN-CANNED-WITH MILK	CUP	248	191	7	15	0.5	12	4.6	4.5	1.6
SOUP-CREAM OF CHICKEN-CANNED-WITH WATER	CUP	244	117	3	9	0.5	7	2.1	3.3	1.5
SOUP-CREAM OF MUSHROOM-CANNED-WITH MILK	CUP	248	203	6	15	0.5	14	5.1	3	4.6
SOUP-CREAM OF MUSHROOM-CANNED-WITH WATER	CUP	244	129	2	9	0.9	9	2.4	1.7	4.2
SOUP-CREAM OF POTATO-CANNED-WITH MILK	CUP	248	148	6	17	0.5	6	3.8	1.7	0.6
SOUP-CREAM OF SHRIMP-CANNED-WITH MILK	CUP	248	164	7	14	0.2	9	5.8	2.7	0.3
SOUP-ESCAROLE-CANNED-READY TO SERVE	CUP	248	27	2	2	*	2	0.5	0.8	0.4
SOUP-GAZPACHO-CANNED-READY TO SERVE	CUP	244	57	9	1	*	2	0.3	0.5	1.3
SOUP-LENTIL WITH HAM-CANNED-READY TO EAT	CUP	248	139	9	20	*	3	1.1	1.3	0.3
SOUP-MINESTRONE-CANNED-PREPARED-WATER	CUP	241	82	4	11	1.9	3	0.6	0.7	1.1
SOUP-ONION-CANNED-PREPARED WITH WATER	CUP	241	58	4	8	*	2	0.3	0.7	0.7
SOUP-ONION-DEHYDRATED-PACKET	SERVING	39	115	5	21	2.2	2	0.5	1.4	0.3
SOUP-ONION-DEHYDRATED-PREPARED-WATER	CUP	246	27	1	5	0.4	1	0.1	0.3	0.1
SOUP-OYSTER STEW-CANNED-PREPARED-MILK	CUP	245	134	6	10	*	8	5.1	2.1	0.3
SOUP-OYSTER STEW-CANNED-PREPARED-WATER	CUP	241	58	2	4	*	4	2.5	0.9	0.2
SOUP-PEA GREEN-CANNED-PREPARED WITH MILK	CUP	254	239	13	32	2.8	7	4	2.2	0.5

t = Trace of nutrient present   ** = Not available*

MAG, magnesium; **IRON,** iron; **ZINC,** zinc; **VITA,** vitamin A; **VITC,** vitamin C; **THIA,** thiamin; **RIBO,** riboflavin; **NIAC,** niacin; **VB6,** vitamin B-6; **FOL,** folate; **VB12,** vitamin B-12; **CALC,** calcium; **PHOS,** phosphorus; **SEL,** selenium; **VE-a,** alpha tocopherol equivalents.

CHOL (mg)	SOD (mg)	POT (mg)	MAG (mg)	IRON (mg)	ZINC (mg)	VITA (RE)	VITC (mg)	THIA (mg)	RIBO (mg)	NIAC (mg)	VB6 (mg)	FOL (μg)	VB12 (μg)	CALC (mg)	PHOS (mg)	SEL (μg)	VE-a (mg)
0	1029	32	6	0.4	0.1	0	0	0.01	0.02	0.6	0.03	3	0	3	20	*	0
0	1005	38	7	0.4	0.1	0	0	0.01	0.03	0.7	0.04	3	0	4	23	*	0
0	1235	956	60	1.6	0.5	306	28	0.14	0.15	3.8	0.88	54	0	70	90	*	*
0	265	*	*	*	*	*	*	*	*	*	*	*	*	*	*	0	*
39	1829	672	39	1.3	1.1	127	1	0.86	0.77	0.8	0.12	9	0.59	521	302	*	*
0	779	66	9	1.6	0.1	0	0	0.01	0.1	0.9	0.31	2	0	41	188	*	1.4
0	22	3	1	t	t	3	3	0	0.01	0	0.01	1	0	t	1	*	t
0	128	88	*	0.3	*	4	6	0.02	0.01	0.3	*	*	*	6	10	*	*
9	98	11	*	0.1	*	3	0	0	0	0	*	*	*	3	4	*	7
0	690	41	11	0.3	t	0	0	0.01	0.01	0.2	0.02	4	0	5	28	*	0.1
0	4791	216	85	2.8	0.1	0	0	0.03	0.09	1.3	0.14	28	0	113	215	*	1.2
0	65	838	43	1.7	0.6	221	30	0.16	0.14	2.6	0.36	20	0	32	72	2	2.9
0	1482	908	47	1.9	0.6	240	32	0.16	0.14	2.8	0.38	23	0	34	78	*	*
0	1152	900	46	8.5	0.8	242	21	0.18	0.15	3.2	0.43	33	0	42	117	*	*
*	1325	869	46	2.1	0.9	240	25	0.19	0.3	3	0.05	20	0	90	132	*	*
0	1107	931	47	2.2	0.5	233	30	0.18	0.27	3.1	0.33	23	0	32	78	*	*
0	1350	1012	47	2.3	0.6	208	31	0.18	0.33	3	0.65	55	0	42	96	*	*
34	797	443	264	0.3	0.5	92	3	0.08	0.45	0.5	0.07	16	1.06	425	256	*	3.9
33	796	348	38	0.5	0.5	115	2	0.12	0.43	0.7	0.06	12	0.7	288	233	*	3.7
0	147	120	2	0.9	t	5	27	0	0.03	0	0	0	0	15	9	*	0
0	156	54	4	0.1	t	21	2	0.01	0.01	0.2	0.02	1	0	3	8	0	0.3
3	952	403	44	2.1	1	89	2	0.09	0.03	0.6	0.04	32	0.05	81	132	8	*
0	782	130	5	0.4	0	0	0	0.01	0.05	1.9	0.02	5	0.17	14	31	8	*
t	864	15	2	0.1	t	1	0	0.01	0.01	0.1	0.01	1	0.04	2	8	0	t
5	952	99	6	1.1	1.5	63	t	0.07	0.06	1.1	0.04	4	0.2	15	46	8	0.8
14	866	336	5	2.3	2.6	261	7	0.06	0.15	2.7	0.13	13	0.61	31	120	8	*
0	1198	273	42	2.2	1.4	49	1	0.08	0.05	0.5	0.09	25	0.02	45	107	8	*
48	1020	340	20	0.8	0.7	147	1	0.06	0.33	0.5	0.08	10	0.44	288	250	8	0.4
34	860	116	5	0.6	0.4	52	0	0.02	0.07	1.8	0.04	2	0.16	15	60	8	0
1	776	210	2	0.5	0.2	0	0	0.01	0.07	3.4	0.02	5	0.24	9	73	8	*
7	1106	55	5	0.8	0.4	72	t	0.05	0.06	1.4	0.03	2	0.15	17	36	8	0.1
7	36	106	5	1.2	0.4	109	t	0.17	0.14	2.6	0.03	2	0.14	17	36	8	0.1
3	1283	30	8	0.5	0.2	6	t	0.07	0.06	0.9	0.01	2	0	33	33	8	*
30	887	176	8	1.7	1	130	1	0.09	0.17	4.4	0.05	5	0.25	24	113	8	0.1
*	78	264	*	1.8	*	94	2	0.13	0.25	4.8	*	*	*	28	*	8	*
12	888	108	10	1.9	1	586	4	0.02	0.1	4.1	0.05	4	0.31	35	72	8	0.1
13	1035	525	30	2.1	1.4	151	4	0.06	0.08	1.1	0.16	18	0.32	43	148	8	*
2	578	188	12	1.6	1	96	4	0.03	0.04	0.8	0.1	10	4.05	27	42	8	0.2
22	992	300	23	1.5	0.8	40	4	0.07	0.24	1	0.13	10	10.3	187	157	8	0.1
5	915	146	7	1.5	0.8	1	2	0.02	0.04	1	0.08	4	8	44	54	8	0.1
0	636	154	0	0.5	0.4	0	1	0.02	0.03	0.7	0.02	3	0	10	31	8	*
*	33	164	*	0.8	*	93	6	0.1	0.15	1.9	*	*	*	28	*	8	*
10	1234	326	88	1.2	1.5	50	0	0.2	0.07	1.3	0.12	15	0.2	66	88	8	*
22	1041	359	20	0.9	0.9	83	4	0.1	0.28	0.9	0.06	30	0.5	175	153	8	0.8
32	1009	310	22	0.7	0.2	68	1	0.07	0.25	0.4	0.06	9	0.5	186	151	8	1
27	1046	273	18	0.7	0.7	94	1	0.07	0.26	0.9	0.07	8	0.55	180	152	8	0.2
10	986	88	2	0.6	0.6	56	t	0.03	0.06	0.8	0.02	2	0.1	34	37	8	0.2
20	1076	270	20	0.6	0.6	38	2	0.08	0.28	0.9	0.06	10	0.5	178	156	8	1.3
2	1031	101	5	0.5	0.6	0	1	0.05	0.09	0.7	0.02	5	0.05	46	50	*	1.2
22	1060	323	17	0.5	0.7	67	1	0.08	0.24	0.6	0.09	9	0.5	166	160	8	0.1
35	1036	248	22	0.6	0.8	54	1	0.06	0.23	0.5	0.45	10	1.04	164	337	8	3.3
2	3864	265	5	0.7	2.2	217	4	0.07	0.05	2.3	0.22	35	0.5	32	79	8	*
0	1183	224	7	1	0.2	20	3	0.05	0.02	0.9	0.15	10	0	24	37	8	*
7	1319	357	22	2.7	0.7	36	4	0.17	0.11	1.4	0.22	50	0.3	42	184	8	*
2	911	313	7	0.9	0.7	234	1	0.05	0.04	0.9	0.1	16	0	34	55	8	*
0	1053	68	2	0.7	0.6	0	1	0.03	0.02	0.6	0.05	15	0	27	12	8	*
2	3493	260	25	0.6	0.2	1	1	0.11	0.24	2	0.04	6	0	55	126	0	t
0	849	64	5	0.1	0.1	0	t	0.03	0.06	0.5	0	1	0	12	30	*	*
32	1040	235	21	1	10.3	45	4	0.07	0.23	0.3	0.06	10	2.63	167	162	8	*
15	981	48	5	1	10.3	7	3	0.02	0.04	0.2	0.01	2	2.19	22	48	8	*
18	1048	377	55	2	1.8	58	3	0.16	0.27	1.3	0.1	8	0.44	173	238	8	0.2

WT, weight; **KCAL**, kcalories; **PROT**, protein; **CARB**, carbohydrate; **FIBR**, fiber; **FAT**, fat; **SATF**, saturated fat; **MONO**, monosaturated fat; **POLY**, polyunsaturated fat; **CHOR**, cholesterol; **SOD**, sodium; **POT**, potassium;

Food Name	Portion	WT (Gm)	KCAL	PROT (Gm)	CARB (Gm)	FIBR (Gm)	FAT (Gm)	SATF (Gm)	MONO (Gm)	POLY (Gm)
SOUP-PEA GREEN-CANNED-PREPARED/WATER	CUP	250	165	9	27	2.8	3	1.4	1	0.4
SOUP-PEA GREEN-LOW SODIUM-CANNED-WATER	CUP	250	165	9	27	0.8	3	1.4	1	0.4
SOUP-PEA-SPLIT-CANNED-PREPARED-WATER	CUP	253	189	10	28	2.8	4	1.8	1.8	0.6
SOUP-PEPPERPOT-CANNED-PREPARED/WATER	CUP	241	103	6	9	*	5	2.1	2	0.4
SOUP-TOMATO BEEF & NOODLE-CANNED/WATER	CUP	244	139	4	21	1.5	4	1.6	1.7	0.7
SOUP-TOMATO BISQUE-CANNED-PREPARED/MILK	CUP	251	198	6	29	*	7	3.1	1.9	1.2
SOUP-TOMATO BISQUE-LOW SODIUM-WITH WATER	CUP	247	123	2	24	*	3	0.5	0.7	1.1
SOUP-TOMATO RICE-CANNED-PREPARED/WATER	CUP	247	119	2	22	1.7	3	0.5	0.6	1.4
SOUP-TOMATO VEGETABLE-PREPARED FROM DRY	CUP	253	56	2	10	1.1	1	0.4	0.3	0.1
SOUP-TOMATO-CANNED-PREPARED WITH MILK	CUP	248	161	6	22	0.8	6	2.9	1.6	1.1
SOUP-TOMATO-CANNED-PREPARED WITH WATER	CUP	244	85	2	17	0.9	2	0.4	0.4	1
SOUP-TURKEY NOODLE-CANNED-PREPARED/WATER	CUP	244	68	4	9	0.7	2	0.6	0.8	0.5
SOUP-TURKEY NOODLE-LOW SODIUM-WITH WATER	CUP	244	68	4	9	*	2	0.6	0.8	0.5
SOUP-TURKEY VEGETABLE-CANNED-WATER	CUP	241	72	3	9	1	3	0.9	1.3	0.7
SOUP-TURKEY-CHUNKY-CANNED-READY TO SERVE	CUP	236	135	10	14	2.5	4	1.2	1.8	1.1
SOUP-VEGETABLE BEEF-CANNED-LOW SODIUM	SERVING	305	165	12	18	1.2	4	1.1	1	0.1
SOUP-VEGETABLE BEEF-CANNED-WITH WATER	CUP	245	78	6	10	1	2	0.9	0.8	0.1
SOUP-VEGETABLE-CANNED-LOW SODIUM	CUP	240	98	2	14	3.1	0	0	0	0
SOUP-VEGETARIAN-CANNED-PREPARED-WATER	CUP	241	72	2	12	1.2	2	0.3	0.8	0.7
SOUP-VICHYSSOISE-CANNED-PREPARED/MILK	CUP	248	148	6	17	*	6	3.8	1.7	0.6
Sugars & Sweets										
APPLE BUTTER	TBSP	20	37	t	9	0.2	t	t	t	t
CANDY-ALMOND JOY	OUNCE	28.4	151	2	19	0.3	8	1.7	2.5	1.7
CANDY-BIT O HONEY	OUNCE	28.4	121	1	21	*	4	1.7	1.6	0.2
CANDY-CARAMELS-PLAIN/CHOCOLATE	OUNCE	28.4	115	1	22	0.8	3	1.6	1.1	0.1
CANDY-CHOCOLATE COATED PEANUTS	OUNCE	28.4	160	5	11	*	12	4	4.7	2.1
CANDY-CHOCOLATE-SEMISWEET	CUP	170	860	7	97	8.8	61	36.2	19.8	1.7
CANDY-FONDANT-UNCOATED	OUNCE	28.4	105	0	25	0	1	0.1	0.3	0.1
CANDY-FUDGE-CHOCOLATE-PLAIN	OUNCE	28.4	115	1	21	0.4	3	1.3	1.4	0.6
CANDY-GUM DROPS	OUNCE	28.4	100	0	25	0	0	0	0	0
CANDY-HARD	OUNCE	28.4	110	0	28	0	0	0	0	0
CANDY-JELLY BEANS	ITEM	2.8	7	0	3	0	0	0	0	0
CANDY-KIT KAT BAR	ITEM	43	210	3	25	0.6	11	5.6	3.8	0.4
CANDY-LIFE SAVERS	ITEM	2	8	0	2	0	t	0	0	0
CANDY-LOLLIPOP	ITEM	28.4	108	0	28	0	0	0	0	0
CANDY-M & M-PLAIN-PACKAGE	ITEM	45	220	3	31	*	10	*	*	*
CANDY-MILK CHOCOLATE BAR-NO SUGAR	ITEM	10.1	60	1	5	*	4	*	*	*
CANDY-MILK CHOCOLATE WITH ALMONDS	OUNCE	28.4	151	3	15	1.3	10	4.1	3.9	1.4
CANDY-MILK CHOCOLATE WITH PEANUTS	OUNCE	28.4	154	4	13	*	11	5.2	5	1.8
CANDY-MILK CHOCOLATE-PLAIN	OUNCE	28.4	145	2	16	*	9	5.5	3	0.3
CANDY-MILKY WAY BAR	ITEM	60	260	3	43	0.1	9	5.1	3.6	0.3
CANDY-PEANUT BRITTLE	OUNCE	28.4	123	2	20	0.5	4	1.9	1.8	0.6
CANDY-PEANUT BUTTER CUP	PIECE	17	92	2	9	0.8	5	2.8	1.8	0.8
CANDY-SNICKERS BAR	ITEM	57	270	6	33	1.4	13	4.7	5	2
CHOCOLATE-BITTER-FOR BAKING	OUNCE	28.4	145	3	8	4.3	15	8.9	4.9	0.4
COCONUT CREAM-RAW	CUP	240	792	9	16	1.6	83	73.8	3.5	0.9
COCONUT MILK-RAW	CUP	240	552	6	13	1.1	57	50.7	2.4	0.6
HONEY-STRAINED/EXTRACTED	TBSP	21	65	0	17	0.1	0	0	0	0
ICING-CAKE-CHOCOLATE-PREPARED FROM MIX	CUP	275	1035	9	185	*	38	23.4	11.7	1
ICING-CAKE-FUDGE-PREPARED FROM MIX/WATER	CUP	245	830	7	183	*	16	5.1	6.7	3.1
ICING-CAKE-WHITE-BOILED	CUP	94	295	1	75	0	0	0	0	0
ICING-CAKE-WHITE-UNCOOKED	CUP	319	1200	2	260	0	21	12.7	5.1	0.5
ICING-CAKE-WHITE/COCONUT-BOILED	CUP	166	605	3	124	*	13	11	0.9	0
JAM/PRESERVES-STRAWBERRY-LOW CALORIE	TSP	6	8	0	2	0.1	0	0	0	0
JAMS/PRESERVES-REGULAR	TBSP	20	55	0	14	0.2	0	0	0	0
JAMS/PRESERVES-REGULAR-PACKET SIZE	ITEM	14	40	0	10	0.1	0	0	0	0
JELLIES-REGULAR	TBSP	18	50	0	13	0	0	0	0	0
JELLIES-REGULAR-PACKET SIZE	ITEM	14	40	0	10	0	0	0	0	0
MARSHMALLOWS	OUNCE	28.4	90	1	23	0	0	0	0	0
MOLASSES-CANE-BLACKSTRAP	TBSP	20	45	0	11	0	0	0	0	0
MOLASSES-CANE-LIGHT	TBSP	20	50	0	13	0	0	0	0	0
NUTS-COCONUT-DRIED-FLAKED-CANNED	CUP	77	341	3	32	4.4	24	21.6	1	0.3

t = Trace of nutrient present ** = Not available*

MAG, magnesium; **IRON,** iron; **ZINC,** zinc; **VITA,** vitamin A; **VITC,** vitamin C; **THIA,** thiamin; **RIBO,** riboflavin; **NIAC,** niacin; **VB6,** vitamin B-6; **FOL,** folate; **VB12,** vitamin B-12; **CALC,** calcium; **PHOS,** phosphorus; **SEL,** selenium; **VE-a,** alpha tocopherol equivalents.

CHOL (mg)	SOD (mg)	POT (mg)	MAG (mg)	IRON (mg)	ZINC (mg)	VITA (RE)	VITC (mg)	THIA (mg)	RIBO (mg)	NIAC (mg)	VB6 (mg)	FOL (μg)	VB12 (μg)	CALC (mg)	PHOS (mg)	SEL (μg)	VE-a (mg)
0	988	190	39	2	1.7	20	2	0.11	0.07	1.2	0.05	2	0	28	124	8	0.1
0	33	190	39	2	1.7	20	2	0.11	0.07	1.2	0.05	2	0	28	124	8	0.1
8	1008	399	48	2.3	1.3	44	1	0.15	0.08	1.5	0.07	3	0	22	213	8	0.1
10	970	152	5	0.9	1.2	87	1	0.05	0.05	1.2	0.06	10	0.17	23	42	8	*
5	917	221	8	1.1	0.8	53	0	0.08	0.09	1.9	0.09	7	0.19	17	56	8	0.8
22	1108	604	25	0.9	0.6	110	7	0.11	0.27	1.3	0.14	21	0.44	186	174	8	*
4	30	417	9	0.8	0.6	72	6	0.07	0.07	1.2	0.09	15	0	40	60	8	*
2	815	330	5	0.8	0.5	76	15	0.06	0.05	1.1	0.08	14	0	22	33	8	0.8
0	1146	103	20	0.6	0.2	20	6	0.06	0.05	0.8	0.05	10	0	8	29	*	t
17	932	449	22	1.8	0.3	108	68	0.13	0.25	1.5	0.16	21	0.44	159	149	8	*
0	871	263	8	1.8	0.2	69	66	0.09	0.05	1.4	0.11	15	0	12	34	8	2.5
5	815	75	5	0.9	0.6	29	t	0.07	0.06	1.4	0.04	2	0.15	12	48	8	*
5	42	75	5	0.9	0.6	29	t	0.07	0.06	1.4	0.04	2	0.15	12	48	8	*
2	905	175	4	0.8	0.6	244	0	0.03	0.04	1	0.05	5	0.17	17	40	8	0.2
9	923	361	24	1.9	2.1	716	6	0.04	0.11	3.6	0.31	11	2.12	50	104	8	*
6	57	455	8	1.4	1.9	553	11	0.24	0.33	4.2	0.1	13	0.39	49	50	8	5007
5	960	174	5	1.1	1.6	189	2	0.04	0.05	1	0.08	11	0.31	17	42	8	0.3
0	38	185	7	1	0.5	371	3	0.05	0.05	1.2	0.06	11	0	19	35	8	0.5
0	823	209	7	1.1	0.5	300	1	0.05	0.05	0.9	0.06	11	0	21	35	8	0.3
22	1060	323	17	0.5	0.7	67	1	0.08	0.24	0.6	0.09	9	0.5	166	160	8	*
0	0	50	2	0.1	t	0	t	t	t	t	0.01	t	0	3	4	*	t
1	22	114	13	0.3	0.4	3	t	0.02	0.1	0.2	0.02	4	0.18	60	68	1	0.3
*	*	*	*	0.3	*	*	*	0	0.13	1.4	*	*	*	13	*	1	t
0	74	54	1	0.4	0.2	0	0	0.01	0.05	0.1	0.01	2	0.04	42	35	1	t
0	16	143	*	0.4	*	0	0	0.1	0.05	2.1	*	*	*	33	84	1	0.2
0	3	553	192	4.4	2.6	9	0	0.02	0.14	0.9	0.07	5	0	51	255	6	1.2
0	60	1	t	0.3	0	0	0	0	0	0	0	0	0	4	2	1	0
0	54	42	13	0.3	0.1	0	0	0.01	0.03	0.1	0.01	1	0.06	22	24	1	0.2
0	10	1	t	0.1	t	0	0	0	0	0	0	0	0	2	0	1	t
0	9	1	*	0.5	*	0	0	0	0	0	*	*	*	6	2	1	t
0	t	0	*	t	*	0	0	0	*	*	*	*	*	t	t	0	*
3	38	129	19	0.6	0.4	9	0	0.03	0.11	0.1	0.02	3	0.07	65	78	2	0.3
0	1	0	*	t	*	0	0	0	0	0	*	*	*	t	t	0	*
0	*	*	*	0	*	0	0	0	0	0	*	*	*	0	0	1	*
*	*	*	*	*	*	*	*	*	*	*	*	*	*	*	*	2	0.5
*	10	*	*	*	*	*	*	*	*	*	*	*	*	*	*	1	*
5	23	125	27	0.5	0.4	21	0	0.02	0.12	0.2	0.01	4	0.15	65	77	1	0.3
*	19	138	*	0.4	*	15	0	0.07	0.07	1.4	*	*	*	49	83	1	0.3
0	28	109	16	0.3	*	24	0	0.02	0.1	0.1	*	2	*	65	65	1	0.2
4	114	157	20	0.4	0.4	4	t	0.02	0.14	0.3	0.02	4	0.22	79	79	2	0.7
0	9	43	11	0.6	0.3	2	0	0.02	0.01	1.3	0.02	14	0	11	35	1	0.5
3	55	68	15	0.2	0.2	1	0	0.05	0.03	0.8	0.03	17	0.04	15	41	1	0.2
9	145	189	37	0.5	0.6	3	0	0.03	0.1	1.7	0.06	29	0.17	66	102	2	0.6
0	1	235	82	1.9	0.3	6	0	0.01	0.07	0.4	0.01	3	0	22	109	*	0.3
0	10	781	41	5.5	2.3	0	7	0.07	0	2.1	0.07	34	0	26	293	*	1.8
0	37	630	89	3.9	1.6	0	7	0.06	0	1.8	0.08	39	0	39	240	*	1.8
0	1	11	1	0.1	t	0	0	0	0.01	0.1	t	0	0	1	1	1	0
0	882	536	*	3.3	*	174	1	0.06	0.28	0.6	*	*	*	165	305	3	*
0	568	238	*	2.7	*	0	0	0.05	0.2	0.7	*	*	*	96	218	3	*
0	134	17	*	0	*	0	0	0	0.03	0	*	*	*	2	2	1	*
0	156	57	*	0	*	258	0	0	0.06	0	*	*	*	48	38	3	*
0	195	277	*	0.8	*	0	0	0.02	0.07	0.3	*	*	*	10	50	2	*
0	6	5	t	t	t	t	1	t	t	t	t	1	0	1	t	0	t
0	2	18	1	0.2	t	0	0	0	0.01	0	t	2	0	4	2	0	t
0	1	12	1	0.1	t	0	0	0	0	0	t	1	0	3	1	0	t
0	3	14	1	0.3	t	0	1	0	0.01	0	t	t	0	4	1	0	t
0	2	11	1	0.2	t	0	1	0	0	0	t	t	0	3	1	0	t
0	11	2	1	0.5	t	0	0	0	0	0	0	0	0	5	2	0	0
0	18	585	9	3.2	0.1	0	0	0.02	0.04	0.4	0.04	0	0	137	17	13	0.1
0	3	183	9	0.9	0.1	0	0	0.01	0.01	0	0.04	0	0	33	9	13	0.1
0	15	249	38	1.4	1.2	0	0	0.02	0.02	0.2	0.18	5	0	11	79	*	0.5

WT, weight; **KCAL,** kcalories; **PROT,** protein; **CARB,** carbohydrate; **FIBR,** fiber; **FAT,** fat; **SATF,** saturated fat; **MONO,** monosaturated fat; **POLY,** polyunsaturated fat; **CHOR,** cholesterol; **SOD,** sodium; **POT,** potassium;

Food Name	Portion	WT (Gm)	KCAL	PROT (Gm)	CARB (Gm)	FIBR (Gm)	FAT (Gm)	SATF (Gm)	MONO (Gm)	POLY (Gm)
NUTS-COCONUT-DRIED-SHREDDED	CUP	93	466	3	44	3.9	33	29.3	1.4	0.4
NUTS-COCONUT-RAW-SHREDDED	CUP	80	283	3	12	7.2	27	23.8	1.1	0.3
SORGHUM	TBSP	21	55	0	14	0	0	0	0	0
SUGAR-BROWN-PRESSED DOWN	CUP	220	820	0	212	0	0	0	0	0
SUGAR-EQUAL-PACKET SIZE	ITEM	1	4	0	1	0	0	0	0	0
SUGAR-SWEET & LOW-PACKET SIZE	ITEM	1	4	0	1	0	0	0	0	0
SUGAR-WHITE-GRANULATED	TBSP	12	45	0	12	0	0	0	0	0
SUGAR-WHITE-POWDERED-SIFTED	CUP	100	385	0	100	0	0	0	0	0
SYRUP-CHOCOLATE FLAVORED-FUDGE-THICK	FL OZ	38	125	2	20	*	5	3.1	1.6	0.1
SYRUP-CHOCOLATE FLAVORED-THIN	FL OZ	38	83	1	22	0.1	t	0.2	0.1	t
SYRUP-CORN-TABLE BLENDS-LIGHT AND DARK	TBSP	21	60	0	15	0	0	0	0	0
SYRUP-PANCAKE-KARO	TBSP	20.5	60	0	15	0	0	0	0	0
SYRUP-PANCAKE-LIGHT-AUNT JEMIMA	FL OZ	39	60	0	15	0	0	0	0	0
Vegetables										
ALFALFA SEEDS-SPROUTED-RAW	CUP	33	10	1	1	0.7	t	t	t	0.1
AMARANTH-BOILED-DRAINED	CUP	132	28	3	5	12.5	t	0.1	0.1	0.1
AMARANTH-RAW	CUP	28	7	1	1	2.7	t	t	t	t
ARTICHOKES-BOILED-DRAINED	ITEM	120	60	4	13	4	t	t	t	0.1
ASPARAGUS-CANNED-DIETARY PACK-LOW SODIUM	CUP	244	34	4	5	3.9	t	0.1	t	0.2
ASPARAGUS-CANNED-SPEARS-DRAINED SOLIDS	CUP	242	46	5	6	3.5	2	0.4	0.1	0.7
ASPARAGUS-FROZEN-BOILED-DRAINED-SPEARS	CUP	180	50	5	9	2.2	1	0.2	t	0.3
ASPARAGUS-FROZEN-BOILED-DRAINED-TIPS	CUP	180	50	5	9	2.2	1	0.2	t	0.3
ASPARAGUS-RAW-BOILED-DRAINED-SPEARS	CUP	180	45	5	8	2.2	1	0.1	t	0.2
ASPARAGUS-RAW-BOILED-DRAINED-TIPS	CUP	180	45	5	8	2.2	1	0.1	t	0.2
BALSAM PEAR-LEAFY TIPS-BOILED-DRAINED	CUP	58	20	2	4	1.2	t	t	t	t
BALSAM PEAR-PODS-BOILED-DRAINED	CUP	124	24	1	5	2.5	t	t	t	t
BAMBOO SHOOTS-BOILED-DRAINED	CUP	120	14	2	2	2.2	t	0.1	t	0.1
BAMBOO SHOOTS-CANNED-DRAINED	CUP	131	25	2	4	3.4	1	0.1	t	0.2
BAMBOO SHOOTS-RAW	CUP	151	41	4	8	3.9	t	0.1	t	0.2
BEANS-ADZUKI-BOILED	CUP	230	294	17	57	14.3	t	0.1	7.2	2.1
BEANS-ADZUKI-CANNED-SWEETENED	CUP	296	702	11	163	13.7	t	0	0	0
BEANS-BAKED BEANS-CANNED	CUP	254	236	12	52	19.6	1	0.3	0.1	0.5
BEANS-BAKED BEANS-HOME RECIPE	CUP	253	382	14	54	19.5	13	4.9	5.4	1.9
BEANS-BLACK-COOKED-BOILED	CUP	172	227	15	41	7.2	1	0.2	0.1	0.4
BEANS-FRENCH-COOKED-BOILED	CUP	177	228	13	43	14.9	1	0.1	0.1	0.8
BEANS-GARBANZO-CANNED-RECONSTITUTED	SERVING	28.4	28	1	5	1.4	1	0.1	0.2	0.3
BEANS-GARBANZO-DRY-RAW	CUP	200	720	41	122	*	10	*	*	*
BEANS-GREAT NORTHERN-DRY-COOKED-DRAINED	CUP	180	210	14	38	9.7	1	4.4	5.5	1.7
BEANS-GREEN-CANNED-DIETARY-LOW SODIUM	CUP	136	26	2	6	1.8	t	t	t	0.1
BEANS-GREEN-FROZEN-BOILED-FRENCH STYLE	CUP	135	35	2	8	2.2	t	t	t	0.1
BEANS-KIDNEY-CANNED-DIETARY-LOW SODIUM	CUP	255	230	15	42	12.5	1	0	0	0
BEANS-LIMA-BABY-FROZEN-BOILED-DRAINED	CUP	180	189	12	35	13	1	0.1	t	0.3
BEANS-LIMA-CANNED-DIETARY-LOW SODIUM	CUP	248	186	11	34	10.4	1	0.2	t	0.4
BEANS-LIMA-CANNED-SOLIDS & LIQUIDS	CUP	248	186	11	34	10.4	1	0.2	t	0.4
BEANS-LIMA-FROZEN-BOILED-DRAINED	CUP	170	170	10	32	8.3	1	0.1	t	0.3
BEANS-LIMA-RAW-BOILED-DRAINED	CUP	170	209	12	40	12.2	1	0.1	t	0.3
BEANS-MUNG-SPROUTED-BOILED	CUP	125	26	3	5	2.7	t	t	t	t
BEANS-MUNG-SPROUTED-RAW	CUP	104	31	3	6	1.6	t	t	t	0.1
BEANS-NAVY PEA-DRY-COOKED-DRAINED	CUP	190	225	15	40	9.3	1	0.2	0.1	0.3
BEANS-NAVY-SPROUTED-BOILED	OUNCE	28.4	22	2	4	1.4	t	t	t	0.1
BEANS-PINTO-FROZEN-BOILED	OUNCE	28.4	46	3	9	1.4	t	t	t	0.1
BEANS-RED KIDNEY-CANNED-SOLIDS & LIQUIDS	CUP	255	230	15	42	12.5	1	1.2	3.5	3.1
BEANS-REFRIED	CUP	253	271	16	47	11.6	3	1	1.2	0.3
BEANS-REFRIED-CANNED-SAUSAGE-OLD EL PASO	CUP	200	388	14	26	6	26	6.9	7.9	2.3
BEANS-SHELLIE-CANNED	CUP	245	74	4	15	12	t	0.1	t	0.3
BEANS-SMALL WHITE-BOILED	CUP	179	254	16	46	7.9	1	0.3	0.1	0.5
BEANS-SNAP-GREEN-CANNED-DRAINED-CUTS	CUP	135	27	2	6	1.8	t	t	t	0.1
BEANS-SNAP-GREEN-DIETETIC-LOW SODIUM	OUNCE	28.4	4	t	1	0.4	t	0	0	0
BEANS-SNAP-GREEN-FROZEN-BOILED-CUTS	CUP	135	35	2	8	2.2	t	t	t	0.1
BEANS-SNAP-GREEN-RAW-BOILED	CUP	125	44	2	10	2.3	t	0.1	t	0.2
BEANS-SNAP-YELLOW/WAX-CANNED	CUP	136	27	2	6	1.8	t	t	t	0.1
BEANS-SNAP-YELLOW/WAX-FROZEN-BOILED	CUP	135	35	2	8	2.2	t	t	t	0.1

t = Trace of nutrient present ** = Not available*

MAG, magnesium; **IRON,** iron; **ZINC,** zinc; **VITA,** vitamin A; **VITC,** vitamin C; **THIA,** thiamin; **RIBO,** riboflavin; **NIAC,** niacin; **VB6,** vitamin B-6; **FOL,** folate; **VB12,** vitamin B-12; **CALC,** calcium; **PHOS,** phosphorus; **SEL,** selenium; **VE-a,** alpha tocopherol equivalents.

CHOL (mg)	SOD (mg)	POT (mg)	MAG (mg)	IRON (mg)	ZINC (mg)	VITA (RE)	VITC (mg)	THIA (mg)	RIBO (mg)	NIAC (mg)	VB6 (mg)	FOL (μg)	VB12 (μg)	CALC (mg)	PHOS (mg)	SEL (μg)	VE-a (mg)
0	244	313	47	1.8	1.7	0	1	0.03	0.02	0.4	0.25	8	0	14	99	16	0.7
0	16	285	26	1.9	0.9	0	3	0.05	0.02	0.4	0.04	21	0	12	90	11	0.6
0	2	37	t	2.6	t	0	0	0.03	0.02	0	0	0	0	35	5	26	0.1
0	66	757	44	7.5	0.6	0	0	0.02	0.07	0.4	0.09	0	0	187	42	3	0
0	0	0	0	0	0	0	0	0	0	0	0	0	0	0	0	0	0
0	4	3	0	0	0	0	0	0	0	0	0	0	0	0	0	0	0
0	t	0	0	0	t	0	0	0	0	0	0	0	0	0	0	0	0
0	1	3	0	0.1	0	0	0	0	0	0	0	0	0	0	0	1	0
0	27	107	*	0.5	0.3	18	0	0.02	0.08	0.2	*	*	*	48	60	*	*
0	20	106	21	0.6	0.3	0	0	0.01	0.03	0.2	t	2	0	6	35	*	t
0	15	1	t	0.8	t	0	0	0	0	0	0	0	0	9	3	3	0
0	35	1	t	0.8	t	0	0	0	0	0	0	0	0	9	3	0	0
0	18	7	1	0.1	t	0	0	t	0.01	0	0	0	0	1	4	0	0
0	2	26	9	0.3	0.3	5	3	0.03	0.04	0.2	0.01	12	0	11	23	*	t
0	28	846	73	3	1.2	366	54	0.03	0.18	0.7	0.23	75	0	276	95	*	11.2
0	5	171	15	0.7	0.3	82	12	0.01	0.04	0.2	0.05	24	0	60	14	*	2.4
0	114	425	72	1.6	0.6	22	12	0.08	0.08	1.2	0.13	61	0	54	103	*	0.2
0	849	373	22	1.4	1.2	115	40	0.13	0.22	2.1	0.24	208	0	34	93	3	0.9
0	944	416	24	4.4	1	128	45	0.15	0.24	2.3	0.27	231	0	39	104	9	0.9
0	7	392	23	1.2	1	147	44	0.12	0.19	1.9	0.04	242	0	41	99	7	2.5
0	7	392	23	1.2	1	148	44	0.12	0.19	1.9	0.04	242	0	41	99	7	2.5
0	7	558	34	1.2	0.9	149	49	0.18	0.22	1.9	0.25	177	0	43	110	7	3.6
0	7	558	34	1.2	0.9	149	49	0.18	0.22	1.9	0.25	177	0	43	110	7	3.6
0	8	349	55	0.6	0.2	100	32	0.09	0.16	0.6	0.44	51	0	24	45	*	0.3
0	7	396	20	0.5	1	14	41	0.06	0.07	0.3	0.05	63	0	11	45	*	0.6
0	5	640	4	0.3	0.6	0	0	0.02	0.06	0.4	0.12	3	0	14	24	*	1.2
0	9	105	5	0.4	0.9	1	1	0.03	0.03	0.2	0.18	4	0	11	33	*	1.3
0	6	805	5	0.8	1.7	3	6	0.23	0.11	0.9	0.36	11	0	20	89	*	1.6
0	18	1224	120	4.6	4.1	1	0	0.27	0.15	1.7	0.22	279	0	63	385	*	0.5
0	646	353	91	3.3	4.6	3	0	0.3	0.17	1.9	0.25	316	0	66	220	*	1.9
0	1008	752	81	0.7	3.6	43	8	0.39	0.15	1.1	0.34	61	0	127	264	*	*
13	1068	907	110	5	1.8	t	3	0.34	0.12	1	0.23	122	0.03	155	275	*	0.5
0	1	611	121	3.6	1.9	1	0	0.42	0.1	0.9	0.12	256	0	47	241	*	*
0	11	655	99	1.9	1.1	1	2	0.23	0.11	1	0.19	132	0	111	181	*	*
0	113	55	9	0.7	0.3	1	1	t	0.01	0.1	*	*	0	11	30	*	1
0	52	1594	*	13.8	*	10	*	0.62	0.3	4	*	*	0	300	662	4	6
0	12	749	86	4.9	1.8	0	0	0.25	0.13	1.3	1.01	63	0	90	266	23	0.4
0	3	148	18	1.2	0.4	*	6	0.02	0.08	0.3	*	43	0	32	26	1	t
0	18	151	28	1.1	0.8	72	11	0.07	0.1	0.6	0.08	11	0	61	32	1	0.2
0	10	673	10	4.6	1.9	1	8	0.13	0.1	1.5	1.12	36	0	74	278	5	0
0	52	740	101	3.5	1	31	10	0.13	0.1	1.4	0.21	28	0	50	202	1	0
0	10	668	84	3.9	1.6	43	22	0.07	0.11	1.3	0.15	40	0	70	176	3	1.6
0	618	668	84	3.9	1.6	43	22	0.07	0.11	1.3	0.15	40	0	70	176	4	0.7
0	90	694	58	2.3	0.7	32	22	0.12	0.1	1.8	0.21	111	0	38	153	1	0
0	29	969	126	4.2	1.3	63	17	0.24	0.16	1.8	0.33	45	0	54	221	9	0
0	13	126	18	0.8	0.6	1	14	0.06	0.13	1	0.07	37	0	15	35	*	t
0	6	155	22	0.9	0.4	2	14	0.09	0.13	0.8	0.09	63	0	14	56	*	t
0	13	790	97	5.1	1.8	0	0	0.27	0.13	1.3	1.06	67	0	95	281	21	0.6
0	4	90	32	0.6	0.3	t	5	0.11	0.07	0.4	0.06	30	0	5	29	4	0.1
0	24	183	15	0.8	0.2	0	t	0.08	0.03	0.2	0.06	10	0	15	28	*	t
0	833	673	10	4.6	1.9	1	8	0.13	0.1	1.5	1.12	36	0	74	278	9	0
0	1073	994	99	4.5	3.5	0	15	0.12	0.14	1.2	0.25	211	0	116	213	*	2.1
16	624	600	88	4.2	1.8	0	6	0.29	0.14	0.6	0.31	254	0	88	258	*	1.7
0	818	267	37	2.4	0.7	56	8	0.08	0.13	0.5	0.12	44	0	71	74	*	*
0	4	828	122	5.1	2	0	0	0.42	0.11	0.5	0.23	245	0	131	302	*	0.3
0	339	147	18	1.2	0.4	47	7	0.02	0.08	0.3	0.05	43	0	35	34	1	t
0	t	24	3	0.2	0.1	10	1	0.01	0.01	0.1	*	*	0	7	6	0	t
0	18	151	28	1.1	0.8	72	11	0.07	0.1	0.6	0.08	11	0	61	32	1	0.2
0	4	374	31	1.6	0.5	84	12	0.09	0.12	0.8	0.07	42	0	58	49	1	t
0	341	148	18	1.2	0.4	48	7	0.02	0.08	0.3	0.05	43	0	35	26	1	0.4
0	18	151	28	1.1	0.8	72	11	0.07	0.1	0.6	0.08	11	0	61	32	1	0.2

WT, weight; **KCAL**, kcalories; **PROT**, protein; **CARB**, carbohydrate; **FIBR**, fiber; **FAT**, fat; **SATF**, saturated fat;
MONO, monosaturated fat; **POLY**, polyunsaturated fat; **CHOR**, cholesterol; **SOD**, sodium; **POT**, potassium;

Food Name	Portion	WT (Gm)	KCAL	PROT (Gm)	CARB (Gm)	FIBR (Gm)	FAT (Gm)	SATF (Gm)	MONO (Gm)	POLY (Gm)
BEANS-SNAP-YELLOW/WAX-RAW-BOILED	CUP	125	44	2	10	2.3	t	0.1	t	0.2
BEET GREENS-BOILED-DRAINED	CUP	145	39	4	8	4.4	t	t	0.1	0.1
BEETS-CANNED-DIETARY PACK-LOW SODIUM	CUP	246	71	2	17	2.7	t	t	t	0.1
BEETS-SLICED-BOILED-DRAINED	CUP	170	53	2	11	3.4	t	t	t	t
BEETS-SLICED-CANNED-DRAINED	CUP	170	53	2	12	2.9	t	t	t	0.1
BEETS-WHOLE-BOILED-DRAINED	ITEM	50	16	1	3	1.1	t	t	t	t
BEETS-WHOLE-CANNED	CUP	246	71	2	17	2.7	t	t	t	0.1
BROCCOLI-FROZEN-BOILED-DRAINED	CUP	185	52	6	10	7.3	t	t	t	0.1
BROCCOLI-RAW	CUP	88	25	3	5	2.5	t	t	t	0.1
BROCCOLI-RAW-BOILED-DRAINED	CUP	155	43	5	8	4	1	0.1	t	0.3
BRUSSELS SPROUTS-FROZEN-BOILED	CUP	155	65	6	13	4.5	1	0.1	t	0.3
BRUSSELS SPROUTS-RAW-BOILED	CUP	156	61	4	14	6.7	1	0.2	0.1	0.4
BURDOCK ROOT-BOILED-DRAINED	ITEM	166	146	3	35	*	t	*	*	*
CABBAGE-CELERY-RAW	CUP	76	12	1	2	0.8	t	t	t	0.1
CABBAGE-COMMON-BOILED-DRAINED	CUP	145	31	1	7	4	t	t	t	0.2
CABBAGE-COMMON-RAW-SHREDDED	CUP	90	22	1	5	1.8	t	t	t	0.1
CABBAGE-COMMON-RAW-SLICED	CUP	70	17	1	4	1.5	t	t	t	0.1
CABBAGE-RED-RAW-SHREDDED	CUP	70	19	1	4	1.4	t	t	t	0.1
CABBAGE-SAVOY-RAW-SHREDDED	CUP	70	19	1	4	1.5	t	t	t	t
CABBAGE-WHITE MUSTARD-BOILED	CUP	170	20	3	3	2.7	t	t	t	0.1
CABBAGE-WHITE MUSTARD-RAW	CUP	70	9	1	2	0.7	t	t	t	0.1
CARROT JUICE-CANNED	CUP	246	98	2	23	5.9	t	0.1	t	0.2
CARROT-RAW-SCRAPED-SHREDDED	CUP	110	47	1	11	3.5	t	t	t	0.1
CARROT-RAW-SCRAPED-WHOLE	ITEM	72	31	1	7	2.3	t	t	t	0.1
CARROTS-BOILED-DRAINED-SLICED	CUP	156	70	2	16	5.8	t	0.1	t	0.1
CARROTS-CANNED-DIETARY PACK-LOW SODIUM	CUP	246	57	2	12	2.7	t	0.1	t	0.2
CARROTS-CANNED-SLICED-DRAINED	CUP	146	34	1	8	2.2	t	0.1	t	0.1
CARROTS-FROZEN-BOILED-DRAINED	CUP	146	53	2	12	5.4	t	t	t	0.1
CAULIFLOWER-FROZEN-BOILED	CUP	180	34	3	7	3.2	t	0.1	t	0.2
CAULIFLOWER-RAW-BOILED-DRAINED	CUP	124	30	2	6	2.7	t	t	t	0.1
CAULIFLOWER-RAW-CHOPPED	CUP	100	24	2	5	2.4	t	0	0	0
CELERY-PASCAL-RAW-DICED	CUP	120	19	1	4	1.9	t	t	t	0.1
CELERY-PASCAL-RAW-STALK	ITEM	40	6	t	1	0.6	t	t	t	t
CHARD-SWISS-BOILED-DRAINED	CUP	175	35	3	7	3.7	t	t	0	0.1
CHARD-SWISS-RAW	CUP	36	7	1	1	0.6	t	0	0	0
CHICORY GREENS-RAW-CHOPPED	CUP	180	41	3	8	4.3	1	0.1	t	0.2
CHICORY ROOTS-RAW	ITEM	60	44	1	11	1.4	t	t	t	0.1
CHIVES-FREEZE DRIED	TBSP	0.2	1	t	t	t	t	t	t	t
CHIVES-RAW-CHOPPED	TBSP	3	1	t	t	0.1	t	t	t	t
COLLARDS-FROZEN-BOILED-DRAINED	CUP	170	61	5	12	5.2	1	*	*	*
COLLARDS-RAW-BOILED-DRAINED	CUP	128	35	2	8	2.1	t	t	t	0.1
CORN FRITTER	ITEM	35	132	3	14	0.6	8	2	3.2	1.9
CORN-CREAMED-CANNED-DIETARY-LOW SODIUM	CUP	256	184	4	46	3.1	1	0.2	0.3	0.5
CORN-EAR-FROZEN-BOILED-DRAINED	ITEM	126	117	4	28	2.7	1	0.1	0.3	0.4
CORN-FROZEN-BOILED-DRAINED-KERNELS	CUP	165	134	5	34	3.5	t	t	t	0.1
CORN-KERNELS FROM ONE EAR-BOILED-DRAINED	ITEM	77	83	3	19	2.9	1	0.2	0.3	0.5
CORN-SWEET-CANNED-DRAINED	CUP	165	134	4	31	2.3	2	0.3	0.5	0.8
CORN-SWEET-CANNED-LOW SODIUM	CUP	256	156	5	38	2.1	1	0.2	0.3	0.5
CORN-SWEET-CANNED-VACUUM PACKED	CUP	210	166	5	41	9.5	1	0.2	0.3	0.5
CORN-SWEET-CREAM STYLE-CANNED	CUP	256	184	4	46	3.1	1	0.2	0.3	0.5
CORN-WITH RED AND GREEN PEPPERS-CANNED	CUP	227	170	5	41	5.1	1	0.2	0.4	0.6
CRESS-GARDEN-RAW	CUP	50	16	1	3	0.6	t	t	0.1	0.1
CUCUMBER-RAW-SLICED	CUP	104	14	1	3	1	t	t	t	0.1
CUCUMBER-RAW-WHOLE	ITEM	301	39	2	9	3	t	0.1	t	0.2
DANDELION GREENS-BOILED	CUP	105	35	2	7	4.1	1	0.1	t	0.4
EGGPLANT-BOILED-DRAINED	CUP	96	27	1	6	2.7	t	t	t	0.1
ENDIVE-RAW-CHOPPED	CUP	50	9	1	2	1.2	t	t	t	t
FRIJOLES-BEANS WITH CHEESE	CUP	167	226	11	29	*	8	4.1	2.6	0.7
GARLIC-RAW-CLOVE	ITEM	3	4	t	1	0.1	t	t	0	t
GINGER ROOT-RAW-SLICED	CUP	96	66	2	15	0.7	1	0.2	0.1	0.1
GOURD-WHITE FLOWERED-BOILED	CUP	146	22	1	5	1.6	t	t	t	t
HUMMUS	CUP	246	421	12	50	0	21	3.1	8.8	7.8
JERUSALEM ARTICHOKES-RAW	CUP	150	114	3	26	2	t	0	t	t

t= Trace of nutrient present **= Not available*

MAG, magnesium; **IRON,** iron; **ZINC,** zinc; **VITA,** vitamin A; **VITC,** vitamin C; **THIA,** thiamin; **RIBO,** riboflavin; **NIAC,** niacin; **VB6,** vitamin B-6; **FOL,** folate; **VB12,** vitamin B-12; **CALC,** calcium; **PHOS,** phosphorus; **SEL,** selenium; **VE-a,** alpha tocopherol equivalents.

CHOL (mg)	SOD (mg)	POT (mg)	MAG (mg)	IRON (mg)	ZINC (mg)	VITA (RE)	VITC (mg)	THIA (mg)	RIBO (mg)	NIAC (mg)	VB6 (mg)	FOL (μg)	VB12 (μg)	CALC (mg)	PHOS (mg)	SEL (μg)	VE-a (mg)
0	4	374	31	1.6	0.5	84	12	0.09	0.12	0.8	0.07	42	0	58	48	1	0.4
0	349	1318	99	2.8	0.7	740	36	0.17	0.42	0.7	0.19	21	0	165	60	*	2.2
0	113	349	39	1.7	0.6	2	10	0.03	0.09	0.4	0.14	71	0	34	39	3	0.1
0	83	530	63	1.1	0.4	2	9	0.05	0.02	0.5	0.05	90	0	19	53	1	0.1
0	466	252	29	3.1	0.4	2	7	0.02	0.07	0.3	0.1	51	0	26	29	1	0.1
0	25	156	19	0.3	0.1	1	3	0.02	0.01	0.1	0.02	27	0	6	12	1	t
0	647	349	39	1.7	0.6	2	10	0.03	0.09	0.4	0.14	71	0	34	39	1	0.1
0	44	333	37	1.1	0.6	350	74	0.1	0.15	0.8	0.24	104	0	94	102	3	0.9
0	24	286	22	0.8	0.4	136	82	0.06	0.11	0.6	0.14	63	0	42	58	1	0.4
0	40	453	37	1.3	0.6	215	116	0.09	0.18	0.9	0.22	78	0	71	92	3	0.7
0	36	504	37	1.2	0.6	92	71	0.16	0.18	0.8	0.45	157	0	37	84	1	1.3
0	33	495	31	1.9	0.5	112	97	0.17	0.12	0.9	0.28	94	0	56	87	1	1.3
0	7	597	65	1.3	0.6	0	4	0.07	0.1	0.5	0.46	32	0	82	154	*	*
0	7	181	10	0.2	0.2	91	21	0.03	0.04	0.3	0.18	60	0	59	22	2	0.1
0	28	297	22	0.6	0.2	13	35	0.08	0.08	0.3	0.09	29	0	48	36	3	2.4
0	16	221	14	0.5	0.2	11	43	0.05	0.03	0.3	0.09	51	0	42	21	2	1.5
0	13	172	11	0.4	0.1	9	33	0.04	0.02	0.2	0.07	40	0	33	16	2	1.2
0	8	144	11	0.3	0.1	3	40	0.04	0.02	0.2	0.15	15	0	36	29	2	0.1
0	20	161	20	0.3	0.2	70	22	0.05	0.02	0.2	0.13	56	0	25	29	2	0.1
0	58	631	19	1.8	0.3	437	44	0.05	0.11	0.7	0.28	69	0	158	49	4	1.2
0	46	176	13	0.6	0.1	210	32	0.03	0.05	0.4	0.14	46	0	74	26	2	0.1
0	71	718	34	1.1	0.4	6335	21	0.23	0.14	1	0.53	9	0	59	103	*	t
0	39	355	17	0.6	0.2	3094	10	0.11	0.06	1	0.16	15	0	30	48	2	0.5
0	25	233	11	0.4	0.1	2025	7	0.07	0.04	0.7	0.11	10	0	19	32	2	0.3
0	103	354	20	1	0.5	3830	4	0.05	0.09	0.8	0.38	22	0	48	47	2	0.7
0	96	426	22	1.5	0.7	3239	7	0.05	0.07	1	0.28	20	0	62	49	3	1
0	352	261	12	0.9	0.4	2010	4	0.03	0.04	0.8	0.16	13	0	37	35	2	0.6
0	86	231	15	0.7	0.4	2584	4	0.04	0.05	0.6	0.19	16	0	41	38	3	0.6
0	32	250	16	0.7	0.2	4	56	0.07	0.1	0.6	0.16	74	0	31	43	1	0.1
0	8	400	14	0.5	0.3	2	69	0.08	0.06	0.7	0.25	63	0	34	44	1	t
0	15	355	14	0.6	0.2	2	72	0.08	0.06	0.6	0.23	66	0	29	46	1	t
0	104	344	13	0.5	0.2	16	8	0.06	0.05	0.4	0.1	34	0	48	30	0	0.4
0	35	115	4	0.2	0.1	5	3	0.02	0.02	0.1	0.04	11	0	16	10	0	0.1
0	313	961	150	4	0.6	549	32	0.06	0.15	0.6	0.15	15	0	102	58	70	2.6
0	64	198	31	0.8	0.1	113	6	0.01	0.03	0.1	0.03	3	0	21	12	*	0.5
0	81	756	54	1.6	0.8	720	43	0.11	0.18	0.9	0.19	197	0	180	85	*	*
0	30	174	13	0.5	0.2	1	3	0.02	0.02	0.2	0.15	14	0	25	37	*	0.6
0	t	6	1	t	t	14	1	t	t	t	t	t	0	2	1	*	129
0	t	8	2	t	t	19	2	t	0.01	t	0.01	t	0	2	2	*	t
0	85	427	51	1.9	0.5	1017	45	0.08	0.2	1.1	0.19	129	0	357	46	1	*
0	21	168	9	0.2	0.1	349	16	0.03	0.07	0.4	0.07	8	0	29	10	1	2.9
25	167	47	8	0.6	0.2	14	1	0.06	0.07	0.6	0.02	11	0.06	22	54	*	1.1
0	8	343	44	1	1.4	26	12	0.06	0.14	2.5	0.16	115	0	8	131	1	0.1
0	5	316	37	0.8	0.8	27	6	0.22	0.09	1.9	0.28	38	0	4	95	1	0.1
0	8	228	30	0.5	0.6	41	4	0.11	0.12	2.1	0.16	33	0	4	78	1	0.1
0	13	192	25	0.5	0.4	17	5	0.17	0.06	1.2	0.05	36	0	2	79	1	0.1
0	533	322	33	1.4	0.6	26	14	0.05	0.13	2	0.08	80	0	8	107	1	0.1
0	8	392	41	0.9	0.9	31	17	0.07	0.16	2.4	0.1	98	0	10	131	1	0.1
0	572	390	48	0.9	1	51	17	0.09	0.15	2.5	0.12	104	0	10	134	1	0.1
0	730	343	44	1	1.4	26	12	0.06	0.14	2.5	0.16	115	0	8	131	1	0.1
0	788	347	57	1.8	0.8	52	20	0.05	0.18	2.2	0.22	77	0	11	141	1	0.1
0	8	304	19	0.7	0.1	465	35	0.04	0.13	0.5	0.12	40	0	40	38	*	0.4
0	2	155	11	0.3	0.2	5	5	0.03	0.02	0.3	0.05	15	0	15	18	1	0.2
0	6	448	33	0.8	0.7	15	14	0.09	0.06	0.9	0.16	42	0	42	51	1	0.5
0	46	244	25	1.9	0.3	1229	19	0.14	0.18	0.5	0.17	13	0	147	44	1	2.6
0	3	238	13	0.3	0.1	6	1	0.07	0.02	0.6	0.08	14	0	6	21	*	t
0	11	157	8	0.4	0.4	103	3	0.04	0.04	0.2	0.01	71	0	26	14	*	0.5
36	882	605	85	2.2	1.7	46	2	0.14	0.33	1.5	0.19	111	0.68	188	175	*	*
0	1	12	1	0.1	t	0	1	0.01	t	t	0.04	t	0	5	5	0	0
0	13	398	41	0.5	0.3	0	5	0.02	0.03	0.7	0.15	11	0	17	26	*	0.7
0	3	248	16	0.4	1	0	12	0.04	0.03	0.6	0.06	6	0	35	19	*	*
0	600	428	71	3.9	2.7	5	19	0.23	0.13	1	0.98	146	0	123	275	*	0
0	6	644	26	5.1	0.2	3	6	0.3	0.09	2	0.12	20	0	21	117	*	0.3

WT, weight; **KCAL,** kcalories; **PROT,** protein; **CARB,** carbohydrate; **FIBR,** fiber; **FAT,** fat; **SATF,** saturated fat;
MONO, monosaturated fat; **POLY,** polyunsaturated fat; **CHOR,** cholesterol; **SOD,** sodium; **POT,** potassium;

Food Name	Portion	WT (Gm)	KCAL	PROT (Gm)	CARB (Gm)	FIBR (Gm)	FAT (Gm)	SATF (Gm)	MONO (Gm)	POLY (Gm)
KALE-FROZEN-BOILED-DRAINED	CUP	130	39	4	7	3.8	1	0.1	t	0.3
KALE-RAW-BOILED-DRAINED	CUP	130	42	2	7	4.3	1	0.1	t	0.3
KOHLRABI-BOILED-DRAINED	CUP	165	48	3	11	3.3	t	t	t	0.1
KOHLRABI-RAW	CUP	140	38	2	9	2.5	t	t	t	0.1
LEEKS-BOILED-DRAINED	ITEM	124	38	1	9	4	t	t	t	0.1
LEEKS-RAW	ITEM	124	76	2	18	2.5	t	0.1	t	0.2
LENTILS-SPROUTED-RAW	CUP	77	82	7	17	6.2	t	t	0.1	0.2
LENTILS-WHOLE-COOKED	CUP	198	231	18	40	9.8	1	0.1	0.1	0.3
LETTUCE-BUTTERHEAD-HEAD	ITEM	163	21	2	4	1.6	t	t	t	0.2
LETTUCE-BUTTERHEAD-LEAVES	SLICE	15	2	t	t	0.2	t	t	t	t
LETTUCE-ICEBERG-RAW-CHOPPED	CUP	55	7	1	1	0.6	t	t	t	0.1
LETTUCE-ICEBERG-RAW-HEAD	ITEM	539	70	5	11	5.4	1	0.1	t	0.5
LETTUCE-ICEBERG-RAW-LEAVES	PIECE	20	3	t	t	0.2	t	t	t	t
LETTUCE-LOOSELEAF-RAW	CUP	55	10	1	2	0.8	t	t	t	0.1
LETTUCE-ROMAINE-RAW-SHREDDED	CUP	56	9	1	1	1	t	t	t	0.1
LOTUS ROOT-BOILED-DRAINED	OUNCE	28.4	19	t	5	0.9	t	t	t	t
LOTUS ROOT-RAW	ITEM	115	64	3	20	3.5	t	t	t	t
MISO-FERMENTED SOYBEANS	CUP	275	567	33	77	9.9	17	2.4	3.7	9.4
MUSHROOMS-BOILED-DRAINED	ITEM	12	3	t	1	0.3	t	t	t	t
MUSHROOMS-CANNED-DRAINED	ITEM	12	3	t	1	0.2	t	t	t	t
MUSHROOMS-RAW-CHOPPED	CUP	70	18	1	3	0.9	t	t	t	0.1
MUSTARD GREENS-BOILED-DRAINED	CUP	140	21	3	3	2.7	t	t	0.2	0.1
NATTO-FERMENTED SOYBEANS	CUP	280	468	47	32	9.7	21	4.5	6.8	17.4
NUTS-CHESTNUTS-CHINESE-DRIED	OUNCE	28.4	103	2	23	2.2	1	0.1	0.3	0.1
NUTS-CHESTNUTS-CHINESE-RAW	OUNCE	28.4	64	1	14	2.2	t	t	0.2	0.1
NUTS-CHESTNUTS-ROASTED	OUNCE	28.4	68	1	15	2.2	t	0.1	0.2	0.1
OKRA-RAW-BOILED-DRAINED	CUP	160	51	3	12	2	t	0.1	t	0.1
ONION RINGS-FROZEN-PREPARED-HEATED	ITEM	10	41	1	4	0.4	3	0.9	1.1	0.5
ONIONS-MATURE-BOILED-DRAINED	CUP	210	92	3	21	1.7	t	0.1	0.1	0.2
ONIONS-MATURE-RAW-CHOPPED	CUP	160	61	2	14	2.6	t	t	t	0.1
ONIONS-YOUNG GREEN	ITEM	5	1	t	t	0.1	t	t	0	0
PARSLEY-RAW-CHOPPED	TBSP	4	1	t	t	0.2	t	t	t	t
PARSNIPS-SLICED-BOILED-DRAINED	CUP	156	126	2	31	7.6	t	0.1	0.2	0.1
PEAS-BLACKEYE/COWPEAS-BOILED-DRAINED	CUP	165	179	13	30	15.8	1	0.3	0.1	0.4
PEAS-BLACKEYE/COWPEAS-FROZEN-BOILED	CUP	170	224	14	40	9.8	1	0.3	0.1	0.5
PEAS-BLACKEYE/COWPEAS-RAW-BOILED	CUP	165	160	5	34	11	1	0.2	0.1	0.3
PEAS-EDIBLE PODDED-RAW	CUP	145	61	4	11	3.8	t	0.1	t	0.1
PEAS-GREEN-CANNED-DIETARY-LOW SODIUM	CUP	170	117	8	21	5.8	1	0.1	0.1	0.3
PEAS-GREEN-CANNED-DRAINED	CUP	170	117	8	21	5.8	1	0.1	0.1	0.3
PEAS-GREEN-FROZEN-BOILED-DRAINED	CUP	160	125	8	23	6.1	t	0.1	t	0.2
PEAS-SPLIT-DRY-COOKED	CUP	200	230	16	42	10.5	1	0.1	0.2	0.3
PEAS-SWEET-CANNED IN WATER-DIETETIC	OUNCE	28.4	12	1	2	0.6	t	0	0	0
PEPPERS-HOT CHILI-CANNED	CUP	136	34	1	8	2.1	t	t	t	0.1
PEPPERS-HOT CHILI-RAW	CUP	150	60	3	14	3.6	t	t	t	0.2
PEPPERS-HOT-RED-DRIED	TSP	2	5	0	1	0.7	0	0	0	0
PEPPERS-JALAPENO-CANNED-CHOPPED	CUP	136	33	1	1	2	1	0.1	t	0.4
PEPPERS-SWEET-BOILED-DRAINED	ITEM	73	20	1	5	0.7	t	t	t	0.1
PEPPERS-SWEET-RAW	ITEM	74	20	1	5	1.2	t	t	t	0.1
PIMIENTOS-4 OUNCE CAN OR JAR	ITEM	113	31	1	7	2.6	1	0.1	t	0.4
POI-TARO ROOT PRODUCT	CUP	240	269	1	65	4.8	t	0.1	t	0.1
POTATO CHIPS-SALT ADDED	ITEM	2	11	t	1	t	1	0.2	0.1	0.4
POTATO PANCAKES-HOME RECIPE	ITEM	76	495	5	26	1.4	13	3.4	5.4	2.5
POTATO PUFFS-FROZEN-HEATED	ITEM	7	16	t	2	0.2	1	0.4	0.3	0.1
POTATO SKIN-BAKED	ITEM	58	115	2	27	3	t	t	t	t
POTATO-AU GRATIN-HOME RECIPE	CUP	245	323	12	28	4.4	19	11.6	5.3	0.7
POTATO-AU GRATIN-PREPARED FROM MIX	OUNCE	28.4	26	1	4	0.5	1	0.7	0.3	t
POTATO-BAKED-FLESH & SKIN-WHOLE	ITEM	202	220	5	51	4.9	t	0.1	t	0.1
POTATO-BAKED-PEELED AFTER BAKING	ITEM	156	145	3	34	3.7	t	t	t	0.1
POTATO-BOILED-PEELED AFTER BOILING	ITEM	136	118	3	27	2	t	t	t	0.1
POTATO-BOILED-PEELED BEFORE BOILING	ITEM	135	116	2	27	1.5	t	t	t	0.1
POTATO-CANNED-DRAINED	ITEM	35	21	t	5	0.9	t	t	t	t
POTATO-FRENCH FRIED-PREPARED FROM FROZEN	ITEM	5	11	t	2	0.2	t	0.2	0.2	t
POTATO-FRENCH FRIED-PREPARED FROM RAW	ITEM	5	14	t	2	0.2	1	0.2	0.2	t
POTATO-HASH BROWN-PREPARED FROM RAW	CUP	156	239	4	12	3.1	22	8.5	9.7	2.5

t = Trace of nutrient present ** = Not available*

MAG, magnesium; **IRON,** iron; **ZINC,** zinc; **VITA,** vitamin A; **VITC,** vitamin C; **THIA,** thiamin; **RIBO,** riboflavin; **NIAC,** niacin; **VB6,** vitamin B-6; **FOL,** folate; **VB12,** vitamin B-12; **CALC,** calcium; **PHOS,** phosphorus; **SEL,** selenium; **VE-a,** alpha tocopherol equivalents.

CHOL (mg)	SOD (mg)	POT (mg)	MAG (mg)	IRON (mg)	ZINC (mg)	VITA (RE)	VITC (mg)	THIA (mg)	RIBO (mg)	NIAC (mg)	VB6 (mg)	FOL (µg)	VB12 (µg)	CALC (mg)	PHOS (mg)	SEL (µg)	VE-a (mg)
0	20	417	23	1.2	0.2	826	33	0.06	0.15	0.9	0.11	19	0	179	36	1	10.4
0	30	296	23	1.2	0.3	962	53	0.07	0.09	0.7	0.18	17	0	94	36	1	10.4
0	35	561	31	0.7	0.5	7	89	0.07	0.03	0.6	0.25	20	0	41	74	*	2.7
0	28	490	27	0.6	t	6	87	0.07	0.03	0.6	0.21	23	0	34	64	1	t
0	12	108	17	1.4	0.1	6	5	0.03	0.03	0.2	0.14	30	0	37	21	0	1.1
0	25	223	35	2.6	0.1	12	15	0.07	0.04	0.5	0.29	80	0	73	43	0	1.1
0	8	248	29	2.5	1.2	4	13	0.18	0.1	0.9	0.15	77	0	19	133	8	1
0	4	731	71	6.6	2.5	2	3	0.34	0.15	2.1	0.35	358	0	37	356	20	0.2
0	8	419	21	0.5	0.3	158	13	0.1	0.1	0.5	0.08	119	0	52	38	2	0.9
0	1	39	2	t	t	15	1	0.01	0.01	t	0.01	11	0	5	3	0	0.1
0	5	87	5	0.3	0.1	18	2	0.03	0.02	0.1	0.02	31	0	11	11	0	0.2
0	49	852	49	2.7	1.2	178	21	0.25	0.16	1	0.22	302	0	102	108	5	2.3
0	2	32	2	0.1	t	7	1	0.01	0.01	t	0.01	11	0	4	4	0	0.1
0	5	145	6	0.8	0.2	105	10	0.03	0.04	0.2	0.03	27	0	37	14	0	0.2
0	4	162	3	0.6	0.1	146	13	0.06	0.06	0.3	0.03	76	0	20	25	0	0.2
0	13	103	6	0.3	0.1	0	8	0.04	t	0.1	0.06	2	0	7	22	*	t
0	46	639	27	1.3	0.4	0	51	0.18	0.25	0.5	0.21	15	0	52	115	*	t
0	10030	451	116	7.5	9.1	25	0	0.27	0.69	2.4	0.59	91	0	182	421	*	*
0	t	43	1	0.2	0.1	0	t	0.01	0.04	0.5	0.01	2	0	1	10	1	t
0	51	16	2	0.1	0.1	0	0	0.01	t	0.2	0.01	1	0	1	8	5	t
0	3	259	7	0.9	0.5	0	2	0.07	0.31	2.9	0.07	15	0	4	73	9	0.1
0	22	283	21	1	0.2	424	35	0.06	0.09	0.6	0	103	0	103	58	1	2.8
0	20	697	322	10.4	8.5	0	0	0.07	0.5	1.1	0.36	22	0	103	182	*	t
0	2	206	39	0.7	0.4	9	17	0.07	0.08	0.4	0.19	31	0	8	44	2	0.1
0	1	127	24	0.4	0.2	6	10	0.05	0.05	0.2	0.12	19	0	5	27	2	0.1
0	1	135	26	0.4	0.3	t	11	0.04	0.03	0.4	0.12	21	0	5	29	2	0.1
0	8	515	91	0.7	0.9	92	26	0.21	0.09	1.4	0.3	73	0	101	90	1	1.1
0	38	13	2	0.2	t	2	t	0.03	0.01	0.4	0.01	1	0	3	8	*	0.1
0	6	349	23	0.5	0.4	0	11	0.09	0.05	0.3	0.27	32	0	46	74	7	0.3
0	5	251	16	0.4	0.3	0	10	0.07	0.03	0.2	0.19	30	0	32	53	3	0.5
0	t	13	1	0.1	t	25	2	t	0.01	t	t	1	0	3	2	0	t
0	2	21	2	0.2	t	21	4	t	t	0.1	t	7	0	5	2	0	0.1
0	16	574	46	0.9	0.4	0	20	0.13	0.08	1.1	0.15	91	0	58	108	1	1.6
0	7	693	83	2.4	1.3	105	3	0.11	0.18	1.8	0.08	173	0	46	197	0	0.2
0	9	638	85	3.6	2.4	13	5	0.44	0.11	1.2	0.16	240	0	40	208	*	0.2
0	7	690	86	1.9	1.7	130	4	0.17	0.24	2.3	0.11	210	0	211	84	*	0.2
0	6	290	35	3	0.4	20	87	0.22	0.12	0.9	0.23	61	0	62	77	1	0.2
0	3	294	29	1.6	1.2	131	16	0.21	0.13	1.2	0.11	75	0	34	114	2	t
0	372	294	29	1.6	1.2	131	16	0.21	0.13	1.2	0.11	75	0	34	114	1	t
0	139	269	46	2.5	1.5	107	16	0.45	0.16	2.4	0.18	94	0	38	144	1	0.2
0	8	592	72	3.4	2.1	8	1	0.3	0.18	1.8	0.1	129	0	22	178	3	0.2
0	1	27	5	0.6	0.2	16	3	0.02	0.02	0.2	*	*	0	6	17	0	1
0	1595	254	19	0.7	0.2	83	92	0.03	0.07	1.1	0.21	14	0	10	24	*	0.9
0	10	510	38	1.8	0.5	116	364	0.14	0.14	1.4	0.42	35	0	26	68	*	1
0	20	20	3	0.3	0.1	130	0	0	0.02	0.2	t	t	0	5	4	0	t
0	1990	185	16	3.8	0.3	231	18	0.04	0.07	0.7	0.28	18	0	35	23	0	0.9
0	1	121	7	0.3	0.1	43	54	0.04	0.02	0.3	0.17	11	0	7	13	0	0.5
0	1	131	7	0.3	0.1	47	66	0.05	0.02	0.4	0.18	16	0	7	14	0	0.5
0	35	311	6	1.7	0.2	260	107	0.02	0.07	0.5	0.19	14	0	8	19	*	1
0	28	439	58	2.1	0.5	5	10	0.31	0.1	2.6	0.66	51	0	37	94	*	0.5
0	9	26	1	t	t	0	1	t	0	0.1	0.01	1	0	1	3	0	0.1
93	388	538	24	1.2	0.7	9	t	0.1	0.1	1.6	0.29	22	0.22	21	78	*	1.1
0	52	27	1	0.1	t	t	t	0.01	0.01	0.2	0.02	1	0	2	3	*	0.3
0	12	332	25	4.1	0.3	0	8	0.07	0.06	1.8	0.36	13	0	20	59	*	t
56	1061	970	49	1.6	1.7	93	24	0.16	0.28	2.4	0.43	20	0.49	292	277	*	1.6
*	125	62	4	0.1	0.1	9	1	0.01	0.02	0.3	0.01	2	0	24	27	*	*
0	16	844	55	2.8	0.7	*	26	0.22	0.07	3.3	0.7	22	0	20	115	1	0.1
0	8	610	39	0.6	0.5	0	20	0.16	0.03	2.2	0.47	14	0	8	78	1	t
0	5	515	30	0.4	0.4	0	18	0.14	0.03	2	0.41	14	0	7	60	1	t
0	7	443	26	0.4	0.4	0	10	0.13	0.03	1.8	0.36	12	0	10	54	1	t
0	91	80	5	0.4	0.1	0	2	0.02	0.01	0.3	0.07	2	0	2	10	1	0.1
0	2	23	1	0.1	t	0	1	0.01	t	0.1	0.01	1	0	t	4	0	t
0	11	43	2	0.1	t	0	1	0.01	t	0.2	0.01	1	0	1	6	0	t
0	37	501	31	1.3	0.5	0	9	0.12	0.03	3.1	0.43	12	0	13	66	*	0.3

WT, weight; **KCAL,** kcalories; **PROT,** protein; **CARB,** carbohydrate; **FIBR,** fiber; **FAT,** fat; **SATF,** saturated fat; **MONO,** monosaturated fat; **POLY,** polyunsaturated fat; **CHOR,** cholesterol; **SOD,** sodium; **POT,** potassium;

Food Name	Portion	WT (Gm)	KCAL	PROT (Gm)	CARB (Gm)	FIBR (Gm)	FAT (Gm)	SATF (Gm)	MONO (Gm)	POLY (Gm)
POTATO-HASH BROWN-PREPARED FROM FROZEN	CUP	156	340	5	44	1.5	18	7	8	2.1
POTATO-HUSH PUPPIES	SERVING	78	256	5	35	1.9	12	2.7	7.8	0.4
POTATO-MASHED-FROM DEHYDRATED-WITH MILK	CUP	210	166	4	28	1.2	5	1.4	1.4	1.3
POTATO-MASHED-FROM RAW-WITH MILK	CUP	210	162	4	37	1.2	1	0.7	0.3	0.1
POTATO-MASHED-HOME RECIPE-MILK/BUTTER	CUP	210	223	4	35	3.2	9	2.2	3.7	2.5
POTATO-O'BRIEN-HOME RECIPE	CUP	194	157	5	30	*	2	1.6	0.7	0.1
POTATO-SCALLOPED-HOME RECIPE	CUP	245	211	7	26	4.4	9	5.5	2.6	0.4
POTATO-SCALLOPED-PREPARED FROM MIX	OUNCE	28.4	26	1	4	0.5	1	0.7	0.3	0.1
PUMPKIN PIE MIX-CANNED	CUP	270	281	3	71	*	t	0.2	t	t
PUMPKIN-BOILED-DRAINED-MASHED	CUP	245	49	2	12	6.7	t	0.1	t	t
PUMPKIN-CANNED	CUP	245	83	3	20	5	1	0.4	0.1	t
PUMPKIN-RAW-CUBED	CUP	116	30	1	8	2	t	0.1	t	t
RADISH-DAIKON-SLICED-BOILED-DRAINED	CUP	147	25	1	5	2.9	t	0.1	0.1	0.2
RADISHES-RAW	ITEM	4.5	1	t	t	0.1	t	t	t	t
RUTABAGAS-BOILED-DRAINED	CUP	170	58	2	13	2.5	t	t	t	0.1
SAUERKRAUT-CANNED	CUP	236	45	2	10	6.1	t	0.1	t	0.1
SEAWEED-AGAR-DRIED	SERVING	28.4	87	2	23	0.9	t	t	t	t
SEAWEED-IRISHMOSS-RAW	OUNCE	28.4	14	t	3	1	t	t	t	t
SEAWEED-KELP (KOMBU)-RAW	OUNCE	28.4	12	t	3	1.2	t	0.1	t	t
SEAWEED-LAVER (NORI)-RAW	OUNCE	28.4	10	2	1	1	t	t	t	t
SEAWEED-SPIRULINA-DRIED	OUNCE	28.4	82	16	7	1.4	2	0.8	0.2	0.6
SEAWEED-WAKAME-RAW	OUNCE	28.4	13	1	3	1.2	t	t	t	0.1
SHALLOTS-FREEZE DRIED	TBSP	0.9	3	t	1	0.1	t	t	t	t
SHALLOTS-RAW	TBSP	10	7	t	2	*	t	t	t	t
SOYBEANS-DRY-COOKED	CUP	180	234	20	19	*	10	*	*	*
SOYBEANS-GREEN-BOILED-DRAINED	CUP	180	254	22	20	*	12	1.3	1.3	6.4
SOYBEANS-SPROUTED-STEAMED	CUP	94	76	8	6	1	4	0.5	0.5	2.3
SPINACH-CANNED-DIETARY PACK-LOW SODIUM	CUP	234	45	5	7	5.1	1	0.1	t	0.4
SPINACH-CANNED-DRAINED	CUP	214	50	6	7	6.8	1	0.2	t	0.4
SPINACH-CANNED-SOLIDS AND LIQUIDS	CUP	234	45	5	7	5.1	1	0.1	t	0.4
SPINACH-FROZEN-BOILED-CHOPPED	CUP	205	57	6	11	4.5	t	0.1	t	0.2
SPINACH-LEAF-FROZEN-BOILED-DRAINED	CUP	190	53	6	10	4	t	0.1	t	0.2
SPINACH-RAW-BOILED-DRAINED	CUP	180	41	5	7	4	t	0.1	t	0.2
SPINACH-RAW-CHOPPED	CUP	56	12	2	2	1.5	t	t	t	0.1
SQUASH-ACORN-BAKED	CUP	205	115	2	30	4.3	t	0.1	t	0.1
SQUASH-BUTTERNUT-BAKED	CUP	205	82	2	22	3.5	t	t	t	0.1
SQUASH-HUBBARD-BOILED-MASHED	CUP	236	71	3	15	4.2	1	0.2	0.1	0.4
SQUASH-SUMMER-BOILED-SLICED	CUP	180	36	2	8	2.5	1	0.1	t	0.2
SQUASH-WINTER-BAKE-MASHED	CUP	205	80	2	18	5.7	1	0.3	0.1	0.5
SQUASH-ZUCCHINI-FROZ-BOILED	CUP	223	38	3	8	3.2	t	0.1	t	0.1
SQUASH-ZUCCHINI-ITALIA-CANNED	CUP	227	66	2	16	7	t	0.1	t	0.1
SQUASH-ZUCCHINI-RAW-BOILED	CUP	180	29	1	7	2.3	t	t	t	t
SQUASH-ZUCCHINI-RAW-SLICED	CUP	130	18	2	4	2	t	t	t	0.1
SUCCOTASH-BOILED-DRAINED	CUP	192	221	10	47	14	2	0.3	0.3	0.7
SWEET POTATO-BAKED-PEELED	ITEM	114	117	2	28	3.4	t	t	t	0.1
SWEET POTATO-BOILED-MASHED	CUP	328	344	5	80	9.8	1	0.2	t	0.4
SWEET POTATO-CANDIED	PIECE	105	144	1	29	1.1	3	1.4	0.7	0.2
SWEET POTATO-CANNED-MASHED	CUP	255	258	5	59	4.6	1	0.1	t	0.2
SWEET POTATO-CANNED-VACUUM PACK	CUP	200	182	3	42	4.8	t	0.1	t	0.2
TARO ROOT-COOKED-SLICED	CUP	132	187	1	46	6	t	t	t	0.1
TARO ROOT-RAW-SLICED	CUP	104	111	2	28	*	t	t	t	0.1
TEMPEH-SOYBEAN PRODUCT	CUP	166	330	32	28	*	13	1.8	2.8	7.2
TOFU-FRIED	PIECE	13	35	2	1	0.2	3	0.4	0.6	1.5
TOFU-OKARA	CUP	122	94	4	15	5	2	0.2	0.4	0.9
TOFU-RAW-FIRM	CUP	252	365	40	11	3	22	3.2	4.9	12.4
TOFU-SOYBEAN CURD	PIECE	120	86	9	3	1.4	5	2.6	4.4	4.8
TOMATO JUICE-CANNED	CUP	244	42	2	10	2.9	t	t	t	0.1
TOMATO JUICE-LOW SODIUM	CUP	244	42	2	10	2.8	t	t	t	0.1
TOMATO PASTE-CANNED-LOW SODIUM	CUP	262	220	10	49	11.3	2	0.3	0.4	0.9
TOMATO PASTE-CANNED-SALT ADDED	CUP	262	220	10	49	11.3	2	0.3	0.4	0.9
TOMATO POWDER	OUNCE	28.4	86	4	21	0.7	t	t	t	0.1
TOMATO PUREE-CANNED-LOW SODIUM	CUP	250	103	4	25	5.8	t	t	t	0.1
TOMATO PUREE-CANNED-SALT ADDED	CUP	250	103	4	25	5.8	t	t	t	0.1

t = Trace of nutrient present ** = Not available*

MAG, magnesium; **IRON,** iron; **ZINC,** zinc; **VITA,** vitamin A; **VITC,** vitamin C; **THIA,** thiamin; **RIBO,** riboflavin; **NIAC,** niacin; **VB6,** vitamin B-6; **FOL,** folate; **VB12,** vitamin B-12; **CALC,** calcium; **PHOS,** phosphorus; **SEL,** selenium; **VE-a,** alpha tocopherol equivalents.

CHOL (mg)	SOD (mg)	POT (mg)	MAG (mg)	IRON (mg)	ZINC (mg)	VITA (RE)	VITC (mg)	THIA (mg)	RIBO (mg)	NIAC (mg)	VB6 (mg)	FOL (μg)	VB12 (μg)	CALC (mg)	PHOS (mg)	SEL (μg)	VE-a (mg)
0	54	680	26	2.3	0.5	0	10	0.17	0.03	3.8	0.2	39	0	24	112	1	0.3
135	965	188	16	1.4	0.4	9	0	0	0.02	2	0.1	21	0.18	69	190	*	1.8
4	491	704	34	1.3	0.5	19	6	0.06	0.11	1.7	0.42	15	0	65	92	1	0.1
4	636	628	39	0.6	0.6	4	14	0.19	0.08	2.4	0.49	17	0.11	55	100	1	0.1
4	620	607	38	0.5	0.6	42	13	0.18	0.08	2.3	0.47	17	0	55	97	1	0.1
7	421	516	35	0.9	0.6	93	32	0.15	0.11	2	0.41	16	0.16	70	97	*	*
29	821	926	47	1.4	1	47	26	0.17	0.23	2.6	0.44	21	0	140	154	*	1.1
*	97	58	4	0.1	0.1	6	1	0.01	0.02	0.3	0.01	t	0	10	16	*	*
0	562	373	43	2.9	0.7	2241	9	0.04	0.32	1	0.43	95	0	100	122	*	*
0	3	564	22	1.4	0.6	265	12	0.08	0.19	1	0.11	21	0	37	74	*	2.5
0	12	505	56	3.4	0.4	5404	10	0.06	0.13	0.9	0.14	30	0	64	86	*	2.5
0	1	1	14	0.9	0.4	186	10	0.06	0.13	0.7	0.06	16	0	24	51	1	1.2
0	19	419	13	0.2	0.2	0	22	0	0.03	0.2	0.06	26	0	25	35	1	0.7
0	1	10	t	t	t	t	1	0	t	t	t	1	0	1	1	0	0
0	31	488	36	0.8	0.5	0	37	0.12	0.06	1.1	0.15	26	0	71	83	*	0.3
0	1560	401	31	3.5	0.4	5	35	0.05	0.05	0.3	0.31	56	0	71	47	24	3.9
0	29	320	219	6.1	1.7	0	0	t	0.06	0.1	0.09	165	0	178	15	2	1.6
0	19	18	41	2.5	0.6	3	3	t	0.13	0.2	0.02	52	0	20	45	*	0.3
0	66	25	34	0.8	0.3	3	1	0.01	0.04	0.1	t	51	0	48	12	2	0.2
0	14	101	1	0.5	0.3	148	11	0.03	0.13	0.4	0.05	42	0	20	17	1	0.3
0	298	387	55	8.1	0.6	16	3	0.68	1.04	3.6	0.1	27	0	34	34	2	1
0	248	14	30	0.6	0.1	10	1	0.02	0.07	0.5	t	56	0	43	23	1	0.3
0	1	15	1	0.1	t	51	t	t	t	t	0.02	1	0	2	3	*	*
0	1	33	2	0.1	t	125	1	0.01	t	t	0.04	3	0	4	6	*	t
0	4	972	*	4.9	*	5	0	0.38	0.16	1.1	*	*	0	131	322	*	*
0	25	970	108	4.5	1.6	29	31	0.47	0.28	2.3	0.11	201	0	261	284	90	0
0	9	334	56	1.2	1	1	8	0.19	0.05	1	0.1	75	0	56	127	47	t
0	746	538	131	3.7	1	1505	32	0.04	0.25	0.6	0.19	136	0	194	75	3	t
0	57	740	162	4.9	1	1878	31	0.03	0.3	0.8	0.21	209	0	271	94	2	t
0	746	538	131	3.7	1	1505	32	0.04	0.25	0.6	0.19	136	0	194	75	3	t
0	176	611	141	3.1	1.4	1596	25	0.12	0.34	0.9	0.3	220	0	299	98	2	3.9
0	164	566	131	2.9	1.3	1479	23	0.11	0.32	0.8	0.28	204	0	277	91	2	3.6
0	126	839	157	6.4	1.4	1474	18	0.17	0.43	0.9	0.44	262	0	245	101	2	3.4
0	44	312	44	1.5	0.3	376	16	0.04	0.11	0.4	0.11	108	0	55	27	1	1
0	9	896	87	1.9	0.4	88	22	0.34	0.03	1.8	0.4	38	0	90	93	2	0.2
0	8	582	60	1.2	0.3	1435	31	0.15	0.04	2	0.25	39	0	84	55	2	0.2
0	12	505	32	0.7	0.2	946	15	0.1	0.07	0.8	0.24	23	0	24	33	2	0.3
0	2	346	44	0.6	0.7	52	10	0.08	0.07	0.9	0.12	36	0	48	69	6	0.2
0	2	896	16	0.7	0.5	730	20	0.17	0.05	1.4	0.15	57	0	29	41	6	0.2
0	4	433	29	1.1	0.4	96	8	0.09	0.09	0.9	0.1	17	0	38	56	7	0.3
0	850	622	31	1.5	0.6	123	5	0.1	0.09	1.2	0.35	69	0	39	66	*	0.3
0	5	455	40	0.6	0.3	43	8	0.07	0.07	0.8	0.14	30	0	23	72	6	0.2
0	4	322	29	0.5	0.3	44	12	0.09	0.04	0.5	0.12	29	0	20	42	4	0.2
0	33	787	102	2.9	1.2	56	16	0.32	0.18	2.6	0.22	63	0	33	225	*	0.7
0	11	397	23	0.5	0.3	2487	28	0.08	0.15	0.7	0.28	26	0	32	63	1	5.2
0	42	602	32	1.8	0.9	5594	56	0.17	0.46	2.1	0.8	36	0	70	88	2	15
0	73	198	12	1.2	0.2	440	7	0.02	0.04	0.4	0.04	12	0.03	27	27	1	4.6
0	191	536	61	3.4	0.5	3857	13	0.07	0.23	2.4	0.17	27	0	76	133	2	1.1
0	106	624	44	1.8	0.4	1596	53	0.07	0.11	1.5	0.38	33	0	44	98	2	0.9
0	20	638	40	1	0.4	0	7	0.14	0.04	0.7	0.44	25	0	24	100	*	3.3
0	11	615	34	0.6	0.2	0	5	0.1	0.03	0.6	0.29	23	0	45	87	*	*
0	10	609	116	3.8	3	114	0	0.22	0.18	7.7	0.5	86	1.66	154	342	*	*
0	2	19	8	0.6	0.3	0	0	0.02	0.01	t	0.01	3	0	48	37	0	t
0	11	259	32	1.6	0.7	0	0	0.02	0.02	0.1	0.14	32	0	98	73	*	*
0	35	597	237	26.4	4	43	1	0.4	0.26	1	0.23	74	0	517	479	5	*
0	8	50	115	2.3	1	0	0	0.07	0.04	0.1	0.06	21	0.05	154	151	2	1.1
0	881	537	27	1.4	0.3	137	45	0.11	0.08	1.6	0.27	49	0	22	46	1	0.5
0	24	537	27	1.4	0.3	137	45	0.11	0.08	1.6	0.27	49	0	22	46	1	0.5
0	172	2442	134	7.8	2.1	647	111	0.41	0.5	8.4	1	59	0	92	207	3	*
0	2070	2442	134	7.8	2.1	647	111	0.41	0.5	8.4	1	59	0	92	207	3	4.4
0	38	547	51	1.3	0.5	490	33	0.26	0.22	2.6	0.13	34	0	47	84	*	0.2
0	50	1050	60	2.3	0.6	340	88	0.18	0.14	4.3	0.38	28	0	38	100	3	0.6
0	998	1050	60	2.3	0.6	340	88	0.18	0.14	4.3	0.38	28	0	38	100	3	0.6

WT, weight; **KCAL,** kcalories; **PROT,** protein; **CARB,** carbohydrate; **FIBR,** fiber; **FAT,** fat; **SATF,** saturated fat;
MONO, monosaturated fat; **POLY,** polyunsaturated fat; **CHOR,** cholesterol; **SOD,** sodium; **POT,** potassium;

Food Name	Portion	WT (Gm)	KCAL	PROT (Gm)	CARB (Gm)	FIBR (Gm)	FAT (Gm)	SATF (Gm)	MONO (Gm)	POLY (Gm)
TOMATO-CANNED-DIETARY PACK-LOW SODIUM	CUP	240	48	2	10	1.7	1	0.1	0.1	0.2
TOMATO-COOKED-STEWED-HOME RECIPE	CUP	101	80	2	13	1	3	0.5	1.1	0.9
TOMATO-RED-CANNED-STEWED	CUP	255	66	2	17	2	t	0.1	0.1	0.1
TOMATO-RED-CANNED-WHOLE	CUP	240	48	2	10	1.9	1	0.1	0.1	0.2
TOMATO-RED-CANNED-WITH GREEN CHILIES	CUP	241	36	2	9	0.9	t	t	t	0.1
TOMATO-RED-RAW-BOILED	CUP	240	65	3	14	2.1	1	0.1	0.2	0.4
TOMATO-RED-RIPE-RAW	ITEM	123	26	1	6	1.6	t	0.1	0.1	0.2
TOMATOES-GREEN-RAW	ITEM	123	30	1	6	0.6	t	t	t	0.1
TURNIP GREENS-FROZEN-BOILED	CUP	164	49	5	8	5.1	1	0.2	t	0.3
TURNIP GREENS-RAW-BOILED	CUP	144	29	2	6	4.5	t	0.1	t	0.1
TURNIPS-BOILED-DRAINED-DICED	CUP	156	28	1	8	3.1	t	t	t	0.1
VEGETABLE JUICE-CANNED	CUP	242	46	2	11	2.7	t	t	t	0.1
VEGETABLE JUICE-SNAP E TOM-TOMATO	CUP	243	46	2	9	1.9	0	0	0	0
VEGETABLE JUICE-V8 COCKTAIL-LOW SODIUM	CUP	243	51	0	10	2.7	0	0	0	0
VEGETABLE JUICE-V8-REGULAR	CUP	243	49	0	10	2.4	0	0	0	0
WATERCHESTNUTS-CHINESE-CANNED	CUP	140	70	1	17	*	t	t	t	t
WATERCHESTNUTS-CHINESE-RAW	CUP	124	131	2	30	*	t	t	t	t
WATERCRESS-RAW	CUP	34	4	1	t	0.4	t	t	t	t
YAM-MOUNTAIN-HAWAII-STEAMED	CUP	145	119	3	29	5.6	t	t	t	0.1
YAMS-BOILED OR BAKED-DRAINED	CUP	136	158	2	38	3.3	t	t	t	0.1

t = Trace of nutrient present ** = Not available*

MAG, magnesium; **IRON,** iron; **ZINC,** zinc; **VITA,** vitamin A; **VITC,** vitamin C; **THIA,** thiamin; **RIBO,** riboflavin; **NIAC,** niacin; **VB6,** vitamin B-6; **FOL,** folate; **VB12,** vitamin B-12; **CALC,** calcium; **PHOS,** phosphorus; **SEL,** selenium; **VE-a,** alpha tocopherol equivalents.

CHOL (mg)	SOD (mg)	POT (mg)	MAG (mg)	IRON (mg)	ZINC (mg)	VITA (RE)	VITC (mg)	THIA (mg)	RIBO (mg)	NIAC (mg)	VB6 (mg)	FOL (μg)	VB12 (μg)	CALC (mg)	PHOS (mg)	SEL (μg)	VE-a (mg)
0	31	530	29	1.5	0.4	144	36	0.11	0.07	1.8	0.22	19	0	62	46	2	0.5
0	460	249	15	1.1	0.2	68	18	0.11	0.08	1.1	0.09	11	0	26	38	1	0.3
0	648	609	31	1.9	0.4	140	34	0.12	0.09	1.8	0.04	14	0	84	51	2	0.6
0	391	530	29	1.5	0.4	144	36	0.11	0.07	1.8	0.22	19	0	62	46	2	0.5
0	966	258	27	0.6	0.3	94	15	0.08	0.05	1.5	0.25	22	0	48	34	2	0.5
0	26	670	34	1.3	0.3	178	55	0.17	0.14	1.8	0.23	31	0	14	74	1	0.8
0	11	273	14	0.6	0.1	76	24	0.07	0.06	0.8	0.1	19	0	6	30	1	0.4
0	16	251	12	0.6	0.1	79	29	0.07	0.05	0.6	0.1	11	0	16	34	*	0.5
0	25	367	43	3.2	0.7	1309	36	0.09	0.12	0.8	0.11	65	0	249	56	1	3.7
0	42	292	32	1.2	0.2	792	40	0.07	0.1	0.6	0.26	171	0	197	42	1	3.3
0	78	211	13	0.3	0.3	0	18	0.04	0.04	0.5	0.11	14	0	34	30	1	t
0	883	467	27	1	0.5	283	67	0.1	0.07	1.8	0.34	51	0	27	41	1	0.8
0	1298	688	27	1.9	0.5	103	10	0.1	0.07	2.4	0.34	51	0	37	41	*	0.5
0	58	571	*	1.5	*	437	53	0.05	0.07	1.9	*	*	0	39	*	1	*
0	819	513	27	1.5	0.5	342	49	0.05	0.05	1.7	0.34	51	0	29	41	1	0.8
0	12	164	6	1.2	0.5	1	2	0.02	0.03	0.5	0.22	8	0	6	28	*	*
0	17	724	27	0.1	0.6	0	5	0.17	0.25	1.2	0.41	20	0	14	78	*	*
0	14	112	8	0.1	t	160	15	0.03	0.04	0.1	0.04	3	0	40	20	*	0.3
0	18	717	15	0.6	0.5	0	0	0.13	0.02	0.2	0.3	18	0	11	57	1	6.6
0	11	911	25	0.7	0.3	0	17	0.13	0.04	0.8	0.31	22	0	19	66	1	6.2

APPENDIX B

DIETARY ADVICE FOR CANADIANS

Canada has its own version of RDA, called Recommended Nutrient Intakes (RNI), published by the Minister of National Health and Welfare.

Summary of Examples of Recommended Nutrients Based on Energy Expressed as Daily Rates

Age	Gender	Energy (kcal)	Thiamin (mg)	Riboflavin (mg)	Niacin (Ne)[†]	n-3 PUFA* (g)	n-6 PUFA (g)
Months							
0–4	Both	600	0.3	0.3	4	0.5	3
5–12	Both	900	0.4	0.5	7	0.5	3
Years							
1	Both	1100	0.5	0.6	8	0.6	4
2–3	Both	1300	0.6	0.7	9	0.7	4
4–6	Both	1800	0.7	0.9	13	1.0	6
7–9	M	2200	0.9	1.1	16	1.2	7
	F	1900	0.8	1.0	14	1.0	6
10–12	M	2500	1.0	1.3	18	1.4	8
	F	2200	0.9	1.1	16	1.2	7
13–15	M	2800	1.1	1.4	20	1.5	9
	F	2200	0.9	1.1	16	1.2	7
16–18	M	3200	1.3	1.6	23	1.8	11
	F	2100	0.8	1.1	15	1.2	7
19–24	M	3000	1.2	1.5	22	1.6	10
	F	2100	0.8	1.1	15	1.2	7
25–49	M	2700	1.1	1.4	19	1.5	9
	F	1900	0.8	1.0	14	1.1	7
50–74	M	2300	0.9	1.2	16	1.3	8
	F	1800	0.8[‡]	1.0[‡]	14[‡]	1.1[‡]	7[‡]
75+	M	200	0.8	1.0	14	1.1	7
	F[§]	1700	0.8[‡]	1.0[‡]	14[‡]	1.1[‡]	7[‡]
Pregnancy (additional)							
1st Trimester		100	0.1	0.1	1	0.05	0.3
2nd Trimester		300	0.1	0.3	2	0.16	0.9
3rd Trimester		300	0.1	0.3	2	0.16	0.9
Lactation (additional)		450	0.2	0.4	3	0.25	1.5

From Scientific Review Committee: Nutrition recommendation, *Ottawa, Canada, 1990, Health and Welfare.*
*PUFA, *polyunsaturated fatty acids.*
[†] *Niacin equivalents.*
[‡] *Level below which intake should not fall.*
[§] *Assumes moderate physical activity.*

Summary Examples of Recommended Nutrient Intake Based on Age and Body Weight Expressed as Daily Rates

Age	Gender	Weight (kg)	Protein (g)	Vit. A (RE)*	Vit. D (μg)	Vit. E (mg)	Vit. C (mg)	Folate (μg)	Vit. B_{12} (μg)	Calcium (mg)	Phosphorus (mg)	Magnesium (mg)	Iron (mg)	Iodine (μg)	Zinc (mg)
Months															
0–4	Both	6.0	12[†]	400	10	3	20	25	0.3	250[‡]	150	20	0.3[§]	30	2
5–12	Both	9.0	12	400	10	3	20	40	0.4	400	200	32	7	40	3
Years															
1	Both	11	13	400	10	3	20	40	0.5	500	300	40	6	55	4
2–3	Both	14	16	400	5	4	20	50	0.6	550	350	50	6	65	4
4–6	Both	18	19	500	5	5	25	70	0.8	600	400	65	8	85	5
7–9	M	25	26	700	2.5	7	25	90	1.0	700	500	100	8	110	7
	F	25	26	700	2.5	6	25	90	1.0	700	500	100	8	95	7
10–12	M	34	34	800	2.5	8	25	120	1.0	900	700	130	8	125	9
	F	36	36	800	2.5	7	25	130	1.0	1100	800	135	8	110	9
13–15	M	50	49	900	2.5	9	30	175	1.0	1100	900	185	10	160	12
	F	48	46	800	2.5	7	30	170	1.0	1000	850	180	13	160	9
16–18	M	62	58	1000	2.5	10	40[‖]	220	1.0	900	1000	230	10	160	12
	F	53	47	800	2.5	7	30[‖]	190	1.0	700	850	200	12	160	9
19–24	M	71	61	1000	2.5	10	40[‖]	220	1.0	800	1000	240	9	160	12
	F	58	50	800	2.5	7	30[‖]	180	1.0	700	850	200	13	160	9
25–49	M	74	64	1000	2.5	9	40[‖]	230	1.0	800	1000	250	9	160	12
	F	59	51	800	2.5	6	30[‖]	185	1.0	700	850	200	13	160	9
50–74	M	73	63	1000	5	7	40[‖]	230	1.0	800	1000	250	9	160	12
	F	63	54	800	5	6	30[‖]	195	1.0	800	850	210	8	160	9
75 +	M	69	59	1000	5	6	40[‖]	215	1.0	800	1000	230	9	160	12
	F	64	55	800	5	5	30[‖]	200	1.0	800	850	210	8	160	9
Pregnancy (additional)															
1st Trimester			5	0	2.5	2	0	200	1.2	500	200	15	0	25	6
2nd Trimester			20	0	2.5	2	10	200	1.2	500	200	45	5	25	6
3rd Trimester			24	0	2.5	2	10	200	1.2	500	200	45	10	25	6
Lactation (additional)			20	400	2.5	3	25	100	0.2	500	200	65	0	50	6

From Scientific Review Committee: Nutrition recommendations, *Ottawa, Canada, 1990, Health and Welfare.*

* *Retinol equivalents.*

† *Protein is assumed to be from breast milk and must be adjusted for infant formula.*

‡ *Infant formula with high phosphorus should contain 375 mg calcium.*

§ *Breast milk is assumed to be the source of the mineral.*

‖ *Smokers should increase vitamin C by 50%.*

B

SUMMARY OF THE DESIRED CHARACTERISTICS OF THE CANADIAN DIET

1. **The Canadian diet should provide energy consistent with the maintenance of body weight within the recommended range.** Physical activity should be appropriate to circumstances and capabilities. While the importance of maintaining some activity throughout life can be stressed, it is not possible to specify a level of physical activity appropriate for the whole population. As a general guideline it is desirable that adults, for as long as possible, maintain an activity level that permits an energy intake of at least 1800 kcalories while keeping weight within the recommended range.
2. **The Canadian diet should include essential nutrients in amounts recommended in this report.** While it is important that the diet provide the recommended amounts of nutrients, it should be understood that no evidence was found that intakes in excess of the RNI confer any health benefit. There is no general need for supplements except for vitamin D for infants and folate during pregnancy. Vitamin D supplementation might be required for elderly persons not exposed to the sun, and iron for pregnant women with low iron stores.
3. **The Canadian diet should include no more than 30% of energy as fat (33 g/1000 kcalories) and no more than 10% as saturated fat (11 g/1000 kcalories).** Dietary cholesterol, though not as influential in affecting levels of blood cholesterol, is not without importance. A reduction in cholesterol intake normally will accompany a reduction in total fat and saturated fat. The recommendation to reduce total fat intake does not apply to children under the age of 2 years.
4. **The Canadian diet should provide 55% of energy as carbohydrate (138 g/1000 kcalories) from a variety of sources.** Sources should be selected that provide complex carbohydrates, a variety of dietary fiber, and ***beta-carotene.***
5. **The sodium content of the Canadian diet should be reduced.** The present food supply provides sodium in an amount greatly exceeding requirements. While there is insufficient evidence to support a precise recommendation, potential benefit would be expected from a reduction in current sodium intake.
6. **The Canadian diet should include no more than 5% of total energy as alcohol, or two drinks daily, whichever is less.** The harmful influence of alcohol on blood pressure provides a more urgent reason for moderation. During pregnancy it is prudent to abstain from alcoholic beverages, because a safe intake is not known with certainty.
7. **The Canadian diet should contain no more caffeine than the equivalent of four regular cups of coffee per day.** This is a prudent measure in view of the increased risk for cardiovascular disease associated with high intakes of caffeine.
8. **Community water supplies containing less than 1 mg/liter should be fluoridated to that level.** Fluoridation of community water supplies has proven to be a safe, effective, and economical method of improving dental health.

In essence, suggested actions toward healthful eating as listed in Canada's *Guidelines for Healthy Eating* include the following:

- Enjoy a variety of foods.
- Emphasize cereals, breads, other grain products, vegetables, and fruits.
- Choose low-fat dairy products, lean meats, and foods prepared with little or no fat.
- Achieve and maintain a healthful body weight by enjoying regular physical activity and healthful eating.
- Limit salt, alcohol, and caffeine.

More details are available on RNI and diet recommendations in the 1990 publication entitled *Nutrition Recommendations: The Report of the Scientific Review Committee.*

A separate Canadian food guide, illustrated on the following pages, provides a plan to meet these nutrient needs.

B

Healthy Canada

Health and Welfare Canada | Santé et Bien-être social Canada

CANADA'S

Food Guide

TO HEALTHY EATING

Enjoy a variety of foods from each group every day.

Choose lower-fat foods more often.

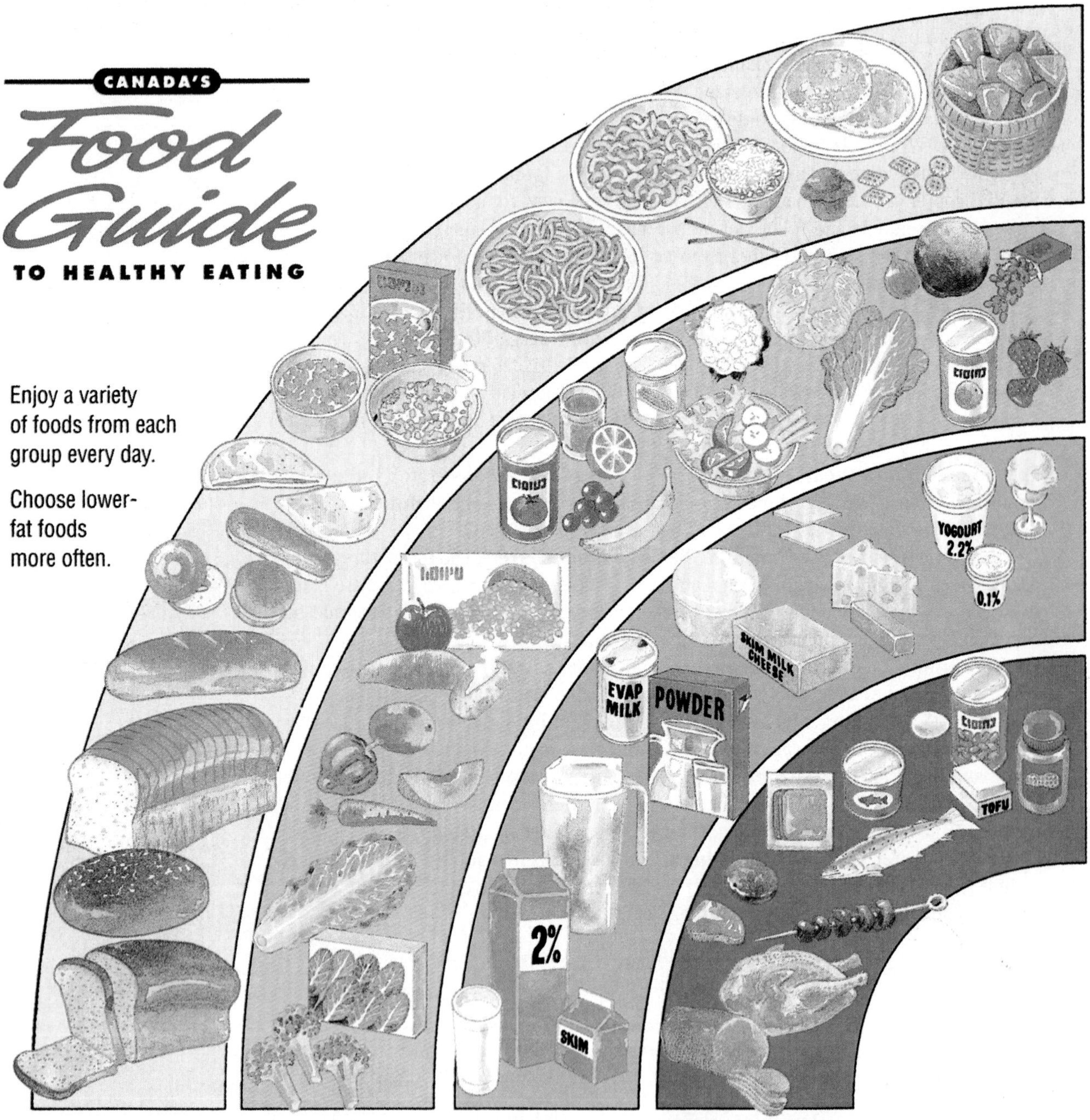

Grain Products
Choose whole grain and enriched products more often.

Vegetables & Fruit
Choose dark green and orange vegetables and orange fruit more often.

Milk Products
Choose lower-fat milk products more often.

Meat & Alternatives
Choose leaner meats, poultry and fish, as well as dried peas, beans and lentils more often.

Canada

CANADA'S
Food Guide
TO HEALTHY EATING

FOR PEOPLE FOUR YEARS AND OVER

Different People Need Different Amounts of Food

The amount of food you need every day from the 4 food groups and other foods depends on your age, body size, activity level, whether you are male or female and if you are pregnant or breast-feeding. That's why the Food Guide gives a lower and higher number of servings for each food group. For example, young children can choose the lower number of servings, while male teenagers can go to the higher number. Most other people can choose servings somewhere in between.

Grain Products
5–12
SERVINGS PER DAY

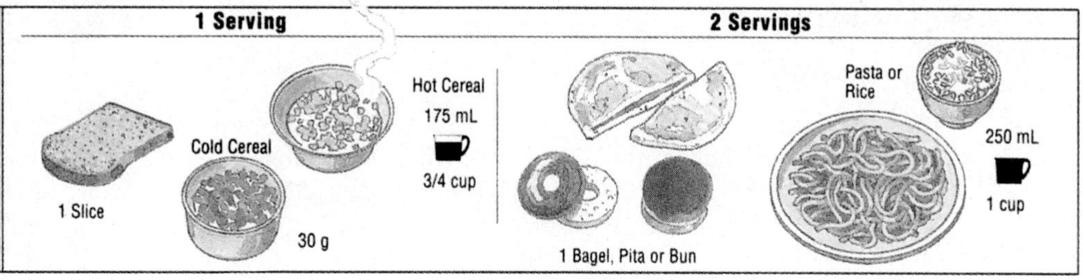

Vegetables & Fruit
5–10
SERVINGS PER DAY

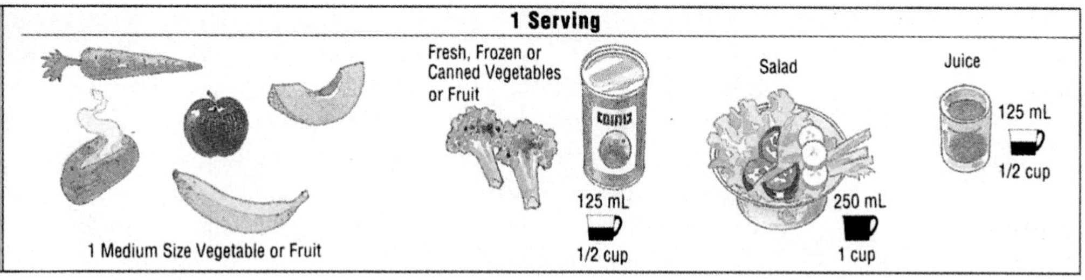

Milk Products
SERVINGS PER DAY
Children 4–9 years: 2–3
Youth 10–16 years: 3–4
Adults: 2–4
Pregnant & Breast-feeding Women: 3–4

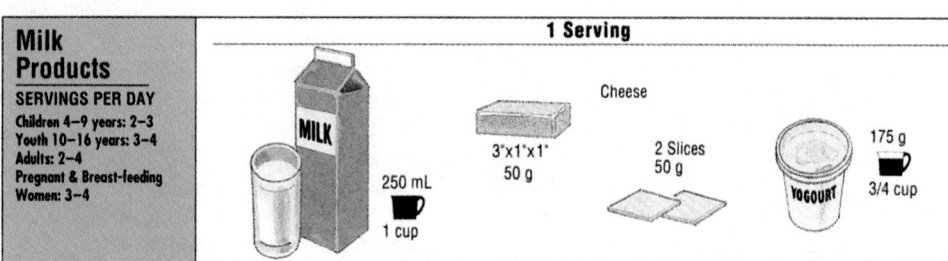

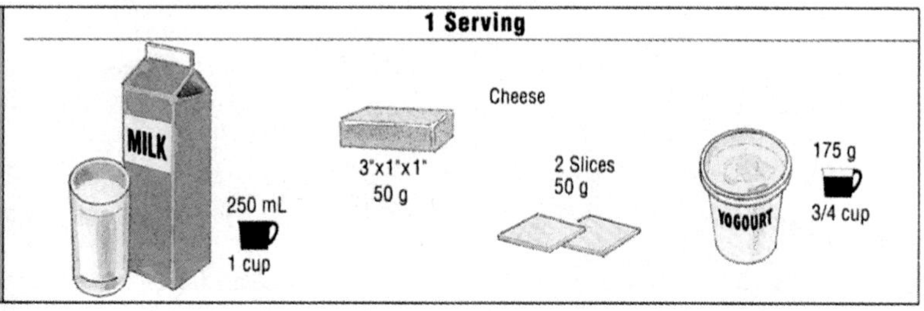

Meat & Alternatives
2-3
SERVINGS PER DAY

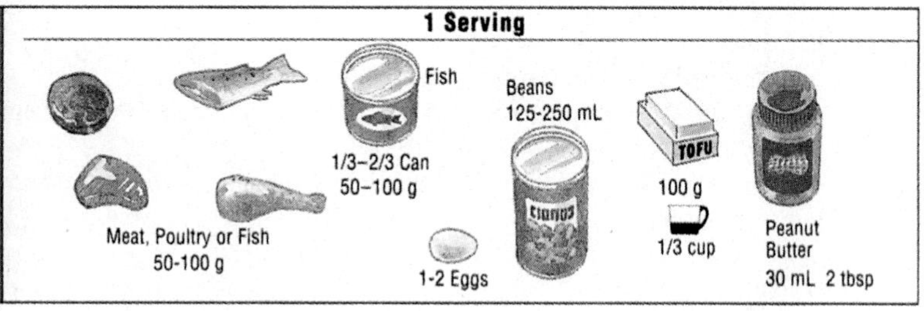

Other Foods

Taste and enjoyment can also come from other foods and beverages that are not part of the 4 food groups. Some of these foods are higher in fat or Calories, so use these foods in moderation.

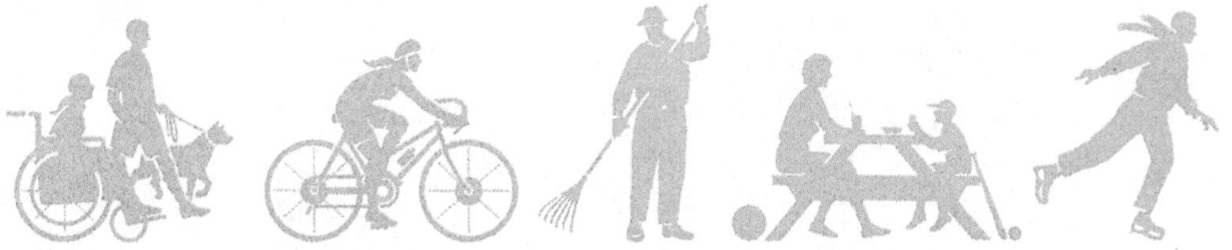

Enjoy eating well, being active and feeling good about yourself. That's VITALITE.

ISBN 0-662-19648-1

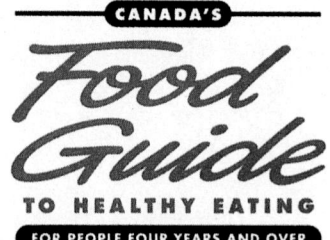

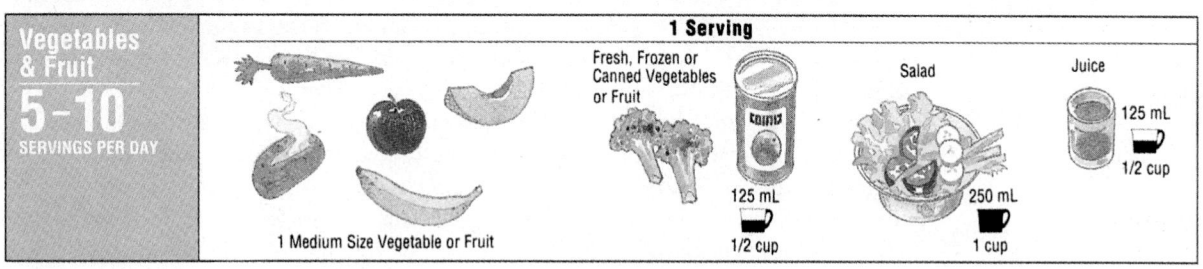

APPENDIX C

DIETARY INTAKE ASSESSMENT

Though it may seem overwhelming at first, it is actually very easy to track the foods you eat. One tip is to record foods and beverages consumed as close as possible to the actual time of consumption.

I. Fill in the food record form that follows. We supply a blank copy (see the completed example in Figure 16-3). Then, to estimate the nutrient values of the foods you are eating, consult food labels and the food composition table in Appendix A or use your Mosby Diet Simple II nutrition software package. If these resources do not have the serving size you need, adjust the value. If you drink ½ cup of orange juice, for example, but a table has values for only 1 cup, halve all values before you record them. Then, consider pooling all the same food to save time; if you drink a cup of 1% milk three times throughout the day, enter your milk consumption only once as 3 cups. As you record your intake for use on the nutrient analysis form that follows, consider the following tips:

- Measure and record the amounts of food eaten in portion sizes of cups, teaspoons, tablespoons, ounces, slices, or inches (or convert metric units to these units).
- Record brand names of all food products, such as "Quick Quaker Oats."
- Measure and record all those little extras, such as gravies, salad dressings, taco sauces, pickles, jelly, sugar, ketchup, and margarine.
- For beverages
  —List the type of milk, such as whole, skim, 2%, evaporated, chocolate, or reconstituted dry.
  —Indicate whether fruit juice is fresh, frozen, or canned.
  —Indicate type for other beverages, such as fruit drink, fruit-flavored drink, Kool-Aid, and hot chocolate made with water or milk.
- For fruits
  —Indicate whether fresh, frozen, dried, or canned.
  —If whole, record as number eaten and size with approximate measurements (such as 1 apple—3 inches in diameter).
  —Indicate whether processed in water, light syrup, heavy syrup, or other medium.
- For vegetables
  —Indicate whether fresh, frozen, dried, or canned.
  —Record as portion of cup, teaspoon, or tablespoon or as pieces (such as 2 carrot sticks—4 inches long, ½ inch thick).
  —Record preparation method.
- For cereals
  —Record cooked cereals in portions of tablespoon or cup (a level measurement after cooking).
  —Record dry cereal in level portions of tablespoon or cup.
  —If margarine, milk, sugar, fruit, or something else is added, then measure and record amount and type.
- For breads
  —Indicate whether whole wheat, rye, white, and so on.
  —Measure and record number and size of portion (biscuit—2 inches across, 1 inch thick; slice of homemade rye bread—3 inches by 4 inches, ¼ inch thick.
  —Sandwiches: list ALL ingredients (lettuce, mayonnaise, tomato, and so on) with amounts.

- For meats, fish, poultry, cheese
  - —Give size (length, width, thickness) in inches or weight in ounces after cooking for meats, fish, and poultry (such as cooked hamburger patty—3 inches across, ½ inch thick).
  - —Give size (length, width, thickness) in inches or weight in ounces for cheese.
  - —Record measurements only on the cooked edible part—without bone or fat that is left on the plate.
  - —Describe how meat was prepared.
- For eggs
  - —Record as soft or hard cooked, fried, scrambled, poached, or omelet.
  - —If milk, butter, or drippings are used, specify kinds and amount.
- For desserts
  - —List commercial brand or "homemade" or "bakery" under brand.
  - —Purchased candies, cookies, and cakes: Specify kind and size.
  - —Measure and record portion size of cakes, pies, and cookies by specifying thickness, diameter, and width or length, depending on the item.

Time	Minutes Spent Eating	M or S*	H†	Activity While Eating	Place of Eating	Food and Quantity	Others Present	Reason for Food Choice

*M or S; *meal or snack.*
†*Hunger (0, none; 3, maximum).*

II. Now complete the nutrient analysis form as shown using your food record. A blank copy of this form also follows for your use. Note that your Mosby Diet Simple II software will create this table for you if you simply enter all food eaten.

Nutrient Analysis Form (Sample)

Quantity	Name	Kcalories	Protein (grams)	Carbohydrate (grams)	Dietary Fiber (grams)	Fat Total (grams)	Saturated Fat (grams)	Monounsaturated Fat (grams)	Polyunsaturated Fat (grams)	Cholesterol (milligrams)	Sodium (milligrams)	Potassium (milligrams)
1 ea.	Egg bagel, 3.5 inch diam.	180	7.45	34.7	0.748	1.00	0.171	0.286	0.400	44.0	300	65.0
1 Tbsp.	Jelly	49.0	0.018	12.7	—	0.018	0.005	0.005	0.005	—	4.00	16.0
1½ cup	Orange juice, prepared fresh or frozen	165	2.52	40.2	1.49	0.210	0.025	0.037	0.045	—	3.00	711
2 ea.	Cheeseburger, McDonald's	636	30.2	57.0	0.460	32.0	13.3	12.2	2.18	80.0	1460	314
1 ea.	French fries, McDonald's	220	3.00	26.1	4.19	11.5	4.61	4.37	0.570	8.57	109	564
1½ cup	Cola beverage, regular	151	—	38.5	—	—	—	—	—	—	15.0	4.00
4 oz.	Pork loin chop, broiled, lean	261	36.2	—	—	11.9	4.09	5.35	1.43	112	88.2	476
1 ea.	Baked potato with skin	220	4.65	51.0	3.90	0.200	0.052	0.004	0.087	—	16.0	844
½ cup	Peas, frozen, cooked	63.0	4.12	11.4	3.61	0.220	0.039	0.019	0.103	—	70.0	134
20 g.	Margarine, regular or soft, 80% fat	143	0.160	0.100	—	16.1	2.76	5.70	6.92	—	216	7.54
2 cup	Iceberg lettuce, chopped	14.6	1.13	2.34	1.68	0.212	0.028	0.008	0.112	—	10.1	177
2 oz.	French dressing	300	0.318	3.63	0.431	32.0	4.94	14.2	12.4	—	666	7.03
1 cup	2% low-fat milk	121	8.12	11.7	—	4.78	2.92	1.35	0.170	22.0	122	377
2 ea.	Graham crackers	60.0	1.04	10.8	1.40	1.46	0.400	0.600	0.400	—	86.0	36.0
	Totals	2584	99.0	300	17.9	112	33.4	44.1	24.8	266	3165	3732
RDA or minimal requirement*		2900	58		—						500	2000
% of RDA		89	170		—						633	187

Values from inside cover. The values listed are for a male aged 19 to 24 years. Note that number of kcalories is just a rough estimate. It is better to base energy needs on actual energy output.

Magnesium (milligrams)	Iron (milligrams)	Zinc (milligrams)	Vitamin A (RE)	Vitamin C (milligrams)	Thiamin (milligrams)	Riboflavin (milligrams)	Niacin (milligrams)	Vitamin B-6 (milligrams)	Folate (micrograms)	Vitamin B-12 (micrograms)	Calcium (milligrams)	Phosphorus (milligrams)	Selenium (micrograms)	Vitamin E (milligrams)
18.0	2.10	0.612	7.00	—	2.58	0.197	2.40	0.030	16.3	0.065	20.0	61.0	5.00	1.80
0.720	0.120	—	0.200	0.710	0.002	0.005	0.036	0.005	2.00	—	2.00	1.00	0.360	0.016
36.0	0.411	0.192	28.5	145	0.300	0.060	0.750	0.165	163	—	33.0	60.0	0.735	0.714
45.8	5.68	5.20	134	4.10	0.600	0.480	8.66	0.230	42.0	1.82	338	410	58.0	0.560
26.7	0.605	0.320	5.00	12.5	0.122	0.020	2.26	0.218	19.0	0.027	9.10	101	0.600	0.203
3.00	0.120	0.049	—	—	—	—	—	—	—	—	9.00	46.0	—	—
34.0	1.04	2.54	3.15	0.454	1.30	0.350	6.28	0.535	6.77	0.839	5.67	277	20.6	0.405
55.0	2.75	0.650	—	26.1	0.216	0.067	3.32	0.701	22.2	—	20.0	115	1.80	0.100
23.0	1.25	0.750	53.4	7.90	0.226	0.140	1.18	0.090	46.9	—	19.0	72.0	3.20	0.400
0.467	—	0.041	199	0.028	0.002	0.006	0.004	0.002	0.211	0.017	5.29	4.06	0.199	2.19
10.1	0.560	0.246	37.0	4.36	0.052	0.034	0.210	0.044	62.8	—	21.2	22.4	0.448	0.120
5.81	0.227	0.045	0.023		—	—	—	0.006	—	—	7.10	3.63		15.9
33.0	0.120	0.963	140	2.32	0.095	0.403	0.210	0.105	12.0	0.888	297	232	5.66	0.080
6.00	0.367	0.113	—	—	0.020	0.030	0.600	0.011	1.80	—	6.00	20.0	1.54	
298	15.4	11.7	607	204	5.52	1.79	25.9	2.14	395	3.65	792	1425	98.2	22.5
350	10	15	1000	60	1.5	1.7	19	2	200	2	1200	1200	70	10
85	154	78	61	340	368	105	132	107	198	180	66	118	140	225

Nutrient Analysis Form

Quantity	Name	Kcalories	Protein (grams)	Carbohydrate (grams)	Dietary Fiber (grams)	Fat Total (grams)	Saturated Fat (grams)	Monounsaturated Fat (grams)	Polyunsaturated Fat (grams)	Cholesterol (milligrams)	Sodium (milligrams)	Potassium (milligrams)
Totals:												
RDA or minimum requirement*												
% of RDA												

**Values from inside cover. The values listed are for a male age 19 to 24 years. Note that number of kcalories is just a rough estimate. It is better to base energy needs on actual energy output.*

Magnesium (milligrams)	Iron (milligrams)	Zinc (milligrams)	Vitamin A (RE)	Vitamin E (milligrams)	Vitamin C (milligrams)	Thiamin (milligrams)	Riboflavin (milligrams)	Niacin (milligrams)	Vitamin B-6 (milligrams)	Folate (micrograms)	Vitamin B-12 (micrograms)	Calcium (milligrams)	Phosphorus (milligrams)	Selenium (micrograms)	Vitamin E (milligrams)

III. Complete the following table as you summarize your dietary intake.

Percentage of Kcalories from Protein, Fat, Carbohydrate, and Alcohol

Intake				
Protein (P):	______ g/day × 4 kcal/g	=	(P)______	kcal/day
Fat (F):	______ g/day × 9 kcal/g	=	(F)______	kcal/day
Carbohydrate (C):	______ g/day × 4 kcal/g	=	(C)______	kcal/day
Alcohol (A):			(A)______	kcal/day*
	Total kcal (T)/day	=	(T)______	kcal/day

Percentage of kcalories from protein:

$\frac{(P)}{(T)}$ × 100 = ______ % of total kcalories

Percentage of kcalories from fat:

$\frac{(F)}{(T)}$ × 100 = ______ % of total kcalories

Percentage of kcalories from carbohydrate:

$\frac{(C)}{(T)}$ × 100 = ______ % of total kcalories

Percentage of kcalories from alcohol:

$\frac{(A)}{(T)}$ × 100 = ______ % of total kcalories

NOTE: The four percentages can total 99, 100, or 101, depending on the way in which figures were rounded off earlier.

**To calculate how many kcalories in a beverage are from alcohol, look up the beverage in Appendix A. Determine how many kcalories are from carbohydrate (multiply carbohydrate grams times 4), fat (fat grams times 9), and protein (protein grams times 4). The remaining kcalories are from alcohol.*

IV. Use the following table to again record your food intake for one day, placing each food item in the correct categories of the Food Guide Pyramid. Note that a food like toast with margarine would contribute to two categories—namely, to the bread, cereals, rice, and pasta group, but also to the fats, oils, and sweets group. You can expect that many food choices contribute to more than one group.

Indicate the number of servings from the Food Guide Pyramid that each food yielded.

Food or Beverage	Amount Eaten	Milk, Yogurt, and Cheese	Meat, Poultry, Fish, Beans, Nuts, and Seeds	Fruits	Vegetables	Bread, Cereals, Rice, and Pasta	Fats, Oils, and Sweets
Group Totals							
Recommend Servings							in moderation
Shortages in number of servings							

V. Evaluation Are there weaknesses suggested in your nutrient intake that correspond to missing servings in the Food Guide Pyramid? Consider improving the latter to aid improving the former.

C

VI. For this same day you keep your food record, also keep a 24-hour record of your activities. Include sleeping, sitting, and walking, as well as the obvious forms of exercise. Calculate your kcalorie expenditure for these activities using Appendix K or your Mosby Diet Simple II software. Try to substitute a similar activity if your particular activity is not listed. Calculate the total kcalories you used for the day (total for column 3). Here is an example of an activity record. A blank form follows for your use. Ask your professor whether you are to turn that in, or the activity printout from the software.

Weight (lb or kg):

	Energy Cost			
Activity	**Time (minutes); Convert to Hours**	**Column 1 kcal/hr (from table)**	**Column 2 Time**	**Column 3 (Column 1 × Column 2)**
Example for 150 lb man: Brisk walking	(30 min) 0.5 hr	299	0.5	150

Weight (lb or kg):

	Energy Cost			
Activity	**Time (minutes); Convert to Hours**	**Column 1 kcal/hr (from table)**	**Column 2 Time**	**Column 3 (Column 1 × Column 2)**

Total kcalories used (from adding all of column 3):

This Appendix is now completed. See whether your professor wants you to complete more work before turning in this assignment.

APPENDIX D

U.S. RDAs, PROPOSED RDIs, DRVs, AND A LABEL READING EXERCISE

D

U.S. Recommended Daily Allowances (U.S. RDAs) These are to be retitled Reference Daily Intakes [RDIs] and used under that name on new food label format through at least December 1993

Vitamins and Minerals	Unit of Measurement	Adults and Children 4 or More Years of Age*	Infants	Children Under 4 Years of Age	Pregnant or Lactating Women
Protein	grams	65†	25†	28	‡
Vitamin A	international units	5000	1500	2500	8000
Vitamin D	international units	400	400	400	400
Vitamin E	international units	30	5.0	10	30
Vitamin C	milligrams	60	35	40	60
Folic acid	milligrams	0.4	0.1	0.2	0.8
Thiamin	milligrams	1.5	0.5	0.7	1.7
Riboflavin	milligrams	1.7	0.6	0.8	2.0
Niacin	milligrams	20	8.0	9.0	20
Vitamin B-6	milligrams	2.0	0.4	0.7	2.5
Vitamin B-12	micrograms	6.0	2.0	3.0	8.0
Biotin	milligrams	0.3	0.05	0.15	0.3
Pantothenic acid	milligrams	10	3.0	5.0	10
Calcium	grams	1.0	0.6	0.8	1.3
Phosphorus	grams	1.0	0.5	0.8	1.3
Iodine	micrograms	150	45	70	150
Iron	milligrams	18	15	10	18
Magnesium	milligrams	400	70	200	450
Copper	milligrams	2.0	0.6	1.0	2.0
Zinc	milligrams	15	5.0	8.0	15

**These U.S. RDA values are on most nutrition labels.*

†If the protein efficiency ratio of the food protein in question is equal to or better than that of casein, U.S. RDA is 45 g for adults, 20 g for children under 4 yrs, and 18 g for infants.

‡Not specified because this U.S. RDA is used only in vitamin and mineral supplements for pregnant or lactating females.

D

(Proposed) Reference Daily Intakes (RDIs)*

Nutrient	Unit of Measurement	Adults and Children 4 or More Years of Age	Children Under Age 4†	Infants‡	Pregnant Women	Lactating Women
Vitamin A	retinol equivalents§	875	400	375	800	1300
Vitamin C	milligrams	60	40	33	70	95
Calcium	milligrams	900	800	500	1200	1200
Iron	milligrams	12	10	8.0	30	15
Vitamin D	micrograms‖	6.5	10	9.0	10	10
Vitamin E	alpha-tocopherol equivalents§	9.0	6.0	3.5	10	12
Vitamin K	micrograms	65	15	7.5	65	65
Thiamin	milligrams	1.2	0.7	0.4	1.5	1.6
Riboflavin	milligrams	1.4	0.8	0.5	1.6	1.8
Niacin	niacin equivalents§	16	9.0	5.5	17	20
Vitamin B-6	milligrams	1.5	1.0	0.5	2.2	2.1
Folate	micrograms	180	50	30	400	280
Vitamin B-12	micrograms	2.0	0.7	0.4	2.2	2.6
Biotin	micrograms	60	20	13	65	65
Pantothenic acid	milligrams	5.5	3.0	2.5	5.5	5.5
Phosphorus	milligrams	900	800	400	1200	1200
Magnesium	milligrams	300	80	50	320	355
Zinc	milligrams	13	10	5.0	15	19
Iodine	micrograms	150	70	45	175	200
Selenium	micrograms	55	20	13	65	75
Copper	milligrams	2.0	0.9	0.6	2.5	2.5
Manganese	milligrams	3.5	1.3	0.6	3.5	3.5
Fluoride	milligrams	2.5	1.0	0.5	3.0	3.0
Chromium	micrograms	120	50	33	13	130
Molybdenum	micrograms	150	38	26	160	160
Chloride	milligrams	3150	1000	650	3400	3400

**The FDA will reconsider these values based on public and industry comments, with final approval set for December 1993.*

†The term "children under age 4" means persons 13 through 47 months of age.

‡The term "infants" means persons not more than 12 months of age.

§1 retinol equivalent = 1 microgram retinol or 6 micrograms beta-carotene; 1 alpha-tocopherol equivalent = 1 milligram d-alpha-tocopherol; 1 niacin equivalent = 1 milligram niacin or 60 milligrams of dietary tryptophan.

‖As cholecalciferol.

Daily Reference Values (DRVs) (to provide intake guidelines for substances not included in the 1989 RDAs)

Food Component	Unit of Measurement	DRV† (2000-kcalorie intake)	DRV (2500-kcalorie intake)
Fat	grams	<65	<80
Saturated fatty acids	grams	<20	<25
Protein	grams	50	65
Cholesterol	milligrams	<300	<300
Carbohydrate	grams	300	375
Fiber	grams	25	30
Sodium	milligrams	<2400	<2400
Potassium	milligrams	3500	3500

†Some DRV standards increase as energy intake increases, such as grams of total fat allowed in a diet.

‡Note that protein content of a food can be expressed as a % of the RDI for protein only if certain guidelines are met (see Chapter 2). Otherwise, intake can be compared with the DRV listed at the bottom of the label.

Label-Reading Exercise

Hone your label-reading skills by completing the following exercise. Choose a label on a cereal box, because these typically give the most breakfast information. Be sure to show your calculations if this is to turned in as part of your class assignments.

What is the weight in ounces of one serving? ______ ounces
Convert the weight to grams. ______ grams

Each serving contains how many grams of dietary fiber? ______ grams
What percentage of the weight of one serving is fiber? ______ % weight

Next, refer to the carbohydrate information on the bottom of the label.
  How many grams of complex carbohydrate are provided per serving? ______ grams
  How many kcalories are provided by starch and related carbohydrates? ______ kcalories

  How many kcalories are provided by sucrose? ______ kcalories
    Approximately how many teaspoons of sucrose is this? (Hint: 5 grams = 1 teaspoon.) ______ teaspoons
    What percentage of the kcalories in this cereal come from sucrose? ______ % kcalories

  How many grams of natural sugar are provided per serving? ______ grams

  Name the sugars provided by the fruit in this cereal. ____________ and ____________

  Name the sugar provided by milk. ____________

How would you classify the carbohydrates in this cereal?
  Circle one and explain:
    Mostly complex
    Mostly complex with simple sugars from fruit in the cereal
    Mostly simple sugars

  Explain: ____
____
____

Refer to the top of the label where two columns, cereal and cereal plus milk, are listed:
  What percentage of the kcalories come from protein? ______ % kcalories
  How many grams of protein are in ½ cup milk? ______ grams
  What type of milk was used for the label information? ____________

Is this cereal high in fat? ____________

What is the major ingredient in this cereal? ____________

Identify at least three vitamins added to the cereal. ____________
____
____

Is much vitamin C normally found in whole-grain cereal products? Yes or No

  Vitamin A? Yes or No

  Calcium? Yes or No

  Fiber? Yes or No

  Thiamin? Yes or No

Who manufactures this cereal? ____

Would you buy or will you continue to eat this cereal based on your evaluation? Why or why not? ____________________

APPENDIX E

THE EXCHANGE SYSTEM

The *exchange system* is a valuable tool for quickly estimating the energy, protein, carbohydrate, and fat content of a food or meal. Using it also creates greater understanding about what one eats. Rather than memorizing the tables of composition of all foods, your work is greatly simplified by using the exchange system because it generalizes those details into a manageable framework.

The exchange system arranges food into six different categories: milk, fruit, vegetables, starch/bread, meat, and fat. These categories are designed so that after noting the proper serving size, each food within a category provides about the same amount of carbohydrate, protein, fat, and kcalories. This equality allows the exchange of foods within a category. Hence the term "exchange system."

USING THE EXCHANGE SYSTEM

Using the exchange system requires knowing what foods are in each group and knowing the serving sizes for each food. We have listed the entire U.S. exchange system in Appendix F. You will need to consult the exchange lists many times before you can apply the system.

Table E-1 shows the carbohydrate, protein, fat, and energy composition of each of the six exchange groups. The starch/bread group has 15 grams of carbohydrate, 3 grams of

TABLE E-1

The Exchange Lists Composition (1986 Edition)

Exchange List	Household Measures*	Carbohydrate (grams)	Protein (grams)	Fat (grams)	Kcalories
Starch/bread	1 slice, ¾ cup raw, or ½ cup cooked	15	3	trace†	80
Meat	1 ounce				
Lean		—	7	3	55
Medium-fat		—	7	5	75
High-fat		—	7	8	100
Vegetable	½ cup cooked	5	2	—	25
Fruit	1 small piece	15	—	—	60
Milk	1 cup				
Skim		12	8	trace	90
Low-fat		12	8	5	120
Whole		12	8	8	150
Fat	1 teaspoon	—	—	5	45

The American Diabetes Association and American Dietetic Association, Exchange Lists for Meal Planning, 1986.
**Just an estimate. See exchange lists for actual amounts.*
†Calculated as 1 gram for purposes of energy contribution

protein, and a trace of fat per exchange. The trace of fat is calculated as 1 gram of fat when the total energy contribution of an exchange is determined. The meat group is divided into three subclasses: lean, medium fat, and high fat. Each exchange has 7 grams of protein. Lean meats contain 3 grams of fat per exchange, medium-fat meats have 5 grams of fat per exchange, and high-fat meats have 8 grams of fat per exchange. Meats have essentially no carbohydrate. The vegetable group contains 5 grams of carbohydrate, 2 grams of protein, and no fat per exchange. The fruit group has 15 grams of carbohydrate per exchange. Fruit has no appreciable fat or protein.

The milk group is divided into three subclasses: nonfat, low-fat, and whole. Each exchange has 12 grams of carbohydrate and 8 grams of protein. Nonfat milk has a trace of fat (calculated as 1 gram when energy content is expressed) per exchange. Low-fat milk has 5 grams of fat per exchange, and whole milk has 8 grams of fat per exchange. Finally, the fat group contains 5 grams of fat per exchange. Fats contain no appreciable amount of carbohydrate or protein.

An exchange from the starch/bread group contains 80 kcalories. Lean meats have 55 kcalories per exchange, medium-fat meats have 75 kcalories per exchange, and high-fat meats have 100 kcalories per exchange. Vegetables have 25 kcalories per exchange. Fruits have 60 kcalories per exchange. Skim milk has 90 kcalories per exchange, low-fat milk has 120 kcalories per exchange, and whole milk has 150 kcalories per exchange. Finally, fat has 45 kcalories per exchange.

TAKING A CLOSER LOOK AT THE EXCHANGE GROUPS

Before you can turn a group of exchanges into a meal plan for 1 day, you first have to see what each exchange group contains. The starch/bread group contains dry cereal, cooked cereal, rice, pasta, baked beans, corn on the cob, potatoes, bread, and tortillas. This list is not the same as that used for the Food Guide Pyramid. The exchange system is not concerned about the origin of the food, animal or vegetable. It is primarily concerned with the nutrient composition in terms of carbohydrate, protein, and fat of each food in a group. For example, the carbohydrate composition of potatoes resembles that of bread more than that of broccoli, although bread is not a vegetable.

The lean meat list contains round steak, lean ham, veal, chicken (without skin), fish, cottage cheese, and 95% fat-free luncheon meat. The medium-fat meat list contains T-bone steak, pork roast, lamb chops, well-drained duck and goose, salmon, mozzarella cheese, and eggs. The high-fat meat list contains prime cuts of beef (marbled), ribs, sausage, fried fish, cheddar cheese, salami, and peanut butter.

The vegetable list contains most vegetables. Some starchy vegetables were listed previously in the starch/bread group. Some vegetables—such as cabbage, celery, mushrooms, lettuce, and zucchini—are free foods: their minimal energy contribution does not count in the calculations. The fruit list contains fruits and fruit juices.

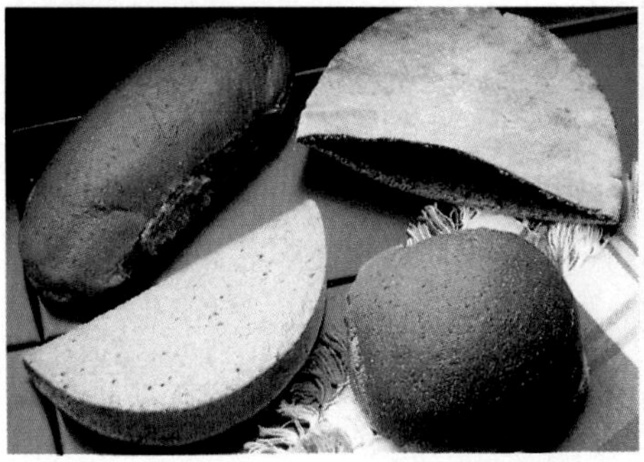

The starch/bread exchange group

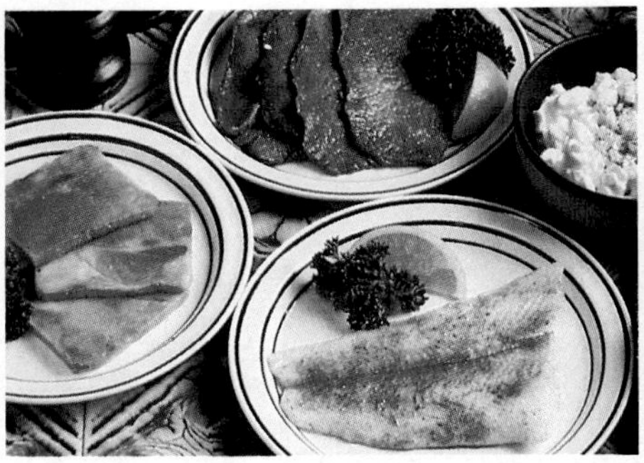

The meat exchange group

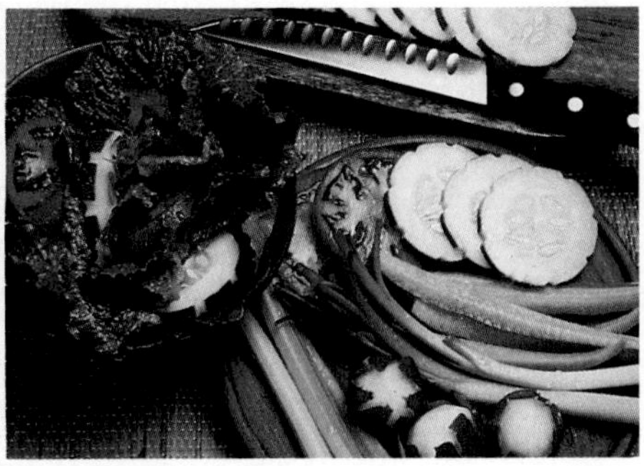

The vegetable exchange group

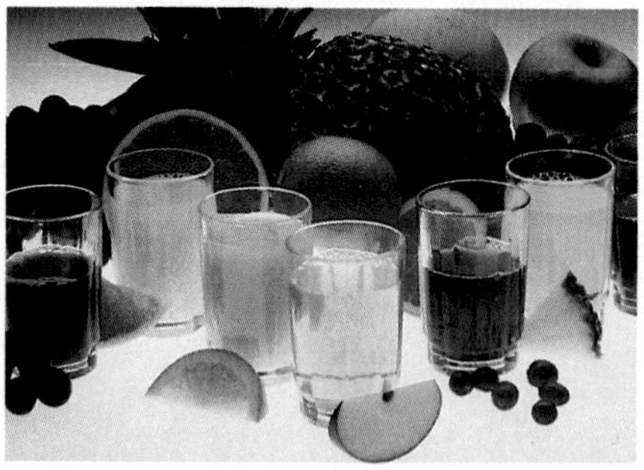
The fruit exchange group

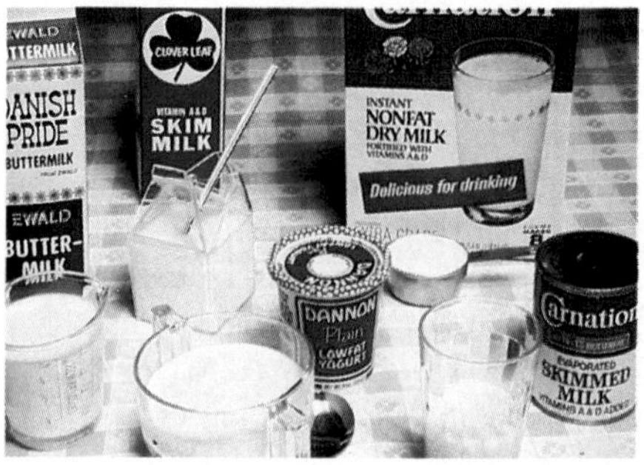

The milk exchange group

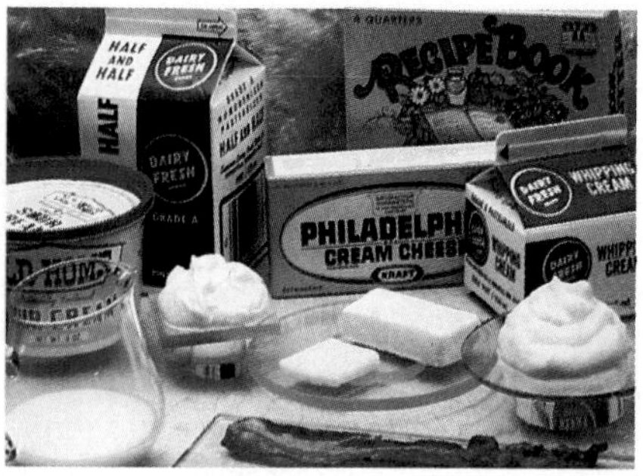

The fat exchange group

The milk exchange list contains milk, plain yogurt, and buttermilk. The amount of fat in a product determines whether the serving is nonfat, low-fat, or whole.

The fat list contains margarine, mayonnaise, nuts and seeds, salad oils, olives, sour cream, and cream cheese. Bacon is considered a fat, rather than a high-fat meat.

Free foods, other than the vegetables already mentioned, include bouillon, diet soda, coffee, tea, dill pickles, and vinegar, as well as herbs and spices.

PUTTING THE EXCHANGE SYSTEM TO WORK

Let's now turn an exchange food plan into 1 day's menu. Let's say we want to consume 2000 kcalories, consisting of 55% energy from carbohydrates, 15% energy from protein, and 30% energy from fat. This can be translated into 2 low-fat milk exchanges, 3 vegetable exchanges, 5 fruit exchanges, 11 bread exchanges, 3 medium-fat meat exchanges, and 8 fat exchanges (Table E-2). Note this is only one of many possible combinations; the exchange system offers great flexibility.

Table E-3 arbitrarily separates these exchanges into breakfast, lunch, dinner, and a snack. Breakfast includes 1 low-fat milk exchange, 2 fruit exchanges, 3 starch/bread exchanges, and 2 fat exchanges. This total corresponds to ¾ cup cold cereal eaten with 1 cup of 1% milk, 2 slices of bread with 2 teaspoons margarine, and 1 cup of orange juice.

Lunch consists of 3 fat exchanges, 4 starch/bread exchanges, 1 vegetable exchange, 2 fruit exchanges, and 1 low-fat milk exchange. This translates into 2 slices of bacon with 1 teaspoon mayonnaise, two slices of bread, and tomato—in other words, a bacon and

TABLE E-2

Exchange Patterns to Get You Started

Kcalories/day	1200	1600	2000	2400	2800	3200	3600
Exchange Group							
Milk (low-fat)	2	2	2	2	2	2	2
Vegetables	2	2	3	3	3	3	3
Fruit	5	4	5	8	8	10	10
Starch/bread	4	8	11	11	15	17	20
Meat (medium-fat)	2	2	3	5	5	7	8
Fat	4	7	8	9	12	12	14

These are just one set of options. More meat could be included if less milk is used, for example. The breakdown is 55% energy as carbohydrate, 30% energy as fat, and 15% energy as protein.

tomato sandwich. Add to this a 9-inch banana (1 exchange equals ½ banana), 16 animal cookies, and 1 cup of 1% milk.

Dinner consists of 3 medium-fat meat exchanges, 1 fruit exchange, 2 vegetable exchanges, 1 fat exchange, and 2 starch/bread exchanges. This total corresponds to a 3-ounce broiled T-bone steak (meat only; no bone), 1 large baked potato (1 exchange equals 1 small baked potato) with 1 teaspoon of margarine, 1 cup broccoli, and 1 kiwi fruit. Coffee, if desired, is not counted because it yields no appreciable energy.

Finally, we have a snack containing two starch/bread exchanges and two fat exchanges. This translates into 1 bagel with 2 tablespoons of cream cheese.

We have listed only one of many possibilities for a day's food plan. Orange juice could be exchanged for apple juice. The banana could be an apple. The tenderloin steak could be 3 ounces of chicken breast with the skin. The choices are endless.

TABLE E-3

Turning an Exchange System Plan into a Menu for 1 Day

Breakfast	
1 low-fat milk exchange	1% milk (put some on cereal), 1 cup
2 fruit exchanges	Orange juice, 1 cup
3 bread exchanges	Cold cereal, ¾ cup Whole-wheat toast, 2 pieces
2 fat exchanges	Margarine on toast, 2 tsp.
Lunch	
4 bread exchanges	Whole-wheat bread, 2 slices Animal crackers, 16
3 fat exchanges	Bacon, 2 slices Mayonnaise, 1 tsp.
1 vegetable exchange	1 sliced tomato
2 fruit exchanges	1 banana (9 inches)
1 low-fat milk exchange	1% milk, 1 cup
Dinner	
3 medium-fat meat exchanges	T-bone steak, broiled, 3 oz.
2 bread exchanges	Baked potato, 1 large
1 fat exchange	Margarine, 1 tsp.
2 vegetable exchanges	Broccoli, 1 cup
1 fruit exchange	1 kiwi fruit
	Coffee (if desired)
Snack	
2 bread exchanges	1 bagel
2 fat exchanges	Cream cheese, 2 Tbsp.
Prescription	Values calculated using a computer and nutrient analysis software
2000	Kcalories 2037
55%	Carbohydrate 55%
15%	Protein 16%
30%	Fat 29%

Note that an exchange list is much easier to plan if you use individual foods as we have. However, the exchange system tables (Appendix F) list some combination foods to help you. Using combination foods, such as pizza or lasagna, just makes it more difficult to calculate the number of exchanges in a serving. For instance, lasagna has meat, vegetable, and starch/bread exchanges. With experience, you will be able to tackle such complex foods. For now, using individual foods makes learning the exchange system much easier.

To recap, Table E-3 lists the original prescription for carbohydrate, protein, fat, and energy intake. The actual percentages of carbohydrate, protein, fat, and kcalories in the diet have also been calculated using a nutrient software package and a computer. Note that the exchange system values closely match the computer analysis shown in the table. The exchange system is a very useful tool for diet planning. If used correctly, there is no easier way to plan a precise menu pattern. Table E-1 gives you a head start in planning diets. Use this table and the following form to plan a day's diet for tomorrow. Then follow the diet you develop. Practicing this system makes it much easier to understand (Figure E-1).

Exchange List	Total Exchanges to be Consumed Daily	Exchanges Consumed at Each Meal		
		Breakfast	Lunch	Dinner
Milk				
Vegetable				
Fruit				
Starch/ bread				
Meat				
Fat				

FIGURE E-1
Record the Exchange System pattern you have chosen in the left-hand column. Then distribute the exchanges throughout the day, noting the food to be used and the serving size.

E

APPENDIX F

EXCHANGE SYSTEM LISTS

Milk Exchange List

Skim milk (12 grams carbohydrate, 8 grams protein, 0 grams fat, 90 kcalories)

1 cup	skim or nonfat milk (½% and 1%)
⅓ cup	powdered (nonfat dry, before adding liquid)
½ cup	canned, evaporated skim milk
1 cup	buttermilk made from skim milk
1 cup	yogurt made from skim milk (plain, unflavored)

Low-fat milk (12 grams carbohydrate, 8 grams protein, 5 grams fat, 120 kcalories)

1 cup	2% milk
1 cup	plain nonfat yogurt (added milk solids)

Whole milk (12 grams carbohydrate, 8 grams protein, 8 grams fat, 150 kcalories)

1 cup	whole milk
1 cup	custard-style yogurt made from whole milk (plain, unflavored)

Vegetable Exchange List

(5 grams carbohydrate, 2 grams protein, 0 grams fat, 25 kcalories)

1 vegetable exchange equals:

½ cup cooked vegetables or vegetable juice

1 cup raw vegetables

artichoke (½ medium)
asparagus
beans (green, wax, Italian)
bean sprouts
beets
broccoli
brussels sprouts
cabbage, cooked
carrots
cauliflower
eggplant
green pepper
greens (e.g., collard)
mushrooms, cooked
onions
pea pods
sauerkraut
spinach, cooked
squash (summer)
string beans (green, yellow)
tomato
tomato juice
turnips
vegetable juice
zucchini

Fruit Exchange List

(15 grams carbohydrate, 0 grams protein, 0 grams fat, 60 kcalories)

1 fruit exchange equals:

1	apple (2 inches in diameter)
4 rings	dried apple
½ cup	apple juice
½ cup	applesauce (unsweetened)
4	apricots, fresh
½ cup	apricots, canned
7 halves	apricots, dried
½	banana, 9 inches
¾ cup	blackberries
¾ cup	blueberries
⅓ melon	cantaloupe (5 inches in diameter)
12	cherries (large, raw)
½ cup	cherries, canned
½ cup	cider
⅓ cup	cranberry juice cocktail
2½ medium	dates
2	figs, fresh (2 inches in diameter)
1½	figs, dried
½	grapefruit
½ cup	grapefruit juice
15	grapes
⅓ cup	grape juice
⅛ melon	honeydew melon (7 inches in diameter; cubes = 1 cup)
1	kiwi (large)
¾ cup	mandarin oranges
½ small	mango
1 small	nectarine (2½ inches in diameter)
1 small	orange (2½ inches in diameter)

$\frac{1}{2}$ cup	orange juice
1 medium or $\frac{3}{4}$ cup	peach, fresh ($2\frac{3}{4}$ inches in diameter)
$\frac{1}{2}$ cup or 2 halves	peach, canned
1 small or $\frac{1}{2}$ large	pear, fresh
$\frac{1}{2}$ cup or 2 halves	pear, canned
$\frac{3}{4}$ cup	pineapple, raw
$\frac{1}{3}$ cup	pineapple, canned
$\frac{1}{2}$ cup	pineapple juice
2	plums (2 inches in diameter)
3	prunes, dried
$\frac{1}{3}$ cup	prune juice
2 tablespoons	raisins
1 cup	raspberries
$1\frac{1}{4}$ cup	strawberries (raw, whole)
2	tangerine ($2\frac{1}{2}$ inches in diameter)
$1\frac{1}{4}$ cups	watermelon (cubes)

Starch/Bread Exchange List

(15 grams carbohydrate, 3 grams protein, 0 grams fat, 80 kcalories)

1 starch/bread exchange equals:

Bread

1 slice (1 ounce)	white (including French and Italian)
1 slice	whole wheat
1 slice	rye or pumpernickel
1 slice	raisin (unfrosted)
2 ($\frac{2}{3}$ ounce)	bread sticks (crisp, 4 inches long, $\frac{1}{2}$ inch wide)
$\frac{1}{2}$ (1 ounce)	bagel, small
$\frac{1}{2}$	English muffin
1 (small)	plain roll
$\frac{1}{2}$ (1 ounce)	frankfurter bun
$\frac{1}{2}$ (1 ounce)	hamburger bun
1	tortilla (6 inches in diameter)
$\frac{1}{2}$	pita (6 inches in diameter)

Cereal/Grains/Pasta

$\frac{1}{2}$ cup	bran flakes
$\frac{3}{4}$ cup	other ready-to-eat unsweetened cereal
$1\frac{1}{2}$ cups	puffed cereal (unfrosted)
$\frac{1}{2}$ cup	cereal (cooked)
$\frac{1}{3}$ cup	rice or barley (cooked)
3 tablespoons	grapenuts
$\frac{1}{2}$ cup	shredded wheat
3 tablespoons	wheat germ
$\frac{1}{2}$ cup	pasta (cooked spaghetti, noodles, macaroni)
$2\frac{1}{2}$ tablespoons	cornmeal (dry)
$2\frac{1}{2}$ tablespoons	flour (dry)

Crackers/Snacks

3	graham ($2\frac{1}{2}$ inch square)
$\frac{3}{4}$ ounce	matzoh (4 inches × 6 inches)
24	oyster
4	rye crisp (2 inches × $3\frac{1}{2}$ inches)
6	saltines
8	animal
5 slices	melba toast
3 cups	popcorn (popped with no added fat)
$\frac{3}{4}$ ounce	pretzels

Dried Beans/Peas/Lentils

1/3 cup	dried beans, such as kidney, white, split, blackeye (cooked)
1/3 cup	lentils (cooked)
1/4 cup	baked beans

Starchy Vegetables

1/2 cup	corn
1	corn on the cob (6 inches)
1/2 cup	lima beans
1/2 cup	peas, green (canned or frozen)
1 small	potato, white (3 ounces, baked)
1/2 cup	potato, mashed
1 cup	winter squash, acorn or butternut
1/3 cup	yam or sweet potato

Starch/Bread Group (With Additional Fat)

1 starch/bread exchange
1 fat exchange

1	biscuit (2 1/2 inches across)
1/2 cup	chow mein noodles
1 (2 ounce)	corn bread (2-inch cube)
6	cracker, round butter type
10 (1 1/2 ounce)	French fries (2 inches to 3 1/2 inches)
1	muffin, plain, small
2	pancake (4 inches in diameter)
1/4 cup	stuffing, bread (prepared)
2	taco shell (6 inches across)
1	waffle (4 1/2 inches square)
4-6 (1 ounce)	whole-wheat crackers (such as Triscuits)

Meat Exchange List

Lean (0 grams carbohydrate, 7 grams protein, 3 grams fat, 55 kcalories)

Beef	1 ounce	baby beef (lean), chipped beef, flank steak, tenderloin, round (bottom, top)
Pork	1 ounce	leg (whole rump, center shank), ham (center slices), USDA good or choice grades such as round, sirloin, and tenderloin
	1 1/2 ounce	95% fat-free luncheon meat
Veal	1 ounce	leg, loin, rib, shank, shoulder, chops, roasts, all cuts except cutlets (ground or cubed)
Poultry	1 ounce	chicken, turkey, cornish hen (without skin)
	3 (1/2 cup)	egg whites, egg substitutes
Fish	1 ounce	fresh or frozen, tuna (in water)
	2 ounces	clams, oysters, scallops, shrimp, crab, lobster
	2 medium	sardines, drained
Cheeses	1/4 cup	cottage
	2 tablespoons	grated parmesan

F

Medium-fat (0 grams carbohydrate, 7 grams protein, 5 grams fat, 75 kcalories)

Beef	1 ounce	all ground beef, roast (rib, chuck, rump), steak (cubed, porterhouse, T-bone), meat loaf
Lamb	1 ounce	leg, rib, sirloin, loin (roast and chops), shank, shoulder
Pork	1 ounce	chops, roast, Boston butt, cutlets
Poultry	1 ounce	capon, duck (domestic), goose, ground turkey, chicken with skin
Veal	1 ounce	cutlets
Organ meats	1 ounce	all types
Fish	¼ cup	tuna (canned in oil), salmon (canned)
Cheeses	¼ cup or 1 ounce	cottage (creamed), mozzarella (made with skim milk), ricotta, Neufchatel
Egg	1	egg
Other	4 ounces	tofu

High-fat (0 grams carbohydrate, 7 grams protein, 8 grams fat, 100 kcalories)

Beef	1 ounce	brisket, corned beef (commercial), chuck (ground commercial), roasts (rib), steaks (club and rib), most USDA prime cuts of beef
Lamb	1 ounce	patties (ground lamb)
Pork	1 ounce	spare ribs, loin (back ribs), pork (ground), country-style ham, deviled ham, pork sausage
Cheeses	1 ounce	all regular cheeses (American, blue, brick, Camembert, cheddar, Gouda, Limburger, Muenster, Swiss, Monterey), all processed cheeses
Cold cuts	1 ounce	bologna, salami, pimento loaf
Frankfurter	1 frank (10/pound)	turkey, chicken
Peanut butter	1 tablespoon	
Sausage	1 ounce	Polish, Italian

Fat Exchange List

(0 grams carbohydrate, 0 grams protein, 5 grams fat, 45 kcalories)

⅛ medium	avocado
1 strip	bacon, crisp
1 teaspoon	butter, margarine
2 tablespoons	cream, light
2 tablespoons	cream, sour
1 tablespoon	cream, heavy
1 tablespoon	cream cheese
Dressing	
1 tablespoon	oil varieties
2 teaspoons	mayonnaise type
2 tablespoons	reduced calorie
1 tablespoon	reduced calorie (mayonnaise type)

Nuts, 6	almonds, whole, dry roasted
2 large	pecans, whole
20 small or 10 large	peanuts, Spanish, whole
10	peanuts, Virginia, whole
2 whole	walnuts
1 tablespoon	cashews, dry roasted
1 tablespoon	seeds (pine nuts, sunflower)
2 teaspoons	pumpkin seeds
1 tablespoon	other
Oil	
1 teaspoon	corn, cottonseed, safflower, soy, sunflower, olive, peanut, canola
Olives	
10 small or 5 large	

Free Foods

A free food is any food or drink that contains less than 20 kcalories per serving. You can eat as much as you want of those items that have no serving size specified. You may eat two or three servings per day of those items that have a specific serving size. Be sure to spread them out through the day.

Drinks:
Bouillon or broth without fat
Bouillon, low-sodium
Carbonated drinks, sugar-free
Carbonated water
Club soda
Cocoa powder, unsweetened (1 tablespoon)
Coffee/tea
Drink mixes, sugar-free
Tonic water, sugar-free

Nonstick pan spray

Fruit:
Cranberries, unsweetened (½ cup)
Rhubarb, unsweetened (½ cup)

Vegetables:
(raw, 1 cup)
Cabbage
Celery
Chinese cabbage
Cucumber
Green onion
Hot peppers
Mushrooms (fresh)
Radishes
Zucchini

Salad greens:
Endive
Escarole
Lettuce
Romaine
Spinach

Sweet substitutes:
Candy, hard, sugar-free
Gelatin, sugar-free
Gum, sugar-free
Jam/jelly, sugar-free (2 teaspoons)
Pancake syrup, sugar-free (1-2 tablespoons)
Sugar substitutes (saccharin, aspartame)
Whipped topping (2 tablespoons)

Condiments:
Catsup (1 tablespoon)
Horseradish
Mustard
Pickles, dill, unsweetened
Salad dressing, low-calorie (2 tablespoons)
Taco sauce (3 tablespoons)
Vinegar

Seasonings:
Basil (fresh)
Celery seeds
Cinnamon
Chili powder
Chives
Curry
Dill
Flavoring extracts (e.g., vanilla, almond, walnut, peppermint, butter, lemon)
Garlic
Garlic powder
Herbs
Hot pepper sauce
Lemon
Lemon juice
Lemon pepper
Lime
Lime juice
Mint
Onion powder
Oregano
Paprika
Pepper
Pimento
Soy sauce
Soy sauce, low-sodium (lite)
Spices
Wine, used in cooking (¼ cup)
Worcestershire sauce

APPENDIX G

THE HUMAN CELL—PRIMARY SITE FOR METABOLISM

The cell is the basic unit of body structure, and it is where most metabolic reactions occur (Figure G-1). The cell is surrounded by a semipermeable membrane that controls the passage of nutrients and other substances in and out of it. Within the cell is fluid called the cytosol. Within the cytosol are small bodies called organelles that perform specific metabolic functions. The names and activities of the various cell parts are given below:

Nucleus: This spherical structure is bound by its own double membrane. Within the nucleus are chromosomes, which are long threads of DNA (also called chromatin) that contain hereditary information for directing cell protein synthesis and cell division. Although most cell types have only one nucleus, muscle cells contain many nuclei.

Mitochondria: These have their own outer membrane, as well as an inner membrane that is highly folded. The mitochondria are the major sites of energy production in the cell. Muscle cells contain many mitochondria.

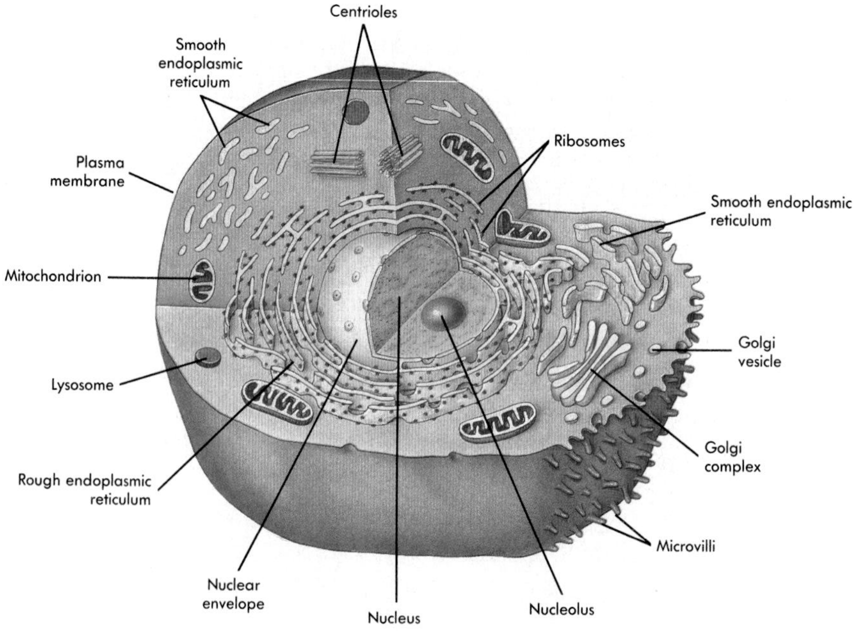

FIGURE G-1
An animal cell. *Almost all human cells contain these various organelles.*

Endoplasmic reticulum: This network of internal membranes serves as a communication network within the cell. Small granules called ribosomes are attached to parts of the outside of the endoplasmic reticulum, which is known as the rough endoplasmic reticulum. Ribosomes are the site for protein synthesis. Fat is synthesized in other areas of the endoplasmic reticulum where there are no ribosomes—namely, the smooth endoplasmic reticulum. In muscles, this organelle (called sarcoplasmic reticulum) plays a key role in muscle contraction.

Golgi complex: This consists of stacks of flattened structures that both package proteins for export from the cell and help form other cell organelles (Figure G-2).

Lysosomes: These small bodies contain digestive enzymes that break down worn-out cell parts and other cell debris. When a lysosome fuses with a particle that is to be digested, the digestive activity begins.

Storage forms of energy: These occur in the cell as glycogen granules and lipid droplets.

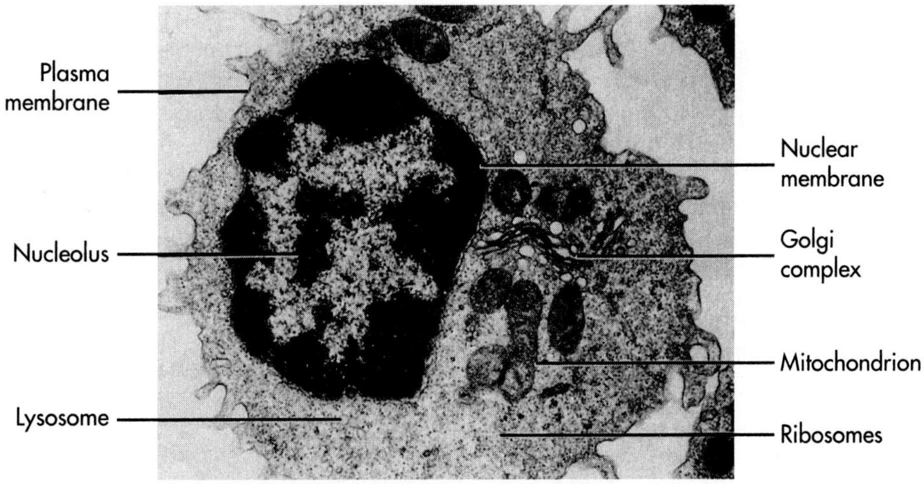

FIGURE G-2

Electron micrograph of a cell, magnified 40,500 times. Our understanding of the structures in cells is based mainly on such pictures as this. (From Raven PH, Johnson GB: Biology, St. Louis, 1992, Mosby–Year Book.)

APPENDIX H

IMPORTANT CHEMICAL STRUCTURES IN NUTRITION

Amino Acids

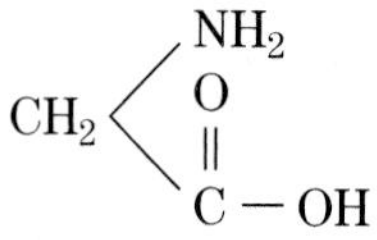

Glycine

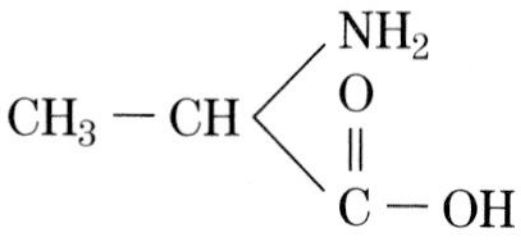

Alanine

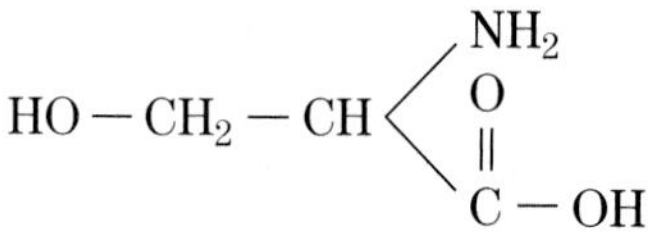

Serine

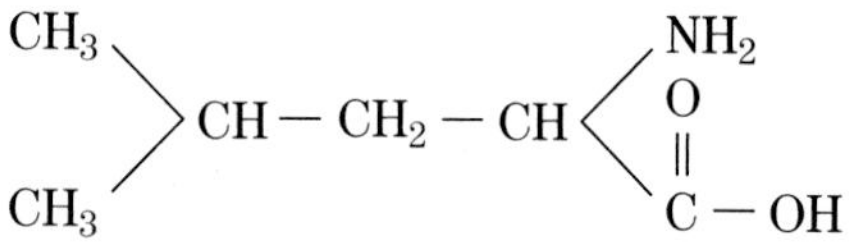

Leucine (essential)

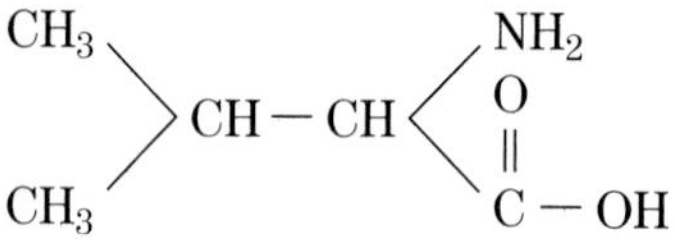

Valine (essential)

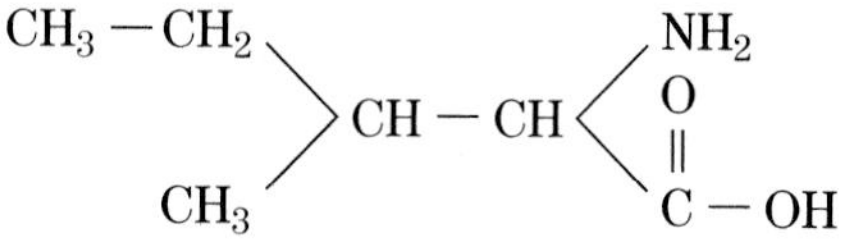

Isoleucine (essential)

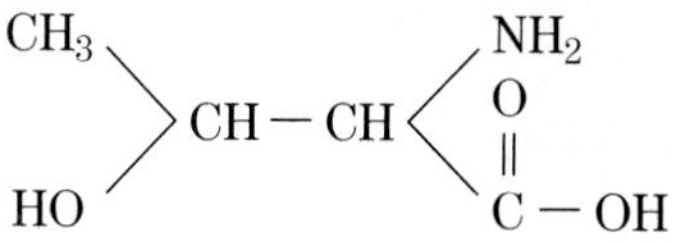

Threonine (essential)

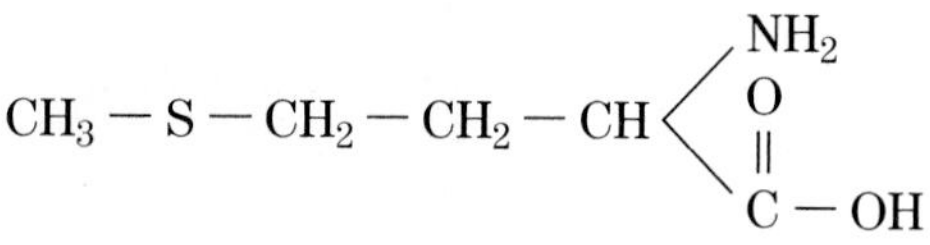

Methionine (essential)

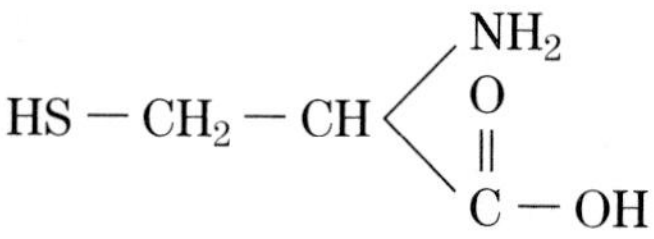

Cysteine

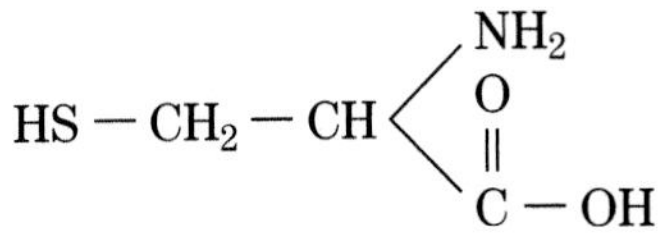

Cysteine

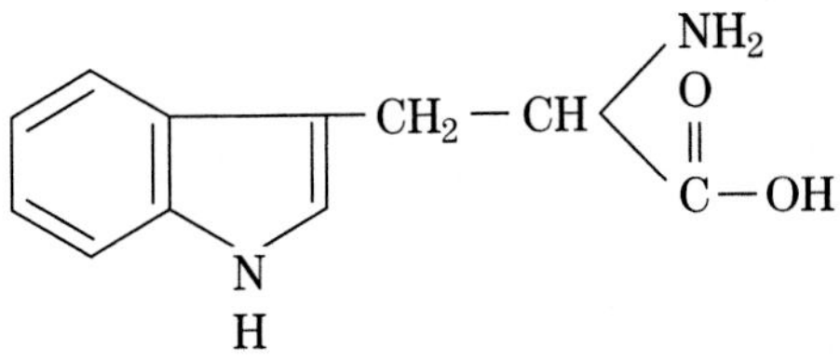

Tryptophan (essential)

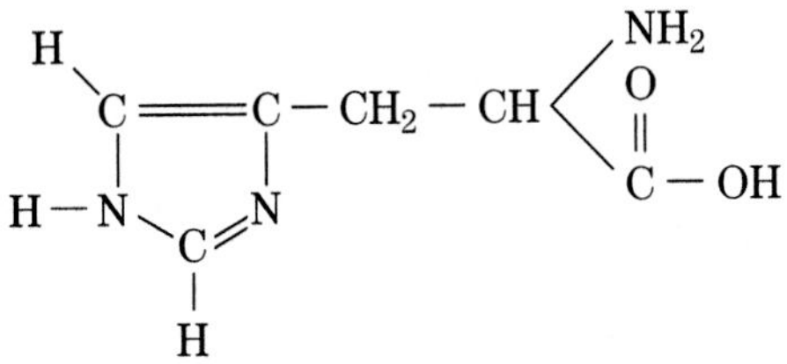

Histidine (essential)

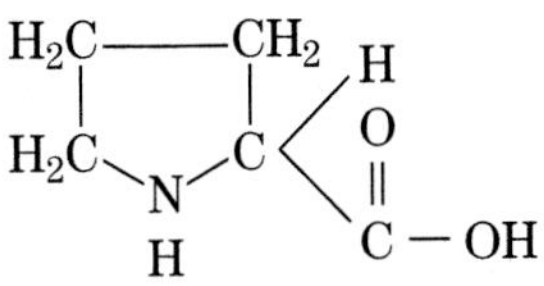

Proline

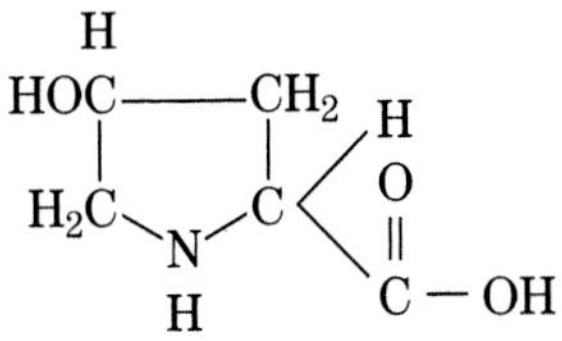

Hydroxyproline

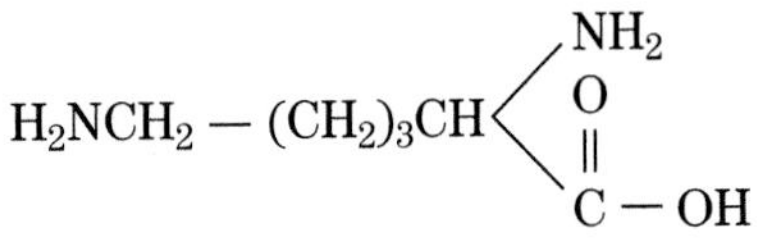

Lysine (essential)

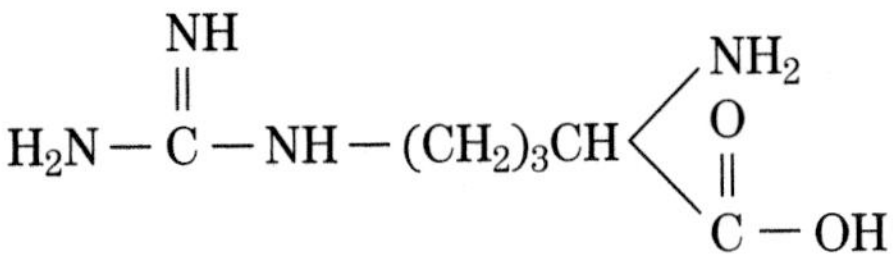

Arginine (essential)

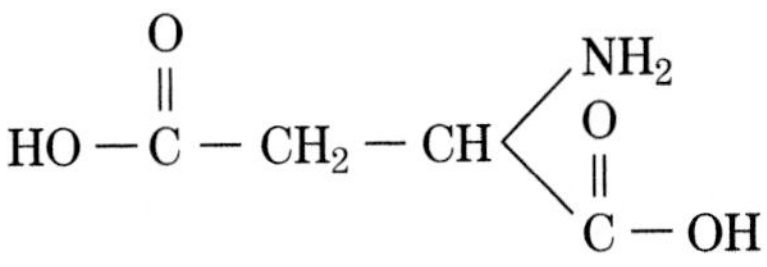

Aspartic Acid

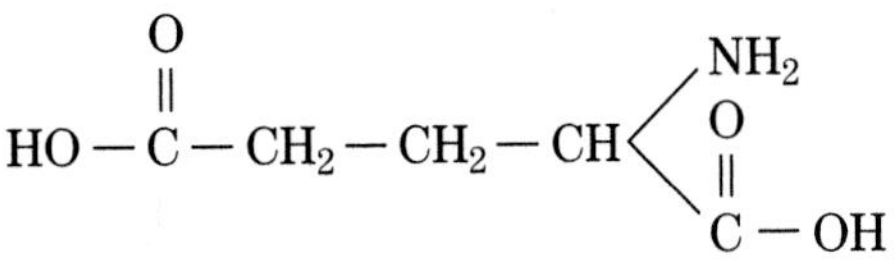

Glutamic acid

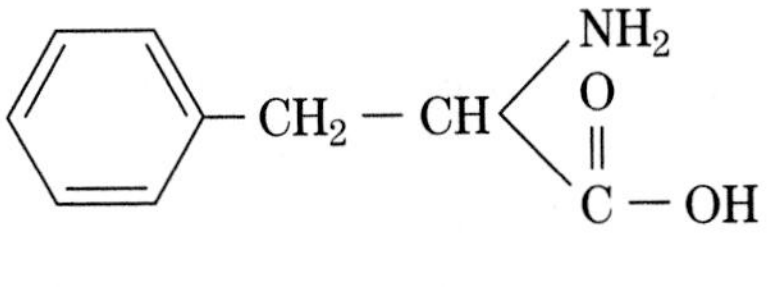

Phenylalanine (essential)

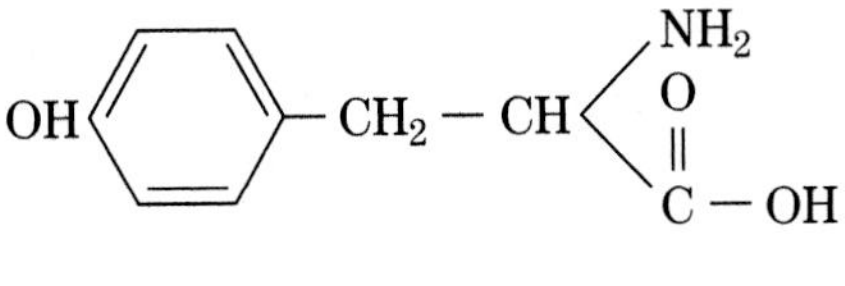

Tyrosine

H

Vitamins

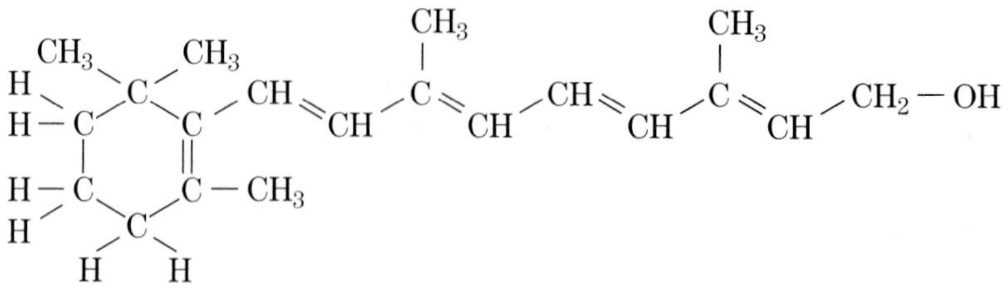

Vitamin A: retinol

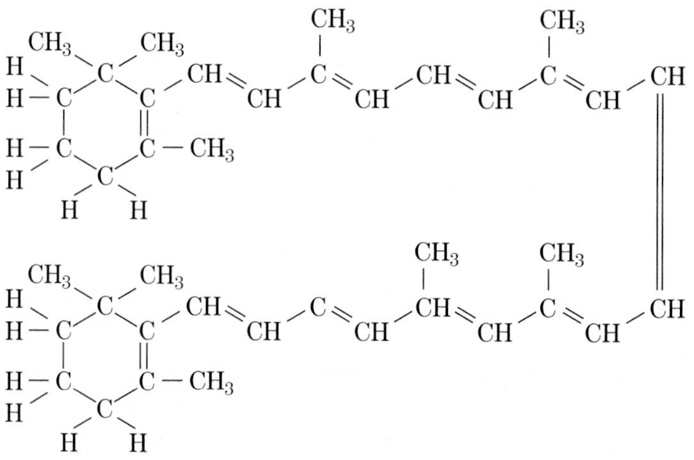

Beta-carotene

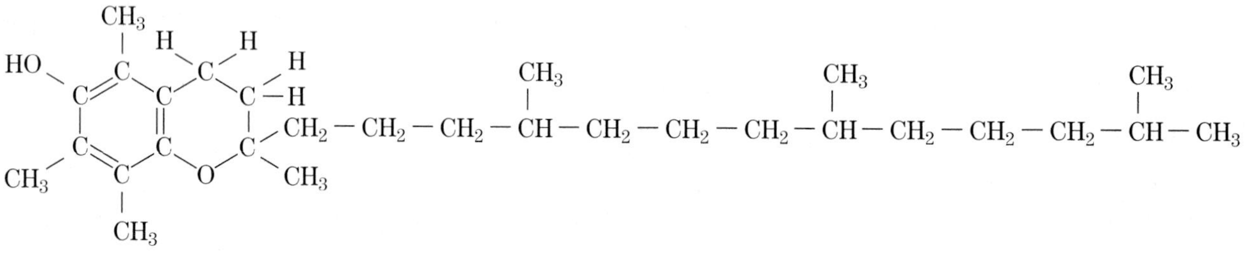

Vitamin E

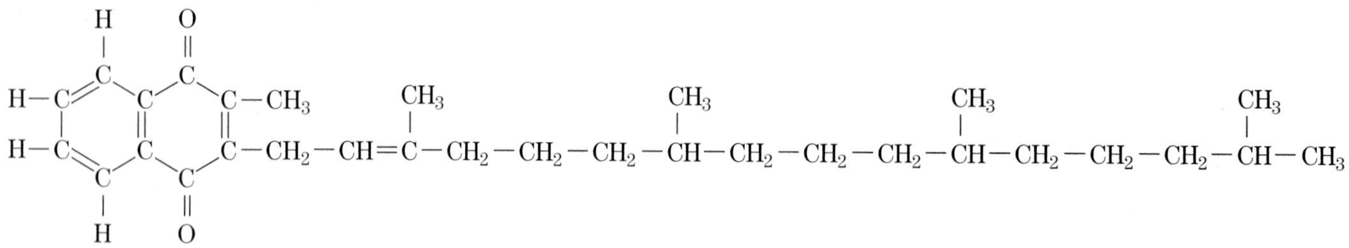

Vitamin K

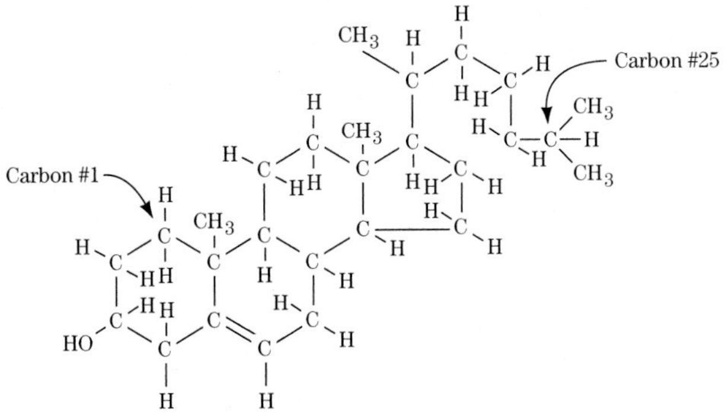

7-dehydrocholesterol

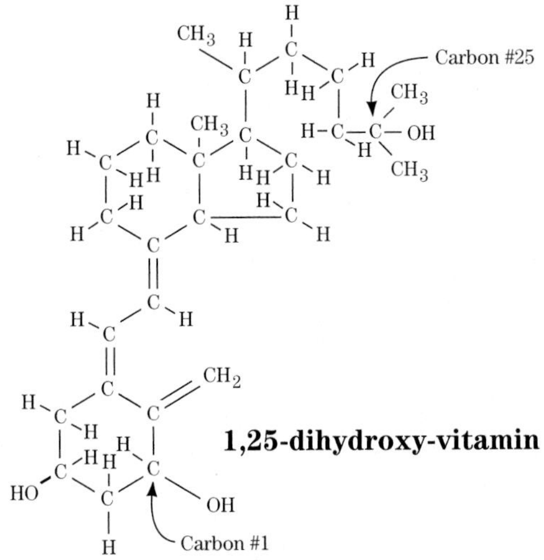

1,25-dihydroxy-vitamin D_3 (calcitriol)

Active vitamin D (calcitriol) and its precursor 7-dehydrocholesterol

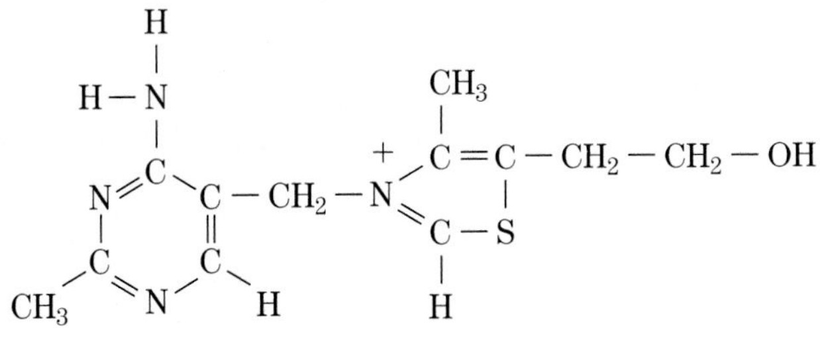

Thiamin

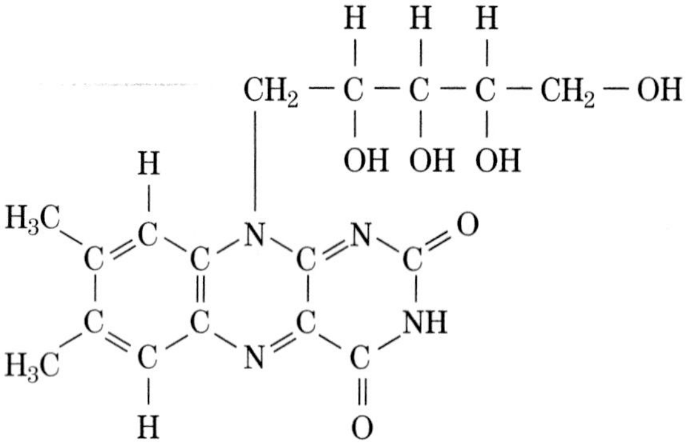

Riboflavin

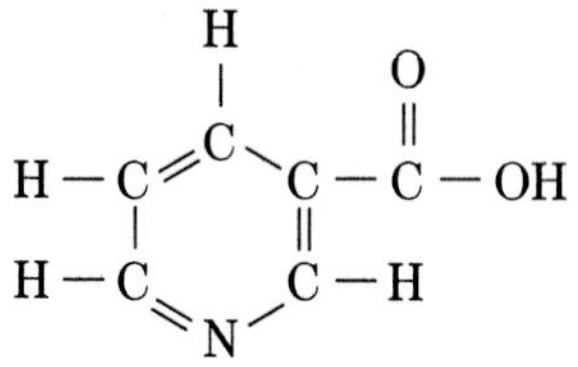

Nicotinic acid

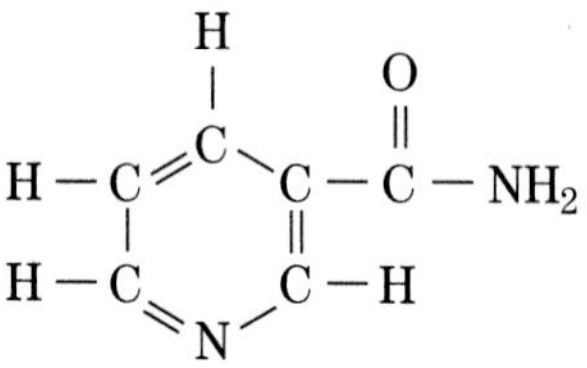

Nicotinamide

Niacin (nicotinic acid and nicotinamide)

H

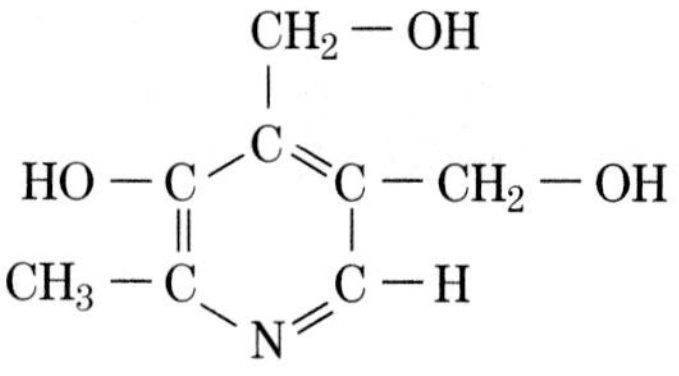

Pyridoxine

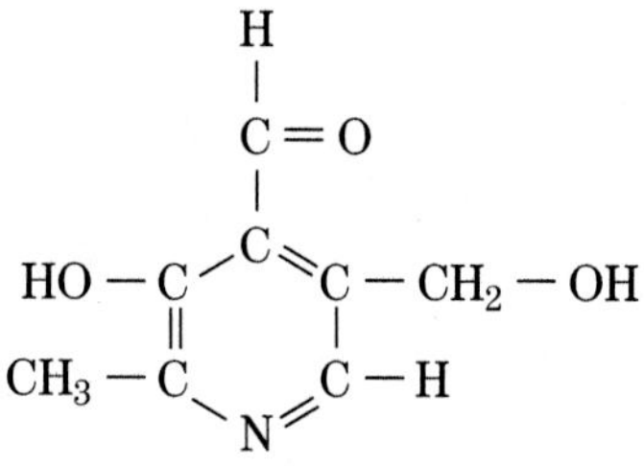

Pyridoxal

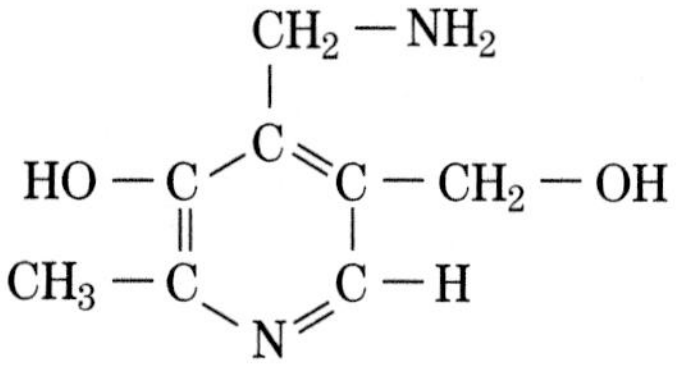

Pyridoxamine

Vitamin B-6 (a general name for three compounds—pyridoxine, pyridoxal, and pyridoxamine).

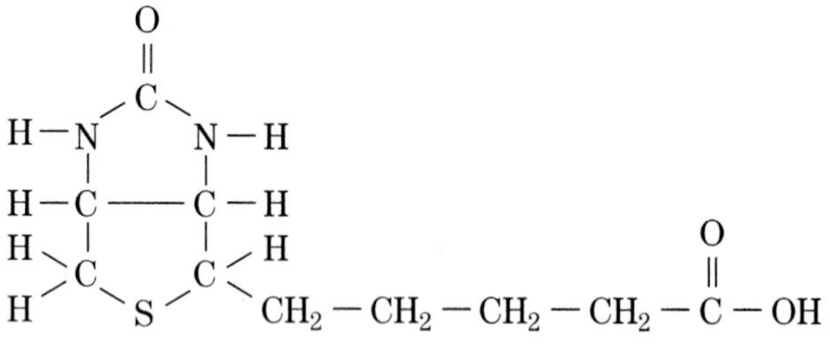

Biotin

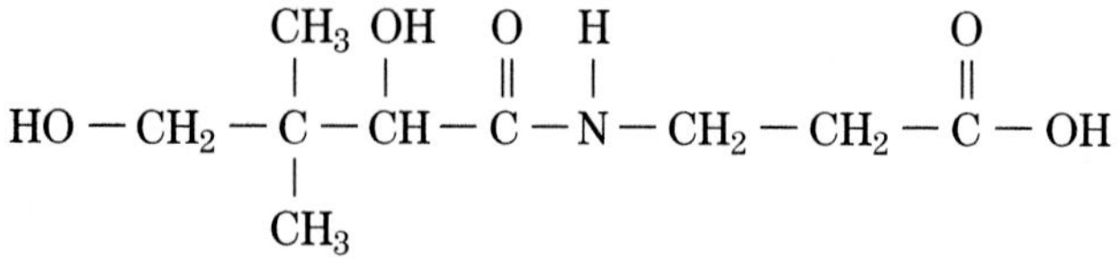

Pantothenic acid

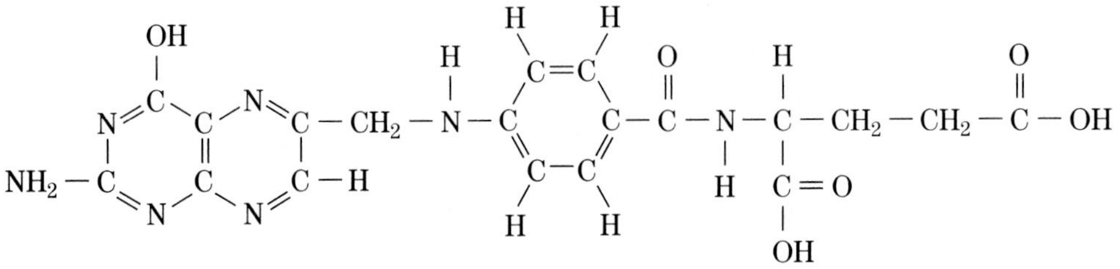

Folate (folacin or folic acid)

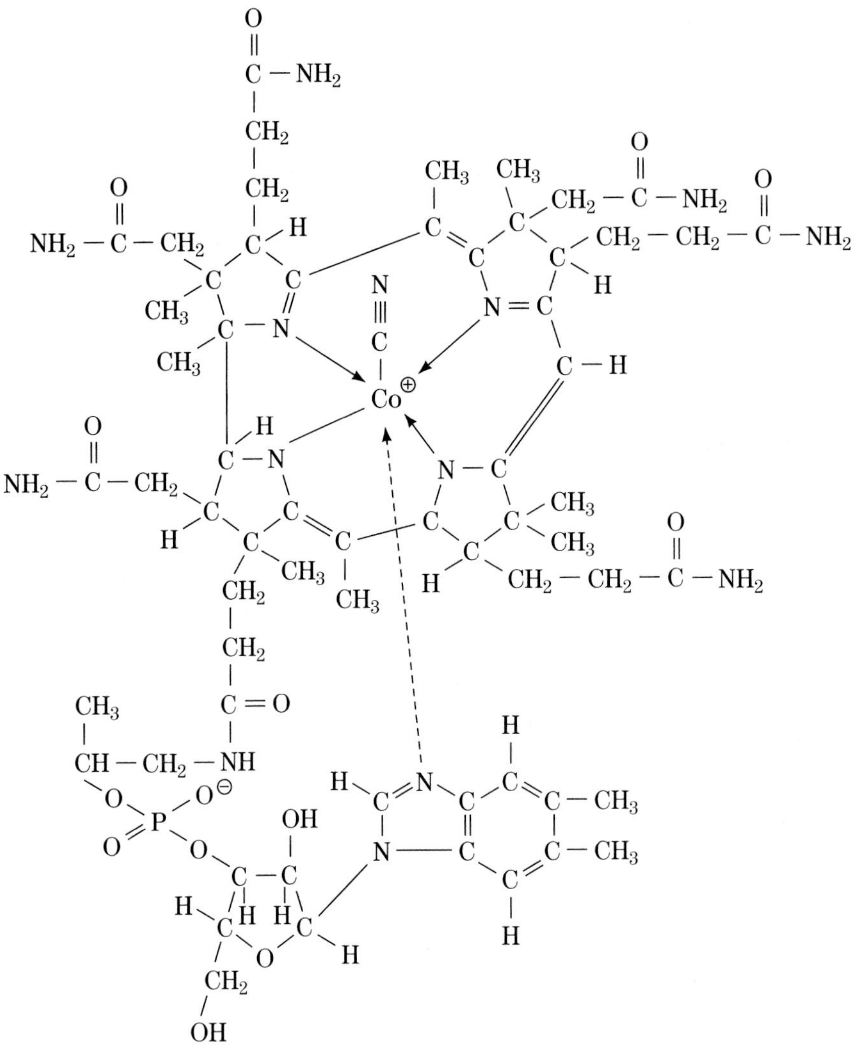

Vitamin B-12 (cyanocobalamin). The arrows in this diagram indicate that the spare electrons on the nitrogens attract them to the cobalt atom.

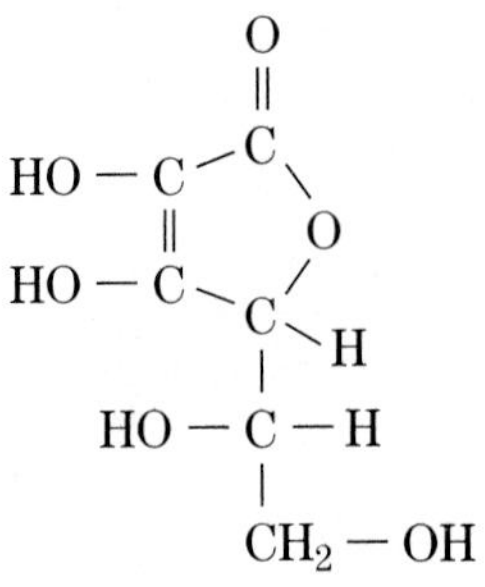

Vitamin C

Vitamin C (ascorbic acid)

H

Ketones

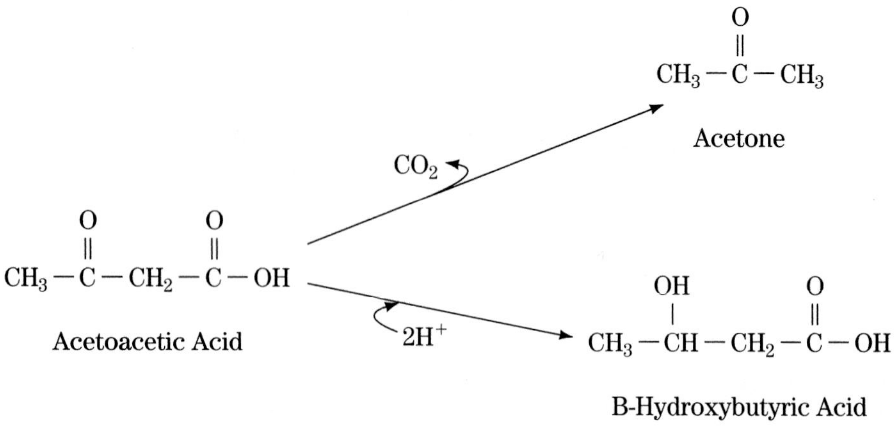

Adenosine Triphosphate (ATP)

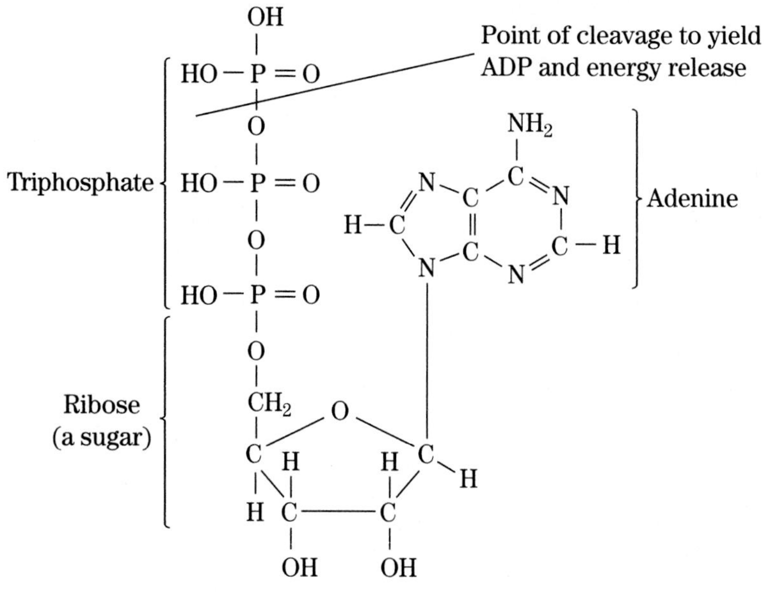

H

APPENDIX I

DETERMINATION OF FRAME SIZE

Method 1

Height is recorded without shoes.

Wrist circumference is measured just beyond the bony (styloid) process at the wrist joint on the right arm using a tape measure.

The following formula is used:

$$r = \frac{\text{height (cm)}}{\text{wrist circumference (cm)}}$$

Frame size can be determined as follows:

Males	Females
r > 10.4 small	r > 11.0 small
r = 9.6-10.4 medium	r = 10.1-11.0 medium
r < 9.6 large	r < 10.1 large

From Grant JP: Handbook of total parenteral nutrition, *Philadelphia, 1980, WB Saunders.*

Method 2

The patient's right arm is extended forward perpendicular to the body, with the arm bent so the angle at the elbow forms 90 degrees, with the fingers pointing up and the palm turned away from the body. The greatest breadth across the elbow joint is measured with a sliding caliper along the axis of the upper arm, on the two prominent bones on either side of the elbow. This is recorded as the elbow breadth. The following tables give the elbow breadth measurements for medium-framed men and women of various heights. Measurements lower than those listed indicate a small frame size; higher measurements indicate a large frame size.

Men		Women	
Height in 1″ Heels	**Elbow Breadth**	**Height in 1″ Heels**	**Elbow Breadth**
5′2″-5′3″	2½-2⅞	4′10″-4′11″	2¼-2½
5′4″-5′7″	2⅝-2⅞	5′0″-5′3″	2¼-2½
5′8″-5′11″	2¾-3	5′4″-5′7″	2⅜-2⅝
6′0″-6′3″	2¾-3⅛	5′8″-5′11″	2⅜-2⅝
6′4″ and over	2⅞-3¼	6′0″ and over	2½-2¾

From Metropolitan Life Insurance Co, 1983.

APPENDIX J

CAFFEINE CONTENT OF FOODS

Beverages	
Carbonated Beverages*	
cherry Coke, Coca-Cola—*12 fl oz (370 g)*	46
cherry cola Slice—*12 fl oz (360 g)*	48
cherry RC—*12 fl oz (360 g)*	12
Coca-Cola—*12 fl oz (370 g)*	46
Coca-Cola Classic—*12 fl oz (369 g)*	46
cola, RC—*12 fl oz (360 g)*	18
Mello Yello—*12 fl oz (372 g)*	52
Mr. Pibb—*12 fl oz (369 g)*	40
Mountain Dew—*12 fl oz (360 g)*	54
pepper type soda—*12 fl oz (368 g)*	37
Pepsi Cola—*12 fl oz (360 g)*	38
Carbonated Beverages, Low-Calorie*	
diet cherry Coke, Coca-Cola—*12 fl oz (354 g)*	46*
diet cherry cola Slice—*12 fl oz (360 g)*	41
diet Coke, Coca-Cola—*12 fl oz (354 g)*	46
diet cola, aspartame sweetened—*12 fl oz (355 g)*	50
diet Pepsi—*12 fl oz (360 g)*	36
diet RC—*12 fl oz (360 g)*	48
Pepsi Light—*12 fl oz (360 g)*	36
Tab—*12 fl oz (354 g)*	46
Coffee	
brewed—*6 fl oz (177 g)*	103
instant powder—*1 tsp (1.8 g)*	57
decaffeinated—*1 rounded tsp (1.8 g)*	2
with chicory—*1 tsp (1.8 g)*	37
prepared from instant powder—*6 fl oz water & 1 tsp powder (179 g)*	57
amaretto, General Foods—*6 fl oz water & 11.5 g powder (189 g)*	60
amaretto, sugar-free, General Foods—*6 fl oz water & 7.7 g powder (185 g)*	60
decaffeinated—*6 fl oz water & 1 tsp powder (179 g)*	2
Francais, General Foods—*6 fl oz water & 11.5 g powder (189 g)*	53
Francais, sugar-free, General Foods—*6 fl oz water & 7.7 g powder (185 g)*	59
Irish creme, General Foods—*6 fl oz water & 12.8 g powder (190 g)*	53
Irish creme, sugar-free, General Foods—*6 fl oz water & 7.1 g powder (185 g)*	48
Irish mocha mint, General Foods—*6 fl oz water & 11.5 g powder (189 g)*	27

From Pennington JAT: Bowes and Church's food values of portions commonly consumed, *ed 16, Philadelphia, 1993, JB Lippincott.*

**Caffeine-free carbonated beverages and most noncola carbonated beverages contain no caffeine.*

Irish mocha mint, sugar-free, General Foods—*6 fl oz water & 6.4 g powder (189 g)*	25
orange cappuccino, General Foods—*6 fl oz water & 14 g powder (191 g)*	73
orange cappuccino, sugar-free, General Foods—*6 fl oz water & 6.7 g powder (184 g)*	71
Suisse mocha, General Foods—*6 fl oz water & 11.5 g powder (189 g)*	41
Suisse mocha, sugar-free, General Foods—*6 fl oz water & 6.4 g powder (184 g)*	40
Vienna, General Foods—*6 fl oz water & 14 g powder (191 g)*	56
Vienna, sugar-free, General Foods—*6 fl oz water & 6.7 g powder (184 g)*	55
with chicory—*6 fl oz water & 1 tsp powder (179 g)*	38
Tea, Hot/Iced	
brewed 3 min—*6 fl oz water (178 g)*	36
instant powder—*1 tsp (0.7 g)*	31
with lemon flavor—*1 rounded tsp (1.4 g)*	25
with sugar & lemon flavor—*3 tsp (23 g)*	29
with sodium saccharin & lemon flavor—*2 tsp (1.6 g)*	36
prepared from instant powder	
1 tsp powder in 8 fl oz water (237 g)	31
Crystal Light—*8 fl oz (238 g)*	11
with lemon flavor—*1 tsp powder in 8 fl oz water (238 g)*	26
with sugar & lemon flavor—*3 tsp powder in 8 fl oz water (259 g)*	29
with sodium saccharin & lemon flavor—*2 tsp powder in 8 fl oz water (238 g)*	36
Candy	
chocolate	
German sweet, Bakers—*1 oz square (28 g)*	8
semi-sweet, Bakers—*1 oz square (28 g)*	13
chocolate chips	
Bakers—*¼ cup (43 g)*	12
German sweet, Bakers—*¼ cup (43 g)*	15
semi-sweet, Bakers—*¼ cup (43 g)*	14
Desserts	
Frozen Desserts	
pudding pops, Jell-O	
chocolate—*1 pop (47 g)*	2
chocolate caramel swirl—*1 pop (47 g)*	1
chocolate fudge—*1 pop (47 g)*	3
chocolate vanilla swirl—*1 pop (47 g)*	2
chocolate with chocolate coating—*1 pop (49 g)*	3
double chocolate swirl—*1 pop (47 g)*	2
milk chocolate—*1 pop (47 g)*	2
Pies	
chocolate mousse, from mix, Jell-O—*⅛ pie (95 g)*	6
Puddings, from instant mix	
chocolate	
Jell-O—*½ cup (150 g)*	5
sugar-free, D-Zerta—*½ cup (130 g)*	4
sugar-free, Jell-O—*½ cup (133 g)*	4
chocolate fudge	
Jell-O—*½ cup (150 g)*	8
chocolate fudge mousse, Jell-O—*½ cup (86 g)*	12
chocolate mousse, Jell-O—*½ cup (86 g)*	9
chocolate tapioca, Jell-O—*½ cup (147 g)*	8
milk chocolate, Jell-O—*½ cup (150 g)*	5
Milk Beverages	
chocolate flavor mix in whole milk—*2-3 tsp powder in 8 fl oz milk (266 g)*	8
chocolate malted milk flavor powder	
in whole milk—*3 tsp powder in 8 fl oz milk (265 g)*	8
with added nutrients in whole milk—*4-5 tsp powder in 8 fl oz milk (265 g)*	5
chocolate syrup in whole milk—*2 Tbsp syrup in 8 fl oz milk (282 g)*	6
cocoa/hot chocolate, prepared with water from mix—*¾ tsp powder in 6 fl oz water (206 g)*	4
Milk Beverage Mixes	
chocolate flavor mix, powder—*2-3 tsp (22 g)*	8
chocolate malted milk flavor mix, powder—*¾ oz (3 t) (21 g)*	8
chocolate malted milk flavor mix with added nutrients, powder—*¾ oz (4-5 tsp) (21 g)*	6
chocolate syrup—*2 Tbsp (1 fl oz) (38 g)*	5
cocoa mix powder—*1 oz pkt (3-4 tsp) (28 g)*	5
Miscellaneous	
baking chocolate, unsweetened, Bakers—*1 oz (28 g)*	25

J

APPENDIX K

TOTAL ENERGY COST OF VARIOUS ACTIVITIES

(Resting energy needs plus any extra energy needed to perform the activity)

	Body Weight		
Activity	**120 Pounds (54 Kilograms) Kcal/Hour**	**150 Pounds (68 Kilograms) Kcal/Hour**	**180 Pounds (82 Kilograms) Kcal/Hour**
Aerobics—heavy	435	544	653
Aerobics—light	163	204	244
Aerobics—medium	272	340	408
Back-packing	489	612	734
Badminton	277	346	416
Ballroom dancing	166	208	249
Basketball—vigorous	544	680	816
Bicycling (5.5 MPH)	163	204	244
Billiards	108	136	163
Bowling	212	265	318
Calisthenics—heavy	435	544	653
Calisthenics—light	217	272	326
Canoeing (2.5 MPH)	179	224	269
Carpentry—general	272	340	408
Circuit training	604	755	906
Cleaning (F)	202	253	303
Cleaning (M)	189	236	284
Climbing (100 FT/HR)	391	489	587
Cooking (F)	146	183	220
Cooking (M)	156	195	235
Cycling (13 MPH)	527	659	791
Disco dancing	326	408	489
Ditch digging—hand	315	394	473
Dressing/showering	85	106	128
Driving	93	117	140
Eating (sitting)	75	93	112
Fencing	239	299	359
Food shopping (F)	202	253	303
Food shopping (M)	189	236	284
Football—touch	380	476	571
Gardening	174	217	261
Gardening—digging	411	514	617
Gardening—raking	176	220	264
Golf	195	244	293
Horseback riding—trotting	277	346	416
Housework—cleaning	217	272	326
Ice skating (10 MPH)	315	394	473

K

Activity	Body Weight: 120 Pounds (54 Kilograms) Kcal/Hour	150 Pounds (68 Kilograms) Kcal/Hour	180 Pounds (82 Kilograms) Kcal/Hour
Jazzercize—heavy	435	544	653
Jazzercize—light	163	204	244
Jazzercize—medium	272	340	408
Jogging—medium	489	612	734
Jogging—slow	380	476	571
Judo	636	795	955
Lawn mowing (hand)	212	265	318
Lawn mowing (power)	195	244	293
Lying—at ease	71	89	107
Piano playing	130	163	195
Racquetball—social	435	544	653
Roller skating	277	346	416
Rowboating (2.5 MPH)	239	299	359
Running or jogging (10 MPH)	718	897	1077
Scull rowing (race)	669	836	1004
Sewing—hand	104	130	156
Shuffleboard/skeet	163	204	244
Sitting quietly	68	85	102
Skiing (10 MPH)	478	598	718
Sleeping	64	80	97
Square dancing	277	346	416
Squash or handball	478	598	718
Swimming (.25 MPH)	239	299	359
Table tennis	282	353	424
Tennis	331	414	497
Volleyball	277	346	416
Walking (2.5 MPH)	163	204	244
Walking (3.75 MPH)	239	299	359
Water skiing	380	476	571
Weight lifting—heavy	489	612	734
Weight lifting—light	217	272	326
Window cleaning (F)	192	240	288
Window cleaning (M)	189	236	284
Wood chopping/sawing	315	394	473
Writing (sitting)	94	118	142

From N^2 Computing, Salem, OR.
M, Male.
F, Female.

APPENDIX K

RECORD # ________

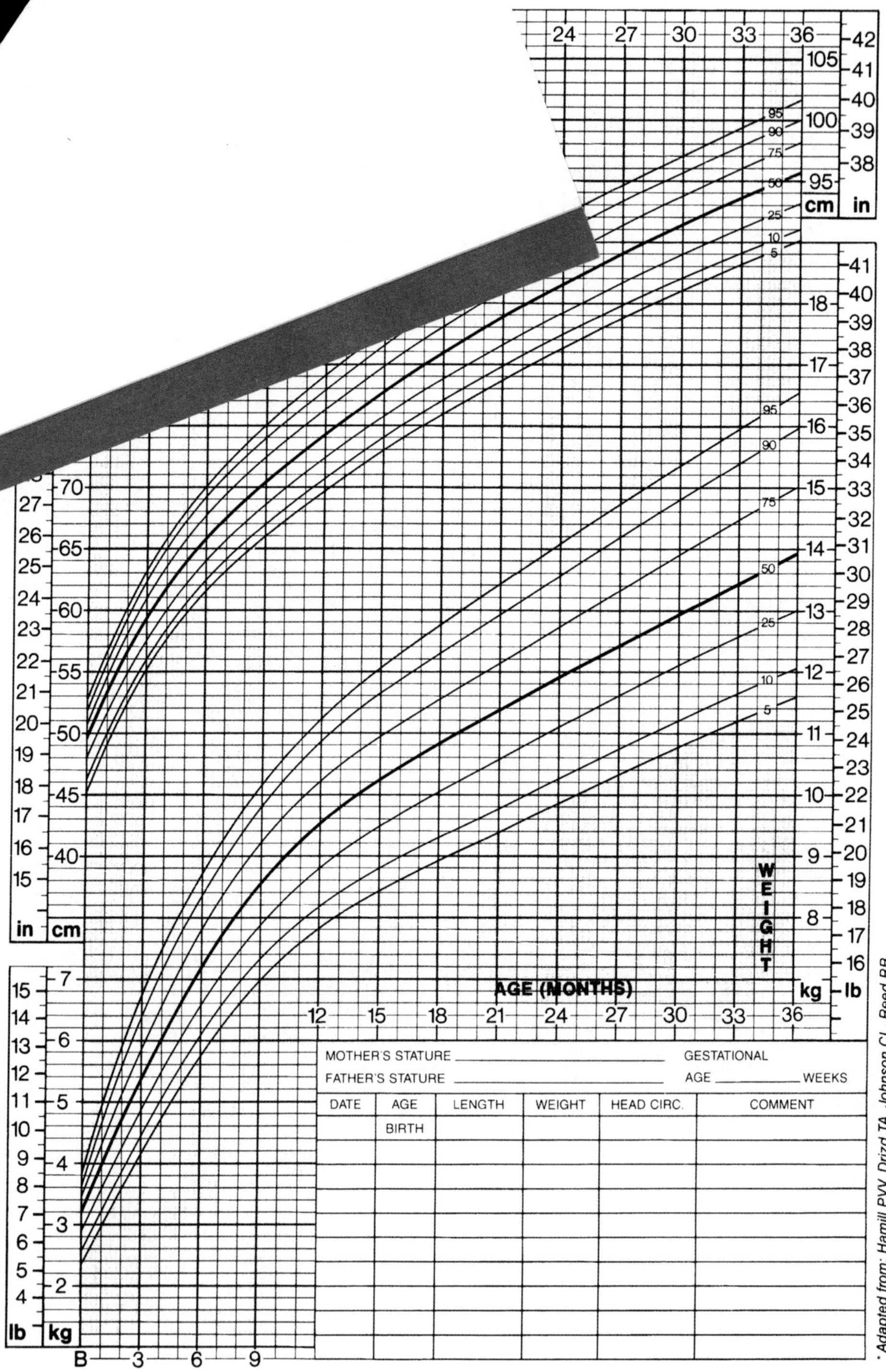

MOTHER'S STATURE ________ GESTATIONAL

FATHER'S STATURE ________ AGE ________ WEEKS

DATE	AGE	LENGTH	WEIGHT	HEAD CIRC.	COMMENT
	BIRTH				

L

* Adapted from: Hamill PVV, Drizd TA, Johnson CL, Reed RB, Roche AF, Moore WM: Physical growth: National Center for Health Statistics percentiles. AM J CLIN NUTR 32:607-629, 1979. Data from the Fels Longitudinal Study, Wright State University School of Medicine, Yellow Springs, Ohio.

BOYS: BIRTH TO 36 MONTHS
PHYSICAL GROWTH
NCHS PERCENTILES*

NAME ____________________ RECORD # ____________

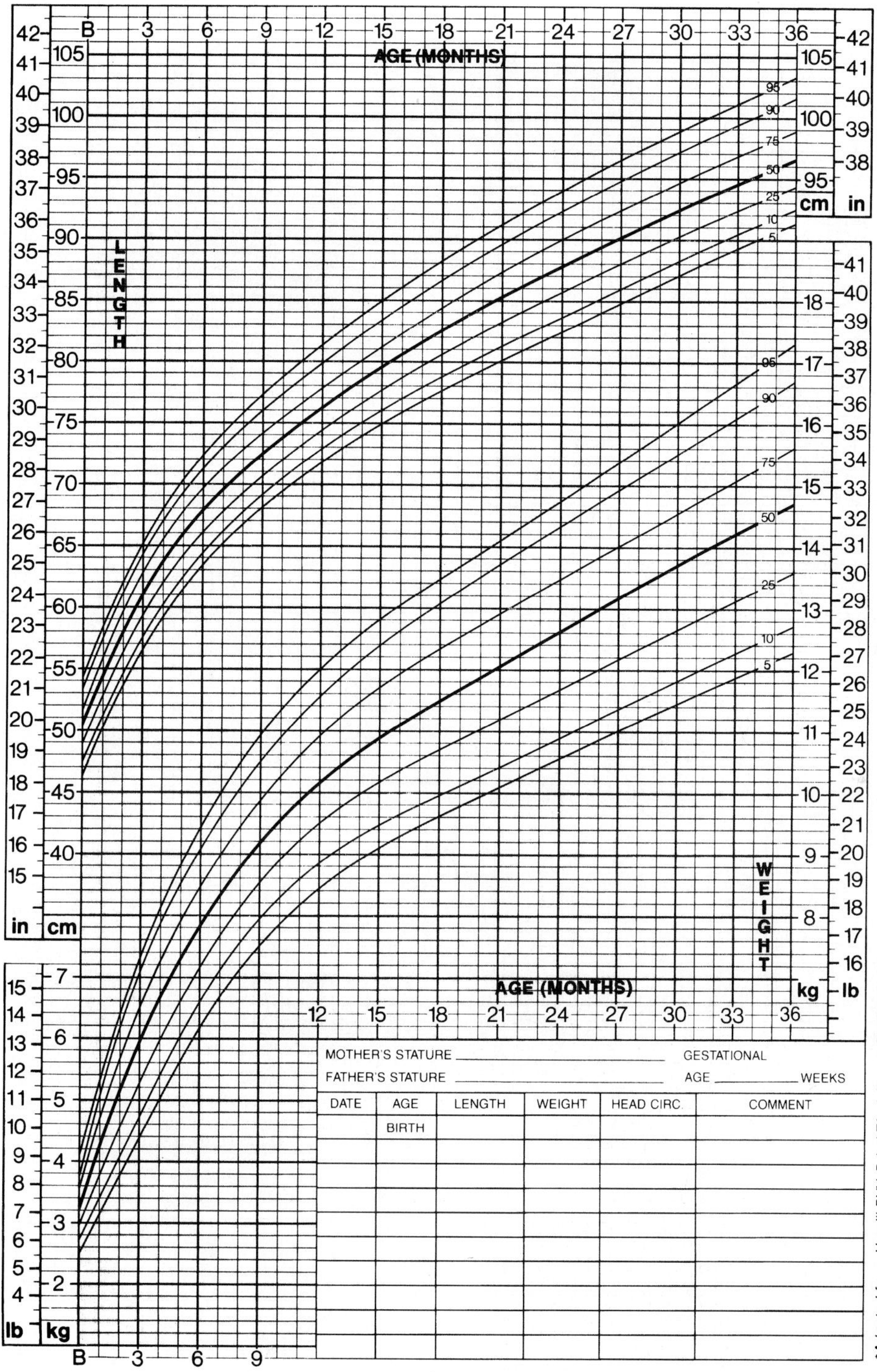

MOTHER'S STATURE ____________ GESTATIONAL
FATHER'S STATURE ____________ AGE ________ WEEKS

DATE	AGE	LENGTH	WEIGHT	HEAD CIRC.	COMMENT
	BIRTH				

*Adapted from: Hamill PVV, Drizd TA, Johnson CL, Reed RB, Roche AF, Moore WM: Physical growth: National Center for Health Statistics percentiles. AM J CLIN NUTR 32:607-629, 1979. Data from the Fels Longitudinal Study, Wright State University School of Medicine, Yellow Springs, Ohio.

L

GIRLS: BIRTH TO 36 MONTHS
PHYSICAL GROWTH
NCHS PERCENTILES*

NAME ______________________ RECORD # ____________

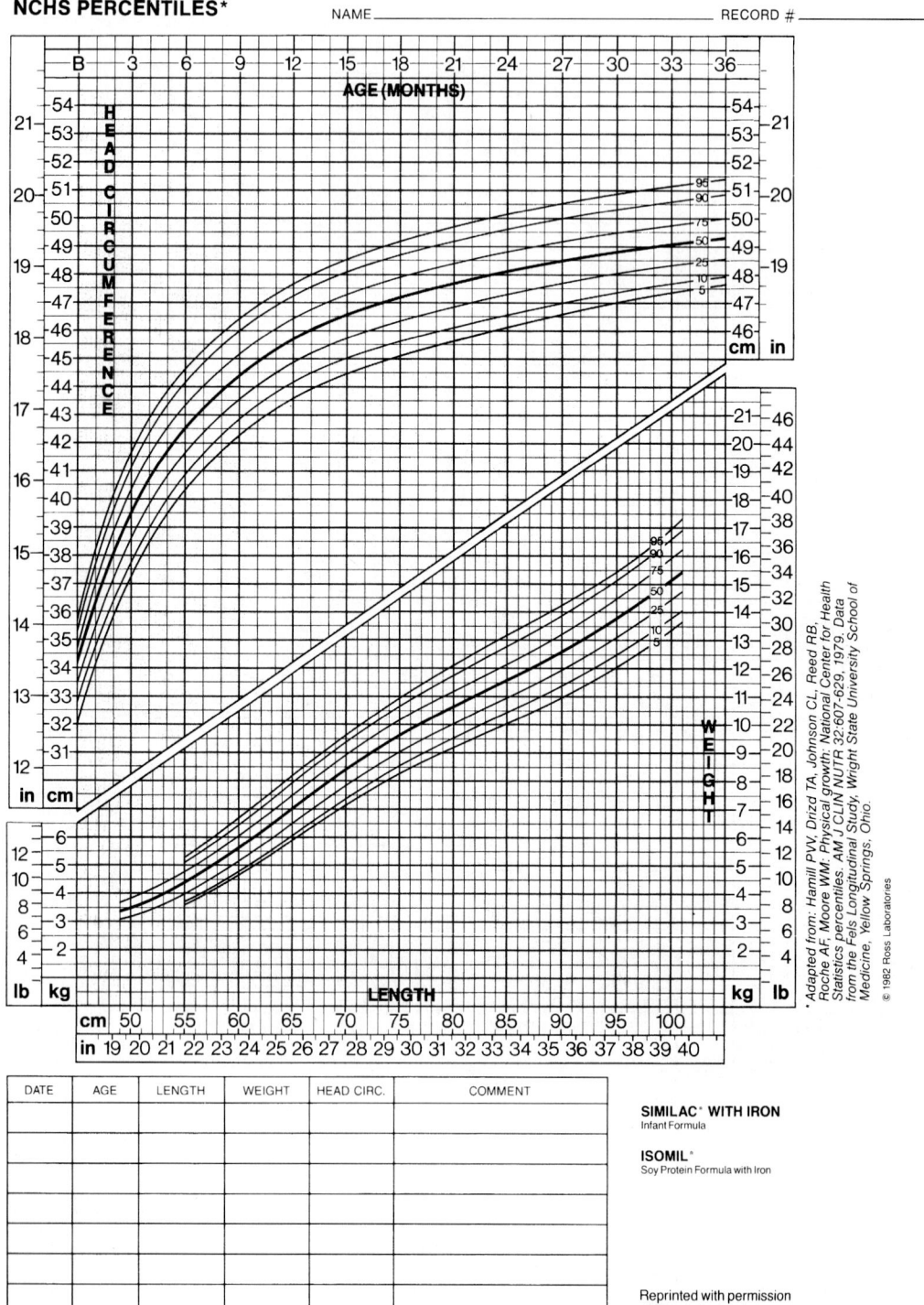

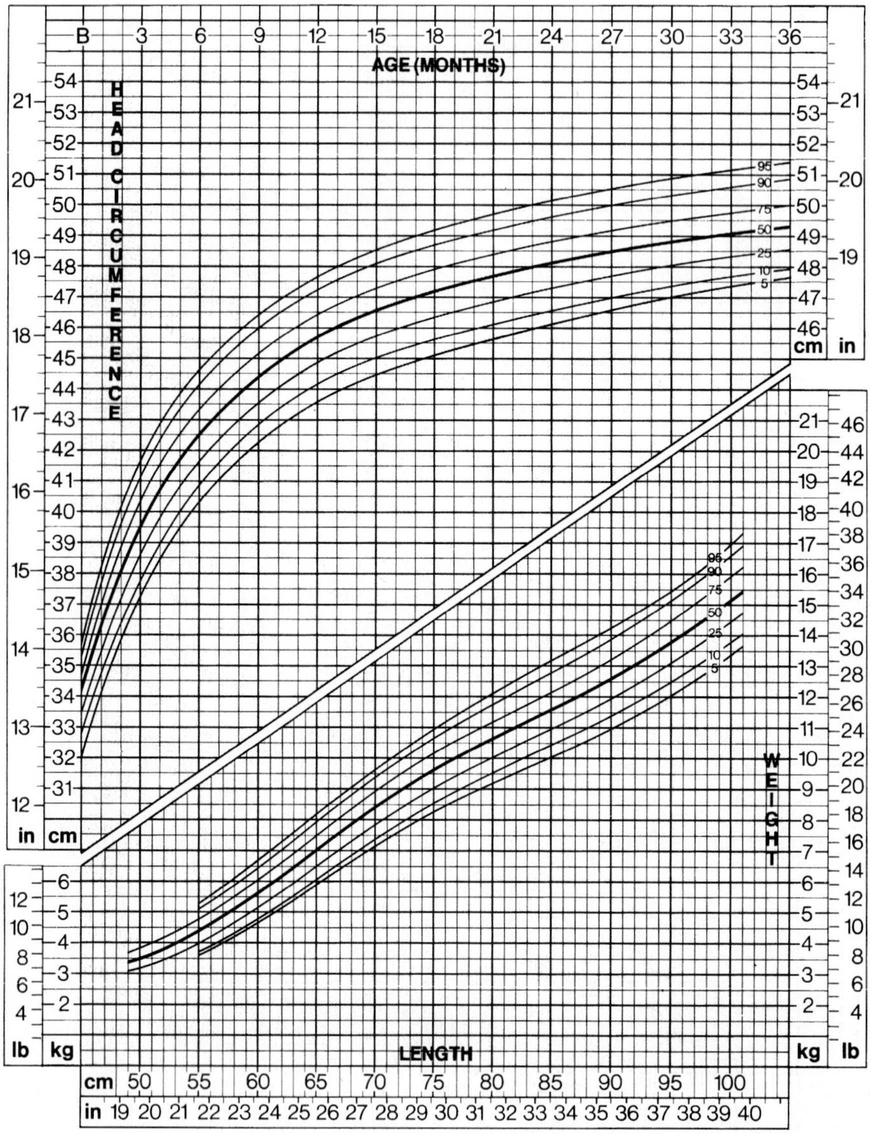

* Adapted from: Hamill PVV, Drizd TA, Johnson CL, Reed RB, Roche AF, Moore WM: Physical growth: National Center for Health Statistics percentiles. AM J CLIN NUTR 32:607-629, 1979. Data from the Fels Longitudinal Study, Wright State University School of Medicine, Yellow Springs, Ohio.

DATE	AGE	LENGTH	WEIGHT	HEAD CIRC.	COMMENT

SIMILAC® WITH IRON
Infant Formula

ISOMIL®
Soy Protein Formula with Iron

Reprinted with permission of Ross Laboratories

L

BOYS: BIRTH TO 36 MONTHS
PHYSICAL GROWTH
NCHS PERCENTILES*

NAME ______________________ RECORD # ____________

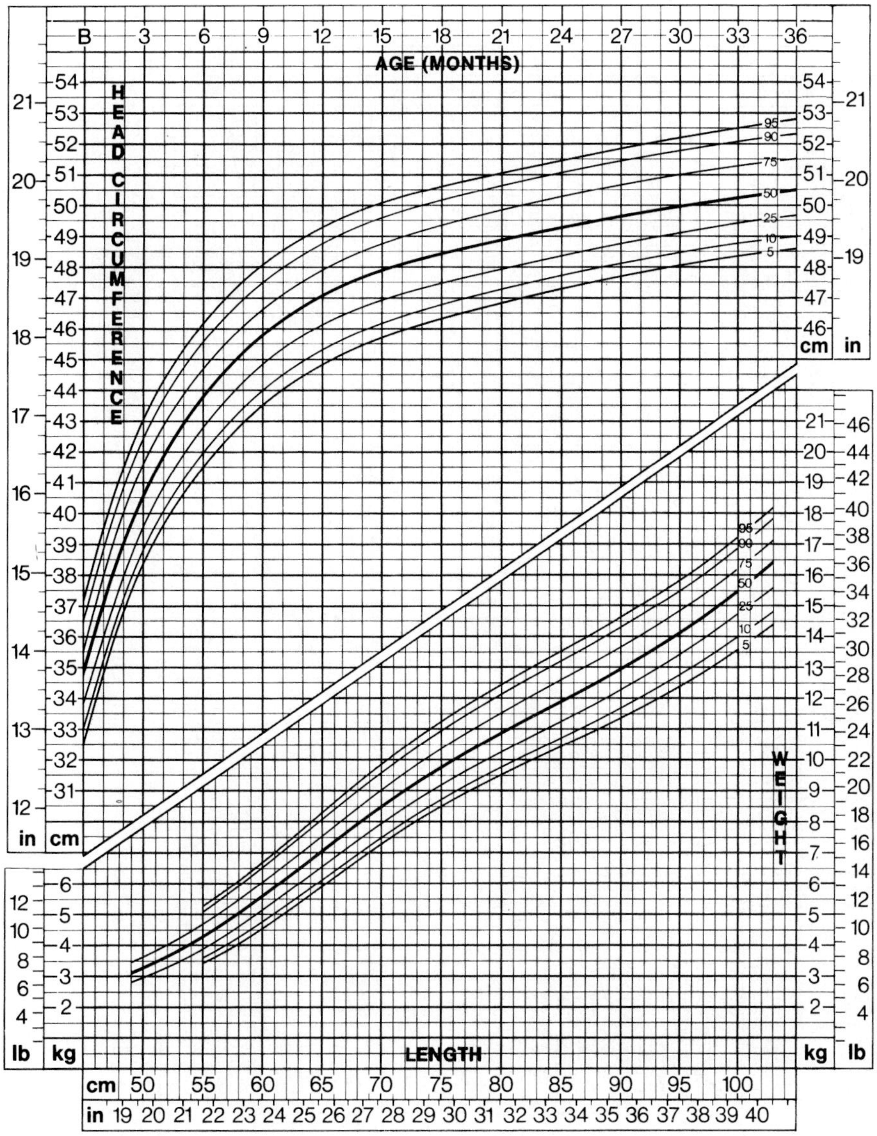

DATE	AGE	LENGTH	WEIGHT	HEAD CIRC.	COMMENT

*Adapted from: Hamill PVV, Drizd TA, Johnson CL, Reed RB, Roche AF, Moore WM: Physical growth: National Center for Health Statistics percentiles. AM J CLIN NUTR 32:607-629, 1979. Data from the Fels Longitudinal Study, Wright State University School of Medicine, Yellow Springs, Ohio.

L

BOYS: PREPUBESCENT PHYSICAL GROWTH NCHS PERCENTILES*

NAME ______________________ RECORD # ____________

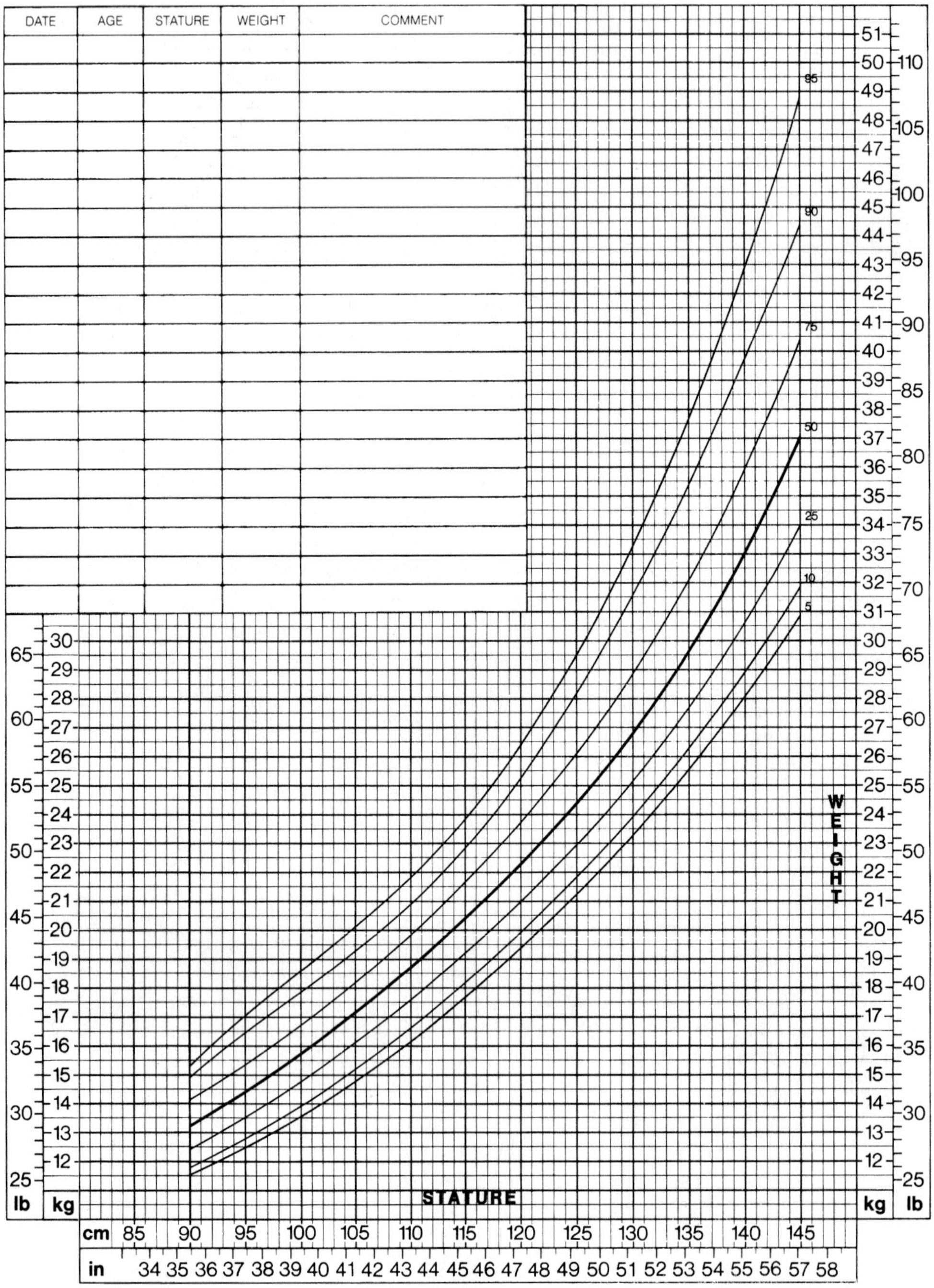

*Adapted from: Hamill PVV, Drizd TA, Johnson CL, Reed RB, Roche AF, Moore WM: Physical growth: National Center for Health Statistics percentiles. AM J CLIN NUTR 32:607-629, 1979. Data from the National Center for Health Statistics (NCHS), Hyattsville, Maryland.

Reprinted with permission of Ross Laboratories

L

GIRLS: PREPUBESCENT PHYSICAL GROWTH NCHS PERCENTILES*

NAME______________________ RECORD #______________

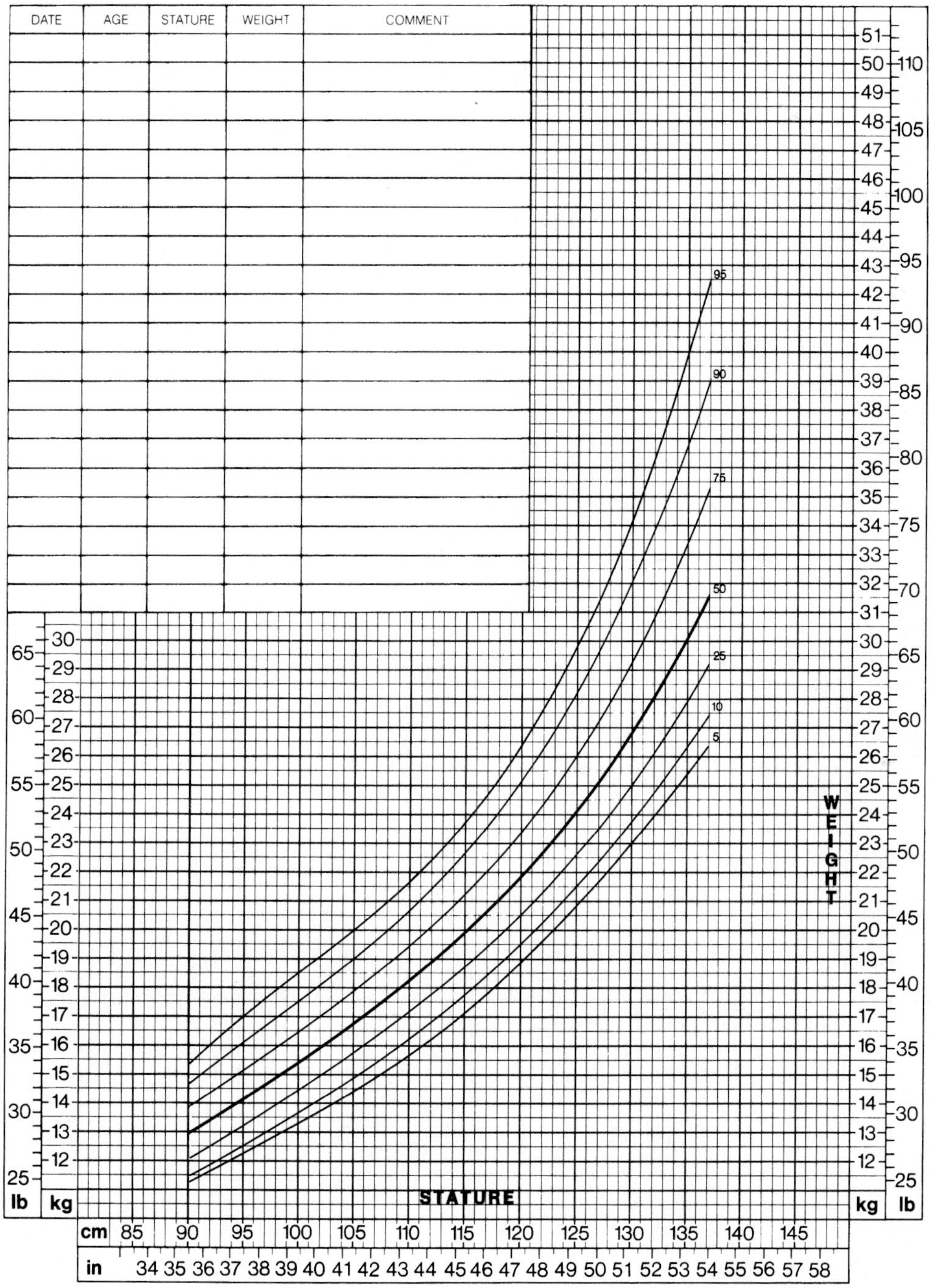

*Adapted from: Hamill PVV, Drizd TA, Johnson CL, Reed RB, Roche AF, Moore WM: Physical growth: National Center for Health Statistics percentiles. AM J CLIN NUTR 32:607-629, 1979. Data from the National Center for Health Statistics (NCHS) Hyattsville, Maryland.

SIMILAC® WITH IRON
Infant Formula

ISOMIL®
Soy Protein Formula with Iron

Reprinted with permission of Ross Laboratories

L

GIRLS: 2 TO 18 YEARS
PHYSICAL GROWTH
NCHS PERCENTILES*

NAME ____________________ RECORD # ____________

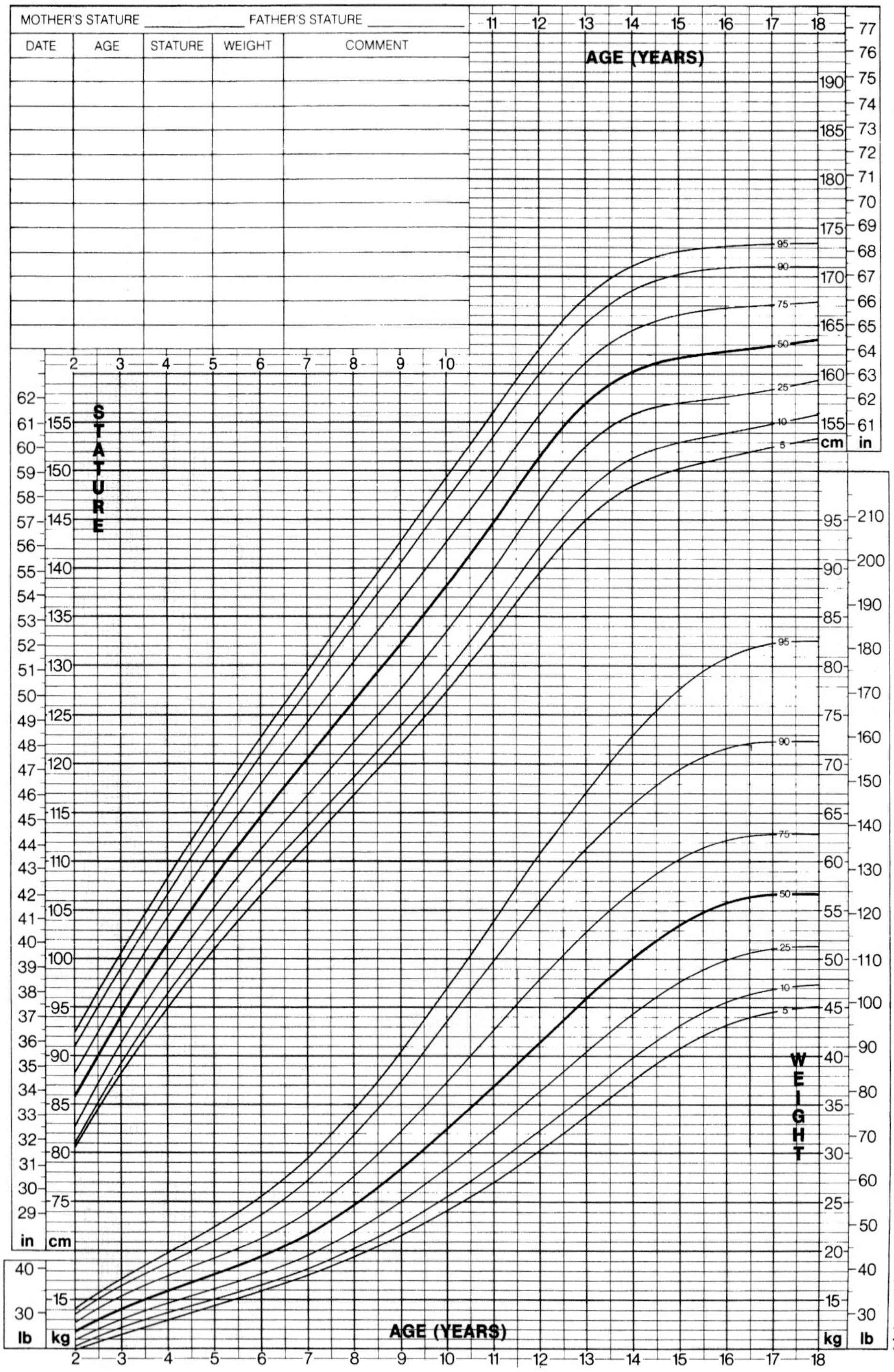

*Adapted from: Hamill PVV, Drizd TA, Johnson CL, Reed RB, Roche AF, Moore WM: Physical growth: National Center for Health Statistics percentiles. AM J CLIN NUTR 32:607-629, 1979. Data from the National Center for Health Statistics (NCHS), Hyattsville, Maryland.

L

BOYS: 2 TO 18 YEARS
PHYSICAL GROWTH
NCHS PERCENTILES*

NAME ____________________ RECORD # ____________

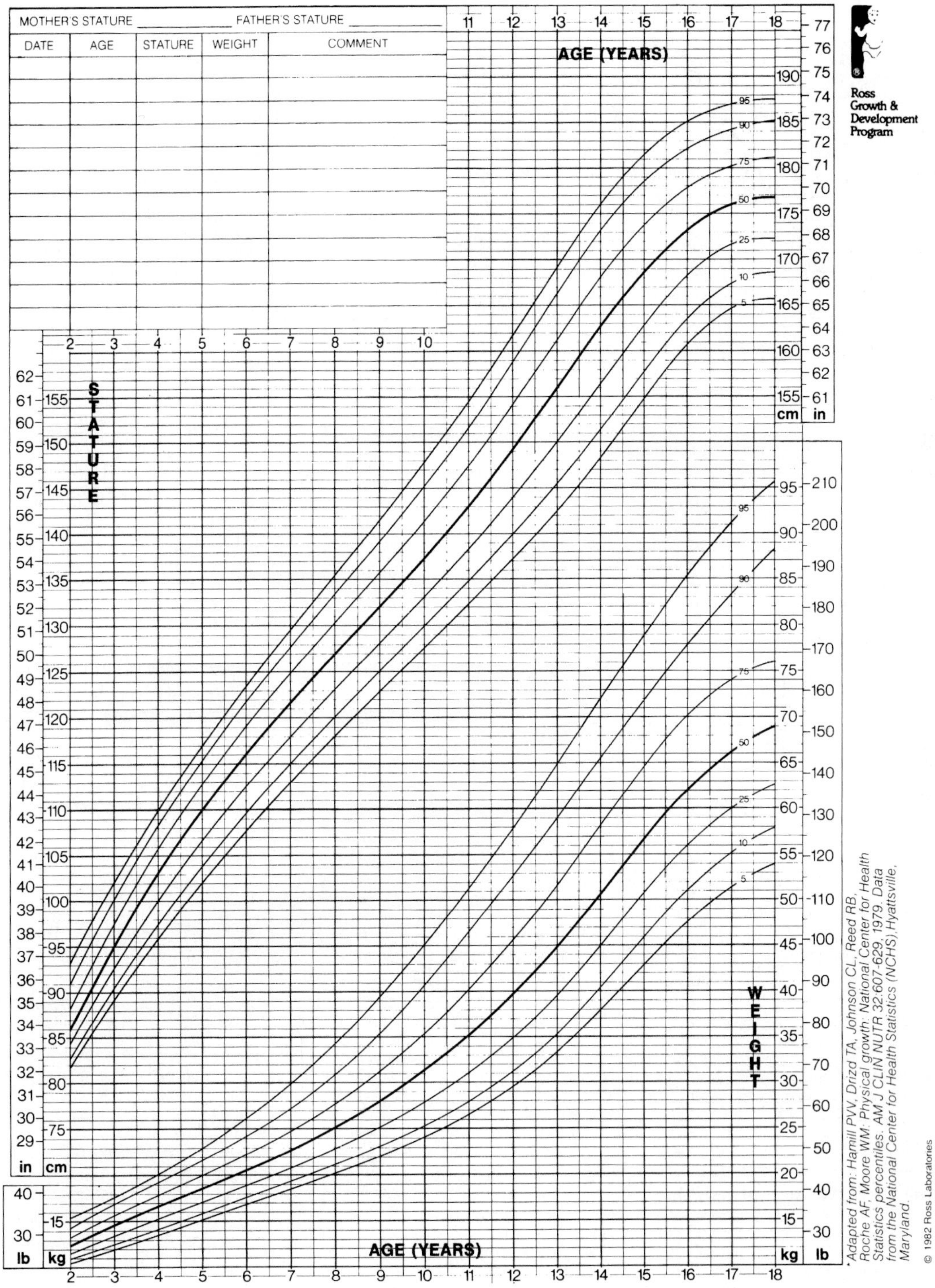

*Adapted from: Hamill PVV, Drizd TA, Johnson CL, Reed RB, Roche AF, Moore WM: Physical growth: National Center for Health Statistics percentiles. AM J CLIN NUTR 32:607-629, 1979. Data from the National Center for Health Statistics (NCHS), Hyattsville, Maryland.

L

APPENDIX M

SAFE FOOD STORAGE

Safe Food Storage and Handling Chart —Refrigerator Storage—

The suggested time aims at maintaining good eating quality and minimizing loss of nutritive value. Suggested maximal times for storing food in refrigerator at 35° F to 40° F

Food	Time	Special Handling
Canned food after opening		
Baby food	2-3 days	*Store covered. Don't feed baby from jar; saliva may liquefy food.*
Fish, seafood, and poultry	1 day	
Fruit	1 week	*Store all canned foods tightly covered. It is not necessary to remove food from can.*
Meats, gravy, broths	2 days	
Pickles, olives	1 month	
Sauce, tomato based	5 days	
Vegetables	3 days	
Cured and smoked meats		
Bacon, corned beef	5-7 days	*Keep wrapped. Store in coldest part of refrigerator or in a meat keeper. Times are for opened packages of sliced meats. Unopened vacuum packs keep for about 2 weeks.*
Bologna loaves	4-6 days	
Dried beef	10-12 days	
Dry and semidry sausage (salami, etc.)	2-3 weeks	
Frankfurters, liver sausage	4-5 days	
Hams (whole, halves)	1 week	
Hams, canned (unopened)	6 months	
Luncheon meat	3 days	
Sausage, fresh or smoked	2-3 days	
Dairy products		
Butter, margarine	1-2 weeks	*Keep tightly wrapped or covered.*
Buttermilk, sour cream, or yogurt	5-14 days	
Cheese		
cottage, ricotta	5 days	*Keep all cheese tightly packaged in moisture-resistant wrap. If outside of hard cheese gets moldy, just cut away mold—it won't affect flavor.*
cream, Neufchatel	2 weeks	
hard and wax-coated cheeses		
large pieces (unopened)	3-6 months	
(opened)	3-4 weeks	
(sliced)	2 weeks	
processed (opened)	3-4 weeks	*Unopened processed cheese need not be refrigerated*
Cream—light, heavy, half-and-half	3 days	*Keep tightly covered. Don't return unused cream to original container. This would spread any bacteria present in leftover cream.*
Dips—sour cream, etc.		
commercial	2 weeks	
homemade	2 days	
Eggs: in shell	3 weeks	
whites	3 days	*Store in covered container.*
yolks	3 days	*Cover yolks with water; cover container.*

M

Safe Food Storage and Handling Chart —Refrigerator Storage—cont'd

The suggested time aims at maintaining good eating quality and minimizing loss of nutritive value.
Suggested maximal times for storing food in refrigerator at 35° F to 40° F

Food	Time	Special Handling
Dairy products—cont'd		
Milk		
evaporated (opened)	4-5 days	
pasturized, reliquefied nonfat dry, skimmed	3-4 days	*Keep containers tightly closed. Do not return unused milk to original container.*
sweetened condensed	4-5 days	*Remove entire lid of can to make pouring easier. Keep covered.*
Fruits and vegetables—fresh		
Fruits		
apples, melons, citrus fruits	1 week	*Do not wash fruit before storing—moisture encourages spoilage. Store in crisper or moisture-resistant bags or wrap. Wrap uncut cantaloupe, honeydew, etc., to prevent odor spreading to other foods.*
berries, cherries	1-2 days	
other fruit	3-5 days	
citrus juices, bottled, frozen, canned	6 days	
Vegetables		
beets, carrots, radishes	2 weeks	*Remove leafy tops; keep in crisper.*
mushrooms	1-2 days	*Do not wash before storing.*
shredded salad greens	1-2 days	*Keep in moisture-resistant wrap or bags.*
peas (in the pod), corn in husks	3-5 days	*Keep in crisper or moisture-resistant wrap or bags.*
other vegetables	3-5 days	*Keep in crisper or moisture-resistant wrap or bags.*
Meat, fish, and poultry—fresh uncooked		
Meats—beef, lamb, pork, and veal—chops	3-4 days	
ground meat, stew meat	1-2 days	
roasts	5-6 days	
steaks	3-5 days	
variety of meats (liver, heart, etc.)	1-2 days	
Fish and shellfish		*Store loosely wrapped. Keep in coldest part of refrigerator or in meat keeper.*
fresh cleaned fish, including steaks, fillets	1 day	
clams, crab, lobster in shell	2 days	*Cook only live shellfish.*
seafood, including shucked clams, oysters, scallops, shrimp	1 day	
Poultry		*Store loosely wrapped. Keep fresh poultry in coldest part of refrigerator or in meat keeper.*
ready-to-cook chicken, duck, turkey	2 days	
Other foods		
Coffee, regular	2 weeks	
Honey, jams, jellies	——	*Refrigeration not needed, but storage life is lengthened if refrigerated.*
Nuts	2 weeks	*Refrigerate nuts after opening.*
Refrigerated biscuits, rolls, pastries, cookie dough	date on label	*Products keep better if stored in back of refrigerator where it is colder.*
Salad dressings (opened)	3 months	*Keep covered.*
Wines, table	2-3 days	*Keep tightly closed.*
cooking	2-3 months	*Keep tightly closed.*

M

Safe Food Storage and Handling Chart
—Freezer Storage—

Suggested maximal times for storing foods in freezer at 0° F.
Longer than recommended storage is not dangerous, but flavors and textures begin to deteriorate.

Food	Time	Special Handling
Dairy products		
Butter, margarine	9 months	*Store in airtight freezer containers or wrapped in freezer wrap.*
Cheese		
cream cheese	1 month	*Thaw in refrigerator.*
hard cheeses	3 months	*Thaw in refrigerator.*
Roquefort, blue, processed	3 months	*Thaw in refrigerator.*
Cream—light, heavy, half-and-half	2 months	*Heavy cream may not whip after thawing. Use for cooking. Thaw in refrigerator.*
Cream, whipped	1 month	
Eggs: whites	1 year	*Store in covered container. Freeze in amounts for favorite recipes.*
yolks	1 year	
Ice cream, ice milk, sherbet	1 month	*Cover surface with plastic wrap or foil after each use to keep from drying.*
Milk	3 months	*Freezing affects flavor and appearance. Use in cooking and baking. Thaw in refrigerator.*
Fruits and vegetables		
Fruits		
berries, cherries, peaches, pears, pineapple, etc.	1 year	
citrus fruit and juice, frozen at home	1 year	
Vegetables		
home frozen	10 months	*Cabbage, celery, salad greens, tomatoes do not freeze successfully.*
purchased frozen	8 months	
Meat, fish, and poultry		
Meats—home frozen		
bacon, frankfurters, ham slices, luncheon meats	1 month	*If meat is purchased fresh on trays and in plastic wrap, check for holes. If none, freeze in this wrap for up to 1 month. For longer storage, over-wrap with foil, plastic wrap or freezer wrap.*
ground beef, lamb and veal	4 months	
ground pork	3 months	
ham, whole	2 months	
roasts		
beef	1 year	
lamb, veal	9 months	
pork	6 months	
sausage, dry, smoked	1 month	*Keep meat purchased frozen in original package.*
sausage, fresh	2 months	*Thaw and cook according to label instructions.*
steaks		
beef	1 year	
lamb, veal	9 months	
pork	6 months	
Fish		
fillets and steaks from "lean" fish—cod, flounder, haddock, sole	6 months	*To home-freeze fish, wrap in foil, plastic wrap, or freezer wrap. Make packages as airtight as possible. Freeze in coldest part of freezer.*
"oily" fish—bluefish, mackerel, perch, salmon	3 months	
breaded fish	3 months	*Keep fish purchased frozen in original wrapping.*
clams, lobster, scallops	3 months	
cooked fish or seafood	3 months	*Thaw and cook according to label directions.*
king crab	10 months	
oysters	4 months	
shrimp, unbreaded	1 year	
shrimp, breaded	4 months	

M

Safe Food Storage and Handling Chart —Freezer Storage—cont'd

Suggested maximal times for storing foods in freezer at 0° F.
Longer than recommended storage is not dangerous, but flavors and textures begin to deteriorate.

Food	Time	Special Handling
Poultry		
chicken, whole or cut-up	1 year	*Cook all thawed poultry within 1 day.*
chicken livers	3 months	
cooked poultry	3 months	
duck, turkey	6 months	
Miscellaneous		
Baked goods		
breads, baked	3 months	*Package foods tightly in foil, plastic wrap, freezer wrap, or watertight freezer containers.*
breads, unbaked	2 months	
cakes		
cheesecake	3 months	
chocolate	4 months	
fruitcake	1 year	
spongecake	2 months	
yellow or pound	6 months	
pies		
cream, custard	8 months	
fruit	8 months	
Main dishes		
meat, fish and poultry pies and casseroles	3 months	*For casseroles, allow head room for expansion. Freeze in coldest part of freezer.*
TV dinners	6 months	
Nuts	3 months	

Safe Food Storage and Handling Chart —Pantry Shelf Storage—

Suggested maximal times for sorting foods in coldest cabinets

Food	Time	Special Handling
Canned and dried food		
Canned pineapple, tomato, sauerkraut	8 months	*Put in airtight container.*
Fruits, canned	1 year	
dried	6 months	
Gravies	1 year	*Refrigerate after opening.*
Meat, fish, poultry	1 year	
Pickles, olives	1 year	
Soups, canned, dried	1 year	
Vegetables, canned, dried	1 year	
Herbs, spices, and condiments		
Catsup (opened)	1 month	
Herbs and spices		
whole spices, herbs	1 year	
ground spices, herbs	6 months	
Tabasco, Worcestershire	2 years +	

M

Safe Food Storage and Handling Chart —Pantry Shelf Storage—cont'd

Suggested maximal times for sorting foods in coldest cabinets

Food	Time	Special Handling
Mixes and packaged foods		
Cakes, prepared	1-2 days	*If butter-cream, whipped-cream, or custard frostings or fillings, refrigerate.*
Cake mixes	1 year	
Casserole mixes	18 months	
Cookies, homemade	1 week	*Put in airtight container.*
packaged	4 months	*Keep box tightly closed.*
Crackers	3 months	*Keep box tightly closed.*
Frosting, in cans or mixes	8 months	
Hot roll mix	18 months	*If opened, put in airtight container.*
Pancake mix	6 months	*Put in airtight container.*
Piecrust mix	8 months	
Pie and pastries	2-3 days	*Refrigerate whipped cream, custard, chiffon fillings.*
Potatoes, instant	18 months	
Toaster pop-ups	3 months	
Staples		
Baking powder	18 months	
Boullion cubes	1 year	
Bread crumbs, dried	6 months	
Cereals, ready-to-eat	4 months	
ready to cook	6 months	
Chocolate, premelted	1 year	
semi-sweet	2 years	
unsweetened	18 months	
Coffee, cans (unopened)	1 month	*Refrigerate after opening.*
Coffee, instant (opened)	2 weeks	*Keep lid tightly closed.*
(unopened)	6 months	
Coffee lighteners (dry) (opened)	6 months	
Condensed and evaporated milk	1 year	*Refrigerate after opening.*
Flour (all types)	1 year	*Put in airtight container.*
Gelatin (all types)	18 months	
Honey, jams, syrups	1 year	
Nonfat dry milk	6 months	*Put in airtight container.*
Pasta	2 years+	*Keep tightly closed.*
Pudding mixes	1 year	
Rice, white	2 years+	*Keep tightly closed.*
Rice mixes	6 months	
Salad dressing (all types)	3 months	*Refrigerate after opening.*
Salad oil	1-3 months	
Shortening, solid	8 months	
Sugar, brown	4 months	*Put in airtight container.*
confectioners	4 months	*Put in airtight container.*
granulated, molasses	2 years+	*Keep tightly covered.*
Tea, bags	18 months	*Put in airtight container.*
instant	3 years	*Keep tightly covered.*
loose	2 years	*Put in airtight container.*
Miscellaneous		
Coconut	1 year	*Refrigerate after opening.*
Instant breakfast	6 months	
Nuts	9 months	*Refrigerate after opening.*
Onions, potatoes, sweet potatoes	2 weeks	*For longer storage, keep below 50° F, but not refrigerated. Keep dry, out of sun.*
Parmesan cheese	2 months	
Peanut butter (opened)	2 months	
(unopened)	9 months	
Soft drinks	3 months	
Whipped topping mix	1 year	

APPENDIX N

COMMON FOOD ADDITIVES

This list identifies the functions of some of the more than 2800 additives all[illegible]

Additive	Function
A	
Acetic acid	pH control‡
Acetone peroxide	mat-bleach-condit§
Apidic acid	pH control‡
Ammonium alginate	stabil-thick-tex*
Annatto extract	color
Arabinogalactan	stabil-thick-tex*
Ascorbic acid	nutrient preservative antioxidant
Azodicarbonamide	mat-bleach-condit§
B	
Benzoic acid	preservative
Benzoyl peroxide	mat-bleach-condit§
Beta-apo-8′ carotenal	color
Beta carotene	nutrient color
BHA (butylated hydroxyanisole)	antioxidant
BHT (butylated hydroxytoluene)	antioxidant
Butylparaben	preservative
C	
Calcium alginate	stabil-thick-tex*
Calcium bromate	mat-bleach-condit§
Calcium lactate	preservative
Calcium phosphate	leavening†
Calcium silicate	anticaking‖
Calcium sorbate	preservative
Canthaxanthin	color
Caramel	color
Carob bean gum	stabil-thick-tex*
Carrageenan	emulsifier stabil-thick-tex*
Carrot oil	color
Cellulose	stabil-thick-tex*
Citric acid	preservative antioxidant pH control‡
Citrus Red No. 2	color
Cochineal extract	color
Corn endosperm	color
Corn syrup	sweetener

Additive	Function
D	
Dehydrated beets	[illegible]
Dextrose	[illegible]
Diglycerides	[illegible]
Dioctyl sodium sulfosuccinate	[illegible]
Disodium guanylate	[illegible]
Disodium inosinate	[illegible]
Dried algae meal	[illegible]
E	
EDTA (ethylenediamine-tetraacetic acid)	[illegible]
F	
FD&C Colors:	
Blue No. 1	colo[illegible]
Red No. 3	color
Red No. 40	color
Yellow No. 5	color
Fructose	sweetener
G	
Gelatin	stabil-thick-tex*
Glucose	sweetener
Glycerine	humectant
Glycerol monostearate	humectant
Grape skin extract	color
Guar gum	stabil-thick-tex*
Gum arabic	stabil-thick-tex*
Gum ghatti	stabil-thick-tex*
H	
Heptylparaben	preservative
Hydrogen peroxide	mat-bleach-condit§
Hydrolyzed vegetable protein	flavor enhancer
I	
Invert sugar	sweetener
Iodine	nutrient
Iron	nutrient
Iron-ammonium citrate	anticaking‖
Iron oxide	color

N

Additive	Function
	...rvative
	antioxidant
	stabil-thick-tex*
	humectant
	preservative
	nutrient
	color
S	
Saccharin	sweetener
Saffron	color
Silicon dioxide	anticaking[‖]
Sodium acetate	pH control[‡]
Sodium alginate	stabil-thick-tex*

...ive	Function
...lfate	leavening[†]
	preservative
	leavening[†]
	stabil-thick-tex*
	pH control[‡]
	preservative
	preservative
	preservative
	preservative
	preservative
	mat-bleach-condit[§]
	preservative
	emulsifier
	humectant
	sweetener
	flavor
	sweetener
	...lor
	pH control[‡]
	antioxidant
	nutrient
	color
...ly defatted ... cottonseed flour	color
...copherols (vitamin E)	nutrient
	antioxidant
Tragacanth gum	stabil-thick-tex*
Turmeric (oleoresin)	flavor
	color
U	
Ultramarine blue	color
V	
Vanilla, vanillin	flavor
Vitamin A	nutrient
Vitamin C (ascorbic acid)	nutrient
	preservative
	antioxidant
Vitamin D (D-2, D-3)	nutrient
Vitamin E (tocopherols)	nutrient
Y	
Yeast-malt sprout extract	flavor enhancer
Yellow prussiate of soda	anticaking[‖]

From Lehmann P: More than you ever thought you would know about food additives, *FDA Consumer reprint, Health and Human Services Publication No. (FDA) 79-2115, 1979.*

*Key to abbreviations: *stabil-thick-tex = stabilizers-thickeners-texturizers; [†]leavening = leavening agents; [‡]pH control = pH control agents; [§]mat-bleach-condit = maturing and bleaching agents, dough conditioners; [‖]anticaking = anticaking agents.*

APPENDIX N

...owed in the U.S. food supply.

Function

color
sweetener
emulsifier
emulsifier
flavor enhancer
flavor enhancer
color
antioxidant

N

APPENDIX O

SOURCES OF NUTRITION INFORMATION

Consider the following reliable sources of food and nutrition information:

Journals That Regularly Cover Nutrition Topics:

*American Family Physician**
American Journal of Clinical Nutrition
American Journal of Epidemiology
American Journal of Medicine
American Journal of Nursing
American Journal of Obstetrics and Gynecology
American Journal of Physiology
American Journal of Public Health
American Scientist
Annals of Internal Medicine
Annual Reviews of Medicine
Annual Reviews of Nutrition
Archives of Disease in Childhood
Archives of Internal Medicine
British Journal of Nutrition
BMJ (British Medical Journal)
Cancer
Cancer Research
Circulation
Diabetes
Diabetes Care
Disease-a-Month
FASEB Journal
*FDA Consumer**
Food Chemical Toxicology
Food Engineering
Gastroenterology
Geriatrics
Gut
Human Nutrition: Applied Nutrition
Human Nutrition: Clinical Nutrition
*Journal of the American College of Nutrition**
*Journal of The American Dietetic Association**
Journal of The American Geriatric Society
JAMA (Journal of the American Medical Association)
Journal of Applied Physiology
*Journal of Canadian Dietetic Association**
Journal of Clinical Investigation
Journal of Food Service
Journal of Food Technology
JNCI (Journal of the National Cancer Institute)
Journal of Nutrition
*Journal of Nutritional Education**
Journal of Nutrition for the Elderly
Journal of Nutrition Research
Journal of Pediatrics
Lancet
Mayo Clinic Proceedings
Medicine and Science in Sports and Exercise
Nature
New England Journal of Medicine
Nutrition
Nutrition Reviews
*Nutrition Today**
Pediatrics
The Physician and Sports Medicine
*Postgraduate Medicine**
Proceedings of the Nutrition Society
Science
*Science News**
*Scientific American**

The majority of these journals will be available in college or university libraries, or in a specialty library on campus, such as one designated for health services or home economics. As indicated, a few journals will be filed under their abbreviation, rather than the first word in their full name. A reference librarian help you locate any of these sources. The asterisked (*) journals are ones we feel you will find especially interesting and useful, because of the number of nutrition articles presented each month or the less technical nature of the presentation.

Magazines for the Consumer That Cover Nutrition Topics:

Better Homes and Gardens
Consumer Reports
Good Housekeeping
Health
Parents
Self

Textbooks and Other Sources for Advanced Study of Nutrition Topics:

Food and Nutrition Board: *Recommended dietary allowances,* ed 10, Washington, DC, 1989, National Academy of Sciences.
Hunt SM, Groff JL: *Advanced human nutrition and metabolism,* St Paul, Minn, 1990, West.
Linder MC: *Nutritional biochemistry and metabolism with clinical applications,* New York, 1991, Elsevier Science Publishing.
Mahan LK, Arlin MT: *Krause's food, nutrition, and diet therapy,* Philadelphia, 1992, WB Saunders.
Murray RK and others: *Harper's biochemistry,* ed 21, Norwalk, Conn, 1993, Appleton & Lange.
Present knowledge in nutrition, ed 6, 1990, The Nutrition Foundation.
Schils ME, Olson JA, Shike M: *Modern nutrition in health and disease,* ed 8, Philadelphia, 1994, Lea & Febiger.
Woteki CE, Thomas PR: *Eat for life,* Washington, DC, 1992, National Academy Press.

Newsletters That Cover Nutrition Issues on a Regular Basis:

Contemporary Nutrition
General Mills, Inc.
Production Manager
P.O. Box 1112, Department 65
Minneapolis, MN 55440
(inexpensive)

CNI Nutrition Week
Community Nutrition Institute
2001 S. St. N.W.
Washington, D.C. 20009

Dairy Council Digest
National Dairy Council
6300 River Rd.
Rosemont, IL 60018
(inexpensive)

Dietetic Currents
Ross Laboratories
Director of Professional Services
625 Cleveland Ave.
Columbus, OH 43216
(free)

Environmental Nutrition
52 Riverside Dr.
New York, NY 10024

Food and Nutrition News
National Livestock and Meat Board
444 Michigan Ave.
Chicago, IL 60610
(free)

Harvard Medical School Health Letter
Department of Continuing Education
25 Shattuck St.
Boston, MA 02115

Healthline
830 Menlo Ave. #100
Menlo Park, CA 94025

National Council Against Health Fraud Newsletter (NCAHF)
P.O. Box 1276
Loma Linda, CA 92354

Nutrition Forum
George Stickley Co.
210 Washington Square
Philadelphia, PA 19106

Nutrition & the M.D.
P.O. Box 2160
Van Nuys, CA 91404

Nutrition Research Newsletter
P.O. Box 700
Pallisades, NY 10964

Tufts University Diet & Nutrition Letter
P.O. Box 10948
Des Moines, IA 50940

Professional Organizations with a Commitment to Nutrition Issues:

American Academy of Pediatrics
P.O. Box 1034
Evanston, IL 60204

American Cancer Society
777 Third Ave.
New York, NY 10017

American Dental Association
211 E. Chicago Ave.
Chicago, IL 60611

American Diabetes Association
2 Park Ave.
New York, NY 10016

American Dietetic Association
216 W. Jackson Blvd.
Suite 800
Chicago, IL 60606

American Geriatrics Society
770 Lexington Ave.
Suite 400
New York, NY 10021

American Heart Association
7320 Greenville Ave.
Dallas, TX 75231

American Home Economics Association
2010 Massachusetts Ave. N.W.
Washington, D.C. 20036

American Institute of Nutrition
9650 Rockville Pike
Bethesda, MD 20014

American Medical Association
Nutrition Information Section
535 N. Dearborn St.
Chicago, IL 60610

American Public Health Association
1015 Fifteenth St. N.W.
Washington, D.C. 20005

American Society for Clinical Nutrition
9650 Rockville Pike
Bethesda, MD 20014

The Canadian Diabetes Association
123 Edward St.
Suite 601
Toronto, Ontario M5G 1E2 Canada

The Canadian Dietetic Association
480 University Ave.
Suite 601
Toronto, Ontario M5G 1V2 Canada

The Canadian Society for Nutritional Sciences
Department of Foods and Nutrition
University of Manitoba
Winnipeg, Manitoba, R3T 2N2 Canada

Food and Nutrition Board
National Research Council
National Academy of Sciences
2101 Constitution Ave. N.W.
Washington, D.C. 20418

Institute of Food Technologies
221 N. LaSalle St.
Chicago, IL 60601

National Council on the Aging
1828 L St. N.W.
Washington, D.C. 20036

National Institute of Nutrition
1335 Carling Ave.
Suite 210
Ottawa, Ontario K1Z 0L2 Canada

Nutrition Foundation, Inc.
1126 Sixteenth St. N.W.
Suite 111
Washington, D.C. 20036

Nutrition Today Society
428 E. Preston St.
Baltimore, MD 21202

Society for Nutrition Education
1736 Franklin St.
Oakland, CA 94612

Professional or Lay Organizations Concerned with Nutrition Issues:

Bread for the World
802 Rhode Island Ave. N.E.
Washington, D.C. 20018

Center for Science in the Public Interest (CSPI)
1755 S. Street N.W.
Washington, D.C. 20009

California Council Against Health Fraud, Inc.
P.O. Box 1276
Loma Linda, CA 92354

Children's Foundation
1420 New York Ave. N.W.
Suite 800
Washington, D.C. 20005

Food Research and Action Center (FRAC)
1875 Connecticut Ave. N.W. #540
Washington, D.C. 20009

Institute for Food and Development Policy
1885 Mission St.
San Francisco, CA 94103

La Leche League International, Inc.
9616 Minneapolis Ave.
Franklin Park, IL 60131

March of Dimes Birth Defects Foundation
(National Headquarters)
1275 Mamaroneck Ave.
White Plains, NY 10605

Overeaters Anonymous (OA)
2190 190th St.
Torrance, CA 90504

Oxfam America
115 Broadway
Boston, MA 02116

Local Resources for Advice on Nutrition Issues:

Cooperative extension agents in county extension offices
Dietitians (Contact the state or local Dietetics Association.)
Nutrition faculty affiliated with departments of food and nutrition, home economics, and dietetics
Registered Dieticians (RDs) in city, county, or state agencies

Government Agencies That Are Concerned with Nutrition Issues or That Distribute Nutrition Information:

United States
The Consumer Information Center
Department 609K
Pueblo, CO 81009

Department of Agriculture (USDA)
Extension Services
3 South Building
Room 6007
Washington, D.C. 20250

Food and Drug Administration (FDA)
5600 Fishers Lane
Rockville, MD 20852

Food and Nutrition Information and Education Resources Center
National Library of Congress
Beltsville, MD 20705

Human Nutrition Research Division
Agricultural Research Center
Beltsville, MD 20705

Office of Cancer Communications
National Cancer Institute
Building 31
Room 10A18
90 Rockville Pike
Bethesda, MD 20205

National Agricultural Library
10301 Baltimore Blvd.
Room 304
Beltsville, MD 20705

National Center for Health Statistics
3700 East-West
Hyattsville, MD 20782

U.S. Government Printing Office
The Superintendent of Documents
Washington, D.C. 20402

Canada
Department of Community Health
1075 Ste-Foy Rd.
Seventh Floor
Quebec, Quebec G1S 2M1

Home Economics Directorate
880 Portage Ave.
Second Floor
Winnipeg, Manitoba R3G 0P1

Nutrition Programs
446 Jeanne Mance Building
Tunney's Pasture
Ottawa, Ontario K1A 1B4

Nutrition Services
P.O. Box 488
Halifax, Nova Scotia B3J 3R8

Nutrition Services
P.O. Box 6000
Fredericton, New Brunswick E3B 5H1

Public Health Resource Service
15 Overlea Blvd.
Fifth Floor
Toronto, Ontario M4H 1A9

United Nations
Food and Agriculture Organization (FAO)
North American Regional Office
1325 C St. S.W.
Washington, D.C. 20025
or
Via della Terma di Caracella
0100 Rome, Italy

World Health Organization (WHO)
1211 Geneva 27
Switzerland

Trade Organizations and Companies that Distribute Nutrition Information:

American Egg Board
1460 Renaissance St.
Park Ridge, IL 60068

American Institute of Baking
P.O. Box 1148
Manhattan, KS 66502

American Meat Institute
P.O. Box 3556
Washington, D.C. 20007

Best Foods
Consumer Service Department
Division of CPC International
International Plaza
Englewood Cliffs, NJ 07632

Borden Farm Products
Bordon Co.
Consumer Affairs
180 E. Broad St.
Columbus, OH 43215

Campbell Soup Co.
Food Service Products Division
375 Memorial Ave.
Camden, NJ 08101

Del Monte Teaching Aids
P.O. Box 9075
Clinton, IA 52736

Fleischman's Margarines
Standard Brands, Inc.
625 Madison Ave.
New York, NY 10022

General Foods Consumer Center
250 North St.
White Plains, NY 10625

General Mills
P.O. Box 113
Minneapolis, MN 55440

Gerber Products Co.
445 State St.
Fremont, MI 49412

H.J. Heinz
Consumer Relations
P.O. Box 57
Pittsburgh, PA 15230

Hunt-Wesson Foods
Education Services
1654 W. Valencia Dr.
Fullerton, CA 92634

Kellogg Co.
Department of Home Economics Services
Battle Creek, MI 49016

Mead Johnson Nutritionals
2404 Pennsylvania Ave.
Evansville, IN 47721

National Dairy Council
6300 N. River Rd.
Rosemont, IL 60018-4233

Oscar Mayer Co.
Consumer Service
P.O. Box 1409
Madison, WI 53701

Pillsbury Co.
1177 Pillsbury Building
608 Second Ave. S.
Minneapolis, MN 55402

The Potato Board
1385 S. Colorado Blvd.
Suite 512
Denver, CO 80222

Rice Council
P.O. Box 22802
Houston, TX 77027

Ross Laboratories
Director of Professional Services
625 Cleveland Ave.
Columbus, OH 43216

Sunkist Growers Consumer Service
Division BB, P.O. Box 7888
Valley Annex
Van Nuys, CA 91409

Vitamin Nutrition Information Service (VNIS)
Hoffmann-LaRoche
340 Kingsland Ave.
Nutley, NJ 07110

United Fresh Fruit and Vegetables Association
727 N. Washington St.
Alexandria, VA 22314

GLOSSARY

The Following Medical Terms and Combining Forms Are Used Frequently in the Study of Nutrition.

Term	Meaning
a-	without, from
acyl	a carbon chain
aden-, adeno-	gland
-algia	pain
aliment	food
-amine	containing nitrogen
andr-, andro-	man or male
ap-, apo-	detached
arteri-, arterio-	artery
arthr-, arthro	joint
-ase	enzyme
-blast	immature form, embryonic, growing
brady-	slow
buli-	ox (as in the animal)
cancr-, carcino-	malignant tumor
cardi-, cardio-	heart
centi-	divided into 100 parts
chol-, chole-, cholo-	bile, gall
cholecyst-	gallbladder
chondr-, chondrio-, chondro-	cartilage
chrom-, chromo-	color, colored
-clast	something that breaks
col-, coli-, colo-	colon
cyan-, cyano-	blue
cyt-, cyto-	cell
derm-, dermato-	skin
dextr-, dextro-	right, on or toward the right
duoden-, duodeno-	duodenum
dys-	difficult, painful
ect-, ecto-	without, outside, external
-ectomy	excision of
-ein	a protein
em-	blood
-emia	in blood
encephal-, encephalo-	brain
end-, endo-, ent-, ento-	within
enter-, entero-	intestine
erythr-, erythro-	red
esophag-, esophago-	esophagus
eu-	well, easy, good
gastr-, gastri-, gastro-	stomach
gen-	to become or produce
gloss-, glosso-	tongue
gluco-, glyc-, glyco-	sugar
gyn-, gyne-, gyneco-	woman or female (especially female reproductive organs)
hem-, hemat-	blood

Term	Meaning
hepat-, hepato-	liver
hex-, hexa-	six
hist-, histo-	tissue
homeo-, homoeo-, homoio-	sameness, similarity
hydr-, hydro-	water
hyp-, hypo-	under, beneath, deficient
hyper-	excessive, above, beyond
hyster-, hystero-	uterus
idio-	one's own, peculiar to; separate, distinct
ile-, ileo-	ileum
inter-	between, among
intra-	within, during, between layers of
-itis	inflammation of
jejun-, jejuno-	jejunum
kilo-	1000 times
lact-, lacti-, lacto-	milk
leuc-, leuk-	white, colorless
lev-, levo-	left
lip-, lipo-	fat, lipid
lith-, litho-	stone
lymph-, lympho-	waterlike
-lysis	destruction
mal-	bad, badly
malac-, malaco-	soft, a condition of abnormal softness
mega-, megalo-	large, great
meta-	after, later; change, exchange
metallo-	containing metal
micro-	divided into 1 million parts
milli-	divided into 1000 parts
mono-	one
morph-, morpho-	form, shape
my-, myo-	muscle
myel-, myelo-	marrow; spinal cord
nas-, naso-	nose, nasal
necr-, necro-	dead
nephr-, nephro-	kidney
neur-, neuro-	nerve
-oid	formed like
olig-, oligo-	few, scant
-ol	alcohol
-oma	tumor
ophthalm-, ophthalmo-	eye, eyeball
-orex	mouth
-orexis	desire, appetite
-ose	sugar, carbohydrate
-osis	action, process, result, usually discussed
ost-, oste-, osteo-	bone
ot-	ear
ovari-, ovario-	ovary
ovi-, ovo-	eggs
pan-	all
pancreat-, pancreato-	pancreas
para-	beside
parieto-	wall of a cavity
path-, patho-	disease
ped-	child; foot
-penia	without, lack of
-phobia	fear of

Term	Meaning
-plasm	formative, formed; cell or tissue substance
pneum-, pneumo-, pneumono-	lung
-poiesis	production
poly-	many, much
post-	after
pre-	before
prot-, proto-	first
pseud-, pseudo-	false
pulmo-, pulmon-, pulmono-	lung
pyel-, pyelo-	pelvis
pyr-	fever, fire
rect-, recto-	rectum
reni-, reno-	kidney
rhin-, rhino-	nose
-rrhagia	rupture; excessive fluid discharge
-rrhea	flow, discharge
-sate	to fill
scler-, sclero-	hard, hardness
-scopy	viewing
seb-, sebi-, sebo-	hard fat; sebum, sebaceous glands
semi-	half
-soma, somat-, somato-	body
-stasia, -stasis	slowing or stopping of
stenosis	narrowing of
stomat-, stomato-	mouth, stoma
-stomy	surgical opening
sub-	under, below
super-	over, above
tachy-	swift, fast
thi-, thio-	containing sulfur
thromb-, thrombo-	blood clot
tox-, toxi-, toxo-	poison
trache-, tracheo-	trachea
-trophy	growth, mutation
ure-, urea-, ureo-	urine
uter-, utero-	uterus
vas-, vaso-	blood vessel
ven-, veni-, veno-	vein
vita-	life
xer-, sero-	dry

GLOSSARY TERMS

absorptive cells (ab-sorp-tiv) A class of cells that line the villi (fingerlike projections in the small intestine) and participate in nutrient absorption.
acesulfame-K (ay-see-sul-fame) An artificial sweetener that yields no energy to the body; it is 200 times sweeter than sucrose.
achlorhydria (ay-clor-high-dre-ah) A state of reduced acid production by the stomach, primarily resulting from loss of the acid-producing cells in the stomach; a condition associated with aging.
acquired immunodeficiency syndrome (AIDS) A disease characterized by poor function of one class of white blood cells (called helper T lymphocytes). The resulting poor immune function leaves the person quite susceptible to infection, which can in turn result in rapidly failing health and death.
active absorption Absorption using a carrier and expending energy. In this way the absorptive cell absorbs nutrients, such as glucose, when a high concentration of the nutrient is already present in the absorptive cells.
ad libitum (ad-lib-eh-tum) At one's desire or pleasure.
adenosine triphosphate (ATP) (ah-den-o-sin try-fos-fate) The main energy currency for cells. ATP energy is used to promote ion pumping, enzyme activity, and muscular contraction.
adipose (fat) cells (add-ih-pos) A grouping of fat-storing cells.
adipsin (ah-dip-sin) A protein that appears to be made by fat cells and that acts as a communication link between these cells and the brain.
adult-onset obesity Obesity that develops in adulthood; characteristically, the individual has a normal number of adipose cells, but each cell is enlarged because of fat storage.
aerobic (air-row-bic) Requiring oxygen.
alcohol (al-co-hall) Ethyl alcohol or ethanol. An energy-yielding substance found in beer, wine, and distilled spirits.
aldosterone (al-dos-ter-own) A powerful hormone produced by the adrenal glands that acts on the kidneys to cause sodium reabsorption and, in turn, water conservation.
alimentary canal (al-ih-men-tah-ree) Another name for the gastrointestinal (GI) tract.
alkaline (basic) pH (al-kah-line) A pH greater than 7. Baking soda in water yields an alkaline pH.
allergy (al-er-jee) An immune response that occurs when immune bodies (antibodies) react with a foreign substance (antigen).
alpha-linolenic acid (al-fah lin-oh-len-ik) A fatty acid with 18 carbon atoms and three double bonds; omega-3.
alveoli (al-ve-o-lye) The small air sacs of the lungs.
amino acid (ah-mee-noh) The building block for proteins; amino acids have a carbon in the center with a nitrogen and other atoms attached.
amniotic fluid (am-nee-ott-ik) The fluid that surrounds and protects the fetus in the uterus.
amylase (am-uh-lace) Starch-digesting enzymes from the salivary glands or pancreas.
amylopectin (am-ih-low-pek-tin) A branched-chain polysaccharide made of glucose units.
amylose (am-uh-los) A straight-chain digestible polysaccharide made of glucose units.
anabolism (an-ah-bol-iz-um) The process of building compounds.
anaerobic (an-ah-row-bic) Not requiring oxygen.
anaphylactic shock (an-ah-fih-lak-tic) A severe allergic response that results in greatly lowered blood pressure, as well as respiratory and gastrointestinal distress.
androgen (an-dro-jen) A general term for hormones that stimulate development in male sex organs; testosterone is an example.
anemia (a-knee-me-a) Poor oxygen-carrying ability of the blood, caused by a reduction in the number of healthy red blood cells.
anergy (an-er-jee) Lack of an immune response to foreign compounds entering the body.
animal model A disease in animals that duplicates human disease and thus can be used to further understand human diseases.
anorexia nervosa (an-oh-rex-ee-uh ner-voh-sah) An eating disorder involving a psychological loss of appetite and self-starvation, resulting in part from a distorted body image and various social pressures associated with puberty.
anthropometry (an-throw-pom-eh-tree) The measurement of weight, lengths, circumferences, and thicknesses of the body.
antibody (an-tih-bod-ee) Blood proteins that inactivate foreign proteins found in the body. This helps prevent infection.
anticarcinogens (an-tie-car-sin-o-gins) Compounds that potentially inhibit the development of cancer.
antidiuretic hormone (ADH) (an-tie-dye-your-ret-ik) A hormone secreted by the pituitary gland that acts on the kidneys to decrease water excretion.
antioxidant (an-tie-ox-ih-dant) A compound that can donate electrons to electron-seeking (oxidizing) compounds. This reduces the destructive nature of oxidizing compounds.
apolipoproteins (ape-oh-lip-oh-pro-teens) Proteins embedded in the outer shell of lipoproteins.
appetite (ap-peh-tight) The psychological or external drive to find and eat food, often in the absence of hunger.
arachidonic acid (air-ah-kih-don-ik) A fatty acid with 20 carbon atoms and four double bonds; omega-6.
areola (ah-ree-oh-lah) The circular dark area of skin at the center of the breast.
arithmetic ratio A group of numbers in which the difference between each number is the same.
arthritis (arth-rite-us) Inflammation at a point where bones join; the disease has many possible causes.
aseptic processing (ah-sep-tik) A method by which food and its container are sterilized simultaneously; this process allows manufacturers to produce boxes of milk that can be stored at room temperature. Variations of this process are also known as ultra-high-temperature (UHT) packaging.

aspartame (ah-spar-tame) An alternate sweetener made of two amino acids (part of proteins) and methanol; it is 200 times sweeter than sucrose.
atherosclerosis (ath-er-oh-scleh-roh-sis) A buildup of fatty material (plaque) in the arteries, including those surrounding the heart.
atom The smallest combining unit of an element.
autodigestion (auto-dye-jes-chun) Literally, self-digestion. The stomach limits autodigestion by covering itself with a thick layer of mucus and by producing enzymes and acid only when needed for digestion of food.
autoimmune (auto-im-mune) Immune reactions against normal body cells; self against self.
avidin (av-ih-din) A protein found in raw egg whites that can bind biotin and inhibit its absorption. Cooking destroys avidin.
bacteria A group of single-cell microorganisms, some of which cause disease; some bacteria produce toxins that lead to ill health in humans.
baryophobia (bear-ee-oh-fo-bee-ah) A poor rate of growth in children associated with parents' underfeeding them in an attempt to prevent obesity and heart disease.
basal metabolism (bay-sal) The minimal energy the body requires to support itself when resting and awake. It amounts to roughly 1 kcalorie per minute, or about 1400 kcalories per day.
behavior chains Activities linked in a person's lifestyle, such as snacking while watching television.
behavior contract A written agreement that lists intended changes in behavior, plans for reinforcement, and witnesses to monitor progress.
beriberi (bear-ee-bear-ee) A thiamin-deficiency disorder characterized by muscle weakness, loss of appetite, nerve degeneration, and sometimes edema.
beta-carotene (beta-care-oh-teen) An orange pigment found in many fruits and vegetables, such as peaches and carrots. The body can use beta-carotene to make vitamin A.
BHA and BHT Butylated hydroxyanisole and butylated hydroxytoluene; two common synthetic antioxidants that are added to foods.
bile A substance that is made in the liver and stored in the gallbladder. Bile is released from there into the small intestine to aid fat absorption.
bioavailability The degree to which an ingested nutrient is absorbed and so is available to the body.
biochemical changes Nutritional deficiency symptoms observed in the blood or urine, such as low levels of nutrient by-products or low enzyme activities. These indicate reduced biochemical functioning in the body.
bioelectrical impedance (im-pee-dance) A method of estimating total body fat by measuring the impedance (resistance) of a low-energy electrical current by the body.
biotechnology The use of advanced scientific techniques to alter and, ideally, improve characteristics of animals and plants.
blood doping A technique by which an athlete's red blood cell count is increased. Blood is taken from the athlete. The red blood cells are concentrated by removing fluid from the athlete's blood sample; the red blood cells are then later reintroduced into the athlete.
body mass index Weight (in kilograms) divided by height squared (in meters); a value of 30 or higher generally indicates obesity.
bomb calorimeter (kal-oh-rim-eh-ter) An instrument used to determine the kcalorie content of a food.
bond A sharing of electrons, charges, or attractions used to link two atoms.
brown adipose tissue (add-ih-pos) A specialized form of fat storage that produces large amounts of heat by metabolizing energy-yielding nutrients without synthesizing much usable energy for the body. Much of the energy released simply forms heat.
buffer A compound that can cause a solution to resist changes in acid-base balance.
bulimia (boo-leem-ee-uh) An eating disorder in which large quantities of food are eaten at one time (binging) and then purged from the body by vomiting, use of laxatives, or other means.
calcitriol (kal-sih-try-ol) The active hormone form of vitamin D. A cholesterol-like substance is part of its structure.
cancer (can-sir) A condition characterized by uncontrolled growth of body cells.
carbohydrate loading The process of consuming a very high carbohydrate diet for about 3 days before an athletic event to try to increase muscle glycogen stores.
carbohydrates (kar-bow-high-drates) Compounds containing carbon, hydrogen, and oxygen atoms; known as sugars and starches.
carcinogens (car-sin-oh-gins) Compounds that have the potential to cause cancer.
cardiac output The amount of blood pumped by the heart.
cardiovascular Pertaining to the heart and blood vessels.
cariogenic (care-ee-oh-jen-ik) A substance, often rich in carbohydrates, that promotes dental caries (e.g., caramels and raisins).
carnitine (car-nih-teen) A compound used to shuttle fatty acids into the cell mitochondria, allowing the fatty acids to be burned for energy.
carotenoids (care-ah-ten-oids) Pigment substances in plants that often can form vitamin A. Beta-carotene is the most active form.
casein (kay-seen) A protein found in milk that forms curds; it tends to be difficult for infants to digest.
cash crops Crops grown by a country specifically for export rather than to feed the country's citizens (e.g., coffee, tea, cocoa, and bananas).
catabolic (cat-ah-bol-ik) Breaking down compounds.
catalyst (cat-uhl-ist) A compound that speeds reaction rates but is not altered by the reaction.

cell A minute structure; the living basis of all plant and animal organization. Cells can both take up compounds from their environment and excrete compounds into it.

cell membrane An outer barrier found in animal cells. It is composed mostly of fats and proteins and surrounds each body cell.

cellulose (sell-you-los) A straight-chain polysaccharide of glucose molecules that is undigestible; part of insoluble fiber.

Celsius A centigrade measure of temperature; to convert Fahrenheit temperatures to Celsius, use this formula: (degrees Fahrenheit − 32) ÷ 1.8.

centimeter A measure of length in the metric system; 100 centimeters equal 1 meter.

cerebrovascular accident (CVA) (se-ree-bro-vas-cue-lar) Death of part of the brain tissue as a result of a blood clot.

chain breaking Breaking the link between two or more behaviors that encourage overeating, such as snacking while watching television.

chemical reaction An interaction between two chemicals that changes both participants.

cholecystokinin (CCK) (koh-lee-sis-toe-ky-nin) A hormone that stimulates the release of enzymes from the pancreas and bile from the gallbladder.

cholesterol (koh-les-te-rol) A waxy fat, made only by animals, that is found in all body cells. Its structure contains multiple chemical rings.

chronic (kron-ik) Long standing, developing over time; slow to develop or resolve. When referring to disease, this indicates that the disease progress slows and tends to remain once it has developed, as with heart disease.

chylomicrons (kye-lo-my-krons) Dietary fats that are surrounded by a shell of cholesterol, phospholipids, and protein. Chylomicrons are made in the intestine after fat absorption and travel through the lymphatic system to the bloodstream.

chyme (kime) A mixture of stomach secretions and partly digested food.

cirrhosis (sir-roh-sis) A loss of functioning liver cells, which are replaced by nonfunctioning connective tissue. Any substance that poisons liver cells, such as alcohol, can lead to cirrhosis.

clinical symptom Generally, a change in health status noted by the individual (e.g., stomach pain) or during a physical examination.

Clostridium botulinum (claw-strid-ee-um bot-you-ly-num) A bacterium that can cause a fatal type of food-borne illness.

coenzyme (koh-en-zime) The active form of many vitamins; coenzyme forms aid enzyme function.

cognitive restructuring Changing one's frame of mind regarding something, such as eating. For example, instead of using a difficult day as an excuse to overeat, substituting other pleasures for rewards, such as a relaxing walk with a friend.

colic (call-ik) Periodic crying in a healthy infant, apparently as a result of gas buildup in the intestinal tract.

collagen (call-a-gin) The major protein form found in connective tissue, cartilage, and bone. Vitamin C aids in its synthesis.

colon (ko-lon) Another name for the large intestine.

colostrum (ko-lahs-trum) The first milk secreted during late pregnancy and the first few days after birth. This thick fluid is rich in immune factors and protein.

complementarity of proteins The ability of two food protein sources to make up for each other's insufficient contribution of specific essential amino acids, such that together they yield a sufficient amount of all nine and so provide high-quality protein for the diet.

constipation A condition of infrequent bowel movements.

contingency management Forming a plan of action for responding to an environment in which overeating is likely, such as when snacks are within easy reach at a party.

cortical bone (kort-ih-kal) Dense compact bone that composes the outer surface and shaft of a bone.

cortisol a hormone produced naturally in the human body; among other functions, cortisol increases blood glucose, promotes protein metabolism, and suppresses the immune and inflammatory responses.

covalent bond (ko-vay-lent) A union of two atoms formed by the sharing of electrons.

cretinism (kreet-in-ism) The stunting of body growth and mental development that results from inadequate maternal intake of iodide during pregnancy.

crude fiber The remains of dietary fiber after acid and alkaline treatment; this consists primarily of cellulose and lignins.

cystic fibrosis (sis-tik figh-bro-sis) A disease that, among other effects, often leads to overproduction of mucus, which can invade the pancreas and decrease the production of enzymes. The subsequent lack of lipase enzyme contributes to severe malabsorption of fat.

Daily Reference Values (DRVs) New reference values for nutrients on food labels; are set by FDA for nutrients that don't have an RDA; will be listed with RDIs under "Daily Values" on food labels.

deamination (dee-am-ih-na-shun) The removal of an amino group from an amino acid.

Delaney Clause A clause in the 1958 Food Additives Amendment of the Pure Food and Drug Act; it forbids the intentional (direct) addition to foods of a compound that has been shown to cause cancer in animals or humans.

dementia (de-men-shah) A general loss or decrease in mental function.

denature (dee-nay-ture) Alteration of a protein's three-dimensional structure, usually as a result of treatment by heat, enzymes, acid or alkaline solutions, or agitation.

dental caries (kare-ees) Sites of erosion on the tooth surface. Caries is caused by the acid produced when bacteria on the tooth's surface metabolize sugar.

deoxyribonucleic acid (DNA) The site of hereditary information in cells; DNA directs the synthesis of cell proteins.

dermatitis (derm-a-tite-us) Inflammation of the skin.

diabetes (dye-uh-beet-eez) A disease characterized by high blood sugar levels that are caused by insufficient action of the hormone insulin.

diastolic blood pressure (dye-ah-stol-ik) The pressure in the bloodstream when the heart is between beats.

dietary fiber Substances in food (essentially all from plants) that are not digested by the processes in the stomach and small intestine.

dietary goals Specific goals for nutrient intake set in 1977 by a committee of the U.S. Senate.

dietary guidelines General goals for nutrient intake and diet composition set by the U.S. Department of Agriculture and the Department of Health and Human Services.

digestibility (dye-jes-tih-bil-it-ee) The proportion of food substances eaten that can be broken down in the intestinal tract and absorbed into the bloodstream.

digestion (dye-jes-tjun) The process by which food is broken down into forms that can be taken up by the GI tract.

diphosphoglycerate (dye-foss-foe-gliss-er-ate) A compound used in the red blood cells that is involved in the release of oxygen from hemoglobin.

direct calorimetry (cal-oh-rim-eh-tree) A method of determining energy use by the body by measuring heat that emanates from the body.

disaccharides (dye-sack-uh-rides) A class of sugars formed by linking two monosaccharides.

diuretic (dye-your-et-ik) A substance that increases the flow of urine.

diverticulae (dye-ver-tik-you-lay) Pouches that protrude through the wall of the large intestine. Diverticulosis is the condition of having many diverticulae in the colon.

diverticulitis (dye-ver-tik-you-lite-us) An inflammation of the diverticula caused by acids produced by bacterial metabolism inside the diverticula.

double-blind study An experiment in which the subjects and researchers are unaware of the actual subject assignment and outcomes until the study is completed.

ecosystem A "community" in nature that includes plants and animals and the environment associated with them.

ectomorph (ek-toh-morf) A body type associated with very long, thin bones and very long, thin fingers.

edema (uh-dee-muh) The buildup of excess fluid in the spaces surrounding cells.

eicosanoids (eye-koh-san-oyds) Hormonelike compounds synthesized from polyunsaturated fatty acids; this class of compounds includes prostaglandins, thromboxanes, and leukotrienes.

eicosapentaenoic acid (EPA) (eye-koh-sah-pen-tah-no-ik) An omega-3 fatty acid with 20 carbon atoms and five double bonds; present in fish oils.

electrolytes (ih-lek-tro-lites) Compounds that break down into ions in water and thus can conduct an electrical current.

elimination diet A restrictive diet that systematically tests foods that may cause an allergic response by first eliminating suspected foods and then adding them back one at a time.

embryo (em-bree-oh) The developing human life form during the second to eighth week after conception.

emulsifier (ee-mull-sih-fye-er) A substance that can suspend fat in tiny droplets within a watery fluid.

endomorph (en-doh-morf) A body type characterized by short, stubby bones, a short trunk, and very short fingers.

endorphins (en-dor-fins) Natural body tranquilizers that may be involved in the feeding response, as well as in pain reduction.

enriched A term generally meaning that the vitamins thiamin, niacin, and riboflavin and the mineral iron have been added to a grain product to improve nutritional quality.

enzyme (en-zime) A compound that speeds the rate of a chemical process but is not altered by the process. Almost all enzymes are proteins.

epidemiology (ep-uh-dee-me-oll-uh-gee) The study of how disease rates vary between different population groups, such as the rate of stomach cancer in Japan compared with that in Germany.

epinephrine (ep-ih-nef-rin) A hormone also known as adrenaline; it is released by the adrenal gland (located near the kidneys) and various nerve endings in the body. Epinephrine increases glycogen breakdown in the liver, among other functions.

epithelial cells (ep-ih-thee-lee-ul) The surface cells that line the outside of the body and all external passages within it.

equilibrium (ee-kwih-lib-ree-um) In nutritional terms, a state in which nutrient intake equals nutrient losses; this allows the body to maintain a stable condition.

ergogenic (ur-go-jen-ic) Work producing.

essential Having no obvious, external cause.

essential amino acids The amino acids that cannot be synthesized by humans in sufficient amounts and therefore must be included in the diet; there are nine essential amino acids. These are also called *indispensable* amino acids.

essential fatty acids Fatty acids that must be present in the diet to maintain health; these are linoleic acid and alpha-linolenic acid.

esterification (e-ster-ih-fih-kay-shun) The process of attaching fatty acids to a glycerol molecule. Removing a fatty acid is called deesterification; reattaching a fatty acid is called reesterification.

Estimated Safe and Adequate Daily Dietary Intake (ESADDI) Nutrient intake recommendations, made by the National Academy of Sciences' Food and Nutrition Board, that give a range for intake of some nutrients because not enough information is available to set a recommended daily allowance (RDA).

exchange system A grouping of foods in six lists. When the serving size for any food in a list is consumed, all foods within the list yield a similar amount of carbohydrate, fat, protein, and energy.

experiment A test conducted to examine the validity of a hypothesis.

failure to thrive Inadequate gains in height and weight in infancy, often resulting from inadequate food intake.

famine A time of massive starvation, often associated with crop failures, war, and political strife.

fasting hypoglycemia (high-po-gligh-see-me-uh) Low blood sugar that follows a day or so of fasting. This is a rare disorder, generally caused by cancer in the pancreas.

fatty acids Acids found in fat; they are composed of carbon atoms linked to hydrogen atoms, with an acidic chemical group at one end.

fat-soluble vitamin Vitamins that dissolve in such substances as ether or benzene. These vitamins are A, D, E, and K.

feeding center A group of cells in the hypothalamus that cause hunger when stimulated. These cells are also known as the lateral feeding centers.

ferritin (ferr-ih-tin) A protein compound that serves as the storage form of iron in the blood and tissues.

fetal alcohol syndrome (FAS) A group of physical and mental abnormalities in an infant caused by the mother's consumption of alcohol during pregnancy.

fetus (feet-us) A developing infant inside its mother from 8 weeks after conception to birth.

fluoroapatite (fleur-oh-app-uh-tite) Tooth crystals containing fluoride ions that are relatively acid resistant.

food diary A written record of sequential food intake for a period of time. Details associated with the food intake are often recorded as well.

Food Guide Pyramid A dietary planning tool that recommends food choices from milk and milk products; meat, fish, poultry, and beans; vegetables; fruits; and breads and cereals.

food intolerance An adverse reaction to food that does not involve allergic mechanisms.

food sensitivity A mild reaction to a substance in food that might be noticed as slight itching or redness of the skin.

fore milk The first breast milk delivered in the nursing session.

fortified A term generally meaning that vitamins, minerals, or both have been added to a food product in excess of what was originally found in the product.

fraternal twins Infants that develop from two separate ova and sperm and therefore have separate genetic identities, although they develop simultaneously in the mother.

fructose (frook-tose) A monosaccharide with six carbons found in fruits and honey.

fungi Simple parasitic life form, including molds, mildews, yeasts, and mushrooms; live on dead or decaying organic material.

galactose (gah-lak-tose) A six-carbon monosaccharide; an isomer of glucose.

galactosemia (gah-lak-toh-see-mee-ah) A disease characterized by the buildup of the monosaccharide galactose in the bloodstream, resulting from the liver's inability to metabolize galactose. If present at birth and left untreated, galactosemia results in severe growth and mental retardation.

gastrin (gas-trin) A hormone that stimulates the secretion of enzymes and acids in the stomach.

gastrointestinal (GI) tract (gas-troh-in-tes-tin-al) The main sites in the body used in nutrient digestion and absorption. It consists of the mouth, esophagus, stomach, small intestine, large intestine, rectum, and anus.

gastroplasty (gas-troh-plas-tee) Surgery performed on the stomach to limit its volume to approximately 50 milliliters, about the size of a shot glass.

generally recognized as safe (GRAS) A group of food additives that in 1958 were considered safe; thus manufacturers have been allowed to use them when needed in food products.

genes The hereditary material on chromosomes that makes up DNA. Genes provide the blueprints for the production of cell proteins.

genetic engineering Alteration of genetic material in plants or animals with the intent of improving growth, disease resistance, or other characteristics.

geometric ratio A group of numbers in which the division of each number by the one to the left of it yields the same number.

gestation (jes-tay-shun) The time of fetal growth from conception to birth; a period of about 40 weeks after a woman's last normal menstrual period.

gestational diabetes (jes-tay-shun-al) A high blood glucose level that develops during pregnancy but returns to normal after birth. One cause is production of hormones by the placenta that antagonize the action of the hormone insulin.

glucagon (gloo-kuh-gon) A hormone made by the pancreas that stimulates the liver to break down glycogen into glucose; this raises the blood glucose level. Glucagon also performs other functions.

gluconeogenesis (gloo-ko-nee-oh-jen-uh-sis) The production of new glucose molecules by metabolic pathways in the cell. Amino acids are usually the source of the carbon atoms for these new glucose molecules.

glucose (gloo-kos) A six-carbon carbohydrate found in blood; in table sugar it is linked to another sugar called fructose.

glucose polymer A carbohydrate source used in some sports drinks that consists of grouping of a few glucose molecules.

glycerol (gliss-er-ol) A three-carbon alcohol used to form triglycerides.

glycogen (gligh-ko-jen) A carbohydrate made up of several units of glucose containing a highly branched structure; sometimes known as animal starch. Glycogen is the storage form of glucose, which is synthesized in the liver and muscles.

glycolysis (gligh-coll-ih-sis) The pathway that results in the breakdown of glucose into two three-carbon molecules.

glycosylation The process by which glucose is attached to other compounds, such as proteins.

goiter (goy-ter) An enlargement of the thyroid gland (located in the neck area) often caused by insufficient iodide in the diet.

goitrogens (goy-troh-jens) Substances in food that interfere with the absorption and use of iodide; they therefore may cause goiter if consumed in large amounts.

gram A measure of weight in the metric system; 28 grams equal 1 ounce, and 1 kilogram equals 2.2 pounds.

green revolution A period in the 1960s when much emphasis was placed on improving strains and cultivation practices of cereal grains, such as rice, wheat, and corn.

growth hormone A pituitary hormone that produces body growth and the release of fat from storage, among other effects.

gums A group of soluble fibers containing chains of galactose, glucuronic acid, and other monosaccharides; gums are characteristically found in matter exuded from plant stems.

hazard The chances that injury will result from use of a substance.

heart attack A rapid fall in heart function caused by reduced blood flow through the heart's blood vessels. Often part of the heart dies in the process.

heart disease A disease characterized by the deposition of fatty material in the blood vessels in the heart. The fatty materials reduce blood flow through the blood vessels supplying the heart.

heartburn A pain emanating from the esophagus as a result of stomach acid backing up into the esophagus and irritating the tissue in that organ.

hematocrit (hee-mat-oh-krit) The percentage of blood that is made up of red blood cells.

heme iron (heem) Iron provided from animal tissues as hemoglobin and myoglobin. Approximately 50% of the iron in meat is heme iron; it is readily absorbed.

hemicellulose (hem-ih-sell-you-los) A group of insoluble fibers containing the monosaccharides xylose, galactose, and glucose, as well as other monosaccharides linked in an indigestible fashion.

hemochromatosis (heem-oh-krom-ah-tos-sis) A disorder of iron metabolism characterized by increased iron absorption and deposition in the liver tissue; this eventually poisons the liver cells.

hemoglobin (heem-oh-glow-bin) The iron-containing protein in red blood cells that carries oxygen to the cells and carbon dioxide away from the cells. Hemoglobin also gives blood its red color.

hemolysis (hee-mol-ih-sis) Destruction of red blood cells. The red blood cell membrane breaks down, allowing cell contents to leak into the fluid portion of the blood.

hemorrhoids (hem-or-oyds) Swollen veins of the rectum and anus; they often protrude into the anus.

hemosiderin (heem-oh-sid-er-in) An insoluble iron-protein compound found in the liver. Hemosiderin stores increase as the amount of iron in the liver exceeds the storage capacity of ferritin.

herbicide (erb-ih-side) A compound that reduces the growth and reproduction of plants.

high-density lipoprotein (HDL) (lip-oh-pro-teen) A lipoprotein synthesized by the liver and small intestine that picks up cholesterol from dying cells and other sources and transfers it primarily to the other lipoproteins in the bloodstream. A low HDL level increases the risk for heart disease.

high-fructose corn syrup A corn syrup that is 40% to 90% fructose.

high-quality (complete) protein Protein that contains ample amounts of all nine essential amino acids.

hind milk (hynd) The milk secreted at the end of a nursing session; it is higher in fat than fore milk.

hormone (hore-moan) A compound secreted into the bloodstream that acts to control the function of distant cells.

hospice Hospital care that emphasizes comfort and dignity in death.

hunger The physiological or internal drive to find and eat food.

hydrogenation (high-draw-je-nay-shun) The addition of hydrogen atoms to the double bonds of polyunsaturated and monounsaturated fatty acids to reduce the extent of unsaturation; this process turns liquid vegetable oils into solid fats.

hydrophilic (high-dro-fill-ik) Attracts water (literally means "water loving").

hydrophobic (high-dro-fo-bik) Repels water (literally means "water fearing").

hydroxyapatite (high-drox-ee-app-uh-tite) A compound composed of calcium and phosphate that is deposited into the bone protein matrix to give bone strength and rigidity.

hyperactivity A poorly defined term generally used to label inattention, irritability, and excessively active behavior in children.

hyperglycemia (high-per-gligh-see-me-uh) A high blood glucose level; that is, above 140 milligrams per 100 milliliters of blood.

hypertension (high-per-ten-shun) A condition also known as high blood pressure in which blood pressure remains persistently elevated, especially when the heart is between beats.

hypoglycemia (high-po-gligh-see-mee-uh) A low blood glucose level; that is, below 40 to 50 milligrams per 100 milliliters of blood.

hypothalamus (high-po-thall-uh-mus) A grouping of cells at the base of the brain. These cells participate in many body functions, such as regulating hunger.

hypothesis (high-poth-eh-sis) An "educated guess" by a scientist to explain a phenomenon.

identical twins Two infants who develop from a single ovum and sperm and consequently have the same genetic makeup.

ileum The last portion of the small intestine.

in utero (in you-ter-oh) "in the uterus"; that is, during pregnancy.

incidental food additives Additives introduced into food products indirectly from environmental contamination of ingredients or during the manufacturing process.

indirect calorimetry (kal-oh-rim-eh-tree) A method of estimating energy use by the body by measuring oxygen uptake and then using formulas to convert that gas usage into energy use.

infectious disease (in-fek-shus) Any disease caused by invasion of the body by microorganisms, such as bacteria, fungi, or viruses.

infrastructure The basic framework of a system or organization. For society, this includes roads, bridges, telephones, and other basic technologies.

inorganic (in-ore-gan-ik) Chemical compounds that contain no carbons linked to hydrogens in the structure.

insensible Not consciously perceived by the individual, such as the water lost with each breath.
insoluble fibers (in-sol-you-bul) Fibers that mostly do not dissolve in water and are not digested by bacteria in the large intestine. These include cellulose, some hemicellulose, and lignins.
insulin (in-suh-lin) A hormone produced by the beta cells of the pancreas. Insulin increases the synthesis of glycogen in the liver and the movement of glucose from the bloodstream into body cells.
insulin-dependent diabetes A form of diabetes prone to ketosis; it requires insulin therapy.
intentional food additives Additives knowingly (directly) incorporated into food products by manufacturers.
intermediate-density lipoprotein (IDL) (lih-poh-pro-teen) The product formed after a very-low-density lipoprotein (VLDL) has had most of its triglyceride removed.
international unit (IU) A crude measure of vitamin activity, often based on the growth rate of animals. Today these units have been replaced by more precise milligram and microgram quantities.
intracellular fluid Fluid contained within a cell.
intravenous (in-trah-veen-us) Introduced directly into the bloodstream.
intrinsic factor A proteinlike compound produced by the stomach that enhances absorption of vitamin B-12.
ion an atom with an unequal number of electrons and protons. If the number of electrons exceeds the number of protons, the ion is negative. If the number of protons exceeds the number of electrons, the ion is positive.
irradiation (ir-ray-dee-ay-shun) A process whereby radiation energy is applied to foods, creating compounds within the food that destroy cell membranes, break down DNA, link proteins, limit enzyme activity, and alter a variety of other proteins and cell functions that can lead to food spoilage. This process does not make the food radioactive.
isomer (eye-so-mer) Different chemical structures for compounds that share the same chemical formula.
kcalories or kilocalories (kay-kal-oh-rees) A measure of the energy content in foods. A kcalorie is the heat needed to raise the temperature of 1000 grams (1 liter) of water 1° Celsius. This is the same as raising the temperature of about 4 cups of water 2° Fahrenheit.
ketone (kee-tone) Incomplete breakdown products of fat containing three or four carbons.
ketone bodies Products of acetyl-CoA (fat) metabolism containing three to four carbon atoms: acetoacetic acid, beta-hydroxybutyric acid, and acetone. These contain a ketone group, hence the name.
ketosis (kee-toe-sis) The condition of having high levels of ketones in the bloodstream.
kidney nephrons (nef-rons) A unit of kidney cells that filter wastes out of the bloodstream and dispose these wastes into the urine.
kilogram A measure of weight in the metric system; 1 kilogram equals 1000 grams.
kjoule (kay-jool) A measure of work in which 1 kjoule equals the work needed to move 1 kilogram a distance of 1 meter with the force of 1 newton; 1 kcalorie equals 4.18 kjoules.
kwashiorkor (kwash-ee-or-core) A disease occurring primarily in young children when disease and infections add to the high nutrient demands of growth; if the child then consumes insufficient energy and protein, kwashiorkor may result. Edema, moderate weight deficit, and weakness are common symptoms.
lactation (lak-ta-shun) The period after childbirth during which milk is produced in the woman's breasts.
lactic acid (lak-tik) A three-carbon acid formed during anaerobic cell metabolism; a partial breakdown product of glucose; also called lactate.
lacto-ovo-vegetarian A semivegetarian food plan in which a person consumes plant products, dairy products, and eggs.
lacto-vegetarian (lak-toe ve-jah-tear-ree-an) A semivegetarian food plan in which milk products, as well as vegetable products, are consumed.
***Lactobacillus bifidus* factor** (lak-toe-bah-sil-us biff-id-us) A protective factor secreted in colostrum that encourages growth of beneficial bacteria in the intestine of an infant.
lactose (lak-tose) A sugar made up of glucose linked to another sugar, called galactose.
lactose intolerance A condition in which lactose digestion is reduced because lactase production declines. Symptoms include gas and bloating after consuming dairy products.
lanugo (lah-new-go) The downlike hair that appears after much body fat is lost as a result of semistarvation. The hair stands erect and traps air, which acts as insulation to the body, replacing that usually supplied by body fat.
larva (lar-vah) An early developmental stage in the life history of some microorganisms, such as parasites.
laxative A medication or other substance that stimulates evacuation of the intestinal tract.
lean body mass The part of the body that is free of all but essential body fat. About 2% of body fat is essential; the rest represents storage and so is not part of lean body mass. Lean body mass includes muscle, bone, organs, connective tissue, skin, and other body parts.
lecithin (less-uh-thin) A phospholipid containing two fatty acids, a phosphate group, and a choline molecule.
let-down reflex A reflex stimulated by infant suckling that causes the release (ejection) of milk from milk ducts in the mother's breasts.
life expectancy The average length of life for a given group of people.
life span The potential oldest age to which a person can survive.
lignin (lig-nin) A group of insoluble fibers made up of a multiringed alcohol (noncarbohydrate) structure.
limiting amino acid The essential amino acid in the lowest concentration in a food in proportion to body needs.
linoleic acid (lin-oh-lay-ik) A fatty acid with 18 carbon atoms and two double bonds; omega-6.
lipase (lye-pase) Fat-digesting enzymes; lipase produced by the pancreas to act in the small intestine is the most important form used in digestion.

lipectomy (lip-eck-toe-mee) Surgical removal of body fat; also known as liposuction.
lipids (lip-ids) Compounds containing carbon, hydrogen, oxygen, and sometimes other atoms. Lipids dissolve in ether or benzene and are commonly known as fats and oils.
lipogenic (lye-poh-jen-ik) Means "creating lipid." The liver is the major lipogenic organ in the body.
lipoprotein (lye-poh-pro-teen) A compound found in the bloodstream containing a core of lipids with a shell of protein, phospholipid, and cholesterol.
lipoprotein lipase (lye-poh-pro-teen lye-pase) An enzyme attached to the outside of the cells that line the bloodstream; it breaks down triglycerides into free fatty acids and glycerol.
liter (lee-ter) A measure of volume in the metric system; 1 liter equals 1.06 quarts.
lobules (lob-you-els) Saclike structures in the breast that store milk.
long-chain fatty acids Fatty acids that contain more than 12 carbon atoms.
low birth weight (LBW) Infant weight at birth of less than 5.5 pounds (2.5 kilograms), usually because of premature birth; these infants have a higher risk of health problems.
low-density lipoprotein (LDL) The product of the VLDL metabolism that contains primarily cholesterol; an elevated level of LDL is strongly linked to heart disease.
low-input sustainable agriculture (LISA) A form of farming that attempts to limit use of purchased materials, such as manufactured fertilizers and pesticides. Use of manure and crop rotation are typical substitutes.
low-quality (incomplete) protein Dietary proteins that are low in or lack one or more essential amino acids.
lower-body obesity The type of obesity, called gynoid, in which fat is stored primarily in the buttocks and thigh area.
lumen (loo-men) The inside cavity of a tube, such as the GI tract.
lymphatic system (lim-fat-ick) The system of vessels that can accept fluid surrounding cells and large particles, such as products of fat absorption. This lymph fluid eventually passes into the bloodstream via the lymphatic system.
macrobiotics (mack-row-by-ah-tiks) A food plan that emphasizes vegetable foods over animal foods, often with heavy use of brown rice.
macrocyte (mac-row-site) A greatly enlarged mature red blood cell; these cells have a short life span.
major mineral A mineral vital to health that is required in the diet in amounts greater than 100 milligrams per day.
malnutrition Failing health that results from a long-standing dietary intake that fails to meet or greatly exceeds nutritional needs.
maltose (mawl-tose) Glucose linked to glucose.
marasmus (mah-ras-mus) A disease caused essentially by starvation; the person does not consume sufficient protein and energy and thus has the equivalent of severe protein-energy malnutrition. The individual will be severely underweight and have little or no fat stores, little muscle mass, and poor strength.
marginal Noticeable but not severe.
mass movements Peristaltic waves that are simultaneously coordinated over a large area of the colon. These contractions move material from one portion of the colon to another and from the colon into the rectum.
meconium (meh-koh-nee-um) The first stool passed by an infant after birth. It has a thick, mucuslike consistency.
medium-chain fatty acids Fatty acids that contain 6 to 10 carbon atoms.
megadose (meg-ah-dose) Intake of a nutrient in amounts greater than 10 times the desired 1989 RDA listed values.
megaloblast (meg-ah-low-blast) A large, immature red blood cell that results from the particular cell's inability to divide when it normally should.
menarche (men-ar-kee) The onset of menses in women, which usually occurs between 10 and 13 years of age.
menopause (men-oh-paws) The cessation of menses in women, which usually begins at about 50 years of age.
mesomorph (mez-oh-morf) A body type associated with average bone size, trunk size, and finger length.
metabolism (meh-tab-oh-liz-um) Chemical reactions that occur in the body, enabling cells to release energy from foods, convert one substance into another, and prepare end products for excretion.
meter (meet-er) A measure of length in the metric system; 1 meter equals 39.4 inches.
micelle (my-sell) A droplet of fat surrounded by a shell of water. Emulsifiers are used to produce micelles.
microgram A measure of weight in the metric system; 1 million micrograms equal 1 gram.
milligram A measure of weight in the metric system; 1000 milligrams equal 1 gram.
minerals Chemical elements used in the body to promote chemical processes and form body structures.
Minimum Requirements for Health (MRH) Nutrient intake standards for sodium, potassium, and chloride, as set by the National Academy of Sciences' Food and Nutrition Board.
miscarriage Loss of pregnancy that occurs before 28 weeks of gestation; also called spontaneous abortion.
mitochondria Main site of energy production in most cells.
molecule (mol-e-kewl) A group of like or unlike atoms that are chemically linked; it is similar to a compound, which is a group of different types of atoms bonded together in definite proportion.
monoglycerides (mon-oh-glis-er-ides) A breakdown product of a triglyceride, consisting of one fatty acid bonded to the carbohydrate glycerol.
monosaccharide (mon-oh-sack-uh-ride) A single sugar, such as glucose, that is not broken down further during digestion.
monounsaturated fatty acid A fatty acid containing one carbon-carbon double bond.

mortality Synonymous with death; rate of death.
mottle (mot-tal) Discoloration or marking of the surface of teeth caused by a high fluoride content.
mucilage (mew-sih-laj) A group of soluble fibers consisting of chains of galactose, mannose, and other monosaccharides; characteristically found in seaweed.
mucus (mew-cuss) A thick fluid, secreted by glands throughout the body, that contains a compound that is both carbohydrate and protein in nature. Mucus acts as a lubricant and a means of protection for cells.
mycotoxins (my-ko-tok-sins) A group of toxic compounds produced by molds, such as aflatoxin B-1, found on moldy grains.
myocardial infarction (my-oh-card-ee-ahl in-fark-shun) Death of part of the heart muscle.
myoglobin (my-oh-glow-bin) An iron-containing compound that transports oxygen and carbon dioxide in muscle tissue.
neural tube defect A defect in the formation of the neural tube occurring during early fetal development. The defect results in various nervous system disorders, such as spina bifida.
neurotransmitter A compound made by a nerve cell that allows communication between it and other cells.
nitrate (nye-trate) A nitrogen-containing compound used to cure meats. It gives meat a pink color and confers some resistance to bacterial growth.
no observable effect level (NOEL) The highest dose of an additive that produces no deleterious health effect in animals.
nonessential amino acids Amino acids that can be synthesized by the body in sufficient amounts; there are about 11 nonessential amino acids. These are also termed *dispensable* amino acids.
nonheme iron Iron provided from plant sources and animal tissues other than in the form of hemoglobin and myoglobin. Nonheme iron is less efficiently absorbed than heme iron.
non-insulin dependent diabetes A form of diabetes in which ketosis is not common, and insulin therapy may be used but is not often required.
nonpolar A compound with no charges.
nucleus (new-klee-us) The core of an atom; it consists of protons and neutrons.
nutrient density The ratio formed by dividing a food's contribution to the needs for a nutrient by its contribution to energy needs. When the contribution to nutrient needs exceeds that of energy needs, the food is considered to have a favorable nutrient density for that nutrient.
nutrients Chemical substances in food that nourish the body by providing energy, building materials, and factors to regulate needed chemical reactions in the body. The body either can't make these substances or can't make them fast enough for its needs.
nutrition The Council on Food and Nutrition of the American Medical Association defines nutrition as "the science of food, the nutrients and the substances therein, their action, interaction, and balance in relation to health and disease, and the process by which the organism (i.e., body) ingests, digests, absorbs, transports, utilizes, and excretes food substances."
nutrition labels A label format that must be included on foods under certain circumstances, such as when nutrients are added to foods or when a nutritional claim is made for the food. The nutrition label must follow specific guidelines set by FDA.
nutritional status The nutritional health of a person as determined by anthropometric measures (height, weight, circumferences, and so on), biochemical measures of nutrients or their by-products in blood and urine, a clinical (physical) examination, and a dietary analysis; these elements can be remembered by the mnemonic ABCD.
obesity (oh-bees-ih-tee) A condition characterized by excess body fat.
oligosaccharides (ol-ih-go-sak-ah-rides) Carbohydrates that contain 3 to 10 monosaccharide units.
omega-6 fatty acid A fatty acid with its first carbon-carbon double bonds starting at the sixth carbon atom from the — CH_3 end.
omega-3 fatty acid A fatty acid with its first carbon-carbon double bond starting at the third carbon atom from the — CH_3 end.
omnivore (ahm-nih-voor) A person who consumes foods from both plants and animals.
opportunistic infections Infections primarily seen in undernourished or otherwise weakened people.
organ A group of tissues designed to perform a specific function (e.g., the heart). An organ contains muscle tissue, nerve tissue, and so on.
organic (ore-gan-ik) Chemical compounds that contain carbons linked to hydrogens in the structure.
organism (ore-gan-ih-zim) A living thing. The human body is an organism consisting of many organs that act in a coordinated manner to support life.
osmosis (oz-mos-is) The passage of solutions across a semipermeable membrane.
osmotic pressure The pressure needed to prevent particles in a solution from drawing liquid across a semipermeable membrane.
osteomalacia (os-tee-oh-mal-ay-shuh) The adult form of rickets, osteomalacia is a weakening of the bones as a result of poor calcium content. The condition is caused by a reduction in the activity of the vitamin D hormone.
osteopenia (os-tee-oh-pee-nee-ah) Decreased bone mass stemming from cancer, hyperthyroidism, or other causes.
osteoporosis (os-tee-oh-po-roh-sis) A bone disease that develops primarily after menopause in women and is characterized by a decrease in bone density.
ostomy (oss-toh-mee) A surgically created short circuit in intestinal flow in which the end point usually opens from the abdominal cavity rather than the anus, as with a colostomy.
outpatient A person treated by medical personnel outside the hospital setting; for example, in a clinic or a physician's office.

overnutrition A state in which nutritional intake exceeds the body's needs.
ovum The egg cell from which a fetus eventually develops if the egg is fertilized by a sperm cell.
oxidize (ox-ih-dize) Generally refers to the loss of an electron or gain of an oxygen atom.
oxidizing compound (ox-ih-dy-zing) A compound capable of capturing an electron from another compound (or supplying oxygen to another compound).
palatable (pal-it-ah-bull) Pleasing to the taste.
passive absorption Absorption that requires (1) permeability of the absorptive surface to the substance and (2) a higher concentration of the substance in the intestinal lumen than in the absorptive cells.
pasteurize (pas-tur-eyes) The process of heating food products to kill pathogenic microorganisms. Under one method, milk is heated at 161° F for a short period of time.
pathway A metabolic progression of individual steps from starting materials to ending products.
pectin (peck-tin) A group of soluble fibers containing chains of galacturonic acid and other monosaccharides; characteristically found between plant cell walls.
peer-reviewed journal A journal that publishes research only after two or three scientists (essentially peers) who were not part of the study agree that it was well conducted and that the results are fairly represented.
pellagra (peh-lahg-rah) A disease resulting from lack of the vitamin niacin in the diet; it is characterized by inflammation of the skin, diarrhea, and, eventually, mental incapacity.
pepsin (pep-sin) A protein-digesting enzyme produced by the stomach.
peptide bond A bond formed to link amino acids in a protein.
peptides (pep-tydes) A few amino acids bonded together (often two to four).
percent A part of the total when the total consists of 100 parts.
peristalsis (pear-ih-stall-sis) A coordinated muscular contraction that is used to propel food down the GI tract.
pernicious anemia (per-nish-us ah-nee-mee-ah) The anemia that results from a lack of vitamin B-12 absorption; it is "pernicious" because of the associated nerve degeneration that eventually can result in paralysis.
pesticide (pest-i-side) A general term signifying that an agent can destroy bacteria, fungi, insects, rodents, or other pests.
pH A measure of the hydrogen ion concentration in a solution.
phenylketonuria (PKU) (fee-null-kee-tone-your-ee-ah) A disease in which the liver cannot readily metabolize the amino acid phenylalanine. Toxic by-products of phenylalanine build up in the body, leading to mental retardation.
phenylpropanolamine (fee-null-pro-pan-awl-ah-meen) An over-the-counter decongestant that has a mild appetite-reducing effect.
phosphocreatine (PCr) A high-energy compound that can be used to reform adenosine triphosphate (ATP) from adenosine diphosphate (ADP).
photosynthesis (foto-sin-tha-sis) The process by which plants use energy from the sun to produce energy-yielding compounds, such as glucose.
physiological anemia The normal increase in blood volume that occurs during pregnancy and dilutes the concentration of red blood cells, resulting in anemia; also called hemodilution.
phytobezoars (fy-tow-bee-zors) A pellet of fiber characteristically found in the stomach.
pica (pie-kah) The practice of eating nonfood items such as dirt, laundry starch, or clay.
placebo (plah-see-bo) A fake medicine used to disguise the roles of participants in an experiment.
placenta (plah-sen-tah) An organ formed only during pregnancy that secretes hormones and makes possible the transfer of oxygen and nutrients from the mother's blood to the fetus and the removal of fetal wastes.
plaque (plack) A cholesterol-rich substance deposited in the blood vessels; it contains various white blood cells, cholesterol and other lipids, and eventually calcium.
polar A compound with distinct positive and negative charges, which act like poles on a magnet.
polysaccharides (paw-lee-sack-uh-rides) Carbohydrates that contain up to 3000 or more glucose units; also known as complex carbohydrates.
polyunsaturated fatty acid A fatty acid containing two or more carbon-carbon double bonds.
portal vein (poor-tall vane) A large vein leading to the liver. Capillary blood vessels from the intestine drain into this vein.
positive balance A state in which nutrient intake exceeds losses, resulting in a net gain of the nutrient in the body (e.g., when tissue protein is gained during growth). The opposite of this state is negative balance, in which losses exceed intake, as with starvation.
pregnancy-induced hypertension A serious disorder, also called toxemia, that can involve high blood pressure, kidney failure, convulsion, and even death of the mother and the fetus. Although the exact cause is not known, good nutrition and prenatal care can prevent or limit the severity of this disorder. Mild cases are known as preeclampsia; more severe cases are called eclampsia.
premature An infant born before 38 weeks of gestation.
premenstrual syndrome (PMS) A disorder found in some women in the days surrounding menstrual periods that is characterized by depression, headache, bloating, and mood swings.
preservatives Compounds that extend the shelf life of food by inhibiting microbial growth or by minimizing the destructive effect of oxygen and metals.
progestins (pro-jes-tins) Hormones, including progesterone, that are necessary for maintaining pregnancy and lactation.
prognosis (prog-no-sis) A forecast of a disease's course and end.
prolactin (pro-lack-tin) A hormone secreted by the mother that stimulates the synthesis of milk.

protein-energy malnutrition (PEM) A condition that results when a person regularly consumes insufficient amounts of energy and protein. The deficiency eventually results in body wasting and an increased susceptibility to infections.
proteins (pro-teens) Compounds made up of amino acids. Proteins contain carbon, hydrogen, oxygen, nitrogen, and sometimes sulfur atoms in a specific configuration. They contain the form of nitrogen most easily used by the human body.
prothrombin (pro-throm-bin) A blood protein needed for blood clotting that requires vitamin K for its synthesis.
psyllium (sil-ee-um) A mostly soluble type of dietary fiber found in the seeds of the plantain plant.
quack (kwak) A person who does not have the medical skills or knowledge he or she claims to have.
R-protein A protein produced by the salivary glands that enhances absorption of vitamin B-12.
radiation (ray-dee-ay-shun) Literally, that which is transmitted from a center in all directions. Various forms of radiation energy include x-rays, ultraviolet rays from the sun, and microwaves.
rancid (ran-sid) Having a disagreeable odor or taste, usually as a result of the breakdown of fat.
reactive hypoglycemia (high-po-gligh-see-mee-uh) Low blood sugar that follows a meal high in simple sugars, with corresponding symptoms of irritability, headache, nervousness, sweating, and confusion.
receptive framework The process by which a person opens and responds to learning more about a problem; it usually involves seeking more information about the issue from books and people.
receptor pathway for cholesterol uptake A process by which LDL molecules (cholesterol containing) are bound by cell receptors, with the incorporation of the LDL molecule into the cell.
Recommended Dietary Allowances (RDAs) Recommended nutrient intakes that meet the needs of essentially all people of similar age and gender. These amounts are established by the Food and Nutrition Board of the National Academy of Sciences.
Recommended Nutrient Intakes (RNIs) The Canadian version of the RDA.
Reference Daily Intakes (RDIs) New term for expressing nutrient content on nutrition labels. Currently U.S. RDA values are used for the RDIs. In the future it is likely that RDI figures will be based on average 1989 RDA values set for a nutrient that is applicable for a particular age-group, such as children over 4 years through adults.
registered dietitian (RD) (dye-eh-tish-shun) A person who has completed a baccalaureate degree program approved by the American Dietetic Association, has participated in a supervised professional practice program, and has passed a registration examination.
reinforcement A reaction by others in response to a person's behavior. Positive reinforcement entails encouragement; negative reinforcement entails criticism or penalty.
requirement The amount of a nutrient required by one person to maintain health; this varies from individual to individual. We do not know our individual requirements for each nutrient.
reserve capacity The extent to which an organ can preserve essentially normal function despite decreasing cell number or cell activity.
resting metabolic rate Essentially the same as the basal metabolic rate, but the individual need not meet the strict conditions for determining a basal metabolic rate. The terms often are used interchangeably.
retinoids (ret-ih-noyds) Chemical forms of preformed vitamin A; one source is animal foods.
reverse transport of cholesterol The process by which cholesterol is picked up by HDL molecules and transferred to other lipoproteins that can dispose of it.
rhodopsin (row-dop-sin) A protein involved in vision; it is made in the eye and incorporates a protein called opsin and a form of vitamin A. It is especially important to night vision.
rickets (rick-its) A deficiency disease characterized by softening of the bones because of poor calcium content. It arises from insufficient vitamin D activity in the body.
risk factor A characteristic or behavior that contributes to the chances of developing an illness.
runner's anemia A condition found in athletes that involves a decrease in the blood's ability to carry oxygen; this may be caused by iron loss through perspiration, destruction of red blood cells from the impact of exercise, or increased blood volume.
saccharin (sack-ah-rin) An alternate sweetener that yields no energy to the body; it is 300 times sweeter than sucrose.
safety The relative certainty that a substance won't cause injury.
saliva (sah-ligh-vah) A watery fluid produced by the salivary glands in the mouth; it contains lubricants, enzymes, and other substances.
salt Generally refers to a mixture of sodium and chloride in a 40:60 ratio.
satiety (suh-tie-uh-tee) A state in which there is no longer a desire to eat.
satiety center A group of cells in the hypothalamus that, when stimulated, cause satiety. These cells are also known as the ventromedial satiety center.
saturated fat (sat-your-ate-ed) A fat containing no carbon-carbon double bonds in its structure; this causes the fat to be saturated with hydrogen atoms.
saturated fatty acid A fatty acid with no carbon-carbon double bonds.
scavenger pathway for cholesterol uptake A process by which LDL molecules (cholesterol containing) are taken up by scavenger cells embedded in the blood vessels.
scurvy (sker-vee) The deficiency disease that results after a few weeks of consuming a diet that lacks vitamin C.
sebum (see-bum) A secretion of the sebaceous glands consisting of fats, waxes, and other substances.
secrete (se-kreet) To produce and then release a substance, generally called a secretion, from a cell in the body.
secretin (see-kreh-tin) A hormone that causes bicarbonate ion release from the pancreas and slow stomach emptying.

self-monitoring A process of tracking foods eaten and conditions affecting eating; these are usually recorded in a diary, along with the location, time, and state of mind. This is a tool to help a person understand more about his or her eating habits.
semiessential amino acids Amino acids that, when consumed, spare the need to use an essential amino acid for their synthesis.
senile Related to old age.
sequesterants (see-kwes-ter-ants) Compounds that bind substances such as free metal ions. In so doing, they reduce the ions' ability to cause rancidity in compounds containing fat.
serotonin (ser-oh-tone-in) A neurotransmitter synthesized from the amino acid tryptophan that appears both to decrease the desire to eat carbohydrates and to induce sleep.
set point A term referring to the close and essentially automatic regulation of body weight. It is not known what cells control the set point nor how it actually functions in weight regulation. There is no doubt, however, that there are mechanisms that help regulate weight.
short-chain fatty acids Fatty acids that contain fewer than six carbon atoms.
sickle cell disease An anemia that results from a malformation of the red blood cell protein hemoglobin, a condition caused by an incorrect amino acid composition in the hemoglobin protein chains. The disease can lead to anemia and episodes of severe bone and joint pain, abdominal pain, headache, convulsions, paralysis, and even death.
slough (sluf) To shed or cast off.
small for gestational age (SGA) (jes-tay-shun-al) Infants born after normal gestation length (38 weeks) but weighing less than 2500 grams (about 5.5 pounds).
sodium bicarbonate An alkaline substance made basically of sodium and carbon dioxide ($NaHCO_3$).
soluble fibers (sol-you-bull) Fibers that either dissolve or swell when in water or are metabolized by bacteria in the large intestine. Soluble fibers include pectins, gums, mucilages, and some hemicellulose.
solvent A substance in which other substances dissolve.
sorbitol An alcohol derivative of glucose that yields about 4 kcalories per gram but that is slowly absorbed from the small intestine; used in some sugarless gums and dietetic foods.
sphincter (sfink-ter) A muscular valve; these valves help control the flow of food in the GI tract.
spontaneous abortion Loss of pregnancy, also called miscarriage, that occurs within 28 weeks of conception.
starch A carbohydrate made up of several units of glucose attached in a form that the body can digest; also a part of complex carbohydrates.
steroids (stare-oydes) A group of hormones and related compounds that are derivatives of cholesterol.
stimulus control Altering the environment to minimize the stimuli for eating; for example, removing foods from sight and storing them in kitchen cabinets.
stress fracture A fracture that occurs from repeated jarring of a bone; commonly occurs in bones of the foot.
stroke The loss of body function that results from a blood clot in the brain, which in turn causes the death of brain tissue.
subjects Participants in an experiment.
sucrose (sue-kros) Fructose linked to glucose.
symptom A change in health status noted by the person with the problem, such as a stomach pain.
synapse (sin-apps) Spaces between nerve cells. One nerve stimulates other nearby cells, including other nerve cells, by releasing chemicals that cross the synapse. These chemicals are what excite neighboring cells.
systolic blood pressure (sis-tol-ik) The pressure in the bloodstream associated with the pumping of blood from the heart.
tetany (tet-ah-nee) A body condition marked by sharp contraction of muscles and failure to relax afterward; usually caused by abnormal calcium metabolism.
theory An explanation for a phenomenon that has numerous lines of evidence to support it.
thermic effect of food The increase in metabolism occurring during the digestion, absorption, and metabolism of energy-yielding nutrients. This effect represents 5% to 10% of kcalories consumed.
"thrifty" metabolism A metabolism that characteristically conserves more energy than normal, such that the risk of weight gain and obesity is enhanced.
tissue A group of cells designed to perform a specific function; muscle tissue is an example.
tocopherols (tuh-koff-er-alls) The chemical name for some forms of vitamin E.
toxic (tok-sick) Poisonous; caused by a poison.
toxicity (tok-sis-ih-tee) The capacity of a substance to produce injury at some level of intake.
toxicology (tok-si-call-oh-gee) The scientific study of harmful substances.
trabecular bone (trah-beck-you-lar) The spongy, inner matrix of bone, found primarily in the spine, pelvis, and ends of bones.
trace mineral A mineral vital to health that is required in the diet in amounts less than 100 milligrams per day.
transamination (trans-am-ih-na-shun) The transfer of an amino group from an amino acid to a carbon skeleton to form a new amino acid.
triglyceride (try-gliss-uh-ride) The major form of lipid in food. It is composed of three fatty acids bonded to the carbohydrate glycerol.
trimester One of the three 13- to 14-week periods that make up a normal pregnancy.
trypsin (trip-sin) A protein-digesting enzyme secreted by the pancreas to act in the small intestine.
ulcer (ul-sir) Erosion of the tissue lining in either the stomach or the upper small intestine; usually referred to as a peptic ulcer.
undernutrition Failing health that results from a long-standing dietary intake that does not meet nutritional needs.
unsaturated fat (un-sat-your-ate-ed) A fatty acid containing one or more carbon-carbon double bonds in its structure; this causes the fat to be less than fully saturated with hydrogen atoms.

upper-body obesity (android) When body fat is stored primarily in the abdominal area; closely associated with a high risk of heart disease, hypertension, and diabetes, and more prevalent among males.

urea (yur-ee-ah) A nitrogen-containing waste product found in urine. Most nitrogen excreted from the body leaves in this form.

U.S. Recommended Daily Allowances (U.S. RDAs) Nutrient standards established by FDA for use on nutrition labels. Generally the four existing versions use the highest nutrient recommendation in the appropriate age and gender category from the 1968 publication of the RDA. The version that includes children over 4 years of age and adults is most commonly seen on nutrition labels.

vegan (veh-gan) A person who consumes no animal products.

vegetarian (veh-jih-tair-ee-un) A person who avoids eating animal products to a varying degree, ranging from eating no animal foods to simply not eating foods from four-footed animals.

very low-calorie diet (VLCD) Also known as a protein-sparing modified fast (PSMF), this diet allows the consumption of 400 to 800 kcalories per day in liquid form. Of this about 30 grams or more is carbohydrate; the rest is mostly protein.

very low-density lipoprotein (VLDL) The lipoprotein that initially leaves the liver; it carries both the cholesterol and lipid newly synthesized by the liver.

villi (vil-eye) Fingerlike protrusions into the small intestine that participate in digestion and absorption of food.

virus Smallest type of infectious agent causing disease in humans; essentially a piece of genetic material surrounded by a coat of protein; viruses reproduce, metabolize, grow, and move with the aid of a living organism.

visual cycle A chemical process in the eye that contributes to vision. Forms of vitamin A are used in the process.

vitamins (vye-ta-mens) Carbon-containing compounds needed in very small amounts in the diet to help promote and regulate chemical reactions and processes in the body.

water Chemical symbol: H_2O. Transparent, tasteless liquid composed of hydrogen and oxygen atoms that is the solvent of life. A daily intake of about 2 liters (2 quarts) via foods and water itself meets adult needs.

water-soluble vitamin Vitamins that dissolve in water; these are the B vitamins and vitamin C.

whey (way) Proteins, such as lactalbumin, found in great amounts in human milk. These are easy to digest.

whole grains Grains containing the entire seed of the plant, including the bran, germ, and endosperm (starchy interior).

xerophthalmia (zer-off-thal-mee-uh) Literally, "dry eye." A cause of blindness that results from a vitamin A deficiency. The specific cause is a lack of mucus production by the eye, a condition that leaves the eye more vulnerable to surface dirt and bacterial infections.

yo-yo dieting The practice of losing weight and then regaining it, only to lose it and regain it again.

CREDITS

Cover: Photography: Kathy Sanders/Sanders Studio, Inc. Computer Imaging: Studio Montage.

Chapter 1 p. 2, Superstock FourByFive; p. 10 (left), Janeart Ltd., Image Bank; (right), John Kelly, The Image Bank; p. 11, James Schnepf, Woodfin Camp and Associates; p. 14, Wolff Communications; p. 15, Reprinted by permission of United Feature Syndicate, Inc.; p. 18, CATHY, copyright 1990, Cathy Guisewite. Reprinted with permission of UNIVERSAL PRESS SYNDICATE. All rights reserved; p. 16, Lawrence Migdale, Stock Boston; p. 19, Daniel MacDonald, The Stock Shop; p. 20, Reprinted with permission of North American Syndicate, Inc.; p. 21, Wolff Communications; p. 22, Tom Ebenhoh, Photographic Resources; p. 28, CLG Photographics, Inc., copyright 1993.

Chapter 2 p. 31, CLG Photographics, Inc.; p. 34, Linsley Photographics; pp. 40-41, Donald O'Connor Graphic Studios; p. 41, Reprinted by permission of United Feature Syndicate, Inc.; p. 42, U.S. Department of Agriculture; p. 52, Reprinted by permission of NEA, Inc.; p. 54, International Diabetes Center, Minneapolis, MN; p. 60, Reprinted by permission of NEA, Inc.

Chapter 3 p. 67, Reprinted with special permission of North America Syndicate, Inc.; p. 68, CLG Photographics, copyright 1993; p. 74, Wolff Communications; p. 78 (left), From Hechtlinger, Adelaide: The Great Patent Medicine Era, Grosset & Dunlap, Inc., 1970; p. 82, Wolff Communications; p. 93, Reprinted by permission of NEA, Inc.

Chapter 4 p. 96, Neil Molinairo; p. 98 (top left), H. Armstrong Roberts; (middle right), Ed Reschke; p. 108, Reprinted by permission of NEA, Inc.; p. 109, from Guthrie, H., Introductory Nutrition, ed. 7, Times Mirror/Mosby College Publishing; p. 110, Science Photo Library, Photo Researchers; p. 112, Lennart Nilsson © Boehringer Ingelheim International GmbH; p. 117, from the Student Study Guide to accompany Wardlaw, G., Insel, P., and Seyler, M., Contemporary Nutrition, Mosby–Year Book; p. 119, Wolff Communications; p. 120, International Diabetes Center, Minneapolis, MN.

Chapter 5 p. 122, CLG Photographics, Inc.; p. 126, Wolff Communications; p. 132, Carolyn Delevitt, The Stock Shop; p. 134, Linsley Photographics; p. 138, ZIGGY, copyright 1990, ZIGGY AND FRIENDS, INC. Distributed by UNIVERSAL PRESS SYNDICATE. Reprinted with permission. All rights reserved; p. 140, THE FAR SIDE by Gary Larson reprinted by permission of Chronicle Features, San Francisco, CA. All rights reserved.

Chapter 6 p. 154, Superstock FourByFive; p. 165, Wolff Communications; p. 166, Wolff Communications; p. 170, C.P. George, H. Armstrong Roberts; p. 174, National Cancer Institute, Bethesda, MD; p. 178, NutraSweet, Monsanto Corp.; p. 188, Benda/Zefa, H. Armstrong Roberts; p. 190, FOX TROT, copyright 1990, UNIVERSAL PRESS SYNDICATE. Reprinted with permission. All rights reserved.

Chapter 7 p. 191, Superstock FourByFive; p. 194, CLG Photographics, Inc.; p. 198, Wolff Communications; p. 199 (left), Bill Longcore, Science Source; (right) Omikron/Science Source; p. 207, Superstock FourByFive; p. 212, FPG International; p. 217, THE FAR SIDE by Gary Larson reprinted by permission of Chronicle Features, San Francisco, CA. All rights reserved; p. 220, Reprinted by permission of NEA, Inc.

Chapter 8 p. 221, James Meyer, The Image Bank; p. 224, Reprinted by permission of United Feature Syndicate; p. 231, Garry Gay, The Image Bank; p. 232, Wally McNamee, Woodfin Camp and Associates; p. 234, George Obrenski, The Image Bank; p. 243, Joe Devenney, The Image Bank; p. 252, CLG Photographics, Inc.

Chapter 9 p. 265, Antonia M. Rosario, The Image Bank; p. 272, CLG Photographics, Inc., copyright 1993; p. 273, Plessner International, The Stock Shop; p. 275, Michael A. Keller, The Stock Market; p. 277, Reprinted with special permission of King Features Syndicate, Inc.; p. 278, from Healthline, Menlo Park, CA; p. 291, Frank Oberle, Photographic Resources; p. 295, from McLaren, Donald S.: A Colour Atlas of Nutritional Disorders, ed. 1, Wolfe Medical Publications, Ltd., 1981.

Chapter 10 p. 310, Don Parks, The Image Bank; p. 314, Reprinted with permission of North America Syndicate, Inc.; p. 317, Reprinted with permission of North America Syndicate, Inc.; p. 319, Medical Graphics Corporation, St. Paul, MN; p. 322, Linsley Photographics, from Payne, W. and Hahn, D., Understanding Your Health, ed. 2, Times Missor/Mosby College Publishing; p. 328, Robert Jones, Jr.; p. 349, CATHY, copyright 1990, Cathy Guisewite. Reprinted with permission of UNIVERSAL PRESS SYNDICATE. All rights reserved.

Chapter 11 p. 351, Wolfgang Filser, The Image Bank; p. 353, CLG Photographics, Inc.; p. 362, Reprinted by permission of NEA, Inc.; p. 362, CLG Photographics, Inc.; p. 369, FPG International.

Chapter 12 p. 379, CLG Photographics, Inc.; p. 384, Paul Buddle, H. Armstrong Roberts; p. 385, FOR BETTER OR FOR WORSE, copyright 1992, Lynn Johnston Prod., Inc. Reprinted with permission of UNIVERSAL PRESS SYNDICATE. All rights reserved; p. 389, CLG Photographics, Inc.; p. 390, CLG Photographics, Inc.; p. 391, Donald O'Connor Graphic Studio; p. 393, Wolff Communications; p. 395, CLG Photographics, Inc.; p. 403, A) Culver Pictures, Inc., B) Kobal Collection, Superstock International Inc.; C) Caron/Gamma Liaison, D) 1991, Sports Illustrated; p. 403 (bottom), Wolff Communications; p. 405, CATHY, copyright 1990, Cathy Guisewite. Reprinted with permission of UNIVERSAL PRESS SYNDICATE. All rights reserved.

Chapter 13 p. 408, Patrick J. La Croix, The Image Bank; p. 412, FOR BETTER OR FOR WORSE, copyright 1990, Lynn Johnston Prod., Inc. Reprinted with permission of UNIVERSAL PRESS SYNDICATE. All rights reserved; p. 413, Wolff Communications; p. 414, CLG Photographics, Inc., copyright 1993; p. 416, Donald O'Connor Graphic Studios; p. 417, CATHY, copyright 1990, Cathy Guisewite. Reprinted with permission of UNIVERSAL PRESS SYNDICATE. All rights reserved; p. 424, CLG Photographics, Inc.; p. 429, William Hubbell, Woodfin Camp and Associates; p. 439, George Steinmetz.

Chapter 14 p. 441, CLG Photographics, Inc.; p. 451, CLG Photographics, Inc.; p. 453, CLG Photographics, Inc.; p. 458, H. Armstrong Roberts; p. 460 (top), David Hundley, The Stock Market; p. 460 (bottom), Reprinted with permission of North America Syndicate, Inc.; p. 464, CALVIN AND HOBBES, copyright 1992, Watterson. Distributed by UNIVERSAL PRESS SYNDICATE. All rights reserved; p. 465, Mike Clemmer, Picture Group; p. 469, CLG Photographics, Inc.

Chapter 15 p. 477, Larry Dale Gordon; p. 480, International Diabetes Center, Minneapolis, MN; p. 482, Reprinted by permission of NEA, Inc.; p. 486, Reprinted by permission of NEA, Inc.; p. 491, John Lawlor, The Stock Market; p. 497, Lynn Johnson, Black Star; p. 501 (top), Ron Chapple, FPG International; (bottom), Miro Vintoniv, The Picture Cube.

Chapter 16 p. 514, Superstock FourByFive; p. 518, ZIGGY, copyright 1991, ZIGGY AND FRIENDS, INC. Distributed by UNIVERSAL PRESS SYNDICATE. Reprinted with permission. All rights reserved; p. 527, CATHY, copyright 1991, Cathy Guisewite. Reprinted with permission. All rights reserved; p. 529, Ellis Herwig, The Picture Cube; p. 536, John H. Anderson, Photographic Resources.

Chapter 17 p. 537, FPG International; p. 543, George Contorakes, The Stock Market; p. 545, ZIGGY, copyright 1989, ZIGGY AND FRIENDS, INC. Distributed by UNIVERSAL PRESS SYNDICATE. Reprinted by permission. All rights reserved; p. 546, CALVIN AND HOBBES, copyright 1993, Watterson. Distributed by UNIVERSAL PRESS SYNDICATE. All rights reserved; p. 547, Stacey Pick, Stock Boston; p. 549, THE FAR SIDE, copyright 1990, FARWORKS, INC. Distributed by UNIVERSAL PRESS SYNDICATE. Reprinted by permission. All rights reserved; p. 553, Karen Kasmauski, Woodfin Camp and Associates; p. 555, Zanetti, The Stock Market; p. 556, J. Barry O'Rourke, The Stock Market; p. 565, Superstock FourByFive.

Chapter 18 p. 568, FPG International; p. 587, Frans Lanting, Minden Pictures; p. 590, Steve McCurry, Magnum Photos; p. 594, Suzanne L. Murphy, FPG International; pg. 596, ZIGGY, copyright 1992, ZIGGY AND FRIENDS, INC. Distributed by UNIVERSAL PRESS SYNDICATE. Reprinted with permission. All rights reserved; p. 600, Jay Freis, The Image Bank.

INDEX

E

F

G

Median Heights and Weights and Recommended Energy Intake

Category	Age (years) or Condition	Weight (kg)	Weight (lb)	Height (cm)	Height (in)	REE[a] (kcal/day)	Average Energy Allowance (kcal): Multiples of REE	Per kg body weight	Per day[b]
Infants	0.0-0.5	6	13	60	24	320		108	650
	0.5-1.0	9	20	71	28	500		98	850
Children	1-3	13	29	90	35	740		102	1,300
	4-6	20	44	112	44	950		90	1,800
	7-10	28	62	132	52	1,130		70	2,000
Males	11-14	45	99	157	62	1,440	1.70	55	2,500
	15-18	66	145	176	69	1,760	1.67	45	3,000
	19-24	72	160	177	70	1,780	1.67	40	2,900
	25-50	79	174	176	70	1,800	1.60	37	2,900
	51+	77	170	173	68	1,530	1.50	30	2,300
Females	11-14	46	101	157	62	1,310	1.67	47	2,200
	15-18	55	120	163	64	1,370	1.60	40	2,200
	19-24	58	128	164	65	1,350	1.60	38	2,200
	25-50	63	138	163	64	1,380	1.55	36	2,200
	51+	65	143	160	63	1,280	1.50	30	1,900
Pregnant	1st Trimester								+0
	2nd Trimester								+300
	3rd Trimester								+300
Lactating	1st 6 months								+500
	2nd 6 months								+500

[a]Resting energy expenditure (REE); calculation based on FAO equations, then rounded. This is the same as resting metabolic rate (RMR).
[b]Figure is rounded.

Metropolitan Life Insurance Company Height-Weight Data

Height-Weight Tables for Adults

Height Ft	Height In	WOMEN Frame* Small	Medium	Large	Height Ft	Height In	MEN Frame* Small	Medium	Large
4	10	102-111	109-121	118-131	5	2	128-134	131-141	138-150
4	11	103-113	111-123	120-134	5	3	130-136	133-143	140-153
5	0	104-115	113-126	122-137	5	4	132-138	135-145	142-156
5	1	106-118	115-129	125-140	5	5	134-140	137-148	144-160
5	2	108-121	118-132	128-143	5	6	136-142	139-151	146-164
5	3	111-124	121-135	131-147	5	7	138-145	142-154	149-168
5	4	114-127	124-138	134-151	5	8	140-148	145-157	152-172
5	5	117-130	127-141	137-155	5	9	142-151	148-160	155-176
5	6	120-133	130-144	140-159	5	10	144-154	151-163	158-180
5	7	123-136	133-147	143-163	5	11	146-157	154-166	161-184
5	8	126-139	136-150	146-167	6	0	149-160	157-170	164-188
5	9	129-142	139-153	149-170	6	1	152-164	160-174	168-192
5	10	132-145	142-156	152-173	6	2	155-168	164-178	172-197
5	11	135-148	156-159	155-176	6	3	158-172	167-182	176-202
6	0	138-151	148-162	158-179	6	4	162-176	171-187	181-207

Based on a weight-height mortality study conducted by the Society of Actuaries and the Association of Life Insurance Medical Directors of America, Metropolitan Life Insurance Company, revised 1983.
**Weights at ages 25 to 59 based on lowest mortality. Height includes 1-in heel. Weight for women includes 3 lb. for indoor clothing. Weight for men includes 5 lb. for indoor clothing. (See Chapter 10 for controversy surrounding the use of these tables and Appendix I for determination of frame size.)*